Dermatologic Surgery & Cosmetic Procedures *in* PRIMARY CARE PRACTICE

Dermatologic Surgery & Cosmetic Procedures *in* PRIMARY CARE PRACTICE

Editor

JONATHAN KANTOR, MD, MSCE, MA

Department of Dermatology
Center for Global Health
Center for Clinical Epidemiology and Biostatistics
University of Pennsylvania Perelman School of Medicine
Philadelphia, Pennsylvania
Florida Center for Dermatology, PA
St Augustine, Florida

Mc Graw Hill

New York Chicago San Francisco Athens London Madrid Mexico City
Milan New Delhi Singapore Sydney Toronto

Dermatologic Surgery and Cosmetic Procedures in Primary Care Practice

1 2 3 4 5 6 7 8 9 DSS 25 24 23 22 21 20

ISBN 978-1-260-45395-9
MHID 1-260-45395-2

This book was set in Adobe Garamond Pro by Cenveo® Publisher Services.
The editors were Karen G. Edmonson and Christie Naglieri.
The production supervisor was Richard Ruzycka.
Project management was provided by Revathi Viswanathan, Cenveo Publisher Services.
The designer was Mary McKeon.
The cover designer was W2 Design.

Library of Congress Control Number: 2019955327

For Bella. "Thou thy self dost give invention light." —Shakespeare

Contents

List of Videos

Videos can be accessed via the following link: mhprofessional.com/dermsurgery

Credits for Figures and Tables

The following figures have been used with permission from these McGraw Hill publications:

Goldman GD, Dzubow LM, Yelverton CB. *Facial Flap Surgery*. New York: McGraw Hill; 2013:

Chapter 20: Figures 20-1, 20-4, 20-6, 20-10, 20-17, and 20-18

Kantor J. *Atlas of Suturing Techniques: Approaches to Surgical Wound, Laceration, and Cosmetic Repair*. New York: McGraw Hill; 2016:

Chapter 5: Figures 5-1, 5-2, 5-3, 5-4, 5-6, 5-7, 5-8, 5-9, 5-10, 5-11, 5-12, 5-13, 5-14, 5-15, 5-16, 5-17, 5-18, 5-19, 5-20, 5-21, 5-22, 5-23, 5-24, and 5-25

Chapter 10: Figures 10-1, 10-2, 10-3, 10-4, 10-5, 10-6, 10-7, 10-8, 10-9, 10-10, 10-11, 10-12, 10-13, 10-14, 10-15, 10-16, 10-17, 10-18, 10-19, 10-20, 10-21, 10-22, 10-23, 10-24, 10-25, 10-26, 10-27, 10-28, and 10-29

Chapter 16: Figure 16-37

Kantor J. *Dermatologic Surgery.* New York, NY: McGraw Hill; 2018:

Chapter 1: Chapter opener figure, Figures 1-1, 1-3, 1-4, 1-5, 1-6, 1-8, 1-9, 1-10, 1-11, 1-12, 1-13, 1-14, 1-15, 1-16, 1-17, 1-18, 1-19, 1-20, 1-21, 1-22, 1-23, 1-24, 1-25, 1-26, 1-27, 1-28, 1-29, 1-30, and 1-31

Chapter 2: Chapter opener figure, Figure 2-1

Chapter 3: Chapter opener figure

Chapter 4: Chapter opener figure, Figures 4-1, 4-2, 4-3, 4-4, 4-5, 4-6, 4-7, 4-8, 4-9, 4-10, 4-11, 4-12, 4-13, 4-14, 4-15, 4-16, 4-17, 4-18, 4-19, 4-20, 4-21, and 4-22

Chapter 5: Chapter opener figure

Chapter 6: Chapter opener figure

Chapter 7: Chapter opener figure, Figure 7-1

Chapter 8: Chapter opener figure, Figures 8-1 and 8-2

Chapter 9: Chapter opener figure, Figures 9-1, 9-2, 9-3, 9-4, 9-5, 9-6, 9-7, 9-8, 9-9, 9-10, 9-11, 9-12, 9-13, 9-14, and 9-15

Chapter 10: Chapter opener figure, Figure 10-30

Chapter 11: Chapter opener figure, Figures 11-3, 11-4, 11-5, 11-6, 11-7, 11-8, 11-9, 11-10, 11-11, and 11-12

Chapter 12: Chapter opener figure, Figures 12-1, 12-2, 12-3, 12-4, 12-5, and 12-6

Chapter 13: Chapter opener figure, Figures 13-1, 13-2, 13-3, 13-4, and 13-5

Chapter 14: Chapter opener figure, Figures 14-1, 14-2, 14-3, 14-4, and 14-5

Chapter 16: Chapter opener figure, Figures 16-1, 16-2, 16-3, 16-4, 16-5, 16-6, 16-7, 16-8, 16-9, 16-10, 16-11, 16-12, 16-13, 16-14, 16-15, 16-16, 16-17, 16-18, 16-19, 16-20, 16-21, 16-22, 16-23, 16-24, 16-25, 16-26, 16-27, 16-28, 16-29, 16-30, 16-31, 16-32, 16-33, 16-34, 16-35, 16-36, 16-38, 16-39, and 16-40

Chapter 17: Chapter opener figure, Figures 17-1, 17-2, 17-3, and 17-4

Chapter 18: Chapter opener figure, Figures 18-1, 18-2, 18-3, 18-4, 18-5, 18-6, 18-7, 18-8, and 18-11

Chapter 20: Chapter opener figure, Figures 20-2, 20-3, 20-5, 20-7, 20-8, 20-9, 20-11, 20-12, 20-13, 20-14, 20-15, 20-16, 20-19, 20-20, and 20-21

Chapter 21: Chapter opener figure, Figures 21-1, 21-2, 21-3, 21-4, 21-5, 21-6, 21-7, 21-8, 21-9, 21-10, 21-11, and 21-12

Chapter 22: Chapter opener figure, Figures 22-1, 22-2, 22-3, 22-4, 22-5, 22-6, 22-7, 22-8, 22-9, 22-10, 22-11, 22-12, 22-13, 22-14, and 22-15

Chapter 23: Chapter opener figure, Figure 23-1
Chapter 24: Chapter opener figure, Figures 24-1, 24-2, 24-3, 24-4, 24-5, 24-6, 24-7, 24-8, 24-9, 24-10, 24-11, 24-12, 24-13, and 24-14
Chapter 25: Chapter opener figure, Figures 25-1, 25-2, 25-3, 25-4, 25-5, 25-6, 25-7, 25-8, 25-9, 25-10, 25-11, 25-12, 25-13, 25-14, 25-15, 25-16, and 25-17
Chapter 26: Chapter opener figure, Figures 26-1, 26-2, 26-3, 26-4, 26-5, 26-6, 26-7, 26-8, 26-9, 26-10 and Table 26-9
Chapter 27: Chapter opener figure, Figures 27-1 and 27-5
Chapter 28: Chapter opener figure, Figures 28-1, 28-2, 28-3, and 28-4
Chapter 29: Chapter opener figure, Figures 29-1, 29-2, 29-3, 29-4, 29-5, 29-6, 29-7, 29-8, 29-9, 29-10, 29-11, 29-12, 29-13, 29-14, 29-15, 29-16, 29-17, and 29-18
Chapter 30: Chapter opener figure, Figures 30-1 and 30-2
Chapter 31: Chapter opener figure, Figures 31-1, 31-2, and 31-3
Chapter 32: Chapter opener figure, Figures 32-1, 32-2, 32-3, 32-4, 32-5, 32-6, 32-7, 32-8, 32-9, and 32-10
Chapter 33: Chapter opener figure, Figures 33-1, 33-3, 33-4, 33-5, 33-6, 33-7, 33-8, 33-9, 33-10, 33-11, 33-12, 33-13, and 33-14
Chapter 34: Chapter opener figure, Figures 34-1, 34-2, 34-3, and 34-4
Chapter 35: Chapter opener figure, Figures 35-1, 35-2, 35-3, 35-4, 35-5, 35-6, 35-7, 35-8, 35-9, and 35-10

Foreword

Sitting at home in the midst of COVID-19, I take a respite from the world of "tele-everything" to contemplate the disrupted world around me. I'm now a dean of a school of public health, and in the midst of this public health crisis, the critical themes that resonate now include the need for us to communicate clearly, to share what we know and don't know, and to see the importance of working together to better the situation and to serve others. What a perfect time to be writing a foreword for this tome—*Dermatologic Surgery and Cosmetic Procedures in Primary Care Practice*—by my friend and colleague Jonathan Kantor. For this work is in essence a clear communication and a sharing of knowledge, with the goal of serving our patients.

Without a doubt, Jonathan and his team have both the expertise as well as the experience to author this book, as it is based on a well-regarded previous work written specifically for the specialist. But it goes well beyond expertise. Jonathan Kantor was quoted in *Dermatology* (Volume 26, Issue 6, June 2018) as saying, "Dermatology is not just about treating skin disease; it is also about serving our patients, our colleagues, and the field in general . . . ." With this complete work, he and his colleagues take these words and make them real.

I've worn many different hats in my professional career, including those of dermatology, public health, occupational and preventive medicine, refugee health, disaster response, counterterrorism and emerging threats, health communication, and public health policy. But the roots of my career stem from primary care. Originally trained as a family physician, I took on the overwhelming role of caring for the whole person and was proud to be part of a specialty that was solely devoted to primary care. Family physicians take on about 20% of all office visits, with 192 million visits annually. Add to that the primary care fields of pediatrics, internal medicine, and obstetrics and gynecology and you have built the critical base of the pyramid of medical care that fulfills the general medical needs of specific patient populations.

It is this group of medical colleagues to which this book is directed. With the full understanding that one does not become an expert by reading a book, the primary care physician is still in a position of being that first entry point for a patient seeking care. It's about access, and the world of primary care needs to understand the role and importance of both dermatologic surgery and cosmetic procedures and their place in the general medical needs of the patient. This book provides the primary care world with an expansion of knowledge and could lead to the seeking out of further training for the good of the patients we are all honored to serve.

As a family physician, I knew what I was capable of and what I was trained to do. That capability expanded further with book knowledge, mentorship, and hands-on training in many different areas. By taking this path, I was able to serve my patients and "do good" but also to know my limitations and "do no harm."

Boris D. Lushniak, MD, MPH, FAAD, FACPM
Dean and Professor, University of Maryland School of Public Health, College Park, Maryland
Rear Admiral (Retired), US Public Health Service
US Surgeon General (Acting 2013–2014),
US Deputy Surgeon General (2010–2015)

Preface

Welcome to *Dermatologic Surgery and Cosmetic Procedures in Primary Care Practice*!

It is with great pleasure—and a healthy dose of excitement—that I compose this preface. This book was designed to fill a gap, providing a specialist perspective on procedures for a nonspecialist audience. With the democratization of knowledge and the push to promote best practices, my hope is that this book fits squarely within such a framework, as it is (to my knowledge) the first time a book of this kind was created from the perspective of a surgical dermatologist for the benefit of a nonspecialist audience of primary care practitioners.

This book benefits from including the broadest range of techniques for the clinician, including chapters on ethics, photodynamic therapy, body contouring, sclerotherapy, neck rejuvenation, and hand rejuvenation—all approaches that have never before been explored in a text for this audience—not to mention the most detailed chapters on excisions and linear repairs, flaps, anatomy, and suturing techniques ever presented to a nonspecialist audience.

Where to start? Each chapter begins with an infographic page designed to summarize key takeaway points and outline important areas for the clinician, including both beginner tips and expert tips—as well as billing tips and words of warning. I have chosen to include a fairly comprehensive head and neck anatomy chapter at the beginning of this book; while some readers may be tempted to elide over it, its focus on three-dimensional anatomy and tissue planes should be of particular interest to both those who perform repairs on the head and neck as well as those using soft-tissue fillers, where a detailed understanding of anatomy is of critical value. At the very least, it should serve as a useful reference point.

The key chapters in this book for the clinician looking to incorporate straightforward procedures into daily primary care practice are those on biopsy approaches (Chapter 11), suturing techniques (Chapter 10), and excisions and linear repairs (Chapter 16). While clinicians often think that they need to incorporate cosmetic procedures to survive and thrive financially, this is often not the case, and the nonfinancial rewards of performing medically necessary procedures with skill and finesse on grateful patients cannot be overstated.

Many of the chapters in this book are closely based on similar sections in my (much longer!) textbook for the specialist, *Dermatologic Surgery*. Indeed, the impetus for this book was in part the warm reception of that text and the numerous requests to create a similar textbook sized, priced, and geared for a less specialized audience.

I would be remiss in not thanking not only the authors of the original chapters in the full-length textbook (some of whose work has largely been re-created here verbatim), but also the section editors from the first edition of *Dermatologic Surgery*—John G. Albertini, Jeremy S. Bordeaux, Leonard M. Dzubow, Naomi Lawrence, and Stanley J. Miller. That original team includes some of the luminaries of the field who are not only experts in their respective areas but also helped forge many of the techniques described in this book.

For cosmetic procedures, I have largely eschewed cookbook approaches based on device type, particularly for devices where in-class heterogeneity means that the required training performed by the manufacturer (with their associated charts, protocols, and tables) is likely more useful to the practicing clinician than any chapter could hope to be. Instead, the book focuses on approaching *problems* as a cosmetic patient comes to the office, with concerns regarding dyspigmentation, wrinkling, hand appearance, and the like. Even with the chapters on botulinum toxin and fillers, the goal is to move beyond the plain vanilla techniques taught by trainers and on to an appreciation of the finesse needed to elegantly meet and exceed patients' expectations through a three-dimensional understanding of volumizing.

On a global level, the primary care clinician should always pause before any procedure—and cosmetic procedures in particular—to decide whether they are comfortable and expert enough to perform the procedure in a competent and expeditious way. Patient care is the ultimate arbiter of appropriateness, and there is no substitute for training, mentorship, and experience. Performing a straightforward procedure that goes according to plan can be done by anyone; preparation for the exceptional circumstance when things deviate from the expected is when training and experience truly kick in. It is important to have a mentor (or ideally a team of mentors) and a backup plan in the event that a procedure does not go as planned. Dermatologists and plastic surgeons have the luxury of years of graded and supervised training, and while some primary care clinicians have similar experience, this is not always the case. Unfortunately, bad things can happen to good patients—and clinicians. An untoward outcome at the hands of someone specialized in these techniques may be perceived by the patient as an unavoidable risk of the procedure, while for a clinician with less training or experience, the default may be to assume the worst and that a true medical error occurred. Therefore, seeking out as much training and experience as possible before embarking on procedures is always the best approach for clinician and patient alike.

Finally—and importantly—a special and heartfelt thank you goes out to the brilliant Karen Edmonson of McGraw Hill, who has consistently gone above and beyond on our books; she is a model editor, scholar, and friend, and without her, this book would not be a reality.

Jonathan Kantor, MD, MSCE, MA

Acknowledgments

Much of the work in this textbook is derivative from chapters in the original *Dermatologic Surgery* manuscript. Some chapters are reproduced almost verbatim, while others are largely unrecognizable. My deep and heartfelt thanks goes out to the brilliant chapter authors from the original textbook:

From Surgical Anatomy, Surface Anatomy, and Cosmetic Subunits: Nirusha Lachman, Wojciech Pawlina, Basel Sharaf, Kevin N. Christensen; from Wound Healing and Surgical Wound Dressings: Amy Vandiver, Luis Garza; from Preoperative Evaluation, Patient Preparation, and Informed Consent: Dori Goldberg, Amanda Auerbach, James Bota, Mary E. Maloney; from Surgical Instrument Selection: Michael S. Lehrer, Ashish C. Bhatia, Aashish Taneja; from Antibiotics: Pre- and Postoperative Considerations: Allen F. Shih; from Billing and Financial Considerations in Dermatologic Surgery: Alexander Miller, Ann F. Haas; from Local Anesthesia, Regional Nerve Blocks, and Postoperative Pain Management: David T. Harvey, Emma Elizabeth Harvey; from Superficial Biopsy Techniques: Dirk M. Elston; from Cryosurgery: Carolyn Stull, Clifford Perlis; from Electrosurgery and Hemostasis: Michael Frank, Anthony V. Benedetto; from Incision and Drainage: Sirunya Silapunt, Michael R. Migden; from Approach to Dysplastic Nevi: Lauren C. Strazzulla, Caroline C. Kim; from Approach to Cysts and Lipomas: Rebbecca J. Larson, Amy J. Schutte, Sandra Lee; from Approach to Nonmelanoma Skin Cancer: Alex M. Glazer, Aaron S. Farberg, Darrell S. Rigel; from Flaps and Advanced Techniques: Cassandra J. Simonetta, Jennifer A. Fehlman, Ian A. Maher, Jeremy R. Etzkorn, Michael P. Rabinowitz, Ilya Lim, Renelle Pointdujour-Lim, Thuzar M. Shin, Joseph F. Sobanko, Christopher J. Miller, Luke Nicholas, James Bota, Mary E. Maloney, Dori Goldberg, Joy Kunishige, John A. Zitelli; from Nail Procedures: Molly Hinshaw, Katherine Garrity, Bertrand Richertl; from Managing Surgical Complications: Eileen Axibal, Ramin Fathi, Mariah Ruth Brown; from The Cosmetic Consultation: Kathryn J. Tan, Heidi A. Waldorf; from Botulinum Toxin: Douglas C. Wu; from Fillers: Amelia K. Hausauer, Derek H. Jones, Shino Bay Aguilera, Sean Brabch, Peter L. Mattei, Luis Soro, Emily Tongdee, Vince Bertucci, Mohammad Almohideb, Kucy Pon; from Chemical Peels: Min Deng, Brandon Coakley, Naomi Lawrence, Patrick K. Lee, Seemal R. Desai, Rashmi Sarkar, Pallavi Ailawadi, Kevin Prier; from Lasers for Pigmented Lesions and Tattoos: Adele Haimovic, Deborah S. Sarnoff; from Lasers for Erythema and Telangiectasias: Margaret A. Weiss, Anne M. Mahoney; from Laser Resurfacing: Marc Z. Handler, David J. Goldberg; from Laser and Light-Based Approaches to Hair Removal: Jared Jagdeo, Melissa Shive, George Hruza; from Body Contouring Devices and Noninvasive Fat Removal: Mark S. Nestor, Alexandria B. Glass Michael H. Gold; from Photodynamic Therapy for Acne, Actinic Keratoses, and Nonmelanoma Skin Cancer: Jill S. Waibel, Ashley Rudnick; from Sclerotherapy and Management of Varicose Veins: Neil Sadick; from Approaches to Neck Rejuvenation: Hayes B. Gladstone, Shannon Humphrey; and from Approaches to Hand Rejuvenation: Isabela T. Jones, Ross C. Radusky, Sabrina G. Fabi.

PART I

Fundamentals

Surgical Anatomy, Surface Anatomy, and Cosmetic Subunits

1

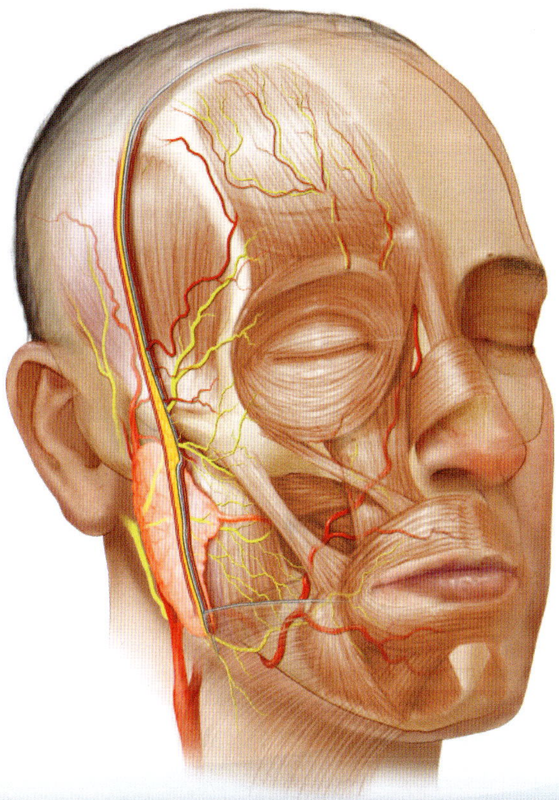

SUMMARY

- Conceptualizing superficial anatomy as a three-dimensional layered system helps understand the course and location of important neurovascular structures as they travel in a stepwise pattern in and between the muscular, bony, and fascial planes to reach their terminal areas of supply and innervation.
- When approaching anatomically susceptible regions ("danger zones"), understanding the depth, course, and relation of these structures as they traverse anatomical boundaries provides the key to successful surgery.

Beginner Tips

- Striated muscles of the face (muscles of facial expression) produce movement of the overlying soft tissue by creating tension transmitted by fibrous strands (retinacula) that connect the SMAS to the skin.
- Facial nerve branches, while generally protected by the SMAS, are surgically vulnerable as they reach areas of transition along their course toward their final destination.
- The forehead and temple are functionally related to the scalp and through SMAS can easily glide over the skull.

Don't Forget!

- The key area of anastomosis between the external and internal carotid arteries is located above the medial canthal tendon where the angular artery communicates with the dorsal nasal branch of the ophthalmic artery.
- Both the facial artery and the marginal branch of the facial nerve lie deep to the fibers of the platysma.

Expert Tips

- The internal carotid artery via its ophthalmic branch supplies a central triangular area including the eyes, superior nose, and central portion of the forehead.
- The angular artery and vein cross the medial canthal tendon and contribute to an important site of anastomosis just superior to the tendon between branches of the external carotid (facial artery) and internal carotid (ophthalmic artery).
- Nasal blood supply is mainly from the angular artery externally and the sphenopalatine artery internally, with smaller contributions from the superior labial and ophthalmic arteries.
- The parotid gland is contained within a shiny, tight fascial sheath (the parotid fascia), which helps differentiate it from fat.

Pitfalls and Cautions

- Erb's point, located 6 cm below the midpoint of a line connecting the angle of the mandible with the mastoid process, provides a landmark for the exit point of the superficial cervical nerves and the accessory nerve (cranial nerve XI).
- The mandibular branch of the facial nerve crosses over the facial artery about 5 to 10 mm above the point at which the facial artery crosses the mandible.

1 Surgical Anatomy, Surface Anatomy, and Cosmetic Subunits

INTRODUCTION

Understanding fundamental anatomy is crucial before embarking on any skin surgery—or any interventional procedure. Although head and neck anatomy is more subtle and complex than that of the trunk and extremities, even those restricting their practice to nonfacial areas need to understand the complex interactions between tissue planes in order to yield the best possible results—and confer the lowest possible risk of adverse events. Importantly, the head and neck display significant variation in skin thickness, texture, color, amount of subcutaneous fat, and laxity, and if these differences are ignored, this may lead to the blunting of natural contours and a suboptimal outcome.

Naturally occurring lines divide the face into areas referred to as cosmetic units and subunits. Surgical repair for an ideal cosmetic outcome should be based on preservation of the subunits by maintaining incision lines along or within these lines as much as possible (**Figure 1-1**).

KEY PRINCIPLES FOR UNDERSTANDING FACIAL ANATOMY

Skin Tension Lines of the Face

Striated muscles of the face (muscles of facial expression) produce movement of the overlying soft tissue by creating tension transmitted by fibrous strands (retinacula) that connect the superficial musculoaponeurotic system (SMAS) to the skin. In younger patients, this tension is opposed by elastic fibers within the skin. With progressive aging, however, changes in the configuration of collagen fibers and the decreased ability of the elastic fibers to resist this tension result in the formation of wrinkle lines along these retinacula attachments. Relaxed skin tension lines (RSTLs), therefore, run perpendicular to the underlying muscle fibers; for example, wrinkle lines on the forehead run horizontally because the frontalis muscle contracts vertically.

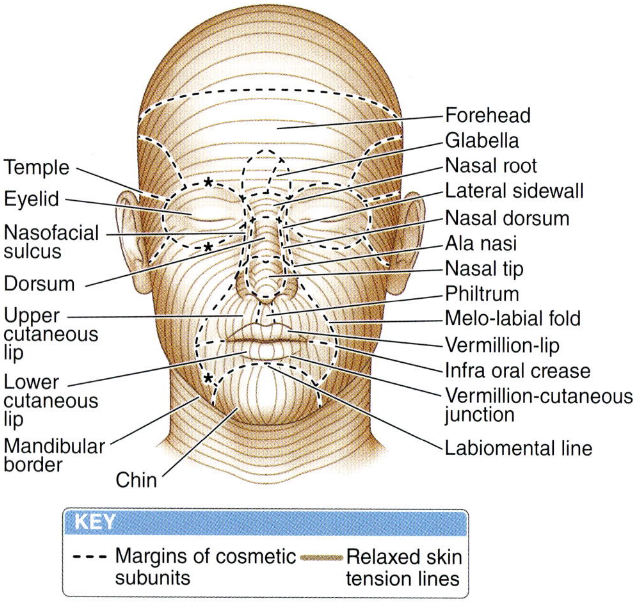

FIGURE 1-1 Diagram illustrating cosmetic subunit boundaries and relaxed skin tension lines.

Understanding the profiles of RSTLs is a key element in surgical planning with the goal of minimizing visible scarring. Techniques for scar reduction have been well described in the literature, and one principle is to align the long axis of the repair within or as close as possible to the RSTL to promote merging of the scar into the wrinkle line. Having patients perform exaggerated facial expressions will expose these lines, while gentle manipulation of the skin may also highlight RSTLs; for this reason, it is important to always touch and move the skin prior to initiating a repair (**Figure 1-1**).

UNDERSTANDING THE FASCIAL PLANES OF THE FACE AND NECK

The anatomy of the face and its subunits presents itself through a distinct arrangement of fascial planes that enclose subcutaneous tissue, superficial muscles, nerves, and blood vessels. Deconstructing the complex relationships that exist between these planes provides a view of the course and relations of vascular networks and important traversing branches of the superficial motor and sensory nerves. Understanding and predicting the trajectory of the branches of an intricate plexus of motor and sensory nerves within the muscular architecture is crucial to minimizing complications associated with dermatologic surgery.

A few basic concepts are strategic to predicting potential challenges that accompany surgical manipulation of the superficial face:

1. The face can be dissected through principal fascial planes that consist of skin, subcutaneous fibroadipose layer, SMAS, space containing traversing nerves and retaining ligaments, and deep fascial layer (**Figure 1-2**).[1,2]
2. Muscles of facial expression are not set within the same architectural plane. They attach to the dermis and are reinforced by retaining ligaments while maintaining an arrangement within a stepped configuration (**Figure 1-3**).[2]
3. Exiting branches of the facial nerve are the principal motor suppliers of the muscles of facial expression and they tend to innervate these muscles through their deep surfaces, overlying muscles only as they traverse from their points of origin to innervation (**Figure 1-4**).[3,4]
4. Facial nerve branches exit the parotid fascia along its anterior margin, often networking as they travel from a deep to superficial plane, while still lying deep to the SMAS plane (**Figure 1-5**).[5]
5. Facial nerve branches divide into a variable number of rami and, in the mid-lateral face, form a plexus of interconnected communications that include connections between the facial nerve and the trigeminal nerve branches (**Figure 1-6**).[5,6]

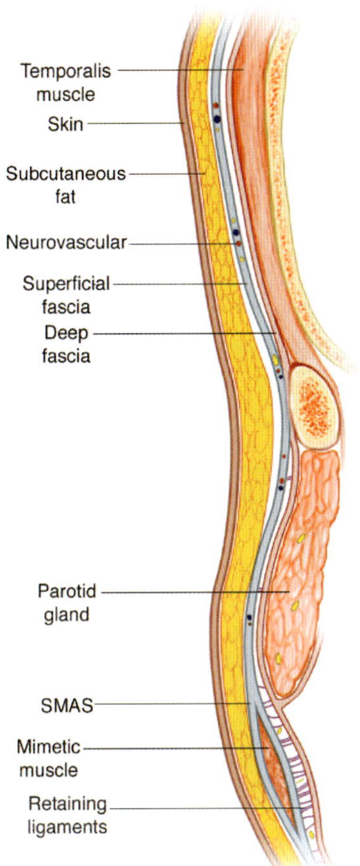

FIGURE 1-2 Conceptual illustration demonstrating layers of the face from superficial to deep. (Used with permission of Mayo Foundation for Medical Education and Research. All rights reserved.)

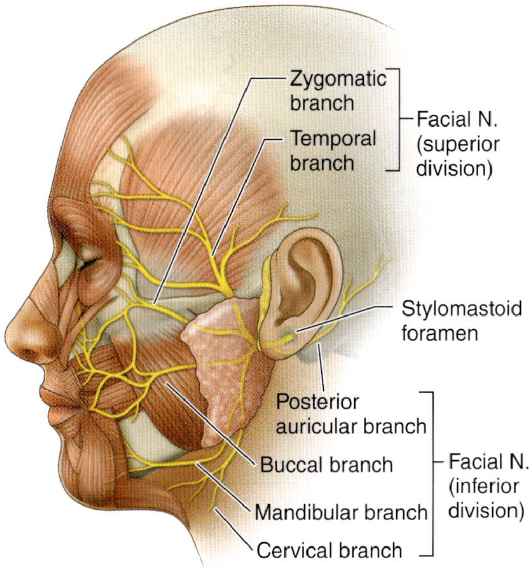

FIGURE 1-4 Diagram illustrating standard pattern of distribution of branches of the facial nerve.

6. While the SMAS splits to enclose muscles of facial expression, it remains continuous with fascia of the platysma, superficial parotid fascia, galea aponeurotica, and superficial temporal fascia (temporoparietal fascia) (**Figure 1-2**).[7]
7. While the superficial temporal vessels are contained within the SMAS, the sub-SMAS plane remains relatively avascular (**Figure 1-7**).[7]
8. Trigeminal nerve branches travel in a plane above the SMAS and then exit the supraorbital, infraorbital, and mental foramina and travel in a deep to superficial direction toward the skin, where they lie within the subcutaneous fibroadipose layer (**Figure 1-8**).[4,8-10]

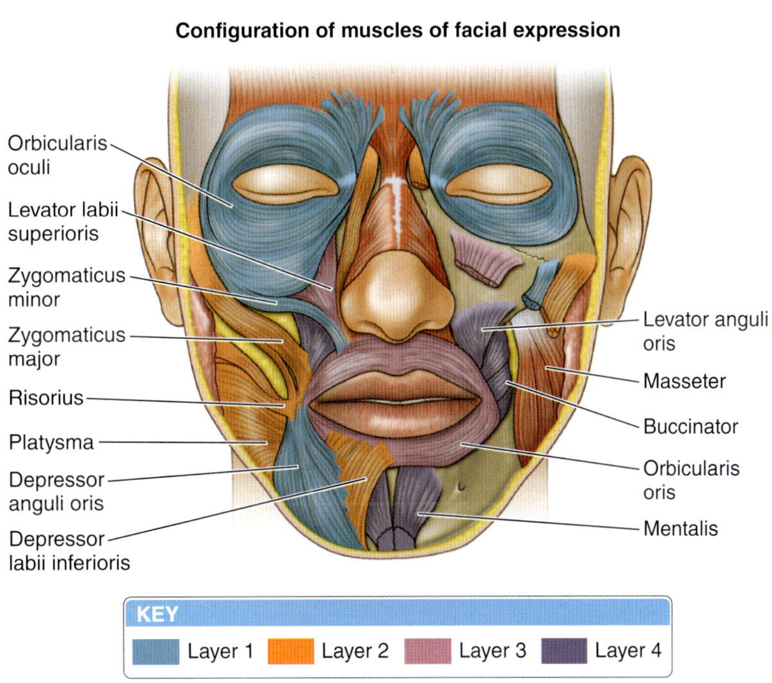

FIGURE 1-3 Diagram illustrating stepped configuration and arrangement of muscles of facial expression (mimetic muscles).

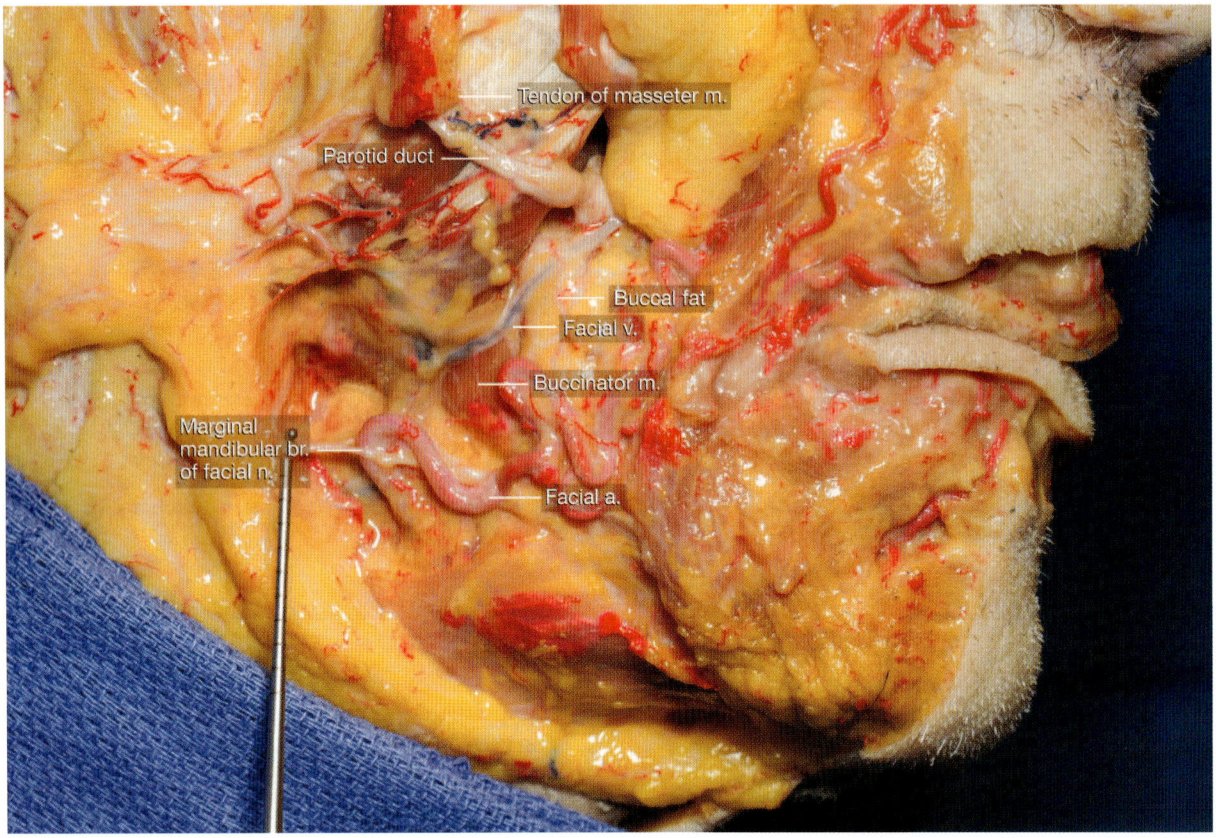

FIGURE 1-5 Deep dissection of facial nerve with reflected upper portion of parotid gland.

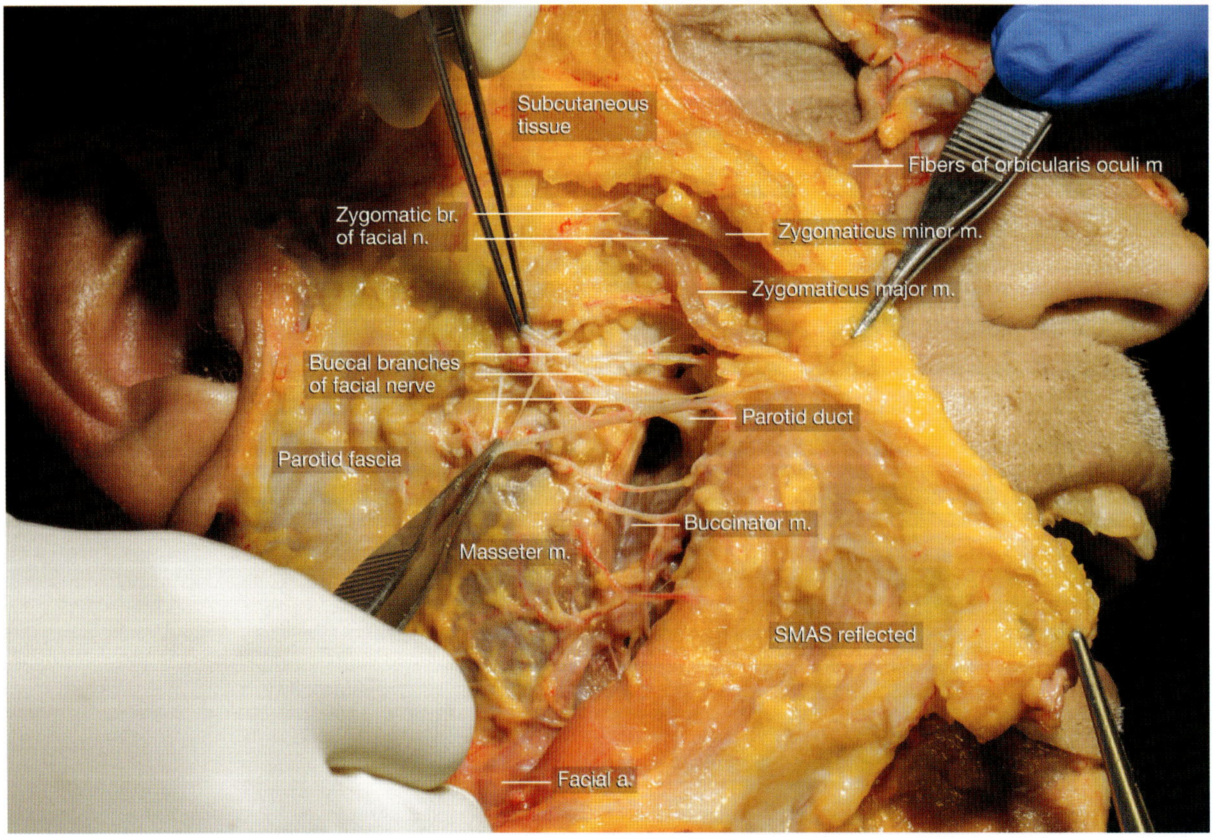

FIGURE 1-6 Dissection of facial nerve deep to SMAS.

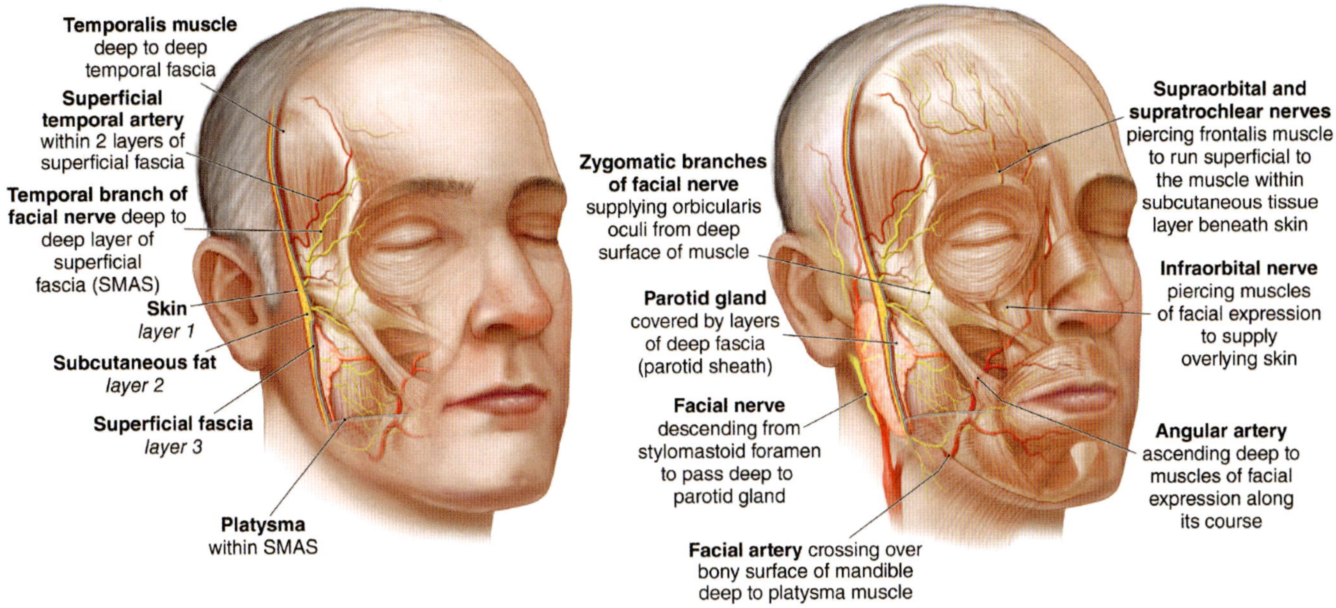

FIGURE 1-7 Conceptual illustration demonstrating relationship of structures within layers of the face from superficial to deep. (Used with permission of Mayo Foundation for Medical Education and Research. All rights reserved.)

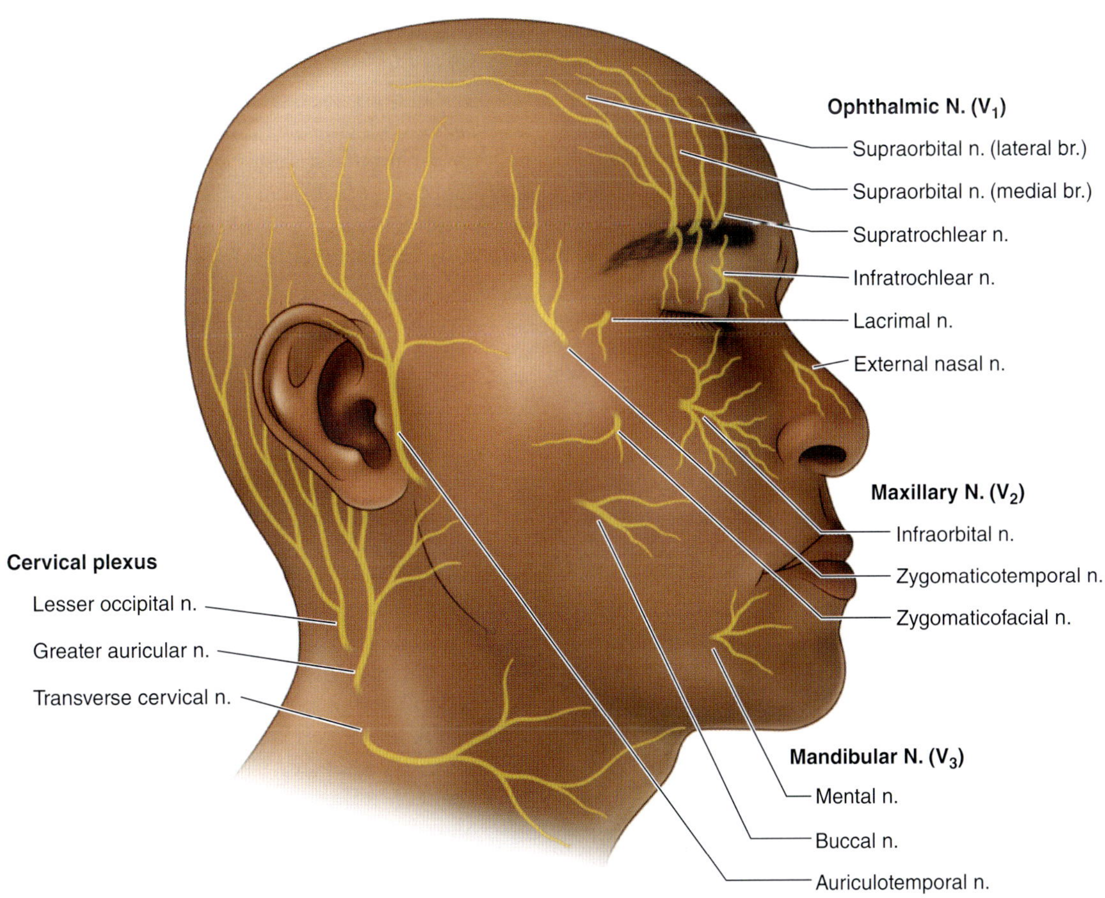

FIGURE 1-8 Diagram illustrating distribution patterns of sensory branches of the trigeminal nerve.

9. The facial artery and its branches travel deep to the SMAS and run along a superficial course to cross palpable bony boundaries or penetrate the SMAS (**Figure 1-7**).[11,12]
10. The thickness of the subcutaneous layer varies significantly and displays fat compartments that are predictable and distinct within cosmetic subunits. The layer is more uniform in thickness over the scalp, while compaction of the subcutaneous tissue around the eyelids and lips appears to make this layer almost nonexistent.[1,2,13,14]

TOPOGRAPHIC FRAMEWORK OF THE SUPERFICIAL FACE

1. Skin
2. Subcutaneous plane
3. SMAS
4. Soft tissue spaces, facial ligaments, deep portions of the muscles of facial expression, and segments of the facial nerve branches traversing toward points of innervation
5. Deep fascia overlying the superficial muscles of mastication (deep temporal fascia, masseteric fascia), periosteum, and parotid fascia

SURGICALLY RELEVANT ANATOMY WITHIN COSMETIC UNITS

1. Forehead

KEY STRUCTURES AND ANATOMIC POINTS

- Muscles acting on the forehead and eyebrow: frontalis, corrugator supercilii, and procerus.
- The forehead and temple are functionally related to the scalp and through SMAS can easily glide over the skull.
- The supraorbital and supratrochlear neurovascular bundles supply this region.

The forehead extends from the hairline to the eyebrows in a vertical direction and ends laterally at the temporal ridges. Skin of the forehead varies in dermal thickness, decreasing as it extends superiorly toward the hairline. In addition, while more taut in younger individuals, skin of the forehead in older patients tends to be more mobile, usually as a result of chronological or actinic damage. Beneath the skin, the subcutaneous layer is minimal, usually not more than about 1 mm thick. Just deep to the subcutaneous tissue, the SMAS encloses the frontal or anterior belly of the occipitofrontalis muscle with its vertically oriented fibers. As the thickness of the muscle tends to decrease with age, these fibers can be rather sparse in older patients, making the traversing neurovascular structures easier to reach.

Between the left and right anterior bellies of occipitofrontalis, a fascial extension known as the galeal median raphe is present. The galeal raphe is devoid of muscle fibers and does not usually contain any significant associated neurovascular structures. Inferiorly, superolateral fibers of the orbicularis oculi can be visualized as they interface with the medially located fibers of procerus and corrugator supercilii.

It is helpful to remember that the frontalis muscle is enveloped by superficial and deep investing layers of the SMAS and periosteum. The supratrochlear and supraorbital nerves are important structures that provide sensory innervation to the scalp and skin. They exit the supraorbital foramen within a neurovascular bundle above the orbital rim (**Figure 1-9**).

The forehead receives vascular supply centrally from the right and left supratrochlear and supraorbital arteries and bilaterally by the anterior branch of the temporal arteries. These vessels are located in the subcutaneous tissue and are predictable in their location (**Figures 1-10 and 1-11**).

2. Temple

KEY STRUCTURES AND ANATOMIC POINTS

- The superficial temporal artery travels within the layers of the superficial temporal fascia.
- Rich anastomosis occurs between branches of the superficial temporal artery and supraorbital artery.
- The auriculotemporal nerve runs deep and posterior to the superficial temporal artery.
- The frontal branch of the facial nerve is most vulnerable as it crosses the zygomatic arch as a single trunk en route to the deep surfaces of the frontalis muscle.

The temporal fossa contains a relatively sparse amount of subcutaneous tissue devoid of muscles of facial expression, with the exception of traversing fibers of the orbicularis oculi muscle and even fewer fibers of the anterior auricular muscle. Two distinct layers of fascia are contained within this unit: the deep temporal fascia, which is a continuation of the investing fascia containing the deeper temporalis muscle as it becomes continuous with the periosteum of the skull; and the superficial temporal fascia, which is a continuation of the SMAS as it connects to the galea aponeurotica (**Figure 1-12**). In this region, the superficial temporal fascia is of anatomic and subsequent surgical importance as it contains within its layers key vascular and neural structures as they traverse between the fascial layers. The superficial temporal artery along with its branches and sensory nerves, including the auriculotemporal nerve, can be accessed within the layers of the superficial temporal fascia (**Figure 1-12**). The motor branches of the facial nerve remain deep to the superficial temporal fascia as they course toward the deep surface of the orbicularis oculi and frontalis muscles (**Figure 1-6**). The superficial temporal fascia forms a continuous layer with the galea aponeurotica but splits medially to enclose the frontalis and orbicularis oculi muscles and laterally the superficial periauricular fibers. Inferiorly, the superficial temporal fascia is adherent to the zygomatic arch. Immediately adjacent to the superficial layer of the superficial temporal fascia, the subcutaneous fatty layer separates it from the overlying dermis. Fibrous septa create a more taut area as one moves toward the scalp, with relatively greater laxity just above the zygomatic arch. Numerous cutaneous vessels and nerves lie in this interval between the fat and fascia, which is important to remember when undermining in this area. The deep layer of the superficial temporal fascia glides over the loose connective tissue of the deep

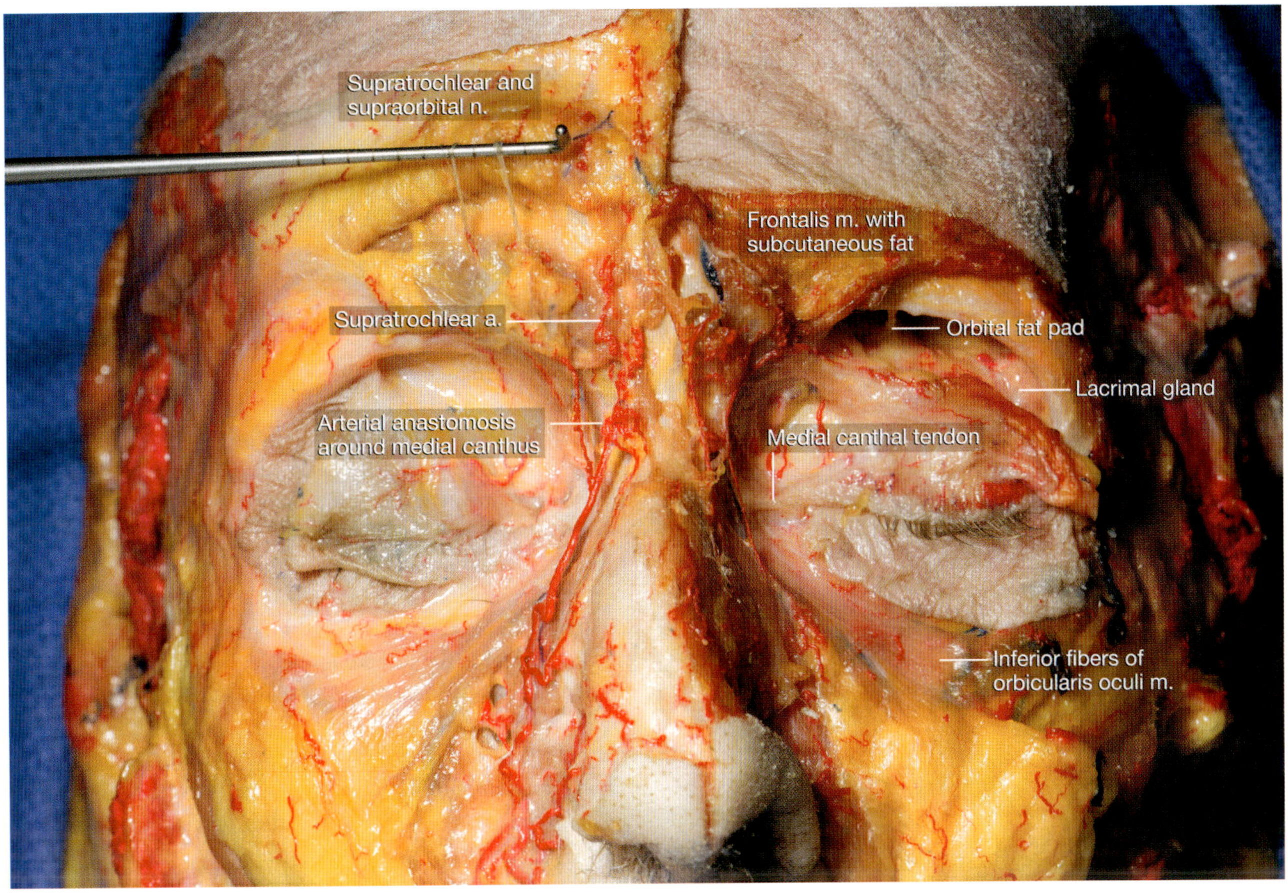

FIGURE 1-9 Anterior view of dissection of the upper face highlighting supratrochlear and supraorbital nerves.

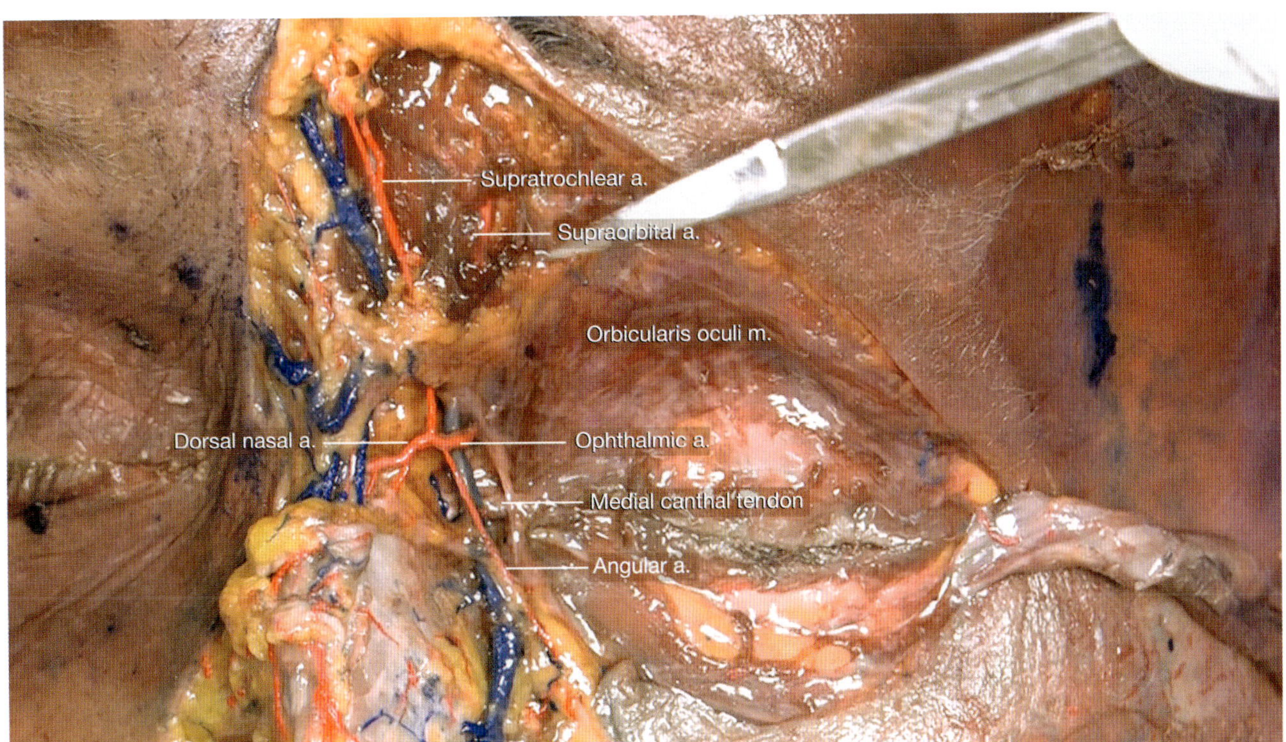

FIGURE 1-10 Anatomy of anastomosis around the medial canthus of the left eye.

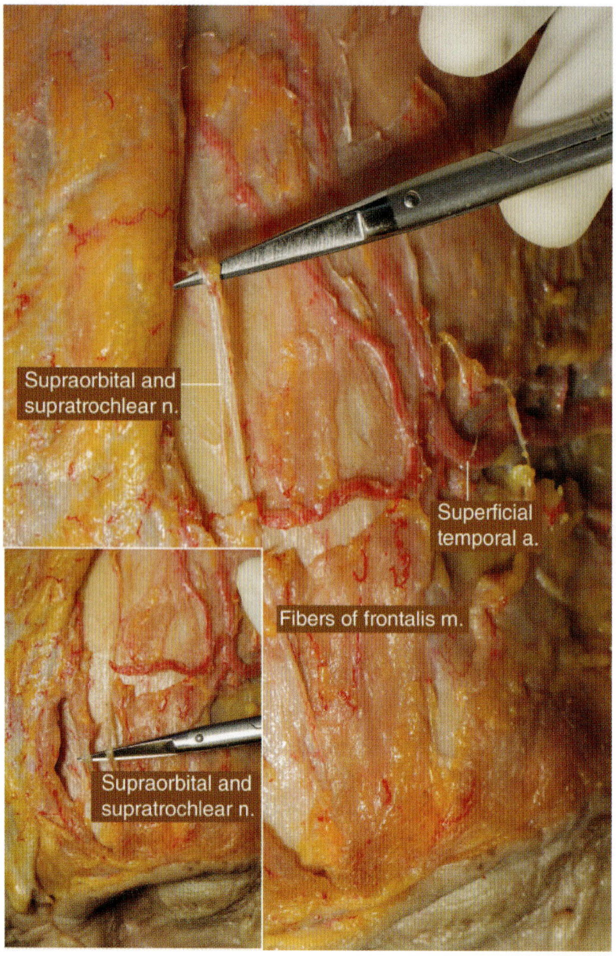

FIGURE 1-11 Supraorbital and supratrochlear nerves coursing over fibers of frontalis muscle.

temporal fascia, deep to which the temporalis muscle can be visualized (**Figure 1-12**).

The primary source of vascular supply to the temple comes from the superficial temporal artery, a terminal branch of the external carotid artery. The superficial temporal artery emerges from the superior pole of the parotid gland as it pierces the parotid fascia anterior to the tragus (**Figure 1-12**). Inferior to it, the transverse facial artery runs below and in line with the zygomatic arch. The artery is accompanied by corresponding veins and usually divides anteriorly into anterior and posterior branches, with two or sometimes three significant-sized pedicles. The anterior branch follows a distinct tortuous course, especially prominent in elderly patients, to supply the temple and the temporal scalp region. Branches anastomose freely with the posterior parietal branches as well as contributions from the supraorbital artery. From an anatomic standpoint, it is important to note that while the superficial temporal artery lies within the layers of the superficial temporal fascia, the corresponding veins are located within the subcutaneous layer. As the arteries continue toward the scalp, they also come to lie within the subcutaneous plane just above the superficial temporal fascia.

Sensory innervation to the temple is achieved via the maxillary and mandibular divisions of the trigeminal nerve. The auriculotemporal nerve (**Figure 1-13**) travels posterior and deep to the superficial temporal artery and branches as it runs within the same fascial plane as the artery as they proceed toward the scalp. The skin adjacent to the lateral canthus is supplied by a branch of the maxillary artery, with the zygomaticotemporal nerve emerging from the lateral orbital wall. Additionally, the zygomaticotemporal nerve innervates an area of scalp between the territories of the auriculotemporal and supraorbital nerves (**Figure 1-8**). Emerging from the superior pole of the parotid gland, the temporal branch

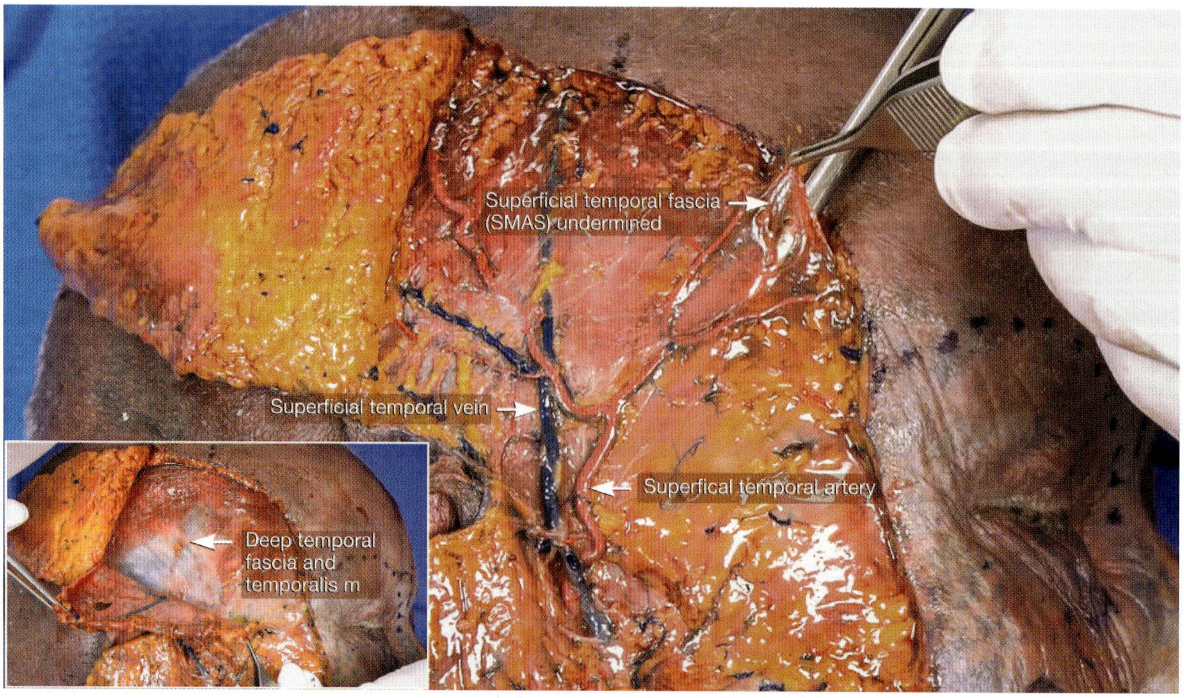

FIGURE 1-12 Dissection of superficial temporal fascia reflected to show superficial temporal vessels.

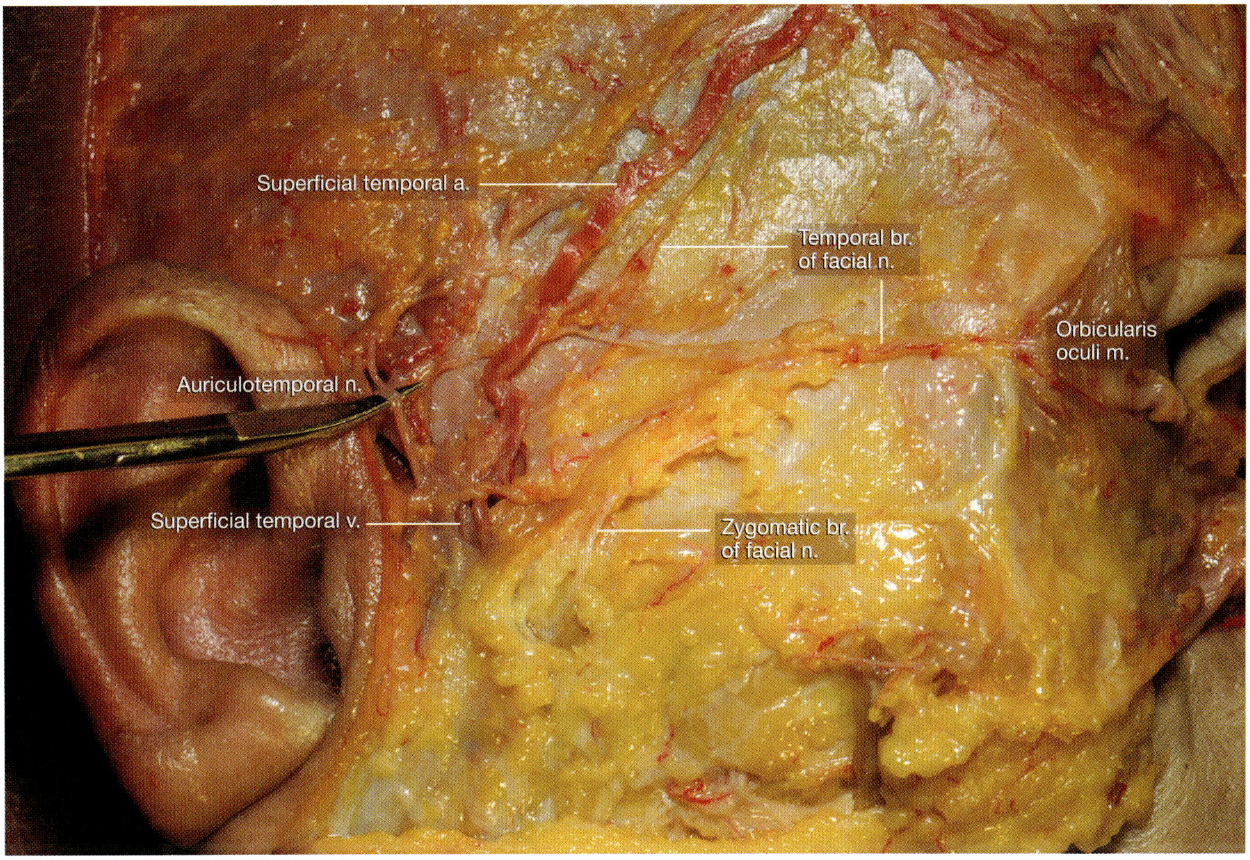

FIGURE 1-13 Dissection of temporal region highlighting the auriculotemporal nerve.

of the facial nerve crosses superficial to the zygomatic arch as a single branch within the superficial temporal fascia, increasing its vulnerability to surgical injury (**Figure 1-14**). With the use of surface anatomic landmarks, the temporal branch may be visualized along a line 0.5 cm below the tragus to a point approximately 1.5 cm superior to the lateral edge of the eyebrow. The temporal branch of the facial nerve supplies the frontalis muscle from the deep lateral edge with few branches contributing to fibers of orbicularis oculi and those of surrounding muscles of facial expression.

3. Superficial Orbital Region and Eyelid

KEY STRUCTURES AND ANATOMIC POINTS

- Skin of the eyelids is very thin with only a thin fascial layer between it and fibers of the orbicularis oculi muscle. There is no fat beneath the dermis.
- Lacrimal canaliculi are deep to the medial canthal tendon.
- The angular artery and vein cross the medial canthal tendon and contribute to an important site of anastomosis just superior to the tendon between branches of external carotid (facial artery) and internal carotid (ophthalmic artery).

The orbital rim is formed laterally by the zygomatic process of the frontal bone and the frontal process of the zygomatic bone. The frontal bone forms the superior orbital margin as well as the roof of the orbit, with the superciliary arch of the frontal bone defining the superior orbital rim.

Along the mid-pupillary line, the superior orbital rim presents a notch, sometimes a foramen (>25%), known as the supraorbital notch/foramen, through which the supraorbital vessels and nerves are transmitted (**Figure 1-9**).

The medial orbital margin is formed by the maxillary process of the frontal bone along with the frontal process of the maxillary bone. The maxillary bone forms the floor of the orbit and the infraorbital rim. The lateral canthus lies in contact with the sclera, whereas the medial canthus is separated from the sclera by the caruncle and the lacrimal lake. The caruncle contains sweat and sebaceous glands, whereas the lacrimal lake provides a collection area for tear fluid before passing through the lacrimal canaliculi.

The skin around the eyelids is very thin, with only a thin fascial layer between it and the fibers of the orbicularis oculi muscle. Unlike the usual anatomic relationship of skin to subcutaneous tissue, there is no fat beneath the dermis. Understanding this arrangement provides insight into the depth of dissection as the subdermal space is approached. There are no significant superficial nerves or vessels in this subfascial space. Additionally, skin over the tarsal plates is tightly adherent, whereas the preseptal area allows for greater mobility. Another point of importance when understanding the layers of tissue around the eye is to

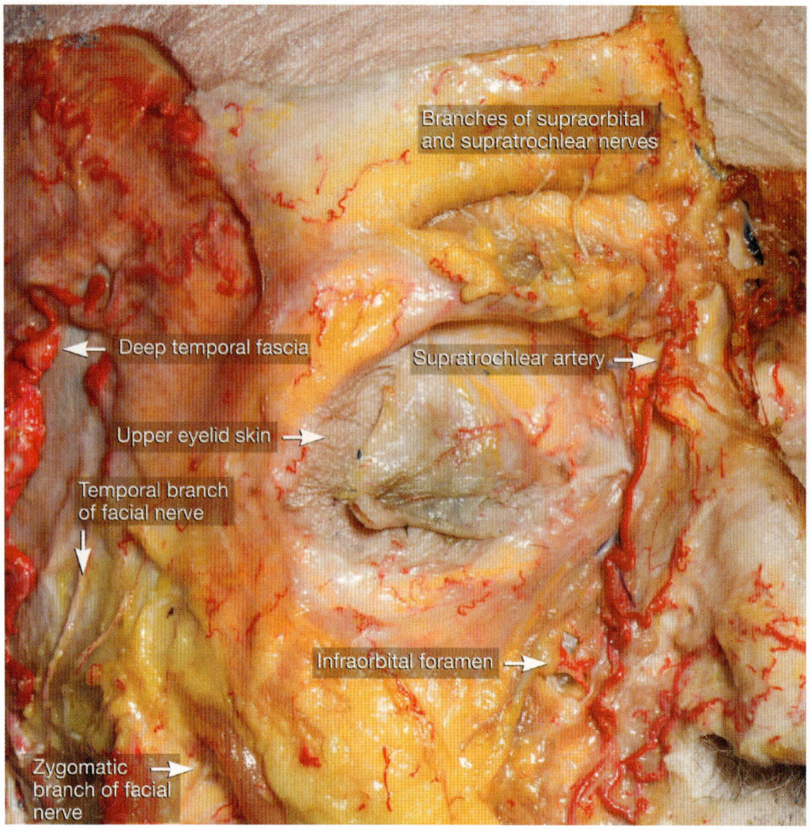

FIGURE 1-14 Dissection demonstrating relationship between superficial temporal artery and temporal branch of the facial nerve.

remember that the region over the orbital septum, just proximal to the tarsal region, presents with several layers. Following the skin, subcutaneous tissue orbicularis oculi, and orbital septum, there is a layer of orbital fat followed by the aponeurosis of the levator palpebrae superioris, Muller's muscle, and then conjunctiva (**Figure 1-15**).

The orbicularis oculi and levator palpebrae superioris muscles are two predominant muscles of surgical concern. The orbicularis oculi is best described as two parts: the orbital portion and the palpebral portion. These portions of the muscle contract independently, the orbital portion under voluntary control and the palpebral fibers under both voluntary and involuntary control. The upper portion is innervated by the temporal branch of the facial nerve, whereas the lower fibers are innervated by the zygomatic branch of the facial nerve. The action is to tightly close the lids together. The orbital fibers attach to the orbital rim and blend in with the surrounding muscles of facial expression—the frontalis superiorly and the procerus medially. Corrugator supercilii lies beneath the medial aspect of the orbital fibers, and its origin from the medial orbital crest and insertion into the upper medial portion of the eyebrows bring the eyebrows medially.

The palpebral portion of the orbicularis oculi overlies the pretarsal and preseptal regions. Preseptal fibers cover the orbital septum of both upper and lower lids. It is important to note that the upper and lower preseptal fibers attach to the respective areas of the medial canthal tendon, and this arrangement has significant impact on the functioning of the lacrimal canaliculi. The continuation of these fibers laterally toward the lateral canthal tendon helps in bringing the lids together to produce winking and blinking actions. The pretarsal portion is attached firmly to the tarsal plate. Their connections maintain a similar anatomic arrangement as the medial and lateral preseptal muscles and are connected to the medial and lateral canthal tendons. The palpebral muscle unit is an important contributor to the mechanism of tear movement.

The medial canthal area is frequently a site for surgical excisions. Several important anatomic structures should be considered when working around this area. The lacrimal canaliculi are deep to the medial canthal tendon. However, they are secured at a deeper plane and relatively protected by an undisrupted tendon. The angular artery and vein traverse the area on their ascent within the nasolabial groove. They cross the medial canthal tendon and contribute to an important site of anastomosis just superior to the tendon between branches of the external carotid (facial artery) and internal carotid (ophthalmic artery) (**Figure 1-9**).

The upper lid has two fat pads, the pre-aponeurotic and nasal units,[15] and it may be difficult to distinguish between them and the lacrimal gland, which lies in a lateral position on the upper lid. The lower lid contains a nasal, central, and lateral fat pad. Their connection to the orbital septum laterally and via its fascia to the inferior oblique muscle medially makes the muscle susceptible

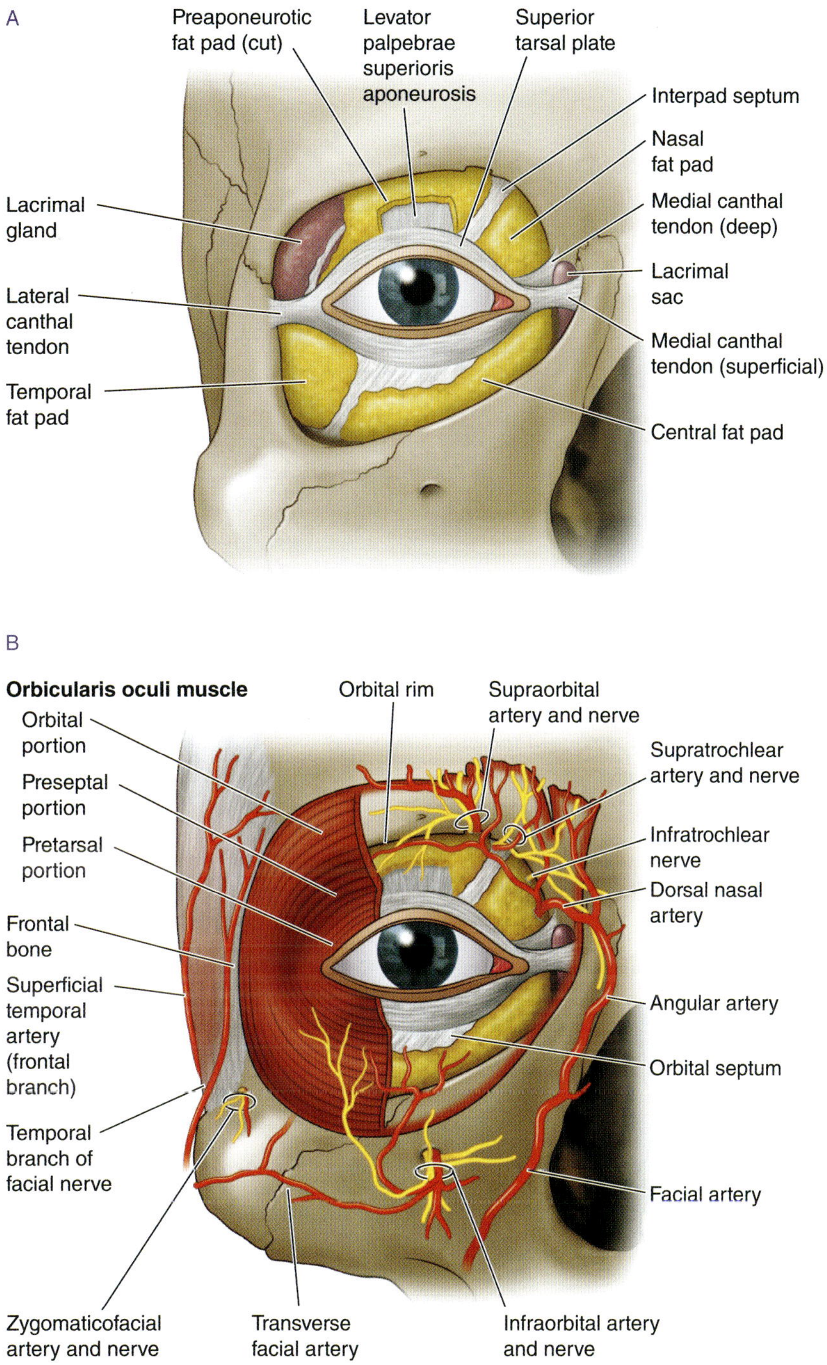

FIGURE 1-15 Diagram illustrating basic anatomy of the eye.

to injury (**Figure 1-15**). The levator palpebrae superioris and its aponeurosis are responsible for raising the eyelid and are innervated by the oculomotor nerve. It is important to remember that the muscle arises in the apical region of the orbit and continues in its superior most location in an anterior direction. It is easily identifiable during dissection as it exists as a well-defined flat or sometimes more bulky muscle. As it approaches anteriorly, it divides into an aponeurosis and posteriorly reflects into Muller's tarsal muscle. Fibers also attach to the orbicularis oculi and are connected to the overlying skin by fibrous strands. The lower lid is retracted by the extraocular inferior rectus muscle and also contains a tarsal muscle.

The tarsal plates are dense fibrous tissue plates that begin at the lacrimal puncta medially and extend to the lateral commissures. Numerous meibomian sebaceous glands are embedded vertically within the tarsal plates.[4,15]

As previously mentioned, arterial supply to the eyelids is derived from extensive anastomosis between the internal and

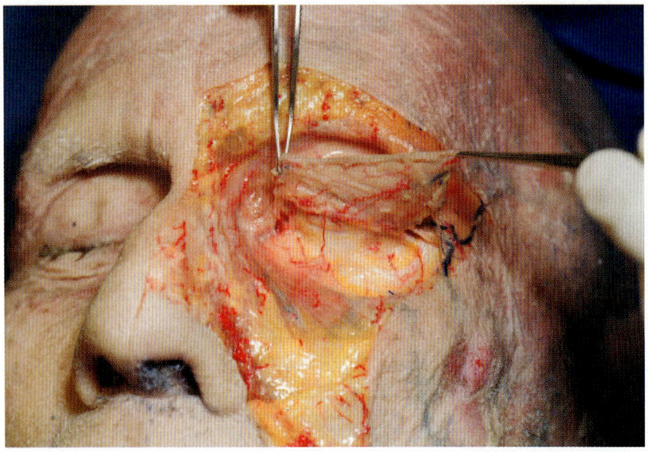

FIGURE 1-16 Dissection demonstrating arterial arcades around the eyelids.

external carotid arteries. Branches from the ophthalmic, facial, and superficial temporal arteries perfuse both the upper and lower lids. Additionally, the maxillary artery via the infraorbital artery also contributes to the extensive vascularity, as its branches anastomose with the ascending branches of the transverse facial, facial, and angular arteries. The main venous drainage of the eyelids occurs via the superficial temporal, angular, and facial veins. Both arterial and venous systems present as vascular arcades along the upper and lower lids (**Figure 1-16**).

4. Nose

KEY STRUCTURES AND ANATOMIC POINTS

- The nose is divided into root, dorsum, lateral walls, tip, alae, and columella.
- Most of the alae are composed of skin and fibrofatty tissue.
- Blood supply is mainly from the angular artery externally and the sphenopalatine artery internally, with smaller contributions from the superior labial and ophthalmic arteries.
- Sensory innervation is derived from infraorbital branch of the maxillary nerve and infratrochlear and external nasal branches of the anterior ethmoidal nerve (ophthalmic nerve).

The challenge with conducting surgery on the nose is twofold. First, the nose presents with complex anatomy consisting of skin, cartilage, and nasal mucosa within a rather small anatomic boundary. Second, the mid-face location of the nose places a premium on cosmetic outcome, which reinforces the importance of thoroughly understanding the anatomy that will facilitate effective surgical repair and outcome. In its simple description, the nose may be divided into the root, dorsum (bridge), lateral side walls, and lobule (**Figure 1-17**). The lobule is further divided into the nasal tip, the infra-tip, and the alae. When viewed from below, the infra-tip lobule presents a soft triangular area anteriorly, a columella that extends inferiorly and separates two nostrils bound by the nostril sills, and laterally the alar base and rim. Together, the bony pyramid, septum, alar cartilages, and cartilaginous vault form the main structural support of the nose.

The nasal bones articulate along the midline and with the frontal processes of the maxillae laterally. Superiorly, the nasal bones articulate with the nasal processes of the frontal bone and inferiorly with the perpendicular plate of the ethmoid bone. Nasal bones are thickest superiorly but thin out inferiorly where they may be easily damaged. There is overlap between these lower borders and the upper borders of the lateral cartilages. Skin over the bony pyramid is loose, fairly mobile, and can be easily undermined.[15,16]

The lateral cartilages are a continuation of the nasal bones, being overlapped superiorly by these bones and inferiorly by the upper border of the lateral crura of the alar cartilages. Ligamentous tissue connects both these overhangs.

The nasal septum consists of bone, cartilage, and soft tissue, which includes all of its articulating craniofacial bony structures. A septal or quadrangular cartilage anchors to the perpendicular plate of the ethmoid bone and maintains structural integrity of the bony septum. The membranous septum, a soft tissue composite, consists of two layers of vestibular skin separated by loose connective tissue. Depressor septi muscle traverses the membranous septum and attaches to the inferior border of the septal cartilage.[4,15]

The lobule is the most mobile portion of the nose due to the lack of any fixed cartilaginous joints. The support of the lobule comes from the paired alar cartilages suspended by soft-tissue ligaments. The soft-tissue portion of the ala does not contain cartilage but rather is structurally maintained by a thickened dermis with no underlying subcutaneous fat, making detecting a good dissection plane challenging in this area.

The key muscles around the nose include procerus, levator labii superioris alaeque nasi, nasalis, and depressor septi muscles. Procerus extends from the frontalis muscle across the root of the nose and blends in with the transversely positioned nasalis muscle. It is important to remember that the plane deep to nasalis is continuous with the subgaleal plane, which maintains a bloodless field of dissection. The levator labii superioris alaeque nasi arises from the maxilla and sends fibers to the medial upper lip and the lateral ala. The most medial portion of these muscle fibers is referred to as the depressor septi, which pulls down on the septum and keeps the airways patent (**Figure 1-18**).

The nose receives a rich blood supply, which is a surgical advantage and allows for versatility in flap design and orientation. While blood supply is mainly from the angular artery externally and the sphenopalatine artery internally, with smaller contributions from the superior labial and ophthalmic arteries, the largest vascular contribution is derived from the external carotid system. The superior and inferior labial arteries are branches off the facial artery, and they continue along the lateral aspects within the nasolabial grooves as the ascending angular artery en route to the medial canthal anastomotic site. The angular artery gives off many small branches to the sidewalls, ala, and dorsum, and forms free and contralateral anastomoses terminating through a connection with the dorsal nasal artery (**Figure 1-19**). This point of

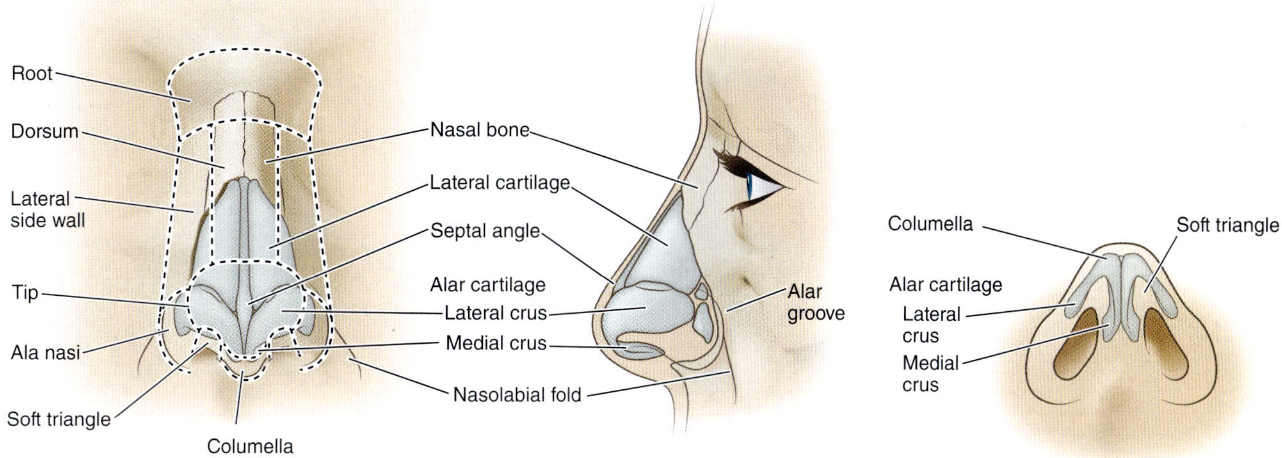

FIGURE 1-17 Diagram illustrating basic anatomy of the nose.

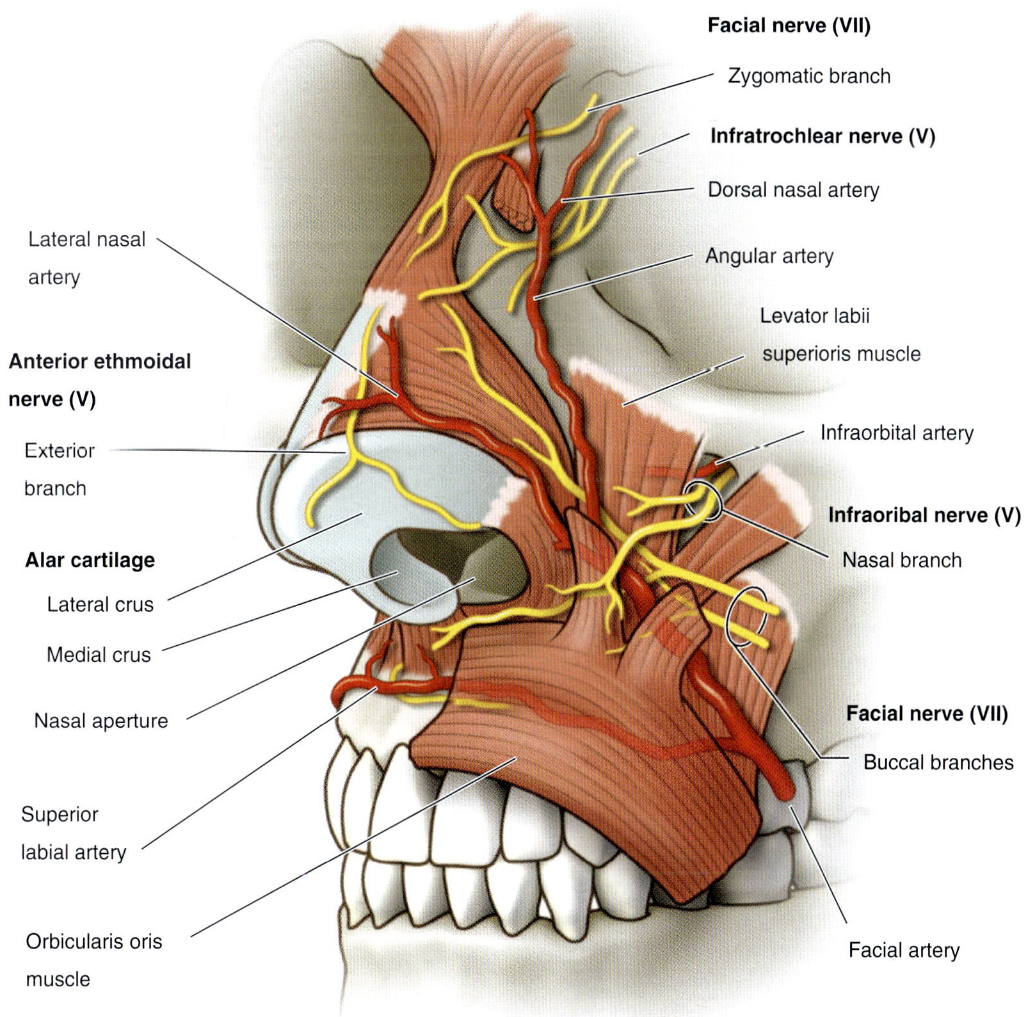

FIGURE 1-18 Diagram illustrating deeper anatomy around the nose.

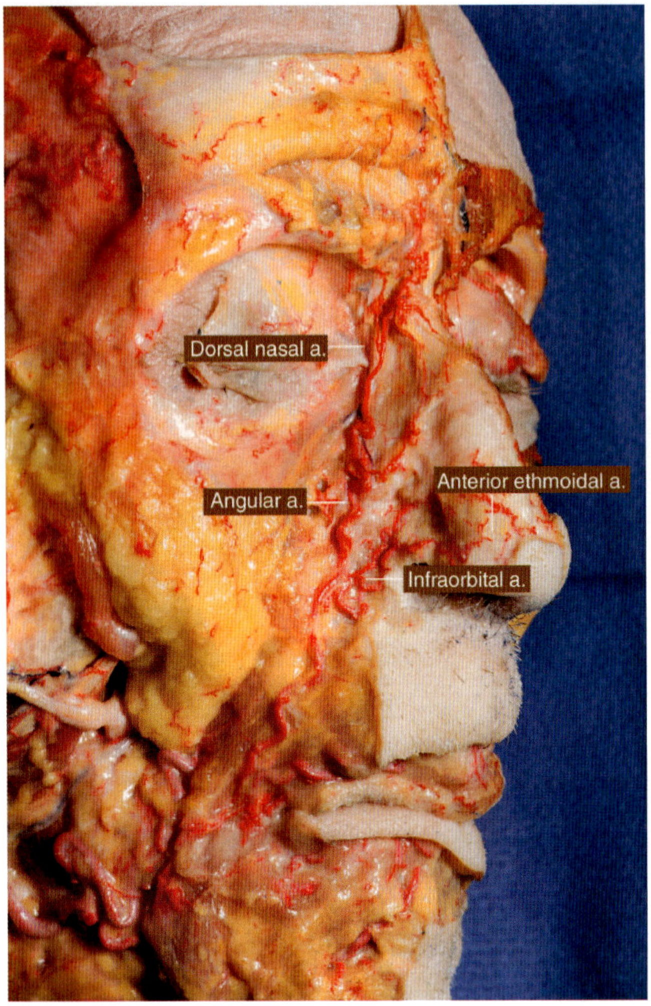

FIGURE 1-19 Dissection demonstrating ascent of the facial and angular artery within the nasolabial region.

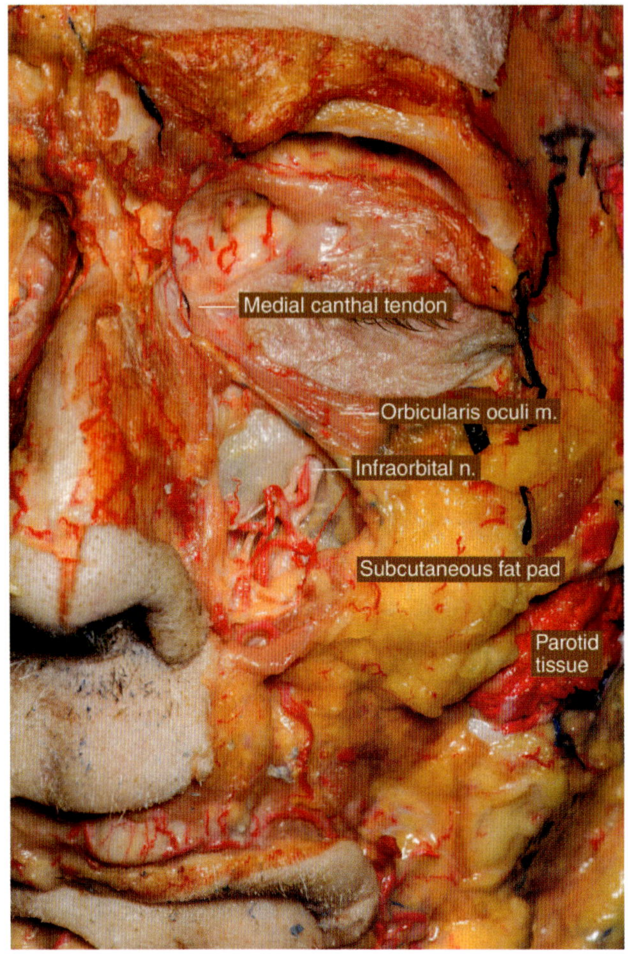

FIGURE 1-20 Dissection of the anterior left cheek highlighting the infraorbital nerve.

anastomosis is highly predictable, and its consistent presentation makes it a very viable pedicle for flap construction. The glabella and mid portion of the forehead are supplied by the supratrochlear artery, a branch of the ophthalmic artery that is also a reliable vascular pedicle in nasal reconstruction of the dorsum and tip of the nose (**Figure 1-20**). Deep to the nasal bone, the external nasal artery emerges onto the dorsum of the nose (**Figure 1-21**). It is usually accompanied by the external branch of the anterior ethmoidal nerve, which supplies sensory innervation to the dorsum and tip of the nose. The infraorbital artery also contributes to vascular anastomosis around this area. Venous drainage follows the pattern of arterial supply and does not display any anatomy of significance.

Sensory innervation to the nose is achieved through branches of the ophthalmic and maxillary divisions of the trigeminal nerve. The ophthalmic division supplies the area along the midline of the nose, whereas the maxillary division via the infraorbital nerve (**Figure 1-20**) innervates the alae, lower lateral walls, and columella. The root and upper nasal bridge along with the upper lateral walls are supplied by the infratrochlear nerve that approaches the nose in a medial direction from above the medial canthal tendon.

5. Ear

KEY STRUCTURES AND ANATOMIC POINTS

- The external ear is divided into the auricle (pinna), the external auditory meatus and canal, and the external surface of the deeper-set tympanic membrane.
- Blood supply to the ear is derived from superior and inferior auricular branches of the superficial temporal artery and the deep auricular branch of the maxillary artery.
- The external ear receives a rich sensory innervation from overlapping cranial and cervical nerves.
- The auriculotemporal nerve travels posterior to the superficial temporal vessels and supplies the anterior portion of the auricle and anterior helix.
- The auriculotemporal nerve lies posterior to the superficial temporal artery and vein and exits the superior parotid fascia as it traverses the parotid gland.
- The mastoid area is supplied by C2, C3 ventral rami derived via the lesser occipital nerve. Concha is supplied by variable overlapping innervation from cranial nerves VII, IX, and X, which also supply the posterior aspect of the external meatus and tympanic membrane and posterior auricular sulcus.

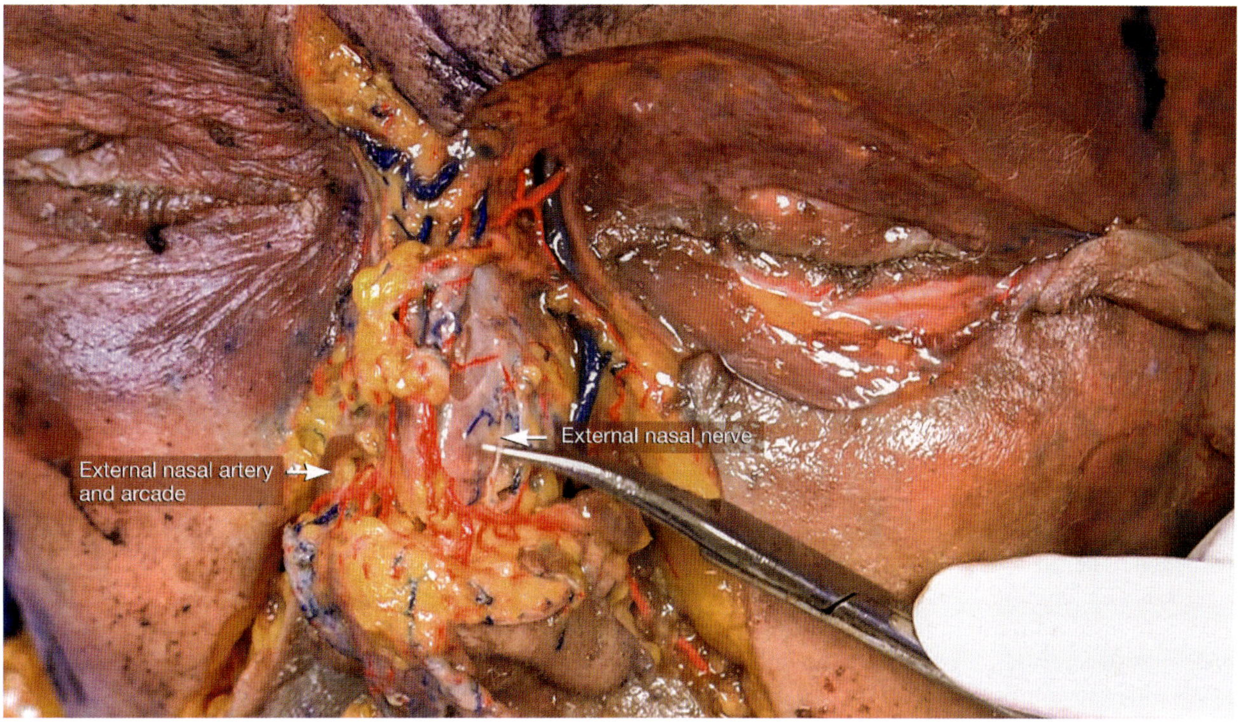

FIGURE 1-21 Superficial dissection of anterior nose demonstrating the external nasal nerve and vessels.

Understanding the architecture of the ear is essential to repairing both large and small defects. When undermining, when performing a primary closure, or during mobilization, knowledge of the variation in skin thickness, elasticity, relationship to the underlying cartilage, and pattern of perfusion helps in producing the most effective repair.

The external ear is divided into the auricle (pinna), the external auditory meatus and canal, and the external surface of the deeper-set tympanic membrane.[15] The auricle consists of a complex cartilaginous framework that is thrown into folds and grooves. The cartilage is covered by tightly bound skin with very little subcutaneous tissue, often with no subdermal fat at all. While the skin is tight anteriorly, posteriorly it offers a little more flexibility. The most inferior portion of the auricle, the lobule, has no cartilaginous base and consists of subcutaneous fat and skin. There are two distinct curves that extend superior to the lobule: (1) the outer helix, an anteriorly curved fold that continues posterosuperiorly from the lobule toward the upper limit of the tragus where it blends in with the crus of the helix; and (2) the antihelix, separated from the helix by a groove known as the scaphoid fossa. The tragus, an anterior extension of the auricular cartilage, is separated from the antitragus by the intertragal space. A deep concave groove referred to as the concha leads to the external auditory meatus. The concha is further subdivided into a more superior impression, the cymba, and an inferior, larger impression, the cavum (**Figure 1-22**).[4,9,15]

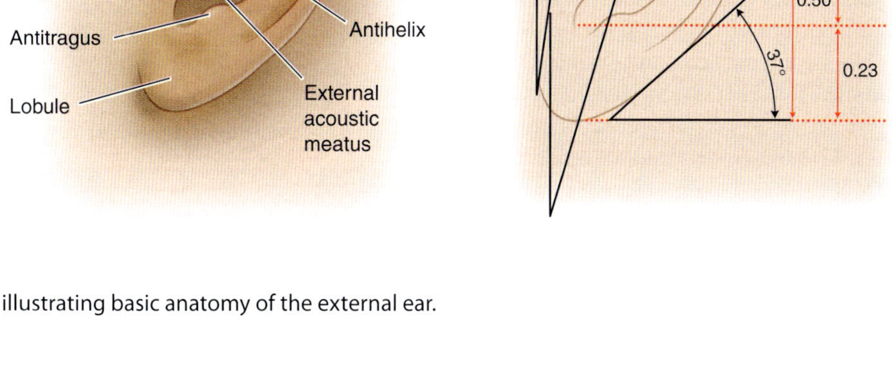

FIGURE 1-22 Diagram illustrating basic anatomy of the external ear.

While variations exist, in its standard anatomic position, the ear is situated laterally and lies somewhat between the eyebrows and base of the nose with the helix protruding beyond the antihelix. Ligamentous fibers connect the auricle to the skull and contain rudimentary intrinsic muscles. Extrinsic muscles are of little clinical significance, but it is helpful to note that these muscles of facial expression—the anterior, posterior, and superior auricular muscles—are contained within the SMAS and innervated by branches of the facial nerve.

The length of the external auditory meatus and canal measures 2.5 to 3.5 cm. The canal itself has both bony and cartilaginous parts.[15] Laterally, the cartilaginous component is continuous with the auricular cartilage, while medially, it is attached to the bony meatus. The cartilaginous portion is mostly present in the inferior aspect of the canal. Superiorly, the canal is bound by the squamous temporal bone. The true bony portion of the canal tunnels between the squamous and tympanic parts of the temporal bone. Around the lateral portion of the external meatus, the skin is thicker, with sebaceous, cerumeniferous glands and hair. The bony portion contains a very thin layer of epithelium and is devoid of hair and glands. Of particular clinical interest are the fissures within the cartilaginous portion of the canal. These randomly arranged fissures, known as fissures of Santorini, offer potential avenues for developing skin cancers to spread into surrounding tissue.

The rich blood supply to the ear is derived from superior and inferior auricular branches of the superficial temporal artery and the deep auricular branch of the maxillary artery. Additionally, the posterior auricular artery, a branch of the external carotid artery, supplies the posterior aspect of the ear. Arterial branches are arranged as a single layer of vessels within the skin as a consequence of the sparsity of subcutaneous fat. The venous pattern corresponds with the arterial supply, and drainage is via the superficial temporal and retromandibular veins.

The external ear receives rich sensory innervation from overlapping cranial and cervical nerves. The mandibular division of the trigeminal nerve gives off the auriculotemporal nerve, which travels posterior to the superficial temporal vessels and supplies the anterior portion of the auricle and anterior helix. Additionally, the auriculotemporal nerve supplies the anterior and superior walls of the auditory canal as well as a portion of the external surface of the tympanic membrane (**Figure 1-13**). Injury to the auriculotemporal nerve may be limited by recalling that it lies posterior to the superficial temporal artery and vein and that inferiorly it exits the superior parotid fascia as it traverses the parotid gland. The great auricular nerve (C2, C3 ventral rami) supplies most of the medial surface of the auricle as well as the posterior portion of the lateral surface of the auricle. This will include most of the helix and antihelix. The mastoid area is also supplied by C2, C3 ventral rami, but its innervation is derived via the lesser occipital nerve. The concha, however, is supplied by variable overlapping innervation from cranial nerve VII, and the meatus is innervated by cranial nerves IX and X.[4,9,15] These cranial nerves also supply the posterior aspect of the external meatus and tympanic membrane and posterior auricular sulcus.

6. Lips and Chin

KEY STRUCTURES AND ANATOMIC POINTS

- Orbicularis oris muscle has no bony attachment and is innervated by the buccal branch of the facial nerve through its deep surfaces.
- Blood supply is derived from superior and inferior labial arteries arising from the facial artery.
- Innervation of the upper lip is achieved via the infraorbital nerve (V_2), and innervation of the lower lip is achieved via the mental nerve (V_3).
- Redundancy of skin as well as mucosa around the commissural junction enables mobility and flexibility when the mouth is opened.
- Sensory innervation to the chin is supplied by the mental nerve branches (V_3).
- Lip depressor muscles and mentalis are innervated by the marginal mandibular branch of the facial nerve.

Surgery of the lips lends itself to both cosmetic and functional importance. Disruption of the architectural contour of the lips has far-reaching consequences for the patient, making preservation and restructuring of the anatomy of utmost importance. While not often considered, the lip constitute more than just the vermillion.[15] It extends superiorly to the nose and inferiorly to the chin, corresponding with the circularly arranged fibers of the orbicularis oris muscle. The boundary line of the upper lip lies at the junction of the columella, nasal sill, and alar crease below the base. Laterally the upper lip extends to the nasolabial fold, a point at which the lip elevators insert into the orbicularis oris fibers. The upper lip is divided by a vertically placed philtrum bound by phitral columns on either side and inferiorly by a downward arch referred to as Cupid's bow. The vermillion is composed of a modified mucosal membrane with a rich underlying vascular supply. There are no underlying sweat, salivary, or sebaceous glands.[4,15] A redundancy of skin as well as mucosa around the commissural junction enables mobility and flexibility when the mouth is opened. A group of muscles of facial expression for elevation, depression, and retraction insert deep to the commissural skin.

The underlying anatomy of the lip is not complex and contains the orbicularis oris fibers covered by mucous membrane (toward the oral cavity) and skin. The muscle fibers have a very close relationship with the dermis via muscular slips, limiting the ease with which dissection and reflection of the skin is possible. Bulging of the muscle fibers creates a corresponding surface marking known as the "white roll" or "white line" along the vermillion-cutaneous junction.[4,9,15] Orbicularis oris muscle has no bony attachments and is circumferentially arranged to facilitate sphincteric action.

Motor innervation of the orbicularis oris is derived from the buccal branch of cranial nerve VII. Most of the angle elevators as well as the lip itself are supplied by the buccal branch. As the buccal branches exit the parotid fascia, they flank the parotid duct as they travel medially toward the orbicularis fibers to then pass deep to the muscle, innervating it from the deep surface (**Figure 1-23**). The marginal mandibular branch of cranial nerve VII contributes to the depressors, again passing through the deep surface of the muscles. Sensory nerves are abundant and derived from the infraorbital branch of the maxillary nerve (cranial nerve [CN] V) (**Figure 1-24**)

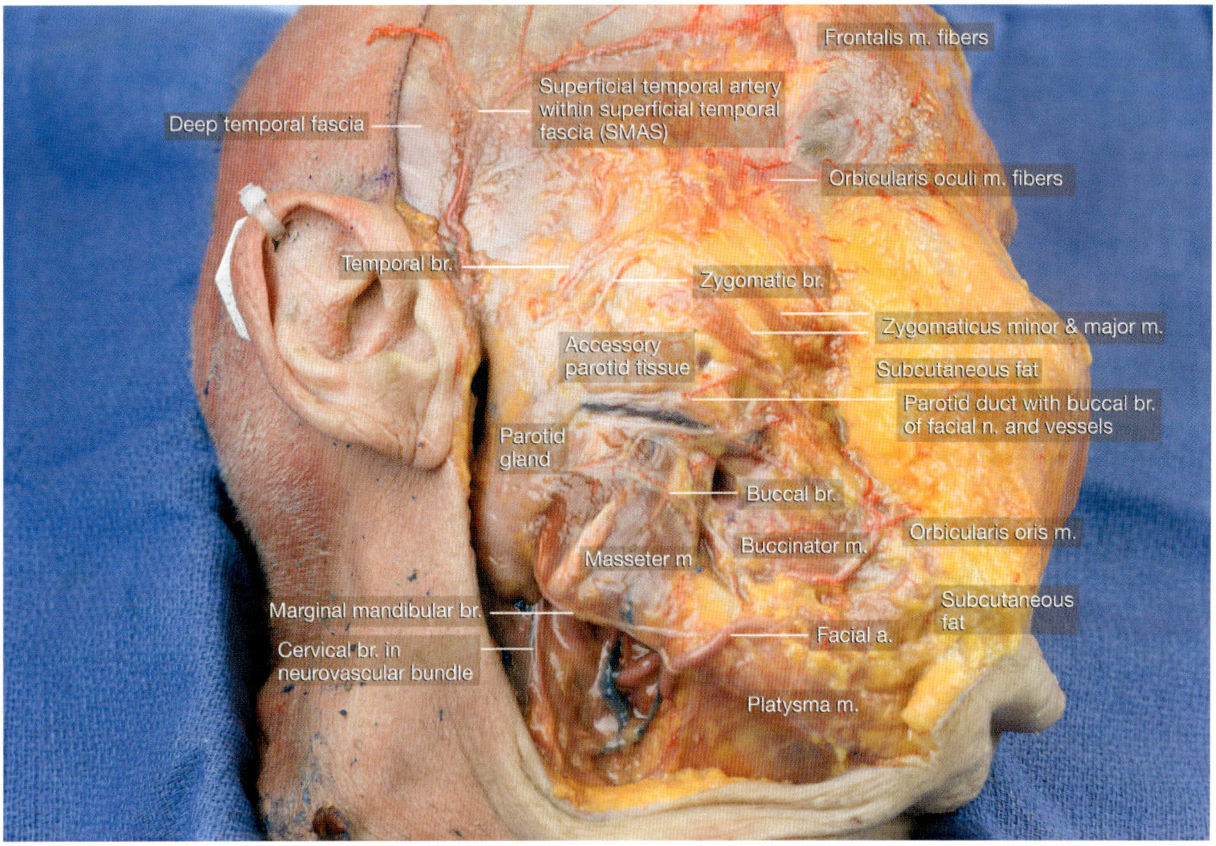

FIGURE 1-23 Dissection of the lateral face with skin and subcutaneous layers reflected medially.

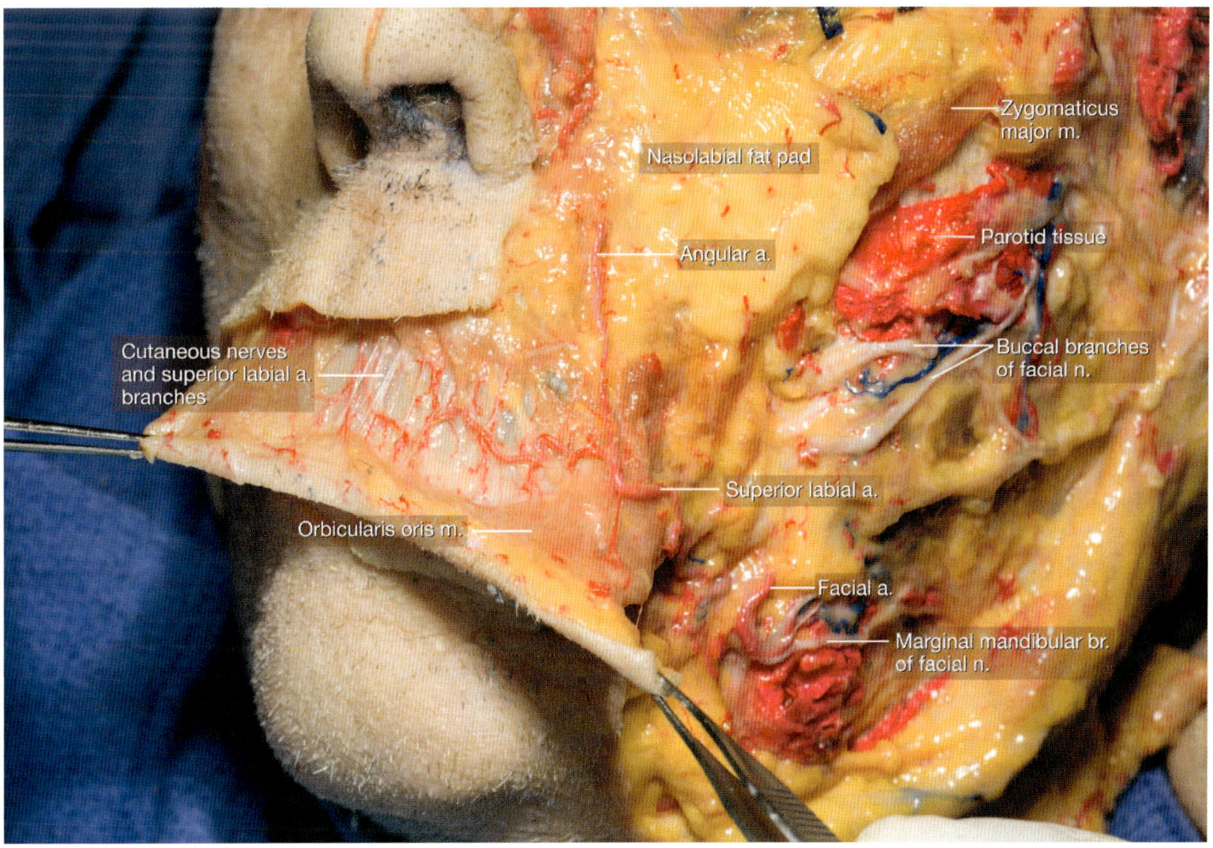

FIGURE 1-24 Anterolateral view of lower face with skin and subcutaneous tissue over upper lip reflected inferiorly.

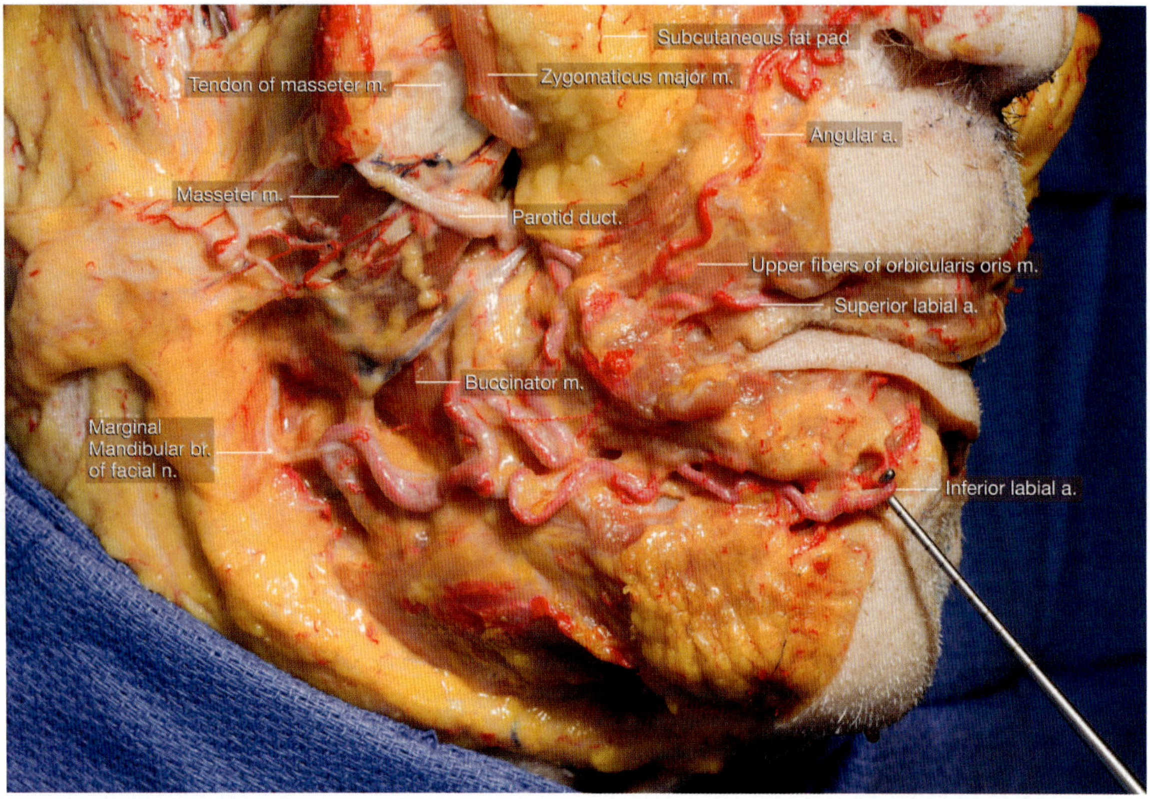

FIGURE 1-25 Lateral view of dissection of regional anatomy around the mid cheek and mandibular region.

reaching the upper lip and from the mental nerve (terminal branch of the inferior alveolar nerve CN V) reaching the lower lip. Numerous small branches are encountered upon reflection of the skin. The main nerve trunks, however, may be accessed at the infraorbital foramen and the mental foramen. The infraorbital and mental foramina are generally located in a fixed position relative to the alae and oral commissure, respectively.

Blood supply to the lips is achieved through an anastomotic arterial arcade formed by the superior and inferior labial arteries (**Figures 1-24 and 1-25**). These branches arise from the facial artery around the angle of the mouth. However, often the inferior labial artery may originate at a lower point, as the facial artery crosses over the angle of the mandible. With this branching pattern, the inferior labial artery may lie lower than its normal position and ascend toward the midline of the chin. Both the superior and inferior labial arteries are often highly tortuous, especially in older individuals, and run deep to the fibers of orbicularis oris. Skin over the lips is supplied by vertically ascending and descending branches off the arcades.

The chin is a relatively fixed anatomic structure that is composed mostly of muscles of facial expression acting on the lower lip. The chin extends from the mentolabial crease to the most inferior point along the midline of the mandible. In older individuals, RSTLs are visible and can be distinguished between (1) the radially extending lines around the lower lip area with diagonal extensions toward the angles of the mouth and (2) the variable lines around the mental region that are determined by the shape of the chin.[15] As the muscles of facial expression insert directly into the skin, very little subcutaneous tissue is found in this area. Creating a dissection plane is somewhat difficult as the taut insertion of the muscles limits undermining in this region.

Muscles of the chin include overlapping fibers of the orbicularis oris muscle that mingles with fibers of the platysma and other surrounding regional muscles. Laterally, the depressor anguli oris attaches to the medial aspects of the mandible and the oral commissure to pull the angle of the mouth downward. On the front of the mandible, the depressor labii inferioris is partially overlapped by the depressor anguli oris. Two slips of the mentalis muscle arise from the mandibular midline and insert onto the skin of the chin, maintaining a variable gap between them (**Figure 1-3**). All these muscles are supplied by the marginal mandibular branch of the facial nerve. The marginal mandibular nerve is easily visualized as it passes along the bony margin to enter the chin deep to the angle of the mouth. Since the marginal mandibular nerve is often seen as a single exposed trunk before branching to supply these muscles, injury to the trunk will result in unopposed action of the antagonists of these muscles (**Figure 1-26**).

The mental nerve exits the mental foramen as a terminal branch of the inferior alveolar nerve. It is a purely sensory nerve and displays a tuft-like branching pattern. With aging, mandibular bone resorption may change the relative location of the mental foramen, bringing it a little higher toward the superior margin due to the decreasing height of the alveolar processes.

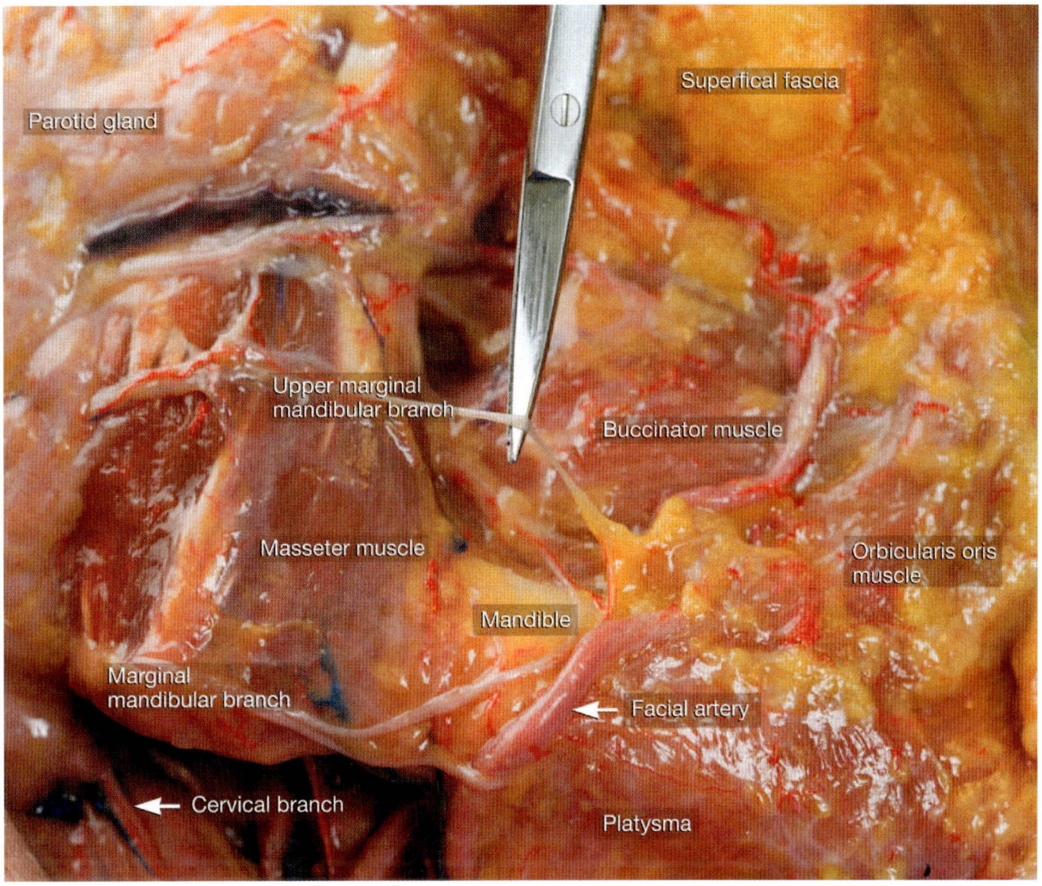

FIGURE 1-26 Dissection highlighting the marginal mandibular branch of the facial nerve and its relationship to the facial artery.

7. Cheek

KEY STRUCTURES AND ANATOMIC POINTS

- The anterior region includes the buccinator muscle, buccal fat pad, buccal branches of the facial nerve, and downward traversing parotid duct.
- The parotid region is dominated by the parotid gland and underlying deep masseter muscle.
- The parotid duct and facial artery are easily identifiable landmarks in this region.
- The marginal mandibular nerve is a key structure in the mandibular region as it consistently crosses the facial artery deep to the fibers of platysma.

Anatomically, the cheek extends from the anterior border of the ear, limited medially by the nose, lips, and chin, and from the mandible up to the zygomatic arch and orbital rim. However, to best appreciate the cosmetic unit of the cheek, it is best described in three regions: the anterior, mandibular, and masseter-parotid regions.[4,9,15]

The *anterior region* contains many of the muscles of facial expression. The risorius is very superficial and of variable size, sometimes even absent. The zygomaticus major and minor as well as the levator labii superioris and the levator labii superioris alaeque nasi originate from the zygomatic bone and orbital rim and are overlapped by fibers of the orbicularis oculi muscle. When reflecting the skin over this region, zygomaticus minor is seen more superficially than the rest of the muscles, with only a few millimeters of subcutaneous tissue overlying it (**Figures 1-6 and 1-23**). Since the facial nerve branches maintain their course and innervation deep to the muscles, injury to these branches is less likely provided that the plane of dissection remains superficial to the muscle plane.

Along the medial aspect of the anterior cheek, the facial artery can be seen anterior to the facial vein after crossing the mandible to ascend toward the angle of the mouth where it gives off the labial branches and subsequently traverses the nasolabial grove as the angular artery. Within the nasolabial groove, the angular artery can be accessed with little difficulty by dissecting within the subcutaneous tissue and overlying muscle slips of the zygomaticus major and minor muscles (**Figure 1-19**). The angular artery then terminates at the medial canthus just above the medial canthal tendon by anastomosing with the ophthalmic branch of the internal carotid artery (**Figure 1-19**). The deepest structures in this region of the cheek are the buccinator and levator anguli oris muscles. Unlike the other muscles of facial expression, the buccinator is a relatively fleshy muscle. It lies within a drop-down plane covered by a significant amount of fatty tissue, often referred to as the buccal fat pad (**Figure 1-25**). The buccinator is pierced by the parotid duct as well as blood vessels and buccal branches of the maxillary nerve en route to supply sensory innervation to the buccal mucosa.[4,9,15] The buccal fat pad itself lies technically in the medial cheek. This fatty mass is well defined and contained by a thin layer of fascia, and on its surface, the facial nerve branches can be visualized crossing over the fat pad still deep to the SMAS (**Figure 1-6**). Superiorly, the infraorbital nerve branches out as a leash of nerves to supply sensory innervation to the medial cheek. The supraorbital foramen is easily palpated on most individuals.

The *masseter-parotid region* offers a very important anatomic landmark—the deeply set masseter muscle. A muscle of mastication supplied by the trigeminal nerve, the masseter can be easily visualized and palpated when the jaw is clenched. Its strong attachments extend between the zygomatic arch and ramus of the mandible, and its anterior musculotendinous border provides an important landmark for key facial structures. The posterior half of the masseter is covered by the parotid gland. Contained within its own fascia, the parotid gland, wedged along the preauricular mandibular region, is separated from the masseteric fascia, which is a continuation of the superficial layer of deep cervical fascia. The lower anterior portion of the masseter may be overlapped by fibers of the platysma in most individuals.

When visualized on unembalmed cadaveric specimens, the parotid gland displays a yellowish color, very similar to the living patient. It may sometimes be confused with subcutaneous fat as it is relatively close to the skin itself (**Figure 1-23**). Unlike the subcutaneous tissue, however, the parotid gland is contained within a shiny, tight fascial sheath, the parotid fascia, which may help in differentiating it from fat. On the anterior border of the gland, the parotid duct can be located as it travels horizontally and then downward into the buccal fat. It consistently crosses over the masseter muscle before turning sharply toward the buccinator to pierce it and enter the oral cavity opposite the upper second molar. From its surface anatomy, the parotid duct may be located in the region of intersection between the tragolabial line[15] and the anterior edge of the masseter muscle and, additionally, along the zygomatic arch about 2 cm below it. The parotid duct is a prominent structure and provides a reliable anatomic landmark. As the parotid duct lies deep to the SMAS, it is crossed by fibers of the zygomatic branch of the facial nerve and also flanked by the upper and lower buccal branches of the facial nerve (**Figures 1-5, 1-6, and 1-23**).

The transverse facial artery, arising from the external carotid artery, passes parallel to the parotid duct between it and the zygomatic arch. It also crosses over the anterior margin of the masseter muscle. The superficial temporal artery exits the parotid fascia below the zygomatic arch just anterior to the tragus (**Figure 1-27**).[4,9,15] It passes posterior and deep to the parotid gland as one of the terminal branches of the external carotid artery. The facial artery and vein (posterior to the artery) also travel beneath the SMAS as they cross over the mandible. The facial artery and vein can be located just anterior to the masseter muscle. The facial artery, which travels in a tortuous ascending course, is often more prominently tortuous in older individuals. The mandibular branch of the facial nerve crosses over the facial artery about 5 to 10 mm above the point at which the facial artery crosses the mandible.

The mandibular region extends from the anterior margin of the masseter muscle to the chin. Three predominant muscles are

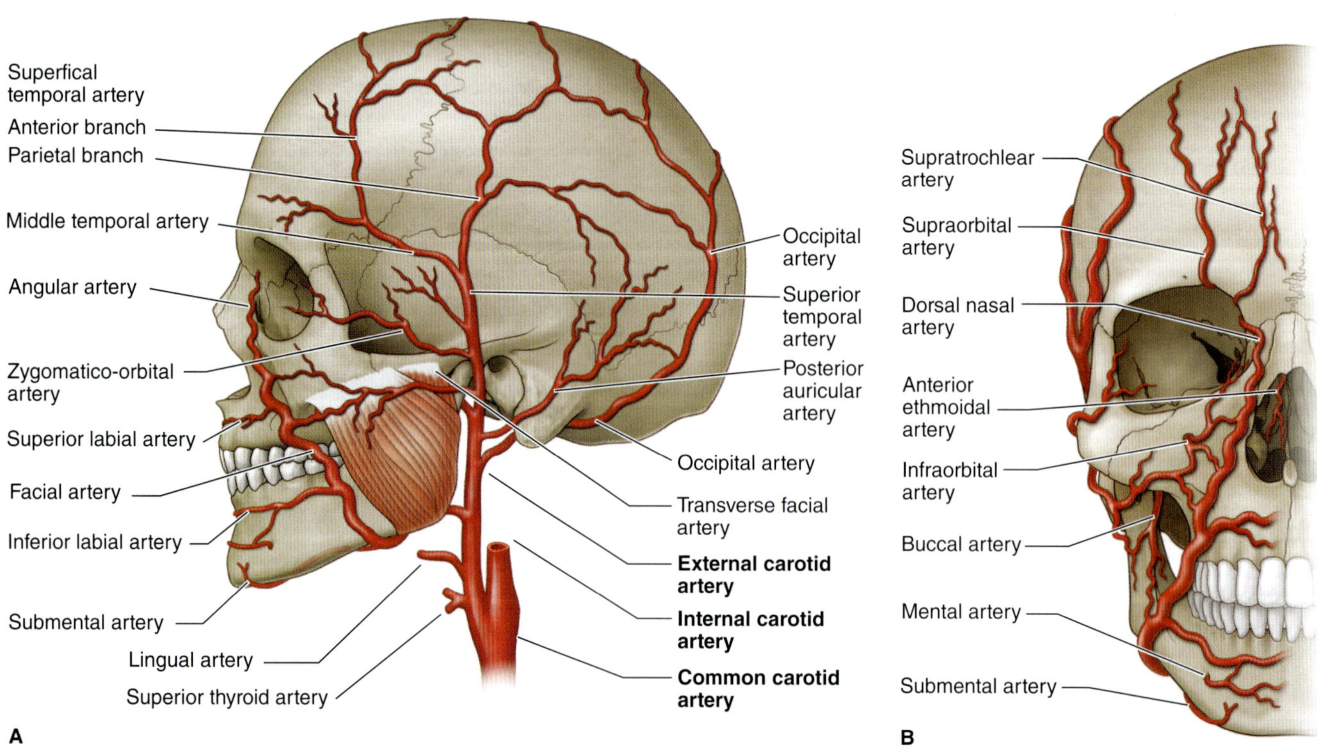

FIGURE 1-27 Diagram illustrating the arterial pattern and supply to the face.

encountered after reflecting the skin in the region. The platysma lies within the superficial fascia and inserts into the skin of the lower lip, blending in with the fibers of the orbicularis oris muscle. The depressor anguli oris, which originates on the mandible and inserts onto the angle of the mouth, also sends fibers that blend in with those of the platysma and orbicularis oris.

Both the facial artery and the marginal branch of the facial nerve lie deep to the fibers of the platysma. In most individuals, the marginal branch of the facial nerve maintains a course above the mandibular rim, crossing the facial artery to supply the depressors of the lips and the mouth. While there are usually two branches, the mandibular branch of the facial nerve can exist as a single nerve or have as many as four branches (**Figure 1-26**).

SURGICAL CONSIDERATIONS

Muscles of the Face

The muscles of facial expression and the superficial group of muscles of mastication form the basis for the muscular framework of the face (**Figure 1-3**). Muscles of facial expression lie at varying depths just deep to subcutaneous tissue. They attach from the facial skeleton to the overlying dermis in a three-dimensional configuration from deep to superficial.[2,3,6,14,17] Seen from this four-layered overlaying construct, the deepest muscles include buccinator, mentalis, and levator anguli oris. At the next level, the orbicularis oris and levator labii superioris can be visualized, followed by the more superficial depressor labii inferioris, risorius, platysma, zygomaticus major, and levator labii superioris alaeque nasi. Fibers of the depressor anguli oris, zygomaticus minor, and orbicularis oculi can be identified most superficially. All the muscles (except for the deepest layer) are innervated by branches of the facial nerve passing through their deep surfaces.[4,9]

Branches of the Facial Nerve

Facial nerve branches, while generally protected by the SMAS, are surgically vulnerable as they reach areas of transition along their course toward their final destination.

Injury to the facial nerve and its branches during surgical exposure has been a topic of detailed discussion.[2,5,6,18-23] A few key points can help guide dissection around facial nerve branches: (1) Facial nerve exits its intracranial course through the stylomastoid foramen and immediately gives off the posterior auricular nerve, which passes behind the ear toward auricularis posterior and the occipital belly of occipitofrontalis muscles. (2) At the posteromedial surface of the parotid gland, just before this point or within the gland, the facial nerve branches into a superior temporofacial and inferior cervicofacial division. (3) Facial nerve divides and reconnects through an extensive branching pattern before it exits the parotid fascia along the medial margin to give rise to five main trunks: temporal, zygomatic, buccal, mandibular, and cervical.[4,9,20] (4) Main branches lie within the parenchyma of the parotid gland and are not at risk for injury during superficial surgical procedures unless the parotid gland or parts of it have been resected (**Figure 1-4**). (5) Vulnerability to injury of the facial nerve branches increases as they travel toward their areas of innervation. (6) Facial nerve branches are most susceptible to injury in their transition from layer 5 (deep fascial plane) to layer 4 (soft-tissue spaces).[2,18,20] (7) Along their course, branches of the facial nerve lie deep to the SMAS and can be safely encountered as long as the plane of dissection is maintained above the SMAS (**Figure 1-6**).

Anatomic Points of Consideration to Limit Vulnerability of Facial Nerve Branches to Injury

1. Temporal branches emerge from the upper margin of the parotid fascia and cross the zygomatic arch. Usually three to four branches supply frontalis and parts of orbicularis oculi (**Figures 1-4, 1-6, and 1-14**).
2. Zygomatic branches cross the zygomatic arch and bone and are in direct contact with periosteum. As they cross the bony eminence, they lie directly under the skin with no subcutaneous protection (**Figures 1-4, 1-6, and 1-23**).
3. Buccal branches flank the parotid duct along its upper and lower margins. Keeping the parotid duct in view helps maintain a safe zone, limiting injury to the buccal branches as they travel toward the buccinator, nasalis muscle fibers, and the upper portions of the orbicularis oris muscle (**Figures 1-5 and 1-23**).
4. The marginal mandibular branch travels frequently as a single branch, and often as two branches running above, along, or about 1 cm below the inferior border of the mandible. It consistently crosses over the facial artery, making it vulnerable to injury once the facial artery is approached. The platysma offers a layer of protection over the marginal mandibular branches and the mandible-traversing portion of the facial artery (**Figure 1-26**).
5. The cervical branch is located deep to the platysma as it descends from the lower border of the parotid gland maintaining its position on the deep surface of the muscle. It is only vulnerable to injury if the fibers of platysma are reflected (**Figure 1-23**).

Anatomic Points of Consideration to Avoid Injury and Maximize Vascular Sources for Reconstruction

The superficial arterial supply to the face includes a rich anastomotic network of branches originating from the external and internal carotid arteries. Through extensive anastomoses, these major vascular trunks provide reliable pedicles and contribute to the microvascular infrastructure of the superficial face. The external carotid artery includes a vast network of arborizing, anastomotic, and tortuous arteries varying in size and depth within the fascial planes. The internal carotid artery via its ophthalmic branch supplies a central triangular area including the eyes, superior nose, and central portion of the forehead.[4,9] The key area of anastomosis between external and internal carotid arteries is located above the medial canthal tendon where the angular artery communicates with the dorsal nasal branch of the ophthalmic artery (**Figure 1-19**).

The superficial temporal artery ascends behind the temporomandibular joint, anterior to the tragus and auriculotemporal nerve. It crosses the zygomatic arch and branches over a wide surface deep to the skin and within the layers of the superficial temporal fascia. The supraorbital and supratrochlear arteries run along the same territory as a neurovascular bundle with the supraorbital and supratrochlear nerves. The larger supraorbital artery usually anastomoses with the superficial temporal artery (**Figure 1-12**).

The anastomosis of the angular branch of the facial artery with the dorsal nasal artery above the medial canthal ligament is an area of surgical importance (**Figures 1-10 and 1-19**). While the course of the facial artery within the nasolabial fold is well known, its infrequent course outside the fold has been documented. The artery has been recorded passing through the fold in up to 90% of individuals, and at least 5 mm outside the territory or crossing it in up to 45% of individuals.[10,24,25] In the nasolabial region, the facial artery along with its superior and inferior labial arteries may not always maintain a submuscular position. Lee et al[24] provide anatomic evidence for the vessels traveling superficial to the surrounding muscles of facial expression and sometimes looping deep and superficial to the muscle fibers.

Anatomy of the Neck

Understanding the superficial anatomy of the neck begins with the ability to visualize key structures bound by palpable landmarks. The topographic anatomy of the neck is marked by consistent musculoskeletal structures that present triangular spaces seen from the anterior and lateral aspects (**Figure 1-28**). Surgical approaches to the neck can be enhanced by keeping the following anatomic points in perspective:

1. The most prominent landmark in the neck, the sternocleidomastoid muscle (SCM), provides the primary boundary for differentiating the anterior and posterior triangles.
2. The most superficial muscle of the neck, the platysma, is invested by superficial cervical fascia (continuous with the SMAS), creating a thin muscular veil over the superficially traversing cutaneous nerves.
3. Superficial cervical nerves, the great auricular, lesser occipital, and transverse cervical nerves, are encountered at the posterior border of the SCM when platysma muscle is reflected.
4. Erb's point, located 6 cm below the midpoint of a line connecting the angle of the mandible with the mastoid process, provides a landmark for the exit point of the superficial cervical nerves and the accessory nerve (CN XI).[26]
5. The external jugular vein travels along a vertical course on the superficial surface of SCM anterior to the great auricular nerve to the base of the neck where it pierces the deep cervical fascia.

Triangles of the Neck

The triangles of the neck are formed by visible and palpable landmarks of its musculoskeletal framework. The anterior triangle is bound posteriorly by the anterior margin of the SCM, superiorly by the inferior margin of the mandible, and anteriorly by the

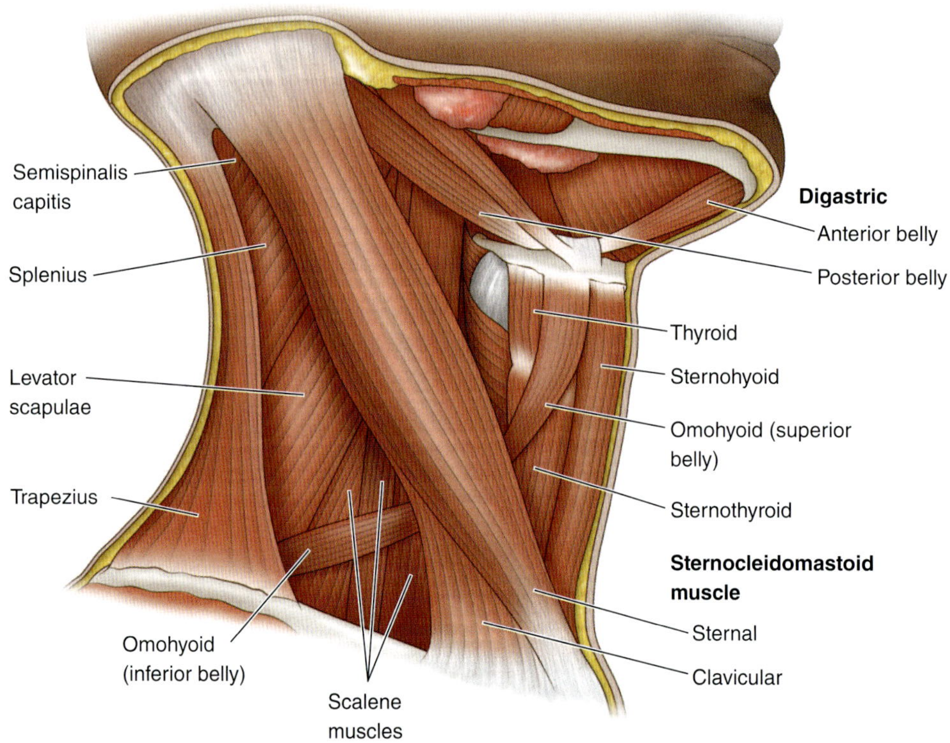

FIGURE 1-28 Diagram illustrating the anatomic boundaries and structures within the posterior triangle of the neck.

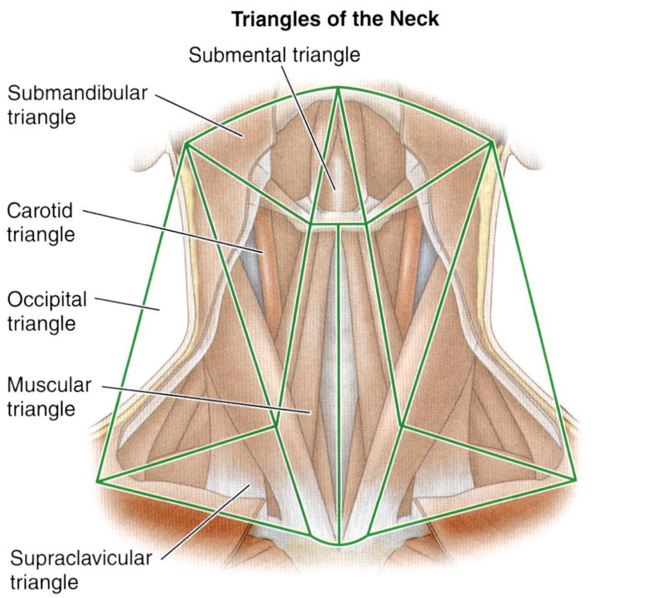

FIGURE 1-29 Diagram illustrating the subdivisions of the triangles of the neck.

sternohyoid and sternothyroid muscles. The posterior triangle is bound anteriorly by the posterior border of the SCM and posteriorly by the anterior border of the trapezius muscle and lateral portion of the clavicle (**Figure 1-28**).

The anterior triangle may be further subdivided by the posterior and anterior bellies of the digastric muscle and hyoid bone into the submental, submandibular, carotid, and muscular triangles (**Figure 1-29**).

- Submental triangle: The flat mylohyoid muscle forms the floor, with the nerve to mylohyoid running along this surface; it contains few structures of significance other than subcutaneous fat, fascia, and lymph nodes.
- Submandibular triangle: The submandibular gland is the most prominent structure. It contains lymph nodes and the proximal portion of the facial artery as it courses between the parts of the submandibular gland; the low-hanging marginal mandibular branch of the facial nerve passing below the mandibular margin must be considered within this space.
- Carotid triangle: The carotid sheath containing the common carotid artery, internal jugular vein, and vagus nerve fills the space. The ansa cervicalis (branch of cervical plexus) motor contribution to strap muscles loops over the anterior surface of the carotid sheath; internal and external carotid arteries originate within this triangle; and the hypoglossal nerve may be seen as it travels along the uppermost portion of the triangle from posterior to anterior.
- Muscular triangle: Contains the strap muscles (infrahyoid), including sternohyoid, sternothyroid, omohyoid, and thyrohyoid muscles, and traversing muscular branches of the cervical nerves.

The posterior triangle (**Figure 1-28**) can be further divided anatomically by the inferior belly of the omohyoid into the occipital and supraclavicular triangles. However, these divisions are rarely differentiated clinically. The deepest aspect of the posterior triangle, the floor, is formed by the parallel arrangement of deeper, smaller neck muscles. Superiorly, the triangle contains the splenius capitus. Inferiorly, the levator scapulae (an important muscular landmark for isolation of the accessory nerve) lies above the posterior and middle scalene muscles. It is surgically useful to note that these muscles are covered by the prevertebral fascia (deep cervical fascia) on top of which lies the superficial layer of deep cervical fascia.

In the next layer, two important nervous structures lie over and between the muscles of the floor of the posterior triangle. The proximal portions of the trunks of the brachial plexus lie anterior to the middle scalene muscle and are covered by the overlying prevertebral fascia. Injury to the trunks of the brachial plexus is unlikely as long as the prevertebral fascia remains uninterrupted.

Perhaps one of the most emphasized structures of surgical interest in the posterior triangle is the accessory nerve (CN XI) (**Figure 1-30**). As it descends over the levator scapulae muscle to pass beneath the trapezius muscle, the course of the accessory nerve can be traced along the midline of the posterior triangle. As the accessory nerve contains primary motor fibers to the trapezius muscle, injury during deeper surgical excisions will result

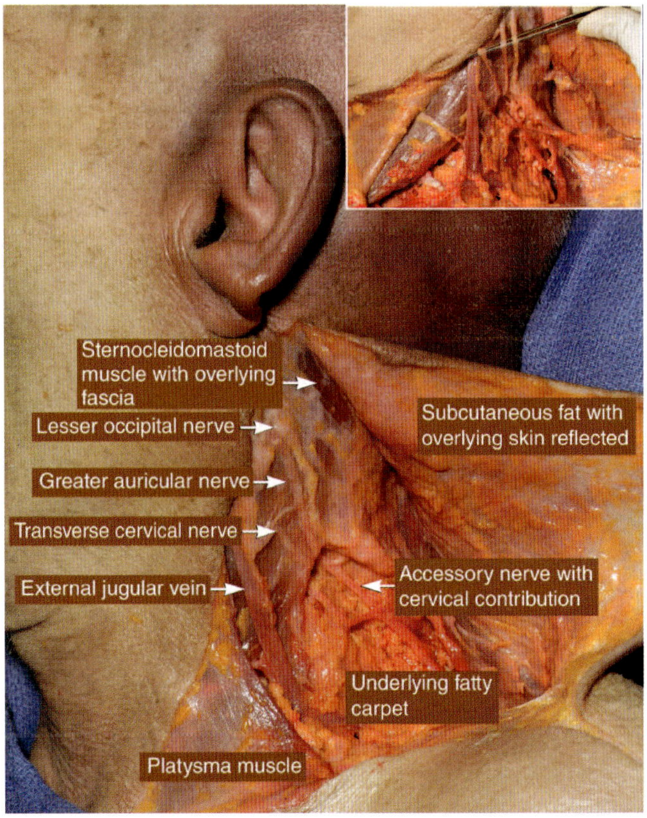

FIGURE 1-30 Superficial dissection of the posterior triangle of the neck with detailed demonstration of the key regional nerves.

in impaired function of the trapezius muscle (symptoms include winged scapula, inability to shrug shoulders, pain, and initiation of arm abduction). The accessory nerve also provides motor innervation to the SCM muscle, but its branches to the SCM are less likely to be injured as they innervate the muscle on its deep surface. In the posterior triangle, the accessory nerve is most vulnerable to injury in the 3- to 4-cm area between the SCM and trapezius muscles. The accessory nerve can be distinguished from the surrounding cutaneous cervical nerves at Erb's point[26] as it passes posteriorly along a diagonal course to become almost vertical within the posterior triangle. The great auricular nerve traverses the SCM, while the lesser occipital nerve remains close to the muscle along its ascent. The transverse cervical nerve passes horizontally across SCM in an anterior direction. During dissection, cervical nerves carrying proprioceptive fibers can be seen in a slightly more superficial plane traveling along the course of the accessory nerve. While the accessory nerve is a superficial structure and very vulnerable to surgical injury, it is still offered a layer of fascial cover as it lies between the prevertebral and superficial layers of deep cervical fascia. A consistent carpet of fatty tissue lies beneath the accessory nerve. The thickness of subcutaneous tissue of the superficial fascia over the nerve can vary between individuals. Additionally, proprioceptive fibers from the cervical plexus can be seen communicating with the accessory nerve and may sometimes be confusing when identifying the accessory nerve itself (**Figure 1-30**).

The layered organization of anatomic structures presents access to safe dissection planes. When performing surgery on the neck, appreciating the organization of the fascia allows the clinician to maintain integral anatomy while safely accessing clinically targeted structures or areas. Fascia of the neck can be differentiated into superficial fascia and deep fascia. The superficial fascia is often synonymous with the subcutaneous tissue, but in the neck, the platysma is contained within it and shares the same relationship that the muscles of facial expression have with the SMAS. The deep cervical fascia, on the other hand, is further separated into three layers. The superficial layer and deep layer completely surround the neck, while the middle layer is discontinuous. The investing layer of deep cervical fascia (superficial) splits to surround the SCM, trapezius, and strap muscles (connecting the sternum to the laryngeal framework). As this layer covers the posterior triangle of the neck, it also forms a fascial layer over the cervical cutaneous and accessory nerves. The deep layer of deep cervical fascia (prevertebral fascia) covers the deeper layer of neck muscles as well as the scalene muscles, thereby also forming the floor of the posterior triangle of the neck (**Figure 1-30**). In the posterior triangle of the neck, the deep layer of deep cervical fascia overlays the trunks of the brachial plexus as well as the phrenic nerve, which travels on the anterior surface of the anterior scalene muscle (**Figure 1-31**). Pretracheal fascia can only be found on the anterior aspect of the neck. It arises from the superficial layer of the deep cervical fascia and overlies the thyroid gland, laryngeal structures, and trachea.

As the plane beneath the platysma is entered, branches of the cervical plexus become distinctly visible. Care should be taken to avoid injury to these nerves; even though their disruption results in nothing more than loss of cutaneous innervation, possible formation of neuromas must also be considered.

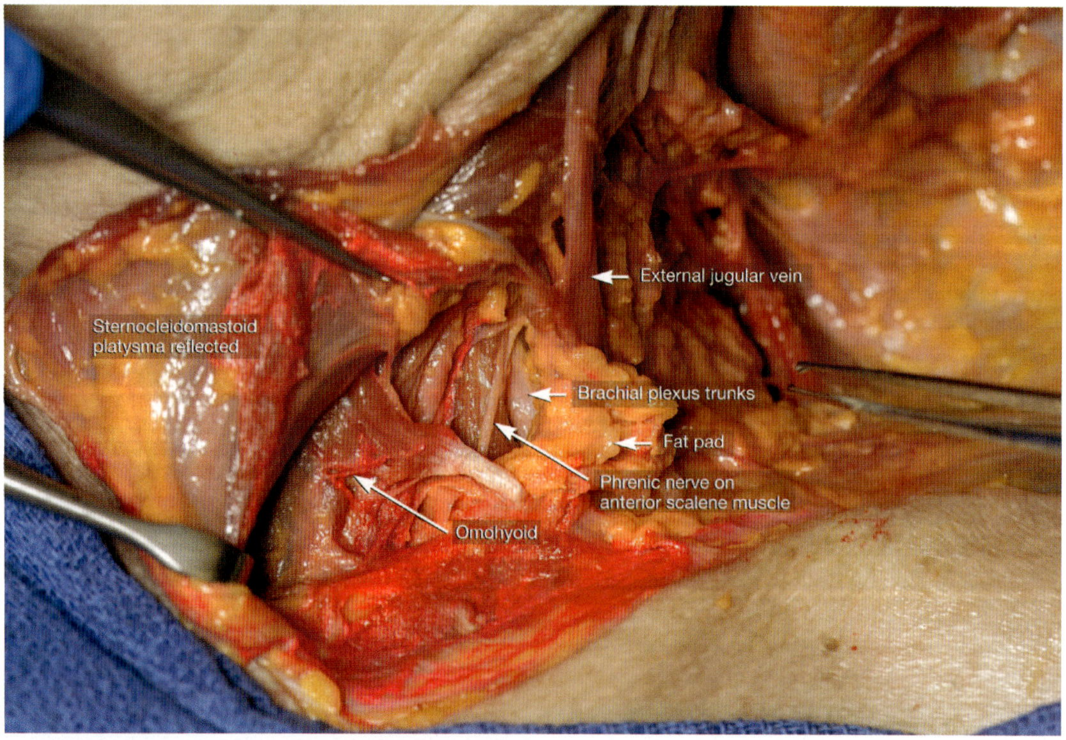

FIGURE 1-31 Deeper dissection of the posterior triangle demonstrating anatomic structures beneath fatty carpet.

The great auricular nerve (**Figure 1-30**), derived from the second and third cervical nerve loops, passes around the SCM almost vertically to the skin of the ear lobe. It can be quite adherent to the overlying fascia and is the largest of the cervical nerves in that region. Additionally, it supplies cutaneous innervation to posterior portion of the ear, inferior parotid, and mastoid areas.

The lesser occipital nerve (**Figure 1-30**), also derived from the second and third cervical nerves, passes close to the posterior edge of SCM in a superior trajectory. It innervates the skin behind the ears and parietal scalp.

The transverse cervical nerve (**Figure 1-30**) arises from second and third cervical nerves and passes horizontally across the SCM. It fans out to supply the skin over the anterior aspect of the neck.

Additionally, the supraclavicular nerves (usually three to four branches) arise from the third and fourth cervical nerves to pass inferiorly and supply skin over the supraclavicular triangle, sternum, deltoid region, lateral clavicle, and upper posterior trapezius area.

CONCLUSIONS

Understanding the complexity of head and neck anatomy is of critical importance before beginning procedures in these delicate areas. The goal of this chapter is not to incite every primary care provider performing procedures to become an anatomist; rather, it is to highlight the richness and variety of anatomic considerations in the head and neck region, which hopefully will also serve as a reminder for those situations where referral may be the best treatment.

Visualization of head and neck anatomy as a layered system should strengthen the reader's understanding of the course and location of important neurovascular structures as they travel in a stepwise pattern in and between the muscular, bony, and fascial planes to reach their terminal areas of supply and innervation. This is particularly important since standard descriptions of the neurovascular distribution and patterns provide a limiting two-dimensional view of structures traveling within a three-dimensional configuration. When approaching anatomically susceptible regions, keeping perspective on strong understanding of depth, course, and relations as these structures traverse anatomic boundaries[6,8,27] provides the key to successful surgery.

REFERENCES

1. Delmar H. Anatomy of the superficial parts of the face and neck. *Ann Chir Plast Esthet*. 1994;39:527-555.
2. Mendelson B, Wong CH. Anatomy of aging face. In: Neligan PC, Warren RJ, Van Beek A, eds. *Plastic Surgery*. 3rd ed. London, United Kingdom: Elsevier Saunders; 2013:78-92.
3. Marur T, Tuna Y, Demirci S. Facial anatomy. *Clin Dermatol*. 2014;32:14-23.
4. Standring S. Section 4: head and neck. In: Standring S, ed. *Gray's Anatomy: The Anatomical Basis of Clinical Practice*. 40th ed. Edinburgh, United Kingdom: Churchill Livingstone/Elsevier; 2008:467-495.
5. Zani R, Fadul R Jr, Da Rocha MA, Santos RA, Alves MC, Ferreira LM. Facial nerve in rhytidoplasty: anatomic study of its trajectory in the overlying skin and the most common sites of injury. *Ann Plast Surg*. 2003;51:236-242.
6. Roostaeian J, Rohrich RJ, Stuzin JM. Anatomical considerations to prevent facial nerve injury. *Plast Reconstr Surg*. 2015;135:1318-1327.
7. Ghassemi A, Prescher A, Riediger D, Axer H. Anatomy of the SMAS revisited. *Aesthetic Plast Surg*. 2003;27:258-264.
8. Randle HW, Salassa JR, Roenigk RK. Know your anatomy. Local anesthesia for cutaneous lesions of the head and neck – practical applications of peripheral nerve blocks. *J Dermatol Surg Oncol*. 1992;18:231-235.
9. Sinnatamby CS. Chapter 6: head and neck and spine. In: Sinnatamby CS, ed. *Last's Anatomy: Regional and Applied*. 12th ed. Edinburgh, United Kingdom: Churchill Livingstone/Elsevier; 2011:329-454.
10. Yang HM, Won SY, Kim HJ, Hu KS. Sihler staining study of anastomosis between the facial and trigeminal nerves in the ocular area and its clinical implications. *Muscle Nerve*. 2013;48:545-550.
11. Coscarella E, Vishteh AG, Spetzler RF, Seoane E, Zabramski JM. Subfascial and submuscular methods of temporal muscle dissection and their relationship to the frontal branch of the facial nerve. Technical note. *J Neurosurg*. 2000;92:877-880.
12. Ishikawa Y. An anatomical study on the distribution of the temporal branch of the facial nerve. *J Craniomaxillofac Surg*. 1990;18:287-292.
13. Erdogmus S, Govsa F. The arterial anatomy of the eyelid: importance for reconstructive and aesthetic surgery. *J Plast Reconstr Aesthet Surg*. 2007;60:241-245.
14. Turvey TA, Golden BA. Orbital anatomy for the surgeon. *Oral Maxillofac Surg Clin North Am*. 2012;24:525-536.
15. Salasche SJ, Bernstein G, Senkarik M. *Surgical Anatomy of the Skin*. Norwalk, CT: Appleton and Lange; 1998:151-269.
16. Chow S, Bennett RG. Superficial head and neck anatomy for dermatologic surgery: critical concepts. *Dermatol Surg*. 2015;41(Suppl 10):S169-S177.
17. Ouattara D, Vacher C, de Vasconcellos JJ, Kassanyou S, Gnanazan G, N'Guessan B. Anatomical study of the variations in innervation of the orbicularis oculi by the facial nerve. *Surg Radiol Anat*. 2004;26:51-53.
18. Larrabee WF Jr, Henderson JL. Face lift: the anatomic basis for a safe, long-lasting procedure. *Facial Plast Surg*. 2000;16:239-253.
19. Brown SM, Oliphant T, Langtry J. Motor nerves of the head and neck that are susceptible to damage during dermatological surgery. *Clin Exp Dermatol*. 2014;39:677-682.
20. Gosain AK. Surgical anatomy of the facial nerve. *Clin Plast Surg*. 1995;22:241-251.
21. Kwak HH, Park HD, Youn KH, et al. Branching patterns of the facial nerve and its communication with the auriculotemporal nerve. *Surg Radiol Anat*. 2004;26:494-500.
22. Liebman EP, Webster RC, Berger AS, DellaVecchia M. The frontalis nerve in the temporal brow lift. *Arch Otolaryngol*. 1982;108:232-235.
23. Odobescu A, Williams HB, Gilardino MS. Description of a communication between the facial and zygomaticotemporal nerves. *J Plast Reconstr Aesthet Surg*. 2012;65:1188-1192.

24. Lee JG, Yang HM, Choi YJ, et al. Facial arterial depth and relationship with the facial musculature layer. *Plast Reconstr Surg.* 2015;135(2):437-444.

25. Koh KS, Kim HJ, Oh CS, Chung IH. Branching patterns and symmetry of the course of the facial artery in Koreans. *Int J Oral Maxillofac Surg.* 2003;32(4):414-418.

26. Tubbs RS, Loukas M, Salter EG, Oakes WJ. Wilhelm Erb and Erb's point. *Clin Anat.* 2007;20:486–488.

27. Carlson KC, Roenigk RK. Know your anatomy: perineural involvement of basal and squamous cell carcinoma on the face. *J Dermatol Surg Oncol.* 1990;16:827-833.

Wound Healing and Surgical Wound Dressings

2

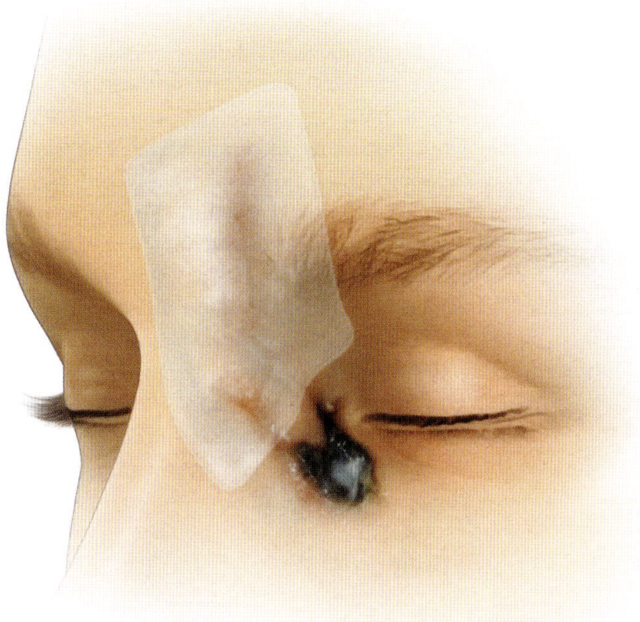

SUMMARY

- Acute postsurgical wounds follow an orderly progression in healing, from hemostasis/inflammation to proliferation, and on to maturation and remodeling.
- Minimizing tension during primary wound closure will help limit the proliferative phase of wound healing and decrease chances of keloid formation.
- Simple wound dressings, such as polymer films, are generally adequate for most postoperative wounds.

Beginner Tips

- Avoid dressing a wound with gauze directly adjacent to the wound bed, as it has a tendency to become incorporated into the wound.
- An ounce of prevention truly is worth a pound of cure; pay attention to meticulous suturing and wound closure, and dressing choice will be far less important.
- Be sure to affix the pressure dressing to the surrounding skin and not to the polymer film, or when the pressure dressing is removed the film will be as well.

Pitfalls and Cautions

- Wound debridement is of vital importance, but can be painful. In general, the removal of necrotic tissue is fairly painless, though pretreatment with local anesthetics may be desirable.
- Expensive wound dressings and devices generally add little (other than expense) to the healing of well-sutured operative wounds.

Expert Tips

- While polymer films, such as Tegaderm, may work well for wounds closed with buried sutures alone, nylon sutures that will require removal in under a week may be best dressed with nonadherent pads.

Patient Education Points

- When using clear polymer films, advise patients that they will likely see some serous drainage or even frank bleeding under the dressing. A small amount of eschar present under the film is not concerning.
- Patient education regarding leg elevation and compression after lower leg procedures is of vital importance.

Don't Forget!

- When using a polymer film dressing, some moisture under the dressing is desirable, but excess serous drainage may lead to maceration.
- Most surgical wounds do not require topical antibiotic dressings or ointments.

Billing Pearls

- While wound dressings are incorporated as part of any surgical procedure, debridement may be separately billable using the debridement codes (11042 series). Wound debridement performed during the postoperative global period, however, cannot be billed separately.

2 Wound Healing and Surgical Wound Dressings

INTRODUCTION

A working understanding of the fundamentals of the wound healing process, as well as available wound dressings, is critical for the primary care practitioner embarking on performing skin procedures. Acute wounds are created with every surgical procedure, and what patients are interested in the most—outcomes—are generally dependent not only on the care and skill of the individual practitioner, but on the natural wound healing process as well.

The healing process is highly dependent on a patient's underlying health status, and complications such as surgical site infections, chronic wound development, and keloid scarring are common. In the United States, over 70 million surgeries are performed a year, with an estimated 38 million patients requiring acute postsurgical wound care.[1]

BASIC BIOLOGY OF WOUND HEALING

Three Phases of Acute Wound Healing

The biological process of healing an acute wound is coordinated across many cell types and physiologic systems. It is classically described as consisting of three phases: an initial response in which hemostasis and inflammation dominate, followed by a proliferative phase and, finally, by a period of maturation and remodeling (**Table 2-1**).[2-4]

Hemostasis and Inflammation: In the initial phase of wound healing, local injury triggers recruitment of inflammatory cells. Wounding is accompanied by vascular injury and exposure of subendothelial collagen, which activates the intrinsic clotting cascade to aggregate platelets and form a fibrin clot. The damaged parenchymal cells and activated platelets then release multiple cytokines and growth factors, including platelet-derived growth factor (PDGF) and transforming growth factor-β (TGF-β), which attract inflammatory cells and fibroblasts to the site of injury. The established fibrin clot then serves as a scaffold for recruited cells. Following coagulation, cells migrate to the site of injury in waves. Neutrophils arrive first and play an antimicrobial role, phagocytizing bacteria or other foreign particles. Next, monocytes from the bloodstream enter the wound site and are activated by platelet-released factors and the extracellular matrix (ECM) to release multiple factors necessary for a continued inflammatory response and recruitment of fibroblasts, including colony-stimulating factor-1 (CSF-1), tumor necrosis factor-α (TNF-α), PDGF, and nitric oxide.[5,6]

TABLE 2-1 • The Acute Wound Healing Process

Hemostasis/ Inflammation	Proliferation	Maturation/ Remodeling
Hours	Days	Weeks

Proliferation: During the proliferative phase of wound healing, granulation tissue and a new epithelial layer are formed. Granulation tissue begins forming 2 to 4 days after wounding when fibroblasts from neighboring dermal tissue are activated by release of growth factors including PDGF and epidermal growth factor (EGF). These cells replicate and migrate into the matrix produced by the initial clot. Triggered by interactions with the clot, they secrete enzymes that break down the existing matrix and produce type III collagen to build a new matrix. Also during this period, angiogenesis is initiated, stimulated by factors released by macrophages and epidermal cells in response to damage and local hypoxia (**Figure 2-1**).

Reepithelialization is initiated soon after wounding when epidermal cells at the wound edge dissolve their basement membrane connections, alter their integrin presentation and cytoskeleton, and begin migrating into the wound site, separating the clot products from underlying viable tissue.[7-9] Next, the remaining epidermal cells at the wound margin proliferate and migrate over the provisional matrix. Once an intact cell layer is formed by proliferation and migration, basement membrane attachments and integrin expression revert to baseline state.

Maturation and Remodeling: For wounds in which the edges were not approximated by external means, a process of wound contracture occurs over 2 to 3 weeks following wounding. This process is mediated both by fibroblasts moving on the collagen matrix and the presence of specialized myofibroblast cells, which can be detected beginning 6 days after wounding.[10] After contracture is complete, the wound remains weak, reaching approximately 20% of its final strength.[11] Over the next several weeks, the matrix undergoes a slower process of remodeling during which matrix metalloproteinases breakdown the existing type III collagen ECM and fibroblasts synthesize the stronger type I collagen.[12] By 3 months after wounding, the scar tissue will reach its maximum strength of approximately 80% of the tensile strength of normal tissue.[11]

Factors Affecting Wound Healing

The ability of the carefully orchestrated process of wound healing to proceed in a timely and organized manner is highly dependent on optimal physiologic status. The level of bacteria, moisture balance, and tissue oxygenation all have large impacts on a wound's ability to heal. Regarding bacteria, it is the level and type of bacterial burden that determine whether infection will spread and inhibit healing. A bacterial load of greater than 10^5 per gram of tissue impairs closure regardless of method, as does the presence of any level of β-hemolytic *Streptococcus*.[13] When the load is

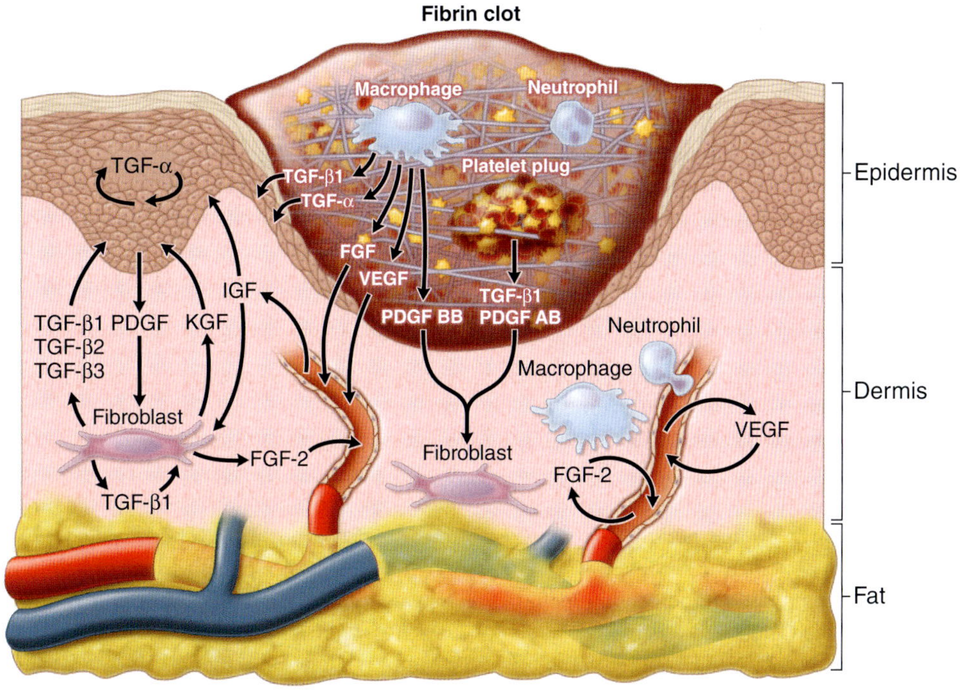

FIGURE 2-1 Overview of proliferative phase wound healing activity.

elevated, the inflammatory stage is prolonged and bacteria excrete enzymes that disrupt formation of ECM.

The impact of oxygenation varies throughout healing. While initial localized hypoxia stimulates proliferation, prolonged hypoxia is detrimental, triggering endothelial cell apoptosis and diminishing the essential activity of both neutrophils and fibroblasts.[14,15] Coupled with the importance of maintaining perfusion, local edema and elevated tissue pressures play a detrimental role in wound healing by creating local ischemia. Pressure-related ischemia is a detrimental factor for healing in patients with low oncotic pressures, in patients with venous-related edema and lymphedema, and in tissues that sustain elevated pressure during activity, such as bony prominences or feet.[16]

Evidence has shown that sufficient moisture is also necessary for proper healing. Excessive drying can lead to eschar formation and necrosis, whereas maintaining a moist environment facilitates the action of cytokines and formation of a preliminary ECM.[17-19] However, excessive moisture can also be detrimental, leading to maceration of surrounding tissue and preventing appropriate formation of granulation tissue.[20]

Patient Factors

The ability of a wound to heal is strongly affected by the patient's underlying nutritional status, age, and health status and the underlying integrity of the wound site. It is important to consider these factors when evaluating a patient's potential for healing and need for specialized wound care. Healing-related factors to consider in a patient's initial history and physical are noted in **Table 2-2.**

Malnutrition has a negative effect on multiple processes of wound healing. The amino acids methionine and arginine are specifically implicated in cellular proliferation, matrix building, and angiogenesis. Multiple trace metals and vitamin C are all implicated in collagen synthesis, supporting the observation that patients with poor nutrition status have lowered ability to rebuild an ECM.[21]

TABLE 2-2 • Considerations for Preoperative History and Physical to Predict Wound Healing

Healing-Focused History and Physical
History
Prior surgeries with prolonged healing
Prior keloid scarring
Prior lymph node dissection
Prior radiation
Recent HbA1c
Nutritional history
Use of steroids
Smoking history
Family history of prolonged healing
Dermatologic conditions
Physical
Body mass index
Perfusion distal to wound site
Local edema
Quality of scarring throughout body

Obesity and hyperglycemia are also detrimental to healing. Obese individuals experience a higher rate of wound dehiscence, surgical site infection, and pressure ulcers,[22] which is attributed to reduced perfusion of adipose tissue and systemic inflammation.[23,24] Patients with diabetes also have pathologic inflammation in normal tissue, coupled with decreased migration of inflammatory cells, fibroblasts, and keratinocytes impairing progression of wound healing.[25,26] Many diabetics also have vascular abnormalities, leading to impaired delivery of nutrients and oxygen.[25,27] Recent glycemic status, as measured by HbA1c, is inversely correlated with rate of wound healing.[28]

Increasing age is associated with characteristic changes in the healing process that result in delayed healing. Delays have been documented in inflammatory response, collagen synthesis, and reepithelialization, along with decreased turnover and remodeling.[29-31] Much of this change has been linked to changes in sex hormones. Wounds in elderly individuals have altered expression of estrogen-regulated genes, and improvement in wound healing is seen with estrogen supplementation in both aged men and women.[32,33]

Other patient factors that can impair wound healing include cigarette smoking and steroid use (**Table 2-3**). Cigarette smoking has a major negative impact on wound healing across all demographics, with two-pack-per-day smokers having a six times greater risk of skin graft necrosis than nonsmokers.[34] Nicotine decreases proliferation of fibroblasts, macrophages, and endothelial cells and decreases tissue oxygenation.[35] Taking systemic glucocorticoid steroids negatively impacts wound healing by decreasing the necessary inflammatory response and decreasing fibroblast response. Wounds heal with incomplete granulation tissue and less contracture.[36]

Complicated Wound Healing

Chronic Wounds: Wounds are considered chronic when they fail to heal for more than 42 days or exhibit frequent recurrence in the same location. These are most commonly seen in situations with multiple systemic risk factors for wound healing. Approximately 90% are either pressure ulcers, venous ulcers, or diabetic ulcers, although an estimated 20% of acute wounds with significant tissue loss transition into a chronic pattern, so clinicians working with surgical wounds should be aware of the behavior associated with chronic wounds.[37,38] Histologically, chronic wounds are associated with increased presence of inflammatory cells and inadequate ECM formation.[39] Derangements in moisture balance, bacterial burden, and perfusion are all implicated in pathogenesis. Exudate from chronic wound shows increased proteolytic activity, degrading growth signals, and ECM components.[40,41] As chronic wounds progress, bacterial burden and necrotic tissue burden increase, stimulating further inflammatory signaling. Significant tissue edema is often present, decreasing perfusion and inhibiting wound healing.[37]

TABLE 2-3 • Factors Affecting Wound Healing

Risk Factor	Mechanism
Obesity	Decreased perfusion of adipose tissue and increased inflammation
Malnutrition	Amino acid, vitamin, mineral, and cofactor unavailability
Diabetes	Pathologic inflammation and decreased migration
Age	Decreased estrogen levels
Cigarette smoking	Decreased tissue oxygenation
Steroid use	Decreased inflammatory and fibroblast response

Keloid Scarring: Keloid scars arise when the proliferative phase of wound healing is prolonged, without appropriate negative feedback and remodeling. These scars grow outside the initial margin of the wound, can become large, and are often associated with pain, pressure, and pruritus. They do not spontaneously regress. Histologically, these have few organized bundles of collagen, with unorganized deposition of both collagen type I and type III.[42,43] The likelihood of a patient forming keloid scars after wounding appears to have a strong genetic contribution and is particularly enriched within the African American population.[44,45] The altered pathophysiology underlying keloid scarring centers on overactivation of fibroblasts in the proliferative stage. This is thought to be mediated by TGF-β and PDGF signaling,[46,47] as well as increased vascular endothelial growth factor (VEGF) signaling from keratinocytes overlying the scar.[48,49] Recent work shows that increased fibroblast activation and inflammation may also be due to the effects of tension on a healing wound, mediated by fibroblast focal adhesion kinase (FAK) mechanotransduction.[50]

CLINICAL IMPLICATIONS

While many factors affecting healing may be out of the clinician's control at the time of a procedure, a clinician can have a large impact on healing outcome through appropriate wound care, including closure design and tension minimization, management of bacterial burden, wound dressing, and monitoring. The proper choices for each of these parameters depend largely on the type and location of the initial wound.

Wound Closure

The main types of closure used in dermatologic procedures are primary closure and closure by secondary intention. For primary closure, the dermis is approximated immediately after a procedure. For closure by secondary intention, a wound is left open to heal spontaneously. Delayed primary closure refers to leaving a wound open for initial care and approximating the dermal edges at a later time.

Primary closure using sutures, staples, or surgical glue is the first choice for wounds that are clean and have sufficient tissue for approximation. For these wounds, the processes of reepithelialization and wound contracture are less necessary for healing. This method often requires the least complex wound care and heals more quickly and with less pain. Wounds closed in this manner have reduced scarring.[51]

Closure by secondary intention is appropriate for most wounds that do not meet criteria for primary closure or grafting, such as contaminated wounds or those with significant tissue destruction, or in cases where shallow wounds would be expected to heal fairly quickly. This process often requires more involved care during the healing process. While it is generally thought that healing by secondary intention is more likely to leave a prominent scar, cosmetically favorable healing through secondary intention has been reported in many instances, particularly on concave body surfaces such as the nasolabial fold, canthus, ears, and temples.[51,52]

Hemostasis

Hemostasis is essential for wound healing, as the activation of the coagulation cascade and formation of a clot play an essential role in initiating the healing cascade. While hemostasis is an important goal at the end of surgery, some bleeding at the time of dressing and wound care is frequently seen. The main options for hemostasis in open or actively bleeding small wounds are caustic agents, physical agents, and physiologic agents. Caustic agents include aluminum chloride, ferric sulfate, silver nitrate, and zinc chloride. These work by local tissue destruction, initiating coagulation and forming a small eschar. Aluminum chloride is most commonly used and is desirable because it does not leave residual skin pigmentation. Noncaustic agents include physical agents, gelatin, cellulose, p-GlcNAc, and microfibrillar collagen, which promote clot formation by forming a mesh for further clotting. These approaches may promote a granulomatous foreign body reaction and thus should be avoided in the setting of infection or near the eyes in particular. Physiologic agents include epinephrine and cocaine, which induce vasoconstriction, as well as topical thrombin, fibrin sealant, and platelet gels.[53]

Management of Bacterial Burden

Surgical site infections (SSIs) are generally uncommon in dermatologic surgery, and their frequency can range from 3% to 28% depending on the body site involved. SSIs are more frequently seen in the distal lower extremities.[54] The most commonly isolated organism in SSIs is *Staphylococcus aureus*, much of which is from an endogenous origin.[55] The skin resident *Staphylococcus epidermidis* can also lead to pathogenic infection when it adopts different virulence factors.[56] Although less common, wound infections with gram-negative bacteria and β-hemolytic streptococci are observed, often in the lower extremities, and can be particularly destructive.

The majority of dermatologic surgeries do not require systemic antibiotic prophylaxis unless the wound appears dirty or the patient has a particularly high risk for infection.[57] If prophylaxis is desired because of patient risk factors or wound location, a single preoperative dose is recommended. If the wound does appear infected or dirty, a 7- to 10-day course of systemic antibiotics is merited. Antibiotics should be chosen based on suspected pathogen.[57] Antibiotic choices and protocols are discussed in detail in Chapter 6.

If a wound appears heavily contaminated or has a large burden of devitalized tissue that may serve as a nidus for infection, it is important to remove as much of this as possible by debriding the wound before dressing. There are multiple options for debridement. The first-line option, sharp debridement, involves use of instruments to remove material with local anesthetic (**Figure 2-2**). It is most effective and targeted but can be painful and is not always well tolerated. Other options include autolytic debridement, in which a moist environment is created to facilitate digestion of necrotic tissue by endogenous enzymes, or enzymatic debridement using laboratory-produced collagenase or papain. Autolytic debridement carries a risk of overhydration and maceration, whereas enzymatic debridement is expensive and thus not a first-line choice. Surgical debridement under anesthesia may be performed as well. Recently, other options, such as cold helium plasma with radiofrequency, have also been explored.[58] Hydrosurgery offers a less damaging option in which a saline beam is applied tangentially to the wound, but this technique also requires anesthesia and is not widely available.[59]

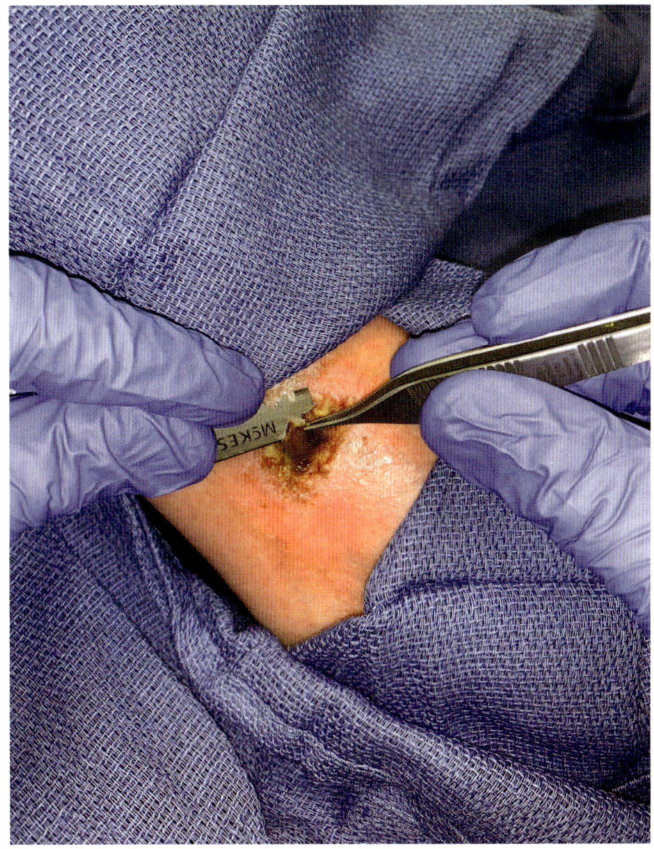

FIGURE 2-2 Sharp debridement can be performed with a surgical blade, scissors, a curette, or—as seen here—with a razor blade used for shave biopsies.

WOUND DRESSINGS

Once hemostasis is achieved and bacterial burden is managed, the clinician must decide whether to dress a wound and, if dressing is desired, what type to use. Dressings can serve multiple functions including protection, hemostasis, compression, and moisture regulation. However, the time spent changing dressings and cost of advanced dressings must be weighed against their benefit in each circumstance. For acute surgical wounds closed by primary intention without infection or excess exudate, there is no evidence that use of a dressing or choice of specific dressing has an impact on time of healing, prevention of infection, pain, or scarring.[60] Given the role of tension in scarring and fibrosis, novel dressings that externally reduce tension may show potential for decreasing scarring, although these benefits may be nonexistent if a wound is well sutured with minimal tension.[61] Cost and ease of use should always be considered when deciding on dressing choice.

For wounds healing by secondary intention, the level of bacterial burden, amount of exudate, and patient preference guide dressing choice. Dressings vary based on degree of occlusion, permeability/moisture, absorption, adherence, compression, and maintenance involved.

Antimicrobial Dressings

The use of local antimicrobials following a procedure is not recommended for general prevention of SSIs. They are no more effective at preventing SSIs than petroleum, and topical antibiotics can increase the frequency of resistant organisms within a wound.[62,63] If a local antimicrobial is desired due to risk of local infection, iodine- or silver-based solutions or dressings are often chosen because they provide broad coverage and are associated with lower levels of bacterial resistance than topical antibiotic ointments. Iodine-based options include povidone-iodine, available as an impregnated tulle, or cadexomer iodine, a starch that absorbs fluid while slowly releasing iodine and is useful for exudative wounds. These should not be used in patients with thyroid conditions due to low levels of systemic absorption. Silver-based antimicrobials are available as a topical cream (silver sulfadiazine) or impregnated in a variety of dressings, including foam, gauze, and nanocrystalline preparations for slow release. Silver sulfadiazine cream is less favorable for use in most settings because it stains skin and forms a pseudo-eschar. Specific silver-impregnated dressings should be chosen based on other desired dressing properties. On a practical level, many clinicians use mupirocin ointment as the antibacterial ointment of choice, although contact allergy and even anaphylaxis have been reported.

Occlusive Dressings

Given the importance of maintaining a moist and relatively sterile environment for healing, occlusive dressings are the first choice for noninfected, nonischemic wounds. These dressings maintain a moist environment, preventing drying and eschar formation, which are detrimental for reepithelialization. As compared to basic gauze dressings, occlusive dressings increase reepithelization and collagenization and decrease rates of SSIs.[19,64,65] Occlusive dressings range widely in their indications, degree of permeability to air and water, level of fluid absorbency, and adherence (**Table 2-4**).

Polymer films, such as Tegaderm and Opsite, represent the classic occlusive dressings. These adhere to healthy skin but not to the wound site. They are semipermeable, allowing air and water vapor exchange, and they are clear, allowing visual monitoring of the wound. These provide no cushioning or absorbency and thus are appropriate for shallow wounds with low exudate only, such as seen in most surgical site repairs. ***Polymer foams***, such as Allevyn and Lyofoam, consist of an absorbent surface in contact with a semipermeable backing to prevent leakage. These are appropriate for heavily exudative wounds. They are nonadherent and require another layer of dressing. ***Hydrocolloids***, including Exuderm, Duoderm, and Comfeel, consist of multiple layers.

TABLE 2-4 • Types and Properties of Occlusive Dressings

Type	Characteristics	Advantages	Disadvantages	Indications	Maintenance
Hydrogels	Semipermeable, nonadherent	Pain relief, nontraumatic removal, allows autolytic debridement	Risk of infection, may overhydrate	Dry, painful wounds	Change every 1-3 days
Polymer films	Transparent, semiocclusive, adherent	Protects from infection	Fluid trapping, can strip skin	Wounds with little exudate, closed wounds	Leave in place for 7 days or until fluid leaks
Hydrocolloids	Opaque, impermeable, adherent, absorbent, occlusive	Protects from infection, allows autolytic debridement	Malodorous discharge, fluid trapping/can overhydrate	Low exudate	Leave in place for 7 days or until fluid leaks
Polymer foams	Opaque, absorbent, occlusive, nonadherent	Cut to shape, thermal insulation	Can be incorporated into wound if dry	Light to moderate exudate, sloughy wounds	Must change every 3 days or incorporated into wound
Alginates	Nonadherent, highly absorbent, hemostatic	Helpful in hemostasis	Malodorous	Wounds with heavy exudate or moderate bleeding	Change when soaked in exudate

When placed on a wound, the bottom layer forms a gel. This moisturizes the wound bed, promoting autolytic debridement. The top layer is adherent and virtually impermeable, providing protection to the wound during daily activity. ***Hydrogels***, such as Restore Hydrogel, SAF-Gel, and CuraGel, consist of a matrix of insoluble polymers and water, allowing them to both donate moisture to a dry wound surface and absorb wound exudate. They are commonly used to promote autolytic debridement. ***Alginates***, including Sorbsan and Kaltostat, are produced from salts of alginic acid found in brown seaweed. These dressings partially dissolve upon contact with a wound bend when sodium ions from the wound are exchanged with calcium ions from the dressing, forming a highly absorptive gel appropriate for wounds with high levels of exudate.

Specific indications and restrictions of each type of occlusive dressing are detailed further in **Table 2-5**.

TABLE 2-5 • Dressing Choice Based on Wound Characteristics

Wound Characteristics	Dressings to Consider
Primarily closed	Polymer film or petroleum
Dry, necrotic	Hydrogel or hydrocolloid, debride when hydrated
Sloughing	Debridement, cadexomer iodine or silver-based dressing
Shallow	Hydrocolloid
With exudate	Alginate
Deep, nongranulating	Synthetic dermal matrix or bilayer
Red, granulating	
Wounds with deep sinuses	Alginate ribbon or hydrogel
Deep cavity	Foam, foam in plastic pouch
Shallow, heavy exudate	Alginate sheet
Shallow mild exudate	Foam
Shallow nonexudative	Hydrocolloid
Pink, epithelializing	
Heavy exudate	Alginate
Mild exudate	Hydrocolloid
Nonexudative	Film
Infected	
Heavy exudate	Negative-pressure wound therapy, hydroconductive dressing
Mild exudate	Silver- or iodine-based dressing
Edematous	Compressive dressing
Ischemic	Hyperbaric oxygen therapy

Long-Term Monitoring

Most dermatologic surgery wounds will be followed in the outpatient setting; therefore, instructing patients in proper wound care is essential for optimal healing. Patients with wounds closed primarily should not shower for the first 48 hours and should avoid bathing or showering for more than 10 minutes throughout healing. Patients with wounds requiring complex dressing should cover dressings with a water-impermeable barrier during bathing. Patients with superficial wounds should avoid direct UV exposure to the wound during healing, as exposure may increase the risk of hyperpigmentation.[66]

Throughout the healing process, clinicians should monitor for evidence of nascent infection and wound dehiscence. If signs of acute infection such as increased purulent discharge, erythema, or warmth are present, wounds should be swabbed and cultured. Empiric topical or systemic antibiotics should be initiated, and mechanical, surgical, or autolytic debridement should be performed based on the extent of infection. If superficial wound dehiscence develops in a primarily closed surgical wound, debridement of necrotic tissue should be performed. Following this, wounds with only superficial dehiscence can be left to close by secondary intention, while those with larger dehiscence should be addressed with negative-pressure dressing or tension-relieving approaches such as tape, glue, or sutures.[67]

CONCLUSIONS

Wound care and dressing choice play an important role in dermatologic procedures, as even the best-designed closure can be undone by less-than-optimal wound care. Patient education is of paramount importance because even a fully healed wound will only retain 80% of the tensile strength of its preinjury period. Wound dressing choice following an uncomplicated surgical procedure should be kept as straightforward as possible. For sutured wounds repaired with absorbable sutures alone, using a simple polymer film dressing may allow the patient to return quickly to their normal activities and concomitantly minimize the need for re-dressing at home.

REFERENCES

1. Sen CK, Gordillo GM, Roy S, et al. Human skin wounds: a major and snowballing threat to public health and the economy. *Wound Repair Regen.* 2009;17:763-771.
2. Gilmore MA. Phases of wound healing. *Dimens Oncol Nurs.* 1991;5:32-34.
3. Witte MB, Barbul A. General principles of wound healing. *Surg Clin North Am.* 1997;77:509-528.
4. Singer AJ, Clark RA. Cutaneous wound healing. *N Engl J Med.* 1999;341:738-746.
5. Rappolee DA, Mark D, Banda MJ, Werb Z. Wound macrophages express TGF-alpha and other growth factors in vivo: analysis by mRNA phenotyping. *Science.* 1988;241:708-712.
6. Albina JE, Henry WL Jr, Mastrofrancesco B, Martin BA, Reichner JS. Macrophage activation by culture in an anoxic environment. *J Immunol.* 1995;155:4391-4396.

7. Larjava H, Salo T, Haapasalmi K, Kramer RH, Heino J. Expression of integrins and basement membrane components by wound keratinocytes. *J Clin Invest.* 1993;92:1425-1435.

8. Goliger JA, Paul DL. Wounding alters epidermal connexin expression and gap junction-mediated intercellular communication. *Mol Biol Cell.* 1995;6:1491-1501.

9. Gabbiani G, Chaponnier C, Huttner I. Cytoplasmic filaments and gap junctions in epithelial cells and myofibroblasts during wound healing. *J Cell Biol.* 1978;76:561-568.

10. Darby I, Skalli O, Gabbiani G. Alpha-smooth muscle actin is transiently expressed by myofibroblasts during experimental wound healing. *Lab Invest.* 1990;63:21-29.

11. Levenson SM, Geever EF, Crowley LV, Oates JF 3rd, Berard CW, Rosen H. The healing of rat skin wounds. *Ann Surg.* 1965;161:293-308.

12. Ehrlich HP, Krummel TM. Regulation of wound healing from a connective tissue perspective. *Wound Repair Regen.* 1996;4:203-210.

13. Robson MC. Wound infection. A failure of wound healing caused by an imbalance of bacteria. *Surg Clin North Am.* 1997;77:637-650.

14. Allen DB, Maguire JJ, Mahdavian M, et al. Wound hypoxia and acidosis limit neutrophil bacterial killing mechanisms. *Arch Surg.* 1997;132:991-996.

15. Steinbrech DS, Longaker MT, Mehrara BJ, et al. Fibroblast response to hypoxia: the relationship between angiogenesis and matrix regulation. *J Surg Res.* 1999;84:127-133.

16. Mrdjenovich DE. Off-loading practices for the wounded foot: concepts and choices. *J Am Col Certif Wound Spec.* 2010;2:73-78.

17. Winter GD. Formation of the scab and the rate of epithelization of superficial wounds in the skin of the young domestic pig. *Nature.* 1962;193:293-294.

18. Hinman CD, Maibach H. Effect of air exposure and occlusion on experimental human skin wounds. *Nature.* 1963;200:377-378.

19. Alvarez OM, Mertz PM, Eaglstein WH. The effect of occlusive dressings on collagen synthesis and re-epithelialization in superficial wounds. *J Surg Res.* 1983;35:142-148.

20. Okan D, Woo K, Ayello EA, Sibbald G. The role of moisture balance in wound healing. *Adv Skin Wound Care.* 2007;20:39-53; quiz 53-55.

21. Haydock DA, Hill GL. Impaired wound healing in surgical patients with varying degrees of malnutrition. *JPEN J Parenter Enteral Nutr.* 1986;10:550-554.

22. Wilson JA, Clark JJ. Obesity: impediment to postsurgical wound healing. *Adv Skin Wound Care.* 2004;17:426-435.

23. Nieman DC, Henson DA, Nehlsen-Cannarella SL, et al. Influence of obesity on immune function. *J Am Diet Assoc.* 1999;99:294-299.

24. Somm E, Cettour-Rose P, Asensio C, et al. Interleukin-1 receptor antagonist is upregulated during diet-induced obesity and regulates insulin sensitivity in rodents. *Diabetologia.* 2006;49:387-393.

25. Ferguson MW, Herrick SE, Spencer MJ, Shaw JE, Boulton AJ, Sloan P. The histology of diabetic foot ulcers. *Diabet Med.* 1996;13(suppl 1):S30-S33.

26. Delamaire M, Maugendre D, Moreno M, Le Goff MC, Allannic H, Genetet B. Impaired leucocyte functions in diabetic patients. *Diabet Med.* 1997;14:29-34.

27. Hu SC, Lan CE. High-glucose environment disturbs the physiologic functions of keratinocytes: focusing on diabetic wound healing. *J Dermatol Sci.* 2016;84(2):121-127.

28. Christman AL, Selvin E, Margolis DJ, Lazarus GS, Garza LA. Hemoglobin A1c predicts healing rate in diabetic wounds. *J Invest Dermatol.* 2011;131:2121-2127.

29. Swift ME, Kleinman HK, DiPietro LA. Impaired wound repair and delayed angiogenesis in aged mice. *Lab Invest.* 1999;79:1479-1487.

30. Swift ME, Burns AL, Gray KL, DiPietro LA. Age-related alterations in the inflammatory response to dermal injury. *J Invest Dermatol.* 2001;117:1027-1035.

31. Gosain A, DiPietro LA. Aging and wound healing. *World J Surg.* 2004;28:321-326.

32. Hardman MJ, Ashcroft GS. Estrogen, not intrinsic aging, is the major regulator of delayed human wound healing in the elderly. *Genome Biol.* 2008;9:R80.

33. Gilliver SC, Ashworth JJ, Ashcroft GS. The hormonal regulation of cutaneous wound healing. *Clin Dermatol.* 2007;25:56-62.

34. Goldminz D, Bennett RG. Cigarette smoking and flap and full-thickness graft necrosis. *Arch Dermatol.* 1991;127:1012-1015.

35. Silverstein P. Smoking and wound healing. *Am J Med.* 1992;93:S22-S24.

36. Guo S, Dipietro LA. Factors affecting wound healing. *J Dent Res.* 2010;89:219-229.

37. Mustoe TA, O'Shaughnessy K, Kloeters O. Chronic wound pathogenesis and current treatment strategies: a unifying hypothesis. *Plast Reconstr Surg.* 2006;117:S35-S41.

38. Greaves NS, Iqbal SA, Baguneid M, Bayat A. The role of skin substitutes in the management of chronic cutaneous wounds. *Wound Repair Regen.* 2013;21:194-210.

39. Herrick SE, Sloan P, McGurk M, Freak L, McCollum CN, Ferguson MW. Sequential changes in histologic pattern and extracellular matrix deposition during the healing of chronic venous ulcers. *Am J Pathol.* 1992;141:1085-1095.

40. Harris IR, Yee KC, Walters CE, et al. Cytokine and protease levels in healing and non-healing chronic venous leg ulcers. *Exp Dermatol.* 1995;4:342-349.

41. Grinnell F, Ho CH, Wysocki A. Degradation of fibronectin and vitronectin in chronic wound fluid: analysis by cell blotting, immunoblotting, and cell adhesion assays. *J Invest Dermatol.* 1992;98:410-416.

42. Ehrlich HP, Desmouliere A, Diegelmann RF, et al. Morphological and immunochemical differences between keloid and hypertrophic scar. *Am J Pathol.* 1994;145:105-113.

43. Costa AM, Peyrol S, Porto LC, Comparin JP, Foyatier JL, Desmouliere A. Mechanical forces induce scar remodeling. Study in non-pressure-treated versus pressure-treated hypertrophic scars. *Am J Pathol.* 1999;155:1671-1679.

44. Bloom D. Heredity of keloids; review of the literature and report of a family with multiple keloids in five generations. *N Y State J Med.* 1956;56:511-519.

45. Slemp AE, Kirschner RE. Keloids and scars: a review of keloids and scars, their pathogenesis, risk factors, and management. *Curr Opin Pediatr.* 2006;18:396-402.

46. Peltonen J, Hsiao LL, Jaakkola S, et al. Activation of collagen gene expression in keloids: co-localization of type I and VI collagen and transforming growth factor-beta 1 mRNA. *J Invest Dermatol.* 1991;97:240-248.

47. Haisa M, Okochi H, Grotendorst GR. Elevated levels of PDGF alpha receptors in keloid fibroblasts contribute to an enhanced response to PDGF. *J Invest Dermatol.* 1994;103:560-563.

48. Kischer CW, Thies AC, Chvapil M. Perivascular myofibroblasts and microvascular occlusion in hypertrophic scars and keloids. *Hum Pathol.* 1982;13:819-824.

49. Gira AK, Brown LF, Washington CV, Cohen C, Arbiser JL. Keloids demonstrate high-level epidermal expression of vascular endothelial growth factor. *J Am Acad Dermatol.* 2004;50:850-853.

50. Wong VW, Rustad KC, Akaishi S, et al. Focal adhesion kinase links mechanical force to skin fibrosis via inflammatory signaling. *Nat Med.* 2012;18:148-152.

51. Zitelli JA. Wound healing by secondary intention. A cosmetic appraisal. *J Am Acad Dermatol.* 1983;9:407-415.

52. Christenson LJ, Phillips PK, Weaver AL, Otley CC. Primary closure vs second-intention treatment of skin punch biopsy sites: a randomized trial. *Arch Dermatol.* 2005;141:1093-1099.

53. Glick JB, Kaur RR, Siegel D. Achieving hemostasis in dermatology: part II: topical hemostatic agents. *Indian Dermatol Online J.* 2013;4:172-176.

54. Futoryan T, Grande D. Postoperative wound infection rates in dermatologic surgery. *Dermatol Surg.* 1995;21:509-514.

55. National Nosocomial Infections Surveillance (NNIS) report, data summary from October 1986-April 1996, issued May 1996. A report from the National Nosocomial Infections Surveillance (NNIS) System. *Am J Infect Control.* 1996;24:380-388.

56. Cogen AL, Nizet V, Gallo RL. Skin microbiota: a source of disease or defence? *Br J Dermatol.* 2008;158:442-455.

57. Cho CY, Lo JS. Dressing the part. *Dermatol Clin.* 1998;16:25-47.

58. Halim AS, Khoo TL, Saad AZ. Wound bed preparation from a clinical perspective. *Indian J Plast Surg.* 2012;45:193-202.

59. Gravante G, Delogu D, Esposito G, Montone A. Versajet hydrosurgery versus classic escharectomy for burn debridment: a prospective randomized trial. *J Burn Care Res.* 2007;28:720-724.

60. Walter CJ, Dumville JC, Sharp CA, Page T. Systematic review and meta-analysis of wound dressings in the prevention of surgical-site infections in surgical wounds healing by primary intention. *Br J Surg.* 2012;99:1185-1194.

61. Gurtner GC, Dauskardt RH, Wong VW, et al. Improving cutaneous scar formation by controlling the mechanical environment: large animal and phase I studies. *Ann Surg.* 2011;254:217-225.

62. Wu PA, Katz KA, James WD. Topical antibiotic use following dermatologic procedures. *J Am Acad Dermatol.* 2013;68:516-517.

63. Smack DP, Harrington AC, Dunn C, et al. Infection and allergy incidence in ambulatory surgery patients using white petrolatum vs bacitracin ointment. A randomized controlled trial. *JAMA.* 1996;276:972-977.

64. Bolton LL, Johnson CL, Van Rijswijk L. Occlusive dressings: therapeutic agents and effects on drug delivery. *Clin Dermatol.* 1991;9:573-583.

65. Hutchinson JJ, McGuckin M. Occlusive dressings: a microbiologic and clinical review. *Am J Infect Control.* 1990;18:257-268.

66. Due E, Rossen K, Sorensen LT, Kliem A, Karlsmark T, Haedersdal M. Effect of UV irradiation on cutaneous cicatrices: a randomized, controlled trial with clinical, skin reflectance, histological, immunohistochemical and biochemical evaluations. *Acta Derm Venereol.* 2007;87:27-32.

67. Yao K, Bae L, Yew WP. Post-operative wound management. *Aust Fam Physician.* 2013;42:867-870.

3 Preoperative Evaluation, Patient Preparation, and Informed Consent

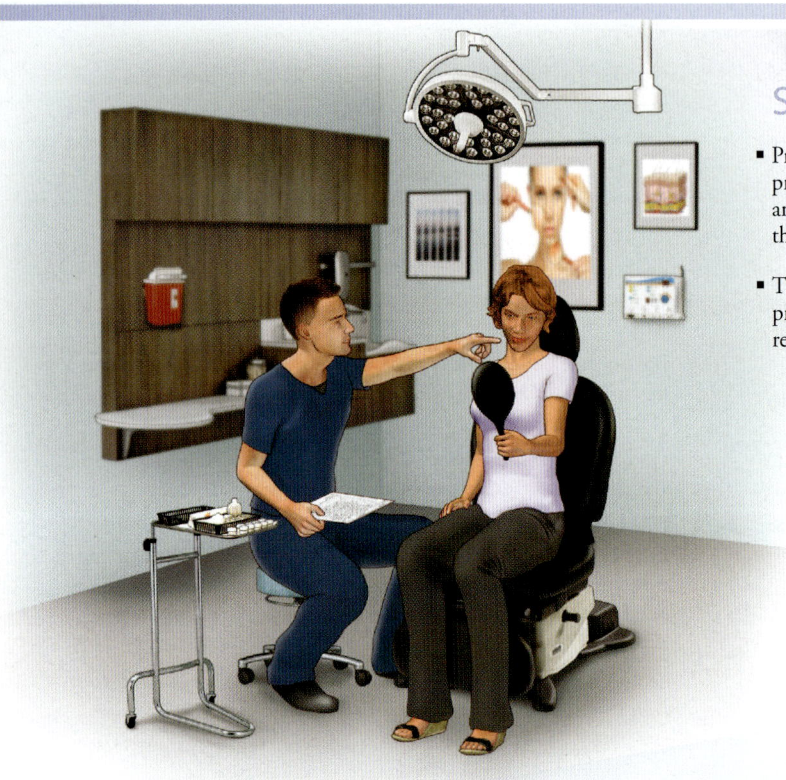

SUMMARY

- Preoperative preparation should include a discussion regarding the procedure; a review of the patient's history, medications, and allergies; any appropriate physical examination; obtaining informed consent through a process; and answering patient and/or family questions.
- The preoperative evaluation ultimately serves as a forum to assess probability of overall success and cement the patient–physician relationship.

Beginner Tips

- From the first moment the patient steps into the office, the front office staff has the opportunity to begin collecting information, such as the patient's mood and degree of anxiety.
- If capacity is ever in question, simple questions like "where do you live?" or "how did you get here?" are innocuous queries that evaluate mental status without prompting any perceived stigmatization.

Expert Tips

- Outline postoperative restrictions ahead of the procedure so that patients avoid conflicts with athletic events as well as allowing them to make any arrangements they may need for home care, child care, time off from work, or transportation to and from the procedure.
- Patient preparation and the informed consent process is a critical part of the surgical procedure.

Don't Forget!

- While a written signature is desirable, the real goal of the consent process is effective communication.
- If an informational packet is provided to help patients prepare, it may include an outline helping them prepare for the pre- and postoperative period.

Pitfalls and Cautions

- Patients who have many questions or voice cosmetic concerns when they are scheduling their procedure are self-identifying as individuals who would benefit from an in-office preoperative consultation.

Patient Education Points

- Without adequate preparation, even mild and expected outcomes, such as edema and ecchymoses, can be a cause for significant concern.
- Make the patient your partner, and use partnering language when discussing the surgical plan.
- Certain subtleties become evident over time, such as personality, forgetfulness, unrealistic expectations, or specific fears that can be noted by the staff and guide the remainder of the visit. These observations can be acted upon early and preemptively, helping to tailor the patient care experience in a positive fashion.
- Some patients under 18 may look older than they are (and vice versa), so it is important when operating on young adults to check their date of birth.
- A full discussion of benefits and risks improves mutual trust and respect between the physician and patient, and ultimately improves patient satisfaction.

Preoperative Evaluation, Patient Preparation, and Informed Consent

3

INTRODUCTION

Evaluating the patient preoperatively, preparing the patient for surgery, and going through the informed consent process are important prerequisites that must be accomplished prior to initiating dermatologic procedures. This is important from an ethical standpoint, but also ultimately yields significant time savings for the clinician, as an informed patient ultimately is less likely to make repeated telephone calls or return visits to the office in the postoperative period. Discussing procedural risks and the possible need for additional surgery or procedures in the postoperative period is always wise, as forewarning and educating patients creates a team atmosphere that ultimately pays significant dividends.

PREOPERATIVE EVALUATION

The preoperative evaluation is most simply thought of as an evaluation of the physical, medical, and emotional preparedness of the patient for a selected procedure. This formal evaluation is generally a multifaceted discussion regarding the procedure; a review of the patient's history, medications, and allergies; any appropriate physical examination; obtaining informed consent through a process; and answering patient and/or family questions. The evaluation can be performed up to several weeks in advance of the surgery, although it may also take place on the same day of the procedure. If a same-day evaluation is chosen, the physician must be prepared to cancel the procedure if it is discovered the operation scheduled is inappropriate for the lesion or the patient is not a good surgical candidate for medical or psychological reasons. There are many factors that should be taken into account when deciding upon the timing of this evaluation, including office setup, physician preference, patient mobility, and travel distance. Nevertheless, the preoperative evaluation ultimately serves as a forum to assess probability of overall success and cement the patient-physician relationship.

Team care is a critical component of the preoperative evaluation. It begins with the very first patient contact and continues up to the initiation of the procedure itself. All members of the team should be empowered and encouraged to have input in this evaluation and have the authority to halt it for any concerns. From the first moment the patient steps into the office, the front office staff has the opportunity to begin collecting information, such as the patient's mood and degree of anxiety. The medical assistants and nursing staff carry this process forward by obtaining a history, complete medication list, and any other standard data points necessary for the field of practice.

Certain subtleties become evident over time, such as personality, forgetfulness, unrealistic expectations, or specific fears that can be noted by the staff and guide the remainder of the visit. These observations can be acted upon early and preemptively, helping to tailor the patient care experience in a positive fashion. Moreover, these initial encounters should serve as a filter for red flags such as abnormal labs or vital signs, concerning new symptoms, or patient aggression/combativeness. Safety is the responsibility of the team, and the clinician, as team leader, must use all information gathered to determine the safest way forward. Overall, the guiding principle is that every person on the care team plays an essential role in the overall patient evaluation and experience. **Table 3-1** provides a list of reasons to delay surgery.

Patient Capacity

Establishing patient decision-making capacity is a cornerstone of the informed consent process and the overall preoperative evaluation. Obtaining an adequate history and providing postoperative instructions are not possible without a patient's ability to accurately understand and make medical decisions on their own behalf. For the vast majority of patients, this is not a problem, but for a few patients, the ability to understand is a significant and delicate issue. Culturally, a stigma is often associated with mental incompetence, and questioning an elderly patient's abilities can

TABLE 3-1 • Reasons to Delay Surgery

Psychological

1. Evidence of medication or drug use that impairs judgment
2. Unavailability of healthcare proxy or guardian when patient is incompetent
3. Indication that the patient does not understand the procedure (negating informed consent)
4. Unrealistic expectations
5. Hostility/anger
6. Evidence of alcohol ingestion/intoxication

Physical Examination

1. Unstable medical condition
    a. Extreme hypertension
    b. New or symptomatic cardiac arrhythmia
2. Fever
3. Acute illness
4. Angina/unstable angina
5. Infection/cellulitis of biopsy site
6. Suggestion of boney involvement

Laboratory Examination

1. International normalized ratio >3.5
2. Thrombocytopenia
3. Metabolic involvement
4. Hypoxia

Miscellaneous

1. Pathology and clinical evaluation do not match
2. Unaccompanied minor without a presigned consent form

interfere with rapport, potentially making the patient angry or defensive. Furthermore, those with functional impairments may hide their diminished capacity well. It is important to understand that competence is a legal term that is commonly confused with capacity—a physician assessment. For informed consent, a patient must be capable of understanding the procedure and relevant information, making a rational choice, and understanding any potential complications or consequences. A patient's family can provide significant insight into capacity and/or competency status. Often the family may be quick to provide information that the patient requires a co-signer or legal guardian present for paperwork, which makes the process straightforward. The dynamics between the patient and the patient's family may also hint at capacity; repeating instructions in different wording, family leading the conversation, and visible frustration may be cues that suggest the need for a more thorough mental status examination. If unaccompanied, the physician should pay close attention to the patient's general hygiene, coordination, and speech patterns. If ever in question, simple questions such as "Where do you live?" or "How did you get here?" are innocuous queries that evaluate mental status without prompting any perceived stigmatization.

During the initial evaluation, it is important for all members of the team to quickly asses the patient's overall state of mind. Is the patient anxious? Confident? Overly worried about cosmetic appearance? With this information, the best support can be offered by the team. Indeed, adequate psychological support cannot be overemphasized for a smooth and successful outcome.

Of course, minors cannot provide true consent for any procedure, although their assent is important. Some patients under 18 may look older than they are (and vice versa), so it is important when operating on young adults to check their date of birth. Be sure any child's parent or legal guardian gives the consent. This can generally be performed with a phone consent as long as it is witnessed by having a staff member join on the phone to verify the consent.

History Review

A standard review of medications, allergies, and past medical history must be obtained for every preoperative evaluation. In particular, the presence of a pacemaker or defibrillator or the use of anticoagulation may impact surgical decision making and techniques, including the type of electrosurgery used, the type of closure chosen, or the type of dressing applied. A history of smoking portends poor wound healing, making a large flap or graft less desirable due to higher risk of failure. A history or alcohol or other substance abuse carries risks of poor wound healing, bleeding, and possible poor compliance with postoperative instructions. A history of radiation treatment to the surgical area increases risks of poor wound healing and tissue mobility. Any positive history should best be shared with the entire team for planning and implementation of the safest care.

Physical Examination

Taking vital signs, including blood pressure, pulse, and respiration rate, is sometimes performed prior to procedures, although doing so is not standard of care for outpatient dermatologic surgery procedures. Elevated blood pressure is common preprocedurally and often is secondary to anxiety or exertion. Repeat measurements are imperative to better delineate "white coat hypertension" or exertional hypertension from more ominous conditions such as hypertensive urgency or emergency. Often patients may abstain from their antihypertensive medications prior to surgery under the misconception that these are anticoagulants. If patients have their medication with them, the physician may consider having them take their scheduled dose and reevaluating after 15 to 20 minutes. Hypertensive urgency is defined as blood pressure greater than 180 mm Hg systolic and greater than 120 mm Hg diastolic in the absence of an acute stressor. A careful review of systems for end-organ damage is necessary, and consideration of procedure abortion and referral to the emergency department is paramount.

Pulse must be evaluated for rate and regularity. Arrhythmias, such as atrial fibrillation, are not uncommon in those on anticoagulants, and a determination of whether such an arrhythmia is well controlled must be made prior to surgery. New or symptomatic arrhythmias are cause for abortion of the procedure and referral to the emergency department.

Any patient showing outward signs of other concerning and acute medical processes, such as shortness of breath, chest pain, or acute neurologic deficit, should be referred to the emergency department immediately.

PATIENT PREPARATION FOR SURGERY

Cognitively preparing patients for surgery helps create a more positive experience for both patient and clinician. This preparation includes elements of informed consent but extends beyond the legal requirements to include patient education about all elements of the procedure from the preoperative to postoperative periods.

Preoperative consultation is one option for cognitively preparing patients for surgery. A clinic visit allows the patient to meet the clinician in advance and discuss all elements of the procedure in detail ahead of time. This is particularly beneficial for planning very complex surgical procedures or with anxious patients or patients having surgery for the first time. When the patient is a child or developmentally delayed adult, preoperative consultation with both the patient and parent or legal guardian present allows proper selection of anesthesia. After a full discussion of the procedure, both the clinician and parent or guardian determine whether local infiltrative anesthesia alone is appropriate or whether the addition of a topical anesthetic, an oral anxiolytic, sedation, or general anesthesia is required to safely and comfortably perform the necessary procedure. This discussion is often helpful for extremely anxious patients as well, who may benefit from an oral anxiolytic such as lorazepam. Obtaining informed consent at the time of preoperative consultation allows the patient to take an anxiolytic prior to surgery, significantly improving the anxious patient's surgical experience. Patients taking anxiolytics should be directed to have someone

SAMPLE EDUCATIONAL HANDOUT OUTLINE FOR PREOPERATIVE PREPARATION

- Preparing for surgery
  - Avoid nonessential aspirin (patients should check with their primary care provider prior to stopping aspirin).
  - Avoid ibuprofen and other nonsteroidal anti-inflammatory drugs (NSAIDs) for at least 24 hours before surgery if possible.
  - No alcohol for 24 hours before surgery.
- Detailed description of the surgery
  - For more complex procedures, a very detailed description of the procedure can be included.
- On the day of surgery
  - Shower/wash the surgical site with soap and water.
  - Do not wear makeup or jewelry on or near the surgery site.
  - Avoid perfume and avoid hair products if the surgical site is the scalp (many hair products are flammable when in contact with cautery).
  - Do not eat or drink anything after midnight the night before (if going to the operating room).
  - Take all of your regular medications (include any exceptions).
  - Inform patients what to bring with them (eg, book, tablet device, friend, snacks) if this is permitted.
- What to expect after surgery
  - Activity limitations.
  - Alcohol and medication restrictions.
  - Wound care instructions will be given after surgery.
  - Follow-up.
- Activity restrictions—It is often helpful to discuss these in front of a family member.
- Wound care—Instructions should be given orally and provided in writing with instructions on who to call with problems or concerns.
- Follow-up—Follow-up appointments should be scheduled if needed, and it is helpful to inform patients if more than one visit will be needed.
- Healing—Preparing patients for what may occur postoperatively can eliminate anxiety and minimize phone calls. Discussing swelling, bruising, scarring, and the potential for scar revision up front will help patients know what to expect as their wound heals.
- Pain management
  - Ice, elevation
  - Recommended analgesics (eg, acetaminophen, NSAIDs, narcotics) with timing and dosage recommendations
  - Elements that may be included when preparing patients

drive them to and from their surgery. Such preoperative consultations can occur by telephone if in-person consultation is not feasible.

Providing patients with an informational packet either by mail or e-mail is a simple and effective way to review the most important elements of surgery. Outlining any restrictions on activities (bending, lifting, housework, sports, etc) as well as the likely duration of these restrictions ahead of time may help patients avoid conflicts with athletic events as well as allow them to make any arrangements they may need for home care, child care, time off from work, or transportation to and from the procedure. The potential timing for follow-up visits should be mentioned as well to prevent patients from scheduling surgery immediately before leaving on a trip (unless proper follow-up can be arranged with another provider or is not needed).

If an informational packet is provided to help patients prepare, it may include an outline helping them prepare for the pre- and postoperative period.

During the preoperative consultation or immediately preceding surgery, a full discussion of the proposed procedure, including the risks and benefits, should be had with the patient. This is largely part of the informed consent process and is critical in preparing a patient for the surgery. Reviewing all other reasonable treatment alternatives and the risks and benefits of these treatment options will help patients identify the best option for them.

Once the treatment modality has been selected, patients will be best prepared if they are walked through the procedure, starting with a description of how they will be positioned, how the site will be prepped and draped, and the use of anesthesia. If an excisional procedure, such as an excision or Mohs surgery, is planned, discussion of possible closures (secondary intention, linear closure, flap or graft, or two-staged closure if this is anticipated) and potential shape and length of the scar line can be had at this time. Patients are often very concerned about how "long" their scar will be. This is an excellent opportunity to educate patients about the cosmetic principles used in designing linear excisions, flaps, and grafts and to discuss the role of hiding incision and scar lines within relaxed skin tension lines and cosmetic boundaries. Understanding that the length of the incision is far less important than the contour and placement of the incision lines and the preservation of symmetry and free margins helps both prepare patients for surgery and instill confidence that their clinician has expertise in the area of wound reconstruction.

If the patient is interested in closure by another surgeon (clinician, plastic surgeon, oculoplastic surgeon, or other subspecialist), this is often revealed during this discussion. This plan is ideally addressed during a preoperative consultation so that such arrangements can be coordinated in advance of the surgery. Patients who have many questions or voice cosmetic concerns when they are scheduling their procedure are self-identifying as individuals who would benefit from an in-office preoperative consultation. Seeing such patients ahead of time to discuss questions and concerns in detail will streamline the actual surgery day and alleviate patient and provider concerns.

Preparing patients for the postoperative period can begin during the preoperative consultation and extend through the end of the surgery. Patients, often nervous about their procedure, may not hear all instructions and can benefit from repetition before and after surgery. Having a friend or family member present to hear instructions is ideal. If the patient is relaxed, reviewing instructions can often occur in part during the surgical procedure as well.

If there will be a pathology result, inform patients when this will be available and how they will receive the result (eg, telephone call, e-mail, postcard, at the follow-up visit). It may be helpful to ask patients if they are comfortable receiving results over the phone and whether or not you can leave a message. It is important to have consent to leave a detailed message on voicemail or with a family member prior to doing so.

INFORMED CONSENT

Obtaining informed consent is one of the most important steps in the preoperative period. It establishes realistic patient expectations and creates a protective legal framework for the physician to operate within. Failure to inform patients adequately of the potential associated risks and expectations can be viewed as negligence, and performing a procedure on patients without their express consent can be considered battery in a court of law, although witnessed verbal consent may be acceptable in some situations. The patient must be provided the information to adequately evaluate a procedure before agreeing to that procedure or surgery. The Joint Commission defines informed consent as agreement or permission accompanied by full notice about the care, treatment, or service that is the subject of the consent.[1]

Before consent can be obtained, the physician must determine whether or not the patient has decision-making capacity. The patient must be over the age of 18 and mentally able to grasp the concepts presented. It is necessary to obtain consent from the healthcare proxy or guardian of mentally incompetent patients. There are many other potential barriers to patient understanding, including ineffective provider communication, lack of patient-provider shared decision making, lack of health literacy, and cultural issues. The clinician must be alert to signs of inadequate patient understanding. Simplification of the content, length, and language may help reduce these communication barriers. A qualified medical interpreter may be used for patients with hearing or visual impairments or limited English fluency, although other technology-based communication approaches may be used as well. Asking patients to summarize the discussion and their decision can also help to highlight those who have failed to understand, and it is up to the physician to uncover the barrier to effective communication and correct it before the procedure is initiated.

Once the clinician has established the patient's competence, the clinician may move on to detail the critical components of informed consent. These include an explanation of the proposed procedure in lay terms, an explanation of the reasonable standard of care, indications for the procedure, common adverse outcomes, unexpected adverse effects, and treatment alternatives, including the expected consequences of no treatment.

Risks to be discussed should include those that either a reasonable physician would disclose or a reasonable patient would think necessary to make an intelligent decision. This means that extremely rare risks need not be discussed, although these standards leave much ambiguity. The clinician should review the likelihood of those risks based on available clinical evidence and their judgment. Risks addressed should include common adverse events (which may be mild), as well as those that are unlikely but severe. Patients should have the opportunity to refuse the procedure if they deem any of those risks intolerable.

For cases in which residents or fellows in training are participating, the attending physician should explain who will be performing the procedure. Patients should be informed that physicians in training will be performing portions of the procedure commensurate with the ability of the resident or fellow and will be under the supervision of the teaching physician. Whether or not the supervising physician will be present during all portions of the procedure should be explained, as this may vary based on the level of competence of the trainee.

While a written signature is required, the real goal of the consent process is effective communication. Inadequate communication was found to be the root cause of the majority of unmet expectations and/or complaints reported to The Joint Commission.[1] Technically, informed consent does not need to be written, but without written documentation, it is difficult to prove the patient's agreement in a court of law. It is generally agreed that a written consent form should be placed into the patient's medical record prior to the procedure. The one exception to this practice would be in an emergent life-threatening condition requiring immediate surgery, in which the principle of implied consent is invoked.

In 2007, the Centers for Medicare and Medicaid Services proposed updated guidelines for participating practitioners obtaining consent.[2] Under these guidelines, consent must be a written document in the patient's medical record and must include additional details, such as the name of the clinician and a reference to the risks, benefits, and alternatives.

CENTERS FOR MEDICARE AND MEDICAID SERVICES GUIDELINES FOR INFORMED CONSENT

- Name of the hospital where the procedure is to take place
- Name of the specific procedure for which consent is being given (now commonly including location)
- Name of the practitioner performing the procedure
- Statement that the procedure, anticipated benefits, risks, and alternatives were explained to the patient or their representative
- Signature of the patient or their representative

CONCLUSIONS

Patient preparation and the informed consent process are critical parts of the surgical procedure. Without adequate preparation, even mild and expected outcomes, such as edema and ecchymoses, can be a cause for significant concern. Working as a team with the patient and appreciating that the patient is indeed the most important person in the room help guide appropriate decision making. A full discussion of benefits and risks improves mutual trust and respect between the physician and patient and ultimately improves patient satisfaction.

REFERENCES

1. The Joint Commission. Informed consent: more than getting a signature. Quick Safety. February 2016. Issue 21. https://www.jointcommission.org/-/media/deprecated-unorganized/imported-assets/tjc/system-folders/joint-commission-online/quick_safety_issue_twenty-one_february_2016pdf.pdf?db=web&hash=5944307ED39088503A008A70D2C768AA. Accessed January 30, 2020.
2. Centers for Medicare and Medicaid Services. CMS memorandum dated April 13, 2007. Revisions to the hospital interpretive guidelines for informed consent. https://www.cms.gov/Medicare/Provider-Enrollment-and-Certification/SurveyCertificationGenInfo/downloads/SCLetter07-17.pdf. Accessed January 30, 2020.

SUGGESTED READINGS

Batuyong E, Birks C, Beischer AD. The use of multimedia as an adjunct to the informed consent process for ankle ligament reconstruction surgery. *Foot Ankle Spec.* 2012;5(3):150-159.

Brandel MG, Reid CM, Parmeshwar N, Dobke MK, Gosman AA. Efficacy of a procedure-specific education module on informed consent in plastic surgery. *Ann Plast Surg.* 2017;78(5 Suppl 4):S225-S228.

Firdouse M, Wajchendler A, Koyle M, Fecteau A. Checklist to improve informed consent process in pediatric surgery: a pilot study. *J Pediatr Surg.* 2017;52(5):859-863.

Fraval A, Chandrananth J, Chong YM, Coventry LS, Tran P. Internet based patient education improves informed consent for elective orthopaedic surgery: a randomized controlled trial. *BMC Musculoskelet Disord.* 2015;16:14.

Hanson M, Pitt D. Informed consent for surgery: risk discussion and documentation. *Can J Surg.* 2017;60(1):69-70.

Kapoor L. Informed consent in aesthetic surgery. *J Cutan Aesthet Surg.* 2015;8(3):173-174.

Koller SE, Moore RF, Goldberg MB, et al. An informed consent program enhances surgery resident education. *J Surg Educ.* 2017;74(5):906-913.

Langerman A. Concurrent surgery and informed consent. *JAMA Surg.* 2016;151(7):601-602.

Newell BL. Informed consent for plastic surgery. Does it cut deeply enough? *J Leg Med.* 2011;32(3):315-335.

Park BY, Kwon J, Kang SR, Hong SE. Informed consent as a litigation strategy in the field of aesthetic surgery: an analysis based on court precedents. *Arch Plast Surg.* 2016;43(5):402-410.

Sarela AI, Thomson M. Balancing law, ethics and reality in informed consent for surgery. *Ann R Coll Surg Engl.* 2014;96(5):329-330.

Siu JM, Rotenberg BW, Franklin JH, Sowerby LJ. Multimedia in the informed consent process for endoscopic sinus surgery: a randomized control trial. *Laryngoscope.* 2016;126(6):1273-1278.

Tipotsch-Maca SM, Varsits RM, Ginzel C, Vecsei-Marlovits PV. Effect of a multimedia-assisted informed consent procedure on the information gain, satisfaction, and anxiety of cataract surgery patients. *J Cataract Refract Surg.* 2016;42(1):110-116.

Wang C, Ammon P, Beischer AD. The use of multimedia as an adjunct to the informed consent process for Morton's neuroma resection surgery. *Foot Ankle Int.* 2014;35(10):1037-1044.

Wollinger C, Hirnschall N, Findl O. Computer-based tutorial to enhance the quality and efficiency of the informed-consent process for cataract surgery. *J Cataract Refract Surg.* 2012;38(4):655-659.

Zhang Y, Ruan X, Tang H, Yang W, Xian Z, Lu M. Video-assisted informed consent for cataract surgery: a randomized controlled trial. *J Ophthalmol.* 2017;2017:9593631.

4 Surgical Instrument Selection

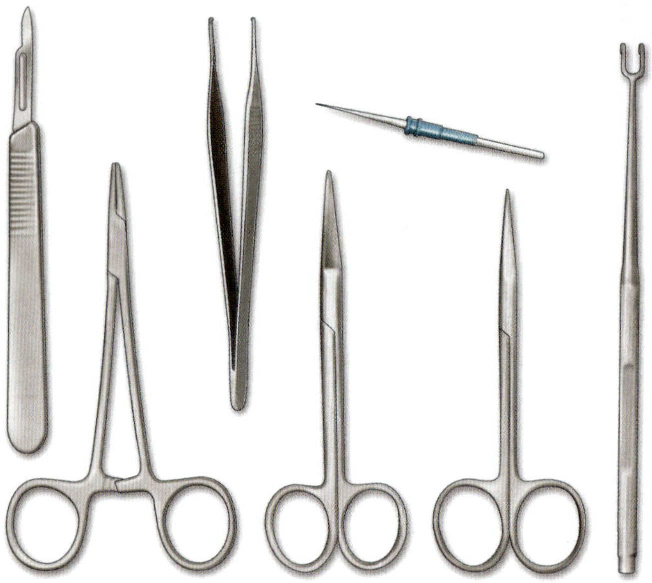

SUMMARY

- Surgical instrument choice may have a direct impact on outcomes, and certainly leads to less traumatic and faster procedures.
- Investing in high-quality instruments is generally a wise decision.
- The highest-quality instruments are the longest lasting, provide the best surgical outcomes, and allow for optimal comfort and speed. Using inadequate instrumentation may lead to need for frequent replacement, poor performance, and tissue damage.
- While the majority of procedures may be completed with a few basic instruments, there is a wide array of available instruments that may be used for specialty procedures.

Beginner Tips

- Consider purchasing instruments at conferences in order to both sample the range of choices and save on costs.
- Surgical packs do not require an exhaustive array of instruments.
- When training staff, including a laminated photograph of the surgical pack above the area where instruments are washed and packaged is a helpful training tool.

Don't Forget!

- Beware the temptation to create overly comprehensive surgical packs. Many accomplished clinicians work with a basic set of high-quality instruments.
- Suture-tying platforms are extremely helpful; it is always preferable to use toothed forceps with platforms rather than nontoothed forceps, as the latter increase the risk of tissue strangulation.

Expert Tips

- Consider color-coding instrument packs for ease of organization and consistency.
- Maintain basic surgical packs and add specialized instrumentation as needed. Instruments used in less than 25% of cases may be kept in separate packs as long as they are easily accessible.
- When using larger-suture needles, such as those on 2-0 suture, be sure to use larger and heavier needle drivers, as fine needle drivers may be loosened by clamping on more robust needles.
- Supercut scissors are denoted by black handles. The upper blades of these scissors are honed with a double, rather than single, bevel, similar to the blade of a high-quality knife or scalpel and the lower jaw is serrated. These scissors optimize tissue cutting in most circumstances, but the sharp blade is easily dulled.
- Some clinicians use a skin hook in place of forceps for skin reflection during suturing to minimize the risk of tissue strangulation.

Pitfalls and Cautions

- Always autoclave instruments in the open position to avoid buckling.
- Avoid using supercut scissors to cut anything but tissue.
- Staff should always be responsible for their own sharps disposal, which should be performed before the used instruments are removed from the room.
- The jaws of a needle driver may be smooth or have fine teeth or ridges. Small teeth may assist in gripping the needle, but may also damage the suture material during handling and tying.
- The most common risk to both clinician and assistant in dermatologic surgery is needle puncture, though the risk of disease transmission is low when using closed-bore sewing needles.

Surgical Instrument Selection

4

INTRODUCTION

Optimal outcomes in dermatologic procedures require selecting the most appropriate surgical instruments. While the majority of procedures may be completed with a few basic instruments, there is a wide array of available instruments that vary broadly in quality and usability.

Modern instruments are made from various metals or alloys, including stainless steel, chromium nickel, and tungsten carbide. In general, the highest-quality instruments are the longest lasting, provide the best surgical outcomes, and allow for optimal comfort and speed. Using inadequate instrumentation may lead to need for frequent replacement, poor performance, and tissue damage. In general, the use of disposable instruments is inadvisable because their quality is so poor as to make them functionally unusable at times.

BIOPSY INSTRUMENTS

Small samples of skin are frequently needed prior to performing comprehensive procedures. While standard instruments such as scalpels may be used, specialty instruments have been developed to simplify biopsy procedures.

Punch biopsy instruments, or punches, are designed with a cylindrical cutting blade attached to a handle (**Figures 4-1 and** 4-2). Although reusable devices were originally used, most have been replaced by disposables. These disposable punches provide both sterility and a razor sharp edge. Useful punches range from 2 to 8 mm in diameter. An elliptically shaped punch has also been developed to facilitate elegant closure. However, many clinicians find this device to be difficult to use, as the punch cannot be rotated to enhance cutting.

A shave biopsy may be performed with any sharp-edged cutting instrument. A double-edged razor blade, snapped in half, provides an extremely sharp and inexpensive tool for shave biopsy. By altering the curvature of the blade between their fingers, the clinician may adjust the depth of the biopsy. Scalpel blades are also readily available and may be stabilized by wrapping the base of the blade in its foil packaging. The Dermablade is a commercially available blade with plastic support handles. This may provide improved grip and safety to the clinician as compared to working with a snapped double-edge blade, though it is significantly more expensive and most experienced practitioners are expert at handling snapped double blades.

CURETTES

The curette is a surgical instrument designed for scraping (**Figures 4-3 and** 4-4). The handle may be of various weights, lengths, and textures. The head, usually crafted from the same piece of metal as the handle, may be round, oval, or cup or ring shaped; ranges from 1 to 10 mm wide; and is sharp on one side. Curettes are most commonly used to remove or destroy benign or malignant lesions. They may also be used to debulk and delineate tumor margins prior to excision. As with other surgical instruments, the most appropriately sized instrument for the procedure should be selected to facilitate destruction while avoiding surrounding tissue damage.

Curettes are available in both disposable and reusable designs. Disposable curettes have a sharper tip and function similarly to a curved scalpel blade. Most clinicians favor the reusable instruments, as their blunter edge provides improved sensory feedback, allowing the clinician to better differentiate between various tissue types.

SCALPELS

Scalpels may be used for cutting, puncturing, dissecting, manipulating specimens, and scraping. They generally consist of a handle and a blade. Both the handle and blade are available in numerous sizes and materials. Selection is based on both clinician preference and the surgical application.

Scalpel blades are disposable, individually wrapped, and presterilized. They may be made of carbon steel or stainless steel. Carbon steel blades are sharper, though they dull more rapidly. Stainless steel blades are not as sharp but last longer. Blades may be coated in silicon or polytetrafluoroethylene to minimize tissue drag and increase longevity. These may be particularly useful in longer procedures or multistaged Mohs surgical procedures.

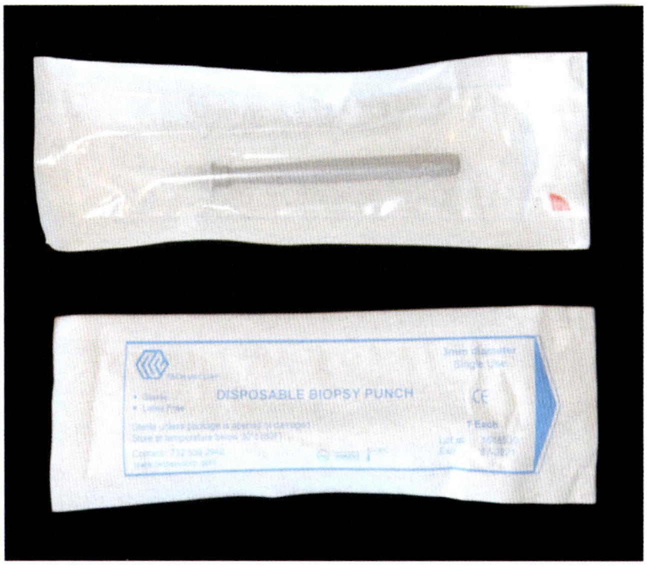

FIGURE 4-1 Punch biopsy instruments are available in an array of sizes and configurations.

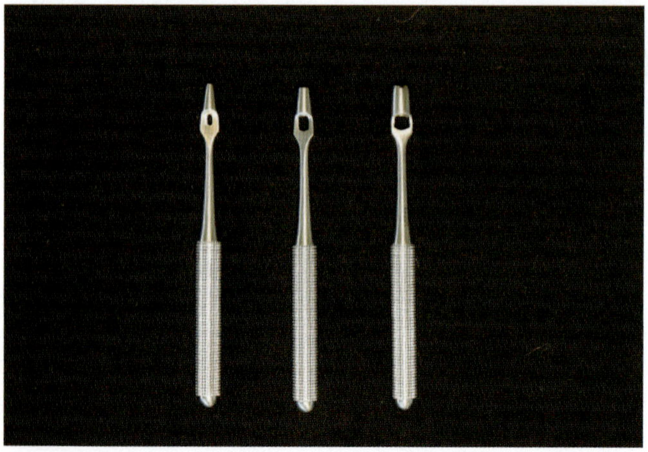

FIGURE 4-2 Some punch devices are autoclavable.

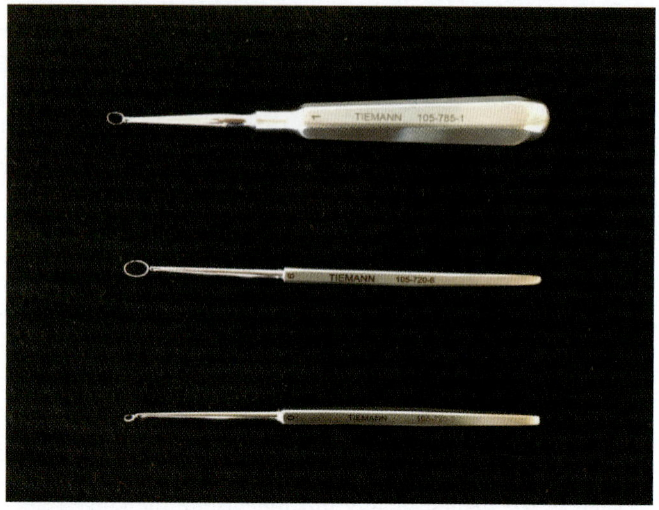

FIGURE 4-4 Larger curettes may be used for thicker tumors.

The most common surgical blades in dermatologic surgery are the 15, 15c, 10, and 11 blades (**Figure 4-5**). These blades are designed to fit a variety of available handles. The 15 blade's small size and gentle curvature make it optimal for the majority of skin procedures. The sharp tip is used to initiate cuts, while the broader belly provides a longer surface for enhanced contact. With the handle held at 30 degrees to the skin, longer smooth cuts may be made. The 15c blade is a smaller variant, used to treat very delicate skin; its sharper carbon blade also dulls faster. The 10 blade also shares a similar shape but is significantly larger, making it optimal for thicker skinned areas such as the back. The 11 blade is triangular with a straight edge that tapers to a sharp point. It is usually used in a stabbing motion for incision and drainage.

Each of the above blades may be fitted interchangeably on a variety of handles (**Figure 4-5**). The flat number 3 handle is the most frequently encountered. It is well suited to the majority of procedures and is available with an imprinted metric ruler.

An alternative handle and blade combination is the miniblade or Beaver system. In this system, smaller blades are inserted into a collet, which is tightened with rotation. Blades are available in a variety of shapes and curvatures. This system may be used in smaller, narrow spaces such as the ear canal or medial canthus.

On a practical level, the primary care clinician can rely on the use of a flat number 3 handle coupled with a 15 blade for almost every closure encountered on a daily basis.

SCISSORS

Surgical scissors come in a great variety of shapes and sizes, each designed for a specific task. Although the choices are dizzyingly extensive, selection of a few optimal pairs of scissors may enhance comfort and surgical outcomes.

The basic anatomy of scissors consists of three parts: the handle, the blade, and the tip. The handle may be long or short. Short-handle scissors are most commonly used by clinicians, as they provide enhanced control when working with delicate tissue. Longer handles provide increased leverage and cutting strength

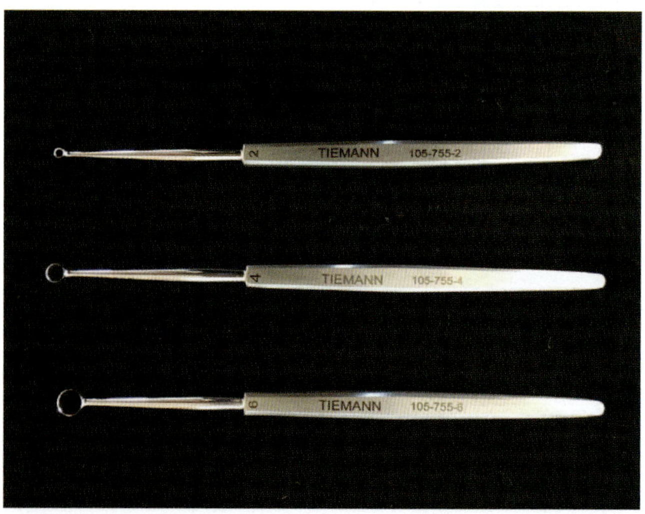

FIGURE 4-3 Curettes are available in various weights, lengths, and textures.

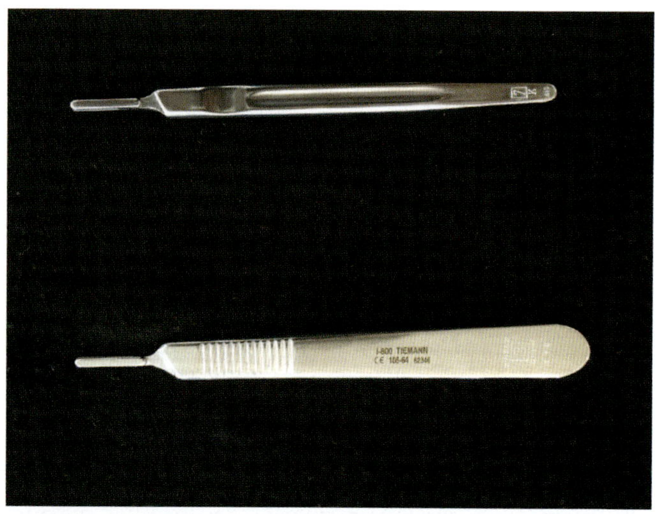

FIGURE 4-5 Surgical blades may be fitted interchangeably on a variety of handles.

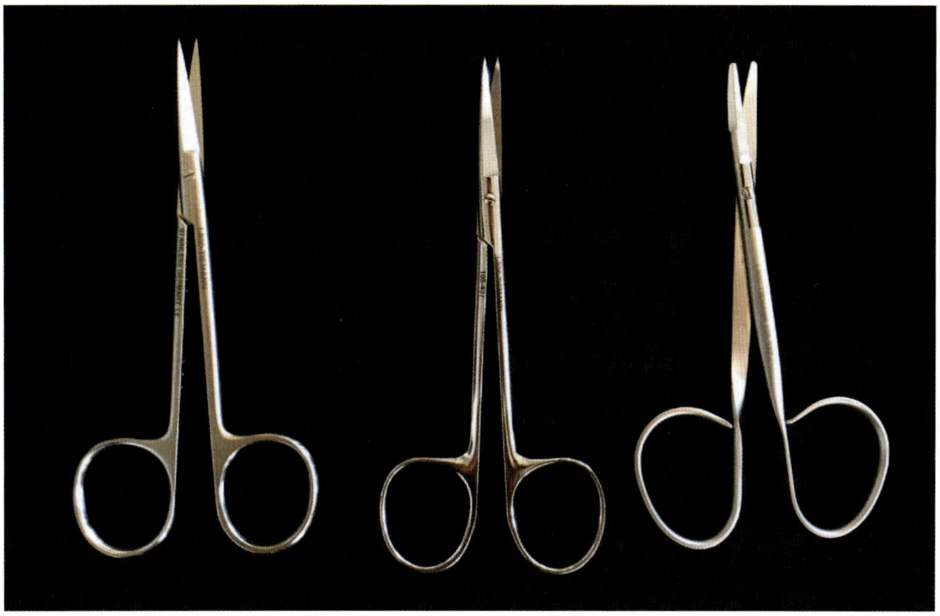

FIGURE 4-6 Numerous scissors are available for use in dermatologic surgery.

and may be necessary when working in cavities, such as when creating a flap for a facelift, or during extensive undermining. Handles are most often straight, although curved or bent handles are available. These alternative shapes may improve visibility or approach for difficult-to-reach areas.

Scissor blades are available in varying shapes and quality. In the most basic design, the blade is formed from the same piece of stainless steel as the handle. Such scissors are inexpensive and well suited for basic procedures, for cutting sutures, and for forming bandages.

The lower blade of a scissor may be serrated to increase stability and reduce slippage. These fine teeth are difficult to visualize but may be easily felt by running the finger gently along the blade. The serrated blade is particularly useful when working with thin skin and for trimming the edges of delicate flaps and grafts. Scissors may be purchased serrated, or this feature may be added after manufacture.

Higher quality scissors may be enhanced with tungsten carbide inserts. This material reinforces the blade, improving cutting and providing a longer life without dulling. Tungsten carbide is brittle and may be damaged if instruments are dropped or mishandled, although the insert may be replaced when dulled or damaged. Surgical instruments with tungsten carbide inserts are identified by their gold handles.

Supercut scissors are denoted by black handles. The upper blades of these scissors are honed with a double, rather than single, bevel, similar to the blade of a high-quality knife or scalpel. The lower jaw is serrated. These scissors optimize cutting in most circumstances. The sharp blade, however, is easily dulled. Supercut scissor should be reserved for tissue and should never be used to cut suture.

Scissor tips may be pointed, blunt, or hooked. Pointed tips are useful for precise trimming and shaping and for aggressive dissection in areas of difficult scissor insertion. Blunt tips are safer for undermining around delicate structures and for freeing flaps and grafts. The single hooked tip may be used to assist with suture removal.

By altering handle, blade, and tip shapes and sizes, many hundreds of scissor designs have been introduced. While a detailed description of each is beyond the scope of this chapter, several common types compose the majority of our armamentarium.

Iris scissors are the most commonly used scissor in dermatologic surgery (**Figure 4-6**). Originally developed for the eyelid, these have wide application for facial and other cutaneous surgery. These usually measure approximately 4 inches, may have straight or curved blades, and may have sharp or blunt tips. Their relatively long handle-to-blade ratio provides excellent accuracy while retaining mechanical advantage. The blepharoplasty scissor is a specialized iris scissor with a gentle curve, blunt tips, tungsten carbide inserts, one serrated blade, and one flattened blade. In addition to its original intention, this scissor may be particularly useful for dissecting cysts and for debeveling and undermining wounds prior to closure.

Gradle and tenotomy scissors have a high handle-to-blade ratio and a small, delicate, sharp tip that is tapered to a fine point with a gentle curve (**Figure 4-7**).

Operating scissors are larger, heavier instruments more commonly used in general surgery. While these have limited use in dermatologic surgery, some may be helpful in larger cases. Mayo scissors are heavy, with a nearly one-to-one handle-to-blade ratio. These may be used for coarse dissection. Metzenbaum scissors are heavier, with a high handle-to-blade ratio for increased leverage and reach.

At the more delicate end of the spectrum are Westcott and Castroviejo scissors (**Figure 4-8**). These spring-loaded instruments are held like a pencil and squeezed closed to cut. The blade reopens when released. They generally have fine, pointed tips and are particularly useful when working with thin periorbital skin.

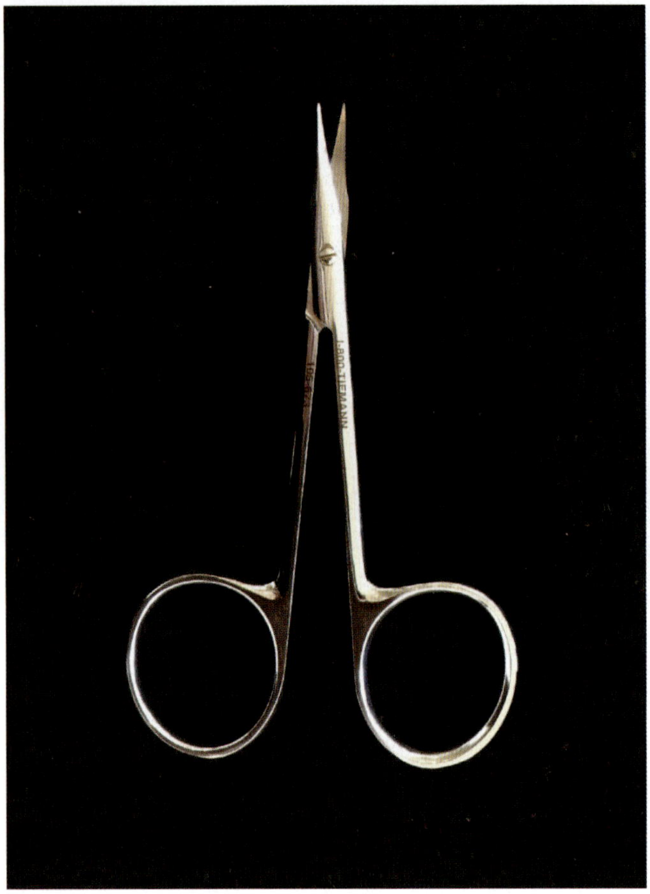

FIGURE 4-7 Gradle scissors have a high handle-to-blade ratio and a small, delicate, sharp tip that is tapered to a fine point with a gentle curve.

The scissors discussed above are intended for tissue and may be damaged when working with other materials. A surgical tray should also contain scissors for cutting suture. Suture-cutting scissors may include a basic stainless steel iris scissor or a standard operating scissor, which is composed of heavier blades with one blunt and one sharp tip. Bandage-cutting scissors tend to be large and have blunt tips to protect the patient's skin during removal of the bandage (**Figure 4-9**). One blade is generally flattened to slide under the dressing without damaging the underlying integument. For suture removal, the Northbent scissor is curved with a hooked blade, the Spencer scissor is straight with a hooked blade, and the O'Brien scissor has a short, angled blade that allows the fine tip to be introduced below suture loops (**Figure 4-10**).

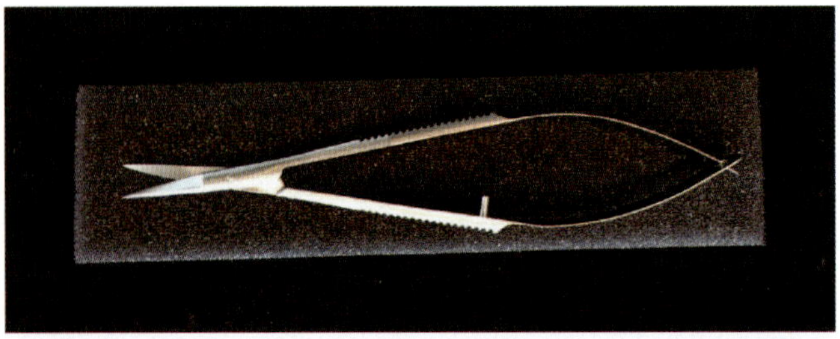

FIGURE 4-8 Castroviejo scissors are spring-loaded and held like a pencil.

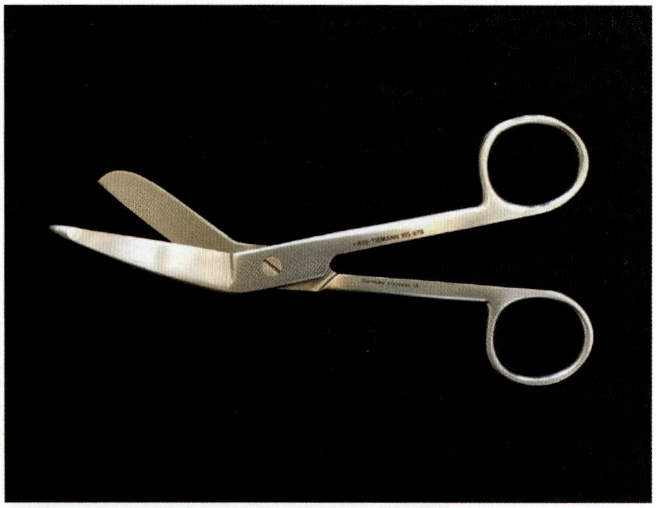

FIGURE 4-9 Bandage-cutting scissors tend to be large and have blunt tips to protect the patient's skin during removal of the bandage.

FORCEPS

Forceps are used to hold or grasp items such as tissue, sutures, or other materials within the surgical field. They are generally held between the thumb and index finger like a pencil. They are pressed to close and are designed to reopen when released. As with other surgical instruments, forceps are available in a variety of sizes and weights. While a matter of personal preference, the most delicate instrument useable for the procedure should usually be selected to avoid tissue damage.

Forceps handles are usually stainless steel. They are available in a variety of weights and lengths. Grips may be ridged or gnarled for improved grip when wet. Handles may also be drilled or fenestrated for weight reduction.

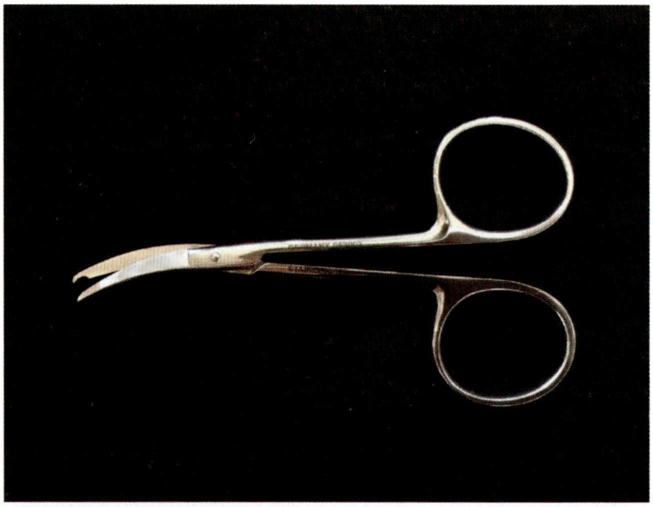

FIGURE 4-10 For suture removal, the Northbent scissor is curved with a hooked blade.

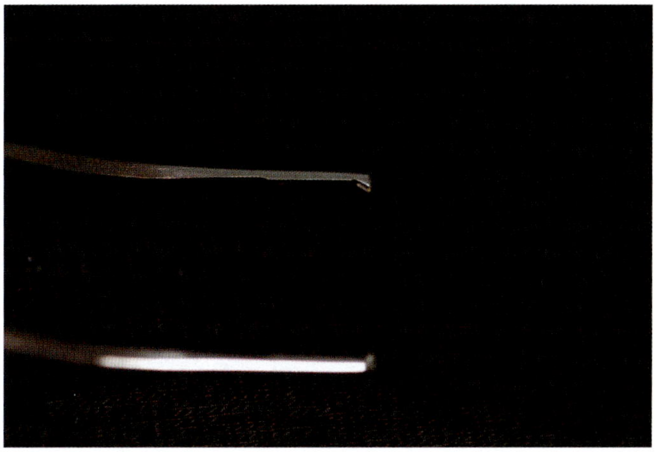

FIGURE 4-11 Some forceps are available with a suturing or tying platform.

Surgical forceps are available with or without teeth. Those without teeth are referred to as dressing or bandage forceps and are, for the most part, not intended to handle the skin. Tissue forceps, on the other hand, have delicate teeth at the tips. When used gently, these tips allow the skin to be manipulated without crushing or leaving marks on the skin. Teeth are available in various weights and sizes to correctly suit the tissue. The most commonly used tooth pattern is 1 × 2, meaning one tooth on one tip that fits between two teeth on the other tip. However, multiple tooth patterns such as 2 × 3 through 8 × 9 are available.

Some forceps are available with a suturing or tying platform (**Figure 4-11**). This is a slightly raised, flattened area placed directly behind the teeth. This platform allows the needle to be gripped securely without twisting or turning. The needle can therefore be passed directly from the needle driver to the forceps without touching the needle with the fingers. This may greatly reduce the risk of needle stick to the clinician. For optimal grip and ease of maintenance, this platform may be constructed of gnarled tungsten carbide. Such forceps are denoted, like all tungsten carbide instruments, with gold handles.

The most common forceps design used in dermatology is the Adson (**Figure 4-12**). These have a broad handle that tapers to a narrow tip. This tip may be serrated, smooth, or toothed; Adson forceps are available with or without tying platforms. Long, heavy handles or lightweight, fenestrated handles are available. By varying these characteristics, Adson forceps suited for nearly all dermatologic surgery procedures have been produced. A common variation is the Brown-Adson forceps, in which a platform of minute teeth is placed at the tip.

For more delicate procedures, small forceps with a longer tip-to-handle ratio are available. Iris forceps are simple and inexpensive and slowly taper from handle to tip. Bishop-Harmon forceps are short, with fenestrated handles and well-defined, long, delicate tips. These are available with or without teeth. Jewelers forceps are similarly delicate, with tapered sharply pointed tips.

Non–tissue handling forceps are also commonly used in dermatologic surgery. Those with smooth tips may be useful for gripping sutures or foreign bodies. The Swiss cilia forceps is short, with a smooth, angled, pointed tip (**Figure 4-13**). This is particularly useful in suture removal. Forceps with serrated tips increase gripping strength and may be used to manipulate gauze within a surgical field. While they may also be used to grasp cysts or lipomas, their use on vital tissue may lead to tissue damage or necrosis.

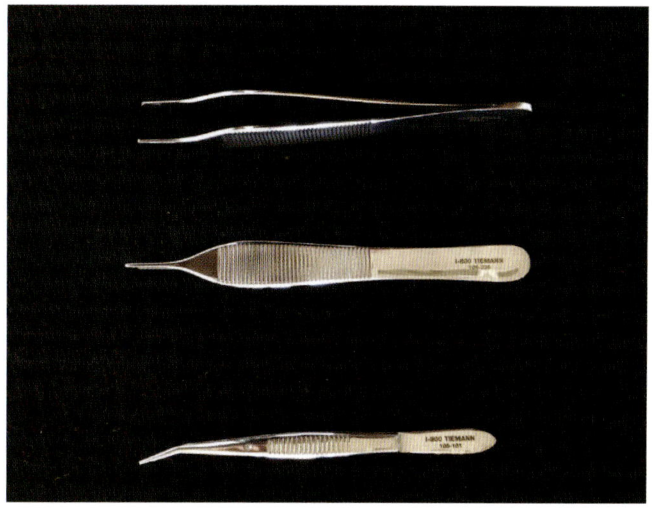

FIGURE 4-12 The most common forceps design used in dermatology is the Adson.

NEEDLE DRIVERS

Needle drivers, or holders, are clamped instruments intended to hold a surgical needle securely when suturing. When closed, a ratchet activates to grip the needle without effort. To release the clamp, the handles are separated laterally. Designed similarly to scissors, these are available in varied weights, handle lengths, tip shapes, and tip materials. While designs vary, the smallest instrument that can be comfortably used to execute the task is recommended. Further, smaller needle drivers are optimized to hold

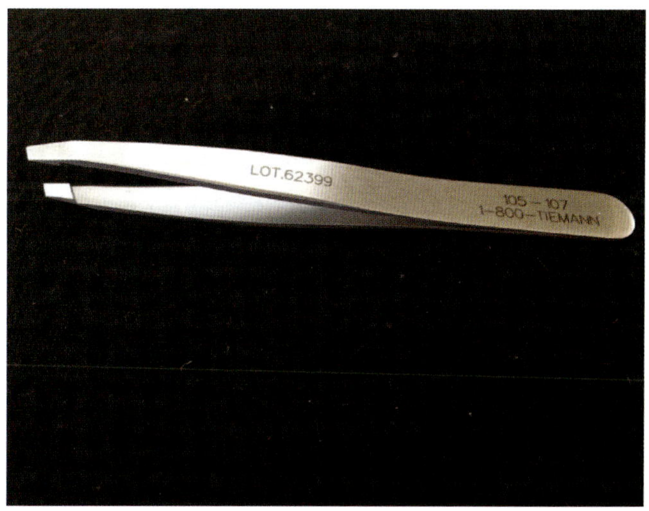

FIGURE 4-13 The Swiss cilia forceps is short, with a smooth, angled, pointed tip.

smaller needles and may be damaged by larger needles, whereas larger drivers are intended to hold larger needles and may bend smaller ones.

The jaws of a needle driver may be smooth or have fine teeth or ridges. Small teeth may assist in gripping the needle but may also damage the suture material during handling and tying. Horizontal ridges may be found in other needle driver jaws. These are intended to keep the surgical needle from twisting. However, fine sutures may pass through these ridges when gripping the suture to perform an instrument tie. Rough-surfaced tungsten carbide inserts are available to improve instrument durability and increase needle grip. These are also replaceable. As usual, these instruments are denoted by gold handles and are more expensive than other options.

The eponymous Webster, Halsey, Baumgartner, Crile-Wood, and Mayo drivers are most commonly used in dermatologic surgery (**Figure 4-14**). These are similarly shaped, with long handles and short tips. They are available in various weights and lengths to optimize needle handling and physician comfort. Most are available with each of the previously discussed tip types.

For more delicate procedures, particularly on eyelids, Castroviejo needle holders may be used. Similar to the Castroviejo scissor, these are delicate spring-loaded instruments. Unlike most needle drivers, these are available in both locking and nonlocking variants.

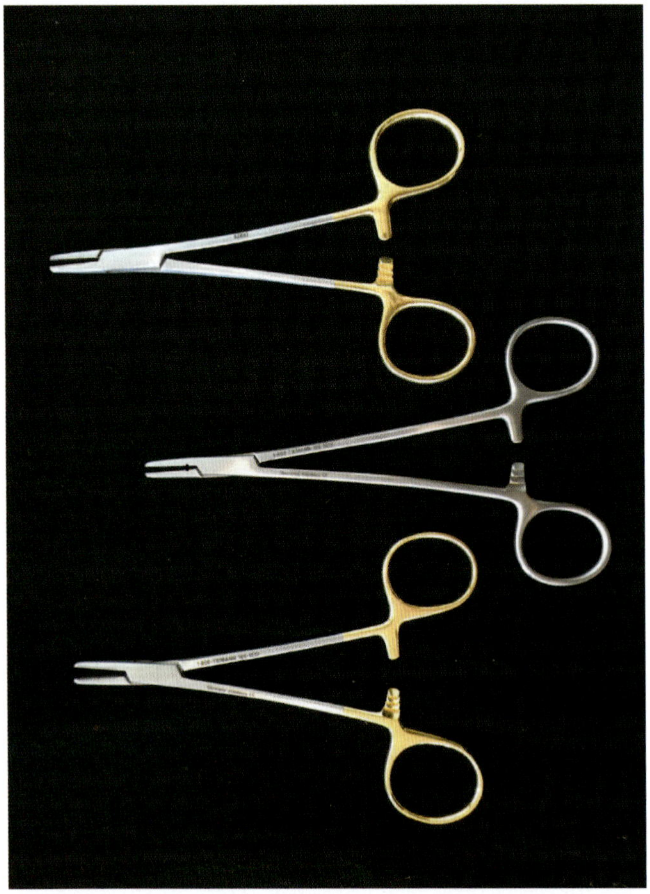

FIGURE 4-14 A variety of needle drivers are available for dermatologic surgery.

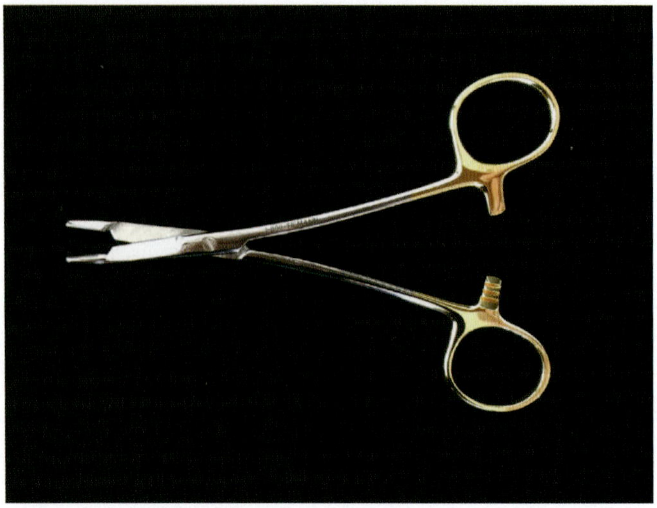

FIGURE 4-15 The Olsen-Hegar needle holder contains a scissor just proximal to the needle holding jaws.

The Olsen-Hegar needle holder contains a scissor just proximal to the needle-holding jaws (**Figure 4-15**). These are often favored by clinicians working without assistance. It may be used to suture and cut suture without changing instruments. However, care must be taken to avoid cutting the suture material accidentally while working.

HEMOSTATS

Hemostats are grasping devices, similar to forceps, but with a ratcheted locking mechanism like a needle driver (**Figure 4-16**). These are used to temporarily clamp bleeding vessels during surgery; vessels can later be sealed with electrosurgery or ligated with sutures before the hemostat is removed. Like needle drivers and forceps, hemostats may vary in length, tip size, curvature, and degree of serration. Common variants include the Jacobsen, Halsted, and Hartman. Small, lightweight hemostats,

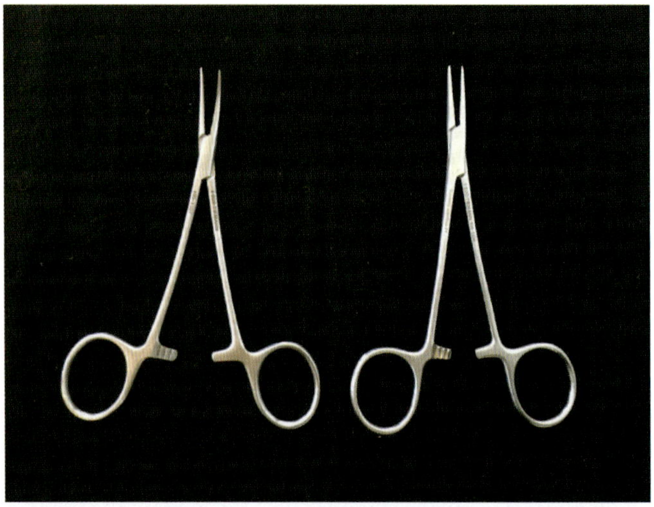

FIGURE 4-16 Hemostats are grasping devices, similar to forceps, but with a ratcheted locking mechanism like a needle driver.

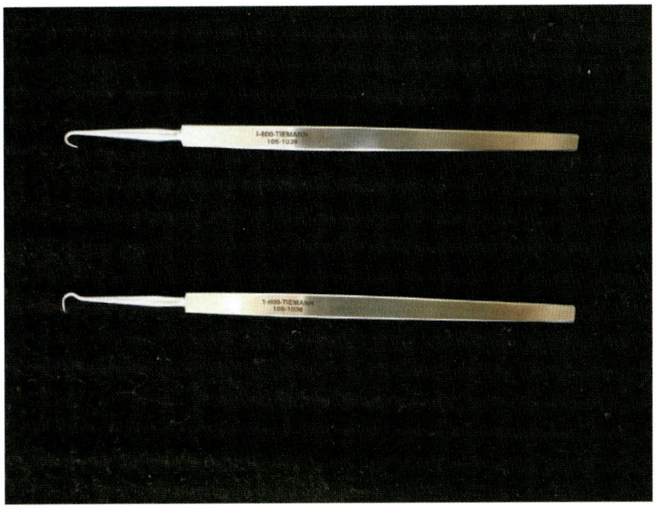

FIGURE 4-17 Skin hooks used in dermatologic surgery are long, tapered instruments with a small, sharp hook at the end.

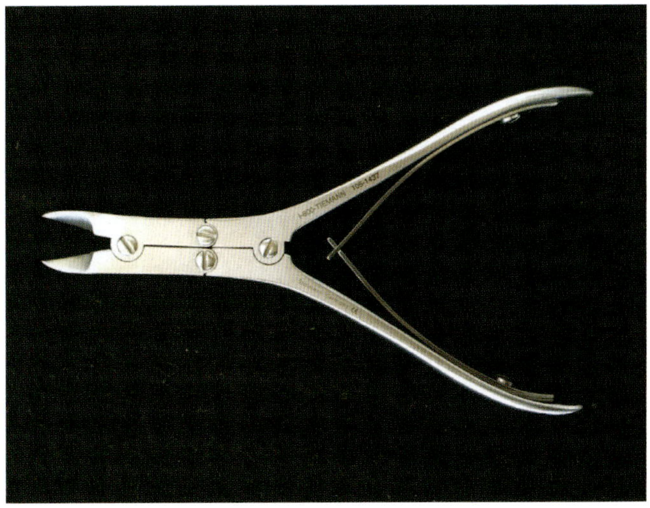

FIGURE 4-18 Double-action nail cutters are also useful in nail procedures and can be used in place of rongeurs when working with superficial bone.

colloquially referred to as "mosquitos," are most often used in dermatologic surgery.

SKIN HOOKS

The skin hooks used in dermatologic surgery are long, tapered instruments with a small, sharp hook at the end (**Figure 4-17**). These are used to delicately manipulate tissue to improve field visualization, assess flap movement, or reflect skin edges during undermining or electrosurgery. Some clinicians use a skin hook in place of forceps for skin reflection during suturing. The chief disadvantage of the skin hook is the sharp tip and resultant risk of puncture injury to the clinician or assistant.

Skin hooks are available in single-, double-, or multi-pronged patterns, with the latter being described as rakes. Larger, wider instruments may be useful when manipulating heavy truncal skin, whereas delicate single-tipped hooks are most useful on the face.

MISCELLANEOUS INSTRUMENTS

The chalazion clamp consists of a flat arm opposed by a ring. As these are clamped down on a mobile, vascular surface such as the lip, eyelid, or earlobe, the ringed arm provides stabilization and hemostasis, while the flat arm provides a backing surface against which the tissue can be cut. The clamp tension is adjusted by a thumbscrew, which can be gradually tightened or released. It is important to release the clamp as soon as possible to avoid tourniquet necrosis. Chalazion clamps are available in a variety of shapes and sizes. Rubber-coated clamps are recommended if electrosurgical instruments are to be used. Double-action nail cutters are also useful in nail procedures and can be used in place of rongeurs when working with superficial bone (**Figure 4-18**).

Periosteal elevators are elongated flat instruments designed to lift the periosteum from the bone (**Figure 4-19**). In dermatologic surgery, they are also frequently used to lift the nail plate off of the nail bed. Bone chisels have a sharpened, flattened head and a broad handle. These may be struck with a small hammer to biopsy bone, usually if invasive neoplasm is suspected during Mohs surgery.

Towel clamps allow sterile drapes to be firmly anchored in place (**Figure 4-20**). They may also be used to keep electrosurgery handles within the operating field. Some clinicians additionally use the towel clip to hold large wounds together prior to suturing or to grip a cyst or lipoma during extirpation.

Corneal shields are available in multiple sizes and may be placed over the eye to protect the cornea during periorbital procedures (**Figure 4-21**). These are available both in plastic, which is both inexpensive and optimal for use during electrosurgery, and in stainless steel. Corneal shield placement requires anesthetic eye drops, careful sizing, and correct technique to avoid corneal irritation or abrasion.

SHARPS SAFETY

The most common risk to both clinician and assistant in dermatologic surgery is needle puncture. Thankfully, the risk of disease transmission is low when using closed-bore sewing needles. Undoubtedly, the most critical protective measure is mandatory glove use when dealing with sharps of any kind.

Loose suture needles on the surgical tray are a common source of needle injury to both the clinician and assistant. Several systems have been developed to minimize risk. Most commonly, all sharps are kept maintained in one area of the tray. In larger cases, however, multiple needles may be used. These may be kept organized with dedicated suture needle boxes, with a disposable foam

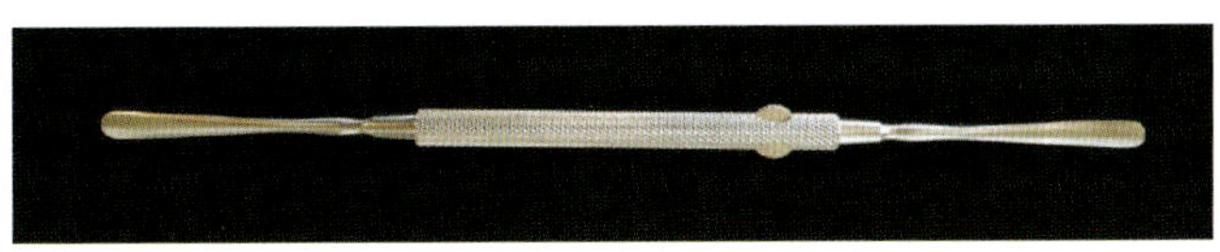

FIGURE 4-19 Periosteal elevators are elongated flat instruments designed to lift the periosteum from the bone.

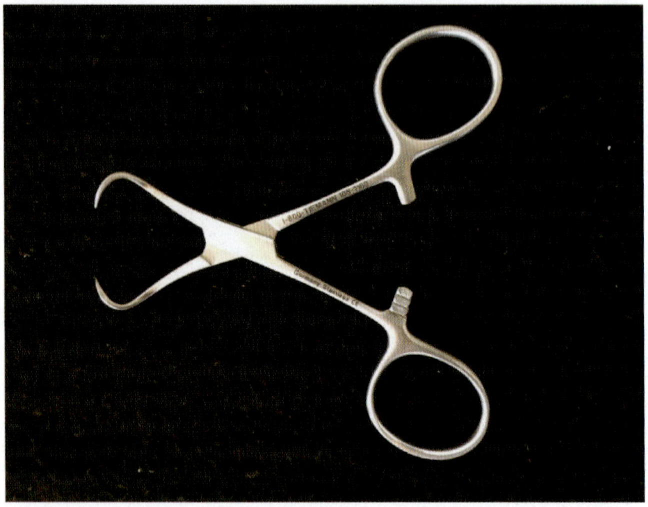

FIGURE 4-20 Towel clamps allow sterile drapes to be firmly anchored in place.

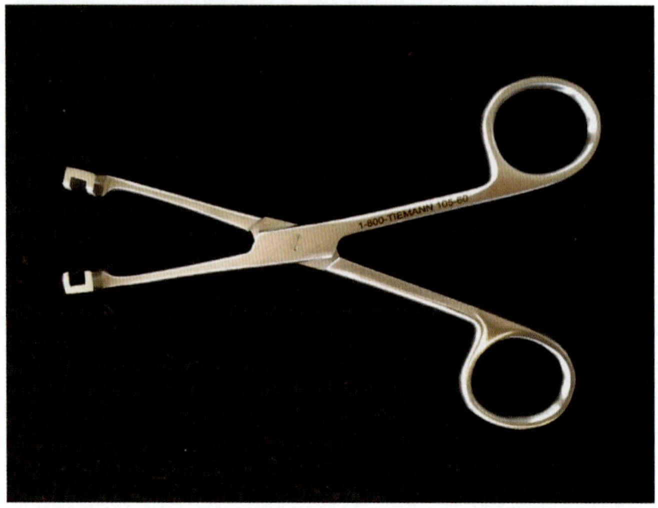

FIGURE 4-22 To avoid scalpel injury at the conclusion of a procedure, a surgical blade remover may be used to separate disposable scalpel blades from the handle.

block or pincushion placed on the field, or by placing a magnet under the surgical tray to attract and organize sharps.

To avoid scalpel injury at the conclusion of a procedure, a surgical blade remover is required to separate disposable scalpel blades from the handle. The most common devices require two hands: one to hold the scalpel, and the other to operate the clamp and remove the blade (**Figure 4-22**). With practice, these are safe, reliable, and cost effective. Counter- or wall-mounted devices have also been created to allow for one-handed operation. With these devices, the scalpel is inserted, blade first, into the machine, and the blade is safely removed. While efficient, these require frequent replacement.

INSTRUMENT MAINTENANCE AND STERILIZATION

Careful instrument maintenance and sterilization are critical to ensure functional equipment and provide patient safety. After surgery, instruments should be cleaned. First, all debris must be removed from the instruments. Organic debris may allow for growth of microorganisms and may interfere with sterilization. This is most commonly performed by soaking followed by hand scrubbing. Ultrasonic cleaning may also be used. Next, instruments should be dried and treated with lubricant such as instrument milk. Instruments are then packed in a self-sealing pouch, metal box, or plastic tray. Instruments should be loosely packed, with needle drivers and scissors in the open position. Surfaces in close contact may not be fully treated during the sterilization process. The pack should then be sterilized by steam autoclave. Although other systems, such as gas, dry heat, and chemical sterilization, are theoretically possible, these are generally less reliable and not frequently used. The autoclave should be routinely tested to ensure adequate sterilization.

With appropriate maintenance, many surgical instruments may last for the career of the clinician. Scissors may be sharpened by the manufacturer or by companies that will provide on-site service. Tungsten carbide inserts in needle drivers, scissors, and forceps may be replaced. Stiff instruments can be lubricated or cleared of mineral deposits with a solution of vinegar and water.

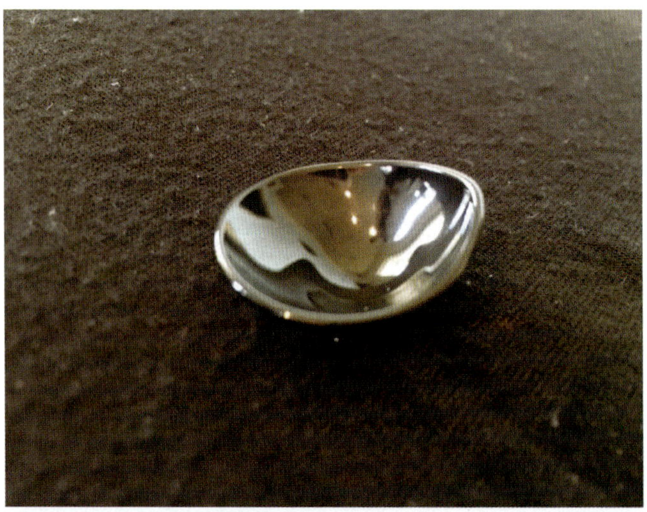

FIGURE 4-21 Corneal shields are available in multiple sizes and may be placed over the eye to protect the cornea during periorbital procedures.

INSTRUMENT PACKS FOR SURGERY

Instruments may be packed and sterilized individually, so that the appropriate instruments may be selected for each surgical case. However, most clinicians find it more convenient to pack multiple instruments together. The most basic surgical kit can be prepared with a scalpel handle, needle driver, scissor, and forceps. Other instruments can be added as needed.

Clinicians vary in their approach to surgical pack preparation. At one end of the spectrum, a clinician may favor a single pack style for all surgical cases, whereas other clinicians use two types of packs (face and body) and still others use three types of packs (face, body, and extremity). Typical surgical kits contain a scalpel handle, needle driver, tissue forceps with tying platform, a tissue-cutting scissor (either blepharoplasty, supercut iris, or both), a skin hook, a hemostat, a suture-cutting scissor, and surgical gauze.

Additional specialty instruments are individually packed and available in the operating room.

CONCLUSIONS

The selection of proper surgical instruments is critical to providing high-quality, safe, and effective care in dermatologic procedures. Individual instrument selection may be based on the scope of procedures to be performed, the expertise and preferences of the individual, and financial limitations. Purchasing the highest-quality instruments and correctly maintaining them should provide long-lasting and efficient instruments.

In choosing instruments, there is no substitute for practical experience because instrument shapes, sizes, and balances vary widely. The clinician should handle and examine a range of choices at conferences or with dealer's representatives. Individual instruments can be purchased and tried before an office is fully equipped. Through experimentation and experience, comfortable and efficient instruments should be found.

A BASIC INSTRUMENT SETUP FOR DERMATOLOGIC SURGERY PROCEDURES

- Blade handle
- Needle driver
- Suture scissors
- Tissue scissors (supercut iris scissors used frequently)
- Forceps (Adson with teeth and platforms used frequently)
- Hooks (optional)
- Hemostat (optional)

SUGGESTED READING

Bernstein G. Choosing the correct surgical instruments. *Adv Dermatol.* 1995;10:245-283.

Bhatia AC, Taneja A. Surgical instruments. In: Vidimos AT, Ammirati CT, Poblete-Lopez C, eds. *Dermatologic Surgery*. Philadelphia, PA: Saunders-Elsevier; 2009:59-71.

Grande DJ, Neuburg M. Instrumentation in dermatologic surgery. *J Dermatol Surg Oncol.* 1989;15:288-297.

Melissa BA, Joseph AK. Instruments and materials. In: Robinson JK, Hanke WC, Sengelman R, Siegle D, eds. *Surgery of the Skin*. London, United Kingdom: Elsevier-Mosby; 2005:59-66.

Neuberg M. Instrumentation in dermatologic surgery. *Semin Dermatol.* 1994;13:10-19.

Olhoffer IH, Goldman G, Leffell DJ. Wound closure materials and instruments. In: Bolognia JL, Jorizzo JL, Rapini RP, eds. *Dermatology*. London, United Kingdom: Mosby; 2003:2248-2252.

Raza SL, Sengelman RD. Instrumentation and sutures. In: Snow SN, Mikhail GR, eds. *Mohs Micrographic Surgery.* Madison, WI: University of Wisconsin; 2004:33-42.

Sebben JS. Sterile technique and the prevention of wound infection in office surgery—part I. *J Dermatol Surg Oncol.* 1988;14:1364-1371.

Watt AM, Patkin M, Sinnott MJ, Black RJ, Maddern GJ. Scalpel safety in the operative setting: a systematic review. *Surgery.* 2010;147:98-106.

Weber LA. The surgical tray. *Dermatol Clin.* 1998;16:17-24.

5 Suture Materials and Needles

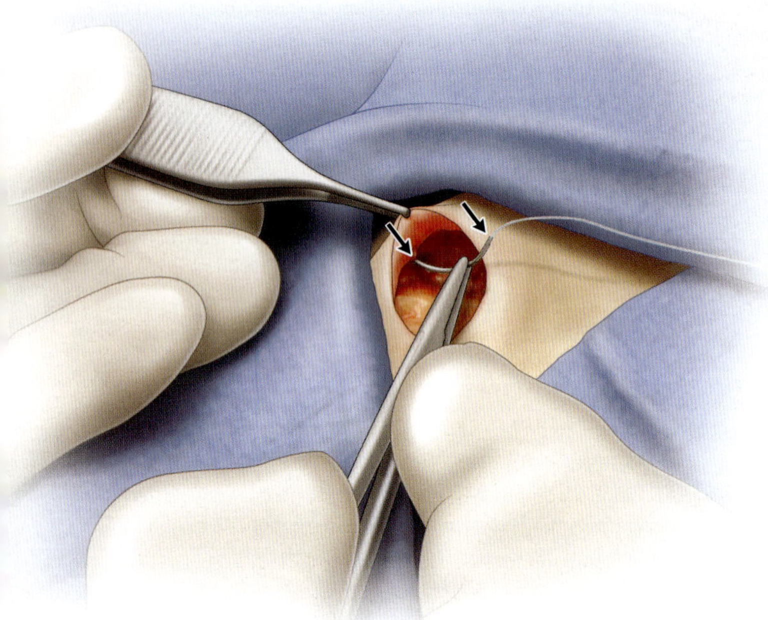

SUMMARY

- Over the past several decades, suture materials have improved dramatically.
- The needle may be as or more important than the suture material itself in promoting an ideal surgical outcome.
- Keep in mind that the greatest differentiator between suture brands is needle quality rather than the suture material itself.
- Knot tying should be performed with an eye to creating a secure knot without adding undue bulk to buried sutures.

Beginner Tips

- Most needles used for skin and soft tissue reconstruction are 3/8 circle in diameter and reverse cutting.

Expert Tips

- A semicircular P-2 needle may be used for narrow closures, such as those sometimes encountered on the nose, and a cutting needle, with the sharp edge on the inside of the curve, may be useful for nasal reconstruction where the thin atrophic dermis may be cut by the superficially running outside edge of a reverse cutting needle.
- Since cutting and reverse cutting needles have a triangular tip, the orientation of the cutting end is indicated by whether the triangle on the box is pointing up (cutting) or down (reverse cutting).
- In order to minimize the risk of needle-stick injury, it is possible to grasp the suture material approximately 6 to 10 cm from the needle swage between the thumb and index finger of the left hand, allowing the needle to drop down below the hand. Since the needle is hanging freely and is not under tension, there is little chance for a needle-stick injury.
- Attention to technique, coupled with choice of a sufficiently large needle for the closure in question, may go a long way to optimizing surgical outcomes.

Don't Forget!

- Any suture, including absorbable sutures, may be used for transepidermal suture placement, which may permit the use of a single suture pack for both buried and epidermal sutures.

Pitfalls and Cautions

- A single click of the needle driver locking mechanism is sufficient for locking the needle, and cranking down on the needle driver excessively will result in a loosening of the locking mechanism, leading to inadvertent suture needle slippage in the future.
- The most frequent error encountered by novice clinicians is using a needle that is too small for a given anatomic location, or using a technique that does not permit the needle to pass naturally and smoothly through tissue.
- When tying a deep suture, it is generally desirable to pull the suture strands together as tightly as possible, secured with a stable knot. For transepidermal sutures, since the goal of suture placement is woundedge apposition, placing the minimal necessary tension across of the surface of the wound is a must; over-tightening these sutures will lead directly to strangulation, necrosis, and—at a minimum—track mark formation.

Suture Materials and Needles

5

INTRODUCTION

Over the past several decades, suture materials have improved dramatically. Three thousand years ago, suture materials were composed of easily processed plant or animal materials affixed to bone or metal. In the middle ages, suture material made from sheep's intestine was introduced, and sterile catgut suture was first used in 1906. In the mid to late 20th century, advances in chemistry and manufacturing led to the production of the first synthetic sutures, and the availability of swaged needles over the past few decades has improved safety for both patient and clinician while improving operative efficiency.

NEEDLES

A wide variety of suture materials are available, all with variable handling characteristics, tissue reactivity, absorption characteristics, and costs. While much attention is paid to suture material, the needle may be as or more important than the suture material itself in promoting an ideal surgical outcome. Needles vary by manufacturer and even by suture material, and using the most appropriate needle for the task is critical. Even the most accomplished clinicians will perform in a less-than-ideal fashion if their instruments or needle choices are flawed.

Most needles used for skin and soft-tissue reconstruction are 3/8 circle in diameter, and most needles used for skin and soft-tissue reconstructions are reverse cutting in nature (**Figure 5-1**). There are, however, important exceptions to this rule. For example, a semicircular P-2 needle may be used for narrow closures, such as those sometimes encountered on the nose, and a cutting needle, with the sharp edge on the inside of the curve, may be useful for nasal reconstruction where the thin atrophic dermis may be cut by the superficially running outside edge of a reverse cutting needle.

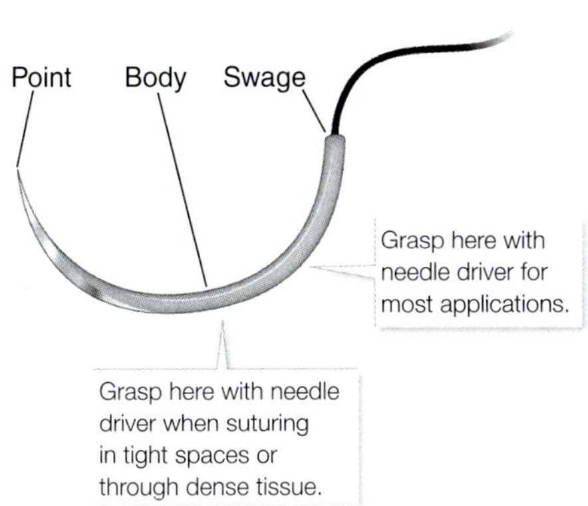

FIGURE 5-1 The suture needle.

The two largest manufacturers of suture material used in cutaneous surgery are Ethicon and Covidien, although many other companies produce high-quality products as well. While suture size is governed by US Pharmacopeia (USP) guidelines (the larger the number of zeros, the smaller the suture), needle size and configuration are largely proprietary. Thus, the clinician must be comfortable understanding the various needle sizes and configurations of the various manufacturers. Suture material packaging does include a cross-sectional image of the needle, permitting some comparison between companies. Of note, Covidien does not (except on its website) refer to any of its needles as reverse cutting; instead, they label cutting needles as conventional cutting and reverse cutting needles as cutting. These distinctions are important when choosing suture, and many suture type and needle combinations are only available with a finite number of permutations. Since cutting and reverse cutting needles have a triangular tip, the orientation of the cutting end is indicated by whether the triangle on the box is pointing up (cutting) or down (reverse cutting).

The material used to make the needles themselves also varies considerably between manufacturers, as proprietary alloys are used to maximize strength and durability. While Ethicon and Covidien products are used most often in skin and soft-tissue reconstruction, many other reputable companies manufacture suture material, and individual preferences may vary widely.

SUTURE MATERIALS

While the needle has a major effect on the ease and efficiency of the surgical procedure, suture material choice also has the potential to impact wound closure significantly. Any suture, including absorbable sutures, may be used for transepidermal suture placement, which may permit the use of a single suture pack for both buried and epidermal sutures.

Many suture characteristics are commonly discussed, including handling, memory, pliability, knot security, tissue reactivity, and others. While there are subtle differences between the handling characteristics of different suture materials, most modern options fall well within the realm of utility, so that while the handling of silk, for example, is clearly superior to the handling of nylon, even nylon handles very well. Similarly, certain materials, such as catgut, may be highly reactive, although the more frequently used formulations, such as chromic gut and fast-absorbing gut, do not lead to enough inflammation to make a marked clinical difference in most situations. For the most part, monofilament sutures lead to less tissue drag and therefore are useful with running techniques, whereas braided sutures provide excellent handling and knot security and are therefore useful for interrupted buried sutures. With improvements in materials, the distinction between outcomes now likely relates

TABLE 5-1 • Frequently Used Suture Materials in Skin and Soft-Tissue Reconstruction

Suture Material Name	Configuration	Handling	Tissue Reactivity	Loss of 50% Strength	Time to Complete Absorption
Absorbable sutures					
Vicryl (polyglactin 910)	Braided, coated	Very good	Moderate	21 days	75 days
Polysorb (glycolide/lactide polymer)	Braided, coated	Very good	Moderate	21 days	75 days
Monocryl (poliglecaprone)	Monofilament	Very good	Moderate	7 days	60 days
Maxon (polyglyconate)	Monofilament	Very good	Moderate	21 days	6 months
PDS I/II (polydioxanone)	Monofilament	Good	Moderate	30 days	6 months
Biosyn (glycomer 631)	Monofilament	Very good	Moderate	21 days	60 days
Caprosyn (polyglytone 6211)	Monofilament	Very good	Moderate	7 days	60 days
Catgut	Braided	Very good	High	Plain: 7 days Chromic: 10 days Fast absorbing: 5 days	Plain: 70 days Chromic: 84 days Fast absorbing: 35 days
Vicryl Rapide	Braided, coated	Very good	Moderate	5 days	42 days
Velosorb Fast	Braided	Very good	Moderate	5 days	42 days
Nonabsorbable sutures					
Monofilament Nylon	Monofilament	Very good	Low		
Prolene, Surgipro (polypropylene)	Monofilament	Good	Low		
Novafil (polybutester)	Monofilament	Very good	Low		
Silk	Braided	Excellent	Moderate		

more to suturing technique than to choice in suture materials (Table 5-1).

Absorbable Sutures

Vicryl (Polyglactin 910): Vicryl is one of the most frequently used suture materials in skin and soft tissue reconstruction. It is a braided, coated suture material that retains its strength for approximately 3 weeks and is completely absorbed in under 3 months. It has excellent handling characteristics and only mild tissue reactivity. Recently a faster-absorbing variation, Vicryl Rapide, was developed, which loses its strength entirely in under 2 weeks and may be seen as an alternative to fast-absorbing gut suture when suture removal is not desired. An antibacterial-coated variation is now also available on the market (Table 5-2).

TABLE 5-2 • Comparison of Frequently Used Suture Materials From Ethicon and Covidien

Ethicon	Covidien	Application
Vicryl	Polysorb	Standard for buried sutures
Vicryl Rapide	Velosorb Fast	Alternative to fast-absorbing gut; excellent for skin grafts or when suture removal is not an option
Monocryl	Biosyn	Monofilament alternative for buried sutures; support is lost faster than Vicryl/Polysorb
PDS I/II	Maxon	Monofilament alternative for buried sutures; support lasts longer than Vicryl/Polysorb
Prolene	Surgipro I/II	Smooth monofilament nonabsorbable suture; excellent choice for running subcuticular sutures if suture removal is planned
Ethilon	Monosof	Standard nonabsorbable monofilament nylon suture for epidermal approximation

Note: This chart does not imply equivalency; it is designed to outline suture materials that are roughly equivalent in terms of application to skin and soft-tissue reconstruction.

Polysorb (Glycolide/Lactide Copolymer): This is a braided absorbable suture, similar to Vicryl. It provides similar handling and knot security while ostensibly providing slightly improved initial tensile strength when compared with Vicryl. Its absorption characteristics are similar to Vicryl. Velosorb Fast has also been developed as an alternative to Vicryl Rapide.

Monocryl (Poliglecaprone): Monocryl, often seen as a monofilament alternative to Vicryl, is another popular suture material choice. It is more expensive than Vicryl, has excellent handling characteristics for a monofilament suture, and loses its strength in less than 1 month, although complete absorption takes 3 to 4 months. As with Vicryl, an antibacterial option is also now available.

Maxon (Polyglyconate): Maxon is a long-lasting monofilament absorbable suture; while it loses some strength already after 3 weeks, it takes 6 months or more for the suture material to be entirely absorbed, making this a good choice when long-term strength retention may be helpful. It has good handling characteristics, although the slow absorption times should be taken into account if dyed suture material is used, as the suture may be visible if placed in a running subcuticular pattern.

PDS (Polydioxanone): PDS I and II are very long-lasting monofilament absorbable sutures. They are useful when long-term strength retention is critical. PDS II was developed as a better-handling alternative to PDS I, which was criticized for its less-than-ideal handling characteristics. It retains strength for an extended period of time, with 50% strength retention at 5 weeks, and may take more than 6 months to absorb.

Biosyn (Glycomer 631): Biosyn is another monofilament absorbable suture. It has very good handling characteristics and outstanding initial tensile strength. It retains its strength for at least 3 weeks and takes up to 4 months to absorb completely. If Biosyn is used for superficial closures, the undyed version may be preferable.

Caprosyn (Polyglytone 6211): Caprosyn is a fast-absorbing monofilament suture, often seen as an alternative to Monocryl. It absorbs completely in 8 weeks, while retaining tensile strength for 7 to 10 days postoperatively. Therefore, it is useful in low-tension closures, such as those on the face, where rapid suture material breakdown is an advantage.

Catgut: Plain gut is derived from bovine or sheep intestines and therefore breaks down by enzymatic degradation, rather than the hydrolysis that breaks down synthetic absorbable sutures. Chromic gut is a longer-lasting version of gut, while fast-absorbing gut is heat treated to speed up absorption. On a practical level, fast-absorbing gut may be useful for closures when transepidermal sutures are desired for wound edge apposition but where suture removal is impractical or inconvenient. Gut does lead to more tissue reactivity than other absorbable sutures and has a tendency toward breakage after multiple passes through tissue.

Nonabsorbable

Nylon: This is a frequently used nonabsorbable suture and provides minimal tissue reactivity coupled with very good handling. While a very good choice for most closures, it does not move through tissue as smoothly as polypropylene, so if buried subcuticular sutures are placed with nonabsorbable suture, the latter would be preferred. Nylon is available either braided or monofilament; the former may confer slightly better handling, though this is outweighed by the ability of monofilament nylon to move easily through tissue.

Polypropylene (Prolene, Surgipro): This is a minimally reactive suture that has the ability to move smoothly through tissue. It does have a fair amount of memory, and therefore may be slightly more challenging to work with than nylon. Extra throws are often advisable during knot tying as well, although this does represent a good option for nonabsorbable subcuticular suturing.

Novafil (Polybutester): This is a very well-handling suture material that also provides significant elasticity. While not as widely used as some other materials, it provides excellent pliability, whereas the elasticity may be helpful in areas where significant wound edema is anticipated, as it will accommodate tissue swelling while maintaining wound edge apposition.

Silk: This is the most highly reactive of the nonabsorbable sutures. However, it is also the gold standard for suture material handling. Its natural softness makes it useful in closures along the lips, where synthetic suture has a tendency to poke against the delicate tissues. Its reactivity, however, makes it less useful on a daily basis for most other surgical sites.

SURGICAL KNOT TYING

Most surgical knots in skin and soft tissue reconstruction are tied using an instrument tie. This is generally the fastest approach and also affords the least amount of suture material waste. Hand tying, using either one- or two-handed ties, may be used rarely in cutaneous surgery and reconstruction.

The distinction in knot tying between transepidermal sutures, where pulling suture tight may lead to strangulation, and buried sutures, where the goal of suture placement is developing directly opposed dermal, muscle, or fascial structures, is critical. When tying a deep suture, it is generally desirable to pull the suture strands together as tightly as possible, secured with a stable knot. For transepidermal sutures, since the goal of suture placement is wound-edge apposition, placing the minimal necessary tension across of the surface of the wound is a must; overtightening these sutures will lead directly to strangulation, necrosis, and—at a minimum—track mark formation. Indeed, while dermal suture placement should be performed as tight as possible, transepidermal sutures should be secured with the minimal possible tension, and indeed, some additional give may be provided by permitting laxity between the first and second throws of the knot, anticipating tissue edema.

Generally, most surgical knots are tied as square knots, so that the two throws occur in opposite directions, locking the

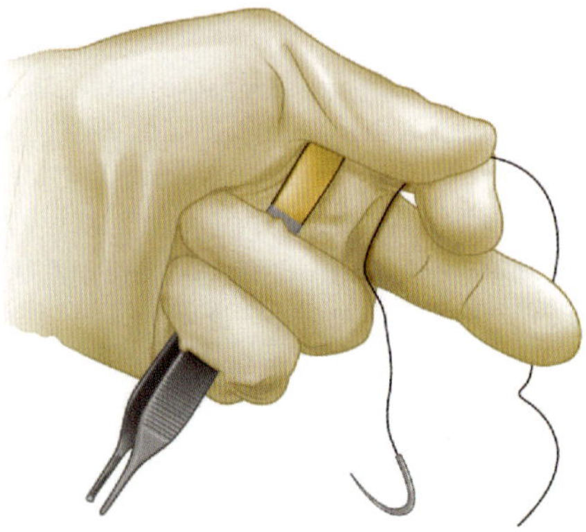

FIGURE 5-2 Grasping the suture material during knot tying; the suture material may be looped around the left hand if needed. Note that the needle hangs freely, without tension.

knot in place. Sometimes, a granny knot is desirable, where the first two throws are in the same direction, as this allows the suture material to be cinched down and tightened. It is critical, however, to follow the granny knot with a throw in the opposite direction so that once the knot is in place it is secured and cannot slip.

Each throw refers to one half knot (ie, a complete twisting of two strands). Thus, to secure a knot, by definition, a minimum of two throws are necessary, and for practical purposes, three throws are used for most braided sutures, while four throws are used for some sutures with a higher risk of knot slippage.

After placement of the suture itself, when beginning an instrument tie, the leading end of suture must be grasped with the nondominant hand. In order to minimize the risk of needle-stick injury, it is possible to grasp the suture material approximately 6 to 10 cm from the needle swage between the thumb and index finger of the left hand, allowing the needle to drop down below the hand. Since the needle is hanging freely and is not under tension, there is little chance for a needle-stick injury (**Figure** 5-2). Excess suture material may be wrapped around the nondominant hand with a gentle turn of the wrist. Some clinicians prefer to hold the needle itself in the nondominant hand (**Figure** 5-3). Recall that when placing a buried suture, the leading and trailing edge of the suture material should be on the same side of the newly created loop prior to initiating a tie.

A single click of the needle driver locking mechanism is sufficient for locking the needle, and indeed, cranking down on the needle driver excessively will result in a loosening of the locking mechanism, leading to inadvertent suture needle slippage in the future. The needle driver may be palmed, where it is locked or released via gentle pressure from the thenar eminence, or may be held with the thumb and fourth finger (**Figures** 5-4 **to** 5-9). When delicately placing fine-gauge sutures in the face, the body of the needle driver may be held with the thumb and first and second fingers and delicately rotated through the skin, permitting precise placement of fine sutures.

When grasping the needle body with the needle driver, the default position is to grasp the needle with the end of the needle driver perpendicular to the body of the needle approximately one-third of the distance from the swage where the suture material is bonded to the needle. When first loading a needle,

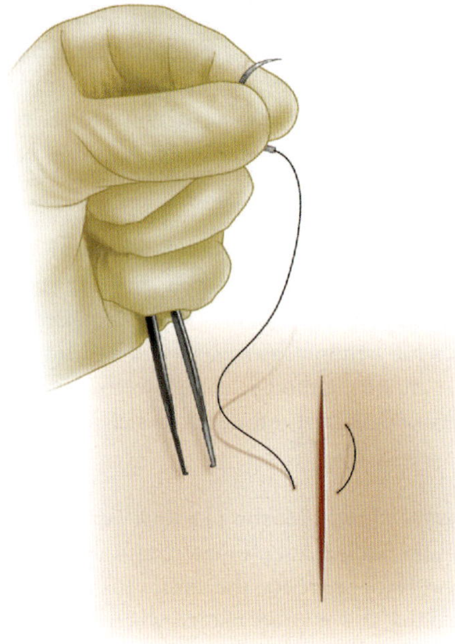

FIGURE 5-3 Grasping the needle during knot tying.

this may be executed by gently pressing the slightly open jaws of the needle driver perpendicularly against the needle and closing the needle driver with a single click. For closures in tight spaces, the needle may be grasped toward the middle or even slightly

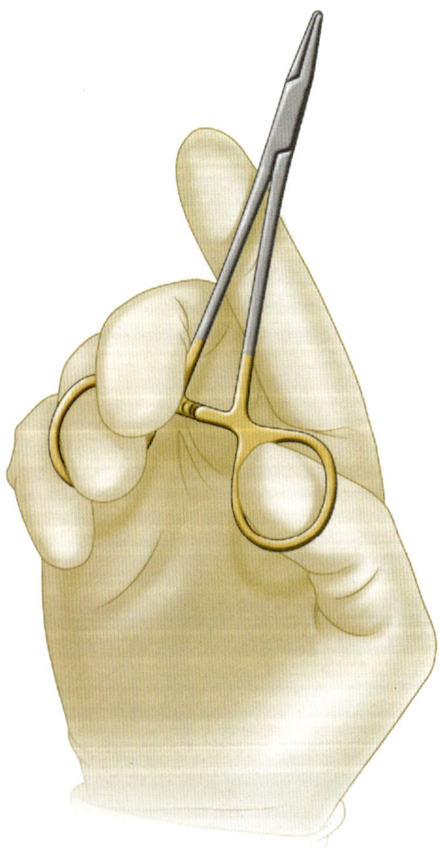

FIGURE 5-4 The basic needle driver grasping position, with thumb and fourth finger in the rings.

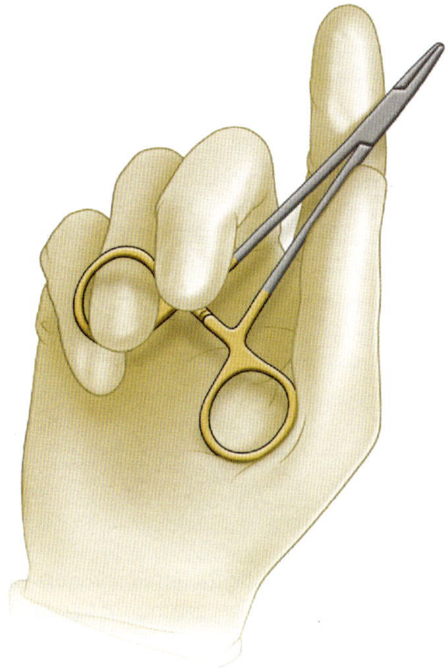

FIGURE 5-5 Palming the needle driver. This is the default position for many clinicians. The fourth finger may rest slightly on the inside of the ring.

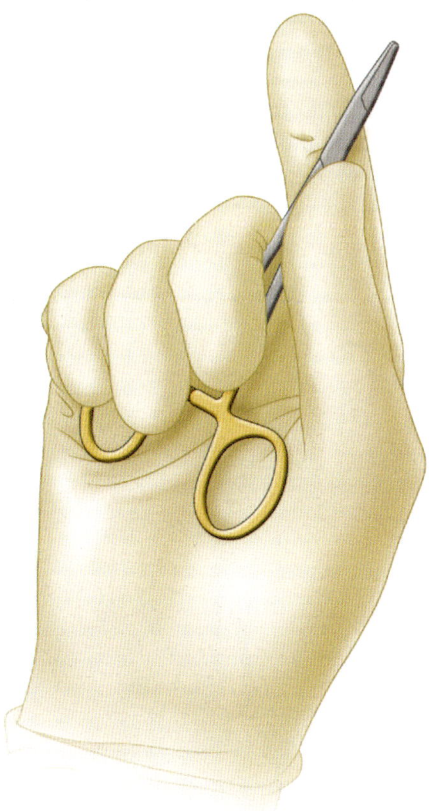

FIGURE 5-6 Palming the needle driver with no fingers in the rings.

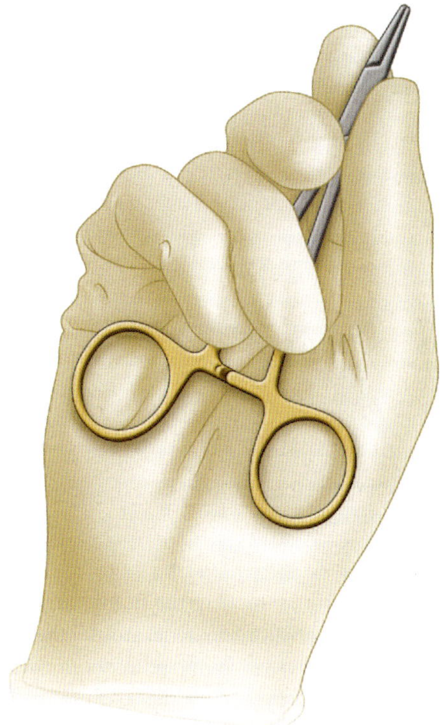

FIGURE 5-7 Needle driver grasping position when performing fine suturing.

distally so that the arc of needle placement is relatively shallow, while for other select closures, such as the running subcuticular technique, the needle may be held at an angle relative to the jaws of the needle driver.

Technique for Performing an Instrument Tie With Nonabsorbable Sutures

a. The leading end of suture material is grasped between the thumb and index finger of the left hand, approximately 6 cm from the needle swage. The needle driver is brought between the leading and trailing strands of suture, and the leading end of suture is wrapped twice around the needle driver.

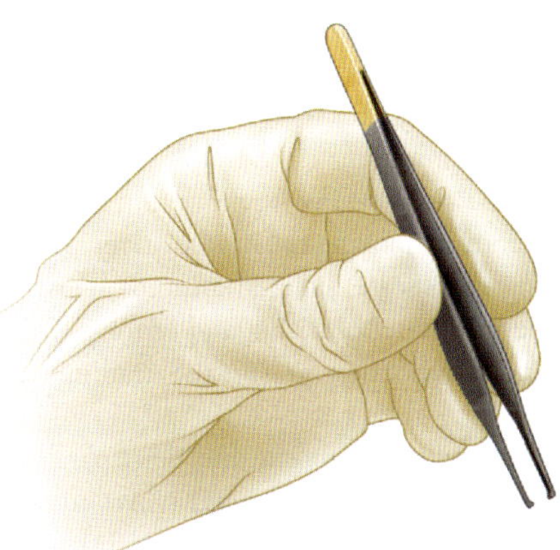

FIGURE 5-8 Holding the forceps for tissue or needle handling.

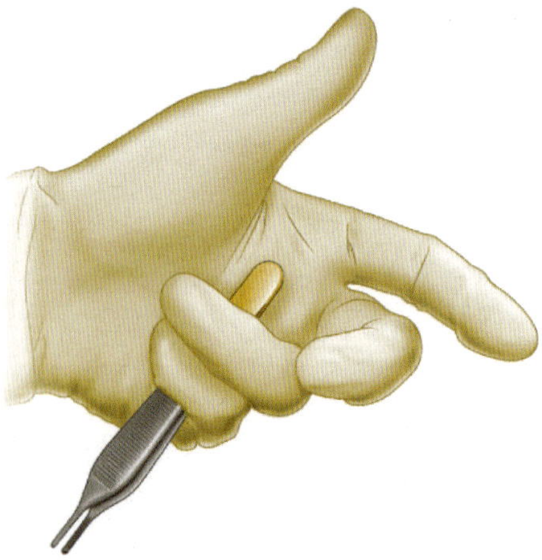

FIGURE 5-9 Palming the forceps to free up the fingers for grasping suture material and knot tying.

This should be done by moving the needle driver around the suture, not moving the suture material around the needle driver, as this will permit better precision and economy of movement.

b. The needle driver then grasps the trailing end of suture material.
c. The hands are pulled in opposite directions, perpendicular to the incised wound edge, so that the right hand moves to the left (where the leading end of suture began) and the left hand moves to the right (where the trailing end of suture began). This should form a surgeon's knot that will be resistant to slippage.
d. The trailing end of suture is released by the needle driver, and the needle driver is then brought from the inside, between the two ends of suture, and the leading end of suture is wrapped once around the needle driver.
e. The hands again move in opposite directions, so that now the right hand moves to the right and the left hand moves to the left. The knot is now locked.
f. For the third (and often final) throw, steps a through c are then repeated. Additional throws may be placed if needed (**Figures 5-10 to 5-17**).

Technique for Performing an Instrument Tie With Buried Sutures

a. The leading end of suture material is grasped between the thumb and index finger of the left hand, approximately 6 cm from the needle swage. The needle driver is brought between the leading and trailing strands of suture, and the leading end of suture is wrapped twice around the needle driver. This should be done by moving the needle driver around the suture, not moving the suture material around the needle driver, as this will permit better precision and economy of movement.
b. The needle driver then grasps the trailing end of suture material.
c. The hands are pulled in opposite directions, parallel to the incised wound edge, so that the right hand moves in the direction of where the leading end of suture began, and the left hand moves in the direction of where the trailing end of suture began. This should form a surgeon's knot that will be resistant to slippage.

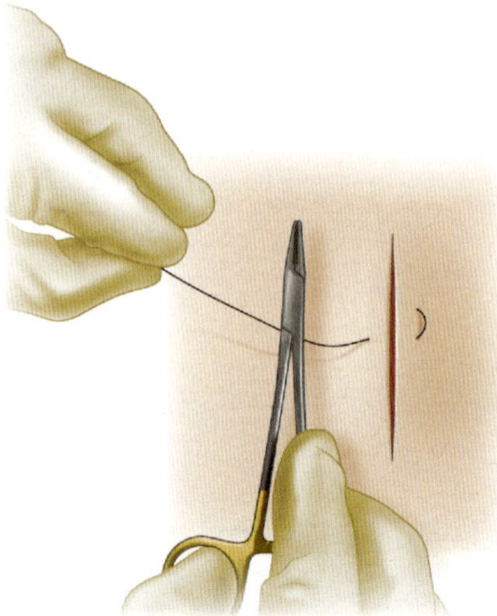

FIGURE 5-10 The instrument tie for nonabsorbable suture material. Step 1: The needle driver is brought between the leading and trailing strands of suture.

d. The trailing end of suture is released by the needle driver, and the needle driver is then brought from the inside, between the two ends of suture, and the leading end of suture is wrapped once around the needle driver.
e. The hands again move in opposite directions parallel to the wound, so that the right hand moves in the direction of where the leading strand began and the left hand moves in the direction of where the trailing strand began. The knot is now locked.
f. For the third (and often final) throw, steps a through c are then repeated. Additional throws may be placed if needed (**Figures 5-18 to 5-25**).

Absorbable suture material is generally trimmed either at the knot (for braided suture material) or with a 1- to 2-mm tail of suture

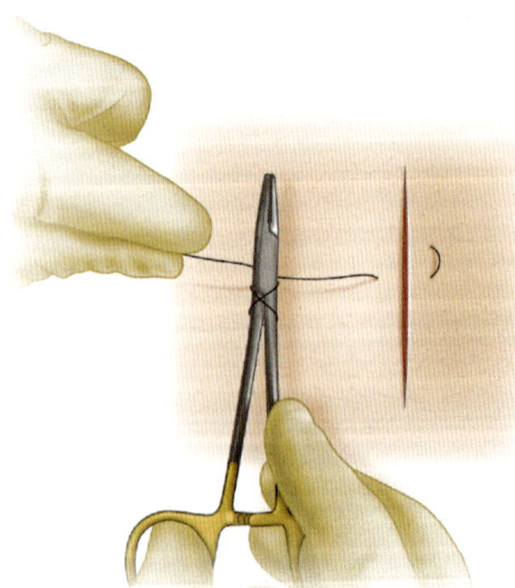

FIGURE 5-11 The instrument tie for nonabsorbable suture material. Step 2: The suture material is looped twice around the needle driver by rotating the needle driver around the suture material.

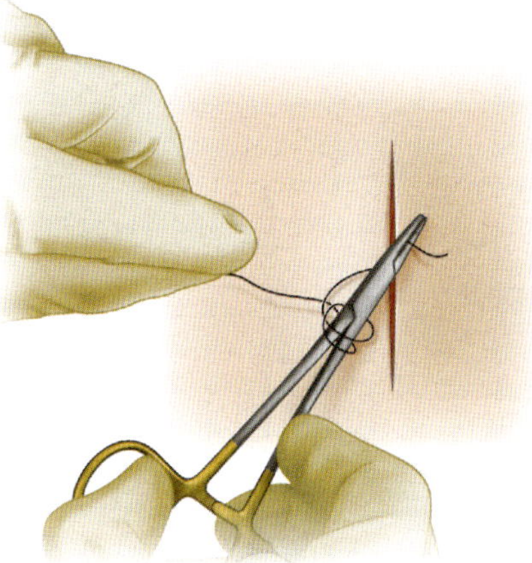

FIGURE 5-12 The instrument tie for nonabsorbable suture material. Step 3: The needle driver is then used to grasp the tail of the suture material.

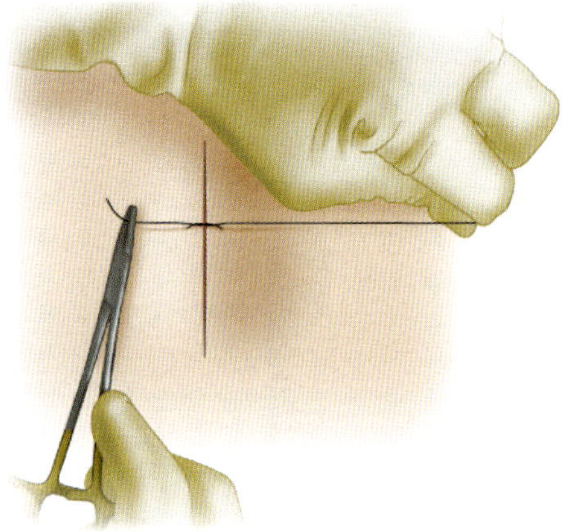

FIGURE 5-13 The instrument tie for nonabsorbable suture material. Step 4: The two ends of suture are pulled in opposite directions, perpendicular to the wound, allowing the knot to lay flat.

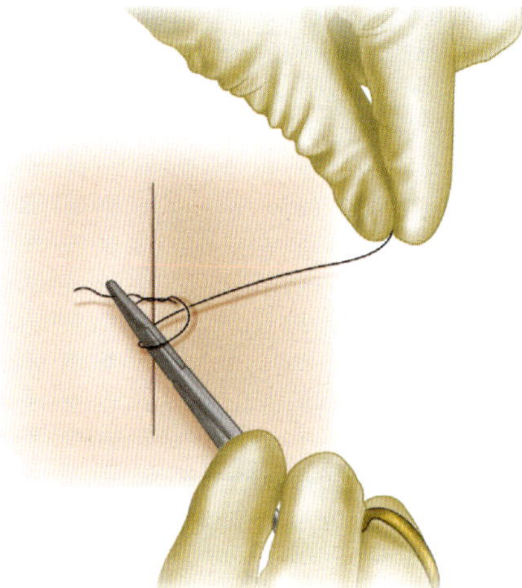

FIGURE 5-14 The instrument tie for nonabsorbable suture material. Step 5: The needle driver is then again brought between the ends of suture, and the leading end of suture material is wrapped once around the needle holder, and the trailing tail is grasped.

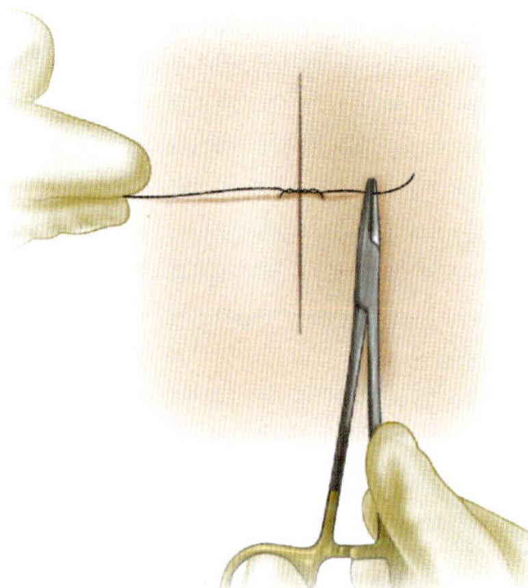

FIGURE 5-15 The instrument tie for nonabsorbable suture material. Step 6: The two ends of suture are again pulled apart, now moving in the direction opposite the prior throw, again perpendicular to the wound edge.

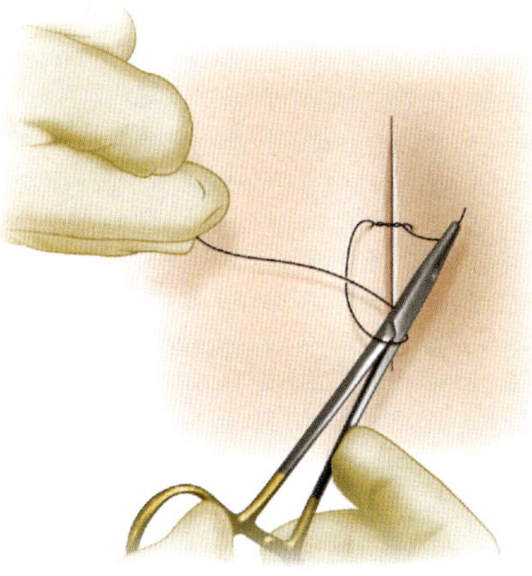

FIGURE 5-16 The instrument tie for nonabsorbable suture material. Step 7: For the third throw, the procedure is repeated again with the needle driver brought between the two strands, the needle driver wraps the leading end of suture around itself once, and the trailing end is grasped.

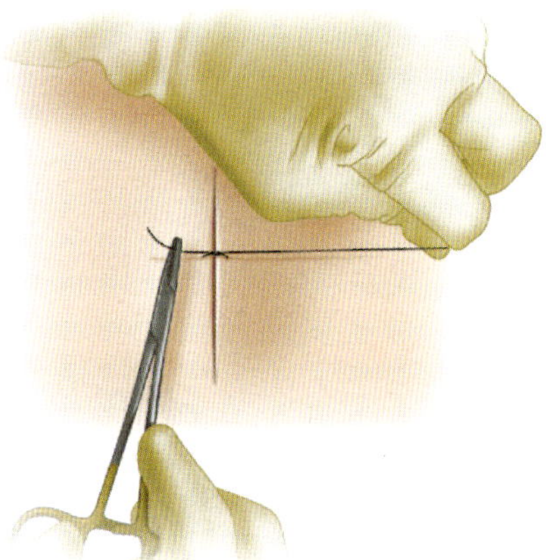

FIGURE 5-17 The instrument tie for nonabsorbable suture material. Step 8: The hands are then pulled in opposite directions, pulling the throw tight and securing the knot. For most braided suture materials, three throws are adequate, whereas for some monofilament sutures, a fourth throw may be added.

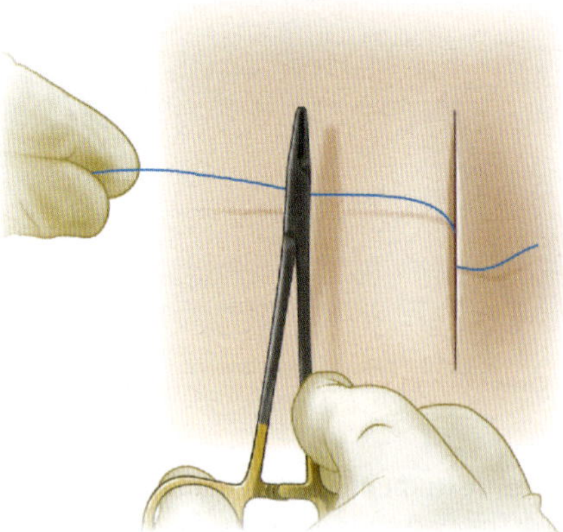

FIGURE 5-18 The instrument tie for absorbable suture material. Step 1: The needle driver is brought between the leading and trailing strands of suture.

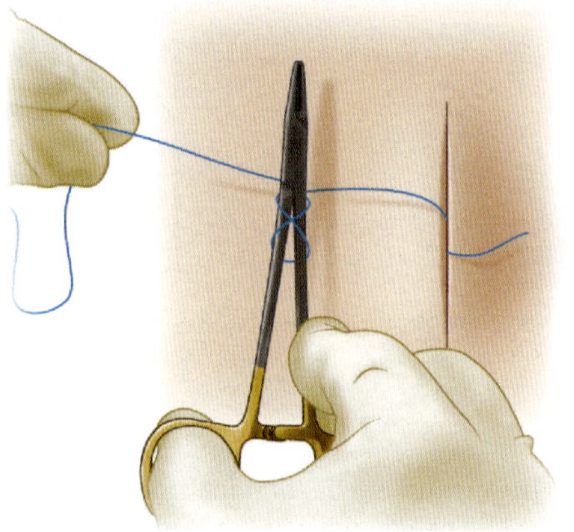

FIGURE 5-19 The instrument tie for absorbable suture material. Step 2: The suture material is looped twice around the needle driver by rotating the needle driver around the suture material.

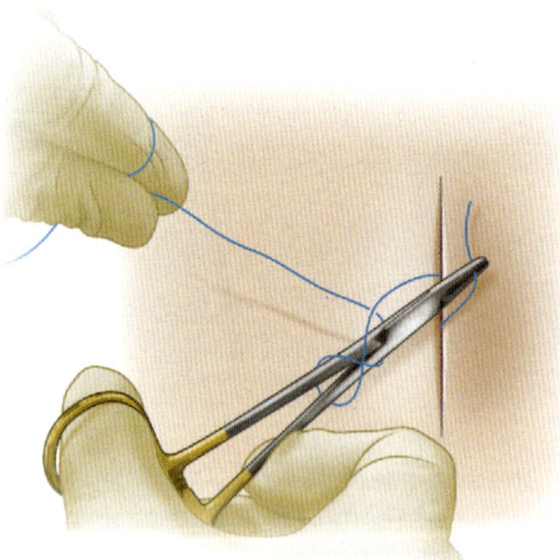

FIGURE 5-20 The instrument tie for absorbable suture material. Step 3: The needle driver is then used to grasp the tail of the suture material.

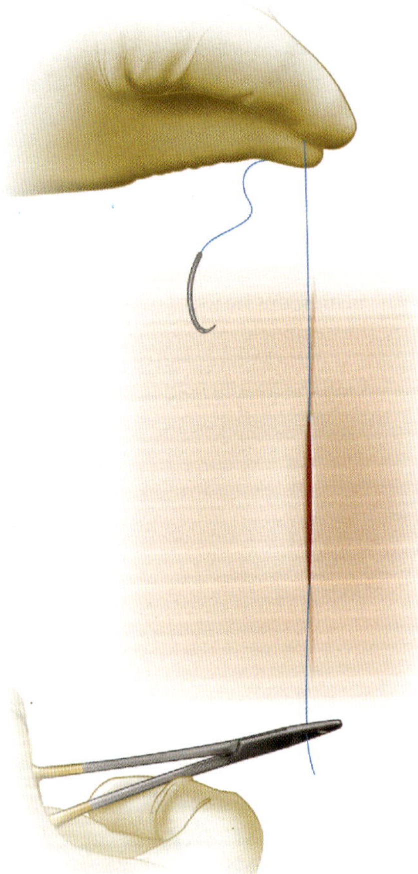

FIGURE 5-21 The instrument tie for absorbable suture material. Step 4: The two ends of suture are pulled in opposite directions, parallel to the wound, allowing the knot to lay flat.

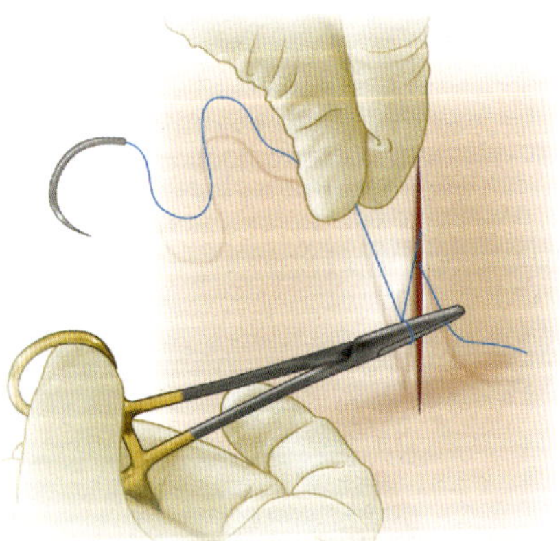

FIGURE 5-22 The instrument tie for absorbable suture material. Step 5: The needle driver is then again brought between the ends of suture, the leading end of suture material is wrapped once around the needle holder, and the trailing tail is grasped.

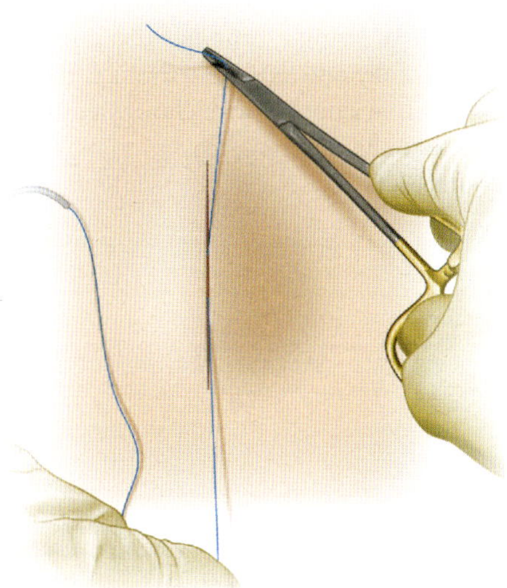

FIGURE 5-23 The instrument tie for absorbable suture material. Step 6: The two ends of suture are again pulled apart, now moving in the direction opposite the prior throw, again parallel to the wound edge.

(for monofilament suture material). Nonabsorbable sutures are generally left with a 3- to 6-mm tail, depending on clinician preference, suture material size, and the anatomic location.

When tying knots with nonabsorbable suture, if there is only minimal tension across the surface of the wound, it is sometimes desirable to leave a gap between the initial surgeon's knot and the square not. To execute this maneuver, the first throw is placed as a surgeon's knot. The next throw is not tightened to lock the surgeon's knot, but rather leaves 1 to 2 mm of space between the surgeon's knot throw and the subsequent throws. This allows for some give so that tissue edema does not cause the suture material to overly constrict the wound edges (**Table 5-3**).

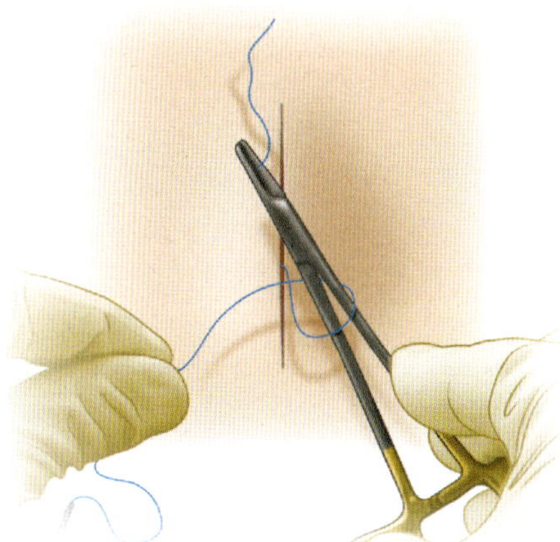

FIGURE 5-24 The instrument tie for absorbable suture material. Step 7: For the third throw, the procedure is repeated again with the needle driver brought between the two strands, the needle driver wrapping the leading end of suture around itself once, and grasping the trailing end.

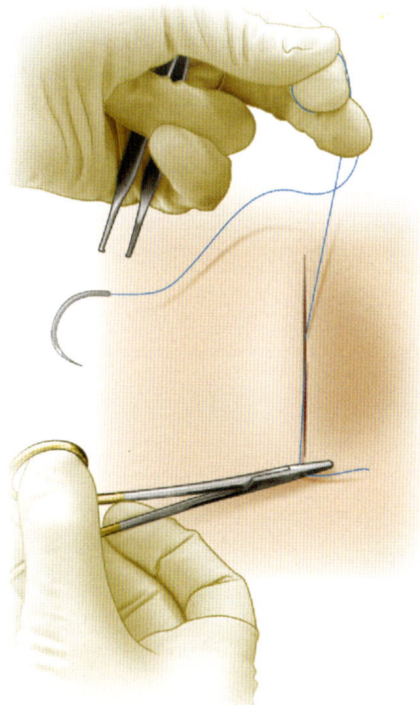

FIGURE 5-25 The instrument tie for absorbable suture material. Step 8: The hands are then pulled in opposite directions, parallel to the wound axis, pulling the throw tight and securing the knot. For most braided suture materials, three throws are adequate, whereas for some monofilament sutures, a fourth throw may be added.

CONCLUSIONS

Historically, much attention has been paid to the various characteristics of suture materials, such as memory and handling, although most modern suture materials are so easy to use that these differences largely become matters of individual taste

TABLE 5-3 • Comparison of Frequently Used Reverse Cutting Needles From Ethicon and Covidien

Ethicon	Covidien
P-1	P-10
P-3	P-13
PS-1	P-14
PS-2	P-12
CP-2	GS-10
FS-1	C-14
FS-2	C-13
P-2	P-21

Note: Comparison does not imply equivalency because the alloy and finish quality within and between companies will vary. All are 3/8 circle in diameter except the P-2/P-21, which are 1/2 circle.

and preference. High-quality suture material used on a high-quality needle permits the facile placement of the large numbers of suture throws that are common in dermatologic surgery. In general, the choice of needle and suture material gauge, rather than suture material itself, may contribute more to the success of an individual procedure. The most frequent errors encountered by novice clinicians are using a needle that is too small for a given anatomic location and using a technique that does not permit the needle to pass naturally and smoothly through tissue. Therefore, attention to technique, coupled with choice of a sufficiently large needle for the closure in question, may go a long way to optimizing surgical outcomes.

Antibiotics: Pre- and Postoperative Considerations

6

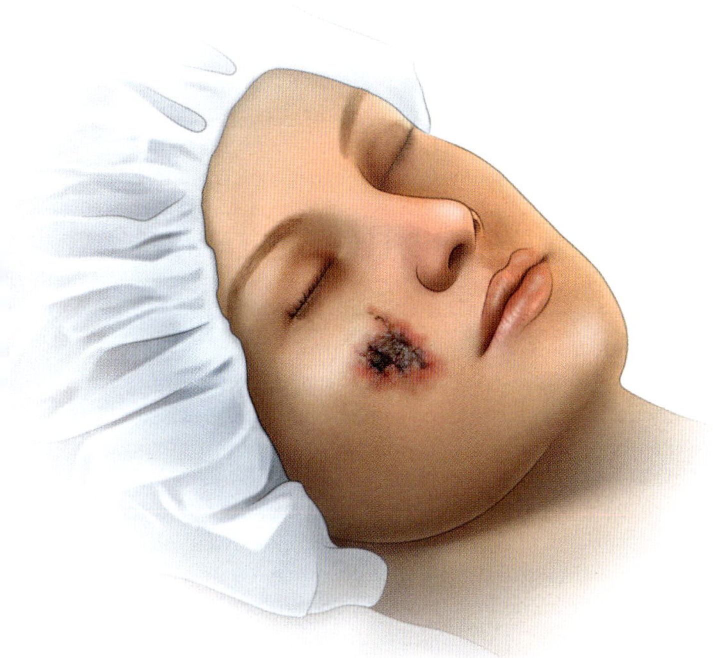

SUMMARY

- The rate of infection after skin surgery is likely between 1% and 4%.
- Antibiotic use in dermatologic surgery has declined markedly over the past several decades, as studies highlighting the baseline low rate of wound infections, coupled with the individual and societal risks associated with widespread antibiotic use, have made the routine prescribing of perioperative antibiotics no longer the standard of care.

Beginner Tips

- The differential diagnosis of postoperative infection includes irritant or allergic contact dermatitis, suture reactions/suture abscesses, filler reactions (if relevant), and inflammatory chondritis.
- Contact dermatitis should be considered, particularly when topical antibiotics or adhesives were used, or when the involved area is geometric.

Pitfalls and Cautions

- While antibiotics are typically given the hour before the procedure, there is ambiguous data about whether prophylactic antibiotic timing affects the risk of superficial skin infection.
- Given the high rate of warfarin and sulfonylurea use in the patient population undergoing dermatologic surgery, systemic antibiotics should be prescribed with extreme caution and an eye to minimizing the risk of drug–drug interactions.

Expert Tips

- Risk factors for infection include patient factors, surgical factors, and surgical site factors.

Don't Forget!

- Cephalexin or dicloxacillin can be used as prophylaxis for wedge excisions of the lip or ear, flaps on the nose, and grafts.
- Clarithromycin, levofloxacin, TMP-SMX, metronidazole, and ciprofloxacin are associated with a higher risk of hypoglycemia in diabetic patients taking sulfonylurea medications.

Patient Education Points

- No rigorous study has demonstrated a robust statistically significant benefit to utilizing any single topical antibiotic preparation, and the American Academy of Dermatology has, therefore, warned against the routine use of topical antibiotics after clean surgical procedures as part of its Choosing Wisely campaign.
- Patients often request perioperative antibiotics under the assumption that these will decrease their risk of developing an infection; therefore, adequate education may be valuable in dissuading patients from this practice and increasing their comfort level.
- It may be helpful to explain to patients that bacteremia is more likely after brushing their teeth than it is postoperatively.

6 Antibiotics: Pre- and Postoperative Considerations

INTRODUCTION

Antibiotic use in dermatologic procedures has declined markedly over the past several decades, as studies highlighting the baseline low rate of wound infections, coupled with the individual and societal risks associated with widespread antibiotic use, have made the routine prescribing of perioperative antibiotics no longer the standard of care. Those performing dermatologic procedures must understand the subtleties of antibiotic choice not only to guide clinical patient management, but also to elegantly explain to patients why they would—or would not—benefit from antibiotic use in the perioperative period. An anxious patient can often be easily calmed by providing a reasoned explanation of the scientific basis of the clinician's decision to decline a patient-suggested antibiotic prescription. Understanding both the scientific literature as well as society-level recommendations regarding antibiotic use is therefore useful both for patient care and patient peace of mind.

EPIDEMIOLOGY

The rate of infection after skin surgery is likely between 1% and 4%,[1-4] varying based on the type of surgery and risk factors for infection. Rates of infection after Mohs micrographic surgery, excisions, full-face carbon dioxide resurfacing, and flaps range from 0.7% to 3%; these numbers generally increase with the complexity of the surgical procedure (**Table 6-1**).[5] The infection rate for Mohs surgery without prophylactic antibiotics has been reported at under 1%.[4] There are significant differences in the rates of infection depending on anatomic site and patient risk factors, with repairs on the genitalia, ears, or lower extremities or in those with other risk factors, such as diabetes, associated with an increased risk of infection.[2]

Despite the low incidence of infections, when they do occur, surgical site infections (SSIs) can lead to severe complications.[6] In dermatologic surgery, serious adverse events occur in only 0.02% of cases, although the rate of postsurgical acute care visits attributed to SSIs in ambulatory surgical centers is around 0.5% in the 30 days after surgery.[7] Moreover, skin surgery infection rates are likely several-fold higher in developing nations, as the burden of overall healthcare-associated infections in resource-limited settings is three times higher than the infection rates in developed countries.[8]

TABLE 6-1 • Incidence of Infections in Dermatology Procedures[5]

Incidence of Infections in Dermatology Procedures	
Procedure	**Overall Infection Rate (%)**
Mohs micrographic surgery	0.7-2.3
Excisions	1.9-2.3
Full-face carbon dioxide resurfacing	1.1-7.6
Flaps	3

Data from Shurman DL, Benedetto AV. Antimicrobials in dermatologic surgery: facts and controversies. Clin Dermatol. *2010 Sep-Oct;28(5):505-510.*

SURGICAL SITE INFECTIONS: CLINICAL FEATURES AND DIAGNOSIS

Surgical sites infections, although generally mild in nature, may lead to severe complications, including bacterial endocarditis and prosthetic joint infection. As defined by the Centers for Disease Control and Prevention, SSIs are infection occurring within 30 days of the procedure, involve only the skin and subcutaneous tissue at the incision, and include one of the following four criteria: purulent drainage from the incision site; positive microbiologic testing from an aseptically obtained specimen; presence of pain or tenderness, localized swelling, erythema, or heat; or diagnosis of SSI by a physician (**Table 6-2**).[9] SSI typically occurs in the first 2 weeks after the procedure.

TABLE 6-2 • Superficial Incisional Surgical Site Infection Definition from the Centers for Disease Control and Prevention, 1999

Superficial Incisional Surgical Site Infection (SSI)
Within 30 days after operative procedure (day 1 = procedure date)
Involves only skin and subcutaneous tissue of incision
One of the following:
1. Purulent drainage from superficial incision
2. Positive microbiologic testing (either culture or non-culture test) from aseptically obtained specimen for purposes of clinical diagnosis or treatment
3. Superficial incision that Is deliberately opened by surgeon and culture- or nonculture-based testing is not performed
AND
At least one of the following: pain or tenderness; localized swelling; erythema; or heat
4. Diagnosis of superficial incisional SSI by a surgeon or attending physician

Adapted with permission from Centers for Disease Control and Prevention (CDC). https://www.cdc.gov/nhsn/pdfs/pscmanual/9pscssicurrent.pdf. *Accessed February 5, 2020.*

TABLE 6-3 • Risk of Surgical Site Infection (SSI) for Wounds Based on Class I, II, III, and IV

	Class I	Class II	Class III	Class IV
Label	Clean	Clean-contaminated	Contaminated	Dirty-infected
Description	Uninfected wounds	Entry in oral cavity, axilla, inguinal area	Acute traumatic wounds that are nonpurulent	Purulent inflammation with necrosis, foreign body
Risk of SSI	<5%	10%	20%-30%	30%-40%
Antibiotics	None	Case-by-case	Antibiotics	Antibiotics

Data from Rossi AM, Mariwalla K. Prophylactic and empiric use of antibiotics in dermatologic surgery: a review of the literature and practical considerations. Dermatol Surg. *2012 Dec;38(12):1898-1921.*

The presentation of SSIs can mimic that of other conditions, and the differential diagnosis may include irritant or allergic contact dermatitis, suture reactions/suture abscesses, filler reactions (if relevant), and inflammatory chondritis. Contact dermatitis should be considered, particularly when topical antibiotics or adhesives were used or when the involved area is geometric. Suture irritation can lead to suture granuloma/suture abscess formation, essentially a foreign body reaction that provokes local inflammation. However, suture granuloma will be culture negative and occurs only in the areas surrounding the suture material itself. If fillers are used, inflammatory reactions to these foreign materials can produce swelling, erythema, and change in color.[10] Filler-induced complications include dermal nodules, abscesses, or delayed hypersensitivity manifesting as erythematous subcutaneous nodules.[11] Detailed patient history can elicit a history of previous soft-tissue augmentation, although patients may not be forthcoming about nonapproved fillers. Biopsy can provide a definitive diagnosis.[12] Finally, in surgical cases involving cartilage, chondritis can mimic SSI with pain, tenderness, and erythema, although it will be culture negative. This is a fairly common phenomenon; in one study, the incidence of inflammatory chondritis after Mohs reconstruction was around 5.6%.[13] The risk of suppurative chondritis, a disfiguring condition involving liquefactive necrosis of the cartilage (particularly involving the ear), can be prevented with perioperative antibiotics with antipseudomonal coverage such as ciprofloxacin.[13]

Delayed reactions should raise the possibility of an infectious process involving biofilms, particularly after procedures involving fillers.[12] Biofilms are polymeric structures produced by bacterial colonies that adhere to surfaces.[14] These self-protective films can thwart normal immune system responses and reduce susceptibility to antibiotics by altering the local microenvironment and employing protective signaling pathways.[15] The National Institutes of Health estimates that up to 80% of human bacterial infections overall are associated with biofilms. Biofilms are associated with particular bacteria, including *Staphylococcus epidermidis*, *Pseudomonas aeruginosa*, *Staphylococcus aureus*, and *Escherichia coli*.[15] Bacteria form biofilms upon lack of prompt antibiotic treatment and inappropriate use of steroids and nonsteroidal anti-inflammatory drugs. These biofilms are often culture negative and need to be further investigated with fluorescence in situ hybridization directed against bacterial DNA.[16]

WOUND CLASSIFICATION AND INFECTION RISK

Wounds can be differentiated into four types—class I, class II, class III, and class IV—based on the degree of contamination and inflammation in the wound (**Table 6-3**).[11] Wounds that are clean and uninfected, without any break in surgical sterile technique, demonstrate less than 5% risk of infection and do not require antibiotics. Class II wounds are clean-contaminated, including wounds that are intended to heal by secondary intention, and entail a 10% risk of SSI. Class III wounds are contaminated and nonpurulent traumatic wounds with an elevated 20% to 30% risk of infection, requiring antibiotics. Class IV wounds include wounds with purulent inflammation or presence of foreign body and are reported to have an infection risk around 30% to 40% and require antibiotics. Almost all dermatologic surgery wounds are class I wounds.

RISK FACTORS FOR INFECTION

Numerous risk factors impact the likelihood that a patient will develop an SSI after surgery (**Table 6-4**).[17] These risk factors can be stratified as patient factors, surgical factors, and surgical site factors. Patient factors include poor nutritional status, immunosuppression, presence of certain comorbidities, concurrent infection, and drug use. Autoimmune diseases, such as rheumatoid arthritis, systemic lupus erythematosus, or drug- or radiation-induced immunosuppression can increase the likelihood of developing a postoperative infection. Concurrent inflammation and infection elsewhere can increase risk of infection as well, and nonemergent dermatologic surgery should be delayed until such conditions are resolved. Comorbidities that increase the rate of SSI include chronic renal disease, peripheral vascular disease, and obesity.[18] Although increased prevalence of comorbidities in older adults may be a confounding factor, increasing patient age is independently associated with increasing infection risk after dermatologic surgery.[19,20] Although well-controlled diabetes mellitus does not lead to increased risk of wound infections, poorly controlled diabetes results in abnormal glucose levels that increase the risk of wound infections.[21] Tobacco use is associated with higher incidence of postoperative complications such as wound dehiscence, flap or graft necrosis, prolonged healing time, and infection.[22] Wound complications after biopsies occur more frequently in smokers and patients taking corticosteroids.[23]

TABLE 6-4 • Risk Factors for Surgical Site Infections

Patient	Surgical Technique	Surgical Site
Nutritional status	Complexity (grafts, flaps, wedge excisions)	Ear
Immunosuppression	Hemorrhage	Groin
Concurrent infection	Longer duration	Axilla
Drug use	Multiple stages	Lower extremity
Tobacco use	Poor tissue handling	Nose
Autoimmune disease	Instrument handling	
Radiation		
Renal disease		
Peripheral vascular disease		
Obesity		
Poorly controlled diabetes		
Advanced age		

Surgical risk factors include high degree of surgical complexity, procedures with greater likelihood of hemorrhage, poor surgical technique, long surgical duration, large postoperative surgical defects,[2] and poor follow-up care. Hemorrhage can lead to local pooling of blood, creating a suitable local environment for the replication of bacteria. It is important that dermal and subcutaneous defects are minimized with close approximation of edges, as the lack of subcutaneous sutures after excisional procedures has been associated with an increased rate of wound complications.[23] During surgery, crush tissue injury from forceps can predispose to local necrosis and subsequent infection. Moreover, longer duration of surgery, including the multiple stages sometimes required for Mohs surgery, may lead to reduced sterility of the surgical site as the patient transfers between the operating area and the waiting room.[4] Longer operative times correlate with increased infection rates, with an approximate doubling of risk with each additional hour of surgery. Poor surgical technique and improper instrument handling and sterilization represent additional potential causes of wound contamination.

More complex dermatologic procedures have higher rates of infection than simpler procedures. Punch and shave procedures of the skin not involving mucous membranes do not require antibiotic prophylaxis. While noninvasive laser treatments also do not require prophylaxis, laser resurfacing and other procedures damaging the epidermis on a larger scale can lead to a larger and deeper wound area. More complex procedures such as grafts, wedge excisions, and flaps are all associated with higher levels of infection risk.[21] While surgical technique is very important, improper wound dressing and inadequate postoperative care could be a source of infection. Despite these risk factors, it is important to remember that the overall rate of infection in dermatologic surgery remains low.

Surgical site factors refer to the anatomic site of the procedure. Different sites can lead to differing levels of immune defense and can be associated with increased prevalence of bacteria. Lack of perfusion and adequate bloody supply can predispose a surgical site to infection. For example, ear procedures involving cartilage, which lacks an intrinsic vascular supply, are associated with a fourfold higher incidence of wound infection compared to Mohs procedures elsewhere.[2] Similarly, suboptimal circulation in the nose[4] and lower extremities, particularly in patients with peripheral arterial disease, may lead to an increased risk of infection.[21] Because the bacterial flora vary by anatomic location, the same surgical procedure can have very different infection rates depending on the surgical site. Surgical sites in areas below the waist, in the groin, and in areas with many sebaceous glands and hair are associated with increased infection.[21]

MINIMIZING RISK OF SSI

Risk of SSI can be reduced through several factors. The National Institute for Health and Clinical Excellence recommends that patients should be informed against removing hair from the surgical site and that patients should shower preoperatively to reduce the bacterial population.[18] It is recommended to remove hair with electric clippers with disposable cartridges instead of a razor because the use of razors may increase infection risk. However, hair removal should be performed when necessary, ideally with scissors.[24]

Cleaning the surgical site before the procedure can be achieved with povidone-iodine, chlorhexidine, or other surgical scrubs. Appropriately prepped surgical sites have a lower rate of infection, although because 20% of skin bacteria reside deep in sebaceous glands and hair follicles, it is not possible to create an entirely sterile field by topical preparation alone.[18] Still, surgical procedures on prepped skin result in a lower rate of bacteremia than brushing teeth.[5] Surgical duration should be minimized because prolonged operating time increases the risk that bacteria may be introduced into the wound. Hands should also be washed prior to the procedure with either alcohol-based hand rubs or aqueous scrubs such as chlorhexidine.[25] Current evidence suggests no difference between alcohol-based rubs with active ingredients and aqueous scrubs such as chlorhexidine in the prevention of SSIs, although chlorhexidine-based aqueous scrubs are more effective than povidone-iodine in reducing the number of bacterial colony-forming units on the hands.[25]

In dermatologic surgery, many procedures do not require true sterile technique, and the majority of studies have not shown any statistically significant difference in infection rate when using nonsterile gloves.[26-28] Low-cost infection protocols that eliminate the use of sterile gloves during the Mohs procedures, sterile gowns, and sterile half-sheet drapes can be implemented without negatively affecting infection risk.[27] Moreover, local anesthesia itself is bacteriostatic and fungistatic, helping prevent bacterial growth.

USE OF PROPHYLACTIC ANTIBIOTICS

Use of antibiotics should consider both the putative benefits of antibiotic prophylaxis and the risks and costs associated with antibiotic use. Except for select circumstances, dermatologic surgery does not require prophylactic antibiotic use. In Mohs surgery, lack of antibiotic prophylaxis does not increase the infection rate.[4]

Goals of Antibiotic Prophylaxis

The goal of antibiotics is to reduce the risk of SSI, hematogenous joint infections, and infective endocarditis. The mechanism of infection is generally hematogenous dissemination and the development of true bacteremia; the overall incidence of postoperative bacteremia in an immunocompetent and noninfected skin site is less than 1%.[29] Antibiotics may decrease the quantity of skin bacteria, but infection risk depends on additional bacterial characteristics such as virulence.[30] Importantly, the latest guidelines continue to narrow the patients appropriate for prophylactic antibiotics. It is important for those performing dermatologic procedures to be aware of new guidelines to avoid the risks of antibiotic overuse and to reserve prophylactic antibiotics for patients deriving maximal benefit.[31]

Risks and Costs of Prophylactic Antibiotics

The costs of antibiotic use include adverse events, drug interactions, financial burden, and societal costs. It is estimated that more than 140,000 visits to the emergency department are attributed to adverse effects of antibiotics annually in the United States, largely from allergic reactions to penicillin and cephalosporins.[32]

Drug-drug interactions are a significant concern, as many antibiotics in common use can interact with other medications. For example, certain antibiotics can slightly increase the risk of supratherapeutic warfarin levels[33] or the risk of hypoglycemia in diabetic patients taking sulfonylurea medications.[34] Indeed, clarithromycin, levofloxacin, trimethoprim-sulfamethoxazole (TMP-SMX), metronidazole, and ciprofloxacin are associated with a higher risk of hypoglycemia compared with noninteracting antimicrobials, with an odds ratio between 2 and 4 in older female adults.[34] Overall, sulfonamides and clindamycin show the highest rates of emergency department visits per number of outpatient prescriptions, averaging one emergency department visit per 500 prescriptions.[32] Because antibiotics adversely affect native bacterial flora, prolonged antibiotic treatment increases the risk of acquired antimicrobial resistance.[35] As such, unnecessary use of antibiotics contributes to worsening antibiotic resistance.[24] Financial costs of antibiotics include the monetary cost for the patient, the cost for treating adverse effects, and the opportunity cost of purchasing and taking the antibiotic.

Antibiotic Prophylaxis for Infective Endocarditis

Antibiotic prophylaxis reduces the risk of infectious endocarditis in patients with high-risk surgical sites or in procedures that involve the mucous membranes such as gingival tissue or oral mucosa.[36] Reasons for prophylaxis for infective endocarditis include patient factors such as prosthetic cardiac valves, history of infective endocarditis, cardiac transplant with valvulopathy, patients with cardiac valve repair with recent prosthetic materials or devices, and unrepaired or residual defect after repair of congenital heart disease (**Table 6-5**).[11,37] Recent prosthetic repairs consist of repaired defects using prosthetic materials during the first 6 months postoperatively, before the prosthetic material is likely endothelialized.[37] Importantly, the high-risk category excludes patients with cardiac pacemakers and internal defibrillators, and prophylaxis is not recommended simply due to increased lifetime risk of developing infective endocarditis.[38]

The 2008 Dermatology Surgery Advisory Statements recommends antibiotic prophylaxis for prevention of infective endocarditis and joint infection only if the procedure occurs on an oral site or site of active skin infection. Any patients fitting these criteria must also satisfy high-risk criteria or have a prosthetic device as defined by the American Heart Association (AHA), American Dental Association (ADA), or American Academy of Orthopedic Surgeons.

Antibiotic Prophylaxis for Prosthetic Joints

The ADA recommends no prophylactic antibiotics prior to surgery for patients with prosthetic joints.[39] Previously, patients were considered high risk for hematogenous joint infection if they underwent joint replacement within 2 years of surgery, had immunosuppression or autoimmune disease such as rheumatoid arthritis or systemic lupus erythematous, or had a history of prosthetic joint infection (**Table 6-5**).[11,40] In addition, previous guidelines indicated the need for prophylaxis when the mucosa are penetrated. However, a thorough evaluation of the literature failed to demonstrate a clinically significant association between dental procedures and prosthetic joint infection in terms of effectiveness of antibiotic prophylaxis.[39] While the risks of antibiotics seem to outweigh their clinically significant benefits, these identified risk factors should be taken into account, along with physician judgement and patient preferences, to determine appropriate therapy.

TABLE 6-5 • High-Risk Patient Characteristics for Infective Endocarditis and Joint Infection

High Risk for Infective Endocarditis
Prosthetic cardiac valves
History of infective endocarditis
Cardiac transplant patients with valvulopathy
Patients with cardiac valve repairs with prosthetic materials or device in the past 5 months
Unrepaired congenital heart defect
Repaired congenital heart defect with residual defect
High risk of hematogenous joint infection
Joint replacement within 2 years of surgery
History of prosthetic joint infection, hemophilia, diabetes mellitus, HIV, malignancy, malnutrition, or immunosuppression

Adapted with permission from Rossi AM, Mariwalla K: Prophylactic and empiric use of antibiotics in dermatologic surgery: a review of the literature and practical considerations. Dermatol Surg. *2012 Dec;38(12):1898-1921.*

TABLE 6-6 • Bacteria Present in Normal Skin Flora in Various Anatomic Locations

Location	Normal Skin Flora	Bacteria
Glabrous	*Staphylococcus aureus, Staphylococcus saprophyticus, Staphylococcus epidermis*	*S aureus*[a], *Streptococcus pyogenes, S epidermis*
Oral or nasal mucosa	*S aureus*, streptococci lactobacilli, corynebacteria, anaerobes	*Streptococcus viridans*, anaerobes (*Peptostreptococcus*)
Intertriginous	*Corynebacterium minutissimum, C lipophilicus, C xerosis, C jeikeium, Acinetobacter* species, *S aureus*	*S aureus*[a], *Escherichia coli, Enterococcus, Bacteroides, Pseudomonas aeruginosa, Corynebacterium, Candida, Serratia*
Sebaceous glands and follicles	*Propionibacterium acnes, P granulosum, P avidum*, Malassezia	*S aureus, Streptococcus*, anaerobic bacteria, *Pseudomonas*, gram-negative species

[a]*S aureus may be found as a natural resident of the skin.*

Data from Rossi AM, Mariwalla K. Prophylactic and empiric use of antibiotics in dermatologic surgery: a review of the literature and practical considerations. Dermatol Surg. *2012 Dec;38(12):1898-1921.*

ANTIBIOTIC SELECTION

Antibiotics should be chosen based on the likely causative pathogens, by considering local skin flora, and keeping in mind patient-specific needs such as allergies and the ability to tolerate oral medications. Wound culture and sensitivities often drive the final selection of the antibiotics. Benefits of antibiotics are weighed carefully against the risks of use. Antibiotics tend to be reserved for specific anatomic sites, complex procedures, and immunocompromised patients.

Skin Flora

Skin is colonized by many bacteria, which may vary by anatomic location (**Table 6-6**).[11] Mucous membrane bacteria tend to be colonized by *E coli*, *Streptococcus viridans*, and peptostreptococci. Intertriginous areas are often moist and macerated, predisposing to the growth of *S aureus* and streptococci. In diabetic patients, streptococcal and coliform bacteria can be found in the perioral area, ear, perineum, and anatomic sites below the waist.

S aureus has become increasingly important in terms of both causing severe SSIs and increasing intractability to antibiotic treatment. *S aureus* is commonly found in the mucosa, including the nasal mucosa (a common colonizing location), oropharynx, and anogenital area.[41] *S aureus* resistance has become more common and, in severe cases, may be associated with mortality rates up to 20%. While methicillin-resistant *S aureus* (MRSA) infections had been separated into those related to healthcare (HC-MRSA) and those that were community acquired (CA-MRSA), distinctions between HC-MRSA and CA-MRSA are currently much less clinically relevant as the evolution of the bacterial species has led to loss of the epidemiologic distinction.[41] The CA-MRSA clones have been increasingly found in hospital and healthcare facilities,[42] leading to increased concern for healthcare providers, as these highly virulent strains can infect otherwise healthy people.[43]

Other skin flora include nonbacterial causes such as *Candida* and less common fungal species such as *Cryptococcus*, *Aspergillus*, and *Mucor*, particularly in the immunosuppressed and immunocompromised population. Patients with skin conditions such as atopic dermatitis carry different bacterial strains. Prolonged antibiotic use may change local skin flora, just as vancomycin can disturb the natural gastrointestinal flora, which secrete antimicrobial peptides and indirectly facilitate the colonization of opportunistic pathogens.[44] Moreover, low-virulence streptococci are a concern for infectious endocarditis, and *S aureus* and *S epidermidis* are a concern for prosthetic joint infections.

With the increased prevalence of antibiotic resistance exemplified by *S aureus* and the slow development of new antibiotics, it is important to follow strict guidelines to prevent worsening resistance.[41]

Antibiotic Selection

In regard to the selection of antibiotics, guidelines are generally derived from the internal medicine and surgery literature because there are few randomized, double-blind studies of antibiotics in dermatologic surgery.[11] The choice of antibiotic use in dermatologic surgery is shown in **Table 6-7**. Cephalosporin and dicloxacillin are systemic agents used for prophylaxis on nonmucosal surfaces to cover gram-positive and gram-negative bacteria. Per AHA guidelines, *S viridans* and peptostreptococci can be treated with amoxicillin. For perineal skin, amoxicillin-clavulanate can be selected to combat potential penicillin-resistant organisms. For *Pseudomonas*, fluoroquinolones such as ciprofloxacin can be used. If a culture is obtainable, antibiotics can be selected based on antibiotic sensitivities. Otherwise, antibiotic use can be tailored to the bacteria most commonly found in the local population, the patient risk factors, the surgical site risk factors, and the surgical risk factors.

An advisory statement has recommended antibiotic therapy based on the procedure type and anatomic location as well as patient allergies to penicillin or inability to tolerate oral antibiotics (**Table 6-7**).[36] Cephalexin or dicloxacillin can be used as prophylaxis for wedge excisions of the lip or ear, flaps on the nose, and grafts. For those with penicillin allergy, clindamycin or azithromycin can be used, and TMP-SMX or levofloxacin may be used for anatomy sites in the groin or lower extremities. For patients who are unable to tolerate oral antibiotics, parenteral antibiotic therapy can be used. Finally, for patients who are unable to tolerate oral antibiotics and who have a penicillin allergy, clindamycin

TABLE 6-7 • Choice of Antibiotics for Prophylaxis in Patients at Risk of Surgical Site Infection

	Antibiotic (adult dose)			
Surgical site	No allergy	Penicillin allergy	Unable to take PO	Unable to take PO with penicillin allergy
Wedge excision of lip or ear, flaps on nose, grafts	Cephalexin or dicloxacillin (2 g PO)	Clindamycin (600 mg PO) or azithromycin/clarithromycin (500 mg PO)	Cefazolin/ceftriaxone (1 g IM/IV)	Clindamycin (600 mg IM/IV)
Groin or lower extremities	Cephalexin or TMP-SMX (2 g PO, double strength) or levofloxacin (1 tablet PO)	TMP-SMX (1 tablet PO, double strength) or levofloxacin (500 mg PO)	Ceftriaxone (1-2 mg IV)	Clindamycin and gentamicin (600 mg/2 mg/kg IV)

IM, intramuscular; IV, intravenous; PO, oral; TMP-SMX, trimethoprim-sulfamethoxazole.
Data from Lee MR, Paver R. Prophylactic antibiotics in dermatological surgery. Australas J Dermatol. 2016;57(2):83-91; Wright TI, Baddour LM, Berbari EF, et al. Antibiotic prophylaxis in dermatologic surgery: advisory statement 2008. J Am Acad Dermatol. 2008;59(3):464-473.

can be used and gentamicin added to cover for the possibility of *P aeruginosa* infection in the groin or lower extremities.[36]

Antibiotics are typically given the hour before the procedure. It is thought that this time permits the antibiotic to travel to the surgical site. Parenteral antibiotics are typically given a half an hour before the procedure. However, there are ambiguous data about whether prophylactic antibiotic timing affects the risk of SSI.[45] For longer procedures, the desired duration of action of the antibiotic should be considered. Blood can neutralize some antiseptics as well. For carriers of *S aureus*, transient decolonization of *S aureus* from the nasal area can significantly reduce the infection rate, and the use of topical mupirocin-chlorhexidine reduces the infection rate by half.[24,46]

For SSIs, wound culture, microscopy, and antibiotic sensitivities should ideally be performed, and antibiotics should be tailored based on the sensitivities.

TOPICAL ANTIBIOTICS

Postoperative topical antibiotics are not recommended for routine dermatologic surgery cases.[47] Numerous studies have evaluated whether the use of topical antibiotic ointment in the postoperative period is associated with a reduction in the already very low baseline risk of SSI in dermatologic surgery procedures, and results have generally suggested that for the majority of wounds, the use of topical antibiotics does not confer a significant advantage. A wide range of topical antibiotic preparations have been explored, including fusidic acid,[48] gentamicin,[49] mupirocin,[50] tobramycin-dexamethasone (combination preparation),[51] bacitracin,[52-54] neomycin-polymyxin (and in combination),[53] and chloramphenicol.[55] No rigorous study has demonstrated a robust statistically significant benefit to using any single topical antibiotic preparation, and the American Academy of Dermatology has therefore warned against the routine use of topical antibiotics after clean surgical procedures as part of its Choosing Wisely campaign.

The use of topical antibiotics may confer a risk to patients as well, since neomycin (11%) and bacitracin (8%) are the two most common causes of allergic contact dermatitis in a general patch-tested US population.[50] Inflammation risk may similarly be higher in patients treated with topical antibiotics rather than petrolatum.[56]

Although routine use of topical antibiotics is inadvisable, select surgical sites at increased risk of infection may benefit from the use of topical antibiotic therapy. One study examining the infection rate in a tropical Australian region found that a single dose of topical chloramphenicol (a topical antibiotic rarely used in the United States but popular in the United Kingdom and elsewhere) resulted in a statistically significant reduction in wound infection rate.[55] That study, however, evaluated wounds that were treated by general practitioners in Australia with a baseline infection rate in the control group of 11%, surgical sites that were possibly prepped with normal saline, and wounds that were closed with a single layer of nonabsorbable sutures; therefore, the generalizability of these findings to the generally low-risk dermatologic surgery population is unknown.

Although there is little evidence to support the practice, many of those performing dermatologic procedures—while eschewing the blanket use of topical antibiotic ointment in all surgical cases—will use these agents on select high-risk cases. Thus, wounds on the ears, nose, genitalia, lower extremities, and some flaps may benefit from the use of topical antibiotic preparations. In the United States, mupirocin is generally favored for its broad coverage and lack of significant risk of contact dermatitis. The effect on wound care compliance of providing patients with a prescription topical ointment has not been explored, although this may arguably represent an additional benefit of topical antibiotic use in select cases. As noted earlier, intranasal topical mupirocin may be useful preoperatively to temporarily decrease the nasal carriage of staphylococcal species.

INTRAINCISIONAL ANTIBIOTICS

Local injection of antibiotic formulations in the perioperative period has been investigated for dermatologic surgery. While local injection of aminoglycosides may be helpful to reduce the infection risk on open fractures,[57] one challenge in dermatologic surgery remains the vanishingly low baseline rate of SSIs, making any effect challenging to detect in a clinical trial setting.

One study demonstrated a statistically significant benefit to local intraincisional clindamycin injection for Mohs micrographic surgery cases.[58] This work was a follow-up to an earlier report on the use of intraincisional nafcillin.[59] The solution for intraincisional clindamycin use was prepared by adding 0.15 mL of clindamycin (150 mg/mL) to a 50-mL bottle containing lidocaine (1%) with epinephrine (1:100,000) buffered with sodium bicarbonate (5 mL of an 8.4% solution). The authors noted that the solution retained its bactericidal properties for at least 1 month after preparation. Given the low cost of clindamycin, it has been advocated as a reasonable approach in select patients and wounds. While this approach is not used broadly for all surgical cases, it may be a useful adjunct for wounds or patients at elevated risk of developing SSI.

CONCLUSIONS

Antibiotic use is a critical part of dermatologic surgery, although *appropriate* antibiotic use remains a significant challenge facing providers and patients. Given the low baseline SSI risk for most dermatologic surgery procedures, antibiotics—whether oral, topical, or intraincisional—are not routinely prescribed. For higher-risk surgical sites or patients with significant risk factors, however, antibiotics may play an important role in decreasing an elevated infection risk. In cases of active infection, antibiotic use, ideally guided by culture and sensitivity results, is warranted. All true abscesses, while rare, require drainage in addition to antibiotic treatment.

REFERENCES

1. Reddy KK, Grossman L, Rogers GS. Common complementary and alternative therapies with potential use in dermatologic surgery: risks and benefits. *J Am Acad Dermatol.* 2013;68(4):e127-e135.
2. Futoryan T, Grande D. Postoperative wound infection rates in dermatologic surgery. *Dermatol Surg.* 1995;21(6):509-514.
3. Cook JL. A prospective evaluation of the incidence of complications associated with Mohs micrographic surgery. *Arch Dermatol.* 2003;139(2):143.
4. Maragh SLH, Brown MD. Prospective evaluation of surgical site infection rate among patients with Mohs micrographic surgery without the use of prophylactic antibiotics. *J Am Acad Dermatol.* 2008;59(2):275-278.
5. Shurman DL, Benedetto AV. Antimicrobials in dermatologic surgery: facts and controversies. *Clin Dermatol.* 2010;28(5):505-510.
6. Awad SS. Adherence to surgical care improvement project measures and post-operative surgical site infections. 2012;13(4):234-237.
7. Owens PL, Barrett ML, Raetzman S, Maggard-Gibbons M, Steiner CA. Surgical site infections following ambulatory surgery procedures. *JAMA.* 2014;311(7):709-716.
8. Allegranzi SB, Bagheri Nejad S, Graafmans W, et al. First global patient safety challenge, WHO patient safety burden of endemic health-care-associated infection in developing countries: systematic review and meta-analysis. *Lancet.* 2011;377(377):228-241.
9. Centers for Disease Control and Prevention. Surgical Site Infection (SSI) Event. 2017;(January):1-14. https://www.cdc.gov/nhsn/pdfs/pscmanual/9pscssicurrent.pdf. Accessed March 20, 2017.
10. Lemperle G, Rullan PP, Gauthier-Hazan N. Avoiding and treating dermal filler complications. *Plast Reconstr Surg.* 2006;118(suppl 3): S92-S107.
11. Rossi AM, Mariwalla K. Prophylactic and empiric use of antibiotics in dermatologic surgery: a review of the literature and practical considerations. *Dermatol Surg.* 2012;38(12):1898-1921.
12. Beer K, Avelar R. Relationship between delayed reactions to dermal fillers and biofilms: facts and considerations. *Dermatol Surg.* 2014;40(11):1175-1179.
13. Kaplan AL, Cook JL, Ratner D, Gloster H. The incidences of chondritis and perichondritis associated with the surgical manipulation of auricular cartilage. *Dermatol Surg.* 2004;30(1):58-62.
14. Rohrich RJ, Monheit G, Nguyen AT, Brown SA, Fagien S. Soft tissue filler complications: the important role of biofilms. *Plast Reconstr Surg.* 2010;125(4):1250-1256.
15. Römling U, Balsalobre C. Biofilm infections, their resilience to therapy and innovative treatment strategies. *J Intern Med.* 2012; 272(6):541-561.
16. Christensen LH. Host tissue interaction, fate, and risks of degradable and nondegradable gel fillers. *Dermatol Surg.* 2009;35:1612-1619.
17. Saleh K, Schmidtchen A. Surgical site infections in dermatologic surgery. *Dermatol Surg.* 2015;41(5):537-549.
18. National Institute for Health and Care Excellence. Surgical site infection: guidance and guidelines. https://www.nice.org.uk/guidance/qs49. Accessed March 15, 2017.
19. Heal CF, Buettner PG, Drobetz H. Risk factors for surgical site infection after dermatological surgery. *Int J Dermatol.* 2012;51(7):796-803.
20. Alam M, Ibrahim O, Nodzenski M, et al. Adverse events associated with Mohs micrographic surgery. *JAMA Dermatol.* 2013;149(12): 1378-1385.
21. Dixon AJ, Dixon MP, Askew DA, Wilkinson D. Prospective study of wound infections in dermatologic surgery in the absence of prophylactic antibiotics. *Dermatol Surg.* 2006;32(6):819-826.
22. Gill JF, Yu SS, Neuhaus IM, Francisco S. Tobacco smoking and dermatologic surgery. *J Am Dermatol.* 2013;68:167-172.
23. Wahie S, Lawrence CM. Wound complications following diagnostic skin biopsies in dermatology inpatients. *Arch Dermatol.* 2007; 143(10):302-303.
24. Lee MR, Paver R. Prophylactic antibiotics in dermatological surgery. *Australas J Dermatol.* 2016;57(2):83-91.
25. Tanner J, Dumville JC, Norman G, Fortnam M. Surgical hand antisepsis to reduce surgical site infection. In: Tanner J, ed. *Cochrane Database of Systematic Reviews.* Chichester, United Kingdom: John Wiley & Sons, Ltd; 2016.
26. Mehta D, Chambers N, Adams B, Gloster H. Comparison of the prevalence of surgical site infection with use of sterile versus nonsterile gloves for resection and reconstruction during mohs surgery. *Dermatol Surg.* 2014;40(3):234-239.
27. Lilly E, Schmults CD. A comparison of high- and low-cost infection-control practices in dermatologic surgery. *Arch Dermatol.* 2012;148(7): 859-861.
28. Rogers HD, Carline JD, Paauw DS. Examination room presentations in general internal medicine clinic: patients' and students' perceptions. *Acad Med.* 2003;78(9):945-949.

29. Carmichael AJ, Flanagan PG, Holt PJ, Duerden BI. The occurrence of bacteraemia with skin surgery. *Br J Dermatol.* 1996;134(1):120-122. http://www.ncbi.nlm.nih.gov/pubmed/8745896. Accessed March 21, 2017.
30. Saleh K, Sonesson A, Persson B, Riesbeck K, Schmidtchen A. A descriptive study of bacterial load of full-thickness surgical wounds in dermatologic surgery. *Dermatol Surg.* 2011;37(7):1014-1022.
31. Bae-Harboe Y-SC, Liang CA. Perioperative antibiotic use of dermatologic surgeons in 2012. *Dermatologic Surg.* 2013;39(11):1592-1601.
32. Shehab N, Patel PR, Srinivasan A, Budnitz DS. Emergency department visits for antibiotic-associated adverse events. *Clin Infect Dis.* 2008;47(6):735-743.
33. Clark NP, Delate T, Riggs CS, et al. Warfarin interactions with antibiotics in the ambulatory care setting. *JAMA Intern Med.* 2014;174(3):409-416.
34. Parekh TM, Raji M, Lin Y-L, Tan A, Kuo Y-F, Goodwin JS. Hypoglycemia after antimicrobial drug prescription for older patients using sulfonylureas. *JAMA Intern Med.* 2014;174(10):1605-1612.
35. Avery CME, Ameerally P, Castling B, Swann RA, Cookson AV, Taylor L. Infection of surgical wounds in the maxillofacial region and free flap donor sites with methicillin-resistant *Staphylococcus aureus. Br J Oral Maxillofac Surg.* 2006;44(3):217-221.
36. Wright TI, Baddour LM, Berbari EF, et al. Antibiotic prophylaxis in dermatologic surgery: advisory statement 2008. *J Am Acad Dermatol.* 2008;59(3):464-473.
37. Alam M, Bastakoti B. Therapeutic guidelines: antibiotic. Version 15. *Aust Prescr.* 2015;38(4):137.
38. Wilson W, Taubert KA, Gewitz M, et al. Prevention of infective endocarditis: guidelines from the American Heart Association. *Circulation.* 2007;116(15):1736-1754.
39. Sollecito TP, Abt E, Lockhart PB, et al. The use of prophylactic antibiotics prior to dental procedures in patients with prosthetic joints: evidence-based clinical practice guideline for dental practitioners—a report of the American Dental Association Council on Scientific Affairs. *J Am Dent Assoc.* 2015;146:11-16.e8.
40. Council on Dental Therapeutics. Management of dental patients with prosthetic joints. *J Am Dent Assoc.* 1990;121(4):537-538. http://www.ncbi.nlm.nih.gov/pubmed/2145346. Accessed March 18, 2017.
41. Del Rosso JQ, Rosen T, Thiboutot D, et al. Status report from the Scientific Panel on Antibiotic Use in Dermatology of the American Acne and Rosacea Society part 3: current perspectives on skin and soft tissue infections with emphasis on methicillin-resistant *Staphylococcus aureus. J Clin Aesthet Dermatol.* 2016;9(6):17-24.
42. Mediavilla JR, Chen L, Mathema B, Kreiswirth BN. Global epidemiology of community-associated methicillin resistant *Staphylococcus aureus* (CA-MRSA). *Curr Opin Microbiol.* 2012;15:588-595.
43. Otto M. Community-associated MRSA: what makes them special? *Int J Med Microbiol.* 2013;303(6-7):324-330.
44. Gallo RL, Nakatsuji T. Microbial symbiosis with the innate immune defense system of the skin. *J Invest Dermatol.* 2011;131(10):1974-1980.
45. Hawn MT, Richman JS, Vick CC, et al. Re: Timing of surgical antibiotic prophylaxis and the risk of surgical site infection. *J Urol.* 2013;190(6):2102.
46. Bode LGM, Kluytmans JAJW, Wertheim HFL, et al. Preventing surgical-site infections in nasal carriers of *Staphylococcus aureus. N Engl J Med.* 2010;362(1):9-17.
47. Kreicher KL, Bordeaux JS. Addressing practice gaps in cutaneous surgery: advances in diagnosis and treatment. *JAMA Facial Plast Surg.* 2017;19(2):147-154.
48. Lee DH, Kim DY, Yoon SY, Park HS, Yoon HS, Cho S. Retrospective clinical trial of fusidic acid versus petrolatum in the postprocedure care of clean dermatologic procedures. *Ann Dermatol.* 2015;27(1):15-20.
49. Campbell RM, Perlis CS, Fisher E, Gloster HM Jr. Gentamicin ointment versus petrolatum for management of auricular wounds. *Dermatol Surg.* 2005;31(6):664-669.
50. Sheth VM, Weitzul S. Postoperative topical antimicrobial use. *Dermatitis.* 2008;19(4):181-189.
51. Andrew R, Luecke G, Dozier S, Diven DG. A pilot study to investigate the efficacy of tobramycin-dexamethasone ointment in promoting wound healing. *Dermatol Ther (Heidelb).* 2012;2(1):12.
52. Draelos ZD, Rizer RL, Trookman NS. A comparison of postprocedural wound care treatments: do antibiotic-based ointments improve outcomes? *J Am Acad Dermatol.* 2011;64(3 suppl):S23-S29.
53. Trookman NS, Rizer RL, Weber T. Treatment of minor wounds from dermatologic procedures: a comparison of three topical wound care ointments using a laser wound model. *J Am Acad Dermatol.* 2011;64(3 suppl):S8-S15.
54. Imber G. The use of bacitracin ointment to avoid shaving the scalp for rhytidectomy. *Plast Reconstr Surg.* 1992;90(2):339-340.
55. Heal CF, Buettner PG, Cruickshank R, et al. Does single application of topical chloramphenicol to high risk sutured wounds reduce incidence of wound infection after minor surgery? Prospective randomised placebo controlled double blind trial. *BMJ.* 2009;338:a2812.
56. Morales-Burgos A, Loosemore MP, Goldberg LH. Postoperative wound care after dermatologic procedures: a comparison of 2 commonly used petrolatum-based ointments. *J Drugs Dermatol.* 2013;12(2):163-164.
57. Lawing CR, Lin FC, Dahners LE. Local injection of aminoglycosides for prophylaxis against infection in open fractures. *J Bone Joint Surg Am.* 2015;97(22):1844-1851.
58. Huether MJ, Griego RD, Brodland DG, Zitelli JA. Clindamycin for intraincisional antibiotic prophylaxis in dermatologic surgery. *Arch Dermatol.* 2002;138(9):1145-1148.
59. Griego RD, Zitelli JA. Intra-incisional prophylactic antibiotics for dermatologic surgery. *Arch Dermatol.* 1998;134(6):688-692.

7 Ethics in Dermatologic Surgery

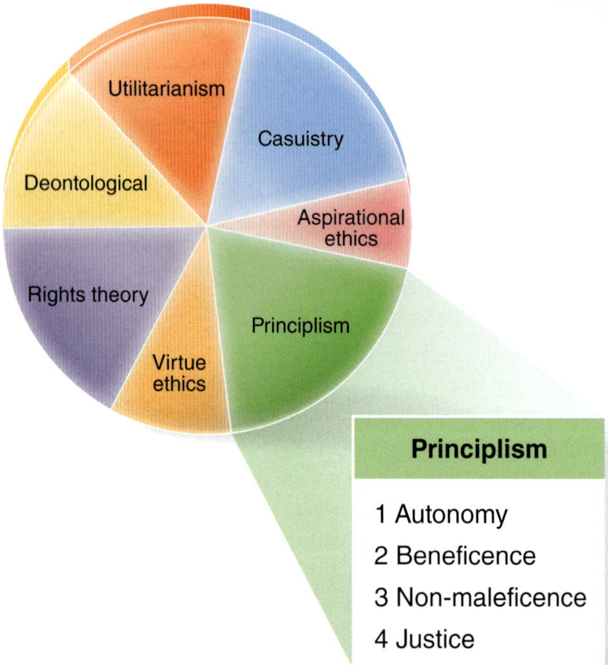

SUMMARY

- Ethical action, like informed consent, is a process.
- Most ethical challenges occur when there are conflicting principles, conflicting duties, or conflicting concepts of to whom the greatest—or least—ethical allegiance is owed.

Beginner Tips

- For centuries, philosophers have struggled with the distinctions between ethics, morality, law, and—more recently—professionalism.
- Ethics reflects a social imperative that is based on moral underpinnings; ethics can therefore be conceptualized as morality in action.

Don't Forget!

- Other approaches to ethical decision-making abound, including utilitarianism, aspirational ethics, casuistry, deontological approaches, rights theory, and virtue ethics.
- While cosmetic dermatology patients may interact with physicians as if they are *consumers*, rather than *patients*, they should still be treated as the latter.

Expert Tips

- Professional morality may be broader and deeper than common morality, as it addresses the moral expectations for a particular group.
- Principlism, perhaps the most popular ethical framework, relies on the (equally weighted) principles of autonomy, beneficence, nonmaleficence, and justice. These four principles are frequently used as a litmus test for ethical legitimacy.
- Morality is a social institution, and the common morality represents the core group of morals that are considered universally binding.

Pitfalls and Cautions

- Keep in mind that there is often more than one reasonable solution to an ethical quandary.
- An action can be legal without being ethical and ethical without being legal.
- Body dysmorphic disorder is a common condition, and identifying such patients is an important challenge for the cosmetic dermatologist, not least because the patient is likely to be dissatisfied after *any* intervention.
- The need for a consistent ethical framework led to the expansion of principlism to the point that the four principles are frequently used as a litmus test for ethical legitimacy, though the challenges of this model of applied ethics may be substantial.

Ethics in Dermatologic Surgery

7

INTRODUCTION

Appreciating and understanding the fundamentals of bioethics is of significant importance for those performing dermatologic procedures, both to better assess and evaluate the nature of ethical challenges and to better engage in informed ethical decision making. The epistemology of bioethics—how we know what falls within the boundaries of ethical actions and what does not—is worth exploring not simply as an intellectual exercise, but as a stepping stone to expanding our understanding of *why* a particular act is or is not the appropriate choice in any given situation.

Despite a 200-year trend of codifying ethical and professional mores, the subjective nature of morality and ethics may be challenging, particularly for physicians, who, as scientists, expect an objective and standardized system rather than a relativistic amalgam of duties and principles.

Ethical challenges may be of several varieties. Sometimes, a true moral or *ethical* dilemma is present, while at others the central challenge is a *practical* dilemma, where a sense of ethical obligation conflicts with either self-interest or pragmatic considerations. Most ethical challenges occur when there are conflicting principles, conflicting duties, or conflicting concepts of to whom the greatest—or least—ethical allegiance is owed.

Ethical action, like informed consent, is a process. Indeed, the very act of expressing concern regarding the ethical implications of an action constitutes a significant step in the right direction, as even professional ethicists may disagree regarding the ideal course of action in complex ethical cases. Real-world ethical challenges generally occur when various ethical imperatives are perceived as being in conflict or when various duties, and those to whom the clinician is responsible, appear to conflict.

HISTORY

Ethics has been a subject of discussion, debate, and deliberation for thousands of years. While the nascence of ethical and moral theories is often ascribed to ancient Greek philosophers, Mesopotamian writings and codes of law—as well as ancient Greek epic poems significantly predating the development of true Greek philosophy and the Old Testament itself—address fundamental ethical issues.[1] Subsequent ancient Greek philosophical writings, particularly those of Plato and Aristotle, formally codified a system of ethical thought.[2]

In ancient Greece, Socrates spoke at length of fundamental principles that would today be considered utilitarian, with a focus on creating the greatest good.[3,4] Aristotle is often considered the father of modern ethics, with his focus on eudaimonia; to Aristotle, appreciating the nature of ethics was a prerequisite to leading the ideal flourishing life.[5-10]

The origins of bioethics as a distinct field of inquiry may be traced to the 1770 publication of John Gregory's *Lectures on the Duties and Qualifications of a Physician* and the subsequent 1803 publication of Thomas Percival's *Medical Ethics* (**Figure 7-1**).[11-14] In Percival's code—later used as a model for the American Medical Association's (AMA) first *Code of Ethics*—he reviewed the ethical underpinnings of practice and duty in an organized fashion. It is no surprise that this occurred in the context of the Industrial Revolution and rapid developments in the field of medicine, when medical care had shifted from a Galenic worldview to a proto-scientific approach to inquiry.[15] Suddenly, the physician had a greater role to play in decisions that could reasonably have a major impact on the patient's life. Moreover, in the post-Enlightenment period, the desires of the patient as an individual also took on a more important role. Further, as society evolved from a medieval feudal system to the beginnings of the modern industrialized world that we know today, obligations—between worker and employer, citizen and country, and physician and patient—took on a more urgent role.[16] Finally, in the United States in the 1820s, with new world medical education

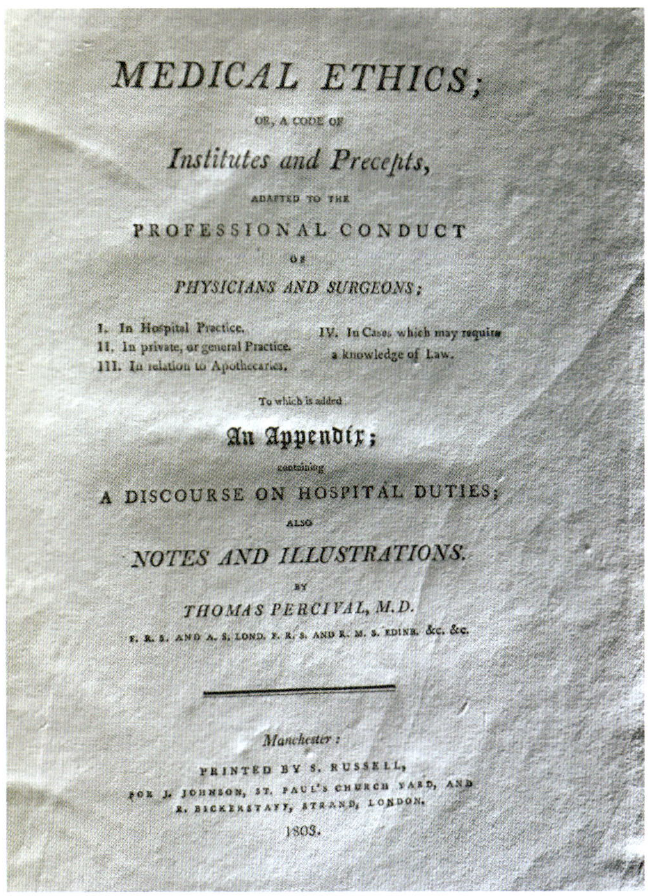
MEDICAL ETHICS;
OR, A CODE OF
Institutes and Precepts,
ADAPTED TO THE
PROFESSIONAL CONDUCT
OF
PHYSICIANS AND SURGEONS;
I. In Hospital Practice.
II. In private, or general Practice.
III. In relation to Apothecaries.
IV. In Cases which may require a knowledge of Law.
To which is added
An Appendix;
containing
A DISCOURSE ON HOSPITAL DUTIES;
ALSO
NOTES AND ILLUSTRATIONS.
BY
THOMAS PERCIVAL, M.D.
F. R. S. AND A. S. LOND. F. R. S. AND R. M. S. EDINB. &c. &c.
Manchester:
PRINTED BY S. RUSSELL,
FOR J. JOHNSON, ST. PAUL'S CHURCH YARD, AND
R. BICKERSTAFF, STRAND, LONDON.
1803.

FIGURE 7-1 First edition of Thomas Percival's medical ethics.

still in its infancy, physicians turned to self-regulation in an attempt to staunch the pressure from charlatans who were felt to be unfairly charging and improperly treating their unwitting patients.[1]

Modern warfare also impacted the perceived need for a robust grounding in medical ethics. From the bloody US Civil War to the trenches of the First World War and the mass slaughter of World War II, the very tools of industrialization that were lauded as harbingers of a truly brave new world were used to take military and civilian lives on a previously unimaginable scale.

With this backdrop, it is no surprise that ethics in medicine took on an even greater urgency in the 20th century. From Tuskegee to Josef Mengele, physicians—long lauded as working in their patients' best interests—were suddenly seen, as industrialization was in the centuries before, to represent a powerful force that could as easily harm as help.

ETHICS, LAW, MORALITY, AND PROFESSIONALISM

For centuries, philosophers have struggled with the distinctions between ethics, morality, law, and—more recently—professionalism. Morals, or common morality, represent a set of behaviors, actions, and imperatives that are so broadly understood to be true that they have been accepted as fundamental and universal. Horace noted over 2000 years ago that laws without morals are useless,[17] and indeed, while moral laws are desirable, only a fraction of moral actions are enumerated in law. Morality, therefore, is a social institution, and the common morality represents the core group of morals that are considered universally binding.

The common morality encompasses not only a set of obligations (do not kill, do not steal), but also a group of ideals and virtues (be charitable, help others when possible). These morals are universally accepted within a society, and their acceptance is often considered a precondition for entry and societal acceptance.[18]

Ethics reflects a social imperative that is based on moral underpinnings; ethics can therefore be conceptualized as morality in action. This is distinct from laws, which are specific rules that have attendant consequences and penalties when they are violated. A particular act may be ethical while being illegal (a woman driving alone in Saudi Arabia) or legal while being unethical (racist speech in the United States).

Professionalism, in contrast, focuses on the role of the physician as professional and expectations that are inherent in this professional role. Professional morality may be broader and deeper than common morality, as it addresses the moral expectations for a particular group.[19-22] Thus the American Academy of Dermatology's (AAD) Ethics Pledge, for example, includes a broader group of commitments than would be expected of a member of the general public.[23] Indeed, biomedical ethics has been codified repeatedly, whether in Percival's book, the AMA's original ethics code (first published in 1847), or the AAD's Ethics Pledge.

ETHICAL FRAMEWORKS

Principlism

Over the past few decades, biomedical ethics, particularly in the United States, has become largely synonymous with principlism.

TABLE 7-1 • Principles of Bioethics

Principle	Definition
Autonomy	Patients should be treated as autonomous agents.
Beneficence	Patients should be treated for their benefit.
Non-maleficence	Patients should not be harmed.
Justice	There should be fairness in ethical action.

Note: All principles are weighted equally.

This ethical framework, stemming largely from the seminal Belmont Report, focuses on four principles considered when evaluating an ethical conundrum (**Table 7-1**).[24] The Belmont Report outlined the principles of respect for persons (autonomy), beneficence (and nonmaleficence), and justice. These principles have been popularized and are now so enmeshed in the modern understanding of bioethics that principlism is in many areas seen as synonymous with bioethics.

First, the principle of autonomy focuses on the premise that individuals should be treated as unique persons and that their individual autonomous choices should be respected. The corollary of this approach is that those with diminished autonomy (children, prisoners, and others) should be entitled to special protection. Second, the principle of beneficence touches on an obligation by physicians to secure the well-being of their patients. In the Belmont Report, its corollary, nonmaleficence, or *not* harming the patient, was included under a single rubric. Finally, the principle of justice touches on an underlying need for fairness.

The need for a consistent ethical framework led to the expansion of principlism to the point that the four principles are frequently used as a litmus test for ethical legitimacy. Still, the challenges of this model of applied ethics may be substantial,[25,26] and some philosophers have argued that the very model of medical ethics appropriating philosophical doctrines is flawed.[11]

Casuistry

The casuistic method involves the extrapolation of the circumstances of one accepted or paradigmatic case to a new circumstance in order to develop a valid ethical decision (**Table 7-2**).[27-30] This approach, rooted in Talmudic and ancient Christian exegesis, is frequently applied today in the field of law. Rather than relying on potentially arbitrary principles, the casuistic approach instead turns to paradigmatic cases where the ethical course of action has either already been determined or is prima facie clear. While this approach is predicated on the proper determination of relevant cases,[31] its advantage is that it is rooted in an intuitive common sense approach to ethics.

Utilitarianism

Unlike principlism, predicated on the inherent value of a set of accepted principles, utilitarianism is a consequentialist approach

TABLE 7-2 • Ethical Approaches

Approach	Definition
Principlism	Four principles determine ethical action.
Casuistry	Prior cases determine ethical action.
Utilitarianism	Maximizing benefits determines ethical action.
Deontological	Rules dictate ethical action.
Rights theory	Respecting the actor's rights determines ethical action.
Virtue ethics	Cultivating virtues determines ethical actions.
Aspirational ethics	Obligations (at a minimum) and supererogation (ideally) determine ethical action.

that aims to do the greatest good for the greatest number—to maximize utility.[32,33] One advantage of utilitarianism is that it does not require the intellectual exercise of accepting four, and only four, principles as the bedrock of ethical action. Still, a utilitarian approach that requires the physician to dispassionately create the most good (or cause the least harm) over all else necessarily creates secondary questions, including perspective (doing the most good for whom?), paternalism (who decides on what is the most good?), and possible ethical conflicts (utilitarianism embodies the idea that the end indeed justifies the means). Other concerns regarding utilitarianism include the demandingness objection (the concept that pure utilitarianism may be too demanding to be adopted on a practical level)[34] and the risks of unjust distribution, as doing the greatest good for the greatest number may consistently marginalize minority groups.

Deontological Approaches

Deontological, or rules-based, ethical approaches are another prism through which ethical action may be viewed.[32,33] Kant's categorical imperative aims to simplify and codify ethical action by stating that one should never act except in such a way that they would wish the maxim driving their actions to become universal. His approach has also been outlined as the unacceptability of treating others as a means alone. This obligation-oriented approach is fundamentally different from the utilitarian approach, where the *outcomes* of the action govern its ethical legitimacy; for the Kantian, the *motives* of the action decide on its ethical grounding.

Another deontological approach is the divine command theory—the idea that while adherence to rules and obligations indeed determines the rightness of an action, the source of such obligations is not a rational actor's decision, but divine law. Thus, religiously rooted ethical frameworks represent a form of deontological ethics; the rightness and morality of an action are determined by whether it was ordered by God.

Rights Theory

Rights theory, the concept that the ethics of an action are determined based on their alignment with a set of human rights, is another approach to bioethics.[35] The idea of moral rights (what the target of action is *owed*) differs fundamentally from the idea of moral obligation (what the actor is *obligated* to do), although in practice ethical actions often align. Since rights represent an entitlement, they may be attractive when trying to protect a group of patients. Yet since rights theory does not address the rights of the community at large, it leads to possible challenges when attempting to formulate a general framework for biomedical ethics that may be applied universally.

Virtue Ethics

Unlike utilitarian and deontological approaches, virtue ethics focuses not on the obligations of an actor, but on the underlying virtues that are cultivated by individual actions.[21,36-45] If an action cultivates virtuous traits, then it is ethical. Like Kant, an Aristotelian virtue ethics approach determines an action's value based on the *motivations* of the actor, not their actions. A virtue ethics approach embodies the idea that character is destiny; obligation-oriented approaches that set out a minimum list of rules and obligations do not, to the virtue ethicist, lead to better behavior. Virtuous judgments, therefore, are seen as the basis of ethical action.

Virtue ethics has been used to delineate a set of ideal virtues—the professional responsibility model—for the physician leader as well.[20] Such virtues include self-effacement, self-sacrifice, compassion, and integrity. Like principlism, virtue ethics may be criticized for its seemingly arbitrary selection of virtues, a shortcoming that becomes particularly apparent when disparate virtues are functionally competing.

Aspirational Ethics

Aspirational ethics is a synthesis of obligation- and virtue-based approaches.[34,46-48] Like obligation ethics, it accepts that there is a set of obligations that may be codified to set a *minimum* level of acceptable behavior. But like virtue ethics, aspirational ethics focuses on cultivating a set of actions that motivate the actor, essentially moving from the normative (what is absolutely required) to the supererogative (what would be ideal).[34,46,47] By combining the strengths of principlism, utilitarianism, and deontological approaches (setting an ethical floor) with the ideals of virtue ethics (aiming for an ethical ceiling), aspirational ethics both guarantees basic safeties and protections while concomitantly promoting growth and excellence.

COMMON ISSUES FACING THOSE PERFORMING DERMATOLOGIC PROCEDURES

Patient Privacy and Autonomy

There is a rich literature on patient autonomy. Various manuscripts have addressed the treatment of the impaired patient, the minor patient, and the prisoner.[49-57] Ethically, the chief challenges associated with privacy and autonomy are when the ethical mandate to maintain privacy conflicts with others.

Regardless of the ethical paradigm used, maintaining patient privacy is an absolute ethical requirement for clinicians. Pragmatically, if patients cannot rely on the privacy of their consultations, the fundamental physician-patient relationship may be undermined.[58-61]

Duty and Honesty

The issue of *duty* is important when considering ethical situations[18,36,62,63]; most clinicians see themselves as obligated exclusively to the patient and perceive that they have a fiduciary duty to their patient alone. In this context, an ethical choice may be interpreted as acceding to the patient's request.

A physician's duty, however, is not only to the patient; it is also to the profession, the healthcare system at large, and the insurer with whom the clinician has a contractual relationship. From a principlist approach, this also touches on the principle of justice. Others have suggested that truth-telling itself is a principle, rather than a virtue.[64] Those performing dermatologic procedures should never take any steps that could erode patients' trust in physicians overall, as our standing—and thus our ability to have patients share openly and honestly—is based on perceived honesty and integrity.[65-71]

Cosmetic Procedures

Patients may present for cosmetic intervention with a variety of concerns, and a reluctance to rely on paternalism, coupled with the economic realities of an out-of-pocket reimbursement schedule, has led to the embrace of a patient-as-client phenomenon. Yet the ethical obligations of the physician remain unchanged, regardless of whether the patient is presenting for cosmetic or medical treatment.

Body dysmorphic disorder is a common condition, and identifying such patients is an important challenge for the clinician, not least because the patient is likely to be dissatisfied after *any* intervention.[72-88] Ethically, performing a procedure on a patient with body dysmorphic disorder, or even a patient with clearly unrealistic expectations, is problematic. From a principlist standpoint, this would violate the principle of nonmaleficence, and from a Kantian perspective, the physician's motivation is likely not the patient's best interests.

Clinical Research

As with other situations resulting from solicitations, it is important to consider the *motivations* for performing clinical research. This Kantian approach is helpful in evaluating the ethical merits of performing this type of work and the appropriate interactions that should take place both with the research sponsor and the clinical trial participants.

Clinical research is a burgeoning area in medicine overall and, indeed, a necessary component in the development of both novel and generic medications.[89-92] While it should not be pursued solely as a potential profit center, fair reimbursement for clinical research work is reasonable and indeed necessary.

Industry Funding

Despite significant efforts to protect medical education from the impact of industry funding and potential bias, a significant proportion of continuing medical education material is industry sponsored, either directly or indirectly.[93-98]

Industry funding is pervasive, as demonstrated by a recent manuscript highlighting the range of payments from pharmaceutical companies to dermatologists.[99] Accepting payments from industry is not ethically fraught per se, although significant evidence has demonstrated that even accepting drug samples has an impact on prescribing patterns.[100,101]

CONCLUSIONS

Those performing dermatologic procedures face ethical challenges on a daily basis. A basic appreciation of the various approaches to ethical decision making is helpful for the practicing clinician as well as the trainee. Ultimately, most ethical guidelines set only a floor for ethical action, limiting frankly unethical actions. Aspiring to a higher level of patient-centered surgical care aids the provider and patient alike.

REFERENCES

1. Leake CD. Percival's code: a chapter in the historical development of medical ethics. *JAMA.* 1923;81(5):366-371.
2. Hamarneh SK. Practical ethics in the health professions. Part I: the Hammurabi and Hippocratic codes. *Hamdard Med.* 1993;36(1):11-24.
3. Pellegrino ED. Socrates at the bedside. *Pharos Alpha Omega Alpha Honor Med Soc.* 1983;46(1):38.
4. Dunea G. Socrates on clinical excellence. *Lancet.* 1973;2(7827):493-494.
5. Saunders J. Bringing back Aristotle. *Indian J Med Ethics.* 2011;8(4):230-233.
6. Allmark P. An argument for the use of Aristotelian method in bioethics. *Med Health Care Philos.* 2006;9(1):69-79.
7. Hauskeller M. Telos: the revival of an Aristotelian concept in present day ethics. *Inquiry (Oslo).* 2005;48(1):62-75.
8. Gillies J, Sheehan M. Practical reasoning and decision making—Hippocrates' problem, Aristotle's answer. *Br J Gen Pract.* 2002;52(479):518-519.
9. Cornell JF. On the relevance of Aristotle's bioethics. *Politics Life Sci.* 1988;6(2):199-201, 226-199.
10. Price AW. Aristotle's ethics. *J Med Ethics.* 1985;11(3):150-152.
11. Baker R, Emanuel L. The efficacy of professional ethics: the AMA Code of Ethics in historical and current perspective. *Hastings Cent Rep.* 2000;30(4 suppl):S13-S17.
12. Namm JP, Siegler M, Brander C, Kim TY, Lowe C, Angelos P. History and evolution of surgical ethics: John Gregory to the twenty-first century. *World J Surg.* 2014;38(7):1568-1573.
13. Stratling M. John Gregory (1724-1773) and his lectures on the duties and qualifications of a physician establishing modern medical ethics on the base of the moral philosophy and the theory of science of the empiric British Enlightenment. *Med Secoli.* 1997;9(3):455-475.
14. Haakonssen L. Medicine and morals in the Enlightenment: John Gregory, Thomas Percival and Benjamin Rush. *Clio Med.* 1997;44:i-x, 1-247.

15. Pellegrino ED. Percival's medical ethics. The moral philosophy of an 18th-century English gentleman. *Arch Intern Med.* 1986;146(11):2265-2269.

16. Thomas Percival (1740-1804) codifier of medical ethics. *JAMA.* 1965;194(12):1319-1320.

17. Horace. *The Odes and Epodes of Horace.* Boston, MA: Ginn & Co; 1896.

18. Horner J. Morality, ethics, and law: introductory concepts. *Semin Speech Lang.* 2003;24(4):263-274.

19. McCullough LB, Grunebaum A, Arabin B, Brent RL, Levene MI, Chervenak FA. Ethics and professional responsibility: essential dimensions of planned home birth. *Semin Perinatol.* 2016;40(4):222-226.

20. Chervenak FA, McCullough LB, Brent RL. The professional responsibility model of physician leadership. *Am J Obstet Gynecol.* 2013;208(2):97-101.

21. McCammon SD, Brody H. How virtue ethics informs medical professionalism. *HEC Forum.* 2012;24(4):257-272.

22. Kinghorn WA. Medical education as moral formation: an Aristotelian account of medical professionalsim. *Perspect Biol Med.* 2010;53(1):87-105.

23. Stoff BK, Scully K, Housholder AL, Fabbro S, Kantor J. The American Academy of Dermatology (AAD) Ethics Pledge: I will put my patients' welfare above all other interests, provide care that adheres to professional standards of practice, provide care for those in need, and foster collegiality through interaction with the medical community. *J Am Acad Dermatol.* 2016;75(2):445-448.

24. Protection of human subjects; Belmont Report: notice of report for public comment. *Fed Regist.* 1979;44(76):23191-23197.

25. Davis RB. The principlism debate: a critical overview. *J Med Philos.* 1995;20(1):85-105.

26. Strong C. Specified principlism: what is it, and does it really resolve cases better than casuistry? *J Med Philos.* 2000;25(3):323-341.

27. Spielthenner G. The casuistic method of practical ethics. *Theor Med Bioeth.* 2016;37(5):417-431.

28. Cudney P. What really separates casuistry from principlism in biomedical ethics. *Theor Med Bioeth.* 2014;35(3):205-229.

29. Iltis AS. Bioethics as methodological case resolution: specification, specified principlism and casuistry. *J Med Philos.* 2000;25(3):271-284.

30. Kuczewski M. Casuistry and principlism: the convergence of method in biomedical ethics. *Theor Med Bioeth.* 1998;19(6):509-524.

31. Beauchamp TL. Reply to Strong on principlism and casuistry. *J Med Philos.* 2000;25(3):342-347.

32. Mandal J, Ponnambath DK, Parija SC. Utilitarian and deontological ethics in medicine. *Trop Parasitol.* 2016;6(1):5-7.

33. Playford RC, Roberts T, Playford ED. Deontological and utilitarian ethics: a brief introduction in the context of disorders of consciousness. *Disabil Rehabil.* 2015;37(21):2006-2011.

34. Kantor J, Lushniak BD. Excellence in medicine and the case for aspirational ethics. *JAMA Dermatol.* 2016;152(9):971-972.

35. Ketchum SA, Pierce C. Rights and responsibilities. *J Med Philos.* 1981;6(3):271-280.

36. Crisp R. The duty to do the best for one's patient. *J Med Ethics.* 2015;41(3):220-223.

37. Chen JY. Virtue and the scientist: using virtue ethics to examine science's ethical and moral challenges. *Sci Eng Ethics.* 2015;21(1):75-94.

38. Misselbrook D. Waving not drowning: virtue ethics in general practice. *Br J Gen Pract.* 2015;65(634):226-227.

39. Misselbrook D. Virtue ethics: an old answer to a new dilemma? Part 2. The case for inclusive virtue ethics. *J R Soc Med.* 2015;108(3):89-92.

40. Misselbrook D. Virtue ethics: an old answer to a new dilemma? Part 1. Problems with contemporary medical ethics. *J R Soc Med.* 2015;108(2):53-56.

41. Han H. Virtue ethics, positive psychology, and a new model of science and engineering ethics education. *Sci Eng Ethics.* 2015;21(2):441-460.

42. Allmark P. Virtue and austerity. *Nurs Philos.* 2013;14(1):45-52.

43. Stovall P. Professional virtue and professional self-awareness: a case study in engineering ethics. *Sci Eng Ethics.* 2011;17(1):109-132.

44. Shelton W. Can virtue be taught? *Acad Med.* 1999;74(6):671-674.

45. Gauthier CC. Teaching the virtues: justifications and recommendations. *Camb Q Healthc Ethics.* 1997;6(3):339-346.

46. Pena A. A critique of the (aspirational) code of ethics. *Am J Bioeth.* 2015;15(5):62-63.

47. Candilis PJ, Martinez R. Commentary: the higher standards of aspirational ethics. *J Am Acad Psychiatry Law.* 2006;34(2):242-244.

48. Kantor J, Lushniak BD. Commentary: ethics in dermatology. *J Am Acad Dermatol.* 2016;75(2):443-444.

49. Buchanan DR. Autonomy, paternalism, and justice: ethical priorities in public health. *Am J Public Health.* 2008;98(1):15-21.

50. Dawson A, Garrard E. In defence of moral imperialism: four equal and universal prima facie principles. *J Med Ethics.* 2006;32(4):200-204.

51. Baumrucker SJ, Easterday J, Stolick M, et al. Ethics roundtable: parental autonomy and the minor patient. *Am J Hosp Palliat Care.* 2017;34(3):287-292.

52. Caenazzo L, Tozzo P, Rodriguez D. Hospitalized hunger-striking prisoners: the role of ethics consultations. *Med Health Care Philos.* 2016;19(4):623-628.

53. Trestman RL. Ethics, the law, and prisoners: protecting society, changing human behavior, and protecting human rights. *J Bioeth Inq.* 2014;11(3):311-318.

54. O'Neill D, Collins R. Medical ethics and prisoners. *Lancet.* 2009;373(9667):896.

55. Pont J. Ethics in research involving prisoners. *Int J Prison Health.* 2008;4(4):184-197.

56. Arboleda-Florez J. The ethics of biomedical research on prisoners. *Curr Opin Psychiatry.* 2005;18(5):514-517.

57. Stone TH. Currents in contemporary ethics. Discerning minimal risk in research involving prisoners as human subjects. *J Law Med Ethics.* 2004;32(3):535-537.

58. Mena MC. EMR push will erode privacy, physician-patient relationship and increase risk. *Tenn Med.* 2009;102(8):9.

59. Coleman PG, Shellow RA. Privacy and autonomy in the physician-patient relationship. Independent contracting under Medicare and implications for expansion into managed care. *J Leg Med.* 1995;16(4):509-543.

60. Sugarman J, Powers M. How the doctor got gagged. The disintegrating right of privacy in the physician-patient relationship. *JAMA.* 1991;266(23):3323-3327.

61. Wilcox DP. The right of privacy and the physician-patient relationship. *Tex Med.* 1985;81(4):84-85.

62. Stoff BK, Bercovitch L, Grant-Kels JM. The case for equal access to urgent dermatology appointments for Medicaid beneficiaries: when professional duty conflicts with economic reality. *J Am Acad Dermatol.* 2015;72(1):181-183.
63. Sokol DK. Law, ethics, and the duty of care. *BMJ.* 2012;345:e6804.
64. Maley A, Swerlick R, Parker D, Stoff B. Should dermatopathologists participate in diagnostic error disclosure to patients? An ethical analysis. *J Am Acad Dermatol.* 2015;72(5):901-904.
65. Sisk B, Frankel R, Kodish E, Harry Isaacson J. The truth about truth-telling in American medicine: a brief history. *Perm J.* 2016; 20(3):74-77.
66. Isaacs D. Telling the truth. *J Paediatr Child Health.* 2016;52(6): 585-586.
67. Madhiwalla N. The ethics of truth telling. *South Asian J Cancer.* 2013;2(2):53-54.
68. Collis SP. The importance of truth-telling in health care. *Nurs Stand.* 2006;20(17):41-45.
69. Sokol DK. How the doctor's nose has shortened over time; a historical overview of the truth-telling debate in the doctor-patient relationship. *J R Soc Med.* 2006;99(12):632-636.
70. Gold M. Is honesty always the best policy? Ethical aspects of truth telling. *Intern Med J.* 2004;34(9-10):578-580.
71. Chiodo GT, Tolle SW. Therapeutic privilege and truth telling. *Gen Dent.* 1994;42(6):504, 506-507.
72. de Brito MJ, Nahas FX, Cordas TA, Tavares H, Ferreira LM. Body dysmorphic disorder in patients seeking abdominoplasty, rhinoplasty, and rhytidectomy. *Plast Reconstr Surg.* 2016;137(2):462-471.
73. Spriggs M, Gillam L. Body dysmorphic disorder: contraindication or ethical justification for female genital cosmetic surgery in adolescents. *Bioethics.* 2016;30(9):706-713.
74. Vashi NA. Obsession with perfection: body dysmorphia. *Clin Dermatol.* 2016;34(6):788-791.
75. Affleck A, Stewart M. Body dysmorphic disorder in dermatology: beware of diagnostic overlabelling. *Clin Exp Dermatol.* 2016;41(2):214-215.
76. Mavrogiorgou P, Bader A, Stockfleth E, Juckel G. Obsessive-compulsive disorder in dermatology. *J Dtsch Dermatol Ges.* 2015;13(10):991-999.
77. Rieder E. Approaches to the cosmetic patient with potential body dysmorphia. *J Am Acad Dermatol.* 2015;73(2):304-307.
78. Sarwer DB, Spitzer JC, Sobanko JF, Beer KR. Identification and management of mental health issues by dermatologic surgeons: a survey of American Society for Dermatologic Surgery members. *Dermatol Surg.* 2015;41(3):352-357.
79. Brunton G, Paraskeva N, Caird J, et al. Psychosocial predictors, assessment, and outcomes of cosmetic procedures: a systematic rapid evidence assessment. *Aesthetic Plast Surg.* 2014;38(5):1030-1040.
80. Winfree WJ, Rouse LE, Brown RS. Body dysmorphic disorder and cosmetic dentistry: diagnostic, management, and ethical issues. *Dent Today.* 2014;33(3):72-74; quiz 75.
81. Ziglinas P, Menger DJ, Georgalas C. The body dysmorphic disorder patient: to perform rhinoplasty or not? *Eur Arch Otorhinolaryngol.* 2014;271(9):2355-2358.
82. Gupta MA, Gupta AK. Evaluation of cutaneous body image dissatisfaction in the dermatology patient. *Clin Dermatol.* 2013;31(1):72-79.
83. Conrado LA, Hounie AG, Diniz JB, et al. Body dysmorphic disorder among dermatologic patients: prevalence and clinical features. *J Am Acad Dermatol.* 2010;63(2):235-243.
84. Goodman MP. Female cosmetic genital surgery. *Obstet Gynecol.* 2009;113(1):154-159.
85. Hill MJ. Body dysmorphic disorder: implications for practice. *Dermatol Nurs.* 2006;18(1):13.
86. Glaser DA, Kaminer MS. Body dysmorphic disorder and the liposuction patient. *Dermatol Surg.* 2005;31(5):559-560; discussion 561.
87. Castle DJ, Phillips KA, Dufresne RG Jr. Body dysmorphic disorder and cosmetic dermatology: more than skin deep. *J Cosmet Dermatol.* 2004;3(2):99-103.
88. Phillips KA, Dufresne RG. Body dysmorphic disorder. A guide for dermatologists and cosmetic surgeons. *Am J Clin Dermatol.* 2000;1(4):235-243.
89. Jones DS, Grady C, Lederer SE. "Ethics and clinical research": the 50th anniversary of Beecher's bombshell. *N Engl J Med.* 2016;374(24):2393-2398.
90. Harnett JD, Neuman R. Research ethics for clinical researchers. *Methods Mol Biol.* 2015;1281:19-30.
91. Woods S, McCormack P. Disputing the ethics of research: the challenge from bioethics and patient activism to the interpretation of the Declaration of Helsinki in clinical trials. *Bioethics.* 2013;27(5):243-250.
92. DeBruin DA, Liaschenko J, Fisher A. How clinical trials really work rethinking research ethics. *Kennedy Inst Ethics J.* 2011;21(2):121-139.
93. Fugh-Berman A, Hogenmiller A. CME stands for commercial medical education: and ACCME still won't address the issue. *J Med Ethics.* 2016;42(3):172-173.
94. Meixel A, Yanchar E, Fugh-Berman A. Hypoactive sexual desire disorder: inventing a disease to sell low libido. *J Med Ethics.* 2015;41(10):859-862.
95. Lineaweaver W. Conflicts of interest, disclosures, CME credits, and censorship. *Ann Plast Surg.* 2015;74(1):1-2.
96. Lo B, Ott C. What is the enemy in CME, conflicts of interest or bias? *JAMA.* 2013;310(10):1019-1020.
97. Davis NL, Galliher JM, Spano MS, Main DS, Brannigan M, Pace WD. Evaluating conflicts of interest in research presented in CME venues. *J Contin Educ Health Prof.* 2008;28(4):220-227.
98. McMahon GT. Accreditation rules safeguard continuing medical education from commercial influence. *J Med Ethics.* 2016;42(3):171.
99. Feng H, Wu P, Leger M. Exploring the industry-dermatologist financial relationship: insight from the open payment data. *JAMA Dermatol.* 2016;152(12):1307-1313.
100. Katz KA, Reid EE, Chren MM. The good, the bad, and the ugly of free drug samples. *JAMA Dermatol.* 2014;150(11):1238.
101. Hurley MP, Stafford RS, Lane AT. Characterizing the relationship between free drug samples and prescription patterns for acne vulgaris and rosacea. *JAMA Dermatol.* 2014;150(5):487-493.

Billing and Financial Considerations in Dermatologic Surgery

8

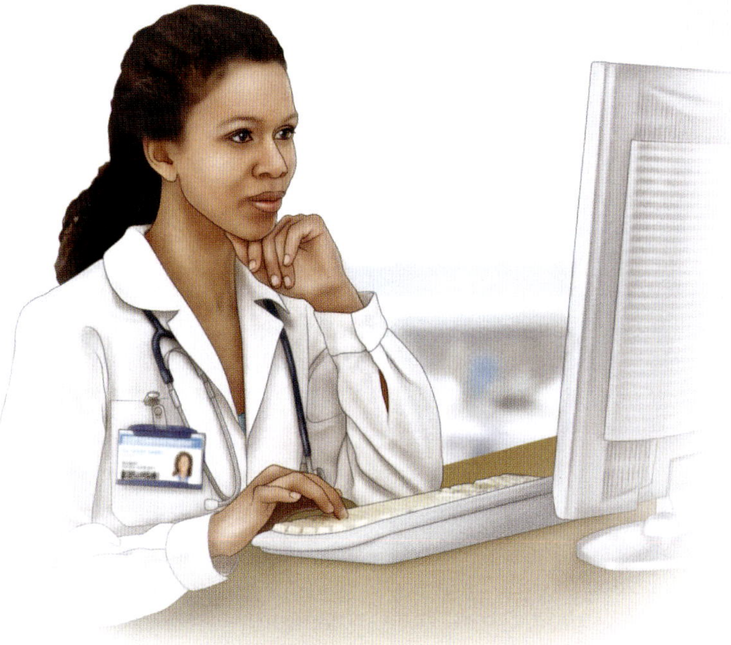

SUMMARY

- The goal of complete and accurate coding is to clearly define to a payer what was performed during a given patient care interaction.
- Each procedural charge submitted to a payer must be correlated with a valid diagnostic code.

Beginner Tips

- Determine the excision code size by adding the maximum lesion diameter to that of the summed narrowest bilateral excision margins.
- If a patient evaluation leads to a 90-day global procedure done on the same day, then the evaluation and management service is separately billable with modifier .57 appended.

Don't Forget!

- When more than one repair of the same type (simple, intermediate, or complex) is done within one anatomical area, sum the lengths of the repairs and bill for one closure, as directed by the site and sum of the of the repair lengths. If repairs of the same type are done in different anatomical code group areas, then bill each one individually
- A Z-plasty generated from the edge of a flap to promote the flap's mobility does not constitute an additional separate flap.

Expert Tips

- Redundant tissue removal (standing cones or dog ears) does not elevate an otherwise linear closure procedure to the level of a flap, though it may turn an otherwise intermediate into a complex linear repair.
- When a defect or a portion of a defect is repaired with a Burow's graft generated from a linear excision and closure adjoining the defect, only the skin graft procedure is billable, as the graft code includes the excision and direct closure of the donor defect. Mohs surgery is still billable separately, though it may be subject to the multiple procedure reduction rule.

Pitfalls and Cautions

- Avoid using "unspecified" (NOS—Not Otherwise Specified) diagnostic codes, highlighted in yellow in the ICD-10 manual, as this indicates that the medical record lacked sufficient information for a more precise code selection. Some insurers may deny claims with "unspecified" codes.
- Excisions of epidermal inclusion and pilar cysts that extend into the subcutaneous space should be coded with the integumentary excision codes, as these entities are of skin, and not subcutaneous, origin.

Patient Education Points

- It is worth explaining to patients that physicians will bill insurance companies as a courtesy to them, but that ultimately it is the patient's responsibility to cover the cost of any procedures performed.
- Explaining that the clinician is bound by the terms of a contract with the insurer helps the patient understand that the clinician is indeed their ally.

8 Billing and Financial Considerations in Dermatologic Surgery

INTRODUCTION

Billing should tell a story, and the goal of billing is not to maximize reimbursement, but to accurately reflect what was done in the office. The goal of complete and accurate coding is to clearly define to a payer what was performed during a given patient care interaction. As this information is typically transmitted electronically via diagnostic, procedural, and modifier codes, it is essential to proper claim adjudication that the codes precisely define what was done and that the patient record support the transmitted billing data.

Although electronic health records and practice management programs may prompt diagnostic and procedure code selections, it is essential to be familiar with optimal diagnostic and procedural code definitions and correlations, as ultimately correct coding is the physician's responsibility. To that end, minimal essential coding sources are the latest International Classification of Diseases, 10th Revision, Clinical Modification (ICD-10-CM) diagnostic coding manual and the Current Procedural Terminology (CPT) manual, both of which are available from the American Medical Association (AMA) and from other sources.

Part of the billing process should also consider whether a given problem and its treatment are considered medically necessary covered services or not medically necessary or not covered. Medicare, for example, excludes coverage for procedures not aimed at improving a patient's health or function, and most private insurers have similar expectations.

ESSENTIALS OF CODING

ICD-10-CM: Diagnostic Coding

Each procedural charge submitted to a payer must be correlated with a valid diagnostic code. The chart record must specify data facilitating precise code selection. This includes a specific diagnosis or tumor type, including anatomic location and laterality. The billing system and/or biller should be able to successfully select an appropriate diagnostic code based on the submitted information. Similarly, insurers, upon chart audit, should be able to readily extract the same information from the patient record.

ICD-10 code selection should be performed to the highest level of specificity available within each code set. If a code listed in the ICD-10 manual is accompanied by an adjacent red box, then the more detailed codes below this listing should be selected, as insurers are unlikely to pay for an inadequately specific diagnosis code. Essential documentation and code selection steps for ICD-10 coding are listed in **Table 8-1**. It is important to note that common tumors (eg, basal cell carcinoma, squamous cell carcinoma, benign nevi) and some rare tumors (eg, Merkel cell carcinoma) have dedicated diagnostic codes, while many others do not. If the tumor diagnosis is known, then select a tumor-specific code. If a specific code is not available, then select an "other specified malignant neoplasm" site-specific code. **Table 8-2** provides a listing of common skin neoplasms and their ICD-10 code series.

When a patient evaluation consists substantially of monitoring for new or recurrent tumor appearance, one may justify the visit with an ICD-10 diagnosis of personal or family skin cancer history, listed in **Table 8-3**.

CODING HINT

Avoid using "unspecified" (NOS—not otherwise specified) diagnostic codes, highlighted in yellow in the ICD-10 manual, as this indicates that the medical record lacked sufficient information for a more precise code selection. Some insurers may deny claims with "unspecified" codes.

Current Procedural Terminology (CPT): Procedural Coding

The CPT manual specifies numerical or alphanumerical codes for medical services. These codes are linked to appropriate ICD-10-CM diagnostic codes for the purposes of transactional record keeping and billing.

Essential to the process is an understanding of the CPT manual, which contains several sets of codes. Category I numerical codes represent the bulk of the manual and are used for specifying most physician services. Category II codes, consisting of four numbers followed by the letter F, are tracking/performance measurement codes and may be used for data collection. They are typically not necessary for billing. These codes are distinct from the "quality" reporting measures (Physician Quality Reporting System [PQRS]) that may be reported for the purpose of avoiding Medicare payment reductions. Category III codes are temporary codes defining emerging technology, services, or procedures. They are sometimes reimbursable, are also used for tracking utilization of the item that they specify, and should be used whenever a service specified by those codes is provided. They are identified by four numbers followed by the letter T. Dermatologic procedures are served by several Category III codes

TABLE 8-1 • Essential ICD-10 Coding Parameters

- Tumor type
  - Specific diagnosis known
    - Use tumor-specific code if available
    - Specific code not available: use "other specified malignant neoplasm" code
  - Uncertain diagnosis: neoplasm of uncertain behavior: D48.5 (skin); D37.01 (lip mucosa)
- Tumor location—always specify
- Laterality—left or right

TABLE 8-2 • ICD-10-CM Codes for Common Cutaneous Neoplasms

Tumor	ICD-10 Code Series
Actinic keratosis	L57.0
Basal cell carcinoma	C44 series
Benign neoplasm, lip mucosa	D10.0
Benign neoplasm, penis	D29.0
Benign neoplasm, scrotum	D29.4
Benign neoplasm, skin	D23 series
Benign neoplasm, vulva	D28.0
Cherry angioma	I78.8
Cyst, eyelid	H02.82 series
Cysts, other, follicular, of skin	L72.8
Epidermal inclusion cyst	L72.0
Hemangioma, skin and subcutaneous	D18.01
Hypertrophic scar	L91.0
Lipoma	D17 series
Malignant melanoma	C43 series
Malignant neoplasm, lip vermilion	C00. series
Malignant neoplasm, type known	C44 series
Mass/swelling	R22 series
Melanoma in situ	D03 series
Merkel cell carcinoma	C4A series
Neoplasm, uncertain behavior	D48.5
Nevus, melanocytic	D22 series
Pilar cyst	L72.11
Port wine stain	Q82.5
Pyogenic granuloma	L98.0
Sebaceous cyst (steatocystoma)	L72.3
Seborrheic keratosis	L82.1
Seborrheic keratosis, inflamed	L82.0
Spider angioma	I78.1
Squamous cell carcinoma	C44 series
Squamous cell carcinoma in situ, penis	D07.4
Squamous cell carcinoma in situ	D04 series
Strawberry angioma	Q82.5
Trichodermal (proliferating pilar) cyst	L72.12
Venous lake	I78.8

(**Table 8-4**). These codes may eventually be changed to Category I codes if their utilization/reporting were to support such a need. Appendix A of the CPT also lists modifier codes, which will be addressed further in this chapter.

TABLE 8-3 • Personal or Family History of Malignant Neoplasm ICD-10 Codes

Z85.42	Personal history of malignant neoplasm of other female genital organs
Z85.49	Personal history of malignant neoplasm of other male genital organs
Z85.818	Personal history of malignant neoplasm of other sites of lip, oral cavity
Z85.820	Personal history of malignant melanoma of skin
Z85.821	Personal history of Merkel cell carcinoma
Z85.828	Personal history of other malignant neoplasm of skin (BCC, SCC, others)
Z85.831	Personal history of malignant neoplasm of soft tissue
Z80.8	Family history of malignant neoplasm of other organs or systems (may be used for specifying family history of melanoma)

BCC, basal cell carcinoma; SCC, squamous cell carcinoma.

COMMON DERMATOLOGIC SURGERY CODES

Most dermatology-related CPT codes appear in the Integumentary System section of the codebook (codes 10030-19499). All of these procedure codes include local anesthesia in their definitions.

Tangential Biopsy: 11102 and 11103

Definition: Removal or sampling skin tissue or mucous membrane for histopathologic examination using a tangential shave approach (the traditional shave biopsy). The depth of the biopsy may extend partially into the skin or through the skin, encompassing underlying subcutaneous or muscle tissue. While the code definition specifies skin or mucous membrane biopsy, there are several other, site-specific biopsy codes that may be used. Since coding should be performed to the most exacting specificity, the site-specific codes (**Table 8-5**) should be used when appropriate.

TABLE 8-4 • Dermatology-Related Category III CPT Codes

0394T	High-dose-rate electronic brachytherapy, skin surface application, per fraction, includes basic dosimetry, when performed
0400T	Multispectral digital skin lesion analysis of clinically atypical cutaneous pigmented lesions for detection of melanomas and high-risk melanocytic atypia; one to five lesions
0401T	Multispectral digital skin lesion analysis; six or more lesions

TABLE 8-5 • Site-Specific Biopsy Codes

CPT Code	Definition
11102	Tangential (shave) biopsy of skin, subcutaneous tissue, and/or mucous membranes
11103	Each separate/additional lesion
11104	Punch biopsy (including simple closure)
11105	Each separate/additional lesion
11106	Incisional biopsy
11107	Each separate/additional lesion
11755	Biopsy of nail unit (plate, bed, matrix, hyponychium, proximal and lateral nail folds)
30100	Biopsy, intranasal
40490	Biopsy of lip mucosa
40808	Biopsy, vestibule of mouth
41100	Biopsy of tongue; anterior two-thirds
41105	Biopsy of tongue; posterior one-third
41108	Biopsy of floor of mouth
54100	Biopsy of penis
56605	Biopsy of vulva or perineum; one lesion
56606	Biopsy of vulva or perineum, each separate additional lesion
67810	Incisional biopsy of eyelid skin including lid margin
69100	Biopsy external ear

CODING HINT

CPT code 67810 is to be used only when lid margin, extending across the lash line to the conjunctival mucosa, is biopsied. Tangential biopsy of the skin of the eyelid is to be coded with 11102 or 11103.

Punch Biopsy: 11104 or 11105

Definition: A biopsy performed using a punch instrument. The same code is used whether or not sutures are placed (do not bill separately for a repair even if the wound is sutured).

Incisional Biopsy: 11106 or 11107

Definition: A wedge-shaped biopsy of tissue (eg, as used to sample a suspected melanoma). This code is rarely used in practice.

CODING HINT

When multiple biopsies are performed, even of different types (tangential/punch/incisional), only a single primary biopsy code should be used, and the other biopsies are coded with their add-on codes. The priority of the primary code is incisional ⟶ punch ⟶ tangential. For example, if two biopsies are performed (one punch and one tangential), the appropriate coding would be 11104 and 11103.

Shaving of Epidermal or Dermal Lesions: 11300-11313

Definition: Removal of epidermal or dermal lesions via a transverse, horizontal incision. Proper codes are determined by the maximum *diameter* of the removed lesion. Depth of lesion removal does not penetrate into the subcutaneous fat. No suturing is required for this coding level. Code selection requires specifying the location and diameter of the lesion. Typical use of a shave code would be to specify tangential removal of a benign nevus, a fibrous papule, a cherry angioma, or a seborrheic keratosis.

CODING HINT

If the depth of lesion removal extends beyond the dermis and into the subcutaneous space, then a shave removal code is not appropriate. Select a biopsy or excision code.

Excisions, Benign and Malignant: 11400-11646

Definition: Full-thickness, through the dermis lesion removal, including margins, and simple closure. The CPT does not require that the closure of a defect be performed in order to qualify for an excision code. The appropriate code is determined by the lesion location and the maximum diameter of the lesion including the narrowest margin required bilaterally. The lesion and margin measurements must be performed prior to the actual excision, because following an excision the tissue tends to rebound away from the excision center, thereby enlarging any diameter measurement (**Figure 8-1**). The integumentary excision codes include local anesthesia and a simple (nonlayered) repair in their definition and valuation. Whenever an intermediate or complex repair is necessary, it is coded in addition to the appropriate excision code.

CODING HINT

Determine the proper code by adding the maximum lesion diameter to that of the summed narrowest bilateral excision margins *prior to excision.*

Several localized special excisional procedures are characterized by their own descriptive excision codes, listed in **Table 8-6**. Note that the excisions in **Table 8-6** include closure, even when

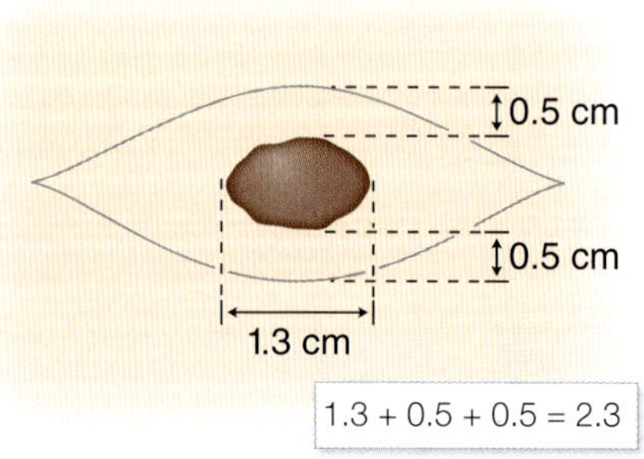

FIGURE 8-1 When billing for an excision, add the largest diameter of the defect as well as any necessary margins.

TABLE 8-6 • Special Excision Procedure Codes

Nail Unit	
11750	Excision of nail and nail matrix, partial or complete, for permanent removal
Nose	
30120	Excision or surgical planing of skin of nose for rhinophyma
Lips	
40500	Vermilionectomy (lip shave), with mucosal advancement
40510	Excision, transverse wedge excision with primary closure
40520	V-excision with primary direct linear closure
40530	Resection of lip, more than one-fourth, without reconstruction
Mouth Vestibule	
40810	Excision of lesions of mucosa and submucosa; without repair
• 40812	With simple repair
• 40814	With complex repair
• 40816	Complex, with excision of underlying muscle
Tongue	
41110	Excision of lesion of tongue without closure
41112	Excision of lesion of tongue with closure; anterior two-thirds
Ear	
69110	Excision external ear; partial, simple repair

not specified, so that separate intermediate or complex repair should not be coded in addition to the excision code.

Soft-Tissue Excision (Musculoskeletal Section of CPT)

Codes specifically dedicated to the excision of subcutaneous and subfascial tumors are grouped in multiple locations within the musculoskeletal section of the CPT, starting with code 21011 for an excision of a subcutaneous tumor less than 2 cm in diameter on the face or scalp and ending with 28041 and 28045 for subfascial tumor excisions on the foot or toe.

These specialized codes are appropriate for resection of typically benign tumors of subcutaneous or subfascial origin, such as lipomas. Code selection is based on tumor location on the body, whether it is subcutaneous or subfascial in origin, and upon its maximum diameter being either above or below a limit specified by an individual code. The medical record should substantiate the depth of excision and the type of tumor excised. Radical resection codes, such as 21015 for face or scalp, are major procedures reserved for aggressive tumor resections, such as deep tissue sarcomas.

CODING HINT

Excisions of epidermal inclusion and pilar cysts that extend into the subcutaneous space should be coded with the integumentary excision codes, as these entities are of skin, and not subcutaneous, origin (CPT Assistant, April 2010).

Repairs

All repair codes include local anesthesia and wound closure with sutures, staples, or tissue adhesives. Closure with adhesive strips only does not merit a repair code and is included in an evaluation and management code. Code selection is based on location and measured length of the repair.

CODING HINT

When more than one repair of the same type (simple, intermediate, or complex) is done within one anatomic area, sum the lengths of the repairs and bill for one closure, as directed by the site and sum of the repair lengths. If repairs of the same type are done in different anatomic code group areas, then bill each one individually.

Simple Repair: 12001-12021

Definition: Single-layer closure for a usually superficial wound. Biopsy and excision codes include a simple repair. These codes would be used for a laceration repair with a single layer of sutures.

Intermediate Repair: 12031-12057

Definition: Specifies "wounds that, in addition to simple repair, require layered closure of one or more deeper layers of subcutaneous tissue and (non-muscle) fascia, in addition to the skin (epidermal and dermal) closure." Typically, the medical record would include a justification for an intermediate repair, such as reducing closure line tension, obliterating dead space, or providing stability to the wound. Rarely, an intermediate repair may be justified when extensive removal of particulate matter is done prior to a single-layer closure (as in some involved laceration repairs). These codes would be used for a laceration repair with two layers of sutures.

Complex Repair: 13100-13153

Definition: These repairs are more involved than a layered closure and include any of the following: scar revision, debridement, extensive undermining, dog-ear correction, stents, or retention suture placement. The most common dermatologic surgical justification for complex repair coding is extensive (broad) undermining, although this definition is not specifically addressed in the CPT or other official publications. The breadth of undermining required to qualify as "extensive" will vary by anatomic site as, for example, what one may consider to be broad undermining on the nose tip would not necessarily be the same as that on a cheek. It is clear, however, that undermining done minimally beyond the wound edges in order to optimize apposition is not extensive undermining. Consequently, undermining alone does not justify a complex repair code. It has to be extensive (broad) and documented as such. In addition, document why extensive undermining was performed, such as due to tension across the wound or to reduce distortion.

CODING HINT

The length of a repair of standing cones (Burow's triangles, "dog ears") is contiguous with the principal repair itself and should be included in the final repair length measurement.

CLINICAL SCENARIO

Your patient returns with a wound dehiscence, which you clean and repair. How do you code for the procedure? If the procedure is, in your judgement (and documented), extensive or complicated, use CPT 13160, *Secondary closure of surgical wound or dehiscence, extensive or complicated.* If it requires a simple closure, use CPT 12020, and if packing was included, then use 12021.

Destruction: 17000-17004, 17100-17111, 17260-17286

The destruction code set is principally stratified into two major sections, one dedicated to the destruction of malignant lesions and the other for benign or premalignant entities. Both categories include destructions by "any method," with examples being laser surgery, electrosurgery, cryosurgery, chemosurgery, and surgical curettage. Specialized destruction categories are dedicated to vascular proliferative lesions (17106-17108) and to the chemical cauterization of granulation tissue (17250). Typically, no tissue is submitted for histopathology prior to the destruction of a benign or premalignant lesion, but there is nothing in the codes prohibiting histopathologic examination, if that were medically necessary. The CPT also offers some special site-specific destruction codes (**Table 8-7**).

Malignant Destruction: 17260-17286

Coding is specified by lesion location and diameter, performed either prior to the destruction, after curettage, or after electrodesiccation or chemical hemostasis. Because curettage may reveal substantial subclinical extension of a tumor, it is best to measure following curettage, as that will yield the most accurate indication of a lesion's diameter. Electrodesiccation can shrink the apparent diameter, so it is prudent to avoid measurements following electrodesiccation, if curettage is first done. It is helpful to identify in the medical record both the lesion diameter and at which point it was measured (eg, following curetting). The depth of curettage is not required to be recorded but can be useful for evaluating the risk of tumor recurrence.

TABLE 8-7 • Site-Specific CPT Destruction Codes

- 40820 Vestibule of mouth, by physical methods
- 46900 Anus, simple; chemical
  - 46910 Simple, electrodesiccation
  - 46916 Simple, cryosurgery
  - 46917 Simple, laser surgery
  - 46922 Surgical excision
- 46924 Anus, extensive[a] (laser, electrosurgery, cryosurgery, chemosurgery)
- 54050 Penis, simple; chemical
  - 54055 Simple, electrodesiccation
  - 54056 Simple, cryosurgery
  - 54057 Simple, laser surgery
  - 54060 Surgical excision
- 54065 Penis, extensive[a] (laser, electrosurgery, cryosurgery, chemosurgery)
- 56501 Vulva, simple (laser, electrosurgery, cryosurgery, chemosurgery)
- 56515 Vulva, extensive[a] (laser, electrosurgery, cryosurgery, chemosurgery)

[a]*"Extensive" is not specifically defined in the CPT.*

CODING HINT

If one first samples presumed malignant tissue for histopathologic evaluation immediately prior to its destruction, then no separate biopsy or shave removal charge is allowed. The removal of the lesion in the setting of its destruction is included in the destruction code set.

Adjacent Tissue Transfer or Rearrangement (Flaps): 14000-14302

Definition: Includes excision of a lesion as well as a repair of the defect by adjacent tissue transfer or rearrangement, with one exception: Mohs surgery–generated excisions are separately billable from any repair code, including flap repairs. The CPT specifies that the extent of undermining to generate tissue motion does not make the procedure a flap. For example, broad undermining of a cheek to facilitate "advancing" it to close a nasofacial sulcus or preauricular defect linearly does not constitute a flap procedure. Proper flap codes are determined by the location of the defect and by the measured square centimeters of the primary defect plus that of the secondary defect created by the raised (detached) portion of the flap. This sum constitutes the "defect" size. The CPT provides code selection based on lesion location and defect surface areas of 10 cm^2 or less, 10.1 to 30.0 cm^2, 30.1 to 60.0 cm^2, any area (14301), and each additional 30.0 cm^2 beyond 60.0, any area (14302).

CODING HINT

Redundant tissue removal (standing cones, Burow's triangles, "dog ears") does not elevate an otherwise linear closure procedure to the level of a flap. (CPT Assistant, April 2014, page 10).

There are flaps (CPT 15570-15738) outside of the adjacent tissue rearrangement section that are used in dermatologic surgery. One should avoid using code 15740 (*Flap; island pedicle requiring identification and dissection of an anatomically named axial vessel*) unless the strict criterion for its use (identifying and dissecting out a named vessel) is met. Just because a named vessel may be identified and contained in the body of a V-Y flap (but not dissected out) does not qualify a repair as an island pedicle flap.

CODING HINT

A bilateral advancement flap constitutes one flap with two sections, just as a bilobed transposition flap is one flap with two lobe components. A Z-plasty generated from the edge of a flap to promote the flap's mobility does not constitute an additional separate flap. In the above cases, one would bill based on the sum of the measured surface areas of the excision defect plus that of all of the raised flap components, including any Z-plasty.

Skin Replacement Surgery (Grafts): 15002-15278

This section has steadily expanded as technology has facilitated the development of skin substitutes. Coding is determined by the type of graft used, the location onto which it is placed, and the square centimeter surface area of the defect covered by the graft. Full-thickness skin graft codes (15200-15261) include excision of the donor skin and direct closure of the donor site. A complicated repair of a surgical defect may require a combination of a flap repair as well as a skin graft. In such cases, both the flap and the graft are separately billable.

CODING HINT

When a defect or a portion of a defect is repaired with a "kite graft" or a Burow's graft generated from a linear excision and closure adjoining the defect, only the skin graft procedure is billable, as the graft code includes the excision and direct closure of the donor defect.

GENERAL CONSIDERATIONS

Global Surgical Periods

Each surgical CPT code is presently assigned a global surgical period, which indicates a time of 0, 10, or 90 days after the procedure during which routine office visits related to the procedure are not billable, as payment for such is included in the surgery valuation. Routine visits include wound checks, patient counseling, bandage changes, and suture removal (**Table 8-8**). Any necessary services provided following a 0-day global procedure are billable. Ten-day global periods include the day of the procedure plus 10 days starting on the day after the procedure. Ninety-day global periods include the day before, the day of, and 90 days starting the day after a surgery. Common dermatologic surgical codes and their global periods are listed in **Table 8-9**.

CODING HINT

If a patient evaluation leads to a 90-day global procedure done on the same day, then the evaluation and management service is separately billable, with modifier .57 appended (see Modifiers, below).

Modifiers

Appendix A of the CPT lists numerical modifiers that are to be appended to CPT codes to distinguish certain services or situations. Whenever an evaluation and management (E/M) encounter or a billable procedure is performed during the global period, one must append an appropriate modifier to the primary billing code to specify that the service provided is unrelated to the global period service (**Table 8-10**).

TABLE 8-8 • Services Included in a Global Period

- Preoperative visits: day of surgery for 10-day global (minor) procedures and day before surgery for 90-day global (major) procedures
- Postoperative complications not requiring a return to the operating room (eg, hemorrhage, infection)
- Postoperative follow-up visits
- Dressing changes, surgical site care, removal of sutures or staples
- Decision to perform a minor (10-day global) procedure made on the day of the procedure

TABLE 8-9 • Common Dermatology-Related Global Periods and CPT Codes

0 Days	10 Days	90 Days
Biopsy (11102-11107)	Destruction (17000-17286)	Flaps (14000-14301; 15570-15760)
Shave removal (11300-11313)	Excisions (11400-11646)	Grafts (15050-15260; 15760)
Debridement (11000-11043)	Repairs (12001-13153)	Tissue expanders
		Mohs surgery (17311-17315)
		Destruction of vascular proliferative lesion (17106-17108)
		Dermabrasion, chemical peel

Therefore, this entails tracking of preceding services and their global periods. Modifier .24 is appended to E/M codes during the global period, and .79 is added to surgical/procedural codes billed during the global period. When a distinct, separately identifiable E/M service is provided on the day of a procedure, one appends modifier .25 to the E/M service code. The patient record should support such a claim. Routine billing of an E/M code along with every procedure will cast one as an outlier biller and is likely to eventually result in insurance company action, such as in the form of a focused chart audit.

Occasionally, one will perform a second procedure, related to the first, during the global period. Typical scenarios include a wide excision of a melanoma within 10 days following an initial diagnostic excision, or a division and inset of an interpolation flap

TABLE 8-10 • Modifiers Commonly Used in Dermatologic Surgery

- 24: Unrelated evaluation and management (E/M) service by the same physician or other qualified healthcare professional during a postoperative period
- 25: Significant, separately identifiable E/M service by the same physician or other qualified healthcare professional on the same day of the procedure or other service
- 57: Decision for surgery (refers to E/M service resulting in a decision to perform a 90-day global surgery the day of or day after the evaluation)
- 58: Staged or related procedure or service by the same physician or other qualified healthcare professional during the postoperative period
- 59: Distinct procedural service (append to distinguish additional procedures performed on same day)
- 76: Repeat procedure or service by the same physician or other qualified healthcare professional
- 79: Unrelated procedure or service by the same physician or other qualified healthcare professional during the postoperative period

during its 90-day global period. Such services require appending a .58 modifier, indicating that the second procedure is a consequence of the first.

Finally, those performing dermatologic procedures frequently perform more than one procedure, such as multiple malignant neoplasm destructions or actinic keratoses destructions along with unrelated lesion biopsies or destructions, during one patient encounter. Insurers must distinguish that the procedures done were separately identifiable and individually payable. Modifier .59 specifies distinct procedural services and should be appended to secondary procedures done on 1 day. Medicare, however, may require a .76 modifier when two or more procedures are done for an identical diagnosis or when the two procedures have the same CPT procedure code. Thus, if a Medicare claim that seems properly coded with a .59 modifier is rejected, one should consider appending a .76 modifier instead.

The choice regarding which code should have no modifier (primary code) and which should have a modifier is based on the National Correct Coding Initiative (NCCI), a project of the Centers for Medicare and Medicaid Services (CMS) dedicated to promoting correct coding and generating guidelines so as to avoid improper payments for Medicare outpatient services. The entity generates a Policy Manual for Medicare Services and quarterly updated procedure-to-procedure (column 1/column 2) edits that specify whether a service paired with another is covered and, if so, which should be subject to the .59 modifier. **Figure 8-2** illustrates the format of the NCCI edits and commonly used edits. The NCCI may be accessed at https://www.cms.gov/Medicare/Coding/NationalCorrectCodInitEd.

GENERAL NCCI EDITS GUIDELINE

- When a malignant destruction is done during the same encounter as a biopsy, append the .59 modifier to the biopsy code.
- When a premalignant destruction (17000) is done during the same encounter as a biopsy (11100), malignant destruction (17260-17286), or benign or malignant excision (11400-11446; 11600-11646), append a .59 modifier to the biopsy, destruction, or excision codes.
- Add-on codes (eg, 11101 and 17003) do not merit a .59 modifier, as only the primary code receives the modifier.

Insurance Coverage Policies

Compulsively correct coding will yield no reimbursement if the procedures that are done are not considered medically necessary or are noncovered services. To that end, it is useful to know whether an insurer is likely to cover a given service. With Medicare, coverage decisions are typically reached in a transparent and reproducible fashion. CMS publishes National Coverage Determinations (NCD) that specify coverage for certain conditions. Specific to dermatology is the actinic keratosis NCD, which states that treatment of actinic keratoses is a covered service. Of greater use and impact are the Medicare Administrative Contractors' Local Coverage Determinations (LCDs), which are coverage documents issued for select conditions or procedures as a consequence of high utilization, as a result of suspected or proven fraud and abuse, due to a perception of overuse, or due to standardize criteria for documentation and coverage. The LCDs specify coverage criteria, covered ICD-10 codes, pertinent CPT codes, and documentation requirements. If one fails to satisfy the LCD requirements, payment may not be forthcoming, or a refund may be requested upon audit. That should be sufficient reason to be familiar with LCD content. The most common LCDs are for Mohs surgery and benign skin lesion treatments. The LCDs can be readily accessed from the relevant Medicare Administrative Contractor (MAC) websites.

Advanced Beneficiary Notice

The Advanced Beneficiary Notice (ABN; form CMS-R-131) is a written notice that the physician must provide to a Medicare fee-for-service patient before delivering services that are usually covered by Medicare but are not expected to be paid in a specific instance for a specific reason, such as "lack of medical necessity." The ABN allows the Medicare beneficiary to be made aware that Medicare likely will not pay, and the beneficiary can decide whether or not to have the procedure done. When an ABN is required and the patient has been properly instructed and has signed the form, you can then receive payment from the patient. If Medicare feels that the ABN is invalid or if you failed to obtain one when indicated, you may be financially liable if Medicare does not pay. If payment was collected from the patient in this instance, the payment must be refunded in a timely manner. Items not covered under Medicare are listed on the CMS website at https://www.cms.gov/Outreach-and-Education/Medicare-Learning-Network-MLN/MLNProducts/Downloads/Items-and-Services-Not-Covered-Under-Medicare-Booklet-ICN906765.pdf.

BILLING HINT

If unsure as to whether a service will be covered by the patient's insurer, have the patient sign a fully filled out ABN, available from the MAC or CMS website, prior to providing the service.

Cosmetic Procedures

Report either ICD-10 code Z41.1 (*Encounter for cosmetic surgery*) for procedures that are strictly cosmetic in nature (eg, nontherapeutic toxin injections or fillers) and then the 17999 CPT code

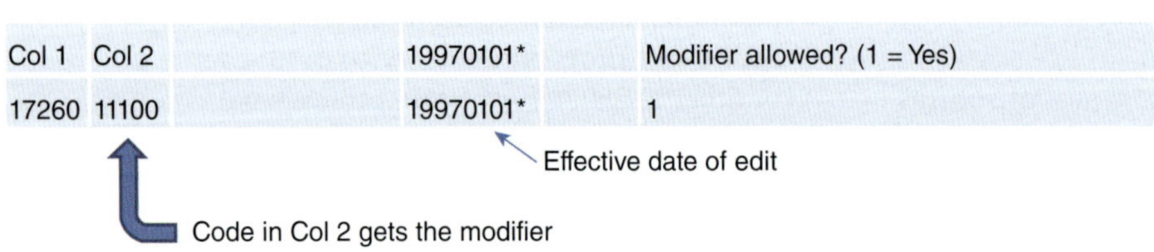

FIGURE 8-2 NCCI edits demonstration. These tables dictate which procedure code receives a modifier for each distinct code pair.

with whatever price was quoted to the patient or code Z41.8 (*Encounter for procedure for purposes other than remedying health state*) when the procedure may not be considered cosmetic in all circumstances but is so in a particular case (eg, nonirritated benign moles or skin tags), whichever is most appropriate, and then the CPT code for whatever procedure was done.

Insurer's Perspectives

Health insurance will typically cover services that are both reasonable and necessary. It is incumbent upon the medical practitioner to record data supporting the decisions for care. If, upon chart audit, such information is not discoverable, a claim may be denied. Each insurer may also have its own requirements for coverage or preferred claims adjudication criteria. Inappropriate denials of claims should be discoverable within one's practice. This requires a feedback and information sharing system between the billing/collections department and those actually doing the charting and generating billing—the medical care providers. This interactive interplay will facilitate discovering and correcting faulty billing patterns and/or record keeping and will stimulate appeals of improperly unpaid or underpaid claims.

Keep in mind that insurers use systems that analyze individual billing patterns, comparing them to a normal distribution curve of billings. If a practice's billing pattern rises to two standard deviations above the norm, then that practice is more likely to catch the insurer's attention and be audited. If exposed to a focused audit, one would have to prove, case by case, why each patient required the complexity of care that they received.

Another subject for insurers' concern is overall cost of care. If a given practice is particularly costly to the system, then that system may want to investigate why, or may even want to drop the practice from its provider panel. It would then be up to the practice to prove why they have the expensive patient care mix and how their practice is essential for the care of the insured patients. Insurers, and particularly MACs, are concerned about "cloning" of chart material, whereby patient data are passed on virtually verbatim from one encounter to the next. Although cloning of individual surgical encounters is less likely, it is possible, particularly via electronic health records system facilitation, to have surgical procedure verbiage that is identical from one to another surgery and from one patient to another. It is helpful to insert case-specific nuances into the surgical report so that all reports do not seem identical. Finally, surgical reports should allow for extraction of pertinent care and billing data.

CONCLUSIONS

Accurate and precise coding and billing require those performing dermatologic procedures to work in a logical and precise fashion. Documenting the medical necessity for every procedure is of paramount importance, and linking each procedure code to the appropriate ICD-10 diagnosis code, as well as to modifiers, if needed, will permit payers to rapidly and reliably decide on the merits of an individual's coding. Attention to detail ultimately results in fewer denials and rejections, a higher paid claims rate, a lower audit rate, and a smoother billing experience overall. Ultimately, it is the practitioner's responsibility to be familiar with the relevant coding, billing, and documentation requirements, and working as a team with the biller and collector will allow clinicians to maintain their focus on the most important goal of all—outstanding patient care.

PART II

Surgical Procedures For Diagnosis, Therapy, and Reconstruction

Local Anesthesia, Regional Nerve Blocks, and Postoperative Pain Management

9

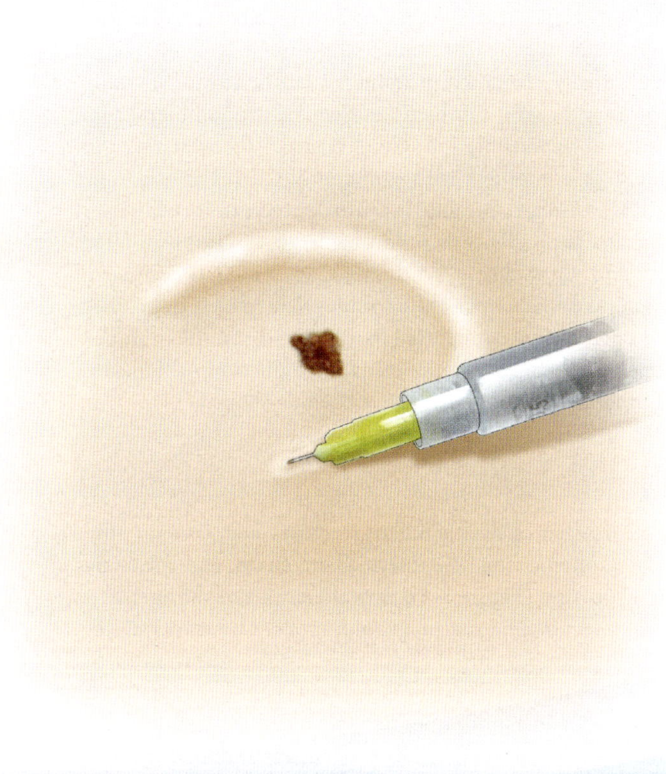

SUMMARY

- Local anesthesia is a critical component of dermatologic surgery, and allows even large procedures to be performed comfortably in an office setting.
- If patients unnecessarily undergo painful procedures, or painful anesthesia injection, this may adversely affect their overall experience and may undermine their confidence in the clinician.

Beginner Tips

- Lidocaine 1% with 1:100,000 epinephrine is the most widely used local anesthetic in dermatologic surgery.
- Use physical and mental distraction liberally and always inject slowly when possible.

Expert Tips

- Lidocaine-allergic patients can usually be treated with either bupivacaine or, for small biopsies, normal saline or cryoanesthesia.
- Patients may complain of an "allergy" to epinephrine; on detailed history, this is often related to intravascular injection during a dental procedure, but patient preference should always be respected.

Don't Forget!

- Concerns regarding digital block-related necrosis due to the addition of epinephrine are probably unfounded, though volume should be minimized when possible.
- Patients should be warned that temporary paralysis may be seen postoperatively; a unilateral facial droop is almost always due to anesthetic effect rather than nerve damage.

Pitfalls and Cautions

- Buffering bupivacaine with sodium bicarbonate is contraindicated due to the risk of precipitation.
- Be cautious when using off-label or compounded topical anesthetics, as these may lead to systemic side effects.

Patient Education

- Topical anesthetics may be applied at home prior to the procedure, though for most patients, a slow local anesthetic injection coupled with distraction leads to only minimal discomfort.
- Local anesthesia is usually instant, while nerve blocks take several minutes to take effect.

9 Local Anesthesia, Regional Nerve Blocks, and Postoperative Pain Management

INTRODUCTION

Local anesthesia is of critical importance in dermatologic surgery. Local anesthesia permits the performance of procedures virtually painlessly through inducing a reversible loss of sensation in a well-circumscribed area of the body. Local anesthetic agents lead to anesthesia by inhibiting excitation of nerve endings or by blocking conduction in peripheral nerves.[1] A thorough understanding of local anesthesia is therefore important to improve the surgical experience for both patient and clinician.

HISTORY

The biological effects of local anesthetics were first recorded in 1860, when Albert Niemann, a graduate student in pharmacology, isolated cocaine from the plant *Erythroxylum coca* and recorded the numbing sensation felt when the substance was placed on his tongue.[2] Niemann did not initially consider the use of cocaine as a surgical anesthetic. Years later, in 1884, a graduate student in Vienna named Sigmund Freud experimented with the effects of cocaine on himself and animals. Freud published a paper called "Uber Coca,"[3] which claimed that cocaine could be used to treat mental disorders. In 1884, Karl Koller, an ophthalmology resident and colleague of Freud, presented the idea of cocaine being used clinically and issued a paper on its use in ophthalmologic surgery.[2] Physicians, at first, were slow to accept the idea of using cocaine for medical purposes but eventually embraced its use. This initial acceptance was followed by scrutiny once the addictive and toxic aspects of cocaine were recognized.

In the early 20th century, several safer anesthetics were developed. In 1904, Alfred Einhorn synthesized an ester of para-aminobenzoic acid (PABA) called procaine.[4] A year later, Heinrich Braun was the first to successfully use it as an anesthetic.[2] Höechst initially promoted procaine under the name Novocain, but soon found that it produced an extreme drop in blood pressure and was responsible for several deaths.[5] To overcome this, procaine was combined with epinephrine. In 1930, a more potent PABA ester, tetracaine, was introduced[5]; unfortunately, it demonstrated a proclivity to produce allergic reactions. In 1943, Lofgren and Lundqvist[2,4] synthesized an amide derivative of diethylaminoacetic acid called lidocaine that proved to be effective and safe.[6] This eventually led to its mainstream use in surgery as a local anesthetic. Since the initial introduction of lidocaine, several other local-acting drugs have been developed.

STRUCTURE

All local anesthetics have similar structures and contain three parts: the aromatic ring, the intermediate chain, and the terminal amine portion (**Figure 9-1**). Any alterations of the anesthetic agent can affect its pharmacologic properties. The aromatic ring, a lipophobic component, is responsible for the diffusion of the anesthetic through cell membranes and nerve sheaths.[6] The intermediate chain binds either an ester or an amide containing between three and seven carbon equivalents and is responsible for its mode of action.[7] Disruption of the intermediate chain is responsible for local anesthetic metabolism and the reversible nature of these agents.[7] The amine terminus can arise in a tertiary form that is lipid soluble or a quaternary form that is water soluble and positively charged.[8] It is this same terminus that is thought to bind to the sodium channel and determine the length of action of the anesthetic.[7]

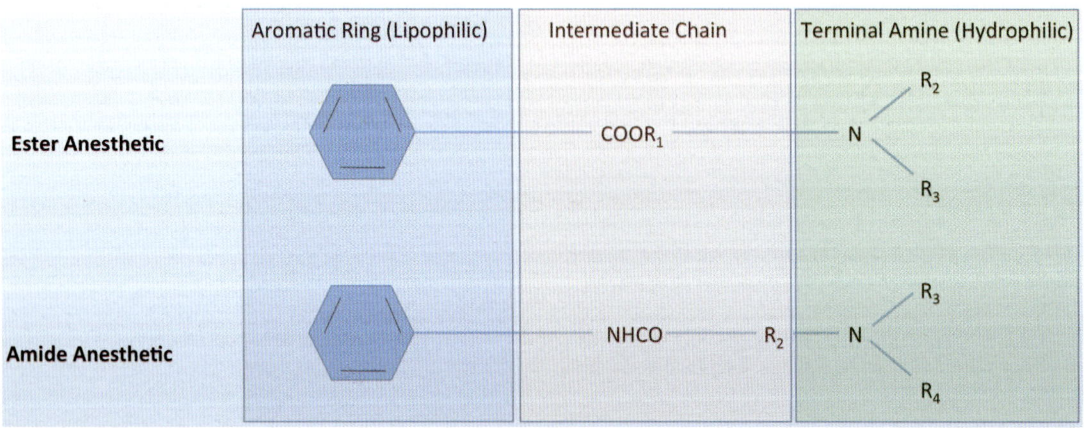

FIGURE 9-1 All local anesthetics have similar structures and contain three parts: the aromatic ring, the intermediate chain, and the terminal amine portion.

TABLE 9-1 • A Comprehensive List of Amide Anesthetics

Generic	Brand
Articaine	Septocaine
Bupivacaine	Marcaine, Sensorcaine
Dibucaine	Nupercainal
Etidocaine	Duranest
Levobupivacaine	Chrocaine
Lidocaine	Xylocaine
Mepivacaine	Carbocaine
Prilocaine	Citanest
Ropivacaine	Naropin
Trimecaine	Mesocain

CLASSIFICATION

Local anesthetics have two main chemical classifications[5] and depend on the structure of the intermediate chain: those that contain an amide group (eg, lidocaine) and those that contain an ester attachment (eg, procaine). This linkage is very important to the anesthetic agent as it defines the pathway by which the molecule is metabolized and excreted.[6]

Amide anesthetics are hepatically metabolized.[5,6] Lidocaine is considered an intermediate potent anesthetic and has a wide range of clinical uses.[9] It exhibits a rapid onset of action, shows no cross-reactivity to ester-type local anesthetics,[5] and is therefore safe to use in patients who are allergic to procaine or tetracaine. Lidocaine comes in 0.5%, 1%, and 2% concentrations and lasts on average for 30 to 400 minutes.[6] Bupivacaine is a high-potency amide anesthetic that lasts for 2 to 6 hours.[6] Longer-lasting effects of bupivacaine have been attributed to its slower elimination time.[10] Lidocaine and bupivacaine in combination have been studied and shown to prolong mean anesthetic duration,[11] as is sometimes required with longer Mohs surgery procedures. A comprehensive list of amide anesthetics is shown in **Table 9-1**.

Ester local anesthetics are metabolized by pseudocholinesterase and excreted in the urine.[6,8] The strength and duration of these agents correlate inversely with their rate of hydrolysis.[6] Patients with atypical[12] or low levels of pseudocholinesterases are prone to a greater risk of inadvertent toxicity.[6] PABA is a major metabolic product of ester anesthetics and a main reason for contact allergies.[8] The most common types of ester anesthetics are benzocaine, procaine, tetracaine, and cocaine.[6] The latter is a highly effective vasoconstrictor and has been used for nasal procedures.[13] Procaine has a rapid onset of action but shorter half-life, lasting for 15 to 30 minutes.[6] Tetracaine is 10 times more potent than procaine and is often used as an ocular anesthetic drop.[14,15] Chloroprocaine was developed to meet the need for a shorter-acting anesthetic agent with a favorable safety profile.[16] It is licensed in Europe for procedures lasting up to 40 minutes. Although less toxic than lidocaine, it is a more painful anesthetic to administer due to its acidic pH.[14]

STRUCTURE AND PHYSIOLOGY

Mechanisms of Action

Local anesthetics work through reversibly impeding nerve depolarization and activation by interfering with Na^+ ion movement across nerve membranes (**Figure 9-2**).[17] Decreased permeability of cell membranes to Na^+ ions prevents the nerve action potential from being reached. In a resting cell, intracellular electric potential is intrinsically negative compared to the extracellular space.[6] The nerve's cell membrane and Na/K ATPase pump help maintain this natural gradient.[6] Although the exact mechanism of sodium channel blockade is unclear, one postulate is that local anesthetics bind to a receptor located on the cytoplasmic portion of the cell membrane.[18] To reach this site, the uncharged form of the anesthetic diffuses though hydrophobic pathways.[14] After binding, the anesthetic induces a conformational change in the receptor and renders it inactive.[19] Local anesthetics preferentially bind to activated sodium channels in rapidly firing neurons, leading to what is termed a "state-dependent" blockade.[20,21]

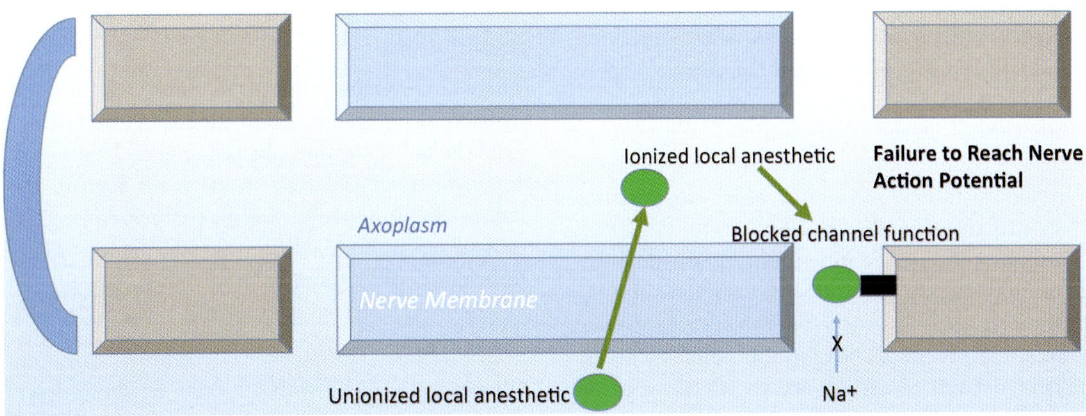

FIGURE 9-2 Local anesthetics work through reversibly impeding nerve depolarization and activation by interfering with Na^+ ion movement across nerve membranes.

TABLE 9-2 • Nerve Fiber Types

A fibers	
Alpha	(Myelinated) Motor Impulses and Proprioception
Beta	(Myelinated) Pressure and light touch
Gamma	(Myelinated) Proprioception and muscle spindle tone
Delta (small)	(Myelinated) Pain and temperature
B fibers	(Myelinated) Preganglionic sympathetic
C fibers (small)	(Unmyelinated) Pain and temperature

Cutaneous nerve fibers vary in size and type.[6] Larger myelinated nerves are usually more difficult to anesthetize than their smaller counterparts.[5] There are three main categories of nerve fibers. They are referred to as A, B, and C (**Table 9-2**). **A** somatic fibers are divided into four subtypes: alpha, beta, gamma, and delta. All A fibers are myelinated,[5] with alpha fibers being responsible for motor impulses and proprioception. Beta fibers are responsible for pressure and light touch, gamma fibers for proprioception and muscle spindle tone, and smaller delta fibers for pain and temperature.[6,14] **B** fibers are myelinated and are preganglionic sympathetic fibers.[5] **C** fibers are the smallest nerves and are unmyelinated.[5] They are responsible for conducting temperature and pain sensation in a manner similar to **A** delta fibers.[5] Due to their smaller size, nerves that conduct the sensations of pain and temperature are affected by local anesthesia before the loss of pressure, vibration, and proprioception.[14] This is why patients may be able to detect light touch during procedures in which they are effectively numbed.[5,14] It is important to understand this principle and be able to readily explain this to patients, preferably prior to surgery, to reduce their anxiety.

Anesthetic Additives

Local anesthetic agents may come premixed or are compounded with additives for additional pharmacologic benefits. It is important to understand how these additives work, what concentrations are safe, and how can they affect anesthesia efficacy.

Epinephrine: Epinephrine is the most common additive used in local anesthesia.[6] It counters the local anesthetic's tendency to induce vascular smooth muscle relaxation, which can promote bleeding.[5] Vasoconstrictive effects occur quickly, with full effects taking 7 to 15 minutes.[5,14] Epinephrine limits anesthetic diffusion and helps to minimize the absorption of anesthetic into the systemic circulation. It also allows less anesthesia to be used to complete the numbing process. A liability for epinephrine use is the potential for delayed bleeding once its effects wear off. Concerns for postoperative hematoma development[14] should be addressed with the patient prior to surgery. Epinephrine is labeled as a Category C drug.

Sodium Bicarbonate

Sodium bicarbonate is a weak base with the molecular formula $NaHCO_3$. When mixed with lidocaine with epinephrine, resultant injections are notably less painful.[22,23] Simple lidocaine with epinephrine has an acidic pH of 3.3 to 5.5,[5] which contributes to patient discomfort. It is usual for clinicians to "buffer" lidocaine with epinephrine with 8.4% solution of $NaHCO_3$ as follows: 1:10 (1 part 8.4% $NaHCO_3$ to 10 parts lidocaine 1% with 1:100,000 epinephrine) or 1:15 (1 part $NaHCO_3$ to 15 parts 1:200,000 epinephrine).[5]

Although patients experience less pain with buffered lidocaine, the addition of $NaHCO_3$ makes the compound less stable, resulting in a shorter action duration.[24] On the positive side, the addition of $NaHCO_3$ allows for faster nerve membrane penetration and a quicker onset of anesthetic effect.[7] In short, there is a double-edged sword when adding sodium bicarbonate to lidocaine, although many clinicians use this additive because of a perceived greater benefit for the patient. Importantly, the use of sodium bicarbonate additives with bupivacaine is contraindicated due to the risk of agent precipitation.[25]

Hyaluronidase

Hyaluronidase is an enzyme that breaks down hyaluronic acid,[5] an acid mucopolysaccharide present in the dermis. When added to local anesthesia, hyaluronidase facilitates diffusion of the anesthetic through soft tissues. This results in a wider field of local anesthesia, faster onset of action, less tissue distortion, and easier tissue undermining.[26] In ophthalmology, hyaluronidase additives allow the clinician to minimize injection sites, decrease the volume of anesthesia used, and lessen the bruising risks for the patient.[5] Doses in cutaneous surgery vary. Some authors recommend that 150 units of hyaluronidase be mixed in 20 to 30 mL of lidocaine for a concentration of 7.5 units/mL.[27]

There are some risks with using hyaluronidase, including decreased anesthetic duration and a greater risk of toxicity due to enhanced absorption.[27] Hyaluronidase also contains the preservative thimerosal,[5] which is a contact allergen. Preoperative skin testing in highly sensitive patients is recommended prior to its use.[5,27] Hyaluronidase should also not be used in those with a documented bee venom allergy.[28]

Triamcinolone

There are several advantages to combining lidocaine with a corticosteroid injectable.[29] This mixture is useful for treating acne cysts, keloid scars, and alopecia areata. Doses vary from 2.5 to 5 mg/mL for facial cysts to 20 to 40 mg/mL for thick keloid lesions. In orthopedic surgery, triamcinolone mixed with lidocaine serves as both a diagnostic and therapeutic tool to evaluate for rotator cuff tendonitis.[30]

Clindamycin

Clindamycin mixed with lidocaine has been described as a way to provide antibiotic prophylaxis. One study examined 1172 wounds treated with 50 mL of 1% lidocaine mixed with epinephrine, 5 mL of 8.4% $NaHCO_3$, and 0.15 mL of 150 mg/mL clindamycin.[31] Culture-positive wound infections were less frequent in the clindamycin group compared to control group. No allergic reactions were reported. More data need to be evaluated before this combination is routinely recommended.

Mixing Two or More Anesthetics

Mixing two or more local anesthetics is a common practice for clinicians.[6,32] Several randomized controlled trials comparing mixtures of local anesthetics have been conducted.[33,34] Combinations studied include bupivacaine and lidocaine, bupivacaine and mepivacaine, and prilocaine and ropivacaine. Evidence suggests that mixing these agents for local infiltration and nerve block anesthesia is safe. There are insufficient data to determine whether any combination results in a faster onset or longer duration of anesthesia, and no strong evidence supports the benefits of mixing anesthetics over the use of a single agent.[28]

Topical Anesthetics

Topical anesthetics play a major role in dermatologic surgical procedures.[5,28,35] From laser hair removal to cosmetic injectables to minor skin surgery, topical anesthesia enhances patient comfort by allowing a "needleless approach" to patient numbing. The limitation of using topical anesthetics is the ability of these agents to penetrate the stratum corneum.[36] For this reason, they work better in thinner skin areas such as the oral mucosa[5] and/or genital skin. Newer delivery systems have enhanced the rate of topical anesthetic absorption and effect.[37] A list of commonly used compounded and standardized topical anesthetics can be found in **Table 9-3**.

TABLE 9-3 • Commonly Used Topical Anesthetics in Dermatologic Surgery

Name (Brand)	Ingredients
EMLA Cream	2.5% lidocaine and 2.5% prilocaine
LMX	4% or 5% lidocaine cream
Pliaglis	7% lidocaine and 7% tetracaine
BLT	20% benzocaine, 6% lidocaine, 4% tetracaine
TAC	0.5% tetracaine, 1:2000 epinephrine, 11.8% cocaine
LET	4% lidocaine, 1:2000 epinephrine, 0.5% tetracaine
Amethocaine gel	4% tetracaine gel
Hurricaine gel	20% benzocaine
Lasergela	10% lidocaine, 10% tetracaine
Lasergel plus 10/10[a]	10% lidocaine, 10% tetracaine, 0.5% phenylephrine
Photocaine gel[a]	6% lidocaine, 6% tetracaine
Betacaine LA ointment[a]	15% lidocaine, 5% prilocaine, phenylephrine
Betacaine Plus ointment[a]	15% lidocaine, 5% prilocaine

[a]Received a warning from the US Food and Drug Administration in 2005.
Adapted with permission from Sobanko JF, Miller CJ, Alster TS. Topical anesthetics for dermatologic procedures: a review. Dermatol Surg. *2012 May;38(5):709-721.*

Topical Benzocaine: Benzocaine is commonly used to numb mucosal surfaces. This ester anesthetic is commercially available as a spray, gel, ointment, and solution, with concentrations ranging from 5% to 20%.[5] Benzocaine has a higher risk of contact sensitization and methemoglobinemia[5,6] and must be used with caution. One common benzocaine product is Hurricane Gel, a 20% gel that is useful for dental procedures and prior to administering intraoral nerve blocks. The gel is applied for 30 to 60 seconds in the desired location.[6] Effects last for up to 15 minutes. Cetacaine is a compound benzocaine product that contains 14% benzocaine, 2% butyl aminobenzoate, and 2% tetracaine. It has a rapid onset of action and has longer-lasting effects (eg, 30-60 minutes).[6,13]

Topical Lidocaine: Lidocaine has been used as a topical anesthetic for many years.[34] It is commercially available as a eutectic combination product or as a solitary agent, with strengths varying from 2% to 30%.[6] Topicaine is a 4% lidocaine microemulsion gel[6,38] that has gained some popularity. It is formulated in cooling penetrating 5% lidocaine gel composed of water, ethanol, glycerin, jojoba oil, aloe vera oil, glycerol monolaurate, benzyl alcohol, carbomer 940, and EDTA.

There is support to suggest that compounded lidocaine mixtures (lidocaine/prilocaine) may have excellent efficacy for certain skin procedures.[39] Delivery systems employing microemulsion gels have been shown to be more effective in reducing pain during cutaneous surgery procedures. LMX is one such product. It has a fast onset of action, requiring only 30 minutes of application time prior to procedures.[6] Studies comparing LMX 5% to EMLA show that both are equally effective for pain reduction.[40,41] One study showed that LMX 5% requires a shorter application time to achieve pain control.[40]

Topical Tetracaine: Tetracaine is an ester anesthetic that comes in a topical cream, gel, and solution.[5] Amethocaine gel is a 4% tetracaine gel that is formulated within a lecithin vehicle, which allows for increased penetration into the skin.[5] When applied for 60 minutes, it has proved superior to other topical anesthetics. This was supported in one study that evaluated pulsed dye laser patients treated with Amethocaine as determined by visual and verbal rating scores.[42] Combination products using tetracaine have also been effective for skin surgery procedures, as noted later.

Lidocaine/Tetracaine Peel: The lidocaine/tetracaine (LT) combination peel consists of a 1:1 eutectic mix of 7% lidocaine and 7% tetracaine.[5] It is constituted in a membranous matrix in which the anesthetic mixture air dries into a flexible membrane. This membrane is then removed just prior to procedure initiation. Application times vary, but recommendations are 20 minutes for nonablative laser treatments, 30 minutes for cosmetic injectable procedures, and 60 minutes for tattoo removal.[43] The LT peel has also been shown to be effective for cryotherapy[5,44] and carbon dioxide laser resurfacing.[45] Studies comparing the LT peel with placebo and EMLA cream have shown that the LT peel may be superior.[45,46] With respect to safety, side effects are limited to local transient erythema.[46] Care must be used when applying any numbing agents around the eyes.

EMLA: EMLA is a 2.5% eutectic mixture of lidocaine and prilocaine that is packaged commercially as a cream or patch.[5] It is one of the most common topical agents used in dermatology and available via prescription. The definition of a eutectic mixture is one in which the ingredients are formulated to melt to liquid phase at room temperature.[35,47] In addition to the two active anesthetic agents, EMLA contains emulsifiers (polyoxymethylene), thickening agents (carboxypolymethylene), and distilled water.[5] It has been effectively used prior to laser surgery, chemical peels, graft procedures, skin biopsies, and electrosurgery procedures.[35,37]

To work effectively, EMLA is usually applied under occlusion with either a plastic wrap or dressing.[6] Numbing effectiveness depends, in part, on the anatomic area being treated and the duration of the occlusion. For example, on the face, anesthesia can occur in 30 minutes or less, whereas on mucous membranes, it only takes 5 to 15 minutes.[6] Most clinicians leave EMLA on the skin for at least 1 hour and, for more painful procedures, 2 to 3 hours with occlusion.[5,35] The maximum effect of anesthesia is reached within 2 to 3 hours after application. EMLA penetrates 3 mm into the skin after 1 hour of application and 5 mm after 2 hours.[35]

Like other amide anesthetics, EMLA should be used cautiously in conditions where the skin integrity is breached, such as in psoriasis or eczema.[48] It is contraindicated in those with liver disease and amide hypersensitivity.[48] Care also must be taken when using EMLA around the eyes.[49]

Pharmacy-Compounded Topical Anesthetics: In some instances, topical anesthetics are compounded by pharmacies for use in dermatology. Standardization of compounded products is difficult because individual pharmacies use different protocols to mix various ingredients in their topical anesthetics.[50,51] Formula standardization should be considered for compounded anesthetics, since the formulations are not regulated by the US Food and Drug Administration and may be inconsistent.[52] Because compounded anesthetics do not require clinical trials, there is a great variability in use.[51] Mixtures are usually made using various concentrations of lidocaine, Betacaine, and tetracaine.[6,51] Care must be taken when using compounded topical anesthetics and choosing the right company to manufacture them. Particulate matter has been shown in one case to cause corneal abrasions due to issues with a particular benzocaine 20%, lidocaine 6%, and tetracaine 4% (BLT) preparation.[52] It is essential that the clinician develop a working relationship with a reputable compounding pharmacy and not exceed the dosages established for traditional topical and/or injectable anesthetic agents. Pharmacy-compounded topical anesthetics should only be used under the direct supervision of a physician and conservatively applied to limited body areas.

Cryoanesthesia

The use of cold as an adjunct can be very helpful in reducing the pain associated with minor procedures such as cosmetic injectables, digital blocks, and wart destruction.[5,6,53] The placement of a cold pack for 5 to 10 seconds prior to cosmetic injectables is a rapid and inexpensive way to provide the patient with increased comfort.

TABLE 9-4 • Cooling Applications Used in Dermatologic Surgery
Ice/cool packs
Liquid nitrogen
Zimmer cooling device (Zimmer Medizin Systems, Irvine, CA) (forced air cooling)
Frigiderm (Delasco, Council Bluffs, IA) (100% dichlorotetrafluoroethane)
Ethyl Chloride (Gebauer Company, Cleveland OH) (50% dichlorodifluoromethane, 50% trichloromonofluoromethane)
Instant Cold Spray (HL Moore, New Britain, CT) (10% isopentane, 90% butane)

Data from Plotkin S. Clinical comparison of preinjection anesthetics. J Am Podiatr Med Assoc. *1998 Feb;88(2):73-79.*

Cryorefrigerant provides another source of effective anesthesia by rapidly cooling the skin.[5,6,54] They are held 6 inches from the target zone and sprayed until the treatment area turns white,[6] usually in 4 to 6 seconds. One should wear a mask and eyewear to avoid inhaling the vaporant and to protect the eyes from inadvertent contact.[5] Ocular exposure from cryorefrigerants and even cryotherapy has been reported to cause pigmentary alterations and scarring.[5,55,56] Those containing ethyl chloride are flammable, so care must be taken around lasers or sources of heat.[5,6,56] Other cooling devices that have been used in dermatology include sapphire cooling laser tips and the Zimmer machine.[5,6] The benefit of these technologies is twofold: they provide anesthesia for the patient and protect against laser-induced thermal injury and blistering. A thorough list of cooling applications is found in **Table 9-4**.

Cryoanesthesia can also be performed effectively using liquid nitrogen; for needle-phobic patients, shave biopsies may be anesthetized using a brief liquid nitrogen spray, although the dermatopathologist should be informed because theoretically freeze artifact could occur.

Iontophoresis

Iontophoresis uses electric current to deliver anesthetic solution into the skin without the pain of a needle.[5] Anesthetic delivery works well, with some studies showing a 20- to 60-fold increase in lidocaine penetration.[57] Although there is a learning curve and expense for the machinery, iontophoresis is a very effective approach to enhance numbing efficacy, especially in the pediatric population.[58]

ANESTHETIC ADMINISTRATION

Local Infiltration

Local anesthesia can be administered either intradermally or subcutaneously. Intradermal injections are superficially placed, create more tissue distortion, have a faster onset of action, and are slightly more painful.[5,6,14] Deeply placed subcutaneous injections are less

TABLE 9-5 • Methods Used to Achieve a More Painless and Comfortable Injection

▪ Supporting the head of the patient while numbing ▪ Talking to and encouraging the patient during local administration ▪ Hiding the needle from the patient's direct view ▪ Playing relaxing music ▪ Having the patient recline comfortably ▪ Using cool compresses, ice, or cryorefrigerants prior to injection ▪ Applying topical anesthetics prior to injection ▪ Using a smaller diameter needle, eg, 30- or 31-gauge needle ▪ Warming the solution prior to injection ▪ Injecting perpendicular to the skin	▪ Injecting slowly ▪ Neutralizing the pH of acidic lidocaine and epinephrine by mixing (10:1) with 8.4% sodium bicarbonate ▪ Employing distraction techniques such as tapping other areas of the skin while actively numbing ▪ Having the patient use a squeeze toy ▪ Holding the patient's hand while the injection is being performed ▪ Stretching the skin taut with the nondominant hand while injecting ▪ In cases where multiple punctures are required, performing needle reentry in areas previously anesthetized ▪ Employing conscious sedation for small children ▪ Utilization of nerve blocks or tumescent anesthesia when large areas of anesthesia are needed

painful and create less tissue distortion than intradermal injections but have a slower onset of action and shorter duration of action.[5,6,14]

It is important to learn proper injection technique to make the experience most comfortable for the patient. Methods to achieve a more painless and comfortable injection experience include those listed in **Table 9-5**. Although studies have been conducted to evaluate pain level with different types of local anesthetics, only a few have had a sufficiently large sample size. One study found that bupivacaine with epinephrine elicited the most discomfort and lidocaine with epinephrine the least.[59] Another prospective, randomized, double-blind study found that 3% mepivacaine and 2% lidocaine with epinephrine induced a similar amount of pain on injection, with the lidocaine group demonstrating a slightly lower, although not clinically significant, amount of moderate pain reported.[60] Further studies would be helpful to explain these differences and standardize recommendations for local anesthetic use.

Field (Ring) Blocks

Field (ring) blocks use local anesthesia that is injected circumferentially around the operative site.[6] Multiple injections are required, with each being placed in an area that was previously anesthetized. Ring blocks are useful in those instances where direct infiltration into the surgical site should be avoided, where nerve blocks are not an option, and for larger surgical areas. In dermatologic surgery, this approach is ideal for the excision of cysts[5,6] and skin cancers[14] and when performing hair transplant procedures.[14] It is important to inject the local anesthetic in both deep and superficial planes to optimize the numbing effect.[5] Ring blocks conserve the total amount of anesthetic that needs to be injected. It is important to wait 5 to 10 minutes after completion of this block to allow for adequate anesthesia and optimal hemostasis. To maximize hemostasis, the central area may be painlessly infused after completing the ring block.

NERVE BLOCKS

Nerve blocks are extremely useful in dermatologic surgery. They help to optimize patient comfort,[14] minimize tissue distortion,[6] and enhance patient safety.[6] Nerve blocks require an in-depth understanding of human anatomy and can be difficult to learn for the novice. Patience and persistence are necessary for the clinician trying to master the art of nerve blocks. They are especially useful for skin procedures of the head and neck, digits, foot, genitals, hand, and lateral thigh regions.[5,6]

Nerve blocks require fewer needle sticks to achieve anesthesia.[6] Selectively using combinations of lidocaine and bupivacaine allows for enhanced anesthetic duration and safety. Sometimes, additional epinephrine or a tourniquet is necessary to enhance hemostasis.[6] Some authors have historically suggested that the use of epinephrine in the digital region poses a risk and should be avoided,[5] although the consensus now is that epinephrine is safe for properly performed digital blocks.[61,62] The risks associated with nerve blocks are rare but can include direct nerve injury, pain, dysesthesia, neuropraxia, infection, and vessel trauma,[6,63] which can cause unwanted bruising and/or hematoma formation.[64,65]

To perform a nerve block, a 30-gauge ½- or 1-inch needle is used. It is important to slowly advance the needle and to aspirate before injecting to avoid direct injection into a blood vessel.[6] The use of topical anesthetics, cryorefrigerants, or distractive vibratory tapping[66] at sites distant to the nerve block area can help with patient comfort. Once the needle is placed in the correct location, small amounts of anesthetic are injected and allowed to diffuse strategically. Nerve size and type tend to correlate with the time to numb.[67] Once a nerve block has been administered, it is important to wait for at least 5 to 10 minutes before proceeding with surgery.[5,6] Repeat injections are sometimes required to complete the block. Patients should be made aware of this before starting their procedure.

HEAD AND NECK NERVE BLOCKS

The head and neck areas of the body have a vast array of nerve and blood vessel structures. The trigeminal nerve (cranial nerve V) and cervical plexus are responsible for the majority of sensory innervation for these areas (**Figure 9-3**).[5,68] The trigeminal nerve can be divided into three main components. These include the ophthalmic branch (V_1), maxillary branch (V_2), and mandibular branch (V_3).[5,6,68] They are responsible for sensation to the forehead, cheeks, conjunctiva, teeth, lips, nose, and chin. There

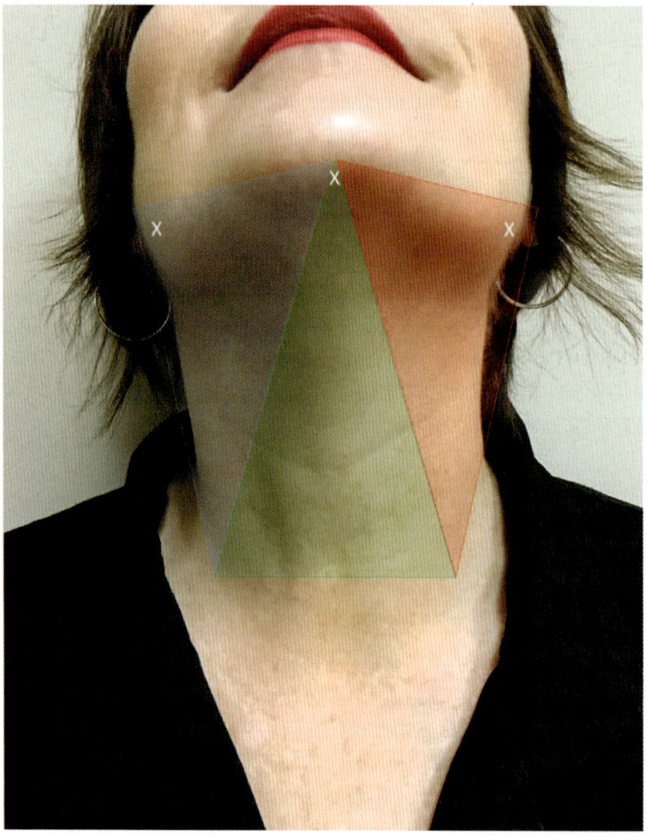

FIGURE 9-3 The neck is divided into the right (*blue*), central (*green*), and left (*red*) submentum.

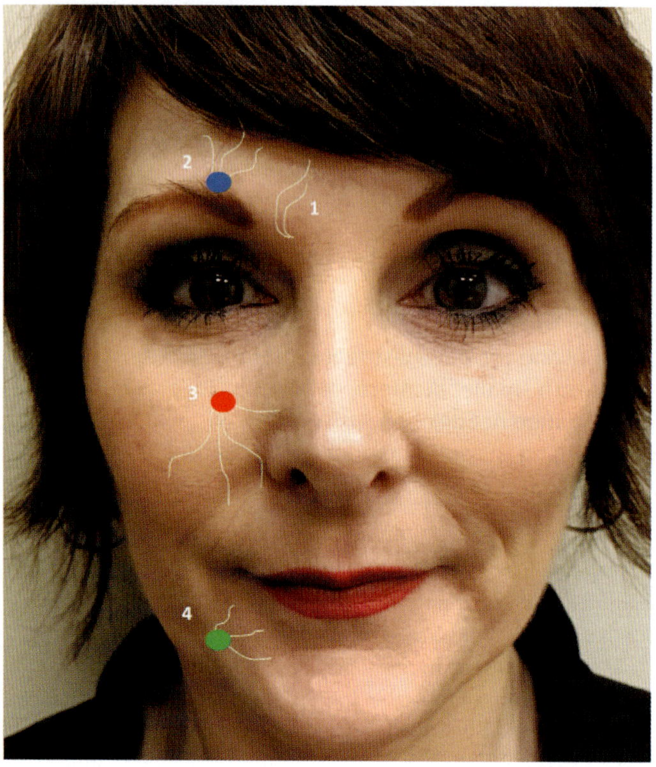

FIGURE 9-4 There are specific facial landmarks that serve to identify where to inject anesthetic to numb certain regions of the face. The supratrochlear (1) and supraorbital (2) nerves, the latter of which emanates from the supraorbital foramen (*blue*), supply sensation to much of the forehead. The infraorbital nerve (3) exits from the infraorbital foramen depicted in *red*. It is located 1 cm below the infraorbital rim and is responsible for innervation of the upper lip and medial cheek. Finally, the mental foramen, seen in *green*, is the exit portal for the mental nerve (4), which innervates the lower lip and chin.

are specific facial landmarks that serve to identify where to inject anesthetic to numb certain regions of the face[68] (**Figure 9-4**). The cervical plexus[69] supplies sensory innervation to the ear, neck, jaw, and posterior scalp.[5,68] This plexus emanates from the anterior rami of four superior cervical nerves.[5] Knowledge of their emergence points is helpful to correctly anesthetize the posterior auricle and angle of the jaw.

Supraorbital and Supratrochlear Nerve Blocks

The supraorbital and supratrochlear nerves provided sensation to the ipsilateral forehead and scalp[5] (**Figure 9-5**). They arise from the ophthalmic branch of V_1.[5,6,68] The supraorbital nerve emanates from the supraorbital notch, which is located on the superior orbital rim near the mid-pupillary line.[5] The supratrochlear nerve is located about 1.2 to 1.7 cm medial to this notch.[5] Both nerves can be blocked simultaneously by palpating the notch, gently pinching up on the skin, and injecting 1 to 2 mL of local anesthetic toward the midline.[14,68,70,71] Care must be taken to aspirate before injecting to avoid inadvertent trauma to the supraorbital and supratrochlear arteries, which run medial to these nerves. The use of cool compresses before injection can also help to minimize this risk by inducing transient vasoconstriction.

Infraorbital Nerve Block

The infraorbital nerve provides sensation to the ipsilateral lower eyelid, nasal sidewall, upper lip, and medial cheek[5,6,14,68] (**Figure 9-5**). It derives from the maxillary branch of V_2 and is the largest branch of the maxillary nerve.[6] Its exit onto the face occurs at the infraorbital foramen, which can be palpated as a notch just medial to the mid-pupillary line, approximately 1 cm below the infraorbital rim.[6,14,68]

The infraorbital nerve can be anesthetized either percutaneously or intraorally.[6] The intraoral approach is considered less painful.[6,14] With this blocking technique, the maxillary gingival sulcus lateral to the canine may be topically numbed[14] with 20% benzocaine left in place for 1 minute. A small bleb of buffered lidocaine is subsequently placed using a 30-gauge 1-inch needle; given the minimal pain associated with this procedure, topical anesthesia is not required. After 10 to 15 seconds, the needle is advanced tangentially above the maxillary periosteum toward the notch. After negative aspiration, 1 to 3 mL of anesthetic is slowly injected. Gentle movement of the lateral upper lip with the nondominant hand can reduce discomfort as the injection is administered. The percutaneous route, like the supraorbital block, is performed by palpating the notch of the foramen, gently pinching up on the skin, and slowly injecting a similar small amount of anesthetic solution. Topical numbing agents and/or cool

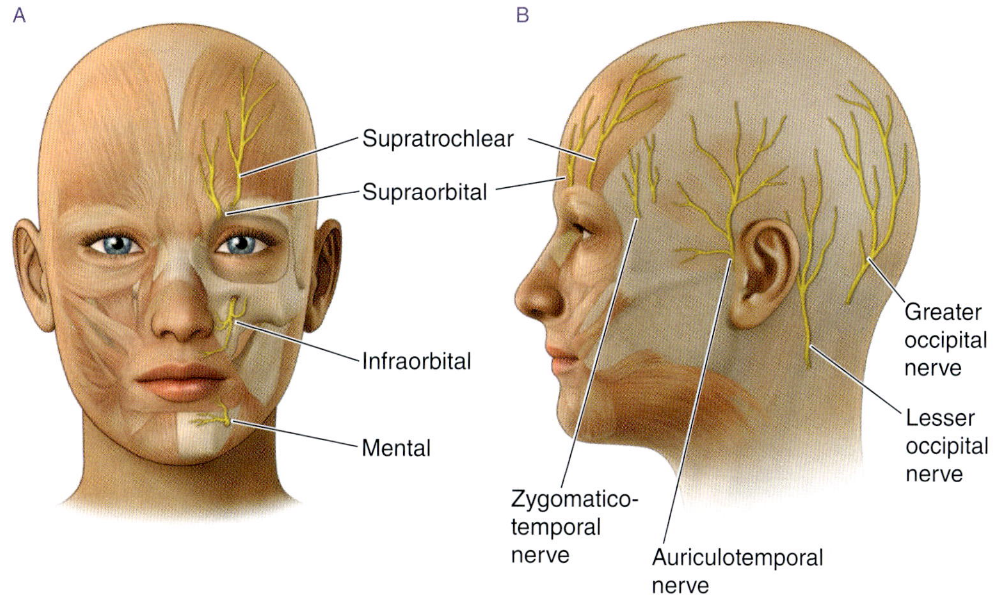

FIGURE 9-5 The supraorbital and supratrochlear nerves provide sensation to the ipsilateral forehead and scalp.

compresses can be employed with the percutaneous approach to optimize patient comfort.

Anterior Ethmoidal (External Nasal) Nerve Block

The external nasal nerve is a branch of the anterior ethmoidal nerve and is located between the upper lateral nasal cartilage and lower border of the nasal bone.[5] Anesthesia of the ipsilateral nasal tip, columella, and nasal dorsum[5] is obtained by injecting 1 to 2 mL of anesthetic at a point between the mobile cartilage and fixed nasal bone periosteum.[68] One way to make this block less painful, as is performed in full-face laser resurfacing cases, is to start with the supraorbital nerve block and gradually advance the anesthesia medially toward the nasal root and lateral mid-nasal sidewall. This may allow for a much better experience for the patient.

Mental Nerve Block

The mental nerve provides sensation to the ipsilateral chin and lower lip, including gingiva and mucosa.[5,14] It is the terminal branch of the mandibular nerve (V_3) and emerges from the mental foramen[6,14] at a point 2.5 cm lateral to midline of the chin.[5,6] With time, as the mandible recedes, the location of the foramen shifts to a point closer to the upper mandibular margin.[5,68]

Like the infraorbital nerve block, the mental nerve block can be performed either intraorally or percutaneously.[5,6] The intraoral approach is considered less painful and uses topical benzocaine gel applied to the gingival sulcus between the first and second premolars.[5] After 60 seconds, a small bleb of buffered lidocaine is placed using a 30-gauge 1-inch needle. To achieve an effective block, 1 to 3 mL of anesthetic is administered per side.

Auriculotemporal Nerve Block

The auriculotemporal (AT) nerve provides sensory innervation to the ipsilateral anterior ear and temple and is another branch of V_3.[6] Its course runs deeper and posterior to the temporomandibular joint (TMJ) before it exits superficially to join a course parallel with the superficial temporal artery.[6] The AT nerve can be blocked with mouth open by palpating the TMJ and injecting just superior to the joint pivot point using 2 to 3 mL of anesthetic[5,6,68] (**Figure 9-6**).

Transverse Cervical and Greater Auricular Nerve Blocks

The transverse cervical and greater auricular nerves provide sensation to the posterior auricle, angle of the mandible, and anterior neck.[6,70] The greater auricular nerve follows the course of the external jugular vein and innervates the posterior auricular area and ipsilateral angle of the jaw.[6] The transverse cervical nerve is located 1 cm inferior to the greater auricular neve and migrates anteriorly, providing sensation to the ipsilateral central mandible and anterior neck.[6,70] Both nerves derive from the cervical plexus and emerge at a well-recognized landmark known as Erb's point.[5,6] To help accentuate accurate injection into this area, the head can be turned 45 degrees against resistance.[5,6] Once Erb's point is identified, 2 to 3 mL of local anesthesia is injected.[68] This will result in numbing of both nerves and an effective field of anesthesia prior to surgery.

EXTREMITY NERVE BLOCKS

Nerve blocks for the extremities are also valuable to know and understand. They are quite effective for hand, foot, and digital numbing[5,6] and are excellent for nail avulsion, wart treatment, and bunion surgery. The following sections will review some of the common extremity nerve blocks that are used in dermatologic surgery.

Digital Blocks

Digital blocks are effective for numbing the nails, toes, and fingers.[5,6] The fingers are innervated by two ventral and two

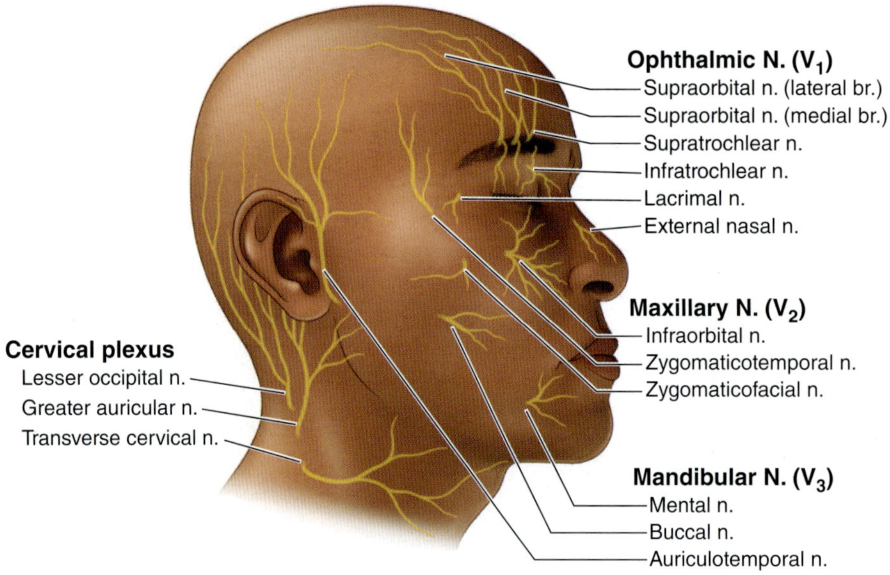

FIGURE 9-6 Auriculotemporal (AT) nerve block. The AT nerve provides sensory innervation to the ipsilateral anterior ear and temple and is another branch of V_3. It can be blocked, with mouth open, by palpating the temporomandibular joint and injecting just superior to the joint pivot point using 2 to 3 mL of anesthetic.

dorsal nerves[14] that run lateral to the digit and usually follow the course of the palmar and dorsal digital arteries[6] (**Figure 9-7**). Proper technique allows the nails and fingers to be rapidly anesthetized. As previously mentioned, the use of epinephrine for digital blocks is no longer controversial as several studies have shown it to be safe.[61,62]

Several digital blocks are available. The most commonly used approach for nail surgery is the distal digital ("wing") block. Its advantages are a quick onset of anesthesia, the use of smaller volumes of anesthetic, and a tumescent effect providing hemostasis. A dorsal approach to finger anesthesia is considered less painful.[5,32] Lidocaine 1% to 2%, buffered, or ropivacaine 0.25% are appropriate choices for this indication; 0.5 mL of anesthetic is injected into a point 5 mm proximal and lateral to the junction of the proximal and lateral nail fold on each side of the digit.

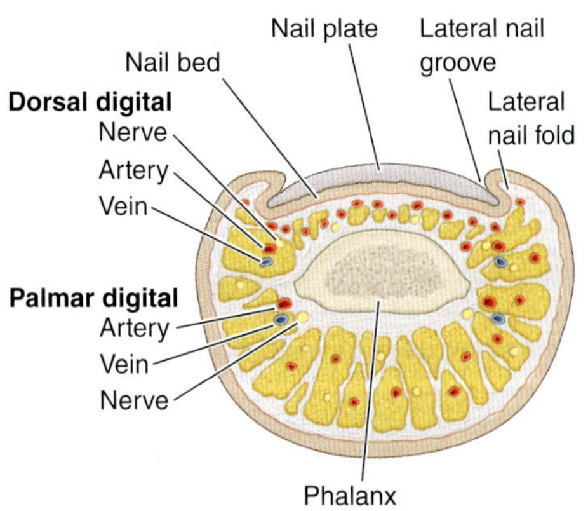

FIGURE 9-7 The fingers are innervated by two ventral and two dorsal nerves that run lateral to the digit and usually follow the course of the palmar and dorsal digital arteries.

If a clinician chooses to use epinephrine in their anesthetic, there should be minimal risk of intra-arterial injection due to the small caliber of arterioles in this anatomic location. If using lidocaine, then the addition of bupivacaine 0.25% to 0.5% will prolong anesthesia for up to 8 to 12 hours.

The proximal digital block is of slower onset, and up to 20 minutes may be needed before complete numbing of the distal tip of the digit takes place. Unlike the distal digital block, it carries a potential risk for damage to the neurovascular bundles. A cryorefrigerant, cold air,[72] or topical anesthetic cream is first applied over the proximal metacarpophalangeal joint at two points lateral to the digit. Approximately 1 mL of anesthetic is injected laterally at the level of the metacarpophalangeal or metatarsophalangeal joints into each side of the digit. Care should be taken to draw back on the syringe before injection to avoid injecting into an arteriole of the common digital artery.

The transthecal block is a useful approach for surgery of fingers 2, 3, and 4. Due to anatomic variation, this approach is not advised for surgery on any other digit. Its advantages are rapid onset (2-5 minutes) and the absence of risk to neurovascular bundles, as the needle is inserted on the palmar aspect of the digit. A rare complication is injury to the flexor tendon that can result in scar or trigger finger.

A digital tourniquet is often employed for additional vasoconstrictive effects. Tourniquet time should be limited to 15 minutes,[5] with no more than 8 mL of anesthesia administered per digit in one setting.[5,14]

Hand and Wrist Blocks

Nerve blocks of the hand and wrist are useful, especially given that multiple injections are required in this sensitive area[5] and topical

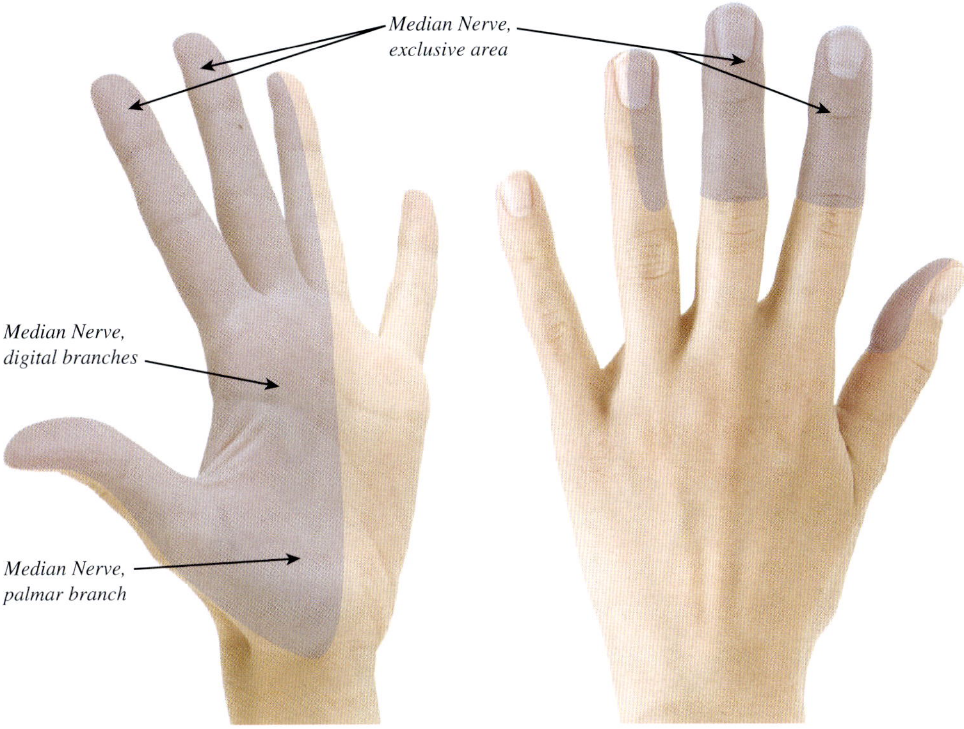

FIGURE 9-8 The median nerve provides sensation to the first three-and-a half fingers on the palmar side and the dorsal second, third, and medial fourth digits.

anesthetics do not work well.[6] The median, ulnar, and superficial radial nerves provide sensory innervation to the hand and wrist.[5]

The median nerve provides sensation to the first three and a half fingers on the palmar side, and the dorsal second, third, and medial fourth digits[5] (**Figure 9-8**). It is located between the palmaris longus and flexor carpi radialis tendons.[73] The injection site for the median nerve is located just below the proximal wrist.[6,73,74] A needle is advanced just medial to the palmaris longus tendon under the flexor retinaculum, and 3 to 5 mL of local anesthetic is used to numb the radial side of the palm.[6,73] As always, it is important to avoid intra-arterial injection when administering anesthesia.[74]

The ulnar nerve provides sensory input to both the palmar and dorsal sides of the fifth digit and lateral half of the fourth digit[5] (**Figure 9-9**). The nerve runs deep to the flexor carpi ulnaris tendon and inserts into the pisiform bone.[73,74] The ulnar block is placed lateral to the flexor carpi ulnaris tendon on the proximal wrist crease.[5] Again, careful injection technique is important because the nerve runs just medial to the ulnar artery.[74] A second approach is to administer the block proximally at the elbow between the epicondyle of the humerus and the olecranon process.[73,74]

The radial nerve provides sensory input to two-thirds of the dorsal hand (**Figure 9-10**).[5] It runs just lateral to the radius and follows a course extending from the wrist to the proximal interphalangeal joint of the second, third, and fourth digits and dorsal side of the first digit.[5] The radial block is performed by injecting lateral to the radial artery and deep to the flexor carpi radialis tendon.[73] It is an effective way to provide anesthesia to the palmar surface of the thumb.[6]

Foot and Ankle Blocks

The posterior tibial, saphenous, sural, and superficial and deep peroneal nerves mediate sensory innervation to the foot and part of the ankle.[5] A thorough understanding of their anatomic routes is important.

The posterior tibial nerve innervates the majority of the plantar surface of the foot, except for its medial aspect.[6] It is anesthetized at the medial malleolus,[5] where the nerve runs posterior to the posterior tibial artery (**Figure 9-11**). The injection is performed with the patient resting supine and the foot externally rotated.[75,76] Three to 5 mL of local anesthetic is injected at the upper portion of the medial malleolus and anterior calcaneal tendon.[5,76]

The saphenous nerve innervates the medial aspect of the plantar foot (**Figure 9-12**). It travels along the medial calf, anterior to the medial malleolus and medial to the saphenous vein.[5] The block is performed by injecting 3 to 5 mL of anesthetic anterior to the medial malleolus and medial to the saphenous vein.[6,75]

The sural nerve is responsible for innervating the lateral aspect of the distal ankle and plantar foot (**Figure 9-12**). It traverses laterally and more superficial than the posterior tibial artery, passing between the Achilles tendon and lateral malleolus on its way to the foot.[5] To block the sural nerve, 3 to 5 mL of local anesthetic is injected between the posterior distal tip of the lateral malleolus and Achilles tendon[76,77] (**Figure 9-13**).

The superficial and deep peroneal nerves arise from the common peroneal nerve[5] (**Figure 9-14**). The superficial peroneal nerve runs initially deep along the anterolateral ankle and then splits superficially into dorsal digital nerves of all but the first web

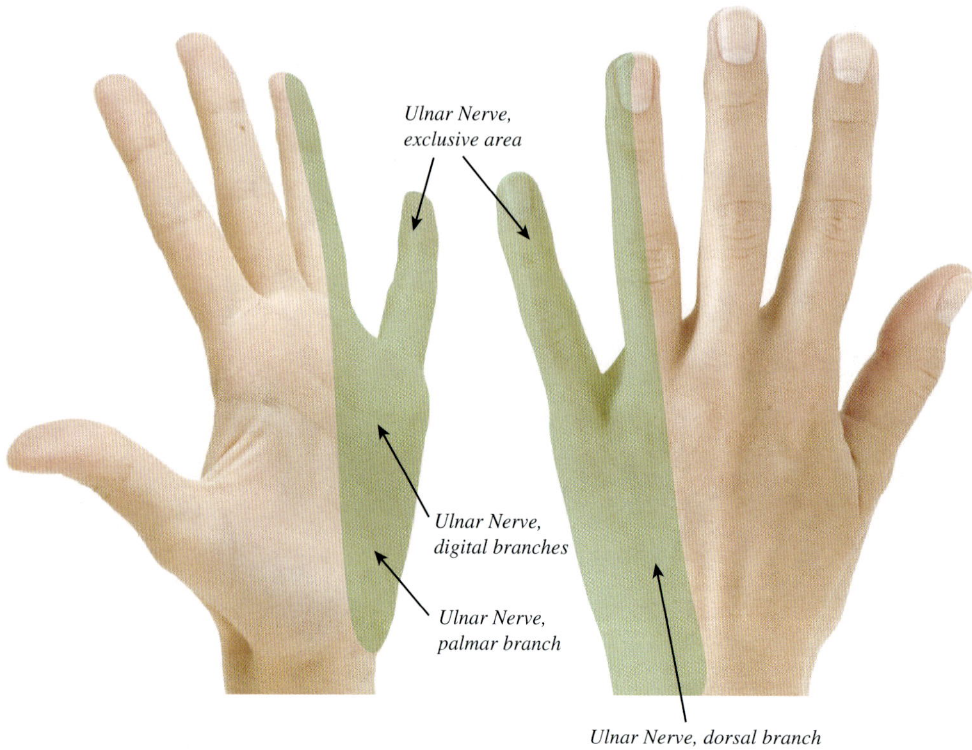

FIGURE 9-9 The ulnar nerve provides sensory input to both the palmar and dorsal sides of the fifth digit and lateral half of the fourth digit.

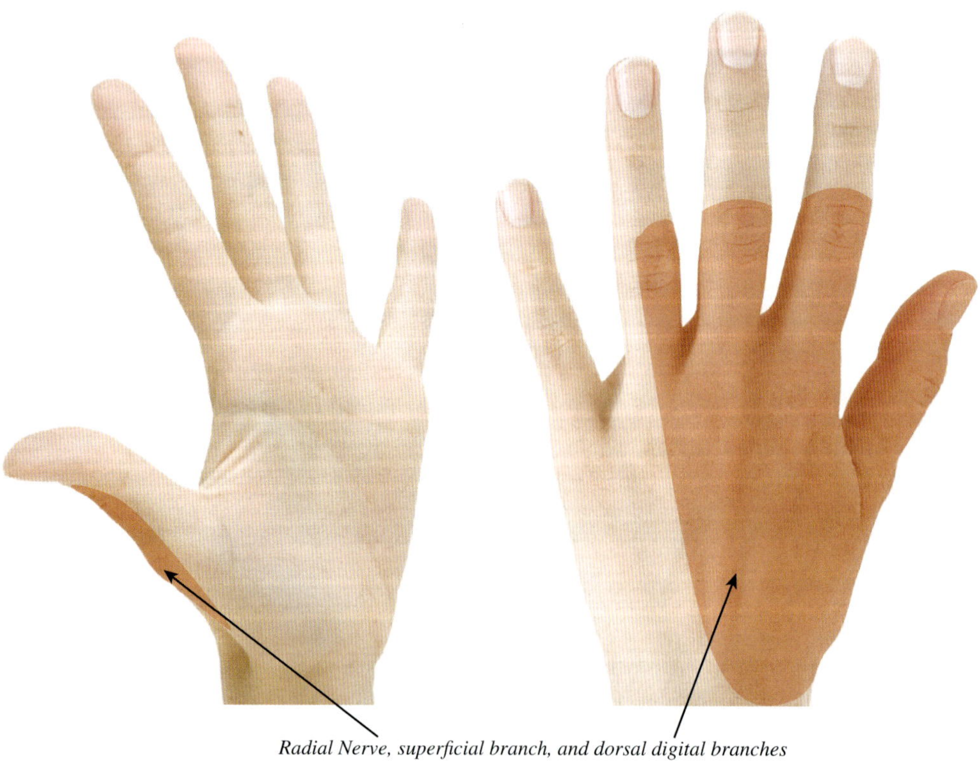

FIGURE 9-10 The radial nerve provides sensory input to two-thirds of the dorsal hand.

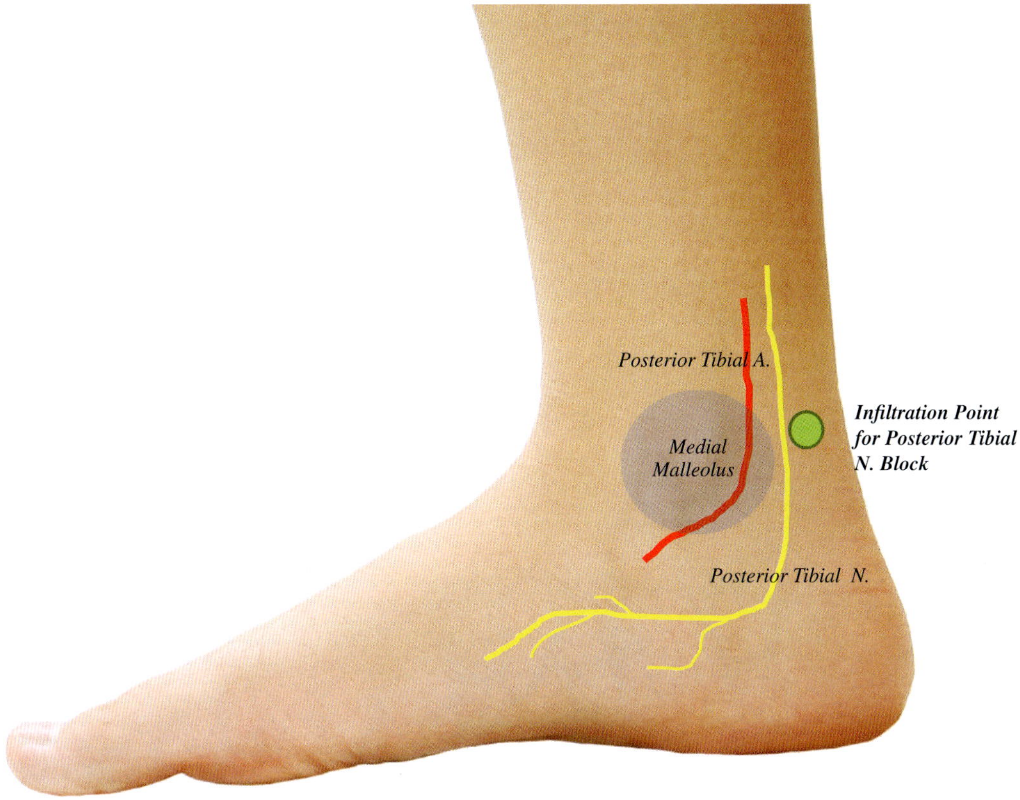

FIGURE 9-11 The posterior tibial nerve innervates the majority of the plantar surface of the foot, except for its medial aspect, and is anesthetized at the medial malleolus, where the nerve runs posterior to the posterior tibial artery.

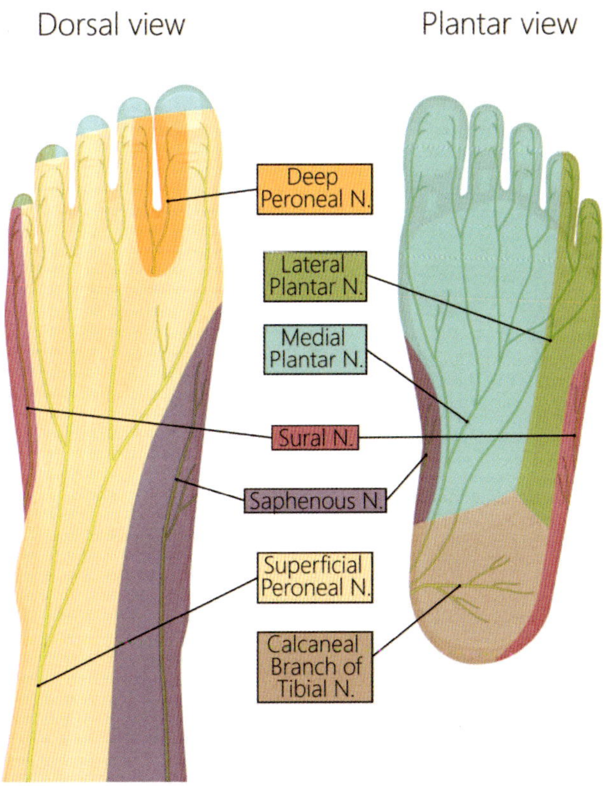

FIGURE 9-12 The saphenous nerve innervates the medial aspect of the plantar foot.

space of the foot.[5,6] It is blocked by injecting 3 to 5 mL of local anesthetic between the anterior tibial surface and lateral malleolus, providing anesthesia to the majority of the dorsal foot.[6,75] The deep peroneal nerve innervates the first web space of the foot[5,6,78] and is located lateral to the extensor hallucis longus tendon and dorsalis pedis artery.[6] It is a rarely blocked nerve because anesthesia to this area can be achieved by local infiltration.[5,6] If a deep peroneal nerve block is required, then 3 mL of anesthetic is injected medial to the dorsalis pedis artery and lateral to the extensor hallucis longus tendon.[6,76]

ADVERSE REACTIONS

Local Adverse Reactions

Adverse reactions to local anesthesia vary in presentation; many reactions are due to improper technique[14] or to added epinephrine,[5] rather than to the anesthetic itself. Swelling, bruising, pain, and temporary disfigurement are some of the most frequently seen adverse reactions.[5,14] Most resolve spontaneously without serious repercussions for the patient.

The use of epinephrine in local anesthetics has been reported to be associated with ischemia in digital areas.[6,62] Those who suffer from collagen vascular disorders, vasospastic diseases, peripheral vascular disease, or uncontrolled hypertension are at somewhat higher risk.[62,79] Digital ischemia has been reported to occur when larger volumes of anesthesia are used even without the addition of

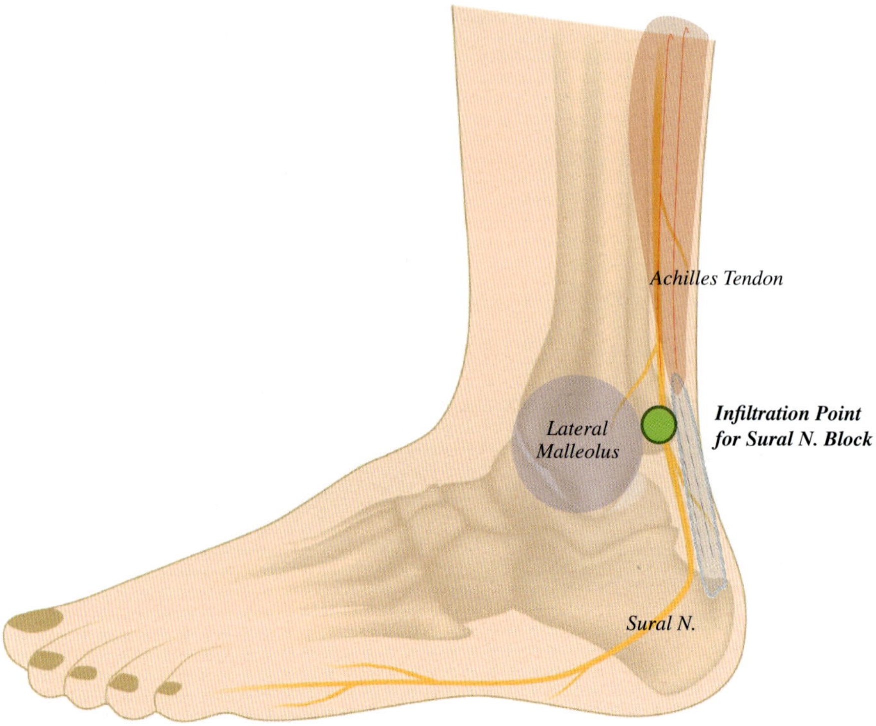

FIGURE 9-13 To block the sural nerve, 3 to 5 mL of local anesthetic is injected between the posterior distal tip of the lateral malleolus and Achilles tendon.

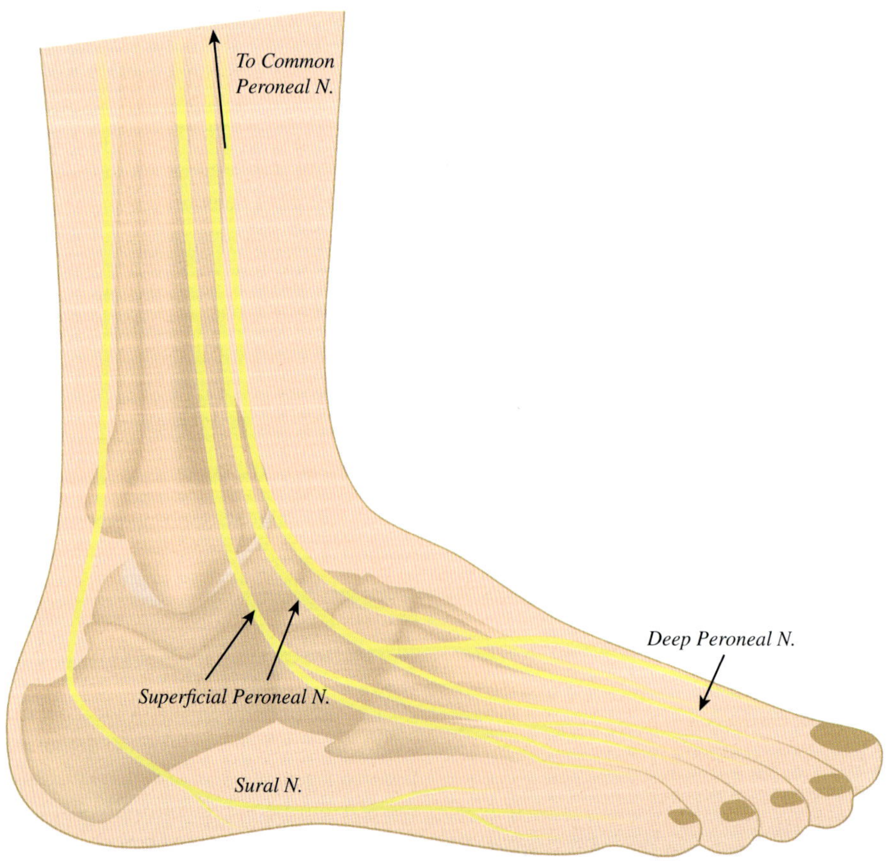

FIGURE 9-14 The superficial and deep peroneal nerves arise from the common peroneal nerve.

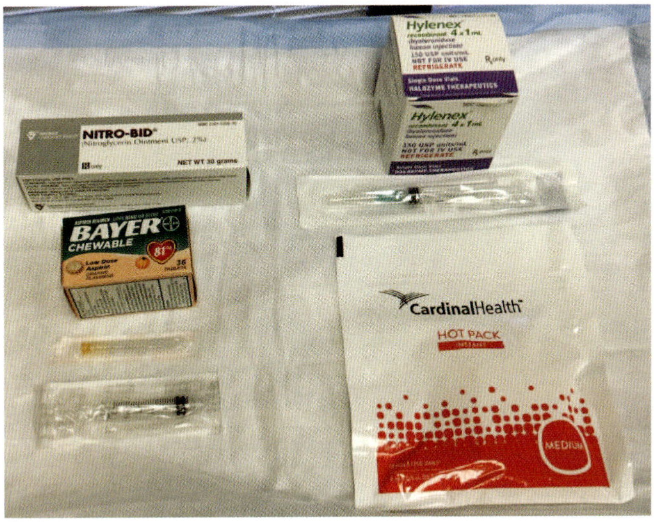

FIGURE 9-15 Filler complication kit.

epinephrine.[79] Reversal can be achieved with topical nitroglycerin and/or injectable phentolamine 0.5 mg/mL.[6,62] The latter is an α-adrenergic blocker that induces vasodilation.[6]

Vascular compromise has also been reported after using cosmetic filler agents containing local anesthetics.[80] Skin necrosis can occur with cosmetic injectables administered in the vascular areas of the glabella, nasal ala, and periocular areas, and it is important to be careful when injecting into these delicate areas.[80,81] The use of cannulas and a retrograde injection technique can minimize the risk of vascular compromise. If ischemia occurs, pain or blanching of the skin is immediately noted. If not quickly treated, pain, cutaneous ulceration, and mottling of the skin can ensue.[80] A post–cosmetic filler injectable kit (**Figure 9-15**) containing hyaluronidase, topical nitroglycerin, thermal warm pack, aspirin, and 27-gauge needle with attached syringe can be helpful to treat such complications[80,81] and should be readily available for clinicians who perform cosmetic injectable procedures. Importantly, these reactions are generally to the filler material rather than its associated anesthetic.

Another rare complication is nerve damage.[5,6,82] This reaction often results from block procedures where the nerve is injured from transection of the sheath, pressure from large volume of anesthesia, direct injection of anesthetic into the nerve, toxicity of the anesthetic agent, or vascular compromise to the nerve structure itself. Pain or paresthesias directly around or distal to the injection site are an early sign that a nerve injury may be occurring.[6] If a patient complains of similar symptoms, then the procedure should be immediately stopped[5] and the patient promptly evaluated.

Chemical burns may be seen with the use of topical anesthetics, especially around the eyes.[6] Many topical anesthetics such as EMLA have an alkaline pH.[6] This allows for easier penetration into the skin. Ocular injuries such as corneal abrasions, ulcerations, erythema, and infections have been reported with the use of these agents.[6,49] It is important to have an eyewash station immediately accessible in case a patient complains of eye burning or tearing from topical anesthetics. An immediate ophthalmologic assessment is important[6] in order to minimize both ocular pain and the risk of permanent blindness.

Lastly, thermal injuries can be seen after procedures that use tumescent anesthesia and/or nerve blocks.[6] Burns from cigarettes and other sources of heat have been reported in patients postoperatively who do not realize that they are still numb.[6,83,84] It is important to educate patients about the duration of their anesthesia prior to discharge from the office in order to minimize the likelihood of this adverse reaction.

Systemic Reactions

Systemic reactions can also occur with topical and local anesthesia. Life-threatening adverse reactions are thankfully rare.[5,6,85] The most common reactions usually involve the central nervous and cardiac systems. One of the most common reactions to local anesthetics is a vasovagal response.[5,7] This is a psychogenic reaction that occurs in response to a patient's general anxiety, fear of needles, pain, or blood. Increased parasympathetic output leads to vagal-induced bradycardia, nausea, diaphoresis, lightheadedness, and hypotension.[5,6] Reversal is accomplished with Trendelenburg positioning,[6,69] cool compresses, fluid intake, hand grip and leg crossing, smelling salts, and rarely midodrine or β-blockers[69] (**Table 9-6**).

Lidocaine Toxicity

The recommended maximum doses of lidocaine are 4.5 mg/kg without epinephrine, 7.0 mg/kg with epinephrine, and 55 mg/kg with tumescent lidocaine solutions[6,28,86] (**Table 9-7**). It is essential that the clinician recognize that higher blood levels of lidocaine

TABLE 9-6 • Treatment of Vasovagal Reaction

- Place in Trendelenburg position
- Smelling salts
- Cool compresses on neck and face
- Intravenous hydration
- Consider β-blockers, midodrine
- Leg compression
- Patient education on how to respond to these reactions, especially if they experience "prodromal" symptoms
- Training exercises "Applied Tension"—tensing muscles in arms, legs, and torso
- Increase salt and fluid intake to increase blood volume (eg, sports drinks) prior to procedure
- Moving/crossing legs and tightening muscles to keep blood pressure from dropping prior to performing procedure
- If a cardiac arrhythmia is found, implantation of a pacemaker may be needed

TABLE 9-7 • Recommended Doses of Lidocaine

Patient Category	Maximum Dose (mg/kg)
Children	
Lidocaine with epinephrine	3.0-4.5
Lidocaine without epinephrine	1.5-2.0
Adults	
Lidocaine with epinephrine	7.0
Lidocaine without epinephrine	4.5
Tumescent anesthesia	55

Data from Avram MR, Avram MM, Ratner D: Procedural Dermatology. *China: McGraw Hill; 2015.*

can be attained from inadvertent vascular injection or rapid drug absorption (eg, in mucous membrane areas).[5] Similarly, one also must be aware that that local anesthetic effects in fair individuals with red hair are difficult to establish. Some authors postulate that this may be due to a mutation in the melanocortin-1 receptor, which may affect neuromodulatory regulation within the central nervous system.[87]

Lidocaine metabolism can also be affected by pseudocholinesterase deficiency, liver disease, and interactions with certain medications.[5,6,14] Lidocaine is an amide anesthetic and is metabolized by the hepatic cytochrome CYP3A4 and CYP1A2 enzymes.[5,6] The use of large lidocaine doses in patients taking medications that inhibit these enzyme systems can lead to an increased risk of toxicity. Common medications including tetracycline, cimetidine, selective serotonin reuptake inhibitors, and fluconazole inhibit CYP3A4, resulting in increased lidocaine levels[6] (**Table 9-8**). β-Blockers can increase lidocaine levels by reducing cardiac and hepatic blood flow.[6] With respect to renal function, no special adjustments need to be undertaken when administering lidocaine.[6]

TABLE 9-8 • Drugs Causing Elevated Lidocaine Levels (Cytochrome P450-3A4 Inhibitors)

- Amiodarone
- Azoles (Fluconazole, Itraconazole)
- Carbamazepine
- Cimetidine
- Clarithromycin
- Chloramphenicol
- Cyclosporine
- Danazol
- Dexamethasone
- Diltiazem
- Erythromycin
- Isoniazid
- Methadone
- Methylprednisolone
- Metronidazole
- Nicardipine
- Nifedipine
- Pentoxifylline
- Propofol
- Propranolol
- Quinidine
- SSRIs
- Tetracycline
- Terfenadine
- Thyroxine
- Valproic acid
- Verapamil

SSRI, selective serotonin reuptake inhibitor.
Reproduced with permission from Robinson J. Surgery of the Skin: Procedural Dermatology, *3rd ed. London: Elsevier/Saunders; 2015.*

TABLE 9-9 • Lidocaine Toxicity Based on Blood Serum Values

Stage	Serum Lidocaine Concentration (μg/mL)	Adverse Effects
I	1-6	Circumoral paresthesia, tinnitus, lightheadedness, agitation, talkative, drowsy, disoriented, metallic taste in mouth
II	6-12	Nausea, vomiting, muscle twitching, tremors, nystagmus, blurred vision, seizures
III	>12	Coma, respiratory arrest, dysrhythmia, cardiac arrest

Signs of Lidocaine Toxicity

Lidocaine toxicity occurs in a concentration-dependent fashion (**Table 9-9**). At lower levels (3–6 μg/mL), toxicity may manifest as circumoral paresthesia, euphoria, anxiety, talkativeness, or blurred vision.[6] As toxicity progresses (5–9 μg/mL), vomiting, tremors, and restlessness ensue.[5,6,28,88] At higher levels of 10 to 26 μg/mL, seizures, cardiopulmonary depression, and cardiac arrest can ensue.[6,85]

When lidocaine toxicity begins to manifest, immediate cessation of drug delivery and basic steps to support the airway and circulation must be undertaken.[5,6] After activating emergency medical services and preparing for possible hospital transport, the initial management plan should be to stop anesthetic delivery, monitor vital signs, maintain ventilation, administer oxygen, and establish an intravenous line.[6] Hypoxia and acidosis decrease the threshold for seizure induction and increase cardiotoxic effects.[89] Seizures are treated with diazepam, propofol, or thiopental sodium.[89] Hypotension is addressed by administering fluid boluses and sometime adding vasopressors such as epinephrine or phenylephrine.[89] Bradycardia may require atropine or inotropic agents. When intubation is required, neuromuscular blockers such as succinylcholine are often employed.[89] An algorithm reviewing the management of local anesthetic–induced systemic toxicity is outlined in **Table 9-10**.[89]

Bupivacaine Toxicity

Bupivacaine is more cardiotoxic than other anesthetic agents and has a greater tendency to induce arrhythmias that are refractory to defibrillation.[89] This may be because it enters the sodium channel rapidly but leaves slowly.[5] It also has the greatest propensity for inducing seizures.[89] In late-trimester pregnancy, cardiotoxicity is more likely due to reduced venous return and increased progesterone levels.[5-7]

Topical Anesthetic Systemic Toxicity

There have been reported adverse effects and even fatalities with the use of topical anesthetics.[28,90,91] Prolonged application with and

TABLE 9-10 • Algorithm to Treat Lidocaine Toxicity

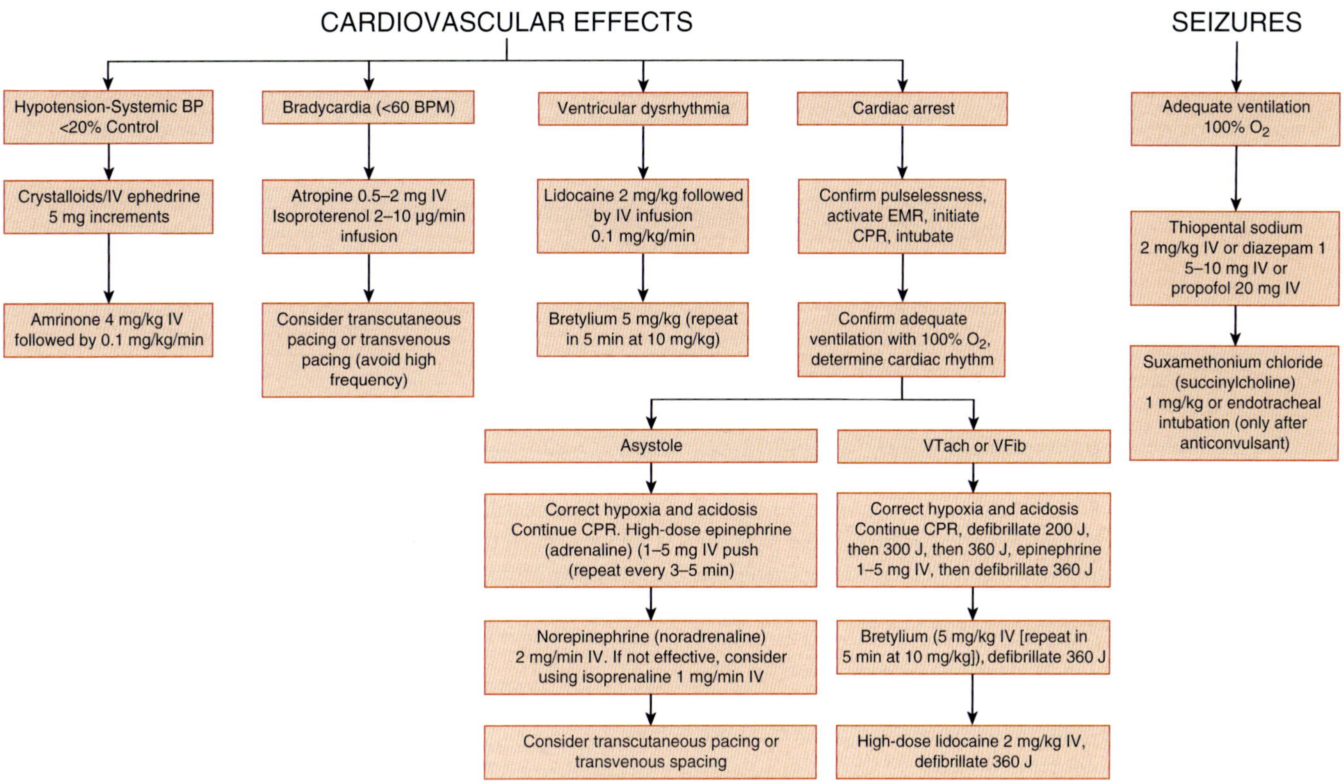

BP, blood pressure; CPR, cardiopulmonary resuscitation; EMR, emergency medical response; IV, intravenous; VFib, ventricular fibrillation; VTach, ventricular tachycardia. Reproduced with permission from Naguib M, Magboul MM, Samarkandi AH, et al. Adverse effects and drug interactions associated with local and regional anaesthesia. Drug Saf. *1998 Apr;18(4):221-250.*

without occlusion, use of inappropriately high concentrations, and application to large surface areas increase the risk of cardiotoxicity and central nervous system toxicity.[90] Usually, the central nervous system is more readily affected by the pharmacologic actions of local anesthesia than the cardiovascular system.[92] As with injected anesthetics, the initial symptoms of topical anesthetic toxicity include lightheadedness, circumoral numbness, diplopia, and tinnitus.[90]

With respect to reported fatalities from topical anesthetics, most reported subjects were young and received topical anesthesia prior to laser hair removal.[6,93-95] Anesthetic application was performed under occlusion for an extended time. Two cases occurred after using compounded creams that were liberally applied to the legs[6,93,94] for greater than 60 minutes under occlusion. Another case involved topical anesthetic application to the back.[95] In some instances, no physician supervision was present, the patients applied the creams themselves, and no pre- and postoperative instructions were reviewed with the patient.

Rapid recognition of anesthetic toxicity is the most important step in managing an accidental overdose. If suspected, the anesthetic must be immediately washed off.[90]

Epinephrine Toxicity

Concentrations of epinephrine greater than 1:100,000 have been reported to induce a higher rate of serious adverse events.[5,8] The maximum dose of epinephrine that one can receive should not exceed 1 mg (1 mL of 1:1000 solution) over a 10-hour period.[5] The clinician should be aware of any patient health risks, such as hyperthyroidism and cardiac disease, which can affect the metabolism and/or sensitivity to epinephrine.[6,14] The most common side effect of epinephrine is transient tachycardia.[14,96] This can progress, in rarer instances, to palpitations, sweating, tremors, pallor, and chest pain.[14,97] Most of these adverse effects occur within 1 to 4 minutes after injection.[14,96]

With respect to pregnancy, animal studies have shown that there is a reduction in uterine blood flow after epinephrine administration.[5,98] Epinephrine is classified as a Category C drug.[5,6,28,99] Pregnancy is considered a relative, although not absolute, contraindication to its use.[5] Nonemergent usage should probably be delayed until after delivery.[5,28,100] Absolute contraindications to epinephrine use include pheochromocytoma, uncontrolled hyperthyroidism,[5] and severe hypertension.[6] A list of relative and absolute contraindications to epinephrine use can be found in **Table 9-11**.

With respect to drug interactions, caution must be used when administering epinephrine-based anesthetics in those who are taking antidepressants and/or β-blockers.[5,6] Epinephrine and propranolol together can result in a life-threatening systemic reaction.[14,101] The injection of epinephrine in a patient

TABLE 9-11 • Absolute and Relative Contraindications to Epinephrine Use

Absolute Contraindications	Relative Contraindications	
Severe Hypertension	β-Blocker Administration	MAO Administration
Uncontrolled hyperthyroidism	Tricyclic antidepressant administration	Phenothiazine administration
Pheochromocytoma	Peripheral vascular disease	Unstable cardiac disease
	Anxiety or psychiatric disorder	
	Pregnancy (when large doses are required)	
	Glaucoma	
	Unstable diabetes mellitus	
	Hypersensitivity to sulfites	Epinephrine allergy

MAO, monoamine oxidase.

receiving propranolol results in unopposed α_1 vasoconstriction activity.[14] This can result in marked hypertension followed by reflex bradycardia, which ultimately can lead to a cardiac or neurologic event.[6,14,101] This reaction has been reported to occur with only 8 mL of lidocaine with 1:200,000 of epinephrine (a very low systemic dose of epinephrine), in a patient taking propranolol (Inderal) 60 mg daily.[101] For smaller dermatologic procedures such as biopsies, this interaction may not be as clinically important.[14] For larger skin surgeries requiring more local anesthesia, it may be advisable to have patients adjust or temporarily wean off their β-blocker as directed by their primary care physician before the scheduled procedure.[14]

Allergic Reactions

Type 1 and 4 hypersensitivity reactions to topical and local anesthetics have been reported but are rare.[6,28] Type 1 reactions are IgE mediated, immediate, and can lead to anaphylaxis.[5] Ester-derived anesthetics are more often associated with allergic reactions than amide anesthetics.[5] There is no cross-reactivity between ester and amide reactions.[6] Ester anesthetics are metabolized to PABA, a common allergen that cross-reacts with thiazides, sulfonylureas, and hair dyes containing para-phenylenediamine (PPD).[6,88] Amide-induced allergic reactions are rare and are likely due to methylparabens found in the preservative.[5,85,88] When a patient has a documented history of procaine or PABA sensitivity, the use of preservative-free lidocaine is recommended.[6,88] If a mild reaction is noted, it can be managed with antihistamines and topical corticosteroids.[5,6] When anaphylaxis is suspected, it should be quickly addressed by activating emergency medical services and administering 0.3 to 0.5 mg of epinephrine subcutaneously along with basic life support measures.[6,102]

There are no specific recommendations to test for allergic reactions to local anesthetics.[5,88] Some authors advise the use of patch tests or intradermal testing with preservative-free lidocaine in high-risk patients.[6,88] Another option is to avoid local anesthetic agents entirely. Nontraditional anesthetics that have been shown to be effective include ice, normal saline, diphenhydramine 1%, bacteriostatic saline,[28] intradermal tramadol, and metoclopramide.[5,103,104] Shave biopsy sites may be easily anesthetized with normal saline or liquid nitrogen. Diphenhydramine is more sedating[5,6] and painful[103] than lidocaine and can rarely lead to skin necrosis.[104] Intradermal tramadol can induce local site skin reactions.[6,105,106] When faced with the dilemma of what is the best anesthetic agent to use in a high-risk patient, it is probably best to consult with an allergist.[5,6] In this way, one can most accurately assess the degree and nature of the allergy, attempt to desensitize the patient to that allergen, and identify the safest anesthetic approach for the patient.

Methemoglobinemia

Methemoglobinemia is the process by which hemoglobin is oxidized to a non–oxygen-carrying state instead of an oxygen-carrying reduced state.[5,6] Benzocaine and prilocaine are most often associated with methemoglobinemia.[6] Infants and children are more susceptible to hemoglobin oxidation given that they may have more susceptible hemoglobin F, have less reductive enzymes, and have a lower body weight.[5,6,89] Other risk factors for methemoglobinemia include glucose-6-phosphate dehydrogenase (G6PD) deficiency, methemoglobin reductase deficiency, and use of medications such as antimalarials and sulfonamides[5,107] (**Table 9-12**). Rare cases have also been reported with EMLA cream.[5,89]

When evaluating and treating methemoglobinemia, it is important to recognize that conventional pulse oximetry is unreliable.[5,6]

TABLE 9-12 • Risk Factors Associated with Methemoglobinemia

- G6PD deficiency
- Methemoglobin reductase deficiency
- Infants and children
  - Less reductive enzymes
  - Hemoglobin F susceptibility
  - Lower weight
- Simultaneous medication ingestion
  - Antimalarials
  - Dapsone
  - Nitrates
  - Phenobarbital
  - Sulfonamides

G6PD, glucose-6-phosphate dehydrogenase.

TABLE 9-13 • Recommended Pediatric Doses for EMLA Cream[a]

Age	Weight (kg)	Max Dose (g)	Max Application Area (cm^2)	Application Time (hours)
0-3 months	<5	1	10	1
3-12 months	5-10	2	20	4
1-6 years	10-20	10	100	4
7-12 years	>20	20	200	4

[a]*For applying to intact skin only. Caution must be taken if applying to injured or inflamed skin as EMLA absorption can vary in these areas.*

The presence of cyanosis without the presence of cardiorespiratory disease is a strong clinical indicator.[6] Actual blood levels of methemoglobin or arterial blood gases are required for accurate diagnosis.[6] Methemoglobin levels below 30% can be managed with observation, oxygen, and the elimination of further local anesthetic delivery.[5,6,102] Higher methemoglobin levels may require intravenous methylene blue administered at 1 to 2 mg/kg.[5,6] In those with G6PD deficiency, methylene blue is contraindicated, although ascorbic acid and/or hemodialysis can be used.[5,6,102,107]

Children

The recommended doses of lidocaine in children over 3 years of age should not exceed 1.5 to 2.0 mg/kg without epinephrine or 3.0 to 4.5 mg/kg with epinephrine.[6,14] The use of preservative-free anesthetic is preferred in neonates with jaundice.[32] This is due to the intrinsic bilirubin displacement properties of parabens found within preservative-containing anesthetics.

Topical anesthetics can induce toxicity in children, and care must be taken when using these agents.[5,51] The recommended pediatric does for EMLA cream can be found in **Table 9-13**.[5,48]

Pregnancy Considerations

Local anesthetics are generally considered safe during pregnancy, despite the fact that they can cross the placenta via passive diffusion.[6] Studies have demonstrated safety with first-trimester lidocaine use with no adverse maternal or teratogenic effects.[100] Lidocaine, etidocaine, and prilocaine are categorized as Category B drugs.[6] Bupivacaine and mepivacaine are classified as Category C because of their potential to induce fetal bradycardia.[6,100] Infant toxicity has also been reported in lactating mothers treated with large volumes of local anesthesia agents.[100]

INTRAOPERATIVE CONSIDERATIONS

For short dermatologic procedures, buffered lidocaine 1% with 1:100,000 epinephrine can be used as a solitary anesthetic. With longer cases, such as Mohs surgery and four-lid blepharoplasty surgery, bupivacaine or etidocaine can be added to maximize anesthetic duration.[5,6] For longer surgeries, buffered lidocaine is administered first in order to provide more comfort for the patient prior to injecting bupivacaine, which is a much more painful and slower-acting anesthetic. Anesthetic is drawn up using an 18-gauge syringe and subsequently injected into the skin using a 30-gauge needle.

Cold compresses prior to injection can also serve to alleviate patient discomfort.[108] Hemostasis can be optimized by waiting for 5 to 10 minutes after injection.[5] For infected sites, larger volumes of local anesthetic may be required because they work less effectively in bacteria-laden acidic environments.[5]

For procedures requiring multiple injections, it is useful to advance the needle in an area that has been previously anesthetized.[6] Puncture number can be reduced by using longer needles or employing cannulas. Ring blocks are a great consideration for cyst removal, incision and drainage procedures, lipoma removal, and scalp and ear procedures.[5,6]

For surgeries involving the face, such as laser resurfacing, or the hand, foot, and digits, nerve blocks are ideal.[5,6,68] They require less anesthetic, create minimal tissue distortion,[5,6] and are often less painful. The disadvantages of nerve blocks are that they take more time to complete[5] and do not provide hemostasis.[6]

Topical anesthesia use is especially effective in mucosal areas or prior to pediatric procedures such as wart or molluscum removal.[5] They can be applied over a treatment site "like cream cheese on a bagel" or under occlusion in limited areas. The removal of skin tags or hemangiomas and incision and drainage procedures are less painful with topical anesthetic formulations. Combined approaches using topical anesthetics with nerve blocks are a great way to help laser resurfacing and dermabrasion patients achieve optimal comfort without the need for general anesthesia.

POSTOPERATIVE CONSIDERATIONS

For postoperative laser resurfacing cases, mix three parts petrolatum with one part topical anesthetic and apply this to a completely treated area while the nerve block is still working (eg, complete the laser procedure on one-half of the face and immediately apply the dilute topical anesthetic agent). With this approach, patients leave the office very comfortable. They are advised to reapply this numbing mixture every 2 to 3 hours for the first 24 hours. After this period, patient discomfort is minimal, and they usually only complain of warmth and swelling, which can be easily managed with cool compresses and oral ibuprofen.

Another postoperative consideration to optimize patient comfort is to inject an additional amount of bupivacaine or tumescent anesthetic solution postoperatively.[6,109,110] This will help the patient gain some added pain relief while they wait for their oral pain medication to take effect (**Table 9-14**).

TABLE 9-14 • Other Postoperative Considerations

- Personally calling patients to ensure a smooth postoperative course and alleviate any concerns that they may have.
- Alternate acetaminophen 500-1000 mg with ibuprofen 600 mg every 4 hours.
- Cool compresses over surgery areas for 5-10 minutes every hour as tolerated.
- For laser resurfacing cases, mix three parts petrolatum with one part topical anesthetic and apply this to a completely treated area while the nerve block is still working. Have patients reapply this mixture every 2-3 hours for the first 24 hours.
- Injecting an additional amount of bupivacaine or tumescent anesthetic solution at the end of the surgery. This will help patients gain some added pain relief as they wait for their oral pain medication to take effect.

CONCLUSIONS

Local anesthesia (along with the advent of antibiotics) represents perhaps the single greatest advance in dermatologic surgery over the past two centuries. Although a wide array of agents are available to the clinician, the workhorse solution of 1% lidocaine with epinephrine is the most frequently used anesthetic agent in dermatologic procedures and is generally safe, effective, and well tolerated by most patients.

REFERENCES

1. McCloud I, Meyers AD. Local anesthetics. *Medscape*. March 18, 2015.
2. Ring ME. The history of local anesthesia. *J Calif Dent Assoc.* 2007;35:275-282.
3. Freud S. Uber Coca. House officer of the General Hospital of Vienna. *Centrallblatt für die ges. Therapie*. 1884;2:289-314.
4. Calatayud J, Gonzalez A. History of the development and evolution of local anesthesia since the coca leaf. *Anesthesiology.* 2003;98:1503-1508.
5. Gharavi NM. Lask GP. Anesthesia and analgesia. Surgical principles. In: Avram MR, Avram MM, Ratner D, eds. *Procedural Dermatology.* New York, NY: McGraw-Hill Education; 2015:33-50.
6. Soriano TT, Breithaupt A, Chestnut C. Anesthesia and analgesia. In: Robinson J, ed. *Surgery of the Skin: Procedural Dermatology.* 3rd ed. London, United Kingdom: Elsevier/Saunders; 2015:43-63.
7. Tetzlaff JE. The pharmacology of local anesthetics. *Anesthesiol Clin North Am.* 2000;18:217-231.
8. Becker DE, Reed KI. Essentials of local anesthetic pharmacology. *Anesth Prog.* 2006;58:98-108.
9. Brunton L, Chabner B, Knollman B. *Goodman and Gillman's the Pharmaceutical Basis of Therapeutics*. 12th ed. New York, NY: McGraw-Hill Medical; 2011:573.
10. Han JW, Nah SK, Lee SY, Kim CY, Yoon JS, Jang SY. A Prospective, Comparative Study of the Pain of Local Anesthesia Using 2% Lidocaine, 2% Lidocaine With Epinephrine, and 2% Lidocaine With Epinephrine-Bupivicaine Mixture for Eyelid Surgery. *Ophthalmic Plast Reconstr Surg.* 2017 Mar/Apr;33(2):132-135. doi: 10.1097/IOP.0000000000000675.
11. Collins JB, Song J, Mahabir RC. Onset and duration of intradermal mixtures of bupivacaine and lidocaine with epinephrine. *Can J Plast Surg.* 2013;21(1):51-53.
12. Covino BG. Local anesthesia. *N Engl J Med.* 1972;286(19):1035-1042.
13. Latorrre F, Klimek L. Does cocaine still have a role in nasal surgery? *Drug Saf.* 1999;20(1):9-13.
14. Grekin RC, Auletta MJ. Local anesthesia in dermatologic surgery. *J Am Acad Dermatol.* 1988;19(4):599-614.
15. Waldman N, Densie IK, Herbison P. Topical tetracaine used for 24 hours is safe and rated highly effective by patients for the treatment of pain caused by corneal abrasions: a double-blind, randomized clinical trial. *Acad Emerg Med.* 2014;21(4):374-382.
16. Forster JG. Short acting spinal anesthesia in the ambulatory setting. *Curr Opin Anaesthesiol.* 2014;27(6):597-604.
17. Covino BG. Pharmacology of local anesthetics. *Br J Anaesth.* 1986;58:701-716.
18. Savarese JJ, Covino BG. Basic and clinical pharmacology of local anesthetic drugs. In: Miller RD, ed. *Anesthesia*. 2nd ed. New York, NY: Churchill Livingstone; 1986:985-1101.
19. Fink BR. The long and short of conduction block. *Anesth Analg.* 1989;658:553-555.
20. Butterworth JF IV, Strichartz GR. Molecular mechanisms of local anesthesia: a review. *Anesthesiology*. 1990;73:711-734.
21. Ragsdale DS, McPhee JC, Scheuer T, Cattarall WA. Molecular determinants of state-dependent block of Na+ channels by local anesthetics. *Science*. 1994;265(5179):1724-1729.
22. Korbon GA, Hurley DP, Williams GS. pH-adjusted lidocaine does not "sting." *Anesthesiology.* 1987;66(6):855-856.
23. McKay W, Morris R, Mushlin P. Sodium Bicarbonate attenuates pain on skin infiltration with or without epinephrine. *Anesth Analg.* 1987;66:572-574.
24. Robinson J, Fernando R, Sun Wai WJ, et al. Chemical stability of bupivacaine, lidocaine and epinephrine in pH adjusted solutions. *Anesthesia.* 2000;55:853-858.
25. Bourget P, Bonhomme L, Benhaman D. Factors influencing precipitation of pH-adjusted bupivacaine solutions. *J Clin Pharm Ther.* 1990;15:197-204.
26. Lewis Smith PA. Adjunctive use of hyaluronidase in local anaesthesia. *Br J Plast Surg.* 1986;39:554-558.
27. Clark LE, Mellete JR. The use of hyaluronidase as an adjunct to surgical procedures. *J Dermatol Surg Oncol.* 1994;20(12):842-844.
28. Kouba DJ, LoPiccolo MC, Alam M, et al. Guidelines for the use of local anesthesia in office-based dermatologic surgery. *J Am Acad Dermatol.* 2016;74:1201-1219.
29. Ono N. Pain free intralesional injection of triamcinolone for the treatment of keloid. *Scand J Plast Reconstr Surg Hand Surg.* 1999;33(1):89-91.
30. Schechtman AD. Letter to editor. Combining triamcinolone and lidocaine for soft tissue injections. *Am Fam Physician.* 2008;77(10):1372.
31. Huether MJ, Griego RD, Broadland D. Clindamycin for intraincisional antibiotic prophylaxis in dermatologic surgery. *Arch Dermatol.* 2002;138(9):1145-1148.

32. Dinehart SM. Topical, local and regional anesthesia. In: Wheeland R, ed. *Cutaneous Surgery*. Philadelphia, PA: WB Saunders; 1994:105-110.
33. Colllins JB, Sing J, Mahibir RC. Onset and duration of intradermal mixtures of bupivacaine and lidocaine with epinephrine. *Can J Plast Surg*. 2013;21(1):51-53.
34. Cuvillon P, Nouvellon E, Ripart J, et al. A comparison of the pharmacodynamics and pharmacokinetics of bupivacaine, ropivacaine (with epinephrine) and their equal volume mixtures with lidocaine used for femoral and sciatic nerve blocks: a double-blind randomized study. *Anesth Analg*. 2009;108(2):641-649.
35. Huang W, Vidimos A. Topical anesthetics in dermatology. *J Am Acad Dermatol.* 2000;43(2):286-298.
36. Adriani J, Dalili H. Penetration of local anesthetics through epithelial barriers. *Anesth Analg*. 1971;50(5):834-841.
37. Friedman PM, Mafong EA, Friedman BS, et al. Topical anesthetics update; EMLA and beyond. *Dermatol Surg*. 2001;27:1019-1026.
38. Kumar M, Chawla R, Goyal M. Topical anesthesia. *J Anesthes Clin Pharm*. 2015;31(4):45-56.
39. Taddio A, Stevens B, Craig K, et al. Efficacy and safety of lidocaine-prilocaine cream for pain during circumcision. *N Engl J Med.* 1997;336(17):1197-1201.
40. Smith DP, Gjellum M. The efficacy of LMX versus EMLA for pain relief in boys undergoing office meatotomy. *J Urol.* 2004;172(4 Pt 2): 1760-1761.
41. Guardiano RA, Norwood CW. Direct comparison of EMLA versus lidocaine for pain control in Nd:YAG 1064 nm laser hair removal. *Dermatol Surg*. 2005;31(4):396-398.
42. Greene JJ, Sidle DM. The hyaluronic acid fillers: current understanding of the tissue device interface. *Facial Plast Surg Clin North Am*. 2015;23(4):423-432.
43. Bryan HA, Alster TS. The S-caine peel: a novel topical anesthetic for cutaneous laser surgery. *Dermatol Surg*. 2002;28:999-1003.
44. McCafferty DF, Woolfson AD, Handley J, Allen G. Effect of percutaneous local anaesthetics on pain reduction during pulse dye laser treatment of portwine stains. *Br J Anaesth*. 1997;78: 286-289.
45. Alster TS, Lupton JR. Evaluation of a novel topical anesthetic agent for cutaneous laser resurfacing: a randomized comparison study. *Dermatol Surg*. 2002;28(11):1004-1006; discussion 1006.
46. Alster TS. The lidocaine/tetracaine peel: a novel topical anesthetic for dermatologic procedures in adult patients. *Dermatol Surg*. 2007;33(9):1073-1081.
47. Juhlin L, Evers H, Broberg F. A lidocaine-prilocaine cream for superficial skin surgery and painful lesions *Acta Derm Venereol.* 1980;60:544-546.
48. Rincon E, Baker RL, Iglesias AJ, Duarte AM. CNS Toxicity after topical application of EMLA cream on a toddler with molluscum contagiosum. *Pediatr Emerg Care*. 2000;16:252-254.
49. Eaglestein NF. Chemical injury to the eye from EMLA cream during erbium laser resurfacing. *Dermatol Surg*. 1999;25:590-591.
50. Railan D, Alster TS. Use of topical lidocaine for cosmetic dermatologic procedures. *J Drugs Dermatol.* 2007;6:1104-1108.
51. Sobanko JF, Miller CJ, Alster TS. Topical anesthetics for dermatologic procedures: a review. *Dermatol Surg*. 2012;38(5):709-721.
52. Greenspan M. BLT topical anesthetics for derm—safety standards. *Linkedin*. November 17, 2016.
53. Kuhwahara RT, Skinner RB. EMLA versus ice as a topical anesthetic. *Dermatol Surg*. 2001;27:495-496.
54. Plotkin S. Clinical comparison of preinjection anesthetics. *J Am Podiatr Med Assoc.* 1998;88:73-79.
55. Tehrani S, Fraunfelder FW. Cryotherapy in ophthalmology. *Open J Ophthalmol*. 2013;3:103-117.
56. White JM, Siegfried E, Boulden M, Padda G. Possible hazards of cryogen use with pulsed dye laser. A case report and summary. *Dermatol Surg*. 1999;25:250-253.
57. Greenbaum SS, Bernstein EF. Comparison of iontophoresis of lidocaine with a eutectic mixture of lidocaine and prilocaine (EMLA) for topically administered local anesthesia. *J Dermatol Surg Oncol.* 1994;20(9):579-583.
58. Galinkin JL, Rose JB, Harris K, Watcha MF. Lidocaine iontophoresis versus eutectic mixture of local anesthetics (EMLA®) for IV placement in children. *Anesth Analg*. 2002;94:1484-1488.
59. Vinycomb TI, Sahlar LJ. Comparison of local anesthetics for digital nerve blocks: a systemic review. *J Hand Surg Am*. 2014;39(4):744-751.
60. Nusstein J, Burns Y, Reader A, Beck M, Weaver J. Injection pain and postinjection pain of the palatal-anterior superior alveolar injection, administered with the Wand Plus system, comparing 2% lidocaine with 1:100000 epinephrine to 3% mepivacaine. *Oral Surg Oral Med Oral Pathol Oral Radiol Endod.* 2004;97(2):164-172.
61. Ilicki J. Safety of epinephrine in digital nerve blocks: a literature review. *J Emerg Med*. 2015;49(5):799-809.
62. Denkler K. A comprehensive review of epinephrine in the finger; to do or not to do. *Plast Reconstr Surg*. 2001;108(1):114-121.
63. Byrne KM, Izzo AJ. Infraorbital nerve block: overview, indications, contraindications. *Emedicine*. March 31, 2016.
64. Upadya M, Upadya GM. Anesthesia for dermatologic surgery. *Indian J Dermatol Venereol Leprol.* 2005;71(3):141-154.
65. Hawkins JM, Moore PA. Local anesthesia: advances in agents and techniques. *Dent Clin North Am*. 2002;46:719-732.
66. Wall PD. The gate control theory of pain mechanisms: a re-examination and re-statement. *Brain*. 1978;101:1-18.
67. Buckenmaier C. *Military Advanced Regional Anesthesia and Analgesia Handbook*. Washington, DC: Government Printing Office; 2009.
68. Eaton JS, Grekin RC. Regional anesthesia of the face. *Dermatol Surg*. 2001;27:1006-1009.
69. Ali Aydin M, Salukhe TV, Wilke I, Willems S. Management and therapy of vasovagal syncope: a review. *World J Cardiol.* 2010;2(10):308-315.
70. Randle HW, Salassa JR, Roenigk RK. Know your anatomy. Local anesthesia for cutaneous lesions of the head and neck – practical applications of peripheral nerve blocks. *J Dermatol Surg Oncol.* 1992;18:231-235.
71. Shin KJ, Shin HJ, Lee SH, Song WC, Koh KS, Gil YC. Emerging points of the supraorbital and supratrochlear nerves in the supraorbital margin with reference to the lacrimal caruncle: implications for regional nerve block in upper eyelid and dermatologic surgery. *Dermatol Surg*. 2016;42(8):992-998.
72. Al-Qarqaz F, Al-Aboosi M, Al-Shiyab D, Al-Dabbagh Z. Using cold air for reducing needle-injection pain. *Int J Dermatol.* 2012;51(7):848-852.
73. Earle AS, Blanchard JM. Regional anesthesia in the upper extremity. *Clin Plast Surg*. 1985;12:97-114.

74. Wilhemi BJ, Moinar JA. Hand anesthesia. *Emedicine (Medscape).* August 12, 2015.

75. Pearce CJ. Hamilton PD. Current concepts review: regional anesthesia for foot and ankle surgery. *Foot Ankle Int.* 2010;31(8):732-739.

76. Cohen SJ, Roenigk RK. Nerve blocks for cutaneous surgery on the foot. *J Dermatol Surg Oncol.* 1991;17:527-534.

77. Sarrafian SK, Ibrahim IN, Breihan JH. Ankle-foot peripheral nerve block for mid and forefoot surgery. *Foot Ankle.* 1983;4:86-89.

78. Wooden SR, Sextro PB. The ankle block: anatomical review and anesthetic technique *AANA J.* 1990;58(2):105-111.

79. Becker DE, Reed KL. Local anesthetics: review of pharmacological considerations. *Anesth Prog.* 2012;59(2):90-101.

80. Darling MD, Peterson JD, Fabi SG. Impending necrosis after injection of hyaluronic acid and calcium hydroxylapatite fillers: report of 2 cases treated with hyperbaric oxygen therapy. *Dermatol Surg.* 2014;40:1049-1052.

81. Monique V, Fabi SG, Carruthers J. Complications in the cosmetic dermatology patient: a review and our experience (part 1). *Dermatol Surg.* 2016;42(1):1-11.

82. Jeng CL, Torrillo M, Rosenblatt MA. Complications of peripheral nerve blocks. *Br J Anaesth.* 2010;10S(Suppl 1):i97-i107.

83. Monique V, Fabi SG, Carruthers J. Complications in the cosmetic dermatology patient: a review and our experience (part 2). *Dermatol Surg.* 2016;42(1):12-20.

84. Grose DJ. Cigarette burn after tumescent anesthesia and intravenous sedation: a case report. *Dermatol Surg.* 2003;29(4):433-435.

85. Faccenda KA, Finucaine BT. Complications of regional anaesthesia: incidence and prevention. *Drug Saf.* 2001;24(6):413-442.

86. Venkataram J. Tumescent liposuction: a review. *J Cutan Aesthet Surg.* 2008;1(2):49-57.

87. Liem EB, Joiner TV, Tsueda K, Sessier DI. Increased sensitivity to thermal pain and reduced subcutaneous lidocaine efficacy in redheads. *Anesthesiology.* 2005;102(3):509-514.

88. McCaughey W. Adverse effects of local anesthetics. *Drug Saf.* 1992;7:178-189.

89. Naguib M, Magboul MM, Samarkandi AH, Attia M. Adverse effects and drug interactions associated with local and regional anesthesia. *Drug Saf.* 1998;18:221-250.

90. Sanko JF, Miller CJ, Alster TS. Topical anesthetics for dermatologic procedures: a review. *Dermatol Surg.* 2012;38(2):709-721.

91. Sabanko JF. Commentary: Serum lidocaine levels and cutaneous side effects after application of 23% lidocaine/7% tetracaine ointment to the face. *Dermatol Surg.* 2013;39(1 part1):92-94.

92. Wagman IH, De Jong RH, Prince DA. Effects of lidocaine on the central nervous system. *Anesthesiology.* 1967;28:155-172.

93. Kaweski S. Plastic Surgery Educational Foundation Technology Assessment Committee. Topical anesthetic creams. *Plast Reconstr Surg.* 2008;121:2161-2165.

94. Press CD, Schraga ED, eds. Topical anesthesia. *Medscape.* November 5, 2015.

95. Scheinfeld N. Legal considerations in the application of topical lidocaine. *Dermatologist.* 2007;15:9.

96. Adriani J. *Labat's Regional Anesthesia: Techniques and Clinical Applications.* 4th ed. St. Louis, MO: Warren H. Green; 1985.

97. Local anesthetics for physicians and dentists. *Med Lett Drugs Ther.* 1971;13(2):5-7.

98. Lawrence C. Drug management in skin surgery. *Drugs.* 1996;52: 805-817.

99. Murase JE, Heller MM, Butler DC. Safety of dermatologic medications in pregnancy and lactation. *J Am Acad Dermatol.* 2014;70:401.e1-401.e14.

100. Richards KA, Stasko T. Dermatologic surgery and the pregnant patient. *Dermatol Surg.* 2002;28:248-256.

101. Foster CA, Aston SJ. Propranolol-epinephrine interaction: a potential disaster. *Plast Reconstr Surg.* 1983;72(1):74-78.

102. Finder RL. Moore PA. Adverse drug reactions to local anesthesia. *Dent Clin North Am.* 2002;46:747-757.

103. Bartfield JM, Jandreau SW, Raccio-Rubak N. Randomized trial of diphenhydramine versus benzoyl alcohol with epinephrine as an alternative to lidocaine local anesthesia. *Ann Emerg Med.* 1998;32:650-654.

104. Dire DJ, Hogan DE. Double blinded comparison of diphenhydramine versus lidocaine as a local anesthetic *Ann Emerg Med.* 1993;22:1419-1422.

105. Altunka H, Ozer Y, Kargi E, Babuccu O. Comparison of local anaesthetic effects of tramadol with prilocaine for minor surgical procedures. *Br J Anaesth.* 2003;90:320-322.

106. Pang WW, Mok MS, Chang DP, Yang TF, Lin CH, Huang MH. Intradermal injection of tramadol has local anesthetic effect: a comparison with lidocaine. *Acta Anaesthesiol Sin.* 1998;38:133-136.

107. Coleman MD, Coleman NA. Drug-induced methemoglobinemia. Treatment issues. *Drug Saf.* 1996;14:394-405.

108. Kelly AP. Hypertrophic scars and keloids section II. In: Gloster HM, ed. *Complications in Cutaneous Surgery.* New York, NY; Springer; 2008:90.

109. Klein JA. The tumescent technique. Anesthesia and modified liposuction technique. *Dermatol Clin.* 1990;8:425-437.

110. Ellis PJ. Liposuction surgery under local anesthesia: limited blood loss and minimal lidocaine absorption. *J Dermatol Surg Oncol.* 1988;14:1145-1148.

Suturing Techniques

10

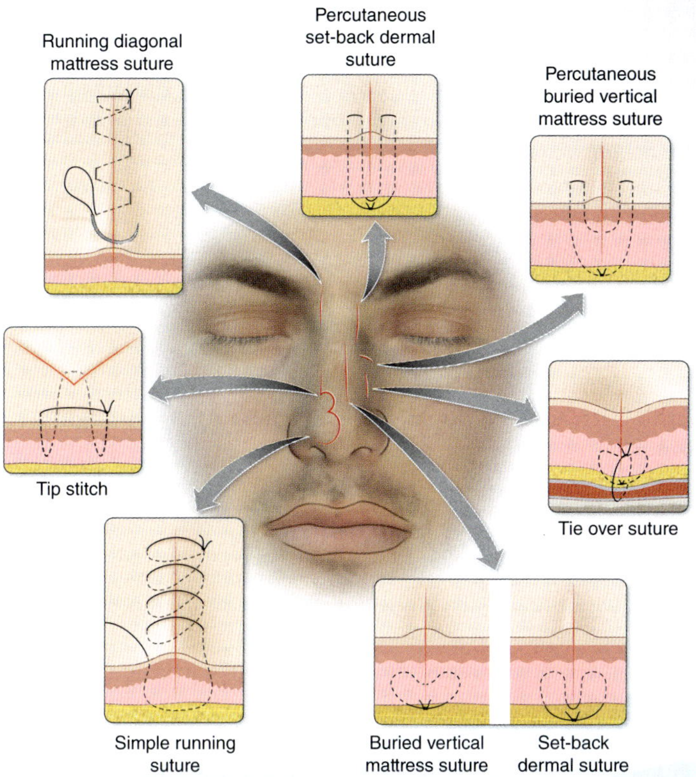

SUMMARY

- While most day-to-day procedures demand only a few suturing techniques, recent evidence has suggested that choice of technique has the potential to impact long-term outcomes.
- Suturing techniques can be dichotomized as buried versus transepidermal techniques, though the use of percutaneous approaches may make this distinction unclear.
- While the clinician does not need to incorporate a vast array of techniques into daily practice, precise placement of sutures coupled with an appreciation of the subtle variations in individual patients that may benefit from particular niche techniques is very helpful and may result in improved surgical outcomes.

Beginner Tips

- Deep suture techniques, such as the buried vertical mattress or set-back dermal suture, are fundamental techniques for all wound closures, as they lead to wound eversion, wound-edge approximation, and shift tension to the dermis.
- Fascial plication sutures are very useful to reduce dead space and reduce tension, and serve to shift tension even deeper, ultimately leading to a possibly improved outcome.

Pitfalls and Cautions

- Pulley variations may be useful for wounds under significant tension, but always using a pulley approach may needlessly increase the amount of suture material left in the wound, leading to an increased risk of foreign body reactions and suture material spitting.
- Fascial plication sutures may increase the risk of pain or infection; if pain after suture placement persists for more than 30 seconds, the suture should be removed.

Expert Tips

- When suturing a tight location, such as the scalp or lower leg, either percutaneous approaches or a buried horizontal mattress suture may be used for the deeper layer of sutures.
- With meticulous suture placement, no transepidermal sutures are needed for many closures, as the deep sutures lead to both tension reduction and wound-edge approximation.

Patient Education Points

- The dramatic eversion seen after dermatologic surgery should be explained to patients ahead of time and reviewed repeatedly.
- Using the analogy of a subcutaneous splint (or cast) may be helpful when explaining that the goal is to reduce tension temporarily but that the eversion will not persist.

Don't Forget!

- When working on the back, use thicker suture such as a 2-0 absorbable suture with a large needle.
- To reduce the risk of suture material spitting, consider using set-back sutures that leave no suture material at the incised wound edge.

Billing Pearls

- An intermediate or complex repair code is predicated on the wound being closed in a layered fashion.
- Fascial plication followed by dermal sutures would be considered a layered closure for these purposes.

10 Suturing Techniques

INTRODUCTION

Suturing techniques have seen a renaissance over the past decades, as clinicians have increasingly appreciated the impact that precisely placed sutures have on surgical outcomes. The rise of evidence-based medicine has led to a boon in suture technique development, as clinicians have become more willing to consider changing the fundamental techniques that were adopted during training in an effort to provide even better patient outcomes.

Even the best-designed repairs can be undone by less-than-optimal suturing techniques and tissue handling. While most day-to-day procedures demand only a very few suturing techniques, recent evidence has suggested that choice of technique has the potential to impact long-term outcomes.[1]

Suturing techniques can be dichotomized as buried versus transepidermal techniques, although the use of percutaneous approaches, discussed in detail later, may make this distinction sometimes unclear. In general, the buried techniques are those that do not require suture removal, while the transepidermal approaches necessitate suture removal unless rapidly absorbing suture materials are used.

BURIED SUTURE TECHNIQUES

The Buried Vertical Mattress Suture

This technique is a common approach widely used by dermatologists and plastic surgeons (**Figures 10-1 through 10-3**).[2]

TECHNIQUE: BURIED VERTICAL MATTRESS SUTURE

a. The wound edge is reflected back using surgical forceps or hooks. Adequate visualization of the underside of the dermis is desirable.
b. While reflecting back the dermis, the suture needle is inserted at 90 degrees into the underside of the dermis 4 mm distant from the incised wound edge.
c. The first bite is executed by following the needle initially at 90 degrees to the underside of the dermis and then, critically, changing direction by twisting the needle driver so that the needle exits in the incised wound edge. This allows the apex of the bite to remain in the papillary dermis while the needle exits in the incised wound edge at the level of the reticular dermis.
d. Keeping the loose end of suture between the surgeons and the patient, the dermis on the side of the first bite is released. The tissue on the opposite edge is then reflected back in a similar fashion as on the first side.
e. The second and final bite is executed by inserting the needle into the incised wound edge at the level of the reticular dermis. It then angles upward and laterally so that the apex of the needle is at the level of the papillary dermis. This should mirror the first bite taken on the contralateral side of the wound.
f. The suture material is then tied using an instrument tie.

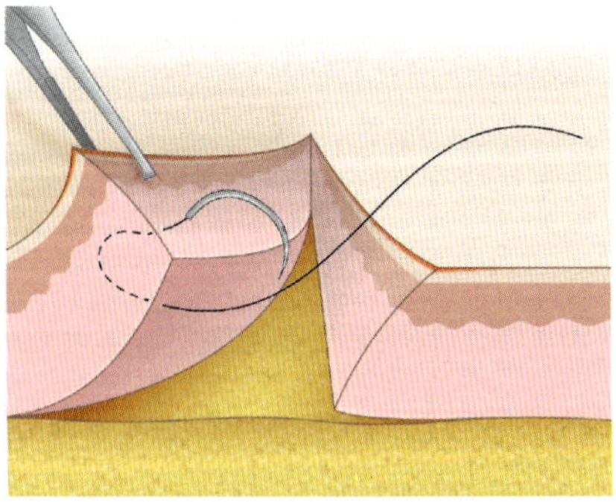

FIGURE 10-1 The needle is inserted through the underside of the dermis and moves upward and outward in the dermis before returning to exit at the incised wound edge.

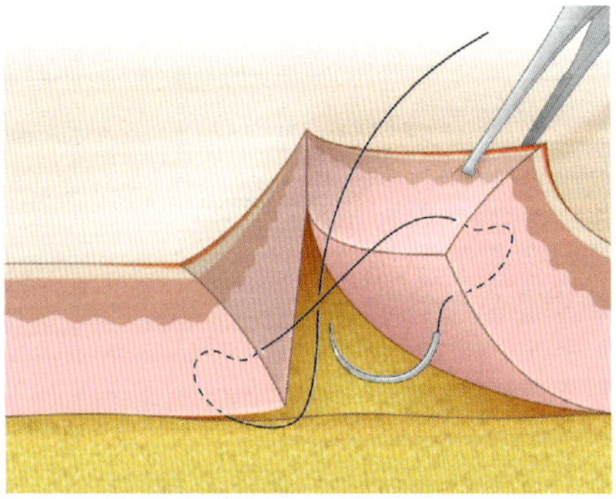

FIGURE 10-2 The needle is then inserted through the incised wound edge before moving upward and outward away from the wound edge and exiting in the deeper dermis.

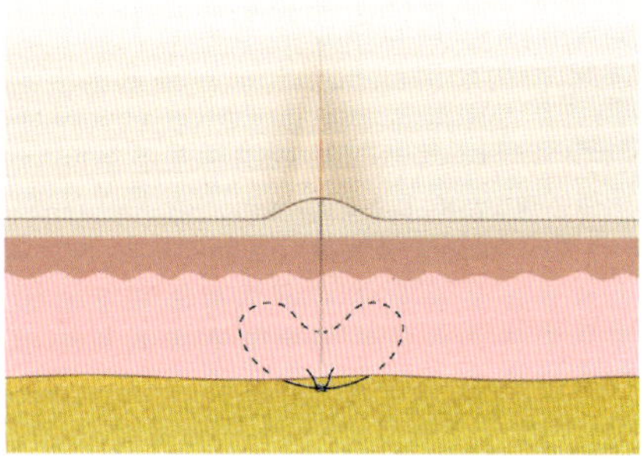

FIGURE 10-3 Lateral view of the buried vertical mattress suture highlighting the heart-shaped path the suture material takes through the dermis.

It requires some practice to master, although once mastered, it is straightforward to execute. The first bite may also be finessed by first reflecting the wound edge back sharply during needle insertion and then returning the edge medially after the apex has been reached. This approach helps to lead the needle in the correct course without an exaggerated change in direction with the needle driver.

When suturing, both the obviously active element (the needle and needle driver, held by the dominant hand) and the ostensibly passive element (the skin, held by forceps or a skin hook) have the potential to move in three dimensions. Thus, changing the way the needle moves through the skin can be accomplished by either adjusting the way the needle is moved through the skin with the dominant hand, adjusting how the skin is held or manipulated by the other hand, or a combination of the two. With experience, a combination is often more effective at creating the vertical mattress suture in an elegant and efficient fashion.

The apex of the needle should be in the papillary dermis; if the needle courses too superficially, dimpling may occur. This technique, if executed appropriately, leads to both excellent wound eversion and outstanding wound edge approximation.

The Set-Back Dermal Suture

This approach is frequently used in areas under significant tension and as an alternative to the buried vertical mattress as a standard buried technique.[3] Since it is easier to place than a buried vertical mattress suture, this technique may be used by budding surgeons, medical students, and residents as the workhorse technique for deep tension-relieving sutures (**Figures 10-4 through 10-6**).

TECHNIQUE: SET-BACK DERMAL SUTURE

a. The wound edge is reflected back using surgical forceps or hooks. Adequate visualization of the underside of the dermis is required.
b. While reflecting back the dermis, the suture needle is inserted at 90 degrees into the underside of the dermis 2 to 6 mm distant from the incised wound edge.
c. The first bite is executed by traversing the dermis following the curvature of the needle and allowing the needle to exit closer to the incised wound edge. Care should be taken to remain in the dermis to minimize the risk of epidermal dimpling. The needle does not, however, exit through the incised wound edge, but rather 1 to 4 mm distant from the incised edge. The size of this first bite is based on the size of the needle, the thickness of the dermis, and the need for and tolerance of eversion.
d. Keeping the loose end of suture between the surgeon and the patient, the dermis on the side of the first bite is released. The tissue on the opposite edge is then reflected back in a similar fashion as on the first side, ensuring complete visualization of the underside of the dermis.
e. The second and final bite is executed by inserting the needle into the underside of the dermis 1 to 6 mm distant from the incised wound edge. Again, this bite should be executed by following the curvature of the needle and avoiding catching the undersurface of the epidermis, which could result in epidermal dimpling. It then exits further distal to the wound edge, approximately 2 to 6 mm distant from the wound edge. This should mirror the first bite taken on the contralateral side of the wound.
f. The suture material is then tied using an instrument tie.

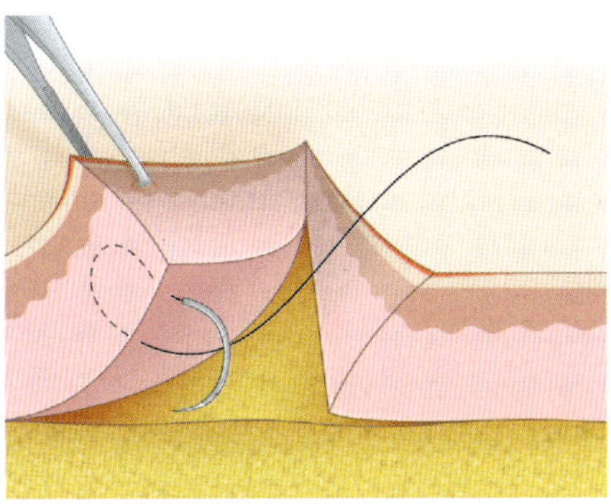

FIGURE 10-4 The needle is inserted through the underside of the dermis, exiting again through the underside of the dermis set back from the wound edge.

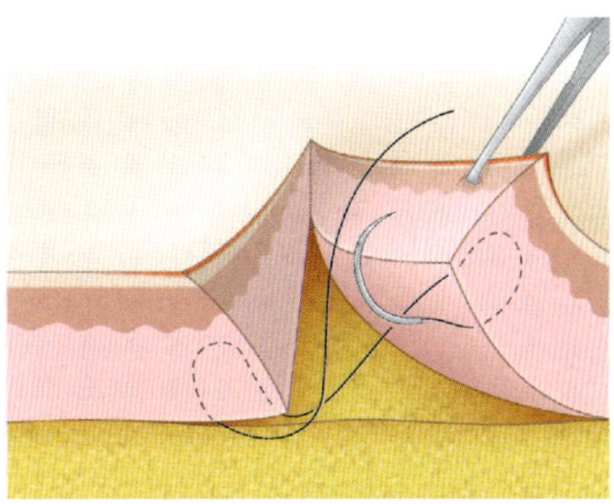

FIGURE 10-5 This is repeated on the contralateral wound edge.

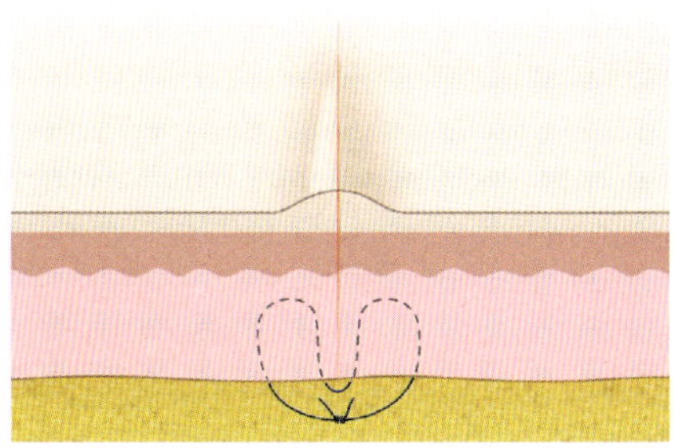

FIGURE 10-6 Cross-sectional view demonstrating the path of the suture material through the dermis and the effect on wound eversion.

This technique was compared with the buried vertical mattress suture in a randomized trial and was found to be superior in terms of eversion and cosmetic outcomes based on both physician and patient assessments.[1]

One of the chief advantages of this technique is its ease of execution; since the suture follows the arc of the needle on the undersurface of the dermis, there is no need to change planes, effect a heart-shaped suture placement, or guarantee that the suture exit point is precisely at the inside edge of the lower dermis, as may be needed with the buried vertical mattress suture.

Accurate suture placement is predicated on having a sufficiently undermined plane, since the entire suture loop lays on the undersurface of the dermis. Therefore, broad undermining is a prerequisite for using this technique, since the first throw of the needle begins 2 to 6 mm distant from the incised wound edge.

This technique may also be used to minimize dead space when excising a space-occupying lesion such as a cyst or lipoma. In this event, taking the first bite set back even further from the incised wound edge will translate into a larger ridge and will simultaneously minimize the laxity in the central portion of the wound as the dermis is pulled taut so that potential dead space is converted to a hypereverted wound ridge, which will absorb with time.

Patients should be cautioned that they might develop a significant ridge in the immediate postoperative period. Depending on the suture material used and the density of the sutures, this ridge may last from weeks to months. Explaining that the technique is akin to placing a subcutaneous splint may help the patient develop reasonable and realistic expectations and reduce anxiety regarding the immediate postoperative appearance of the wound.[4]

A possible complication of hypereversion and an overly broad bite is that the raised ridge may be too large or bulky to be supported by the deep sutures.[5] In this event, the wound edges may paradoxically collapse centrally, leading to the appearance of a dramatically raised ridge with a central valley approximately 1 week postoperatively. As the sutures absorb over time, this will yield a depressed or inverted scar line. This can generally be avoided by not setting back the sutures more than a few millimeters from the wound edge and by placing a sufficient number of sutures so that the body of the ridge may be easily supported.

Suspension Suture

This is a niche technique designed to fix one or both edges of a defect to a deeper structure. This approach has also been referred to as a pexing suture or tacking suture and is used typically in several situations. First, when repairing a defect that crosses a natural sulcus, it is important to tack down the skin overlying the sulcus so that the natural depression is not blunted, or bridged, by the repair. Second, it is used when working near cosmetic subunit boundaries and free margins to avoid functional challenges such as ectropion and eclabium, as well as cosmetic distortion of sensitive areas such as the lip and eyebrows. It is also useful in order to fix a flap in place and minimize tension on the distal portion of the flap. Finally, this approach may also be used to prevent nasal valve collapse in the appropriate setting (**Figure 10-7**).

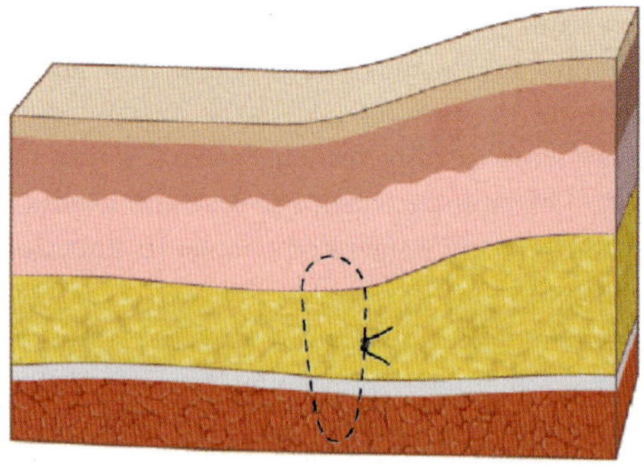

FIGURE 10-7 Overview of the suspension suture technique.

TECHNIQUE: SUSPENSION SUTURE

a. First, the surgeon determines the desired location for fixing the suspension suture, as discussed below. The wound edge is reflected back using surgical forceps or hooks, and adequate visualization of the underside of the dermis is desirable.
b. While reflecting back the dermis, the suture needle is inserted at 90 degrees into the underside of the dermis 2 to 6 mm distant from the incised wound edge.
c. The first bite is executed by traversing the dermis following the curvature of the needle and allowing the needle to exit closer to the incised wound edge. This will minimize the risk of vascular compromise. Care should be taken to remain in the dermis to minimize the risk of epidermal dimpling. The needle does not, however, exit through the incised wound edge, but rather 1 to 4 mm distant from the incised edge or, in select cases, potentially further back from the wound edge.
d. The flap of skin may be gently pulled by the suture material so that the location of the first bite directly overlies the planned fixation point. This permits the surgeon to double-check the final position of the suspension suture. The needle is then blindly inserted through the fat and deeper structures until bone is reached. A 3-mm bite of periosteum is then taken, and the needle is brought back up through the soft tissues into the open center of the wound.
e. The suture material is then tied using an instrument tie. Hand tying may be used as well, which may be useful if the depth of the defect is significant.

This technique is very useful when working around the eyelids and lips, although its use demands familiarity with the underlying anatomy so that no sensitive deeper structures are injured or entrapped during the blind placement of the deep anchoring suture. The deep suture should also be placed parallel to the underlying vascular plexus to similarly mitigate this risk.

Placement is based on several considerations, including the degree of tension across the advanced tissue; the presence of a bony prominence, which can be used easily for suspension purposes; and the absence of underlying nerves, which could inadvertently become strangulated by the anchoring suture.

Pulling on the suture once it is anchored to the periosteum may help assure the surgeon that the suture is indeed tacked down to an immobile surface.

A three-point variation of this approach is possible as well, which allows wound edge approximation and a tacking effect to occur all with one suture placement. This is accomplished by first placing either a buried vertical mattress or set-back dermal suture at the two wound edges and then taking a bite of the underlying periosteum prior to tying the knot. The suture material thus fixes the wound edges together as well as to the underlying anchoring point. This approach, however, may result in suboptimal wound edge eversion and places additional stress on the suture material, increasing the risk of scar spread. Moreover, it is only appropriate if the anchor target lies in the approximate midpoint of the defect, since it recreates a natural sulcus but does not permit differential pull from one side of the defect.

This technique may also be used as an alternative to cartilage grafting when reconstructing the nose. Loss of alar cartilage may lead to nasal valve collapse, which traditionally was addressed by placing an auricular cartilage graft along the reconstructed alar rim in order to maintain valve patency. A simple and elegant alternative is placing a suture in the ala and fixing it to a point superolaterally in the maxillary periosteum, permitting the nasal valve to remain open and potentially obviating the need for a cartilage graft. Since the underside of the dermis is tacked to periosteum, this technique may result in an area of depression at the site of suspension suture placement.

Buried Horizontal Mattress Suture

This is a niche technique, useful when closing narrow wounds or those where there is limited space to insert the needle driver, and when placing a buried suture is desirable. It may be employed in a variety of locations, including the scalp, ears, and lower leg (**Figures 10-8 and 10-9**).

TECHNIQUE: BURIED HORIZONTAL MATTRESS SUTURE

a. The wound edge is reflected back using surgical forceps or hooks. Adequate visualization of the underside of the dermis is desirable.
b. While reflecting back the dermis, the suture needle is inserted into the undersurface of the dermis parallel to the surface of the skin just lateral to the incised wound edge.
c. The first bite is executed by placing gentle pressure on the needle so that it enters the papillary dermis and then relaxing pressure to permit the needle to exit on the undersurface of the dermis.
d. Keeping the loose end of suture between the surgeon and the patient, the dermis on the side of the first bite is released. The tissue on the opposite edge is then reflected back in a similar fashion as on the first side.
e. The second and final bite is executed by inserting the needle into the undersurface of the dermis on the contralateral side, with a backhand technique if desired, and completing a mirror-image loop, so that the needle exits directly across from its original entry point on the contralateral side.
f. The suture material is then tied using an instrument tie.

This technique is useful for narrow or shallow wounds, such as those on the scalp and shins.[6] It may also be used when adding an additional buried suture in an otherwise largely closed wound, where there is insufficient space to insert a vertically oriented buried suture in the narrow space between two other already placed sutures.

The needle driver may also be held like a pencil, and the needle may then be rotated through the dermis while reflecting back with the forceps to permit easy visualization.

Wound edge necrosis has been raised as a potential risk of horizontally oriented suture placement, but in practice, this is only encountered very rarely and as a complication of tightly placed

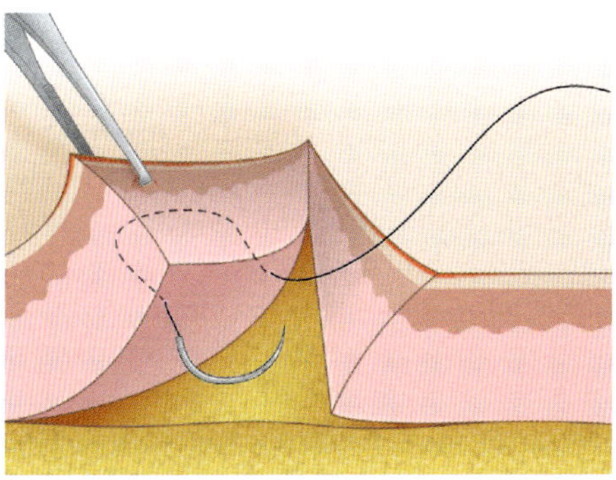

FIGURE 10-8 The needle is inserted through the dermis running parallel to the incised wound edge.

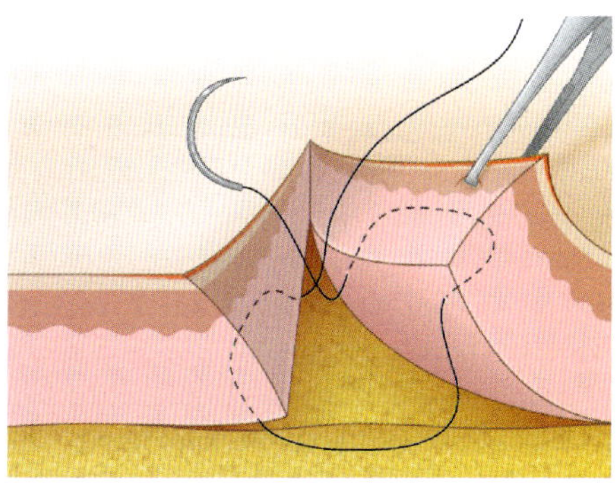

FIGURE 10-9 This procedure is then reversed on the contralateral wound edge.

traditional horizontal mattress sutures, rather than with the buried equivalent. This is likely due to a constrictive effect on the incised wound edge, which is not typically seen with buried sutures.

Fascial Plication Suture

This technique is designed for wounds under marked tension, especially those on the back and shoulders. It can also be used for facial repairs, where grasping the superficial musculoaponeurotic system (SMAS) with this deep suture technique leads to a dramatic reduction in wound size. It is a deep technique, permitting the tension of wound closure to shift from the dermis to the fascia, and concomitantly creating a lower-tension closure. In addition to tension reduction, this approach also leads to an increase in the apparent length-to-width ratio of a fusiform closure and improved dead-space minimization (**Figure 10-10**).

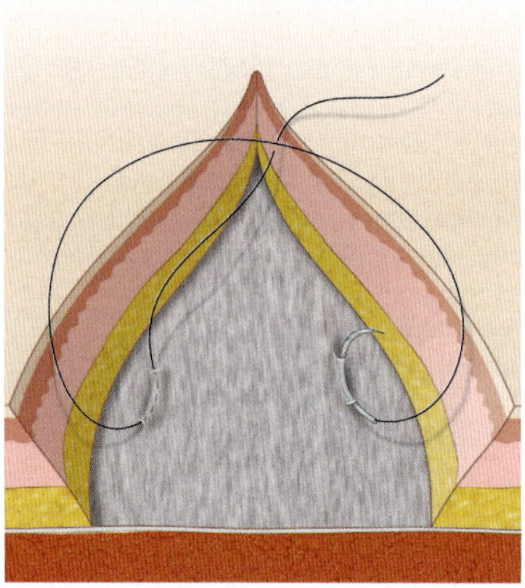

FIGURE 10-10 Overview of the fascial plication suture technique.

TECHNIQUE: FASCIAL PLICATION SUTURE

a. The wound edges are reflected back to permit visualization of the deep bed of the wound. In deep excisions, such as those performed for melanoma or large cysts, the muscle fascia may be directly visible. Otherwise, visualizing the subcutaneous fat is appropriate as well.
b. The suture needle is inserted at 90 degrees through the deep fat 2 to 4 mm medial to the lateral undermined edge of the wound.
c. The first bite is executed by entering the fascia and following the curvature of the needle. The suture material may be gently pulled to test that a successful bite of fascia has been taken.
d. Keeping the loose end of suture between the surgeon and the patient, attention is then shifted to the opposite side of the wound. The second bite is executed by repeating the procedure on the contralateral side.
e. The suture material is then tied using an instrument tie. Hand tying may be used as well, particularly if the wound is deep and the instruments cannot be easily inserted to complete the tie.

This technique is very useful for wounds under marked tension, especially for large defects on the back and shoulders.[7,8] Even a deep, gaping wound can be converted into a manageable fusiform defect with a single well-placed fascial plication suture. It can therefore be conceptualized as an alternative to pulley sutures that affords both a decrease in tension across the wound surface (by shifting tension from the dermis to the fascia) and an increase in the length-to-width ratio of the ellipse.

Indeed, this approach often leads to a more fusiform defect, even when an oval-shaped excision has been performed. Therefore, it may be useful when attempting to keep a defect as short as possible without dog-ear formation. In cases where this approach is anticipated, it may be worthwhile to create a defect with a length-to-width ratio of less than 3:1, as is traditionally employed, as that may be sufficient to lead to a tapered ellipse.

Fascial plication sutures need not be used for all linear closures. This technique is most appropriate for areas under significant tension or large excisions where minimizing the postoperative wound length is desirable. On the face, recruiting the SMAS may be very helpful. When designing the closure of a round defect, the fascial plication suture should be placed prior to removing the dog ears. The risks of fascial plication sutures include possible pain, a theoretically increased infection risk (since the fascial envelope has been pierced by suture), and a theoretical risk of vascular compromise through inadvertent pressure-induced ligation of perforating vessels. In practice, these complications are infrequent, although patients may experience transient pain during needle entry and immediately after the fascial plication suture is tied. If pain persists for more than 5 minutes, the suture should be removed.

Buried Purse-String Suture

This technique is designed to either shrink the size of a defect or obviate it entirely, depending on the degree of tension and the size of the defect. The purse-string effect tends to lead to a slight puckering in the surrounding skin, a feature that may be acceptable (and will likely resolve with time) on areas such as the forearms and back but is less desirable in cosmetically sensitive locations such as the face. The running nature of the technique means that compromise at any point in the course of suture placement may result in wound dehiscence, although for this reason, a larger gauge suture material is generally used (**Figure 10-11**).

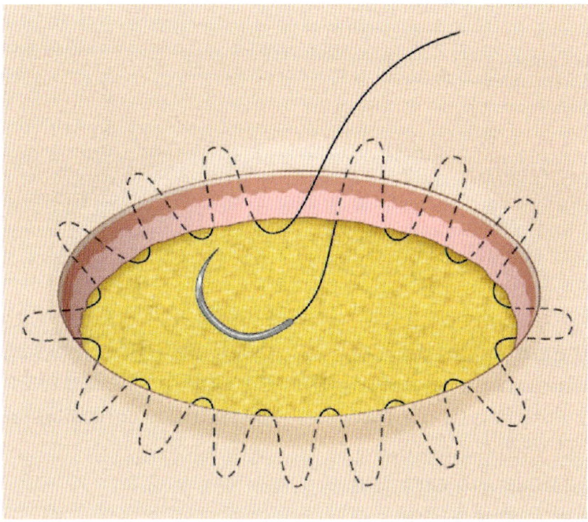

FIGURE 10-11 Overview of the buried purse-string suture technique.

TECHNIQUE: BURIED PURSE-STRING SUTURE

a. The wound edge at the far end of the round- or oval-shaped wound, parallel to the incision line, is reflected back.
b. With the tail of the suture material resting between the surgeon and the far end of the wound, the needle is inserted into the underside of the dermis on the far edge of the wound with a trajectory running parallel to the incision. Generally, this entry point in the dermis should be set back approximately 3 to 6 mm from the epidermal edge, depending on the thickness of the dermis and the anticipated degree of tension across the closure. The needle, and therefore the suture, should pass through the deep dermis at a uniform depth. Bite size is dependent on needle size, although in order to minimize the risk of necrosis, it may be prudent to restrict the size of each bite. The needle should exit the dermis at a point equidistant from the cut edge from where it entered.
c. The needle is then grasped with the surgical pickups and simultaneously released by the hand holding the needle driver. As the needle is freed from the tissue with the pickups, the needle is grasped again by the needle driver in an appropriate position to repeat the above step to the left of the previously placed suture.
d. A small amount of suture material is pulled through and the needle is inserted into the dermis to the left of the previously placed suture, and the same movement is repeated.
e. The same technique is repeated moving stepwise around the entire wound until the needle exits close to the original entry point at the far end of the wound.
f. Once the desired number of throws has been placed, the suture material is then pulled taut, leading to complete or partial closure of the wound, and tied using an instrument tie.

This technique is designed as an efficient method of wound area reduction. In many cases, placing a purse-string suture can effect complete wound closure, and therefore, it represents an alternative to a layered repair of a fusiform incision.

It has been suggested that some defects on the back and extremities, particularly in elderly patients with loose skin, are better closed with a purse-string approach than with a traditional linear closure, since linear closures often heal with a residual scar and require a significantly longer excision line, while the puckering that may be present immediately postoperatively with purse-string closures is likely to resolve with time.[9-14] That said, in the right hands, linear closures on the trunk and extremities often heal with subtle scarring, even when wounds are closed under tension.

On a pragmatic level, this approach is generally used when either a patient is unwilling to undergo a traditional linear closure or when the patient's comorbidities make the additional length of the incision for a linear closure an unrealistic option.

As with linear running dermal techniques, this technique may be used as a modified winch or pulley suture, since the multiple loops help to minimize the tension across any one loop and permit closure of wounds under marked tension. Because each throw is not tied off, however, it is important to adequately secure the knot.

As with other running dermal techniques, this approach leaves a fair amount of absorbable suture material in the dermis. Therefore, foreign-body reactions, suture abscess formation, and infection are possibilities. That said, since the entire suture line is secured with a single knot, and since most of the bulk of any suture line is in the knots, rather than the lengths of suture material between knots, this technique may be less susceptible to suture abscess or suture spitting than others.

The pucker effect of this closure resolves rapidly in atrophic skin, although it can persist in other areas; patients should realize that some degree of residual puckering toward the center of the wound is to be expected. Additionally, this technique may be used to help recreate the nipple-areola complex if full reconstruction is not desired and the nipple is lost to a local tumor.

Since the entire closure is held by a single knot, this approach may be associated with a higher rate of wound dehiscence, as knot failure of failure in the suture material at any point leads to an immediate loss of tension on the closure. Given the concern regarding knot breakage, it may be helpful to attempt to better secure the knot. This may be done by paying particularly close attention to knot tying, tying an extra full knot, adding extra throws, or leaving a longer tail than would traditionally be executed.

A recent study has suggested, however, that the postoperative cosmesis of a purse-string closure is no better than a wound allowed to heal with secondary intention healing.[15]

VARIATIONS

Pulley Variations

Pulley (or double) variations are available for most buried suturing techniques. Typically, pulley variations confer two central advantages: they permit the closure of high-tension wounds, where the mechanics of a pulley allow straightforward wound edge approximation,

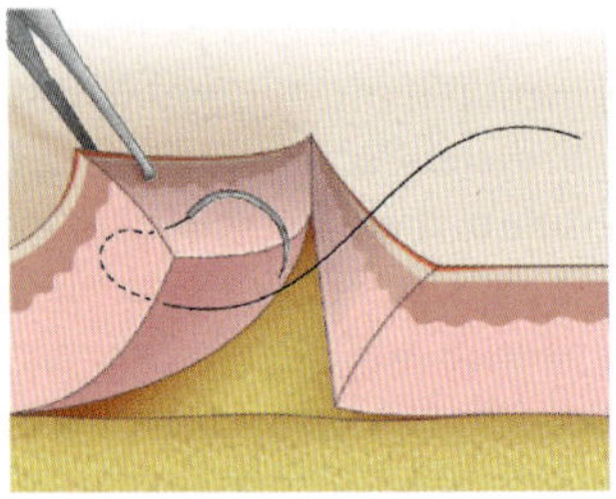

FIGURE 10-12 The pulley buried vertical mattress suture. The needle is inserted through the dermis, angling upward and outward before exiting at the incised wound edge.

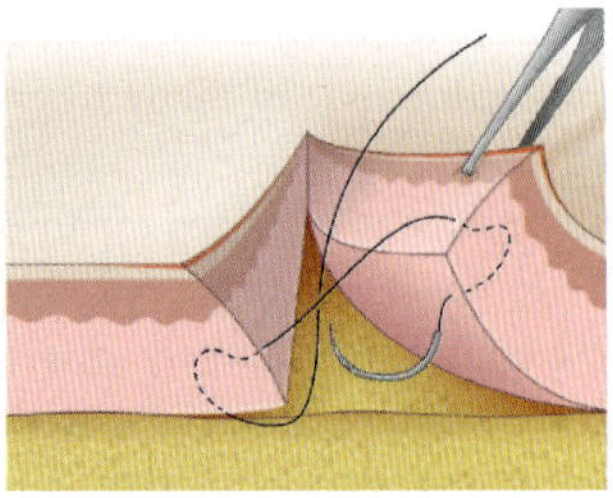

FIGURE 10-13 The needle is then inserted through the incised wound edge on the contralateral side, again moving superolaterally before exiting deep.

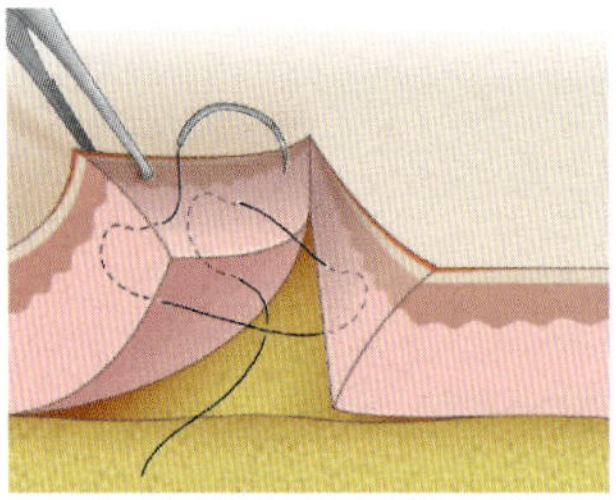

FIGURE 10-14 Keeping the tail of the suture deep to the suture throws and toward the surgeon, the first step is then repeated, with the needle entering deep and exiting at the incised wound edge.

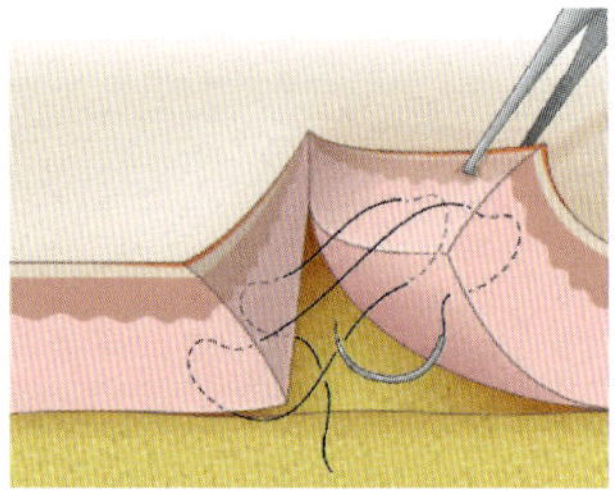

FIGURE 10-15 Again with the tail deep, the needle is inserted through the incised wound edge on the contralateral side.

and they typically lock in place immediately, obviating the need for an assistant. Frequently used approaches include the pulley buried vertical mattress suture[16-19] (**Figures 10-12 through 10-15**) and the pulley set-back suture[20] (**Figures 10-16 through 10-19**).

Running Variations

Running variations of buried sutures permit rapid placement of a long row of buried sutures that are anchored by knots at either end. The speed advantage is offset, however, by the reliance on only two anchor points along an entire wound. Since buried sutures are designed to bear the tension across a wound, relying on a single anchoring suture knot at each end of the wound may be unwise, as a break in suture material anywhere along the suture line (or knot compromise at either end) may result in catastrophic consequences.

Percutaneous Variations

When placing sutures in narrow areas, percutaneous approaches allow the placement of buried sutures when only minimal visualization is possible. This is particularly useful on the tight skin of the scalp and when executing narrow closures on the nose and below the knee. Approaches include the percutaneous buried vertical mattress (**Figure 10-20**), the percutaneous set-back suture (**Figure 10-21**), and the percutaneous horizontal mattress suture (**Figure 10-22**).

TRANSEPIDERMAL SUTURE TECHNIQUES

The Simple Interrupted Suture

This is the standard benchmark suture used for closure and epidermal approximation. It may be used alone in the context of small wounds under minimal to no tension, such as those formed by either a small bunch biopsy or a traumatic laceration. It is also frequently used as a secondary layer to aid in the approximation of the epidermis when the dermis has been closed using a dermal or other deep suturing technique (**Figure 10-23**).

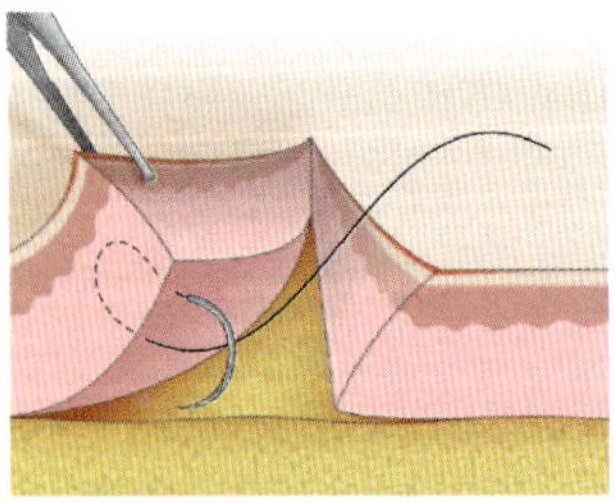

FIGURE 10-16 The pulley set-back dermal suture. The needle is inserted through the underside of the dermis, exiting the underside of the dermis closer to the incised wound edge but still set back from the incised wound edge.

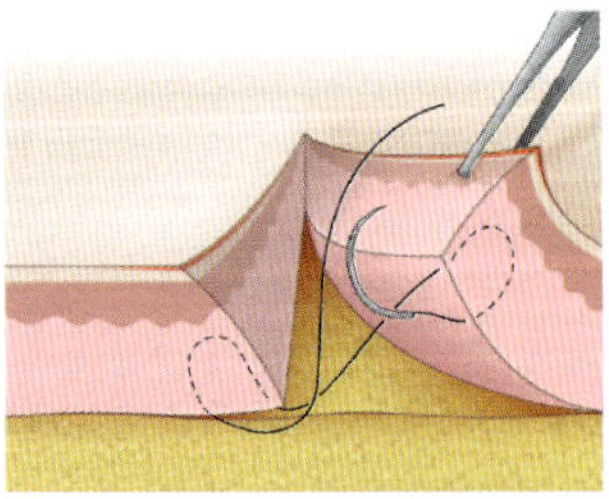

FIGURE 10-17 The needle is then inserted through the underside of the dermis on the contralateral wound edge, exiting further away from the incised wound edge on the undersurface of the dermis.

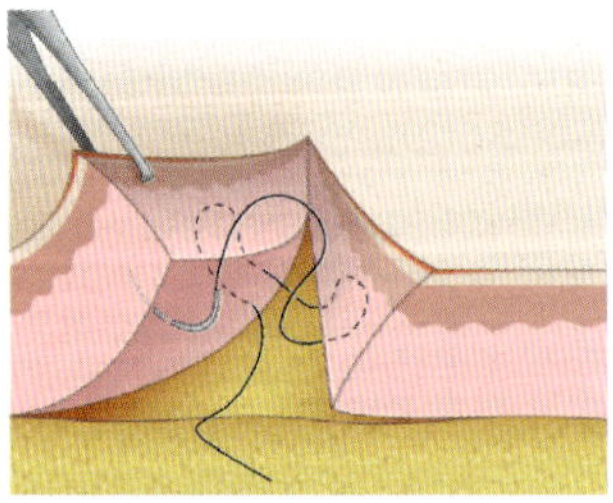

FIGURE 10-18 With the loose end of the suture material deep to the active sutures and resting between the surgeon and the needle driver, the needle is then reinserted through the undersurface of the dermis.

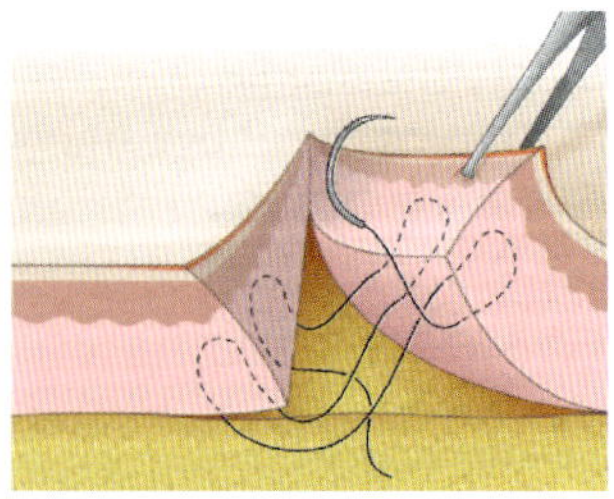

FIGURE 10-19 The procedure is again repeated on the contralateral wound edge.

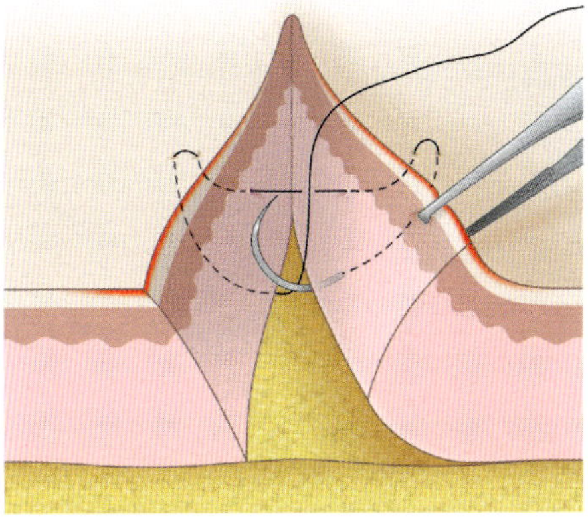

FIGURE 10-20 The percutaneous buried vertical mattress suture.

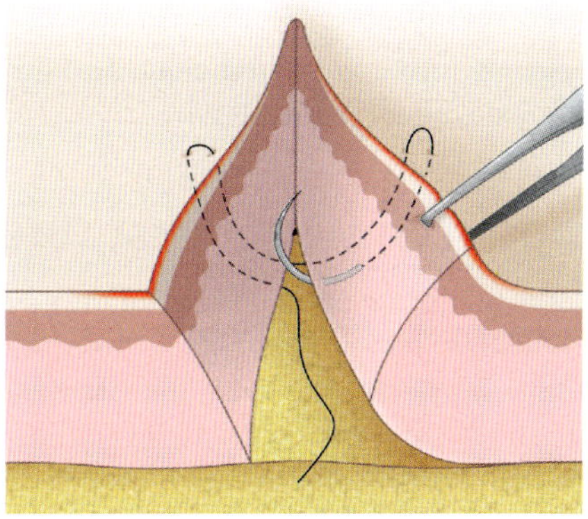

FIGURE 10-21 The percutaneous set-back suture technique.

TECHNIQUE: SIMPLE INTERRUPTED SUTURE

a. The needle is inserted perpendicular to the epidermis, approximately one-half the radius of the needle distant to the wound edge. This will allow the needle to exit the wound on the contralateral side at an equal distance from the wound edge by simply following the curvature of the needle.
b. With a fluid motion of the wrist, the needle is rotated through the dermis, taking the bite wider at the deep margin than at the surface, and the needle tip exits the skin on the contralateral side.
c. The needle body is grasped with surgical forceps in the left hand, with care being taken to avoid grasping the needle tip, which can be easily dulled by repetitive friction against the surgical forceps. It is gently grasped and pulled upward with the surgical forceps as the body of the needle is released from the needle driver. Alternatively, the needle may be released from the needle driver and the needle driver itself may be used to grasp the needle from the contralateral side of the wound to complete its rotation through its arc, obviating the need for surgical forceps.
d. The suture material is then tied off gently, with care being taken to minimize tension across the epidermis and avoid overly constricting the wound edges.

It is important to enter the epidermis at 90 degrees, allowing the needle to travel slightly laterally away from the wound edge before fully following the curvature of the needle when using this technique. This will allow for maximal wound eversion and accurate wound edge approximation. The final cross-sectional appearance of the needle's course should be a flask-like shape, wider at the base than at the surface.

Care should be taken to avoid skimming the needle superficially beneath the epidermis. This results from failing to enter the skin at a perpendicular angle and failing to follow the curvature of the needle. This may result in wound inversion as the tension vector of the shallow bite pulls the wound edges outward and down.

This technique may elicit an increased risk of track marks, necrosis, and other complications when compared with techniques that do not entail suture material traversing the scar line, such as buried or subcuticular approaches. Therefore, sutures should be removed as early as possible to minimize these complications, and consideration should be given to adopting other closure techniques in the event that sutures will not be able to be removed in a timely fashion. Some studies have also demonstrated an increased rate of dehiscence when using interrupted sutures alone without underlying dermal tension-relieving sutures, highlighting that this technique should be used either for wounds under minimal tension or in concert with deeper tension-relieving sutures.[21-26]

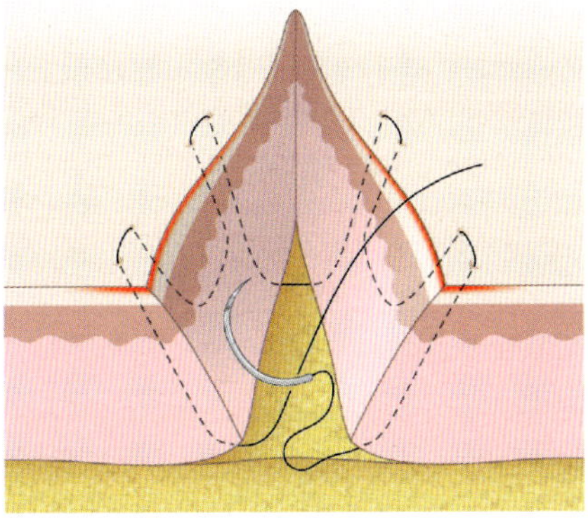

FIGURE 10-22 The percutaneous horizontal mattress suture technique.

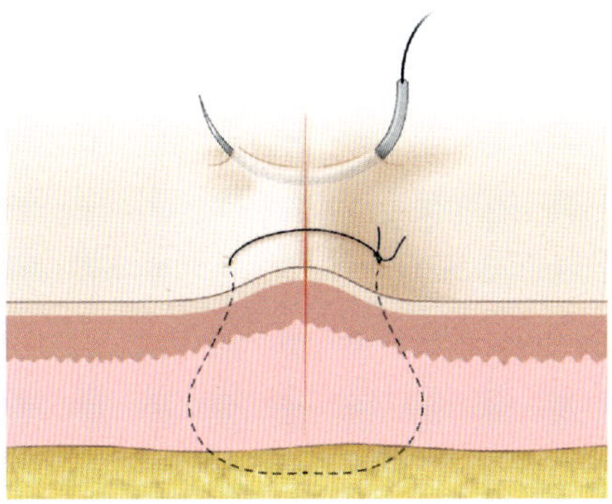

FIGURE 10-23 Overview of the simple interrupted suture technique.

Vertical Mattress Suture

This is a frequently used everting technique used for closure and epidermal approximation (**Figure 10-24**).

TECHNIQUE: VERTICAL MATTRESS SUTURE

a. The needle is inserted perpendicular to the epidermis, approximately 6 mm distant to the wound edge.
b. With a fluid motion of the wrist, the needle is rotated through the dermis, taking the bite wider at the deep margin than at the surface, and the needle tip exits the skin on the contralateral side. (If the needle radius is too small to complete this arc in one movement, this first step may be divided in two, with the needle first exiting between the incised wound edges and then reloaded and reinserted to exit on the contralateral side.)
c. The needle body is grasped with surgical forceps in the left hand and pulled upward with the surgical forceps as the body of the needle is released from the needle driver. Alternatively, the needle may be released from the needle driver and the needle driver itself may be used to grasp the needle from the contralateral side of the wound to complete its rotation through its arc, obviating the need for surgical forceps.
d. The needle is then reloaded in a backhand fashion and inserted at 90 degrees perpendicular to the epidermis approximately 3 mm from the wound edge on the same side of the incision line as the exit point, between the exit point and the incised wound edge.
e. The needle is rotated superficially through its arc, exiting on the contralateral side of the wound 3 mm from the incised wound edge.
f. The suture material is then tied off gently, with care being taken to minimize tension across the epidermis and avoid overly constricting the wound edges.

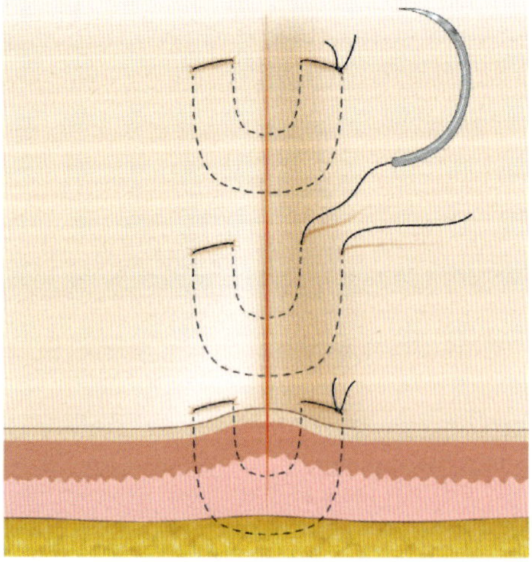

FIGURE 10-24 Overview of the vertical mattress suture.

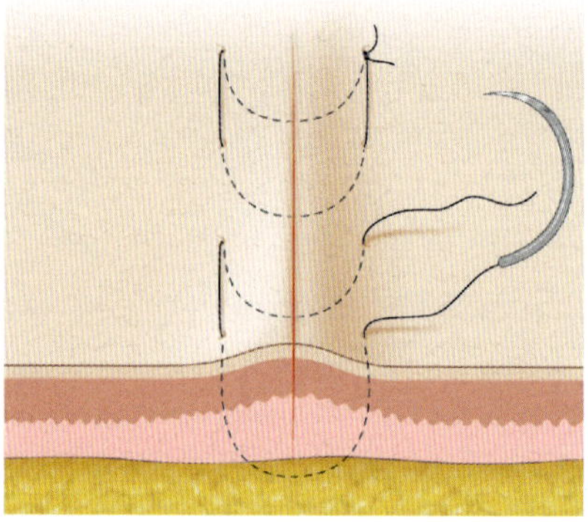

FIGURE 10-25 Overview of the horizontal mattress suture.

This technique is generally used for its pronounced effect on wound eversion. Therefore, although it is appropriate for most skin closures, it should be avoided when either inversion is desired or when exaggerated eversion has already been accomplished with a buried suture.[27-29]

As with the simple interrupted suture, care should be taken to avoid skimming the needle superficially beneath the epidermis. This may result in wound inversion as the tension vector of the shallow bite pulls the wound edges outward and down.

Note that the second throw is placed superficial to the first, deeper far-far suture, leading to a nested placement of the suture material. This leads to both wound eversion as well as wound edge approximation.

The Allgöwer technique involves performing a half-buried vertical mattress suture: the needle is passed from the far entrance point to the interior of the wound. A buried vertical mattress bite is then taken on the contralateral side, and the needle then passes back to the original side, entering near the incised wound edge so that one-half of the wound is closed with a standard vertical mattress suture and the other is closed with a buried vertical mattress.

This technique does not typically permit the same degree of wound edge apposition as can be accomplished with other transepidermal sutures. In the event that deeper sutures were carefully placed, this may not be a significant drawback, since the wound edges may be well aligned from the placement of these deeper sutures. If not, or if there is a need for improved wound edge apposition even after placing the vertical mattress suture, additional interrupted sutures may be helpful.

Horizontal Mattress

This is a frequently used everting technique used for closure and epidermal approximation. This technique may also be used in the context of atrophic skin, as the broader anchoring bites may help to limit tissue tear-through that may be seen with a simple interrupted suture (**Figure 10-25**).

TECHNIQUE: HORIZONTAL MATTRESS

a. The needle is inserted perpendicular to the epidermis, approximately one-half the radius of the needle distant to the wound edge. This will allow the needle to exit the wound on the contralateral side at an equal distance from the wound edge by simply following the curvature of the needle.

b. With a fluid motion of the wrist, the needle is rotated through the dermis, taking the bite wider at the deep margin than at the surface, and the needle tip exits the skin on the contralateral side.
c. The needle body is grasped with surgical forceps in the left hand and pulled upward as the body of the needle is released from the needle driver. Alternatively, the needle may be released from the needle driver and the needle driver itself may be used to grasp the needle from the contralateral side of the wound to complete its rotation through its arc, obviating the need for surgical forceps.
d. The needle is then reloaded in a backhand fashion and inserted at 90 degrees perpendicular to the epidermis proximal (relative to the surgeon) to its exit point along the length of the wound on the same side of the incision line as the exit point.
e. The needle is rotated through its arc, exiting on the right side of the wound (relative to the surgeon) in a mirror image of steps b and c.
f. The suture material is then tied off gently, with care being taken to minimize tension across the epidermis and avoid overly constricting the wound edges.

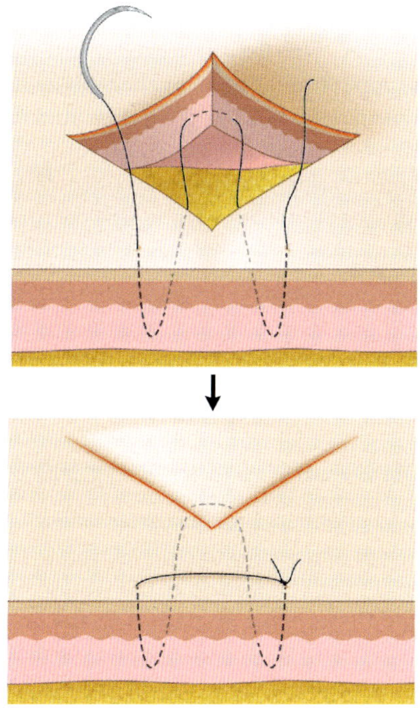

FIGURE 10-26 Overview of the tip stitch.

Since a wide bite of dermis and epidermis is included in the suture arc, it is particularly important to avoid tying the suture material too tight, as this could lead to wound edge necrosis. Some surgeons use bolsters when using this technique under high tension, such as when a 3-0 suture is used on the back, in an attempt to avoid track marks and reduce the risk of tissue necrosis. A wide array of materials may be used for the bolster, including gauze, dental rolls, or plastic tubing. In practice, bolsters are rarely needed with this technique as long as the bulk of the wound tension has been shifted deep using fascial or dermal buried sutures.

Tip Stitch

This technique is designed to bring three ends of tissue together and is often used in the context of a flap, where it permits the tip of tissue to be inset. This approach may be conceptualized as a half-buried horizontal mattress suture (**Figure 10-26**).

The tip stitch is very useful when bringing the tip of a flap into place and is used frequently in this situation.[30-32] Importantly, this technique is designed to gently approximate the tissues so that the flap is properly inset in the surrounding skin. While it bears a technical resemblance to the half-buried horizontal mattress, it is important to appreciate that the tip stitch is *not* designed to work under significant tension, as tension across the suture may lead to necrosis of the delicate and lightly vascularized tip of the flap.

Flap tip necrosis is the greatest risk with this technique, since suture material traverses the dermis containing the tip's vascular supply. This risk may be mitigated by tying the suture relatively loosely so that the tip is not overly constricted when the knot is tied. Additionally, if the bites of dermis are sufficiently set back from the wound edge, a small bite comprising less than half of the dermis in the tip could be taken. This would allow blood supply to the tip even in the context of a relatively tight loop running through the distal flap.

TECHNIQUE: TIP STITCH

a. The flap is brought into place using buried sutures, allowing the tip to rest with only minimal tension in its desired position.
b. The needle is inserted into the distal edge of the distal nonflap section of skin at 90 degrees with a trajectory running toward the planned entry point in the tip.
c. The needle is then grasped with the surgical pickups and simultaneously released by the hand holding the needle driver. As the needle is freed from the tissue with the pickups, the needle is grasped again by the needle driver in an appropriate position to place the next throw.
d. The needle is inserted into the distal portion of the tip at the level of the superficial dermis, which should be the same depth at which it exited in the prior step. Keeping the needle running horizontally, parallel with the skin surface, it is rotated through the dermis of the tip, exiting on the proximal side of the tip at the same depth.
e. The needle is then reloaded in a backhand fashion and inserted into the dermis of the proximal nontip section of skin, exiting parallel to its initial entry point.
f. The suture material is then gently pulled taut and tied using an instrument tie. Care should be taken to minimize tension on this suture to mitigate the risk of flap tip necrosis.

There is sometimes a tendency for the tip to sit deeper than the surrounding tissues. This may be related to the relative upward pull on the nontip sections of skin by the transepidermal sutures.

Finally, while flap tip necrosis is a risk, studies have suggested that the tip stitch provides less vascular constriction than other options, such as placing two vertically oriented sutures at the edges of the tip or a suture directly through the tip itself.[31]

Purse-String Suture

As with its buried variant, this technique is designed to either shrink the size of a defect or obviate it entirely, depending on the degree of tension and the size of the defect (**Figure 10-27**).

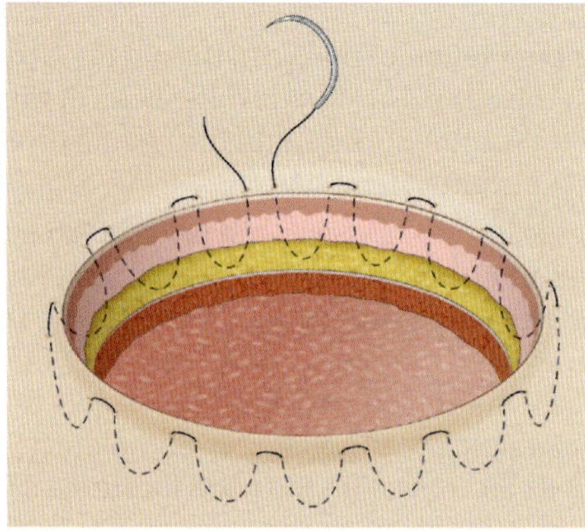

FIGURE 10-27 Overview of the purse-string suture.

TECHNIQUE: PURSE-STRING SUTURE

a. The wound edges are broadly undermined.
b. With the tail of the suture material resting between the surgeon and the far end of the wound, the needle is inserted through the epidermis on the far edge of the wound with a trajectory running parallel to the incision. The entry point in the epidermis should be approximately 3 to 6 mm set back from the epidermal edge, depending on the thickness of the dermis and the anticipated degree of tension across the closure. The needle, and therefore the suture, should pass through the deep dermis into the undermined space at a uniform depth.
c. The needle is then grasped with the surgical pickups and simultaneously released by the hand holding the needle driver. As the needle is freed from the tissue with the pickups, the needle is grasped again by the needle driver in an appropriate position to repeat the above step to the left of the previously placed suture.
d. A small amount of suture material is pulled through and the needle is inserted into the dermis to the left of the previously placed suture, and the same movement is repeated.
e. The same technique is repeated moving stepwise around the entire wound until the needle exits close to the original entry point at the far end of the wound. Once the point closest to the surgeon is reached, it may be more comfortable to shift to a backhand technique.
f. Once the desired number of throws has been placed, the suture material is then pulled taut, leading to complete or partial closure of the wound, and tied using an instrument tie. Alternatively, a hand tie may be used if desired.

For a detailed discussion of the advantages and applications of this technique, see the earlier section on the buried purse-string technique. A monofilament suture is generally used to permit easy pull-through as well as straightforward suture removal.

The purse-string technique may also be used to effect hemostasis in the case of an oozing wound. For wounds in highly vascular areas, such as the scalp, a purse-string suture may be performed distant from the wound edge; small vessels will be captured within the ring of the purse-string suture and compressed when the suture material is tightened, leading to improved hemostasis. A double ring of purse-string sutures may be used as well to take even better advantage of this hemostatic effect.

VARIATIONS

Running

Running suture techniques are frequently used for their rapidity and ease of placement. The classic technique is the simple running suture (**Figure 10-28**), where anchoring sutures are placed at one end of the wound and successive bites are taken moving along the wound. Whether each bite is oriented perpendicularly or diagonally relative to the incision line is largely a point of style.

The running horizontal mattress suture, possibly with intermittent single bites, is another useful technique that leads to excellent wound edge eversion (**Figure 10-29**). A running vertical mattress technique is also possible, although it is used less frequently.

The advantage of running techniques is that they are fairly quick to place, as individual knots are not needed for each suture bite. This is also their central disadvantage, since the entire suture line is secured by only two knots, and if either one is compromised, then the integrity of the repair is lost.

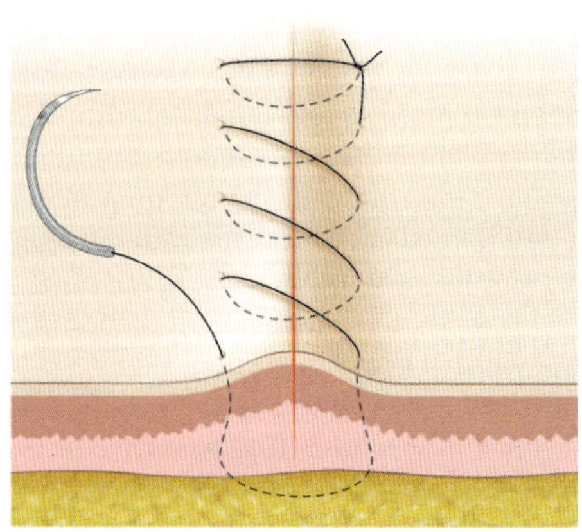

FIGURE 10-28 The simple running suture technique.

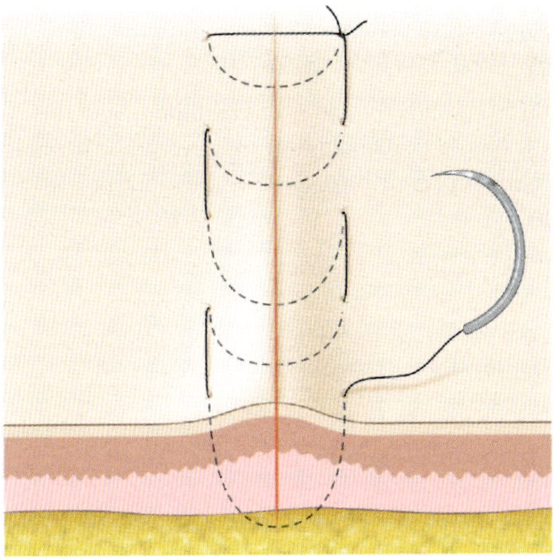

FIGURE 10-29 The running horizontal mattress technique.

Locking

Locking suture techniques, frequently used in concert with running techniques, allow the suture material to be fixed in place. They are frequently used with a simple running suture (the running locking or locked suture), which maintains even tension over each of the suture loops so that bunching and differential tension are less likely.

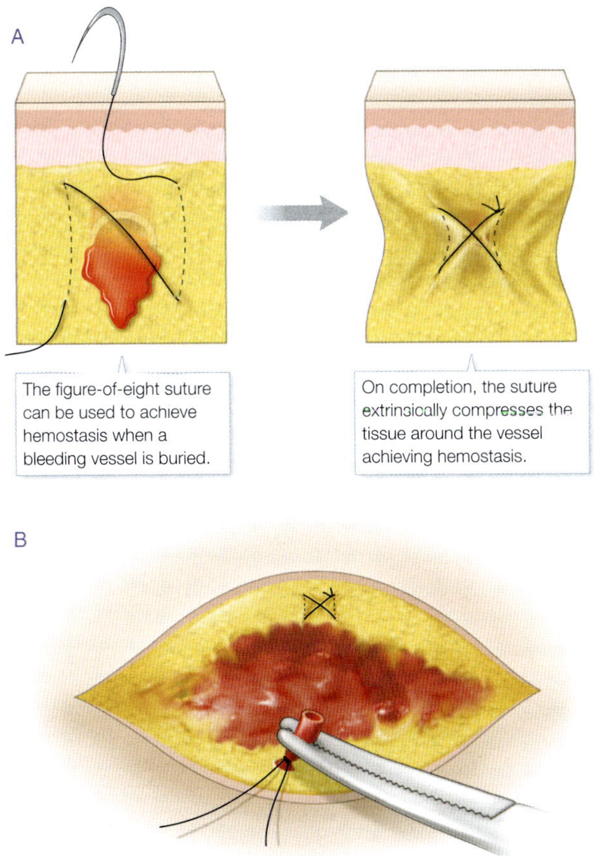

FIGURE 10-30 Approaches to hemostasis using a figure-of-eight suture or direct ligature.

This technique has also been suggested as an adjunct to achieving hemostasis. Other techniques, such as the horizontal mattress suture, may be locked as well, although in practice, this is performed less frequently.

Figure 10-30 shows approaches to hemostasis using a figure-of-eight suture or direct ligature.

CONCLUSIONS

Meticulous suturing technique is the cornerstone of every surgical repair. While the clinician does not need to incorporate a vast array of techniques into daily practice, precise placement of sutures coupled with an appreciation of the subtle variations in individual patients who may benefit from particular niche techniques is very helpful and may result in improved surgical outcomes.

REFERENCES

1. Wang AS, Kleinerman R, Armstrong AW, et al. Set-back versus buried vertical mattress suturing: results of a randomized blinded trial. *J Am Acad Dermatol.* 2015;72(4):674-680.
2. Zitelli JA, Moy RL. Buried vertical mattress suture. *J Dermatol Surg Oncol.* 1989;15(1):17-19.
3. Kantor J. The set-back buried dermal suture: an alternative to the buried vertical mattress for layered wound closure. *J Am Acad Dermatol.* 2010;62(2):351-353.
4. Kantor J. The subcutaneous splint: a helpful analogy to explain postoperative wound eversion. *JAMA Dermatol.* 2014;150(10):1122.
5. Miller CJ, Antunes MB, Sobanko JF. Surgical technique for optimal outcomes: Part II. Repairing tissue: suturing. *J Am Acad Dermatol.* 2015;72(3):389-402.
6. Alam M, Goldberg LH. Utility of fully buried horizontal mattress sutures. *J Am Acad Dermatol.* 2004;50(1):73-76.
7. Kantor J. The fascial plication suture: an adjunct to layered wound closure. *Arch Dermatol.* 2009;145(12):1454-1456.
8. Dzubow LM. The use of fascial plication to facilitate wound closure following microscopically controlled surgery. *J Dermatol Surg Oncol.* 1989;15(10):1063-1066.
9. Zhu JW, Wu XJ, Lu ZF, Cai SQ, Zheng M. Purse-string suture for round and oval defects: a useful technique in dermatologic surgery. *J Cutan Med Surg.* 2012;16(1):11-17.
10. Lin H, Li W. Complete closure using a double purse-string closure for skin defects. *Dermatol Surg.* 2009;35(9):1406-1409.
11. Hoffman A, Lander J, Lee PK. Modification of the purse-string closure for large defects of the extremities. *Dermatol Surg.* 2008;34(2):243-245.
12. Cohen PR, Martinelli PT, Schulze KE, Nelson BR. The purse-string suture revisited: a useful technique for the closure of cutaneous surgical wounds. *Int J Dermatol.* 2007;46(4):341-347.
13. Ciatti S, Greenbaum SS. Modified purse-string closure for reconstruction of moderate/large surgical defects of the face. *Dermatol Surg.* 1999;25(3):215-219; discussion 219-220.
14. Brady JG, Grande DJ, Katz AE. The purse-string suture in facial reconstruction. *J Dermatol Surg Oncol.* 1992;18(9):812-816.
15. Joo J, Custis T, Armstrong AW, et al. Purse-string suture vs second intention healing: results of a randomized, blind clinical trial. *JAMA Dermatol.* 2015;151(3):265-270.

16. Giandoni MB, Grabski WJ, Salasche SJ. Surgical pearl: the dermal buried pulley suture. *J Am Acad Dermatol.* 1994;30(6):1012-1013.
17. Whalen JD, Dufresne RG, Collins SC. Surgical pearl: the modified buried dermal suture. *J Am Acad Dermatol.* 1999;40(1):103-104.
18. Yag-Howard C. Novel surgical approach to subcutaneous closure: the subcutaneous inverted cross mattress stitch (SICM Stitch). *Dermatol Surg.* 2011;37(10):1503-1505.
19. Jeon IK, Kim JH, Roh MR, Chung KY. The subcutaneous inverted cross mattress stitch (SICM stitch) in our experience. *Dermatol Surg.* 2013;39(5):794-795.
20. Kantor J. The pulley set-back dermal suture: an easy to implement everting suture technique for wounds under tension. *J Am Acad Dermatol.* 2015;72(1):e29-e30.
21. Orozco-Covarrubias ML, Ruiz-Maldonado R. Surgical facial wounds: simple interrupted percutaneous suture versus running intradermal suture. *Dermatol Surg.* 1999;25(2):109-112.
22. Koskela A, Kotaluoto S, Kaartinen I, Pauniaho SL, Rantanen T, Kuokkanen H. Continuous absorbable intradermal sutures yield better cosmetic results than nonabsorbable interrupted sutures in open appendectomy wounds: a prospective, randomized trial. *World J Surg.* 2014;38(5):1044-1050.
23. Gurusamy KS, Toon CD, Allen VB, Davidson BR. Continuous versus interrupted skin sutures for non-obstetric surgery. *Cochrane Database Syst Rev.* 2014;2:CD010365.
24. Gurusamy KS, Toon CD, Davidson BR. Subcutaneous closure versus no subcutaneous closure after non-caesarean surgical procedures. *Cochrane Database Syst Rev.* 2014;1:CD010425.
25. McLean NR, Fyfe AH, Flint EF, Irvine BH, Calvert MH. Comparison of skin closure using continuous and interrupted nylon sutures. *Br J Surg.* 1980;67(9):633-635.
26. Pauniaho SL, Lahdes-Vasama T, Helminen MT, Iber T, Makela E, Pajulo O. Non-absorbable interrupted versus absorbable continuous skin closure in pediatric appendectomies. *Scand J Surg.* 2010;99(3): 142-146.
27. Bolster M, Schipper C, Van Sterkenburg S, Ruettermann M, Reijnen M. Single interrupted sutures compared with Donati sutures after open carpal tunnel release: a prospective randomised trial. *J Plast Surg Hand Surg.* 2013;47(4):289-291.
28. Dietz UA, Kuhfuss I, Debus ES, Thiede A. Mario Donati and the vertical mattress suture of the skin. *World J Surg.* 2006;30(2): 141-148.
29. Trimbos JB, Mouw R, Ranke G, Trimbos KB, Zwinderman K. The Donati stitch revisited: favorable cosmetic results in a randomized clinical trial. *J Surg Res.* 2002;107(1):131-134.
30. Bechara FG, Al-Muhammadi R, Sand M, Tomi NS, Altmeyer P, Hoffmann K. A modified corner stitch for fixation of flap tips. *Dermatol Surg.* 2007;33(10):1277-1279.
31. Kandel EF, Bennett RG. The effect of stitch type on flap tip blood flow. *J Am Acad Dermatol.* 2001;44(2, Part 1):265-272.
32. McQuown SA, Cook TA, Brummett RE, Trachy RE. Gillies' corner stitch revisited. *Arch Otolaryngol.* 1984;110(7):450-453.

Superficial Biopsy Techniques

11

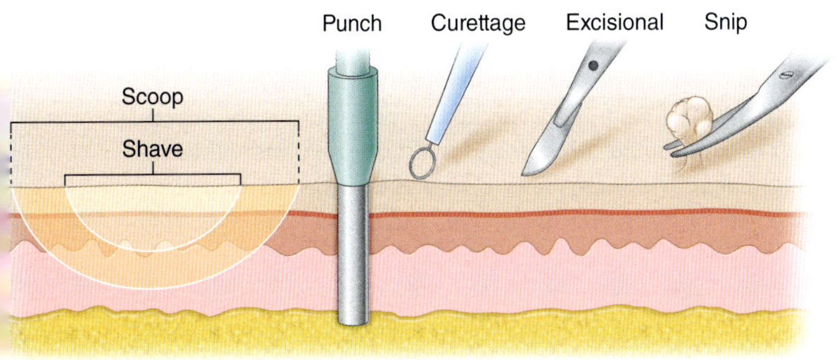

SUMMARY

- The biopsy of tissue for histological examination remains one of the most informative and cost-effective tests in medical practice, and one of the most common procedures performed by those caring for patients' skin.
- In general, all tissue removed during a surgical procedure should be submitted for histopathologic examination.
- Ultimately, the key factor in biopsy success is balancing the need for acquiring an adequate sample for histopathologic evaluation with minimizing the cosmetic and functional sequelae of the biopsy itself on the patient.

Beginner Tips

- Local anesthesia is a prerequisite for a pain-free biopsy; while patients may rarely request that a biopsy be performed without anesthesia, this should be discouraged, particularly as postbiopsy hemostasis may be more painful than the biopsy itself.
- Patients should receive written instructions regarding wound care.
- Shave biopsies are the cornerstone of dermatologic practice, and are useful in most situations when performed appropriately.

Pitfalls and Cautions

- Often the greatest risk associated with a biopsy is not performing it at all; in the hands of experienced clinicians, small biopsies yield nearly undetectable scars, and the diagnostic benefits far outweigh the risks.
- Biopsies from sebaceous skin, such as the nose, may leave pronounced scars that may benefit from later dermabrasion or resurfacing.

Expert Tips

- The "excisional biopsy" that is recommended for pigmented lesions suspicious for melanoma includes a deep shave or scoop biopsy.
- Multiple scouting biopsies may be useful when assessing for lentigo maligna.

Patient Education Points

- Most biopsy sites heal very quickly, but patients should understand that surrounding erythema or excess fibrin formation may be seen, particularly in areas that are subject to friction.
- Preoperative biopsy-site photography may be helpful to reduce the risk of surgical site identification challenges.

Don't Forget!

- When sampling for direct immunofluorescence, a punch biopsy from lower extremity skin should generally be avoided both due to a risk of false-negative results and a slower rate of healing.
- For alopecia, punch biopsy for transverse (horizontal) and vertical sections should ideally be performed.

Billing Pearls

- Biopsy coding is predicated on the assumption that the purpose of tissue removal is for diagnostic purposes.
- Site-specific biopsy codes should be utilized as appropriate.

11 Superficial Biopsy Techniques

INTRODUCTION

The biopsy of tissue for histologic examination remains the most informative and cost-effective test in medical practice and one of the most common procedures performed by clinicians caring for a patient's skin. A range of biopsy techniques are available to the clinician (**Figure 11-1**).

All tissue removed during a surgical procedure should be submitted for histopathologic examination unless specifically exempted by an organization's Tissue Committee policy. Skin tags are sometimes on the exempt list, but caution is advised, as infundibulocystic basal cell carcinoma, neurofibromas, and fibrofolliculomas may have a tag-like appearance. Any unusual-appearing tag should be submitted for examination, even if Tissue Committee policy exempts them, and many prudent clinicians err on the side of sending every piece of removed tissue for evaluation.

ANESTHESIA, PREPARATION, AND POSTOPERATIVE CARE

Prior to any biopsy, local anesthesia should be obtained by the use of lidocaine with epinephrine. The lidocaine is frequently buffered with sodium bicarbonate to reduce the burning sensation during injection. Buffered lidocaine has a finite shelf-life (roughly 1 week), and outdated solutions produce only partial anesthesia with excessive bleeding.

Data vary regarding whether warming or chilling the lidocaine solution results in less pain during injection, with some data favoring either method. Slow injection, vibration, application of an ice cube, or pinching of the skin can all be used to decrease the pain involved with injecting the local anesthetic (**Table 11-1**).

Correct positioning of the patient is essential. If a biopsy site is likely to bleed, a clean barrier should be placed under the affected area. The area should be clean and well organized, with all instruments in place; the biopsy bottle open and labeled with the patient's name, date of birth, and biopsy site; and gauze, hemostatic solution (typically 20% aluminum chloride), white petrolatum, and a band-aid already positioned. The assistant should read the site on each bottle before the specimen is placed into the formalin to assure that it is going into the correct bottle. The specimen should be fully immersed in the formalin solution, and visual inspection by the physician should confirm it is in the bottle before the cap is applied.

Caustic hemostatic agents should be used with extreme caution near the eyes. A cotton-tipped applicator (CTA) should be dipped into the cautery solution and rolled dry so that drips are unlikely. For lesions near the eyes, the patient should be positioned so that gravity and creases will not draw the hemostatic

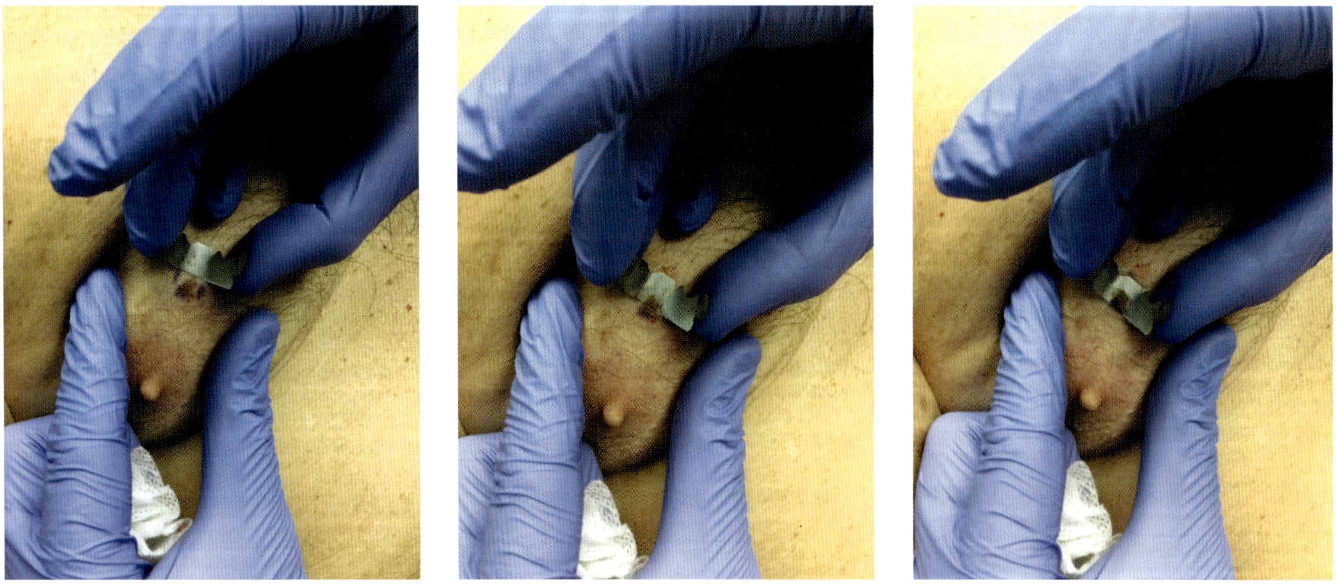

A B C

FIGURE 11-1

a. A shave biopsy is performed from the breast. Note the three-point traction.
b. The blade is gently passed through the lesion superficially using a back-and-forth motion.
c. This continues along the course of the lesion of interest. In general, forceps are not needed for shave biopsies.

TABLE 11-1 • Techniques to Minimize Biopsy-Site Injection Pain
Slow injection
Vibration
Application of an ice cube
Pinching of adjacent skin

solution into the eye. The wound should be blotted dry immediately after the biopsy and a CTA moistened with hemostatic solution rolled gently over the site, rather than twisted into the tissue. The wound surface should then be blotted to remove any excess hemostatic solution, as it will otherwise continue to burn the tissue and produce excess scarring.

Monsel's solution has the potential to cause a visible tattoo and must be used in a precise fashion. The wound must be blotted completely dry and the moistened CTA rolled quickly over the surface to obtain hemostasis. Incorrect application of excessive Monsel's solution to a bleeding wound results in a heavy black crust with continued bleeding through the crust, whereas a barely moistened CTA rolled across a dry wound produces instant hemostasis with little risk of tattoo.

Patients should receive written instructions regarding wound care. Most wounds can be cleaned with soap and water, and then covered with white petrolatum and a bandage. Antibiotic ointments carry a risk of contact allergy and anaphylaxis and make gram-negative wound infection more likely.[1] An exception is often made for wounds with exposed cartilage, which may be treated with topical gentamycin ophthalmic ointment or 0.025% acetic acid compresses twice daily to reduce the risk of *Pseudomonas* chondritis. Most superficial biopsies, however, do not result in exposed cartilage. Patients should be instructed to expect shave biopsy sites to become red around the edges and slightly yellow in the center during wound healing and should be reassured that this does not represent infection.

TECHNIQUE

Shave

Biopsies using a shave technique are commonly used to sample neoplastic lesions, but may also be useful in the setting of inflammatory dermatoses if the key histologic features are present in the epidermis and papillary dermis. Engineered sharps (**Figure 11-2**) can be considered, although currently available engineered sharps are less rigid than traditional double-edged razor blades

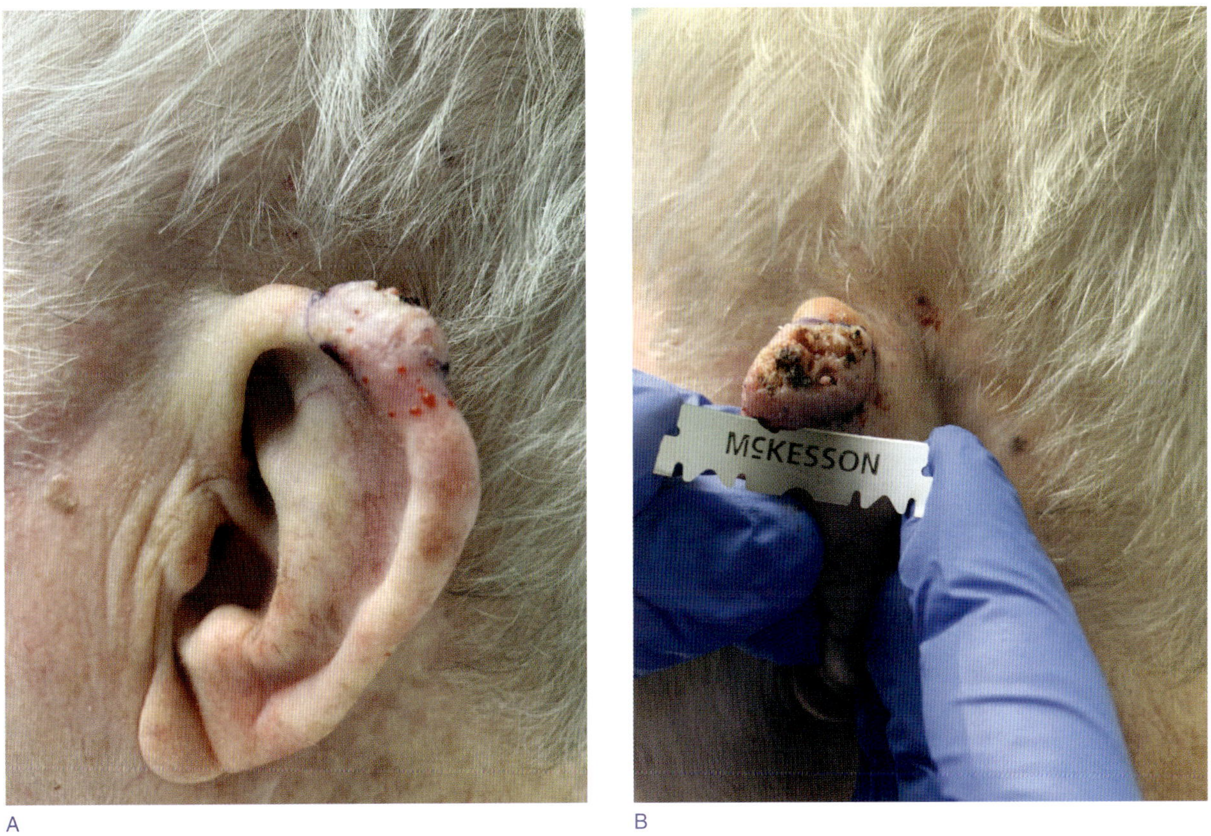

FIGURE 11-2

a. A thick hyperkeratotic plaque is present on the helix.

b. The ear is gently retracted and the blade is inserted at the base of the lesion.

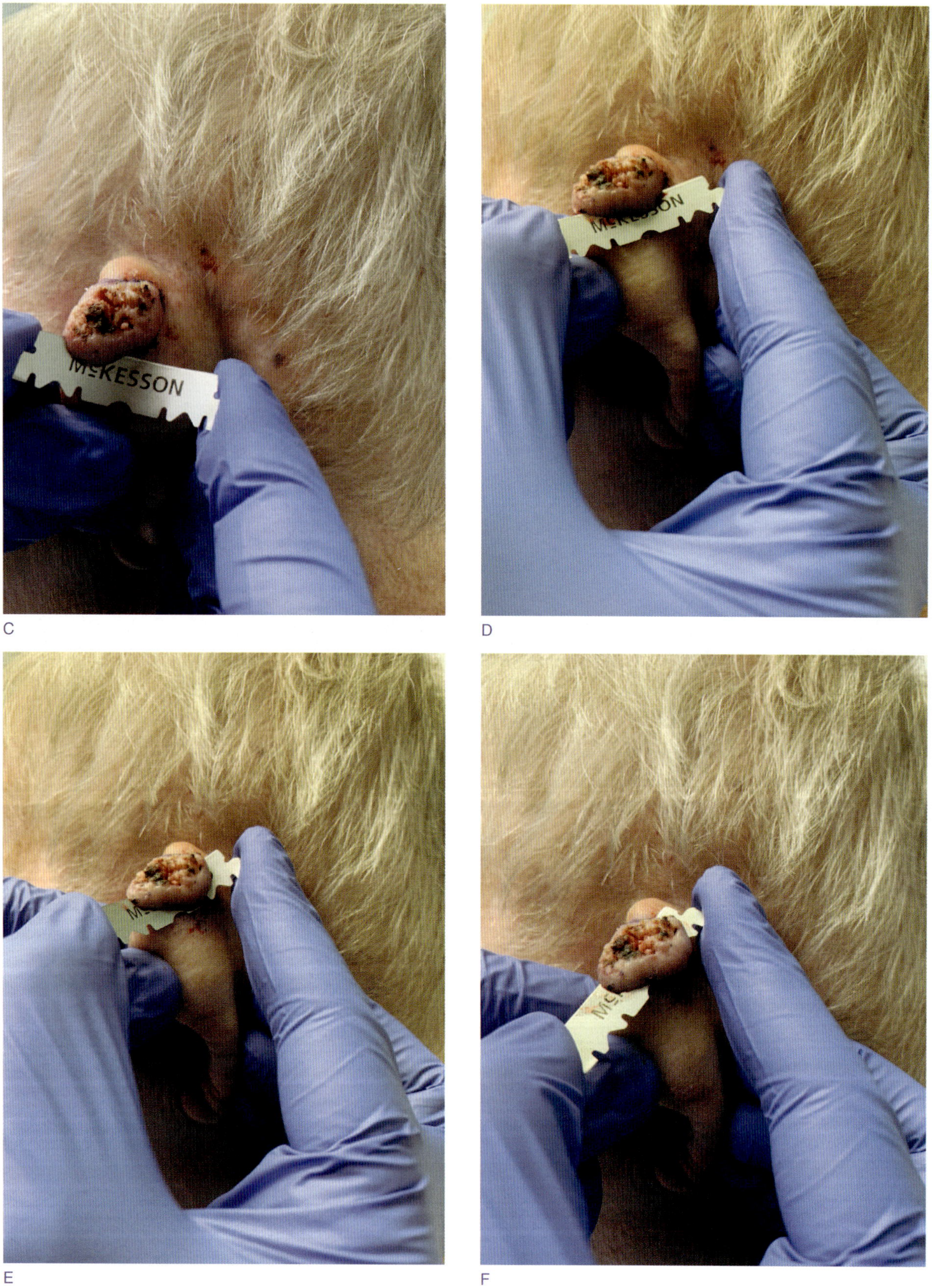

FIGURE 11-2 *(Continued)*

c. A back-and-forth motion is used to incise the base of the lesion.
d. With this large plaque, approaches from several angles are used to free up the plaque from the underlying skin.
e. The same plane is maintained throughout.
f. The plaque is elevated.

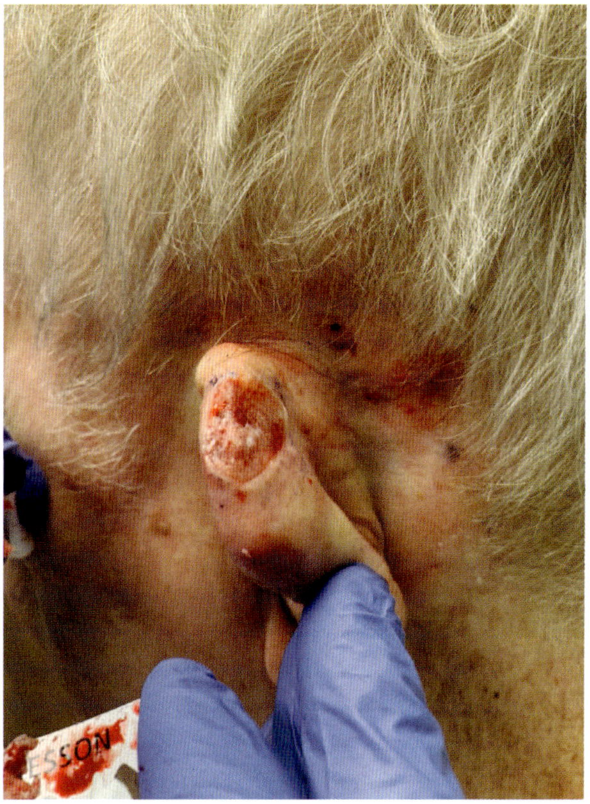

G

FIGURE 11-2 *(Continued)*
g. A smooth base is visible, highlighting the single plane that was used for the biopsy.

and often cannot substitute. Thus, most dermatologists continue to prefer the use of either double- or single-edged razor blades, which are also much less expensive than engineered sharps (**Figure 11-1**). Others prefer the use of a number 15 or number 10 blade followed by curettage to smooth the wound edges.

The Technique: The skin is pulled taut in all directions by the clinician and, if needed, an assistant (**Figure 11-2**). This allows for more precise sampling of the tissue, a smoother wound edge, and quicker sampling. A shave that will not end, producing a tail, is usually the result of failure to pull the skin taut. The blade is initially angled slightly downward to breach the epidermis, carried horizontally to obtain the specimen, and then angled upward to complete the procedure. A fairly rapid but gentle side-to-side motion allows the blade to move smoothly through the tissue without causing ridges. A tumid technique has also been described, which involves ballooning of soft papules such as benign nevi and neurofibromas with a mixture of lidocaine diluted with bacteriostatic 0.9% sodium chloride to create a more rigid structure and facilitate shave removal.[2]

A shave removal is distinct from a shave biopsy since the *intent* is to remove the lesion, rather than sample it. The intention must be clear from the documentation, as this distinction may lead to a coding (and reimbursement) differential (see Chapter 8).

Saucerization

When performed properly, saucerization, or scoop-shave removal, results in an eponymous saucer-shaped specimen with complete extirpation of the lesion (**Figure 11-3**). Saucerization may remain in the dermis or be scooped to subcutaneous tissue.

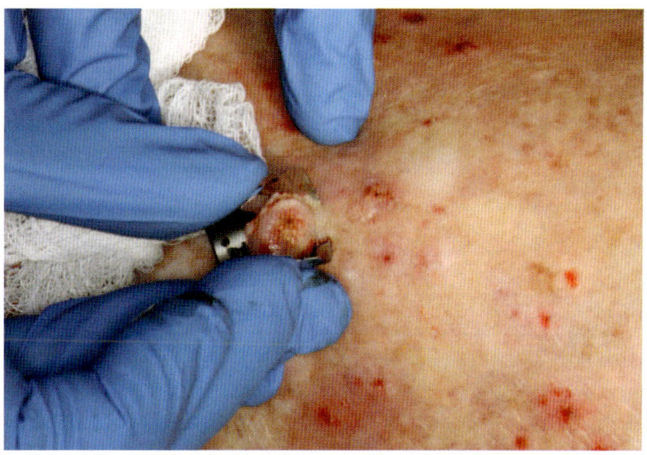

FIGURE 11-3 Saucerization biopsy is essentially a deep shave biopsy. This is a preferred technique for suspicious pigmented lesions.

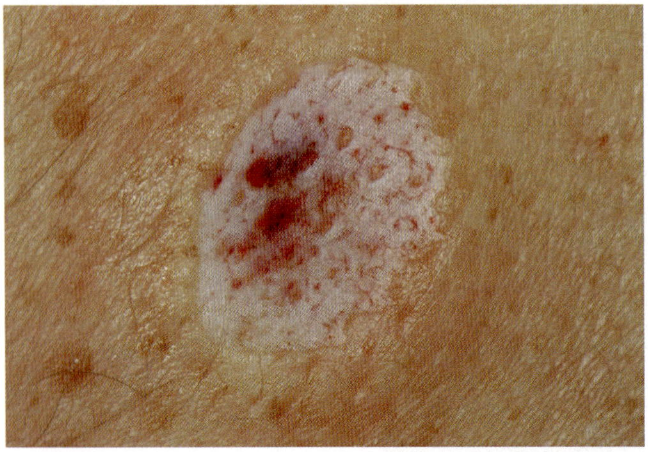

FIGURE 11-4 Often, pinpoint-bleeding dermis is visible immediately after a saucerization biopsy.

The Technique: The overall technique is very similar to a shave biopsy, but the blade is angled more steeply toward the center of the biopsy site and then advanced with a similar rapid but gentle side-to-side motion and a forward scooping motion. Some clinicians prefer to score the skin around the target lesion to aid with an aggressive saucerization. Often, pinpoint-bleeding dermis is visible immediately after a saucerization biopsy (**Figure 11-4**).

Punch

The punch technique can be used to sample an inflammatory process or a lesion or for complete excision of a smaller lesion. Furthermore, lesions slightly larger than 4 mm can often be forced into a 4-mm punch, resulting in satisfactory removal or sampling and a smaller wound.

The Technique: When possible, the skin is pulled taut perpendicular to the skin tension lines, so that the wound created by the punch is oval and aligned with the preferred lines of closure. The punch is twisted gently (**Figure 11-5**) until the full thickness of the metal portion has entered the skin (**Figure 11-6**). The resulting specimen should be removed gently with a needle or by grasping the skin edge with toothed forceps to avoid crushing the specimen (**Figure 11-7**). The resulting defect should then be assessed for the ideal closure vector (**Figure 11-8**). A suture is placed (**Figure 11-9**) and the wound may be closed with either a simple interrupted suture or a cruciate mattress suture (**Figure 11-10**). Other novel punch biopsy devices are available as well.[3]

Snip

A snip biopsy is performed by using surgical scissors, such as gradle scissors, to remove a pedunculated lesion, generally at its base. After local anesthesia is obtained, care should be taken to avoid elevating the target of the biopsy with forceps, as a snip biopsy at the base of a manipulated pedunculated papule will result in a depressed postprocedure scar. Instead, the papule should be snipped at its base in the resting position, which should result in minimal postprocedure scarring.

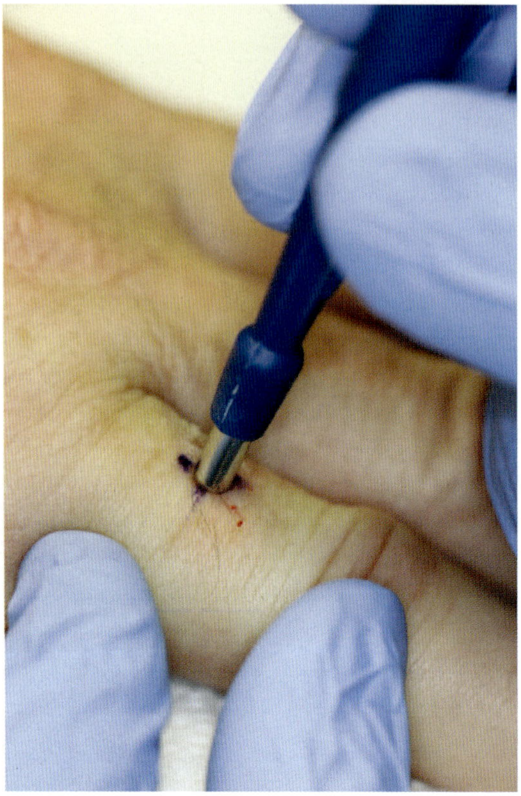

FIGURE 11-5 The punch is twisted gently.

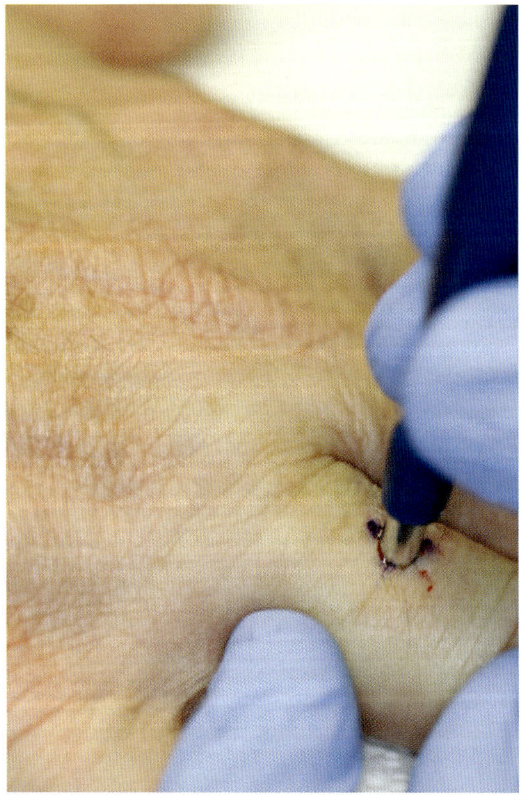

FIGURE 11-6 This continues until the entire device is inserted (when working on the trunk) or once the deep fat has been entered, as seen here.

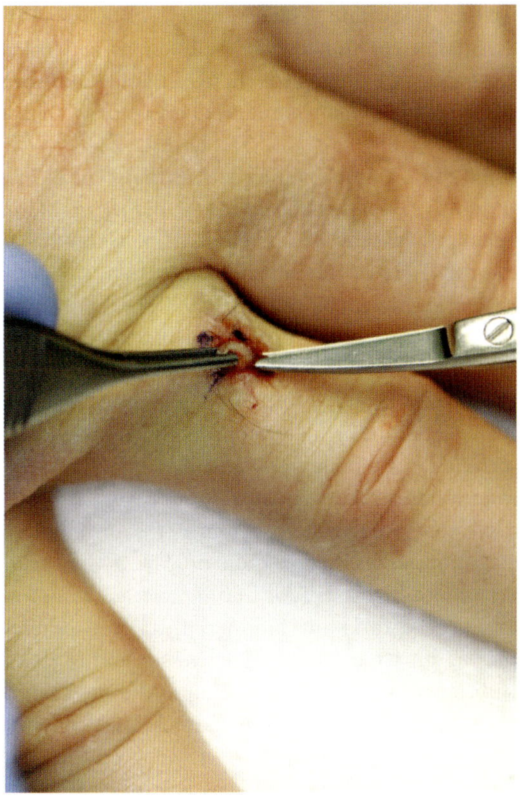

FIGURE 11-7 The specimen is grasped with forceps and elevated, and the base is snipped if needed at the level of the deep fat.

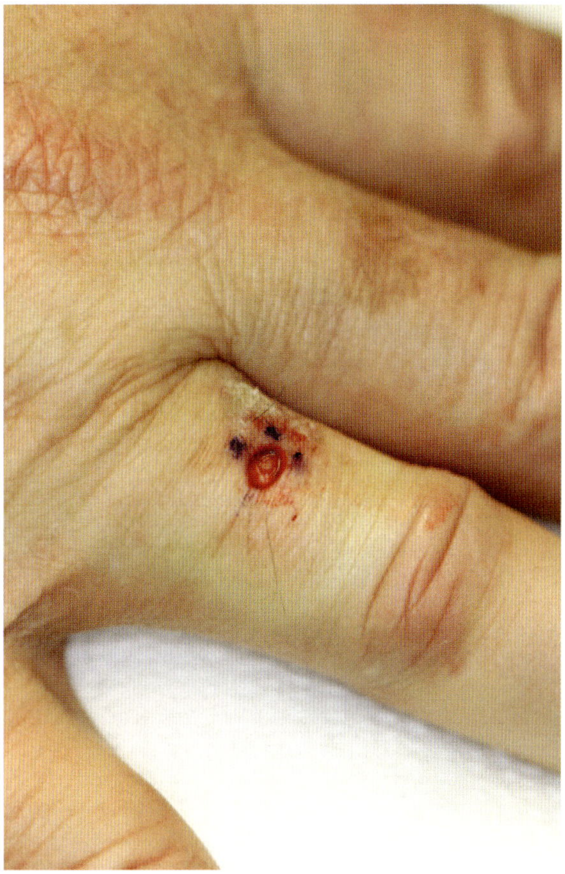

FIGURE 11-8 The resulting oval defect should be assessed for the ideal closure vector.

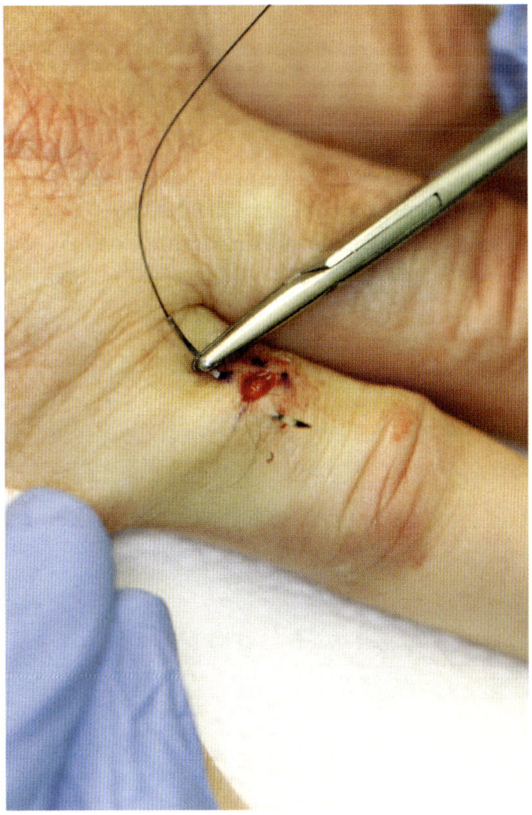

FIGURE 11-9 A suture is placed.

Incisional Biopsy

Incisional biopsies allow the clinician to have full control over the size, shape, and depth of the specimen and are typically followed by straight line closure. Panniculitis is best diagnosed by an incisional biopsy, although double punch and other related techniques have also been used.[4] Large melanocytic lesions are also often approached in this manner.

The Technique: A straight line or elliptical incision is made and the desired portion of tissue is removed (**Figure 11-11**). The resulting defect is then similar to any other created in excisional surgery (**Figure 11-12**), and the wound is closed with simple or layered closure.

Excision

Excision is the most appropriate technique to produce tissue for examination when the lesion is most likely malignant and subtotal excision may compromise diagnosis or outcome.

The Technique: The tissue is removed through to the subcutaneous tissue by means of elliptical, circular, or scooped excision. Undermining is often required to free the wound edges to facilitate closure. The wound is closed with simple or layered closure.

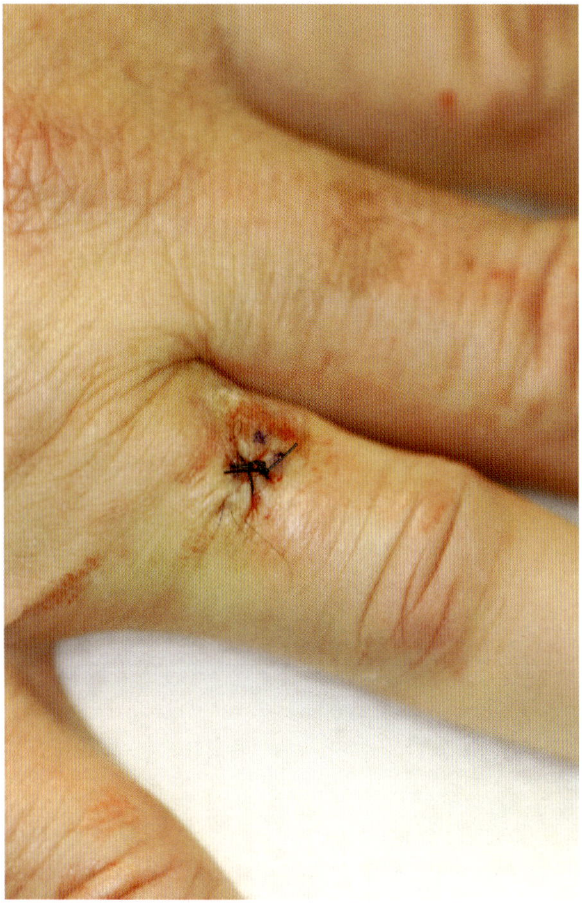

FIGURE 11-10 The cruciate mattress suture, essentially two throws of a simple running suture, is useful for punch biopsy closures.

SPECIAL SITUATIONS AND SPECIAL SITES

Pigmented Lesions

The American Academy of Dermatology (AAD) and the National Comprehensive Cancer Network (NCCN) list narrow excisional biopsy as the preferred technique for sampling lesions suspicious for melanoma. Importantly, saucerization, or a scoop-shave technique, is suitable for thin melanocytic lesions and rarely compromises staging,[5,6] and indeed, the AAD guidelines themselves include saucerization as a technique to accomplish an excisional biopsy.

In a study of 332 melanoma patients, most diagnostic biopsies had positive margins regardless of biopsy technique, but staging changed in only 8% of patients, of whom 59% had a punch biopsy, 15% an incisional biopsy, 15% a shave biopsy, and 11% an excisional biopsy ($P < .0001$). Treatment recommendations changed in 6% of the patients: 2% after excisional biopsy, 5% after shave biopsy, 18% after punch biopsy, and 18% after incisional biopsy ($P < .0001$).[7] These data suggest that the scoop-shave technique on an appropriately chosen lesion can be a prudent choice, but punch biopsy should be discouraged.

Another study of 709 patients showed that shave biopsies resulted in more positive deep margins ($P < .001$). Both shave and punch biopsies resulted in more positive peripheral margins ($P < .001$) and a higher risk of finding residual tumor on wide local excision ($P < .001$), but biopsy type did not confer survival advantage or impact tumor recurrence, suggesting that experienced clinicians should be free to choose the most appropriate technique for a given lesion.[8] Other authors have published data supporting similar conclusions.[9,10]

In the setting of lentigo maligna, it is often impractical to remove the entire lesion, and sampling of the lesion may be more appropriate. A broad area of the dermal-epidermal junction may be demonstrated by a broad, thin biopsy resembling properly cut prosciutto. If the lesion is mottled with many colors, multiple small thin shaves sampling each color may be more appropriate. If a skin crease naturally traverses the area to be sampled, an incisional biopsy can be aligned along the crease.

Immunobullous Disease

In the setting of suspected immunobullous disease, biopsies for direct immunofluorescence (DIF) should be taken from nonbullous lesional skin or perilesional skin within about 1 cm of a bulla. Nonbullous lesional skin has the higher yield.[11] Lower extremity

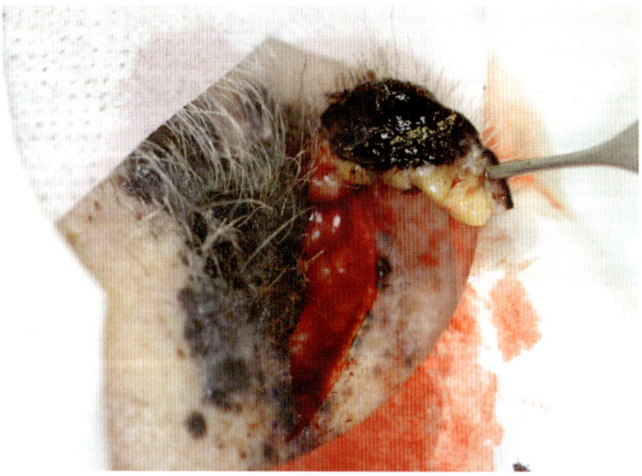

FIGURE 11-11 An incisional biopsy is useful particularly when a deep melanoma is being sampled to assess the depth of invasion.

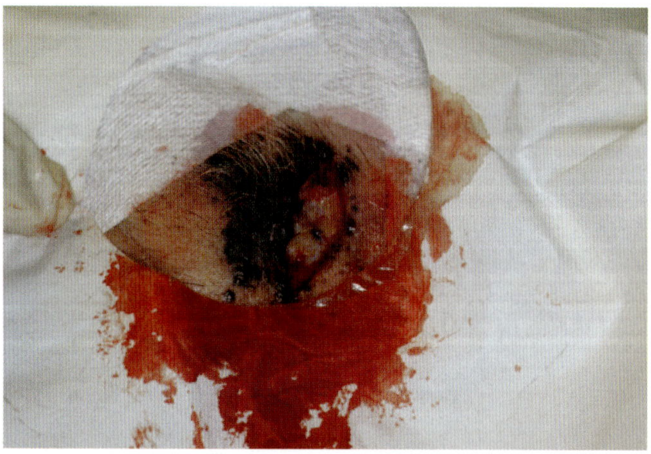

FIGURE 11-12 The resultant defect may then be approached in a similar fashion to any other excisional surgery.

skin should be avoided because of a greater risk of false-negative results.[12,13] Specimens for light microscopy should demonstrate an intact vesicle or bulla whenever possible. For larger lesions, the specimen should contain both portions of the blister and intact skin so that the edge of the blister and a portion of the bulla are biopsied. A punch biopsy or shave excision works well for small vesicles, whereas a scooped shave may be useful to harvest larger bullae intact.

Tissue obtained for DIF should be placed in Michel's medium or Zeus medium.[14,15] Some immunodermatology laboratories prefer specimens transported in saline to reduce background staining. Saline-preserved specimens should be processed within 24 hours. If the specimen is inadvertently placed into formalin, it should immediately be removed and rinsed in normal saline. Brief formalin immersion produces false-negative results for pemphigus, but not for diseases characterized by deposits at the dermal-epidermal junction.[16] In the setting of tense blisters suggesting a subepidermal bullous disease, a single punch technique has been used to obtain both hematoxylin and eosin (H&E) and DIF specimens and provide salt-split skin diagnostic information.[17]

Connective Tissue Disease

In contrast to immunobullous disease, biopsies of suspected connective tissue disease for DIF are best performed on well-established lesions greater than 6 months old. In the setting of systemic lupus erythematosus, the lupus band test performed on normal sun-protected skin has largely been replaced by assays for double-stranded DNA antibodies, which identify the same population at risk for renal disease.

Vasculitis

In the case of suspected vasculitis, biopsies for H&E should be taken from a well-established purpuric lesion (at least 72 hours old), whereas biopsies for DIF should be taken from an acute lesion (<24 hours old). Immunoglobulin A (IgA) vasculitis is more likely to retain positive DIF findings in established lesions when compared with other forms of vasculitis.

Alopecia

To maximize the diagnostic yield in the setting of alopecia, a 4-mm punch biopsy specimen should be obtained from a well-developed lesion, preferably of several months' duration, but still active. Many labs prefer transverse sections, although serial vertical sections are superior in the setting of scarring alopecia. A separate biopsy can be bisected vertically to produce a half punch suitable for DIF and another half punch added to the formalin bottle to provide vertical sections. When biopsies of active lesions prove to be nondiagnostic, a biopsy from a scarred area evaluated with elastic tissue stains or polarized microscopy can provide additional information.[18-21] Both trichoscopy and confocal microscopy can be useful in site selection, directing the clinician to established areas of active inflammation.[22-24] The punch should always enter the scalp at the same angle as the emerging hairs to avoid transecting hair follicles. Hemostasis is more easily obtained with gel foam than with sutures.

Mucosal and Genital Biopsies

The thin skin of the lips has a tendency to retract when a shave biopsy is performed. Therefore, using a tumid-type technique and raising a significant wheal in the target tissue may serve to develop a more rigid substrate for shave biopsy. Alternatively, a chalazion clamp may be used, a snip biopsy may be performed after grasping the target tissue with dressing forceps, or a punch biopsy may be performed in lieu of a shave approach. Similar approaches may be used when performing biopsies on the vulva or shaft of the penis.

CONCLUSIONS

Careful attention to biopsy technique, patient positioning, site selection, and hemostasis will result in better outcomes for the patient and a more efficient practice for the clinician. Ultimately, the key factor in biopsy success is balancing the need for acquiring an adequate sample for histopathologic evaluation and minimizing the cosmetic and functional sequelae of the biopsy itself on the patient.

REFERENCES

1. Kim B, James W. Postoperative use of topical antimicrobials. *Dermatitis*. 2009;20(3):174.
2. Zaiac M, Shah VV, Mlacker S, Bray FN, Alsaidan M. Local anesthesia injection technique for aesthetic removal of dermal nevi. *J Cosmet Dermatol*. 2016;15(4):559-560.
3. AlGhamdi KM. C-punch excision: a novel technique. *Int J Dermatol*. 2016;55(10):1154-1156.
4. Ersoy-Evans S. Surgical pearl: a novel punch biopsy technique for diagnosing panniculitis. *J Am Acad Dermatol*. 2015;72(6):e161-e162.
5. Mendese G, Maloney M, Bordeaux J. To scoop or not to scoop: the diagnostic and therapeutic utility of the scoop-shave biopsy for pigmented lesions. *Dermatol Surg*. 2014;40(10):1077-1083.
6. Saco M, Thigpen J. A retrospective comparison between preoperative and postoperative Breslow depth in primary cutaneous melanoma: how preoperative shave biopsies affect surgical management. *J Drugs Dermatol*. 2014;13(5):531-536.
7. Hicken TJ, Hernández-Irizarry R, Boll JM, Jones Coleman JE. Accuracy of diagnostic biopsy for cutaneous melanoma: implications for surgical oncologists. *Int J Surg Oncol*. 2013;2013:196493.
8. Mills JK, White I, Diggs B, Fortino J, Vetto JT. Effect of biopsy type on outcomes in the treatment of primary cutaneous melanoma. *Am J Surg*. 2013;205(5):585-590.
9. Zager JS, Hochwald SN, Marzban SS, et al. Shave biopsy is a safe and accurate method for the initial evaluation of melanoma. *J Am Coll Surg*. 2011;212(4):454-460.
10. Lowe M, Hill N, Page A, Chen S, Delman KA. The impact of shave biopsy on the management of patients with thin melanomas. *Am Surg*. 2011;77(8):1050-1053.
11. Seishima M, Izumi T, Kitajima Y. Antibody to bullous pemphigoid antigen 1 binds to the antigen at perilesional but not uninvolved skin, in localized bullous pemphigoid. *Eur J Dermatol*. 1999;9(1):39-42.
12. Weigand DA. Effect of anatomic region on immunofluorescence diagnosis of bullous pemphigoid. *J Am Acad Dermatol*. 1985;12(2 Pt 1):274-278.

13. Weigand DA, Clements MK. Direct immunofluorescence in bullous pemphigoid: effects of extent and location of lesions. *J Am Acad Dermatol.* 1989;20(3):437-440.
14. Schmidt E, Zillikens D. Modern diagnosis of autoimmune blistering skin diseases. *Autoimmun Rev.* 2010;10(2):84-89.
15. Patel AN, Simpson RC, Cohen SN. In a patient with an immunobullous disorder, is transportation of the skin biopsy in normal saline adequate for direct immunofluorescence analysis? A critically appraised topic. *Br J Dermatol.* 2013;169(1):6-10.
16. Arbesman J, Grover R, Helm TN, Beutner EH. Can direct immunofluorescence testing still be accurate if performed on biopsy specimens after brief inadvertent immersion in formalin? *J Am Acad Dermatol.* 2011;65(1):106-111.
17. Braswell MA, McCowan NK, Schulmeier JS, Brodell RT. High-yield biopsy technique for subepidermal blisters. *Cutis.* 2015;95(4):237-240.
18. Elston DM, McCollough ML, Warschaw KE, Bergfeld WF. Elastic tissue in scars and alopecia. *J Cutan Pathol.* 2000;27:147-152.
19. Kazlouskaya V, Malhotra S, Lambe J, Idriss MH, Elston DM, Andres C. The utility of elastic Verhoeff–van Gieson staining in dermatopathology. *J Cutan Pathol.* 2013;40:211-225.
20. Fung MA, Sharon VR, Ratnarathorn M, Konia TH, Barr KL, Mirmirani P. Elastin staining patterns in primary cicatricial alopecia. *J Am Acad Dermatol.* 2013;69(5):776-782.
21. Miteva M, Tosti A. Polarized microscopy as a helpful tool to distinguish chronic nonscarring alopecia from scarring alopecia. *Arch Dermatol.* 2012;148(1):91-94.
22. Miteva M, Tosti A. Dermoscopy guided scalp biopsy in cicatricial alopecia. *J Eur Acad Dermatol Venereol.* 2013;27(10):1299-1303.
23. Agozzino M, Tosti A, Barbieri L, et al. Confocal microscopic features of scarring alopecia: preliminary report. *Br J Dermatol.* 2011;165(3):534-540.
24. Jain N, Doshi B, Khopkar U. Trichoscopy in alopecias: diagnosis simplified. *Int J Trichology.* 2013;5(4):170-178.

Cryosurgery

12

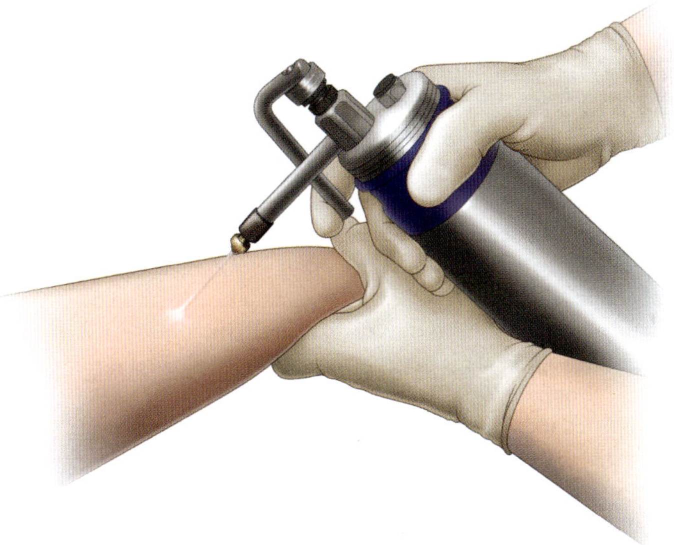

SUMMARY

- Cryosurgery is a versatile technique and the mainstay of the therapeutic armamentarium.
- While used largely for actinic keratoses, cryotherapy may be used for an array of dermatologic conditions.
- Cryosurgery has become a well-established, safe treatment modality for a wide range of conditions, and will likely remain a fixture in dermatologic surgery for years to come.

Beginner Tips

- It is always better to undertreat than overtreat an area. Warn patients that the areas being treated may not resolve and that additional treatments may be needed.
- Localize tissue treatment to the area of concern; it is best to avoid overly broad treatment that only serves to cause more tissue damage.

Pitfalls and Cautions

- Healing time after cryosurgery varies, and patients will almost always have significant edema and erythema in the immediate postprocedure period.
- On the scalp and legs, sites may take significantly longer to heal adequately.

Expert Tips

- Intralesional cryoneedles and other similar approaches may be used to treat larger or more aggressive tumors.
- In such cases, accurately gauging the temperature at the deepest section of the target lesion may be helpful.

Patient Education Points

- When treating actinic keratoses, there is often a field of actinic damage where incipient actinic keratoses are forming. Additional actinic keratoses in this area may be a result of this actinic field injury rather than a recurrence due to inadequate cryosurgery.
- Patients should be told what to expect in the posttreatment period to minimize anxiety.

Don't Forget!

- Melanocytes are highly cold-sensitive, while malignant cells are most resistant to cold-induced damage. Therefore, pigmentation changes are seen frequently with even moderately aggressive cryosurgery.
- Cryosurgery induces tissue necrosis through several pathways, including direct cellular injury, intra- and extracellular ice deposition, and damage to the microcirculatory vasculature.

Billing Pearls

- Cryosurgery coding depends on the lesion and anatomic site being treated. For actinic keratoses, use code 17000 for the first lesion and 17003 for each additional (up to 14), and code 17004 if 15 or more are treated. For warts and other benign lesions, use code 17110 (a single code for up to 14 lesions) or 17111 (15 or more). For genital lesions, use code 54056 for the penis or 56501 for the vulva. For malignant destruction, use the 172XX series.

12 Cryosurgery

INTRODUCTION

Cryotherapy, the application of cold temperatures for therapeutic purposes, has been used for thousands of years. Historical records dating as far back as 2500 BC reveal that the Egyptians used cold to treat injuries and infected wounds.[1] In the 5th century BC, Hippocrates documented the analgesic and anti-inflammatory properties of this modality.[2] However, the technique of cryosurgery, which specifically denotes the use of extreme cold for cellular destruction, has its origin in more modern times. Cryosurgery is a versatile treatment modality that is indicated for the treatment of numerous benign, premalignant, and malignant lesions.

CRYOGENS

Presently, liquid nitrogen is used exclusively in the vast majority of settings. However, prior to its development, several other cryogenic substances were employed for similar purposes. The original cryogen was liquefied air (–190°C), which was composed of approximately 78% nitrogen, 21% oxygen, and 1% argon, with traces of other gases.[2,3] While effective, liquid air was difficult to obtain and was subsequently superseded by solidified carbon dioxide (–78.5°C) in the early 1900s.[4] In the 1920s, liquid oxygen (–182.9°C) became readily available, but its use was limited by safety concerns including flammability.[5] The use of liquid nitrogen (–195.6°C), which remains the most frequently employed cryogen, was first reported in 1950.[3] In contrast to liquid oxygen, liquid nitrogen is inert, and is considered to be both safe and effective.

INSTRUMENTS

There are a variety of methods that may be used to apply liquid nitrogen. The most common of these in dermatologic settings is the use of a handheld spray unit (**Figure 12-1**). These units are available in multiple sizes and with several modifications that allow cryogen delivery to be tailored according to circumstance. Techniques of spray delivery include direct application to the center of a lesion, a spiral pattern that begins in the center and radiates outward, and a "paintbrush" pattern in which the nozzle is moved back and forth from one side to another. Various tips are available for these units (**Figure 12-2**). Devices such as an insulated plastic cone may be used in conjunction with the spray method to increase the concentration of liquid nitrogen applied to a particular location. The cone is placed directly onto the skin and enhances both the rate and depth of freezing. These should generally be avoided by primary care clinicians due to their risk of dramatic tissue damage.

To increase both the depth and lateral extent of freezing, cryoprobes may be used. Cryoprobes are tips cooled by circulating cryogen that can be inserted directly into the skin. They are available in a variety of shapes and sizes and are particularly useful for treating sebaceous hyperplasia and small vascular lesions. Additionally, cryoprobes are well suited to treat small tumors on the eyelid or lip where fine-tuned control of cryogen delivery is essential.[6]

A variation of the probe technique, the intralesional cryoneedle, may be useful for solid masses. This device can be passed through a tumor until the tip reemerges on the opposite side. Liquid nitrogen is circulated through the lumen of the needle, forming an ice cylinder in the surrounding tissue that expands circumferentially. The advantage of this technique is that colder temperatures may be applied directly to deeper structures, rather than the skin surface.[7] This method may be especially useful for the treatment of hypertrophic scars and keloids.[8]

The dipstick method, in which a cryogen-soaked cotton swab is applied directly to the skin, may also be useful. This technique is most suitable for the treatment of benign, superficial lesions, as the maximum depth of freezing achieved is 2 to 3 mm.

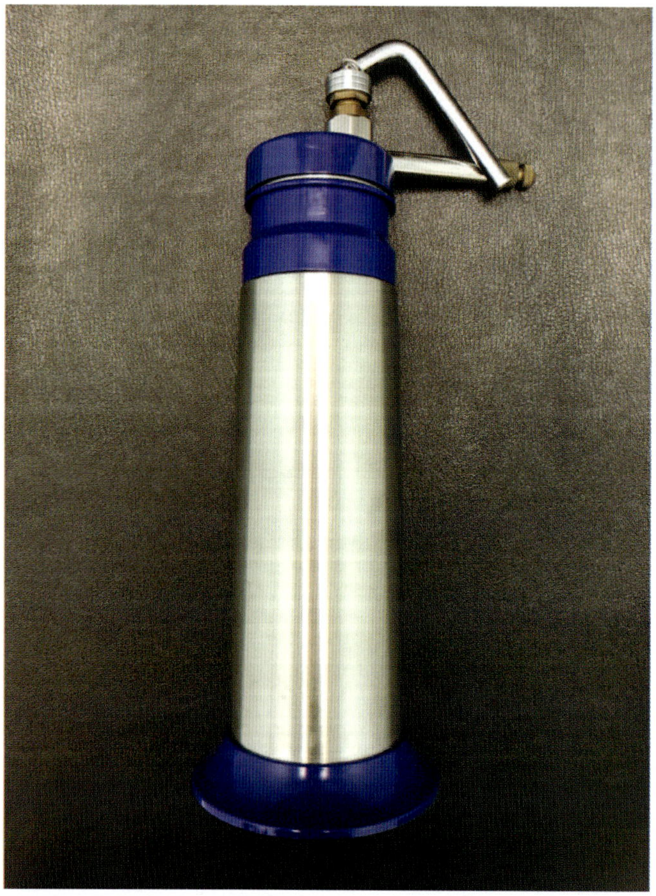

FIGURE 12-1 The liquid nitrogen spray unit.

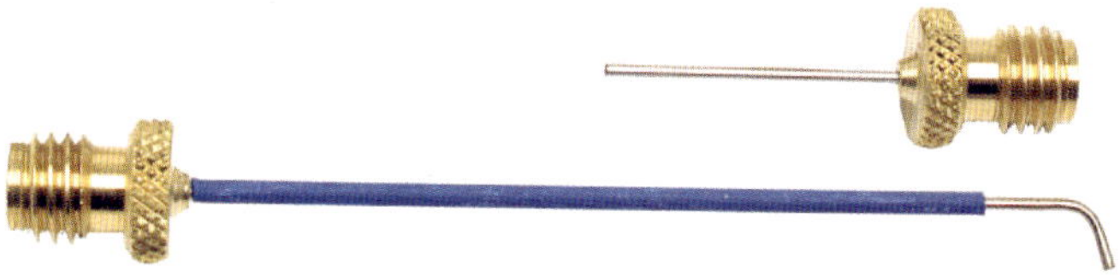

FIGURE 12-2 Various tips are available for the units.

TECHNIQUES

Although there are no absolute contraindications to cryosurgery, some comorbidities are more likely to be associated with adverse outcomes. Some of these include known cold intolerance, cold urticaria, cryofibrinogenemia, cryoglobulinemia, and Raynaud phenomenon. Collagen vascular disease, multiple myeloma, hemodialysis, thrombocytopenia, agammaglobulinemia, and blood dyscrasias of unknown origin have also been noted as relative contraindications.[9]

Several factors affect the amount of tissue destruction achieved with cryosurgery. When tissue is frozen, an ice ball forms that serves as a visible indication of the extent of surface freezing (**Figure 12-3**). However, the depth of freezing, also referred to as the depth dose, may be more difficult to determine. The ice ball maintains a hemispherical shape until it reaches a depth of 5 to 7 mm, at which point it will begin to plateau. For lesions exceeding this depth, a thermocouple may be useful. This device should be inserted into the skin at a 25- to 30-degree angle until the tip reaches the base of the lesion, and will provide a more accurate determination of tissue temperature, although these are rarely used in clinical practice.

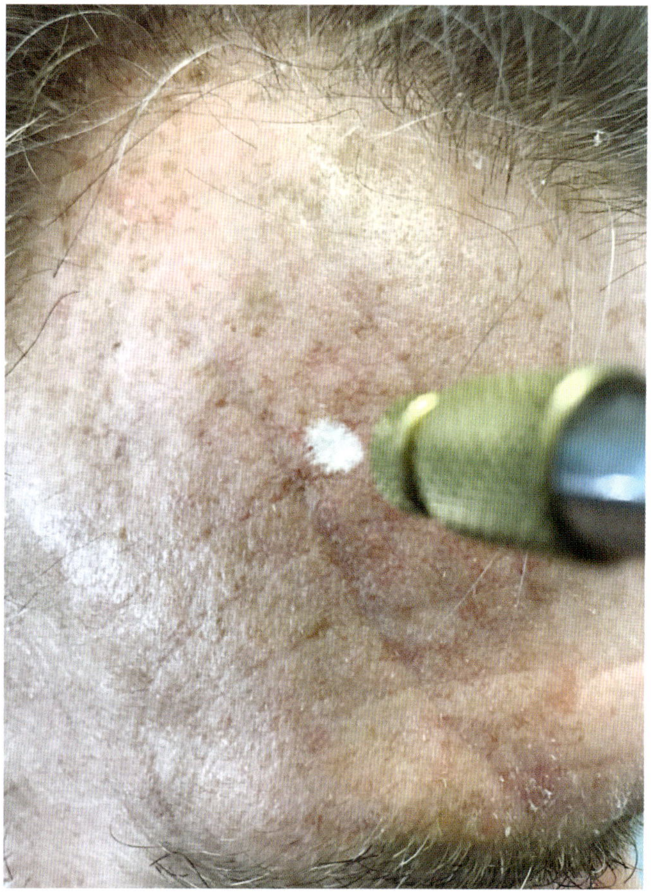

FIGURE 12-3 When tissue is frozen, an ice ball forms that serves as a visible indication of the extent of surface freezing.

The temperature achieved with cryosurgery is directly related to the degree of resultant cellular injury. Melanocytes are the most sensitive to cold and are irreversibly damaged at temperatures ranging from –4°C to –7°C. Keratinocytes are destroyed at temperatures ranging from –20°C to –30°C, and death of fibroblasts occurs between –30°C and –35°C. Malignant cells are the most resistant to cold-induced damage, requiring temperatures below –40°C for destruction.[10] Therefore, when treating a malignancy, a temperature endpoint between –50°C and –60°C is advisable (**Figure 12-4**).

The freeze time, or duration of cooling, is another important consideration. In general, benign lesions require shorter freeze times and may be sufficiently treated with a single freeze-thaw cycle. Malignancies often require a double freeze-thaw cycle and freeze times exceeding 45 seconds.

Additionally, the lateral spread of freeze, or margin of freeze, varies depending on the type of lesion. For benign lesions, margins of 2 to 3 mm are sufficient, whereas malignant lesions may require margins of 5 mm or more.

Certain adverse responses, such as pain and blistering, should be anticipated following cryotherapy; when these become intolerable or progress to longer term effects, they may be considered complications.

In the absence of local anesthetic or preexisting neuropathy, all patients will feel pain during treatment. Many patients will describe burning or stinging pain initially that may progress to a dull throbbing pain. The pain usually resolves spontaneously within minutes. Treatments to certain parts of the body, such as the ear, finger tips, lips, temples, and scalp, may cause more severe pain. Additionally, cryosurgery to the scalp, temple, or forehead may occasionally be associated with migraine-like headaches.[9]

Almost all treated patients will also develop localized edema, blister formation, and erythema (**Figure 12-5**). The amount of edema is related to both the intensity of the treatment and the lesion location. The eyelids, labia minora, lips, and foreskin have more lax skin and therefore develop greater edema.[9]

Hypopigmentation is perhaps the most common complication. One prospective study of 421 actinic keratoses treated with cryosurgery reported hypopigmentation in 29%. The incidence of hypopigmentation increased with the duration of freezing time.[11] This may stem mechanistically from the fact that melanocytes are more cold sensitive than keratinocytes and fibroblasts. Hypopigmentation is especially common in those with darker skin types. Paradoxically, hyperpigmentation may also develop following cryosurgery-induced inflammation.

Sensory and motor neuropathy may also develop following cryosurgery. The extent of neuropathy will depend on the cryosurgery dose and lesion location. One study of sensory neuropathy

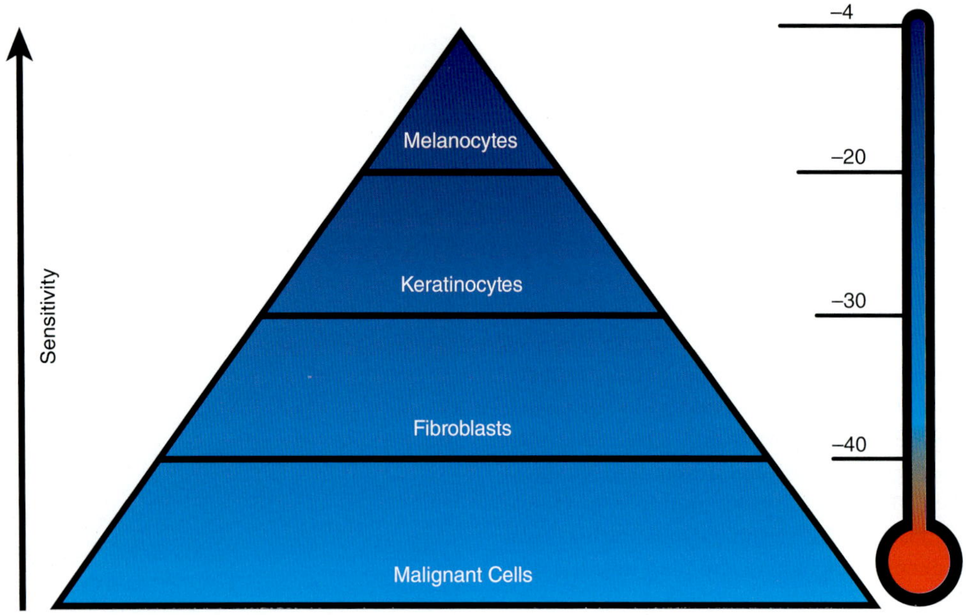

FIGURE 12-4 There is marked variability in the cold sensitivity of different cell types.

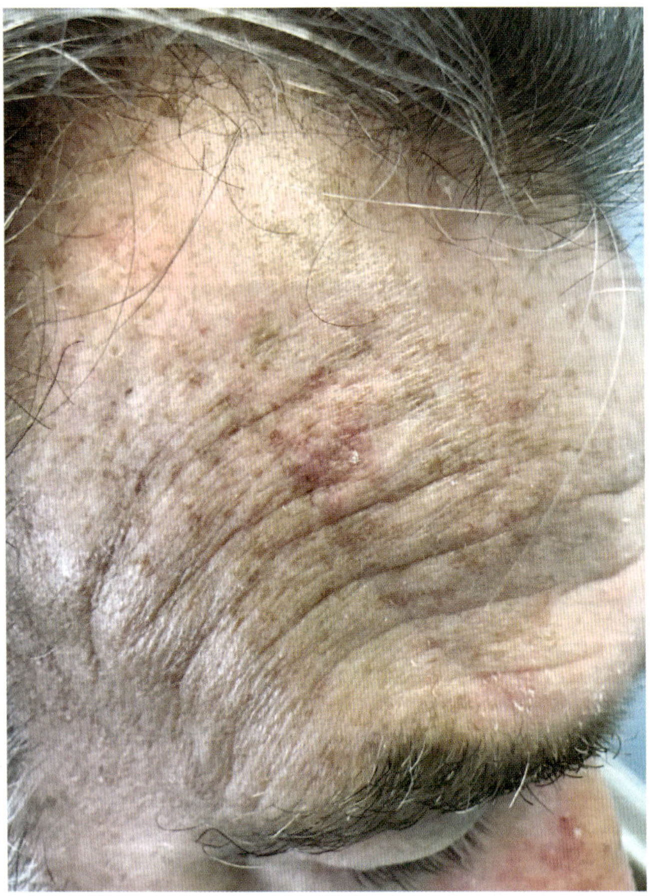

FIGURE 12-5 Almost all treated patients will also develop localized edema, blister formation, and erythema. Note the immediate post-procedure erythema.

associated with cryotherapy revealed complete recovery in all subjects by 18 months.[12] Infection, atrophy, hemorrhage, milia, hypertrophic scarring, bone necrosis, ectropion, and alopecia are additional reported complications.[9]

MECHANISM OF ACTION

Cryoablation induces tissue necrosis through multiple mechanisms including direct cellular injury, apoptosis, vessel thrombosis, and immune response activation. Direct cellular injury occurs through the formation of intracellular and extracellular ice (**Figure 12-6**). Intracellular ice results in the destruction of cell membranes and vital organelles and is maximized by rapid freezing. Extracellular ice alters the osmotic gradient between cytoplasm and extracellular fluid. Together, these changes result in irreversible cell death. Cellular damage continues during the thawing phase, in which the formation of large ice crystals imposes shearing forces on surrounding tissue. To maximize the damage accrued during recrystallization, thawing should proceed as slowly as possible.[13]

In addition to direct cellular injury, cryosurgery also has a destructive effect on microcirculatory vasculature. Freezing causes damage to capillary endothelial cells, resulting in platelet aggregation and thrombosis of papillary dermal vessels. Additionally, freezing destroys mast cell membranes and causes degranulation, which results in histamine-mediated increases in capillary permeability. Subsequent vasodilation results in increased edema and inflammatory cell infiltration.

The immunologic effect of cryosurgery is less well defined. Evidence of a systemic immune reaction is found in reports citing resolution of multiple verruca after cryosurgical treatment of only a few lesions—an abscopal response. This reaction is likely

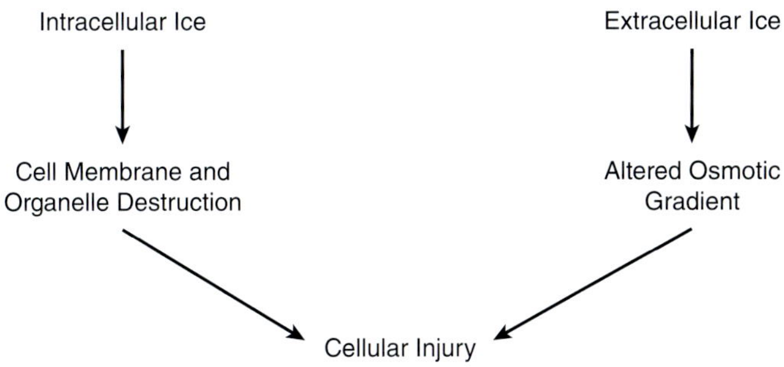

FIGURE 12-6 Direct cellular injury occurs through the formation of intracellular and extracellular ice.

incited by the release of DNA, RNA, uric acid, and other intracellular elements following the destruction of cell membranes. These elements activate toll-like receptors, triggering subsequent immunologic cascades. An innate immune response is generated initially, resulting in early infiltration of granulocytes, monocytes, and macrophages. An adaptive immune response follows, in which dendritic cells travel to regional lymph nodes to undergo maturation and antigen presentation.[10]

INDICATIONS

Cryotherapy has been reported for a broad range of dermatologic conditions including malignant, infectious, autoimmune, and inflammatory conditions.[14] General guidelines recommend a single freeze-thaw cycle for treating benign conditions. This approach is less likely to lead to poor healing or scarring, and treatment can be safely repeated at a later date since the condition is benign. The majority of published findings for treating many of the listed conditions consist of case reports or small uncontrolled series, although larger studies for the treatment of basal cell carcinoma, squamous cell carcinoma, and actinic keratoses have been performed. **Table 12-1** is a summary of benign conditions treated with cryotherapy, and **Table 12-2** is a summary of malignant and premalignant conditions treated with cryotherapy

Warts

Verrucae vulgaris are commonly treated with cryosurgery. A 2014 Cochrane Review analyzed 21 studies of cryosurgery for treating warts.[15] Meta-analysis of cryosurgery versus placebo failed to show a statistically significant difference; 41 (38.3%) of 107 of warts resolved with cryosurgery. However, the largest and most recent of the included studies comparing cryosurgery to placebo did demonstrate a therapeutic advantage to cryosurgery. Thirty (39.5%) of 76 warts in the cryosurgery group responded compared to 13 (15.9%) of 82 warts in the placebo group.[16] Furthermore, treatment intervals every 2, 3, or 4 weeks did not impact cure rates. Aggressive cryotherapy was, however, more effective than gentle cryotherapy. Aggressive cryotherapy was also associated with a higher incidence of pain and blistering.[17] On a practical level, when treating plantar warts, it is often best to first shave the hyperkeratotic portion of the wart flush with the skin

TABLE 12-1 • Benign Conditions Treated With Cryotherapy

Acne	Granuloma annulare	Porokeratosis plantaris discrete
Acne keloidalis	Granuloma faciale	Porokeratosis of Mibelli
Adenoma sebaceum	Granuloma pyogenicum	Prurigo nodularis
Alopecia areata	Hemangioma	Pruritus ani
Angiokeratomas	Herpes labialis	Psoriasis
Angiokeratoma of Fordyce	Idiopathic guttate hypomelanosis	Rhinophyma
Atypical fibroxanthoma	Kyrle disease	Rosacea
Cherry angiomas	Leishmaniasis	Sarcoid
Chondrodermatitis nodularis helicis	Lentigines	Sebaceous hyperplasia
Chromoblastomycosis	Lentigo simplex	Seborrheic keratosis
Clear cell acanthoma	Lichen sclerosus et atrophicus	Solar lentigo
Condyloma acuminatum	Lupus erythematosus	Syringoma
Dermatofibroma	Lymphangioma	Trichiasis
Disseminated superficial actinic porokeratosis	Lymphocytoma cutis	Trichoepithelioma
Elastosis perforans serpiginosa	Molluscum contagiosum	Varicose veins
Epidermal nevus	Mucocele	Venous lake
Erosive adenomatosis of the nipple	Myxoid cyst	Verrucae
Folliculitis keloidalis	Orf	Xanthoma

TABLE 12-2 • Malignant and Premalignant Conditions Treated With Cryotherapy

Actinic cheilitis
Actinic keratosis
Basal cell carcinoma
Bowen disease
Erythroplasia of Queyrat
Keratoacanthoma
Lentigo maligna
Squamous cell carcinoma
Squamous cell carcinoma in situ

(or even deep to the surrounding thickened stratum corneum) using a shave biopsy type technique (no anesthesia is needed as only the stratum corneum is being removed), followed by liquid nitrogen destruction (**Figure 12-7**).

Seborrheic Keratoses

Cryosurgery is a well-described therapy for seborrheic keratoses. It is critical, however, that the clinical, or preferably histologic, diagnosis is confirmed prior to treating with cryotherapy. One study comparing curettage to cryotherapy revealed that 15 (60%) of 25 subjects preferred cryotherapy, whereas 9 (36%) of 25 preferred curettage. Even though cryotherapy was associated with increased pain, subjects preferred this modality largely due to the decreased requirement for postoperative wound care. Self-reported cosmesis was reported to be the same between the two groups. Physician evaluation showed that there was more redness and tendency for hypopigmentation in the curettage group and more frequent residual seborrheic keratoses in the cryotherapy group.[18]

More recently, a randomized prospective trial of 120 seborrheic keratoses compared cryosurgery to an erbium (Er):YAG laser for treating seborrheic keratoses. Following the first treatment session, 100% of the Er:YAG-treated lesions resolved, while only 63.8% of those treated by cryosurgery completely responded. Both groups received topical anesthesia with EMLA cream prior to treatment, and neither group reported severe pain or interrupted therapy due to pain.[19]

Granuloma Annulare

Granuloma annulare is another benign condition effectively treated with cryosurgery. A single freeze-thaw treatment cycle lasting 10 to 60 seconds using either liquid nitrogen or nitrous oxide led to lesion resolution in 25 (80.6%) of 31 patients. All

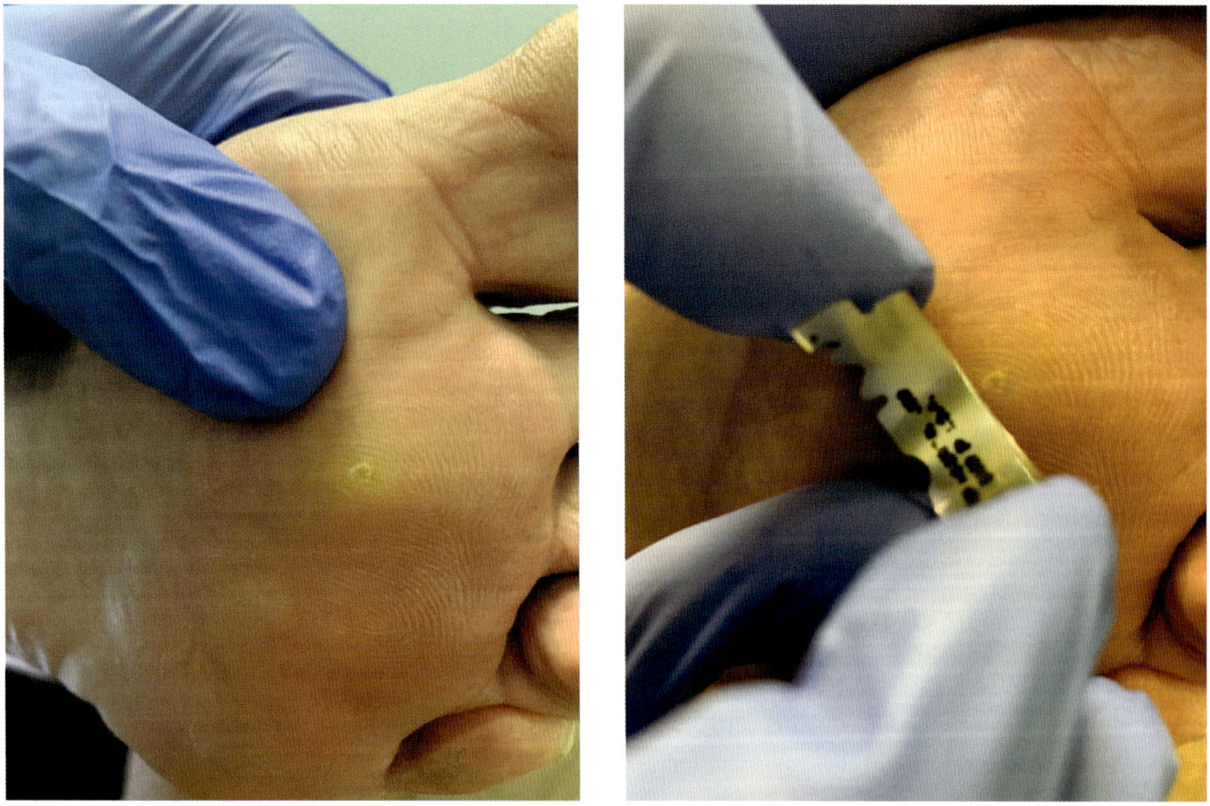

A B

FIGURE 12-7

a. A plantar wart is visible.
b. The blade enters at the base of the wart.

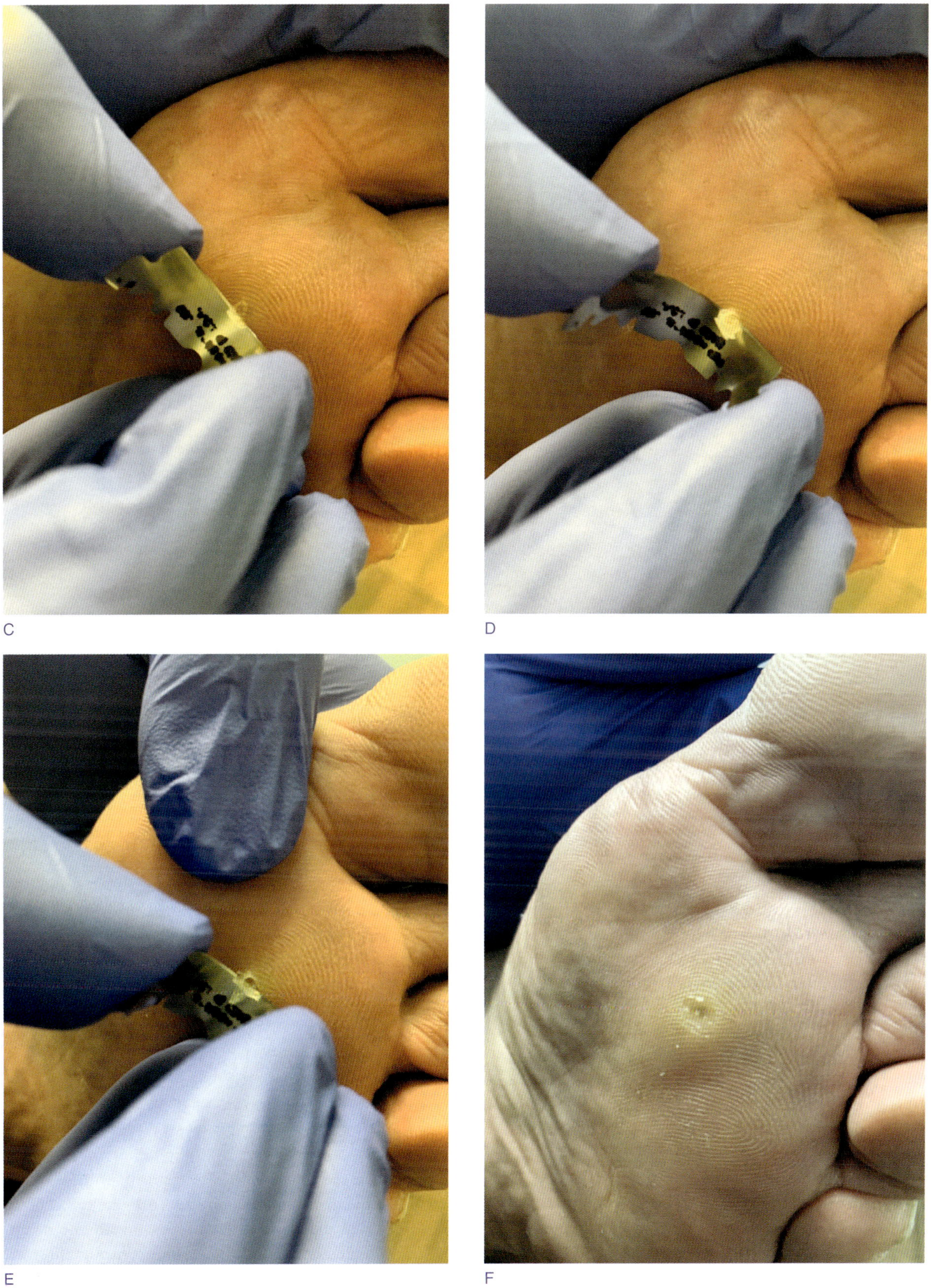

FIGURE 12-7 *(Continued)*
c. A sawing motion is used to remove the hyperkeratotic wart.
d. This continues along the entire lesion.
e. Sometimes a second pass is useful to remove additional hyperkeratotic stratum corneum.
f. The underlying central depression is revealed.

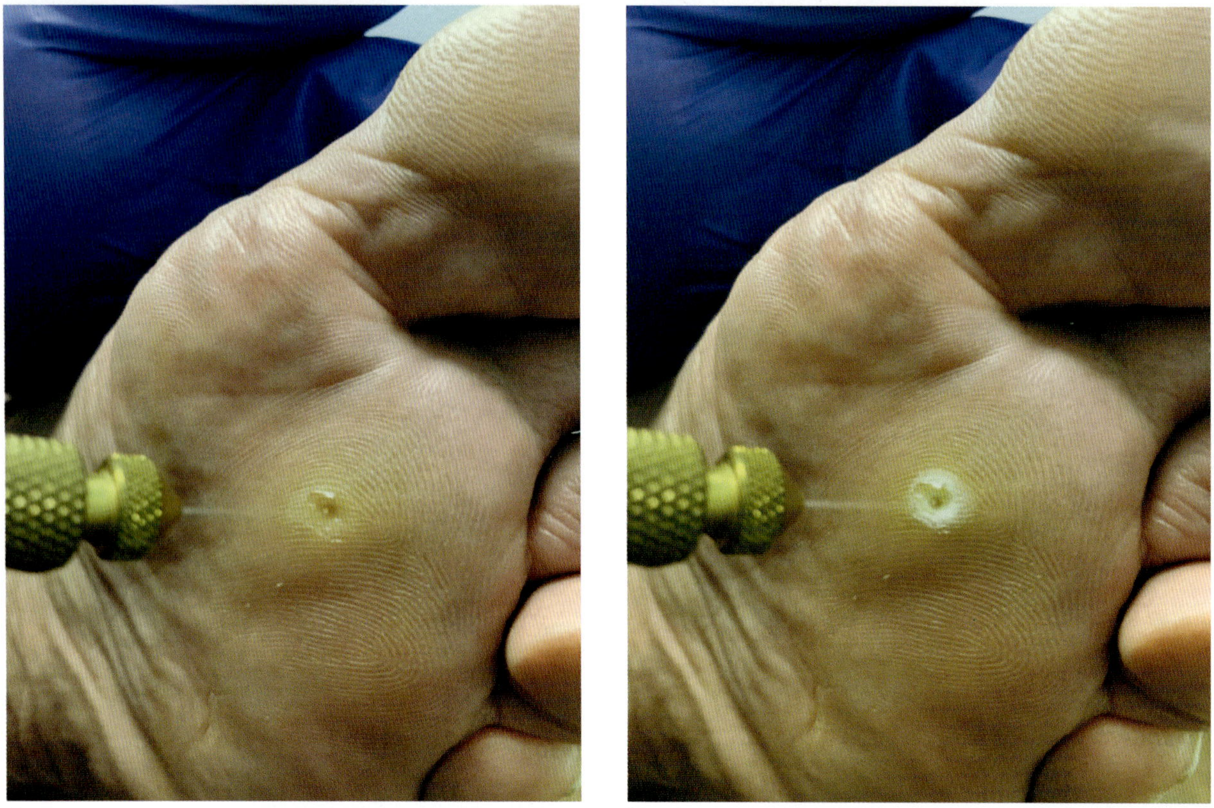

G H

FIGURE 12-7 *(Continued)*
g. Liquid nitrogen is used to destroy the wart.
h. Multiple freeze-thaw cycles may be used.

patients developed blisters within 24 to 48 hours of treatment. Cryoatrophy (14.3%) and dyspigmentation (7.1%) were the most commonly reported adverse effects. Significantly, cryoatrophy developed in 21% of subjects treated with liquid nitrogen and in none of the subjects who received nitrous oxide.[20]

Actinic Keratoses

Actinic keratoses are a well-described and widely practiced indication for cryotherapy.[21] Lesions may be treated with a cryospray or by using a cotton tipped applicator, although the latter is now used infrequently. Cryosurgery is often the treatment of choice for discrete lesions given its quick treatment time, wide availability, and minimal expense. A more recent Cochrane Review from 2012 evaluated various available field and individual lesion therapies for actinic keratoses. Photodynamic therapy, compared to cryotherapy, was more effective and yielded an improved cosmetic outcome for treating individual actinic keratoses.[22] This finding should, however, be weighed against the convenience and cost-effectiveness of cryotherapy in clinical practice as well as patient preferences.

Basal Cell Carcinoma

Much of the primary literature using cryotherapy to treat basal cell carcinoma is over 30 years old. One study of 628 basal cell carcinomas treated between 1980 and 1984 reported a 5-year cure rate of 99%.[23] The authors noted that most of the cancers were "small (<0.5 cm) to medium (0.5–2.0 cm)" or superficial. Additionally, lesions located in critical anatomic locations—such as the medial canthus—were excluded. The treatment technique sometimes included preoperative treatment with a local anesthetic and curettage. Depending on the size and thickness of the tumors, freeze time varied from 40 to 90 seconds, and the authors preferred to include repeated freeze-thaw cycles.

A 2003 review of uncontrolled prospective studies of basal cell carcinomas treated with cryosurgery reported recurrence rates ranging from 0% to 21% for follow-up at 6 months to 10 years.[24] If the single study of 19 patients with eyelid tumors is excluded, the highest reported recurrence rate is 8.2%. Cosmesis was quantitatively evaluated in only two studies but was generally commented on as "acceptable" to "excellent." All studies were assigned a C grade, per Sackett's rules of evidence, indicating lack of randomization, placebo control, or blinding, and were case reports and case series.[25]

In addition to problems with study design noted earlier, at least one author has challenged the previously reported high cure rates for two other reasons.[26] First, previous studies were not stratified based on histologic subtype. In addition, the treatment techniques reported in the initial publications likely differ significantly from how cryotherapy is currently used. Most contemporary dermatologists are unlikely to debulk a tumor with curettage or electrosurgery prior to cryotherapy. Furthermore, contemporary dermatologists probably do not use freeze cycles as long as those previously reported. Accordingly, the cure rates from older studies may not be replicated in contemporary practices. In the United States, cryotherapy is generally not standard of care for basal cell carcinoma.

Squamous Cell Carcinoma

Data on cryotherapy for squamous cell carcinomas are similar to those found for the treatment of basal cell carcinomas in many respects. Pooled analysis of observational studies using cryotherapy reported only one recurrence (0.8%) in 273 patients treated in eight studies.[27] Mean follow-up ranged from 2 to 5 years. A retrospective series of 563 squamous cell carcinomas treated over a 23-year period described a 97% cure rate, although the definition of "cure" was unclear and no follow-up time was reported.[28] Of all the modalities included in the pooled analysis of observation studies for interventions for nonmetastatic cutaneous squamous cell carcinoma, cryotherapy along with electrodessication and curettage had the highest cure rates for squamous cell carcinomas, but most tumors were small and deemed to be low risk.[27] As with the studies on basal cell carcinoma, it is not clear that the techniques employed in the studies—including debulking and prolonged freezing times—are the same techniques employed by contemporary dermatologists. In the United States, cryotherapy is generally not standard of care for squamous cell carcinoma.

Lentigo Maligna

Cryotherapy has also been described for the treatment of lentigo maligna. Although clearly excision is preferable, size, location, and comorbidities sometimes make excisional surgery impractical. At least three small case series describe cryosurgical treatment of lentigo maligna. One series of 30 patients with lesions measuring 1.3 to 4.5 cm treated between 1977 and 1992 reported two recurrences (6.6%).[29] This study used a double freeze-thaw cycle with 1-cm lateral spread. A study of 20 patients reported two recurrences (10%),[30] whereas another study of 20 patients reported three recurrences (15%).[31] Contemporary dermatologists may treat lentigo maligna with cryotherapy less frequently due to both advances in reconstructive techniques as well as concerns with sampling error. Without the opportunity for histologic evaluation, the presence of microscopic foci of lentigo maligna melanoma (which may occur in a significant proportion of cases) cannot be identified, and prognostic outcome cannot be predicted accordingly. In the United States, cryotherapy is generally not standard of care for lentigo maligna.

Kaposi Sarcoma

Kaposi sarcoma, when limited to the skin, may respond well to cryosurgery. A retrospective cohort study of 30 patients was reported in 2013. Patients received two freeze-thaw cycles, lasting 15 to 40 seconds per cycle with a 3-mm margin, every 4 weeks. Nineteen patients (63%) experienced a complete response, eight showed a partial response, and three patients discontinued therapy due to an increasing number of lesions.[32]

CONCLUSIONS

Cryosurgery has become a well-established, safe treatment modality for a wide range of conditions and will likely remain useful for years to come. New developments may include modifications in cryogen delivery methods and the refinement of temperature detection at the surface of the skin. Additionally, other techniques, including fractional cryosurgery, may become more widely employed, expanding the application of cryosurgery to larger tumors.[33,34] For now, the most frequently treated lesions remain actinic keratoses, warts, and seborrheic keratoses. While seemingly benign, aggressive cryosurgery entails a risk of scarring, and therefore, a deft touch is of great value to the patient.

REFERENCES

1. Sguazzi A, Bracco D. A historical account of the technical means used in cryotherapy. *Minerva Med.* 1974;65(70):3718-3722.
2. Korpan NN. A history of cryosurgery: its development and future. *J Am Coll Surg.* 2007;204(2):314-324.
3. Allington HV. Liquid nitrogen in the treatment of skin diseases. *Calif Med.* 1950;72(3):153-155.
4. Kuflik EG, Gage AA, Lubritz RR, Graham GF. Millenium paper: history of dermatologic cryosurgery. *Dermatol Surg.* 2000;26(8):715-722.
5. Kile RL, Welsh AL. Liquid oxygen in dermatologic practice. *Arch Derm Syphilol.* 1948;57(1):57-62.
6. Graham GF. Cryosurgery in the management of cutaneous malignancies. *Clin Dermatol.* 2001;19(3):321-327.
7. Weshahy AH. Intralesional cryosurgery. A new technique using cryoneedles. *J Dermatol Surg Oncol.* 1993;19(2):123-126.
8. Har-Shai Y, Amar M, Sabo E. Intralesional cryotherapy for enhancing the involution of hypertrophic scars and keloids. *Plast Reconstr Surg.* 2003;111(6):1841-1852.
9. Dawber RP. Cryosurgery: complications and contraindications. *Clin Dermatol.* 1990;8(1):108-114.
10. Kasuya A, Ohta I, Tokura Y. Structural and immunological effects of skin cryoablation in a mouse model. *PLoS One.* 2015;10(3):e0123906.
11. Thai KE, Fergin P, Freeman M, et al. A prospective study of the use of cryosurgery for the treatment of actinic keratoses. *Int J Dermatol.* 2004;43(9):687-692.
12. Sonnex TS, Jones RL, Weddell AG, Dawber RP. Long-term effects of cryosurgery on cutaneous sensation. *Br Med J (Clin Res Ed).* 1985;290(6463):188-190.
13. Sabel MS. Cryo-immunology: a review of the literature and proposed mechanisms for stimulatory versus suppressive immune responses. *Cryobiology.* 2009;58(1):1-11.
14. Kuflik EG. Cryosurgery updated. *J Am Acad Dermatol.* 1994;31(6): 925-944.
15. Kwok CS, Gibbs S, Bennett C, Holland R, Abbot R. Topical treatments for cutaneous warts. *Cochrane Database Syst Rev.* 2012;9:CD001781.

16. Bruggink SC, Gussekloo J, Berger MY, et al. Cryotherapy with liquid nitrogen versus topical salicylic acid application for cutaneous warts in primary care: randomized controlled trial. *CMAJ.* 2010;182(15):1624-1630.

17. Connolly M, Bazmi K, O'Connell M, Lyons JF, Bourke JF. Cryotherapy of viral warts: a sustained 10-s freeze is more effective than the traditional method. *Br J Dermatol.* 2001;145(4):554-557.

18. Wood LD, Stucki JK, Hollenbeak CS, Miller JJ. Effectiveness of cryosurgery vs curettage in the treatment of seborrheic keratoses. *JAMA Dermatol.* 2013;149(1):108-109.

19. Gurel MS, Aral BB. Effectiveness of erbium:YAG laser and cryosurgery in seborrheic keratoses: randomized, prospective intraindividual comparison study. *J Dermatol Treat.* 2015;26(5):477-480.

20. Blume-Peytavi U, Zouboulis CH, Jacobi H, Scholz A, Bisson S, Orfanos CE. Successful outcome of cryosurgery in patients with granuloma annulare. *Br J Dermatol.* 1994;130(4):494-497.

21. Lubritz RR, Smolewski SA. Cryosurgery cure rate of actinic keratoses. *J Am Acad Dermatol.* 1982;7(5):631-632.

22. Gupta AK, Paquet M, Villaneuva E, Brintnell W. Interventions for actinic keratoses. *Cochrane Database Syst Rev.* 2012;12:CD004415.

23. Kuflik EG, Gage AA. The five-year cure rate achieved by cryosurgery for skin cancer. *J Am Acad Dermatol.* 1991;24(6 Pt 1):1002-1004.

24. Agnieszka K, Scheinfeld N. Evidence-based review of the use of cryosurgery in treatment of basal cell carcinoma. *Dermatol Surg.* 2003;29(6):566-571.

25. Sacket DL. Rules of evidence and clinical recommendations on the use of antithrombic agents. *Chest.* 1989;95(2 Suppl):2S-4S.

26. Bahner JD, Bourdeau JS. Non-melanoma skin cancers: photodynamic therapy, cryotherapy, 5-flurouracil, imiquimod, diclofenac, or what? Facts and controversies. *Clin Dermatol.* 2013;31(6):792-798.

27. Lansbury L, Bath-Hextall F, Perkins W, Stanton W, Leonardi-Bee J. Interventions for non-metastatic squamous cell carcinoma of the skin: systematic review and pooled analysis of observational studies. *BMJ.* 2013;347:f6153.

28. Graham GF, Clark LC. Statistical analysis in cryosurgery of skin cancer. *Clin Dermatol.* 1990;8(1):101-107.

29. Kuflik EG, Gage AA. Cryosurgery for lentigo maligna. *J Am Acad Dermatol.* 1994;31(1):75-78.

30. Zacarian SA. Cryosurgical treatment of lentigo maligna. *Arch Dermatol.* 1982;118(2):89-92.

31. Bohler-Sommeregger K, Schuller-Petrovic S, Knobler R, Neumann PR. Reactive lentiginous hyperpigmentation after cryosurgery of lentigo maligna. *J Am Acad Dermatol.* 1992;27(4):523-526.

32. Kutlubay Z, Kucuktas M, Yardimci G, Engin B, Serdaroglu S. Evaluation of effectiveness of cryotherapy on the treatment of cutaneous Kaposi's sarcoma. *Dermatol Surg.* 2013;39(10):1502-1506.

33. Goncalves JC. Fractional cryosurgery. A new technique for basal cell carcinoma of the eyelids and periorbital area. *Dermatol Surg.* 1997;23(6):475-481.

34. Goncalves JC. Fractional cryosurgery for skin cancer. *Dermatol Surg.* 2009;35(11):1788-1796.

13 Electrosurgery and Hemostasis

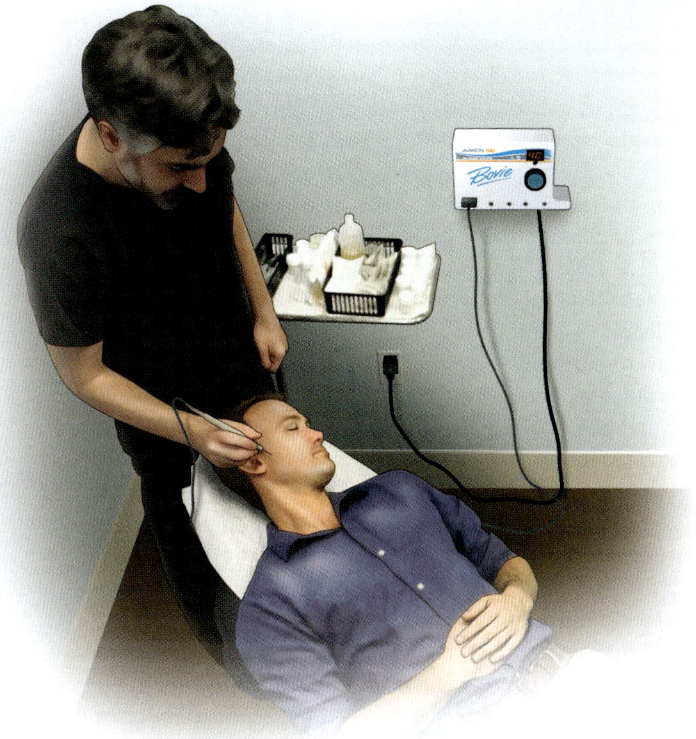

SUMMARY

- Electrosurgery is a workhorse technique with electrocautery and electrodessication representing the most frequently used techniques.
- Monoterminal units that function without a ground may be useful for many applications, but generally cannot be used for high-power applications or electrosection.
- Electrosurgery is a staple of dermatologic surgery practice, whether used for hemostasis, treatment of nonmelanoma skin cancer, or benign lesion desiccation.

Beginner Tips

- For most applications, electrocoagulation is the standard setting, and can be used with a monoterminal unit.
- Generally 40 watts is sufficient for small-vessel coagulation.

Pitfalls and Cautions

- Larger electrosurgical units may generate significantly more power than smaller hyfrecators used in many offices.
- Never overreach by attempting to use electrosurgical approaches on a vessel that should be ligated with suture.

Expert Tips

- Electrosection may be useful for wide undermining.
- Do not use electrosection on any tissue that will be sent for histopathologic analysis in order to minimize the risk of artifact.
- Electrofulguration is an elegant technique in experienced hands to treat seborrheic keratoses, but as no tissue will be available for pathology the diagnosis must be absolutely certain before proceeding.

Patient Education Points

- Cure rates for low-risk nonmelanoma skin cancers with ED&C are very high, but are also highly operator dependent.
- Patients should realize that the tradeoff for a quick ED&C procedure is that the healing time postoperatively may be significantly longer than seen for surgical excisions.

Don't Forget!

- Biterminal units always require that patients be in contact with a grounding plate, and most modern units are well isolated.
- Monoterminal units should never be used on sedated patients.
- Do not attempt to use ED&C to treat areas with a thin dermis, where full-thickness wounds will result.

Billing Pearls

- ED&C coding is based on the site and size of the entire skin cancer that was destroyed.
- Multiple sites treated in the same session would be added together for size, rather than billed individually.

13 Electrosurgery and Hemostasis

INTRODUCTION

For millennia, heat has been used to treat tissue and control bleeding. Over time, the methods used have evolved, with the first widely available commercial electrosurgical unit released in the 1920s. Since then, the units have been refined dramatically, although the basic concept behind electrosurgery has remained the same. Details regarding the physics underpinning electrosurgical devices have been explored at length.[1-3]

Terminology

Electrosurgery refers to the passage of high-frequency alternating electrical current through tissue to achieve a desired surgical effect, such as coagulation or cutting (**Table 13-1**). All true electrosurgical devices use a high-frequency electrical generator and two electrodes. Electric current flows from the active electrode through the patient's body and returns to the electrosurgical generator via the dispersive (return or indifferent) electrode (**Figure 13-1**). When current passes through tissue, the tissue's resistance converts the energy into heat. This differs from electrocautery, which can be conceptualized as a directly heated metallic object, such as a hot iron. In electrocautery, instead of current flowing through the patient's body, electrical current directly heats a metallic probe that is then applied to the tissue (**Figure 13-2**). Since no current passes through the patient, electrocautery is most commonly used when the operative site is near a patient's pacemaker, defibrillator, or deep-brain stimulator, or to limit destruction to only the superficial tissue layers, since no heat is generated in deeper tissue.

In electrosurgery, a small active electrode delivers electrical current to the surgical site. The current is concentrated in a small area providing high current density to induce heating and thermal tissue damage.[4,5] A return electrode attached to the patient's body then collects and disperses this current at a reduced current density that does not induce tissue heating.

Electrocoagulation is the process whereby tissue undergoes thermal denaturation through the heating of tissue below its boiling point.[5] Additional slow heating vaporizes the water content in the coagulated tissue, causing tissue drying, also known as dessication. As superficial coagulated tissues dry out (desiccate), they become less electrically conductive, thereby preventing current from flowing and heating deeper tissue and thereby limiting the depth of coagulation.

In electrosection, tissue adjacent to the electrode is rapidly increased in temperature above its boiling point. This causes a rapid explosive vaporization of the water content in the targeted tissue coupled with tissue fragmentation. This tissue fragmentation permits the electrode to pass through the tissue and function as a cutting instrument.[6-8]

TABLE 13-1 • Common Methods of Electrosurgery and Their Definitions

Method	Definition
Electrosurgery	Electrical current is passed through tissue to achieve a specific surgical effect (eg, cutting or coagulation).
Electrocautery	Electrical current heats a metal probe that is then applied to tissue.
Electrocoagulation (contact coagulation)	Tissue is heated below the boiling point undergoing thermal denaturation.
Electrodesiccation	At the end of coagulation, there is vaporization of the water content and drying of the superficial tissue layers.
Electrofulguration (noncontact or spray coagulation)	Instead of making direct contact with the tissue, the active electrode is held a few millimeters above the tissue and electric current bridges the air gap as a spark.
Electrosection	The tissue is quickly brought to a temperature above its boiling point, causing tissue fragmentation and cutting.
Electrosection, pure cutting	With pure cutting, there is minimal/no coagulation of the incisional wall.
Electrosection, blend cutting	With blend cutting, there is more coagulation of the incisional wall.
Bipolar electrosurgery	There are two active electrodes.
Monopolar electrosurgery	There is one active and one return (dispersive) electrode.
Biterminal electrosurgery	The active and return electrodes are in direct contact with the patient's body.
Monoterminal electrosurgery	While the active electrode is in direct contact with the patient's body, the return electrode is not. It is connected to the earth and the earth acts as the return electrode.

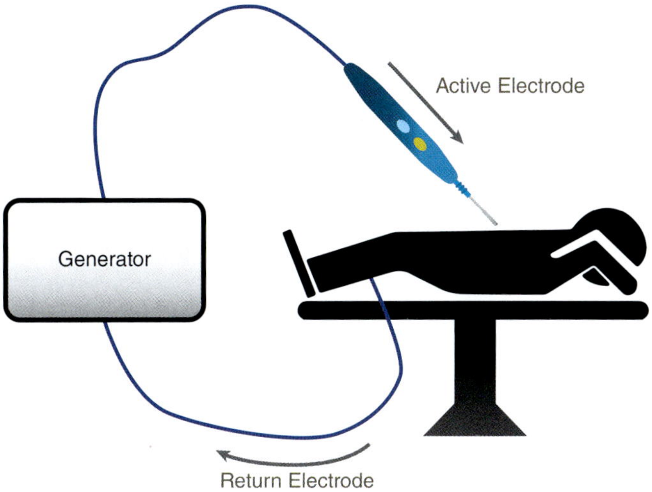

FIGURE 13-1 An electrosurgery unit. Current flows from the generator, through the active electrode, and into the tissue. The tissue's resistance converts this energy into heat. The current then returns to the generator by way of a return (dispersive or indifferent) electrode.

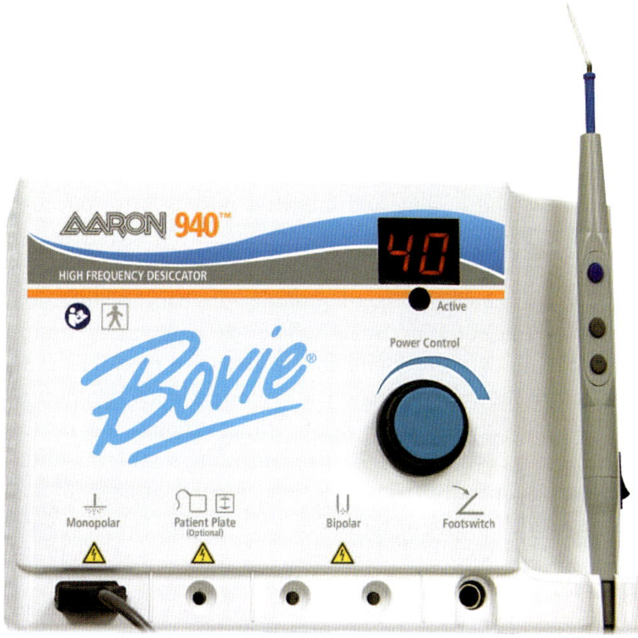

FIGURE 13-3 A simple electrodesiccation unit. This device is appropriate for almost any dermatologic surgery application.

A range of electrosurgical devices are available. These range from simple desiccator units (**Figure 13-3**) to high-powered operating room–ready multifunction devices (**Figure 13-4**).

ELECTROSURGICAL MODALITIES

Electrosection

Electrosection is the cutting of tissue with current rather than a scalpel. The goal in electrosection is for the cutting of tissue to be brisk, with the lowest effective power setting.[7,8] If the power is too low, the cutting process will be slow, resulting in a prolonged contact time with greater heating of the incision walls and therefore higher collateral tissue damage. In order to determine the correct output power for a clean incision, start low and increase the power until maximum cutting speed is achieved. If the power is insufficient, the electrode will not easily glide through the tissue but rather will "stick."[9] If there is arcing or sparking across the tissue surface, the voltage is too high and needs to be reduced. Once the optimal power setting is determined, the same setting can be used for all subsequent patients with only mild fine-tuning required.

Electrosection is infrequently used in dermatologic surgery due to histologic distortion and a lack of evidence that it is superior to scalpel-based surgery. Electrosurgery causes greater collateral tissue damage, and therefore histologic distortion of surgical margins, compared to scalpel surgery. Thermal damage causes carbonization at the excision margin, collagen denaturation, and vessel thrombosis.[10,11] It can cause vacuolar degeneration, along with shriveled and shrunken cell outlines with condensation and elongation of the nuclei and fusion of cells into structureless,

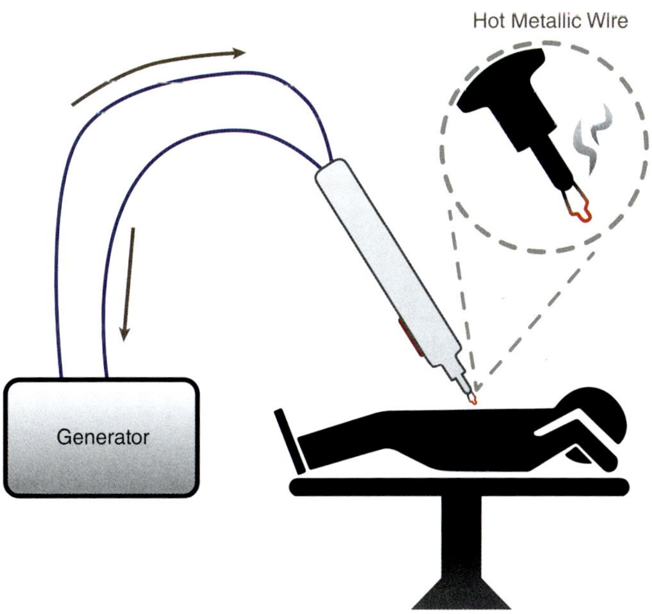

FIGURE 13-2 An electrocautery unit. Unlike in electrosurgery, current simply heats the tip of the electrode, which is then applied directly to the tissue to heat the superficial tissue layers.

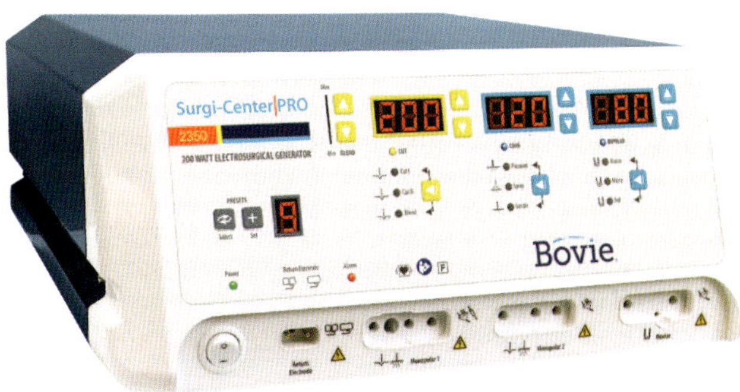

FIGURE 13-4 A high-powered electrosurgical unit.

homogenized masses with a hyalinized appearance.[12] All of these factors may result in false positives due to normal structures mimicking tumor.[13] Therefore, when electrosection is used in the context of dermatologic surgery, it is usually performed as a wide undermining technique for large excisions.

When electrosection units first came to market, reports of impaired wound healing and increased postoperative infection rates discouraged their adoption by clinicians. As such, few data exist comparing electrosection to conventional scalpel surgery with respect to incisional speed, postoperative pain and infection, wound healing, or scar cosmesis. The few randomized control trials that do exist are found in the general surgery literature. Not surprisingly, electrosection is associated with significantly less blood loss and shorter incisional time, although it is unclear whether it is associated with any statistically significant difference in postoperative pain, infection, wound healing, or scar cosmesis.[14,15]

Electrocoagulation

Electrocoagulation can be performed in two manners: contact mode or spray (fulguration) mode. In contact mode, the depth of coagulation is proportional to the size of the electrode tip and its associated power (**Table 13-2**).

For superficial coagulation of small areas (eg, destruction of small seborrheic keratoses or warts), a fine-tipped electrode should be used. The fine tip concentrates the current to a fine point, allowing the clinician to use lower power. When using a fine-tipped electrode, the current density in the tissue rapidly decreases with increasing distance from the electrode. As a result, heat generation is confined to the narrow vicinity of the electrode tip, allowing targeted heating of the superficial lesion while decreasing the chance of dermal heating, damage, and subsequent scarring.[13]

For deeper coagulation, a large-tipped electrode (ie, a ball- or disc-shaped electrode) and higher power should be used. A large-tipped electrode is effective for deep coagulation but not superficial coagulation because unlike with a fine-tipped electrode where current density rapidly decreases with increasing distance from the electrode, current density slowly decreases with distance and thus a larger and deeper area is heated. Large-tipped electrodes are therefore only indicated for deep coagulation (eg, destruction of deep reticular dermis after curettage in the setting of destruction of a nonmelanoma skin cancer).

Electrofulguration

Electrofulguration is useful in the setting of coagulation of large superficial areas (eg, to destroy a large seborrheic keratosis or achieve hemostasis in an oozing field). In electrofulguration, the active electrode is held a few millimeters above the tissue. A spark, or arc of electricity, then jumps from the electrode to the tissue where it moves rapidly from location to location. Unlike using the contact mode, the current is therefore spread superficially over an area larger than just the tip of the electrode.[16]

In electrofulguration, each spark acts like an exquisitely fine electrode. The spark itself is high temperature, so it induces tissue destruction and coagulation at the site of contact. However, the temperature rapidly decreases with increasing distance from the spark itself. Consequently, tissue charring is restricted to superficial tissue. If one wishes to achieve deeper heating and coagulation, this can be achieved by keeping a fulgurating electrode over a confined area for a prolonged period of time. Continuous heating of the superficial layers causes heating of the deeper layers.

TABLE 13-2 • Factors Affecting Depth of Coagulation

Size of the electrode tip
Power setting
Duration the electrode is in contact with the tissue

Electrodessication

During electrocoagulation, especially when performed slowly, the more superficial tissues may dry out. This is called desiccation. This step is important because the current may decrease or stop flowing entirely, limiting the maximum depth of coagulation. When this occurs, a popping sound or sparking may occur through the dried nonconductive layer, exploding and fragmenting the dried layer. Desiccation is not guaranteed and does not always happen, and the time to onset is unpredictable. The timing at which desiccation occurs during the course of coagulation is dependent upon the rate of increase in temperature. This is determined by current density. A low current density can allow for a deeper coagulation before the onset of desiccation.[5] Therefore, in the setting of deep coagulation (eg, after curettage of a malignant lesion), a low power should be used. With no published data, a rule of thumb is to choose a power that can provide desiccation (popping sound) after 4 to 7 seconds to achieve relatively deep destruction.

There are three factors that influence depth of coagulation: the size of the electrode tip, the power setting, and the length of time for which the electrode is in contact with the tissue. The longer the electrode is in contact with the tissue, the more heat is generated and the wider and deeper the tissue damage.

Using a lower power with a longer contact duration is not preferable to adopting a higher power with longer contact duration. Longer contact time conducts more heat, leading to increased collateral tissue damage before the desired outcome is attained.[17,18] This is much the same concept as when choosing pulse duration for a laser. Therefore, to minimize collateral tissue damage, contact time should be minimized or divided into multiple pulses to allow the tissue to cool between pulses.

Bipolar Versus Monopolar Electrosurgery

The prefixes mono- and bipolar refer simply to the number of *active electrodes*. In monopolar electrosurgery, an active electrode transfers current to the tissue where it spreads throughout the body before being collected and returned to the electrosurgery unit by a dispersive (return or indifferent) electrode. Often the dispersive electrode is a plate that the patient either grips or is otherwise in contact with. In bipolar electrosurgery, the active electrode is a pair of forceps. Electrical current flows from the active prong through the grasped tissue and into the dispersive (return) prong where it flows back to the electrical generator. Bipolar electrosurgery may be safer for the patient, since there is less damage to surrounding tissue and lower risk of distant site burns when compared to monopolar electrosurgery.[19,20]

STEP-BY-STEP APPROACH: HEMOSTASIS WITH MONOPOLAR ELECTROCAUTERY

1. Defer hemostasis until the lesion is completely excised and appropriately undermined.
2. In order to achieve complete hemostasis, visualization of the wound bed and undermined surface should be achieved via skin hooks and ample gauze.
3. For electrocoagulation to work effectively, the operative field must be dry, as blood diffuses the current flowing from the electrode. A dry field is best achieved using a two-handed technique. With the nondominant hand, use forceps and a piece of gauze to dry the field and visualize the source of bleeding. With the dominant hand, cauterize the source of bleeding with the active electrode. If possible, an assistant should hold gauze at the dependent area of the wound to absorb any dripping blood.
4. It is easiest to achieve hemostasis by operating in the direction of gravity. For instance, if operating on the neck, work from the superior to the inferior pole.

Biterminal Versus Monoterminal Electrosurgery

The prefixes mono- and biterminal refer to the number of *electrodes in contact with the patient's body*. Bipolar electrosurgery is always biterminal, whereas monopolar electrosurgery may be monoterminal or biterminal.

In monoterminal electrosurgery, there is no dispersive electrode connected to the patient's body. Instead, the return electrode is connected to the earth, often through the power supply cable. These are known as earth-referenced units. These monoterminal units are ubiquitous in medical dermatology suites. However, it is important to note that if an electrically conductive object, such as a metal table or electrocardiogram electrode, makes contact with the patient's body, some current may pass through this object on its return pathway to the ground. If the contact area is small, the current may be concentrated enough to cause a focal burn at the site. Therefore, these devices should only be used on conscious patients who are able to alert the clinician to such complications, and on insulated tables with no exposed metal parts near the patient's body.

The most common electrosurgical unit used in operating rooms today is a floating or isolated biterminal unit. Unlike earth-referenced units, the dispersive electrode is isolated from earth. Therefore, current will only flow if there is a dispersive electrode attached to the patient.[21] As a result, if the patient comes in contact with a conductive environmental object, minimal to no current will pass through that object, and therefore, the risk for burning is minimal. Additionally, the clinician is protected, since one can touch the active electrode, and as long as they do not touch the patient or the dispersive electrode, there is no risk of the clinician sustaining a burn.

STEP-BY-STEP APPROACH: ACHIEVING HEMOSTASIS WITH BIPOLAR ELECTROCAUTERY

1. Dry the field to visualize the sites that are bleeding.
2. Clamp the tines of the bipolar electrode shut, and touch it to the areas that are bleeding.

RISKS AND CAUTIONS

Electrosurgery in the setting of cutaneous surgery is very safe, but it is still not without risk. These risks include burns, infection, ocular injury, and cardiac pacemaker, defibrillator, or deep-brain stimulator malfunction.

Electrical Burns

Electrical burns occur when high current density flows through a small surface area. This usually happens when there is faulty application of the indifferent electrode, the patient makes contact with a metal surface, or there is current channeling to a distant site.

Improper placement of the indifferent electrode includes placing it over a bony prominence, scar tissue, or metal implants, or when too small of a surface area of the indifferent electrode is in contact with the patient. Current becomes concentrated in this small surface area, resulting in high current density. If this high current density is allowed to continue for too long, then an electrical burn occurs. A patient would normally experience pain and discomfort prior to experiencing a focal burn, but if the area is anesthetized, they may not.[5,21-23]

A patient is also at risk for burns if he or she makes contact with a grounded metal object while electrocautery is occurring. This is especially true when the indifferent electrode is broken or improperly placed or when using a monoterminal unit. This is because current seeks any alternative low resistance pathway from the patient to the ground.

Another cause of burns is a phenomenon known as current channeling. This is when current is concentrated as it flows through a small area. For instance, if applying current to a mass with a narrow base or stalk, such as a fibroepithelial polyp, as the current flows into the narrow stalk, it is concentrated. This concentrated current can cause a burn at the site of the base of the lesion.[24,25]

The threat of burns can be mitigated through a few simple precautions. Never leave an active electrode on a patient when not in use. A patient should always be in contact with at least 20 square inches of the indifferent electrode to ensure sufficient current dispersion. This is made easier by flexible indifferent electrodes that conform to the body, the use of protective interface gels, and contact quality monitors. Many modern electrosurgery units have a contact quality monitor for the dispersive electrode. It measures the quality of contact between the patient's skin and the dispersive electrode as well as between the electrode and the generator. However, there is no clinical evidence to support the notion that a contact quality monitor minimizes the risk of burns.[9]

Never use a bent indifferent electrode, as this can create a sharp point that concentrates current. Make sure the patient is not in contact with any metal surfaces. If the patient has any metal in his body, the dispersive pad should be placed between the metal and the surgical site to prevent current from passing through the patient's implanted device. When treating a pedunculated lesion for which there is risk of channeling, use bipolar forceps or wrap a saline-soaked sponge (an electrolyte conductor) around the stalk.[24-26]

Infection Risk

In experimental settings, electrodesiccation has been associated with transmission of human papillomavirus (HPV), hepatitis B virus, and *Staphylococcus aureus*. Some people erroneously think that the heat induced by electrocoagulation sterilizes the electrode tip. This is true in electrocautery where heat is generated in the tip, but not in electrocoagulation where heat is only produced in the tissue. Special precautions in the form of facial masks, protective eye wear, and a smoke evacuator should be used when treating HPV-related lesions, since HPV can become aerosolized in blood microdroplets and in electrosurgical smoke, posing a risk to the patient, physician, and surgical staff (**Figure 13-5**).[27-29]

Eye Injury

When operating in the periorbital area, patients should wear nonmetallic corneal shields, since sparks may arc toward the globe, causing corneal damage and scarring. The corneal shields must be plastic rather than metal to prevent conducting the current toward the globe.[30]

Cardiac Pacemaker, Defibrillator, or Deep-Brain Stimulator Malfunction

Electrosurgery has the potential to interfere with cardiac pacemaker, implantable cardioverter-defibrillator (ICD), or deep-brain stimulator function. Pacemakers are generally classified as fixed rate or demand type. Fixed-rate pacemakers fire at a predetermined rate irrespective of the intrinsic cardiac rhythm. Demand-type pacemakers fire at a predetermined rate only in the absence of intrinsic cardiac rhythm. Demand-type pacemakers are further subdivided into ventricular inhibited or ventricular triggered. The ventricular-inhibited, demand-type pacemaker is the most common pacemaker in the United States.

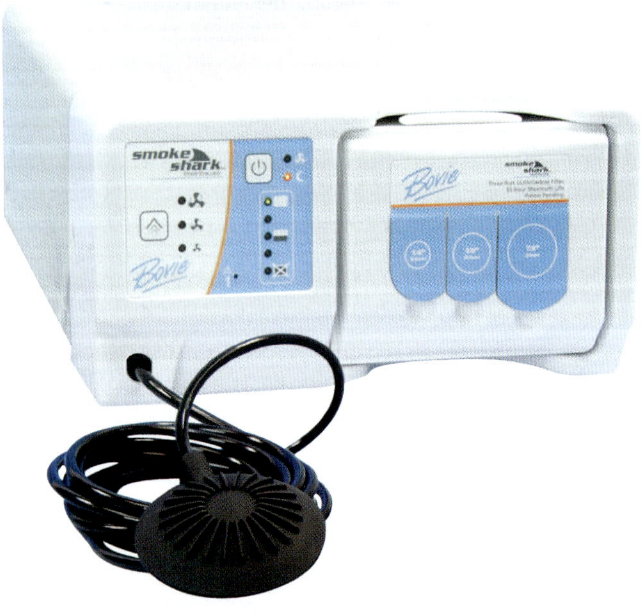

FIGURE 13-5 Smoke evacuation systems are a useful adjunct to electrosurgery.

Since fixed-rate pacemakers fire at a fixed rate regardless of intrinsic cardiac rhythm, they lack sensing circuitry. Consequently, exogenous electrical signals from the active electrode pose no threat to the patient. Conversely, all demand pacemakers contain sensing circuitry and are therefore susceptible to interference from extraneous electrical current. The function of demand pacemakers is to prevent bradycardia and asystole. The ventricular-inhibited pacemakers do this by firing when the patient's intrinsic cardiac rhythm is slower than the preset rate. A ventricular-triggered device fires with each spontaneous heartbeat as well as at a predetermined rate in the absence of intrinsic rhythm.[26,31]

The electromagnetic output of electrosurgery can interfere with the sensing circuitry of demand pacemakers, causing them to erroneously perceive the electrical current from electrosurgery as spontaneous ventricular contraction. In the setting of a ventricular-inhibited pacemaker, the pacemaker perceives this electrical current as a spontaneous heartbeat and erroneously enters stand-by mode. This can cause bradycardia and asystole, leading to syncope, seizure, or death. In a ventricular-triggered device, the electrical current is misread as a spontaneous heartbeat, causing the pacer to falsely stimulate ventricular contraction. This can cause life-threatening tachyarrhythmias or ventricular fibrillation. Although any electrosurgical procedure poses a risk for pacemaker-related complications, electrosection poses the highest risk.[29,31]

An ICD is a device that sends a defibrillatory shock to the heart if it senses tachyarrhythmia or ventricular fibrillation. It is usually inserted into an abdominal or infraclavicular subcutaneous pocket. Electrosurgery can cause an ICD to erroneously shock the heart, which is not only excruciatingly painful to an alert patient but can also induce life-threatening tachyarrhythmias. Electrosurgery can also damage the ICD device itself.[29]

A deep-brain stimulator is an implanted device that generates electrical impulses to control movement disorders such as essential tremor or Parkinson disease. An electrode implanted in the brain is connected to a pulse generator that sits in a subcutaneous pocket in the chest, much like an ICD. As with an ICD, electrosurgery can interfere with functioning of the brain stimulator.

Electrosurgery in the setting of pacemakers, ICDs, or deep-brain stimulators poses life-threatening complications, but how common are they? A survey study of 166 Mohs surgeons with a total of 1959 years of experience examined the number and type of complications due to electrosurgery. The incidence of interference was exquisitely low, with 1.6 cases per 100 years of surgical practice. The incidence of clinical adverse events was even lower at 0.8 cases per 100 years of surgical experience. There was no significant morbidity or mortality. The 25 cases of interference were broken down as follows: eight patients experienced skipped beats, six patients had spontaneous reprogramming of their pacemaker, four patients had their ICD fire, one patient had a shortening of his pacer's battery life, and one patient experienced tachyarrhythmia. Of these 25 cases, 18 of the patients experienced a clinical adverse outcome: six had syncope, five had altered sensorium, three experienced palpitations, three required an outpatient cardiology consult, and one experienced hemodynamic instability.[27] There are only two reports of deep-brain stimulator interference.[32]

Despite these data, several groups, including the American Society of Anesthesiologists, recommend that the patient's cardiologist be consulted prior to using monoterminal electrosurgery and that devices be interrogated within a month after any monoterminal electrosurgical procedure, although the degree to which these suggestions are followed is unknown.[33]

Still, the use of electrosurgery in patients with implanted devices is very safe. This is in part due to the fact that modern-day pacemakers are designed with metallic covers and filters to protect the device from external electrical interference and therefore minimize the risk of malfunction. However, precautions should still be taken. Place the grounding electrode at a site far from the heart and pacemaker and try to avoid having the heart lie directly in the path between the treatment and indifferent electrode. Keep electrosurgical current bursts to less than 5 seconds. If operating near a pacemaker or ICD, using electrocautery or biterminal forceps will avoid or minimize current leakage in the patient. Similar precautions should be taken with patients who have cochlear implants.

STEP-BY-STEP APPROACH: ACHIEVING HEMOSTASIS OF A BLEEDING VESSEL

1. Use gauze to dry the field and visualize the bleeding vessel.
2. Using fine-toothed forceps or a hemostat, grip the vessel and then touch the active electrode to the forceps or hemostat and apply monopolar current through it.
3. If using a bipolar electrode, simply grip the vessel between the two tines and apply current.
4. If a popping sound is heard or a spark is seen, current flow should be stopped and the area reevaluated to ensure satisfactory hemostasis. In order to optimize hemostasis, the surgical field should be dry, as blood will diffuse the current flowing from the electrode.
5. Only small vessels should be cauterized in this fashion; larger or arterial vessels would benefit from direct suture ligation.

Persistent Bleeding

While electrosurgery is well suited to the cauterization of small blood vessels, larger vessels, and even some smaller arterial vessels, may not respond definitively to electrosurgical approaches. This may be immediately obvious, as when persistent bleeding remains even after repeated attempts at electrocoagulation; more insidiously, some larger vessels will initially appear to be effectively treated with electrosurgical approaches only to persist in bleeding in the postoperative period. Therefore, less experienced clinicians should err on the side of ligating larger vessels.

ELECTROSURGERY FOR REASONS OTHER THAN HEMOSTASIS

Electrosurgery and Hair Removal

There are two mechanisms by which hair removal can be achieved through electrosurgery: electrolysis and thermolysis. In electrolysis, a needle electrode is placed into the hair follicle and a direct electrical current (galvanic current) is then applied, resulting in a chemical reaction that destroys the hair follicle. In thermolysis, alternating current is applied and the hair follicle is destroyed through thermal damage. Thermolysis is faster than electrolysis, although there is a greater risk of damage to the dermis and ensuing scar formation.[34,35,36] These are time-consuming but effective methods of hair removal for nonpigmented hairs or in patients with pigmented skin.

Electrosurgery for the Treatment of Malignant Skin Lesions

Electrodessication and curettage (ED&C) is a common and effective treatment for benign and superficially invasive neoplasms.[37-39] In the right setting, it is quick with less morbidity and cost than surgical excision. It involves two to three cycles of curettage followed by electrodessication. The ideal scenario for ED&C is a broad, superficial lesion in an area with thick underlying dermis (eg, the trunk or extremities). ED&C is not an ideal treatment modality for lesions that have the potential for follicular extension, as they are at higher risk for recurrence.[1,40-45]

Basal cell carcinoma is perhaps the most common neoplasm treated by ED&C. Recurrent or micronodular/morpheaform basal cell carcinomas should be treated surgically through excision rather than ED&C because they are at increased risk for having deep dermal infiltration. The cure rates with ED&C are highly operator dependent, with cure rates ranging from 88% to 99%. The studies that report the highest cure rates also use the largest reported safety margins, ranging from 2 to 8 mm.[45] A meta-analysis of basal cell carcinomas treated by ED&C reported a weighted average 5-year recurrence rate of 8%.[46]

One study examined the determinants of 5-year recurrence rates of 2314 primary basal cell carcinomas treated by ED&C between 1955 and 1982. The only variables that impacted occurrence rate were lesion size and location. Patient age, sex, or duration of the lesion had no impact. Researchers divided the body into three categories: high-, middle-, or low-risk anatomic sites. The high-risk sites included the nose, paranasal, nasolabial fold, ear, chin, mandibular, perioral, and periocular areas. Middle-risk sites were the scalp, forehead, pre- and postauricular, and malar areas. Low-risk sites were the neck, trunk, and extremities. Lesions that were treated with ED&C in low-risk areas had a 3% recurrence rate within 5 years regardless of the lesion's diameter. Middle-risk sites had a 5-year recurrence of 5% for lesions less than 10 mm in diameter and a 23% risk for recurrence with lesions 10 mm or larger. High-risk sites had a 5-year recurrence rate of 5% for lesions less than 5 mm and 18% for lesions 6 mm or larger.[47]

Another consideration to take into account when deciding upon whether or not to treat a lesion by ED&C is cosmesis. On the trunk and extremities, ED&C most often results in residual dyspigmented patches, although atrophic, hypertrophic, or keloidal scars can occur. On the face, ED&C often produces a fine white macule or patch, while indurated or depressed circular scars are a risk. For many patients, ED&C offers a cosmetically acceptable scar.[45,47]

STEP-BY-STEP APPROACH: HOW TO PERFORM ELECTRODESSICATION AND CURETTAGE

1. Anesthetize the area with a mixture of 1% lidocaine with epinephrine.
2. With the sharp end of the curette pointing down toward the skin, scrape the affected area to the base, which can be identified by the gritty sensation of the dermis. In the setting of a skin cancer, the cancerous area is more friable compared to normal skin.
3. Dry the base with gauze, and then fully electrodessicate the base with electrosurgery.
4. Recurette the base in a different direction and once again desiccate the base. Repeat for a total of three passes.

Electrosurgery for the Treatment of Benign Epidermal Lesions

Benign skin lesions such as seborrheic keratoses or warts can be treated with superficial coagulation by using a fine-tipped electrode or electrofulguration with very low power. After a quick, gentle treatment, the lesion should be wiped off. If there is any residual lesion left, a subsequent pass of superficial electrocoagulation can be performed. If there is spark formation, this is an indicator of deeper injury. This can be avoided by reducing the voltage, power, or contact time.

CONCLUSIONS

Electrosurgery is a staple of the procedural practice, whether used for hemostasis, treatment of nonmelanoma skin cancer, or benign lesion dessication. A comprehensive appreciation of the underlying principles behind electrosurgery helps the clinician better decide on optimal techniques and approaches for a variety of applications. A simple monopolar plate-free unit, such as the Bovie Aaron 940 desiccator, provides adequate power for the procedural practice with minimal expense and maintenance needs.

REFERENCES

1. Soon SL, Washington CV. Electrosurgery, electrocoagulation, electrofulguration, electrodesiccation, electrosection, electrocautery. In: Robinson JK, Hanke CW, Siegel DM, Fratila A, eds. *Surgery of the Skin: Procedural Dermatology*. 2nd ed. New York, NY: Elsevier; 2010:137-151.
2. Taheri A, Mansoori P, Sandoval LF, et al. Electrosurgery: part I. Basics and principles. *J Am Acad Dermatol.* 2014;70(4):591.e1-14.
3. Taheri A, Mansoori P, Sandoval LF, et al. Electrosurgery: part II. Technology, applications, and safety of electrosurgical devices. *J Am Acad Dermatol.* 2014;70(4):607.e1-12.
4. Christie RV, Binger CA. An experimental study of diathermy: IV. Evidence for the penetration of high frequency currents through the living body. *J Exp Med.* 1927;46:715-734.
5. Brill AI. Electrosurgery: principles and practice to reduce risk and maximize efficacy. *Obstet Gynecol Clin North Am.* 2011;38:687-702.
6. Fante RG, Fante RL. Perspective: the physical basis of surgical electrodissection. *Ophthal Plast Reconstr Surg.* 2003;19:145-148.
7. Sebben JE. Electrosurgery principles: cutting current and cutaneous surgery: part I. *J Dermatol Surg Oncol.* 1988;14:29-31.
8. Sebben JE. Electrosurgery principles: cutting current and cutaneous surgery: part II. *J Dermatol Surg Oncol.* 1988;14:147-150.
9. Van Way CW, Hinrichs CS. Electrosurgery 201: basic electrical principles. *Curr Surg.* 2000;57:261-264.
10. Christie RV, Loomis AL. The relation of frequency to the physiological effects of ultra-high frequency currents. *J Exp Med.* 1929;49:303-321.
11. d'Arsonval A. Action physiologique des courants alternatifs a grande frequence. *Arch Physiol Norm Pathol.* 1893;5:401-408.
12. Elliott JA. Electrosurgery. Its use in dermatology, with a review of its development and technologic aspects. *Arch Dermatol.* 1966;94:340-350.
13. Palanker D, Vankox A, Jayaraman P. On mechanisms of interaction in electrosurgery. *N J Phys.* 2008;10:123022.
14. Pearlman N, Stiegmann G, Vance V, et al. A prospective study of incisional time, blood loss, pain and healing with carbon dioxide laser, scalpel and electrosurgery. *Arch Surg.* 1991;126:1018-1020.
15. Kearns S, Connolly E, McNally S, et al. Randomized clinical trial of diathermy versus scalpel incision in elective midline laparotomy. *Br J Surg.* 2001;88:41-44.
16. Eggleson JL, von Maltzahn WW. Electrosurgical devices. In: Bronzino JD, ed. *The Biomedical Engineering Handbook*. 2nd ed. Boca Raton, FL: CRC Press; 2000.
17. Kalkwarf KL, Krejci RF, Edison AR. A method to measure operating variables in electrosurgery. *J Prosthet Dent.* 1979;42:566-570.
18. Strock MS. The rationale for electrosurgery. *Oral Surg Oral Med Oral Pathol.* 1952;5:1166-1172.
19. Brill AI. Bipolar electrosurgery: convention and innovation. *Clin Obstet Gynecol.* 2008;51:153-158.
20. Rioux JE. Bipolar electrosurgery: a short history. *J Minim Invasive Gynecol.* 2007;14:538-541.
21. The Association of Surgeons in Training website. Principles of electrosurgery. http://www.asit.org/assets/documents/Prinicpals_in_electrosurgery.pdf Accessed June 24, 2016.
22. ECRI. Higher currents, greater risks: preventing patient burns at the return-electrode site during high-current electrosurgical procedures. *Health Devices.* 2005;34:273-279.
23. Edrich J, Cookson CC. Electrosurgical dispersive electrodes heat cutaneous and subcutaneous skin layers. *Med Instrum.* 1987;21:81-86.
24. Bennett R. Electrosurgery. In: Bennet R, ed. *Fundamentals of Cutaneous Surgery*. St. Louis, MO: CV Mosby; 1988;553-590.
25. Schellhammer P. Electrosurgery: principles, hazards, and precautions. *Urology.* 1974;3:261-268.
26. Sebben J. Electrosurgery and cardiac pacemakers. *J Am Acad Dermatol.* 1983;9:457-463.
27. El-Gamal H, Dufrersne R, Saddler K. Electrosurgery, pacemakers, and ICDs: a survey of precautions and complications experienced by cutaneous surgeons. *Dermatol Surg.* 2001;27:385-390.

28. Roenigk R, Roenigk H. Current surgical management of skin cancer in dermatology. *J Dermatol Surg Oncol.* 1990;16:136-151.
29. LeVasseur J, Kennard C, Finley E, et al. Dermatologic electrosurgery in patients with implantable cardioverter-defibrillators and pacemakers. *Dermatol Surg.* 1998;24:233-240.
30. Sebben J. Electrosurgery. In: Ratz J, ed. *Textbook of Dermatologic Surgery*. Philadelphia, PA: Lippincott-Raven; 1998;457-472.
31. Krull E, Pickard S, Hall J. Effects of electrosurgery on cardiac pacemakers. *J Derm Surg.* 1975;1:43-45.
32. Weaver J, Kim S, Torres A. Cutaneous electrosurgery in a patient with a deep brain stimulator. *Dermatol Surg.* 1999;25:415-417.
33. Crossley GH, Poole JE, Rozner MA, et al. The Heart Rhythm Society (HRS)/American Society of Anesthesiologists (ASA) Expert Consensus Statement on the perioperative management of patients with implantable defibrillators, pacemakers and arrhythmia monitors: facilities and patient management this document was developed as a joint project with the American Society of Anesthesiologists (ASA), and in collaboration with the American Heart Association (AHA), and the Society of Thoracic Surgeons (STS). *Heart Rhythm.* 2011;8(7):1114-1154.
34. Wagner RF Jr, Tomich JM, Grande DJ. Electrolysis and thermolysis for permanent hair removal. *J Am Acad Dermatol.* 1985;12: 441-449.
35. Olsen EA. Methods of hair removal. *J Am Acad Dermatol.* 1999; 40(2 Pt 1):143-155.
36. Liew SH. Unwanted body hair and its removal: a review. *Dermatol Surg.* 1999;25:431-439.
37. Sheridan AT, Dawber RP. Curettage, electrosurgery and skin cancer. *Australas J Dermatol.* 2000;41:19-30.
38. Stevinson TR, Swanson NA. Syringoma: removal by electrodesiccation and curettage. *Ann Plast Surg.* 1985;15:151-154.
39. Ghodsi SZ, Raziei M, Taheri A, et al. Comparison of cryotherapy and curettage for the treatment of pyogenic granuloma: a randomized trial. *Br J Dermatol.* 2006;154:671-675.
40. Rodriguez-Vigil T, Vazquez-Lopez F, Perez-Oliva N. Recurrence rates of primary basal cell carcinoma in facial risk areas treated with curettage and electrodesiccation. *J Am Acad Dermatol.* 2007;56:91-95.
41. Reymann F. Treatment of basal cell carcinoma of the skin with curettage. II. A follow-up study. *Arch Dermatol.* 1973;108:528-531.
42. Mitchell JC, Hardie M. Treatment of basal cell carcinoma by curettage and electrosurgery. *Can Med Assoc J.* 1965;93:349-352.
43. Williamson GS, Jackson R. Treatment of basal cell carcinoma by electrodesiccation and curettage. *Can Med Assoc J.* 1962;86:855-862.
44. Zwald F. Immediate curettage and electrodessication following biopsy of suspected basal cell carcinoma at initial visit. *JAMA Dermatol.* 2013;149:981.
45. Goldmann G. The current status of curettage and electrodesiccation. *Dermatol Clin.* 2002;20:569-578.
46. Rowe D, Carroll R, Day C. Long term recurrence rates in previously untreated (primary) basal cell carcinoma: implications for patient follow-up. *J Dermatol Surg Oncol.* 1989;15:315-328.
47. Silverman M, Kopf A, Grin C, et al. Recurrence rates of treated basal cell carcinomas. Part 2: curettage-electrodesiccation. *J Dermatol Surg Oncol.* 1991;17:720-726.

14 Incision and Drainage

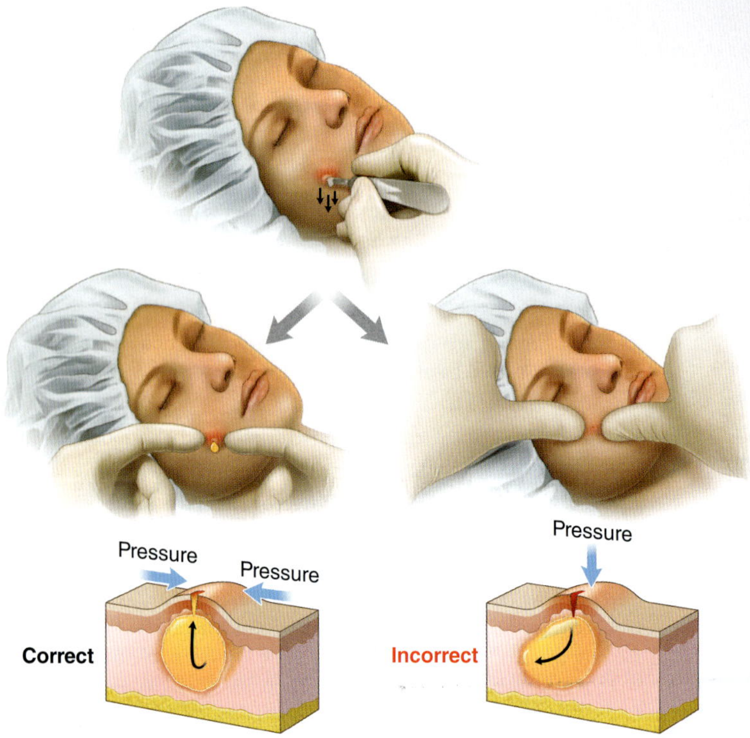

SUMMARY

- I&D may be used to treat various conditions that require the release of enclosed contents, such as hematomas, furuncles, and infected cysts.
- Placing the incision parallel to relaxed skin tension lines may mitigate the appearance of more prominent scars.
- While these procedures are straightforward and can be performed with great rapidity, a poorly performed I&D procedure may serve only to exacerbate an already unpleasant or even dangerous condition.

Beginner Tips

- Choose the most fluctuant area of the lesion, which represents the most liquefied portion of exudate, for easy drainage.
- Choosing the dependent area to facilitate drainage by gravity effect may also reduce the need for manual pressure and attendant patient discomfort.
- Thicker exudate such as blood, coagulum, or mucin requires a longer time to start draining.

Pitfalls and Cautions

- The incision should be stopped as soon as the clinician senses low tissue resistance, in order to avoid tissue damage at the base of lesion.
- Bleeding at incision sites is common. Use external compression to control bleeding.

Expert Tips

- An 18G needle can be useful for I&D on very small lesions. Due to the small opening of this type of incision, thick exudate may not drain out easily. After stabbing, keep the tip of the 18G inside the lesion, push the needle tip laterally to widen the slit-like cut, and wait for exudate to drain.
- Collect fresh, uncontaminated exudate for swab culture to improve the accuracy of culture and sensitivity; avoid collecting the skin surface–contaminated exudate. Allow the exudate to be collected to drain without running on the skin by compressing the lesion and holding the tip of the swab at the proper position and angle.

Patient Education Points

- I&D is a fast and effective procedure, but does not guarantee that a given fluid collection will not recur.
- For inflamed or infected cysts, patients should be warned to expect recurrence, and definitive excisional surgery may be needed in the future.
- I&D requires significant postoperative care, as wounds generally need to be packed or cared for in other ways. Patients should understand that postprocedure management is a process, and drainage may persist for longer than anticipated.

Don't Forget!

- If no or minimal drainage occurs, assess the patency of the incision site.
- Inject lidocaine in the superficial dermis, not into the lesional cavity. Pain with incision may occur when lidocaine injection occurs inside the lesion instead of the dermis and adjacent subcutaneous tissue. A ring block can also be considered.

Billing Pearls

- I&D of an abscess is most frequently coded using CPT code 10060. When draining multiple abscesses, 10061 may be coded, and this code may be used for "complicated" lesions as well, though its use should clearly be justified in the body of the surgical report. Additionally, 10140 may be used for nonabscess I&D. The 10160 code may be more appropriate when performing I&D using an 18G needle alone.

Incision and Drainage

14

INTRODUCTION

Incision and drainage (I&D) is commonly performed in the outpatient setting and is a procedure popular among both patients and clinicians. This approach may be used to treat various conditions that require the release of enclosed contents, such as hematomas, furuncles, infected cysts, and collections of other extraneous substances. While the advantage of I&D is that it is easy to perform, patients should be warned regarding the requirement of postprocedural care. Moreover, since expression of the entire cyst wall is rarely affected when treating inflamed or infected cysts, recurrence of such lesions may be seen (**Tables 14-1 and 14-2**).

Patient Education and Evaluation

Patient evaluation should include inquiry as to history of lidocaine allergy, latex allergy, and hypertrophic scars or keloids. Further, the patient's expectations of the cosmetic outcome should be discussed. Informed consent should be obtained, and the patient should be counseled regarding the risks, benefits, and alternatives of the procedure as well as potential risks of not undergoing the procedure (eg, acute abscesses). Risks include but are not limited to infection (new or worsening of existing infection), bleeding, pain, nerve damage, and scar formation (keloids and hypertrophic scars).

Procedure Overview

All equipment should be placed within reach, ideally on a Mayo stand. Adjust the lighting to allow easy visualization of the abscess; head-mounted lighting works very well.

Choose the incision site in the most fluctuant and prominent part of lesion, where the contents appear most liquefied, in order to permit rapid and effective drainage. In addition, consider starting with the most dependent portion of lesion for the ease of drainage utilizing gravity effect. The patient should be properly positioned so that the area for drainage is fully exposed and easily accessible while ensuring the patient's comfort.

Apply a topical antiseptic (alcohol, povidone-iodine, or chlorhexidine) to the entire lesion and particularly to the area to be incised, followed by application of a sterile drape as indicated. Avoid using chlorhexidine on the ear and periorbital areas.[1]

An absorbent pad, gauze, or chuck is placed to protect other areas from draining exudate. Placement of a cotton ball or dental roll inside the external ear canal is recommended to protect the ear from draining exudate. Gloves, gown, and a face shield should be worn at all times during the procedure to avoid exposure to bodily fluids, particularly from high-pressure abscesses.

Local anesthesia is injected into the selected incision site and around the lesion to minimize both the tenderness associated with pressure as well as the incision proper. This is achieved with infiltration of 1% to 2% lidocaine with or without epinephrine using a 30-gauge needle. Care should be taken to deliver anesthetic solution into the skin overlying the lesion instead of infiltrating lidocaine into the cavity. Needle insertion is just under and parallel to the surface of the skin, and anesthetic is injected into the intradermal and subcutaneous tissues until blanching of the tissue is noted as the anesthetic diffuses. In patients with lidocaine allergy, alternatives can be employed. For a more detailed discussion of anesthetic choices, see Chapter 9.

TABLE 14-1 • Indications for Incision and Drainage

- Hematoma
- Carbuncle or furuncle with fluctuance
- Acute paronychia with abscess
- Inflamed epidermal inclusion cyst
- Dissecting cellulitis with exudate collection
- Hidradenitis suppurativa with abscess
- Pseudocyst of the auricle
- Acne cyst
- Digital mucous cyst
- Mucocele
- Seroma post surgery
- Trapped blood coagulum from sclerotherapy

TABLE 14-2 • Advantages of Incision and Drainage

- Decreases pain associated with tissue expansion from accumulating pus or exudate
- Evacuates the infectious material containing the pathogen
- Enhances antibiotic diffusion into the local tissue, improving their efficacy after release of built-up pus or exudate
- Removes accumulated blood, which may act as a nutritional source for bacterial infection
- May enable visualization of the bleeding site in active hematoma
- Facilitates specimen collection for culture and sensitivity
- Decreases inflammation associated with accumulation of inflammatory exudate.
- Opens and collapses the pocket space, minimizing recollection of the exudate and promoting healing (fibrosis).
- Rapidly decreases the size of lesions, improving their appearance and easing cosmetic concerns

Nerve block or local field block may be required for larger and deeper lesions to ensure the patient's comfort. A ring block may permit anesthesia of the entire target area without directly injecting local anesthetic over the fluctuant mass, which may mitigate the risk of spray back. This approach, however, also does not infiltrate any epinephrine into the area to be incised, so an attendant increased risk of mild bleeding may be anticipated. Adequate anesthesia is essential for complete and thorough drainage. Depending on the patient's pain threshold, ice cubes, ethyl chloride spray, or topical anesthesia may be helpful if applied prior to injecting lidocaine to decrease discomfort delivering local anesthesia. This is particularly important as the acidic environment of infected tissue may make it more difficult to achieve sufficient anesthesia with local agents.

When approaching small digital mucous cysts and trapped blood coagulum following sclerotherapy, I&D may be performed by rapid single puncturing with a needle, and local anesthesia may not be needed. Lidocaine injection may blanch the area or otherwise make these lesions more difficult to visualize for I&D. Ice cubes, ethyl chloride spray, or topical anesthesia instead of lidocaine injection may be better for such lesions. Injectable lidocaine is necessary, however, when I&D of a digital mucous cyst is followed by destruction using electrodesiccation.

INCISION

For smaller lesions, a #11 surgical blade is used to incise the selected and anesthetized area. It is commonly used for I&D due to its sharply pointed tip, which is well suited for a perpendicular stabbing approach into the lesion, although if unavailable, any blade, such as a #15 scalpel blade, will suffice. Following the initial stab to enter the cavity, the incision is extended to create an opening large enough for drainage, which is dependent on the consistency of exudate, and to prevent recurrence of the lesion (recollection). For lesions of larger size and in certain locations (eg, deeper set lesions on the back), a #15 or #10 surgical blade may be used preferentially.

Placing the incision parallel to relaxed skin tension lines may mitigate the appearance of more prominent scars. Care should be taken that the incision length is not too short, restricting the ability of exudate to adequately drain, although an unnecessarily long incision will yield a more prominent scar. Err on the side of creating a shorter incision, as this can always be enlarged if needed.

Care should be taken not to overextend the depth of initial puncture incision, as accidentally stabbing through the base of the lesion's cavity may sever underlying tissue or vessels, increasing the risk of persistent infection or bleeding.[2] Stab incision depth should be designed only to permit the tip of the surgical blade to pass through the skin and the wall of lesion; generally, once this is accomplished, there will be an immediate drop in tissue resistance, and often some of the material to be drained will appear.

Sterile cotton-tipped applicators may be inserted to gently probe the cavity down to its base and facilitate removal of any remaining loculated or congealed fluid. Special care should be taken in making the incision if there are prominent vessels or nerves in the area or when working close to anatomic danger zones. When incision is performed on a highly vascularized area, such as a mucocele on mucosal lip, consider having an assistant apply steady pressure around the lesion while performing I&D for bleeding control and to improve visualization. Care should be taken when incising high-pressure lesions, as the contents may escape explosively in a projectile manner, contaminating the clinician and surrounding area.

Alternative Approaches

Direct puncture with an 18-gauge needle may be used in small lesions that have relatively nonviscous contents, given the relatively large bore size of the 18-gauge needle. Contents of a digital mucous cyst or trapped blood coagulum can be adequately drained when the tip of the 18-gauge needle is kept inside the target space and pushed laterally away from the wound access point in order to open and enlarge the defect. The resulting rounded opening generally permits spontaneous drainage of the exudate. Care should be taken not to remove the needle immediately after puncture so that the nascent skin access point does not reclose. Patience is required with this approach, as it may require 1 to 2 minutes to see the viscous contents slowly drain out while the tip of the needle is kept in place. Importantly, the contents will not rapidly and spontaneously drain. A cotton-tipped applicator is useful to push the lateral wall of the lesion outward immediately after the needle is removed to facilitate complete drainage. I&D of digital mucous cysts may be followed by other treatments such as cryotherapy or injection of sclerosing solution or triamcinolone.[3,4]

Direct puncture with an 18-gauge needle connected to a syringe followed by negative-pressure application by withdrawing the syringe plunger can be used to drain the exudate associated with dissecting cellulitis or trapped blood coagulum of larger veins. The use of duplex ultrasound guidance is particularly helpful in avoiding local arterial injury.

Performing the incision with a punch instrument can be useful because it gives a round-shaped opening for drainage instead of a linear slit. Due to the round-shaped opening, exudate continues to drain at home after the performance of in-office I&D, which may minimize the need to insert wound-packing material. Punch incision is particularly useful in draining thick exudate such as noninflamed epidermal inclusion cysts, as releasing the keratinous content alleviates discomfort from built-up pressure.[5] The size of the punch instrument should be commensurate with the size of the lesion and the thickness of exudate. However, the greater ease of drainage associated with using a larger sized punch instrument should be weighed against the risk of a more substantial postoperative scar. In general, a punch instrument size of 4 mm or less should produce acceptable scar cosmesis.[6]

DRAINAGE

Initially, the exudate may spontaneously drain after incision is performed secondary to built-up pressure. When the lesion is incised at the most fluctuant and dependent area, thin exudate will spontaneously drain out without the need to apply pressure to the lesion, as long as the incised area remains patent.

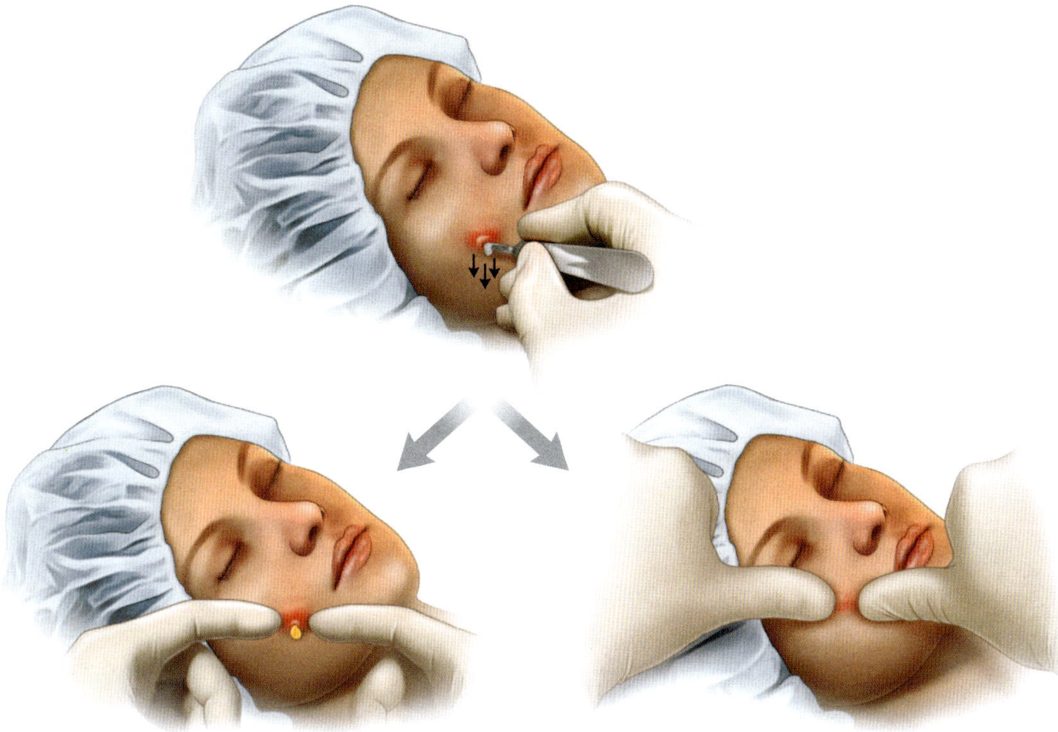

FIGURE 14-1 Incision and drainage on the most dependent portion of a cyst on a patient's cheek in supine position utilizing gravity effect for the ease of drainage. Note that lateral pressure (*left*) results in the extrusion of the contents, whereas downward pressure (*right*) does not.

External pressure may be required in order to definitively drain the remaining exudate, although this may be at the expense of patient comfort. To minimize pain, it is important to apply pressure to the lesion carefully, although often the relief associated with internal pressure reduction outweighs any transient pain associated with the placement of lateral pressure. Pressure is applied gently and slowly from the lateral sides of lesion toward the incision site (**Figures 14-1 to 14-5**). Applying pressure from the top of the lesion at the incision site down to the bottom of the lesion may not result in effective drainage; indeed, the contents may move laterally toward the wall of the fluctuant mass when pressure is applied vertically, and this approach should therefore be avoided. For smaller masses, using a cotton-tipped applicator provides a better focal point of pressure than using a fingertip, which is much larger. If the patient experiences significant discomfort, additional injections of local anesthetic, possibly as a ring block, may be beneficial.

Curved hemostats may be used to enlarge the opening from a narrow slit-like space to a wider exit point, which is especially helpful for thick purulent exudate. The closed tips of curved hemostat clamps are inserted into the incised area and then opened to widen the incised area. The nondominant hand is used to apply pressure to further drain the contents. Hemostats may also be used for careful blunt dissection to break up loculations and facilitate further drainage. Forceps can be used to open the exit for drainage, although they provide only minimal leverage. Care should be taken not to overly stretch and traumatize the skin edges with hemostats or forceps, as this may affect the healing and ultimate cosmesis of the incision site.

When I&D is performed on an acute hematoma, its solidity requires a larger incision and external pressure to remove the clot. Older blood collections can be drained with a shorter incision length or an 18-gauge needle. Attention should be paid to any fresh red blood when I&D is performed on a hematoma, which

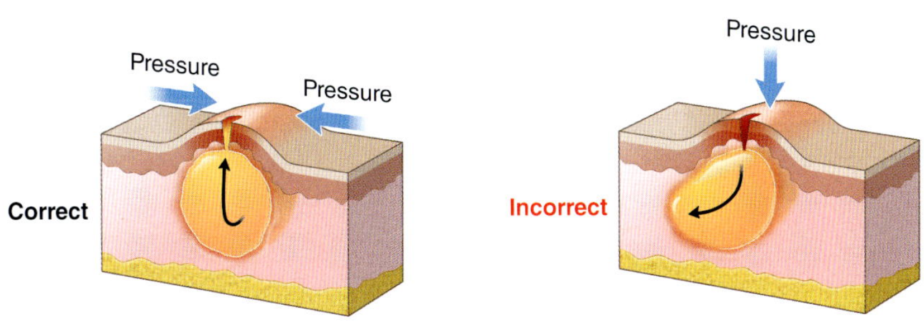

FIGURE 14-2 Pressure is applied gently and slowly from the lateral side of lesion toward the incision site, which moves the contents toward the exit provided by the incision. The contents may move laterally toward the wall of lesion and away from the exit when pressure is applied vertically.

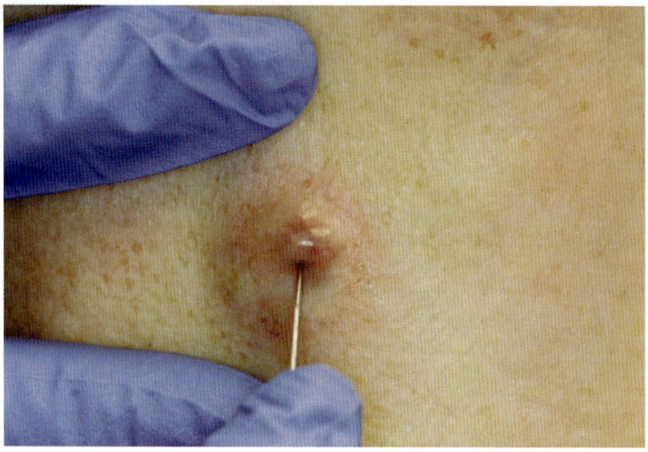

FIGURE 14-3 A small stab incision is made at the inferior pole of the abscess.

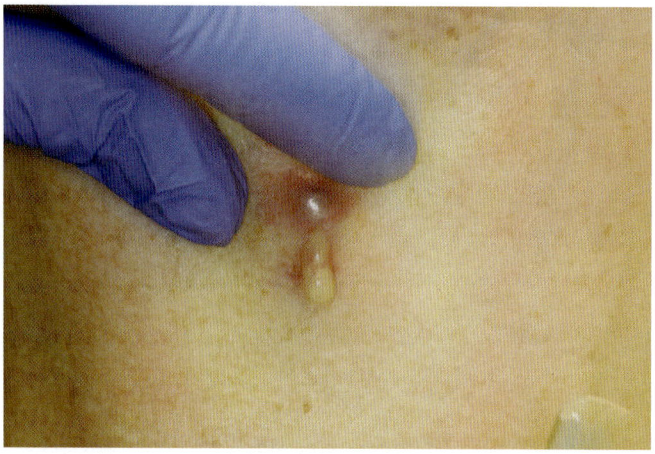

FIGURE 14-4 Gentle lateral pressure is used initially to ensure that contents are effectively extruding through the incision.

may indicate active bleeding that would need to be definitively surgically addressed.

For acute paronychia with an abscess located immediately adjacent to the nail sulcus, the tip of a #11 or #15 surgical blade or 21- or 23-gauge needle may be gently inserted underneath the proximal or lateral nail folds to create an opening for drainage.[7,8] Gentle pressure is applied to extrude the purulent exudate. Care should be taken to point the sharp edge away from the nail and not to insert it too aggressively in order to avoid damaging neurovascular bundles, tendons, or the nail matrix. A piece of gauze may be placed underneath the nail fold to allow continued drainage.[9] For an abscess not located immediately adjacent to the nail sulcus, incision is made directly over the abscess and/or in line with the lateral nail fold to decompress the abscess.[10]

If indicated, swab culture and sensitivities may be sent out using freshly drained exudate. Avoid contacting the tip of the swab with skin or mucosal surface to prevent contamination by normal flora. A sterile syringe may be used to obtain a sample from the interior aspect of the cavity.

Irrigation may be performed to further remove the infectious or inflammatory exudate. The tip of a sterile normal saline-filled syringe is inserted through the incised wound, and the cavity is gently rinsed to thoroughly irrigate the cavity until the effluent is clear. Copious quantities of gauze or absorbent pads should be placed at the site to absorb fluid and minimize splash back over the surrounding area and operator. The nondominant hand may be used to apply gauze to cover the incised area during irrigation. A syringe with a built-in splash shield may also be used. An appropriate incision size will enhance irrigation and prevent excessive buildup of pressure within the lesion.

If further drainage is required, wound-packing material, such as 1/4- or 1/2-inch packing strips with or without iodoform, is gently inserted through the incision site and loosely packed inside the lesional cavity using hemostats or forceps. This will prevent premature closure of the incised wound, which can lead to re-collection. Care should be taken to avoid overpacking the wound, which could cause ischemia of the surrounding tissues and impede the desired drainage.[11]

Electrodesiccation may be performed after I&D of mucoceles or digital mucous cysts to close the dead space and avoid re-collection of the exudate.[12] Any active bleeding points are cauterized.

A pressure dressing may be needed on some lesions in order to collapse the cavity, minimize re-collection of exudate, and minimize dead space, which could lead to reaccumulation. Dissecting cellulitis of the scalp requires pressure dressings and head wraps, as the exudate can rapidly reaccumulate. This pressure dressing may also serve to help control bleeding.

Postprocedure Care

Counsel the patient on local wound care. Change the wound dressing and/or packing every 24 hours and after each shower. Petrolatum may be applied to an incised wound that does not require further drainage in order to promote wound healing.

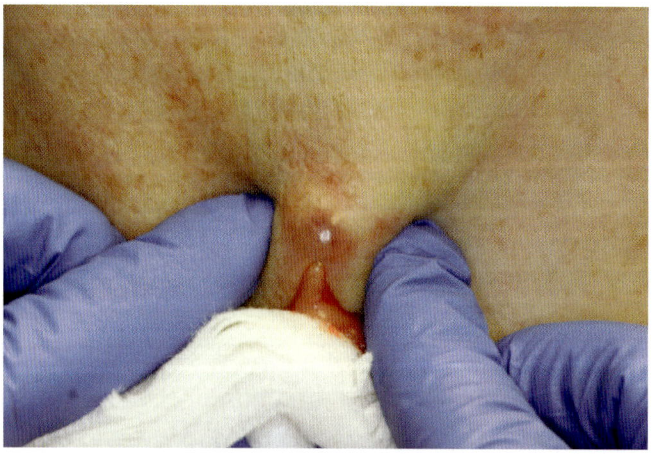

FIGURE 14-5 Firm lateral and upward pressure is applied to force the expulsion of all cyst contents.

Cover the wound with a sterile, nonadherent dressing. Apply several layers of gauze to absorb any persistent drainage, and secure the dressing with surgical tape such as paper tape.

A compression dressing may be applied if indicated.

Counsel patients regarding the likelihood of blood- or exudate-saturated gauze being present during dressing changes.

Antibiotics may be indicated for certain diagnoses, such as hematoma or infection. Preoperative treatment with antibiotics may be a helpful adjunct for the I&D of abscesses in patients who are at increased risk for endocarditis.[13]

Analgesic medications may be helpful if indicated. In general, the majority of pain and discomfort should be significantly relieved after pressure is released following I&D.

Re-counsel the patient regarding the expected scar formation when the incised wound is allowed to heal by second intention, particularly with large hematomas. Also outline the risk of recurrence.

Follow-up may be scheduled within a few days to a week for wound check, dressing change, or packing material removal. Wound packing material is removed when no fresh exudate is visible, and a simple dressing with gauze is then sufficient.

Instruct the patient to call and/or return before the scheduled appointment if there are any signs of worsening or infection such as redness, swelling, tenderness, or fever.

Risks of I&D and Their Management

The potential complications of I&D include inadequate drainage, infection, bleeding, nerve damage, hypertrophic scars, and keloids. Methods to manage these complications are summarized below.

Inadequate Drainage: The drainage exit may close off too soon, resulting in inadequate drainage. This can be prevented by using wound packing material or a punch incision technique or by leaving a cotton-tipped applicator in place during drainage.

Infections: While abscess is one of the most frequently seen indications to perform I&D, local infection can occur in non-infectious indications of I&D as a result of the procedure itself. Purulent drainage, swelling, persistent redness, and delayed healing may be evident, and when these are noted, the patient should undergo evaluation and treatment. Management of these infections includes an appropriate topical and/or systemic antibiotic, daily wound care, and repeat I&D if the site develops an abscess with fluctuance. Responsible organisms vary by anatomic location, although *Staphylococcus aureus* is most commonly seen.

Bleeding: Bleeding is managed by external compression. Appropriate use of hemostatic measures is essential at the site of incision as well as for obtaining adequate hemostasis within an active hematoma requiring I&D.

Hypertrophic Scars or Keloid Formation: Hypertrophic scars may be treated with intralesional corticosteroids, pulsed-dye laser, silicone gel sheeting, cryotherapy, or a combination of these methods.[14] For keloids, these treatments may be combined with surgical excision, intralesional 5-fluorouracil, intralesional interferon, external compression, or a combination of these methods.[13,15-17]

Nerve, Tendon, or Ligament Damage: Paresthesia may occur at the incision site; this should improve with time. Motor nerve damage is extremely rare. A severed tendon or ligament requires referral to the appropriate specialties for evaluation and repair. The risk of this occurring is mitigated by remaining at the appropriate depth during the incision of the lesion. Consider the size and depth of lesion, anatomic location, and length of the sharp used as an incising instrument prior to performing the procedure. A thorough understanding of local anatomy is of vital importance.

CONCLUSIONS

When properly performed, I&D is a useful treatment for abscesses, cysts, hematomas, and numerous other conditions. While these procedures are straightforward and can be performed with great rapidity, a poorly performed I&D procedure may serve only to exacerbate an already unpleasant or even dangerous condition. Therefore, a deep respect for anatomy and an understanding of the appropriate indications and contraindications for this approach remain of vital importance.

REFERENCES

1. Steinsapir KD, Woodward JA. Chlorhexidine keratitis: safety of chlorhexidine as a facial antiseptic. *Dermatol Surg.* 2017;43(1):1-6.
2. Burney RE. Incision and drainage procedures: soft tissue abscesses in the emergency service. *Emerg Med Clin North Am.* 1986;4:527-542.
3. De Berker DA, Lawrence CM. Treatment of myxoid cysts. *Dermatol Surg.* 2001;27(3):296-299.
4. Esson GA, Holme SA. Treatment of 63 subjects with digital mucous cysts with percutaneous sclerotherapy using polidocanol. *Dermatol Surg.* 2016;42(1):59-62.
5. Mehrabi D, Leonhardt JM, Brodell RT. Removal of keratinous and pilar cysts with the punch incision technique: analysis of surgical outcomes. *Dermatol Surg.* 2002;28(8):673-677.
6. Christenson LJ, Phillips PK, Weaver AL, Otley CC. Primary closure vs second-intention treatment of skin punch biopsy sites: a randomized trial. *Arch Dermatol.* 2005;141(9):1093-1099.
7. Shafritz AB, Coppage JM. Acute and chronic paronychia of the hand. *J Am Acad Orthop Surg.* 2014;22(3):165-174.
8. Ogunlusi JD, Oginni LM, Ogunlusi OO. DAREJD simple technique of draining acute paronychia. *Tech Hand Up Extrem Surg.* 2005;9(2):120-121.
9. Canales FL, Newmeyer WL III, Kilgore ES Jr. The treatment of felons and paronychias. *Hand Clin.* 1989;5(4):515-523.
10. Jebson PJ. Infections of the fingertip: paronychias and felons. *Hand Clin.* 1998;14(4):547-555, viii.
11. Fitch MT, Manthey DE, McGinnis HD, Nicks BA, Pariyadath M. Videos in clinical medicine. Abscess incision and drainage. *N Engl J Med.* 2007;357(19):e20.
12. Nallasivam KU, Sudha BR. Oral mucocele: review of literature and a case report. *J Pharm Bioallied Sci.* 2015;7(Suppl 2):S731-S733.
13. Fine BC, Sheckman PR, Bartlett JC. Incision and drainage of soft-tissue abscesses and bacteremia. *Ann Intern Med.* 1985;103(4):645.

14. Berman B, Maderal A, Raphael B. Keloids and hypertrophic scars: pathophysiology, classification, and treatment. *Dermatol Surg.* 2017;43(Suppl 1):S3-S18.
15. Hirshowitz B, Lerner D, Moscona AR. Treatment of keloid scars by combined cryosurgery and intralesional corticosteroids. *Aesthetic Plast Surg.* 1982;6:153-158.
16. Pollack SV, Goslen JB. The surgical treatment of keloids. *J Dermatol Surg Oncol.* 1982;8:1045-1049.
17. Shepherd JP, Dawber RP. The response of keloid scars to cryosurgery. *Plast Reconstr Surg.* 1982;70;677-682.

Laceration Repair

15

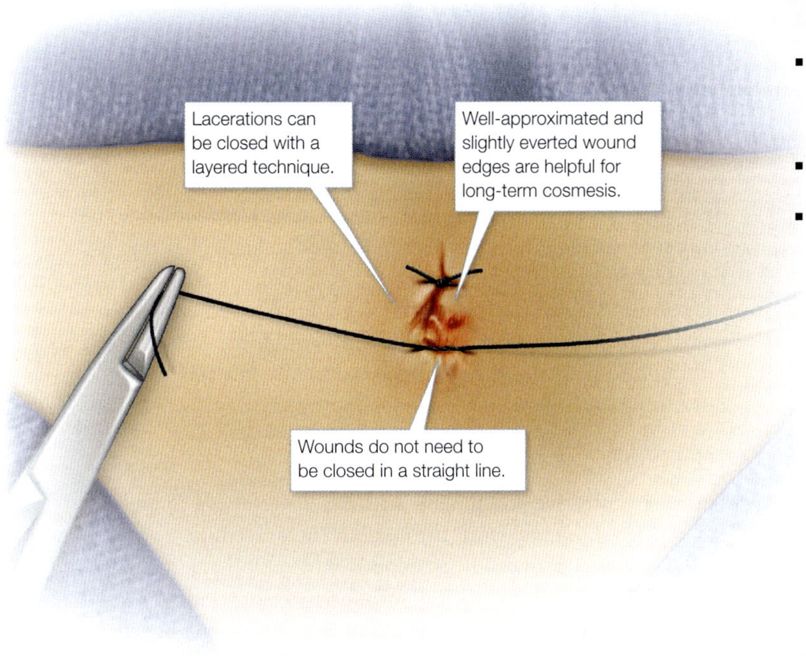

SUMMARY

- Laceration repairs are often the first closures attempted by primary care clinicians. Ensuring that the wound is clean with fresh edges—and that it has been thoroughly anesthetized—is critical.
- Lacerations can be closed with a layered technique.
- Remember to focus on careful technique with well-approximated and slightly everted wound edges for ideal long-term cosmesis.

Beginner Tips

- Ensure that the wound has been thoroughly cleaned and is free from foreign bodies before even considering starting your repair.
- Interrupted sutures have the advantage of resilience in the face of inadvertent suture material breakage.
- Running sutures, while nominally faster to place, will lose all their retention if the suture material breaks anywhere along its course.

Pitfalls and Cautions

- Never close a wound unless you are certain that all debris has been removed.
- In cases of extreme crush injuries, it may be better to debride the devitalized area at the time of the initial repair rather than allow frank necrosis to set in, when an additional procedure will be needed with potentially increased morbidity.

Expert Tips

- It is possible to entirely close a laceration with buried sutures alone.
- Sutures may be spaced closer together where the wound is under the greatest tension, though most lacerations are only under minimal tension.
- Wounds do not need to be closed in a straight line; for shark-fin shaped lacerations, a tip stitch may be useful.

Patient Education Points

- Expect bruising to increase for 2-3 days after the laceration repair, and for forehead or periorbital trauma, patients should expect a black eye that will worsen over several days before improving.
- Minimizing the need for dressing changes can be very helpful for patients, and select wounds can be dressed with adherent film dressings, particularly when no transepidermal sutures are used.

Don't Forget!

- Suture removal can be inconvenient and painful. In select cases, it may be appropriate to close the wound entirely with buried sutures or with fast-absorbing transepidermal sutures (or a combination of the two).
- Avoid nylon sutures around the lips and eyes, where they can poke and represent a source of discomfort for the patient.

Billing Pearls

- Lacerations are generally billed with the simple repair series of codes based on the length of the repair.
- When repairing lacerations with a layered repair including buried sutures, intermediate repair codes can be used.
- Lacerations are almost never be billed as complex closures or as flap repairs.

15 Laceration Repair

INTRODUCTION

Laceration repairs are among the most frequently performed procedures in office practice. The central principles of laceration repair are the same as those for any linear excision and repair: minimize tension, minimize the presence of foreign body material, precisely align wound edges, and minimize dead space and bleeding prior to closure. Because the mechanism of injury is generally traumatic rather than iatrogenic, laceration repairs do entail some added considerations regarding timing from injury to repair and infection risk (and the need for prerepair irrigation).

Mastering laceration repair can increase both the clinician's level of comfort as well as the efficiency of the practice and, most importantly, the ultimate clinical outcome for the patient. It is very helpful to personally see patients back for suture removal to provide a realistic assessment of their healing process as well as active feedback for the clinician. If patients tend to return with similar complications, this is a warning sign for the clinician to seek advice from more experienced colleagues or mentors.

INDICATIONS AND CONTRAINDICATIONS

Repairing a traumatic laceration is similar, in principle, to repairing an excision site, and the repair tray and wound preparation are largely similar (**Table 15-1**). For lacerations, in general, a wound older than 12 hours (or 24 hours on the face) should only be closed with caution due to concerns for infection, and aggressive irrigation should be performed prior to closure. Keep in mind that for patients who are immunosuppressed, these time frames may be shortened. Grossly contaminated wounds and puncture wounds are often left to heal by secondary intention. Wounds with significant tissue loss, crush injury, or injuries to the underlying structures should not be closed primarily. Antiseptic skin preparations, such as chlorhexidine, may be used both before and after irrigation.

The site of the laceration (and the degree of contamination) may have implications for infection risk, since—as with excisions—some body sites, such as the axillae and groin, are at a higher baseline risk for infection.

Tetanus immunization should be administered to patients whose status is unknown. Prophylactic antibiotics are generally only considered for those with grossly contaminated wounds, crush injuries, or baseline immunosuppression.

TABLE 15-1 • Repair Tray for Laceration Repair

Irrigation syringe/bottle with splashguard
Surgical disinfectant (chlorhexidine is ideal if not working around the eyes/ears)
Clean/sterile gloves
Mask with face shield
Nonwoven gauze
3-mL needle with 27-gauge syringe for drawing up anesthetic
30-gauge needle for injecting anesthetic
Suture
Sterile repair kit including: Blade handle Tissue scissors (iris scissors are used frequently) Suture scissors Needle driver Forceps (Adson's with teeth and platforms are generally used) Hooks (optional)

TECHNIQUE

Personal protective equipment, such as gloves and a mask with face shield, should be worn throughout the procedure.

The laceration should be prepped with chlorhexidine, povidone-iodine, or similar topical antiseptics; chlorhexidine should be kept away from the eyes and ear canals but has the benefit of efficacy while still wet (Figures 15-1 to 15-16).

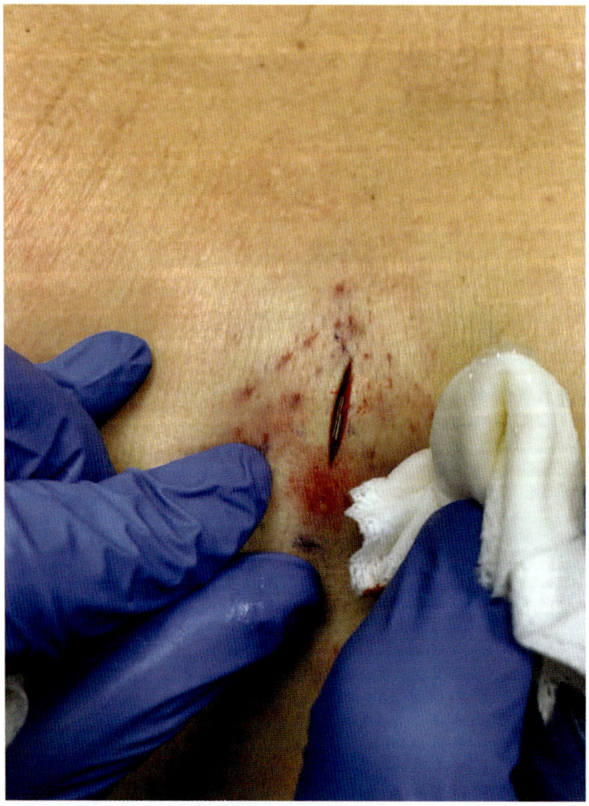

FIGURE 15-1 A laceration is present on the lower back.

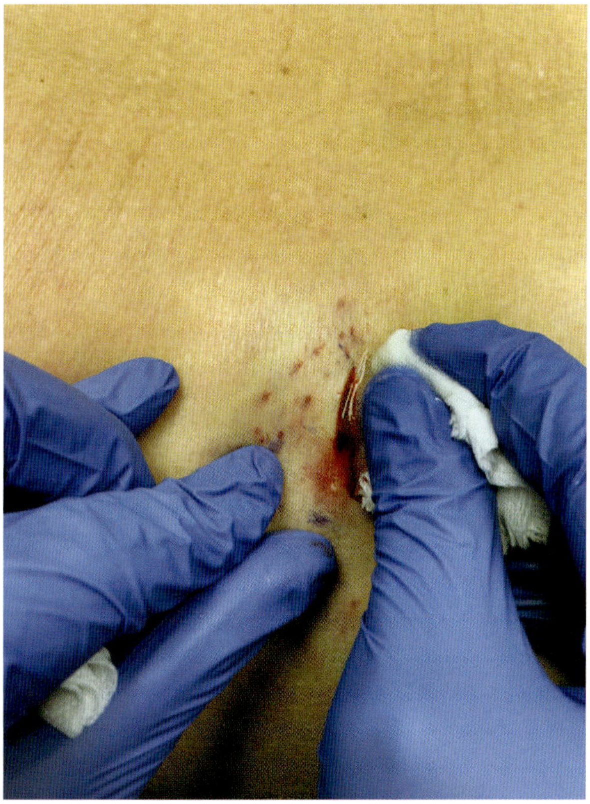

FIGURE 15-2 The area is prepped with chlorhexidine. Lidocaine infiltration is then performed as a ring block.

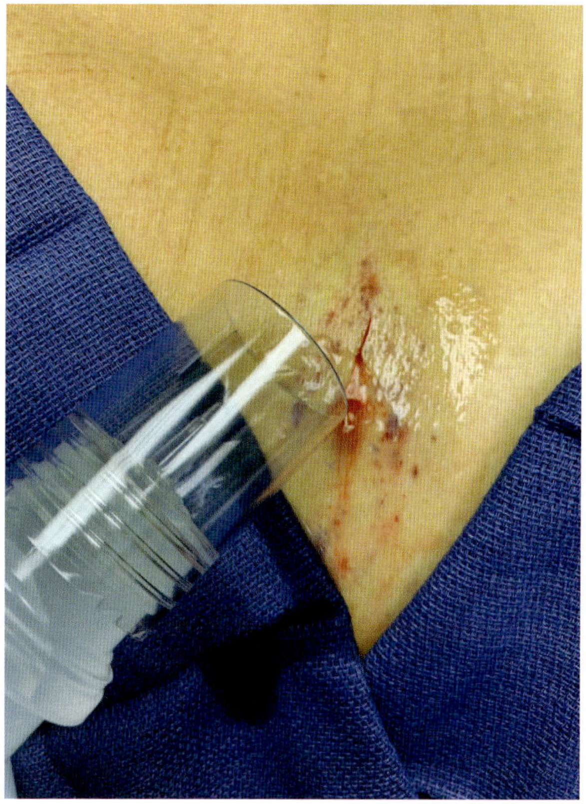

FIGURE 15-3 The area is irrigated.

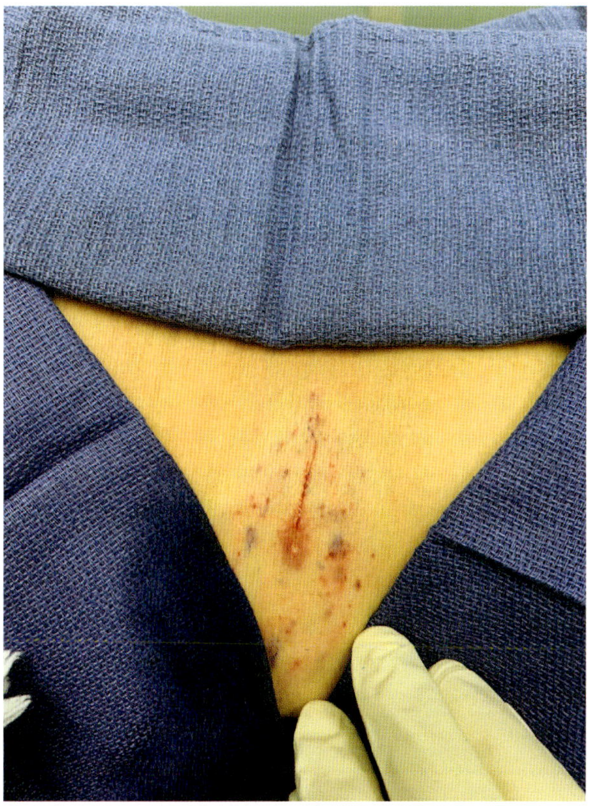

FIGURE 15-4 The area is draped for the laceration repair.

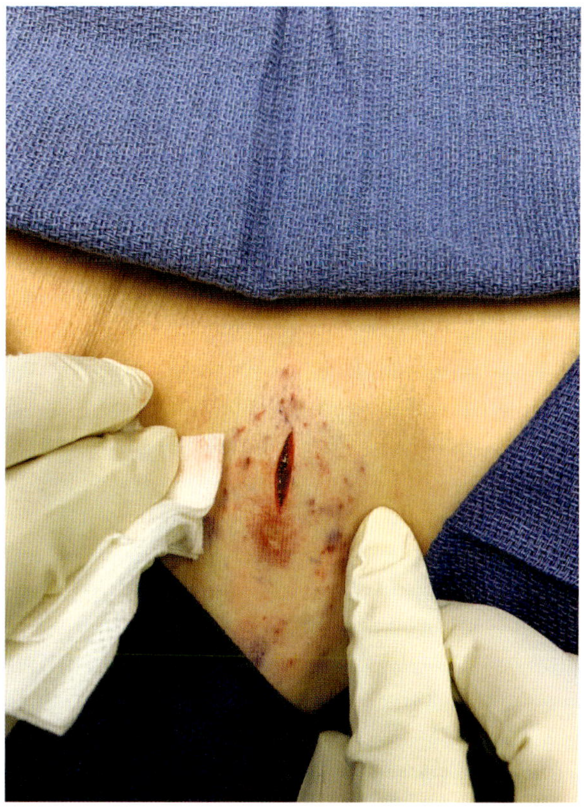

FIGURE 15-5 The wound is gently explored.

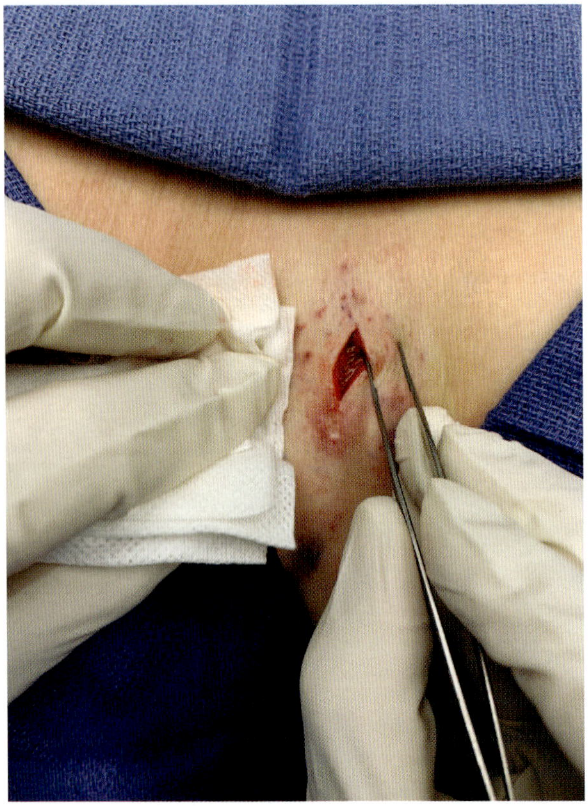

FIGURE 15-6 Forceps are used to explore the lateral extent of the wound.

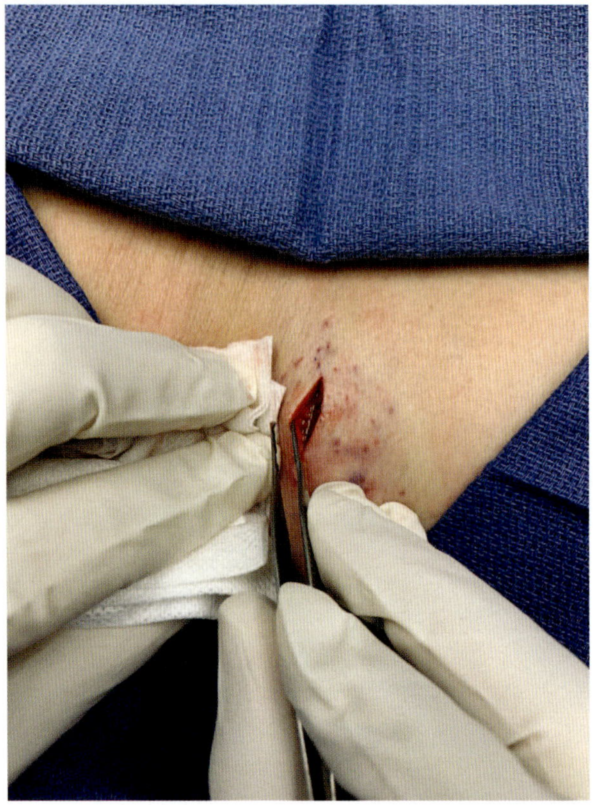

FIGURE 15-7 This is repeated on the other side to inspect for residual foreign body presence.

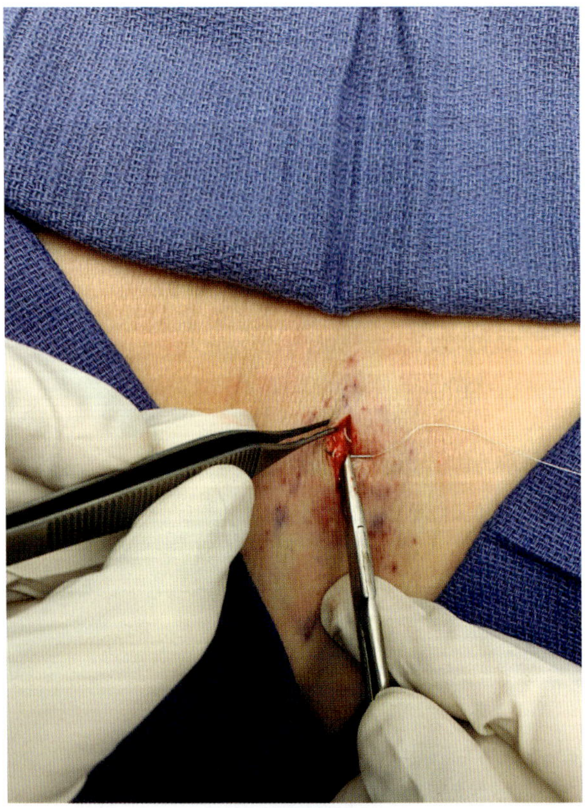

FIGURE 15-8 A deep suture is placed.

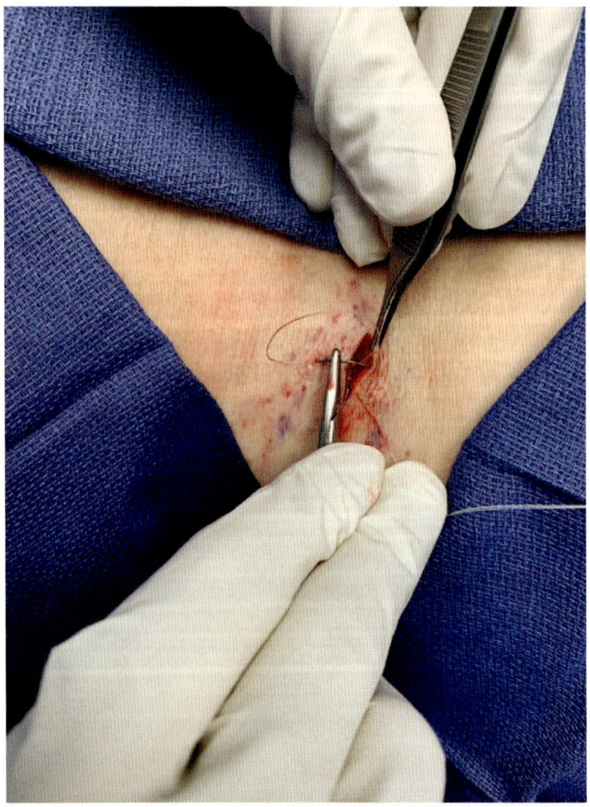

FIGURE 15-9 The suture is completed on the contralateral side (typically a buried vertical mattress or setback suture is best; see Chapter 10 for a full discussion).

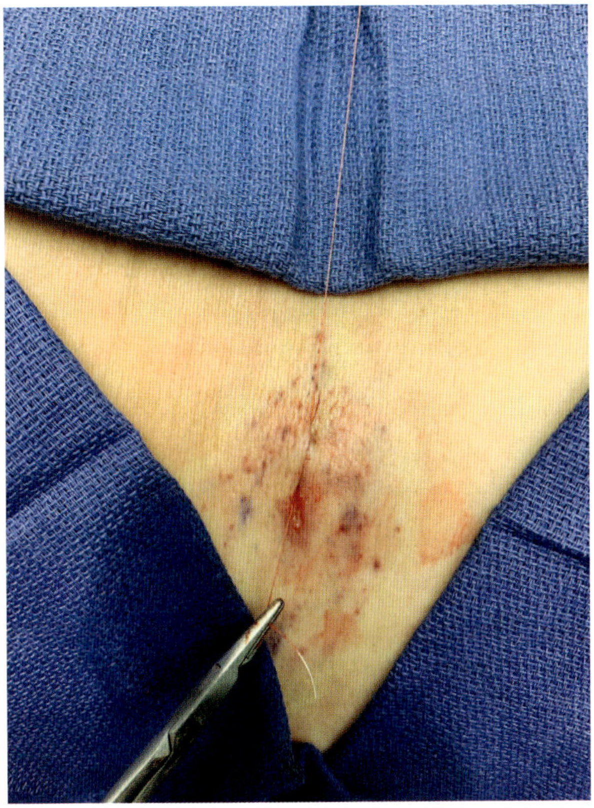

FIGURE 15-10 The suture is tied. Notice the excellent approximation.

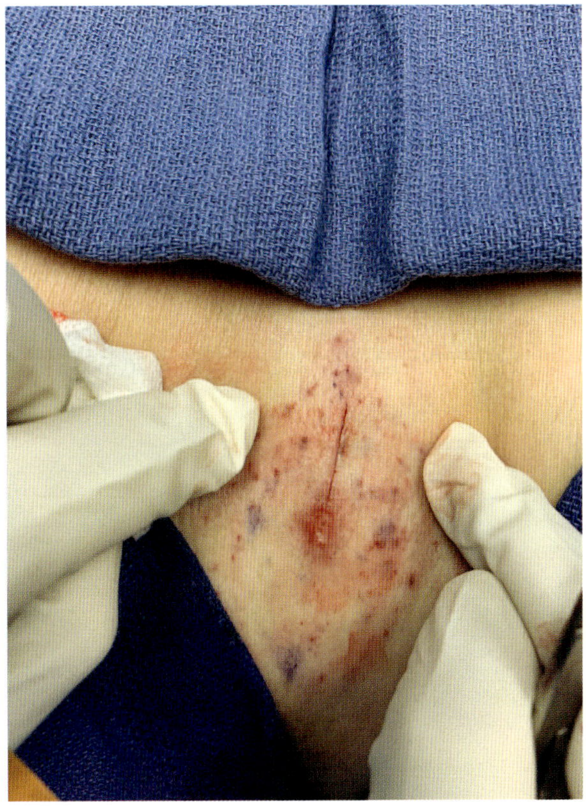

FIGURE 15-11 Even on lateral pressure, the wound remains sealed.

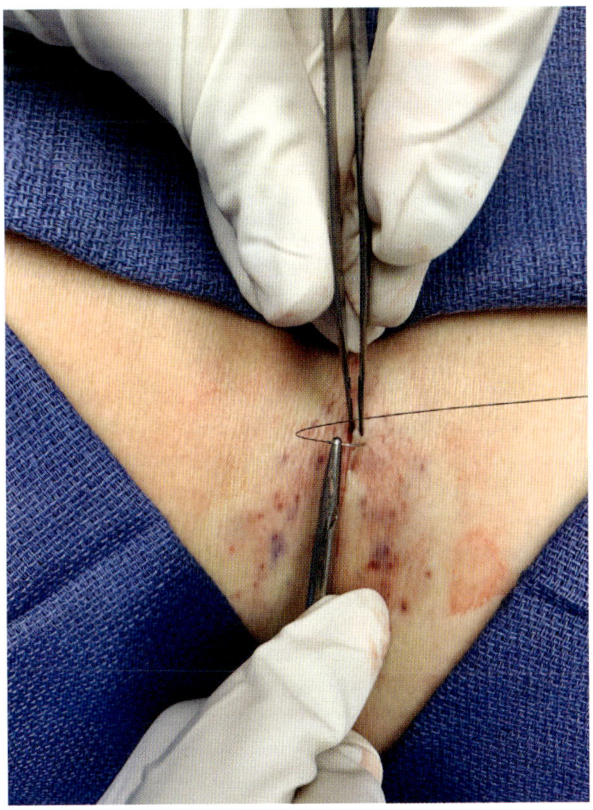

FIGURE 15-12 An interrupted suture is placed. The needle enters at 90 degrees.

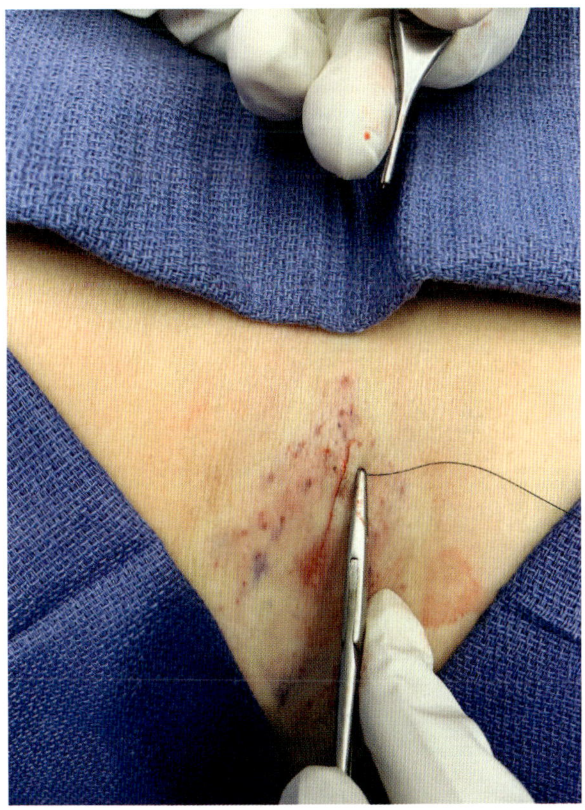

FIGURE 15-13 The bite follows the curvature of the needle.

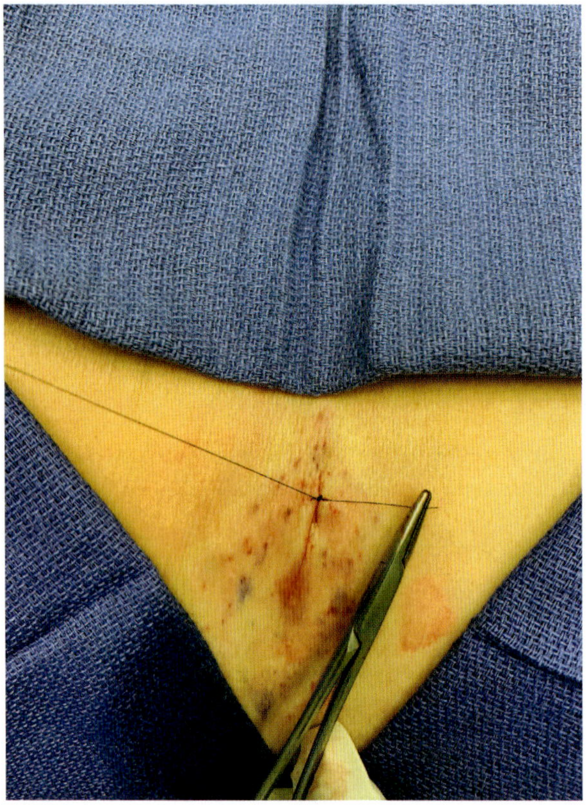

FIGURE 15-14 The suture is tied.

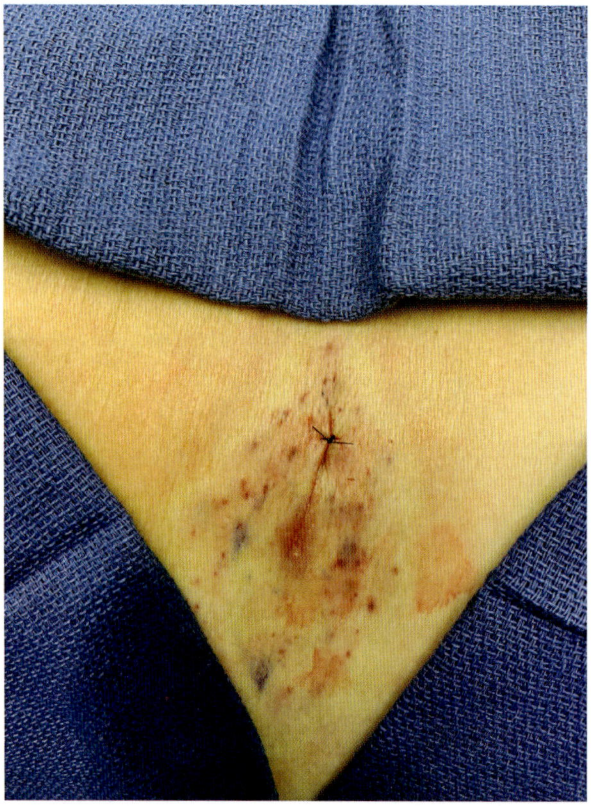

FIGURE 15-15 Appearance after a single suture.

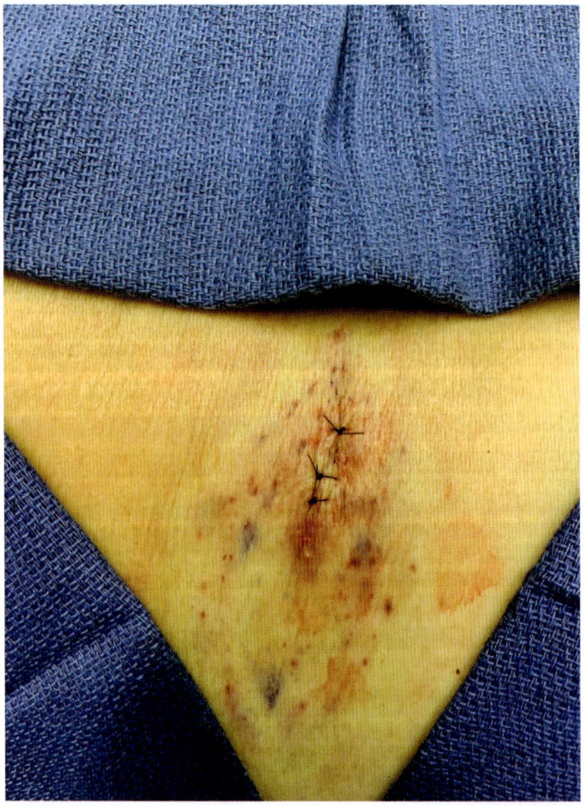

FIGURE 15-16 Additional sutures may be placed as needed. Note that in many cases, no external sutures are needed at all if the buried sutures have led to adequate wound edge approximation.

Once the wound has been prepped, local anesthesia is generally performed using 1% lidocaine with epinephrine (see Chapter 9). Wound irrigation can then be performed, generally with sterile water or saline. A syringe or bottle with splash guard is often used for irrigation to achieve adequate pressure for the removal of gross debris.

After irrigation is complete, the wound should again be prepped and the repair can be initiated. Before starting the repair itself, the wound should be carefully explored gently with forceps (and/or hooks) in order to ensure that no residual foreign body material remains. If devitalized tissue is present, it can be removed through sharp debridement. Laceration repairs should follow similar principles to repairs performed after excisions, including gentle tissue handling and tension reduction. Similarly, the tip of the suture needle should not be grasped with forceps as it can lead to significant dulling, making future bites more challenging (and traumatic to the tissue). As with any repair, the first suture can be placed either at one edge of the wound or at its center. It may be better to start at one edge (the edge furthest away from the clinician) and work proximally in order to minimize tension on any single suture.

Several suturing techniques are useful in repairing lacerations (see Chapter 10). The most common approaches include simple interrupted, vertical mattress, horizontal mattress, and simple running sutures. Depth-correcting sutures can be very useful to minimize the risk of step-off. When buried sutures are placed, the buried vertical mattress is an excellent technique for wounds under minimal tension, whereas the set-back suture is an excellent option for wounds under significant tension (**Table 15-2**).

TABLE 15-2 • Suturing Techniques Frequently Used for Lacerations

	Techniques
Facial skin	Simple interrupted or running
Nonfacial skin	Simple interrupted and/or buried vertical mattress
High-tension areas	Simple interrupted and/or set-back

Sutures may be spaced closer together where the wound is under the greatest tension (generally at its center).

It is possible to entirely close a laceration with buried sutures alone. While there may be a negligibly increased risk of infection when leaving suture material in place, for clean wounds, this is a convenient approach for the patient and may result in a cosmetically more appealing wound.

AFTERCARE

When external sutures are placed, suture removal should be performed as soon as is feasibly possible to minimize the chances of leaving railroad track–like scars (**Table 15-3**). Keep in mind that wounds that include absorbable sutures are likely to fare better than those closed with nonabsorbable sutures alone, since buried sutures slowly absorb over time as wound healing occurs, whereas suture removal leads to an abrupt shift between a wound that is entirely supported by sutures to one that is not supported at all (it is for this reason that the period 24 hours after suture removal is associated with the greatest risk of wound dehiscence).

TABLE 15-3 • Suture Removal Recommendations for Lacerations

	Suture Removal
Facial skin	5-7 days
Nonfacial skin	7-10 days
High-tension areas	10-14 days

Patients often appreciate the option of avoiding a suture removal visit altogether, for both convenience (it saves another visit that may require missing work or school) and comfort (even the gentlest suture removal process can be uncomfortable, or at least stressful, for the patient).

Infection and dehiscence are the primary risks of laceration repair. Other risks include scarring, foreign body retention, and persistent deep structural damage.

CONCLUSIONS

Laceration repairs are frequently encountered in the office, urgent care center, or emergency department. Managing lacerations with finesse can make an important difference both for patient comfort and outcomes. An organized and systematic approach is critical, as this will lead to both more efficient repairs and a less stressful environment for the patient.

16 Layered Excision and Surgical Repairs

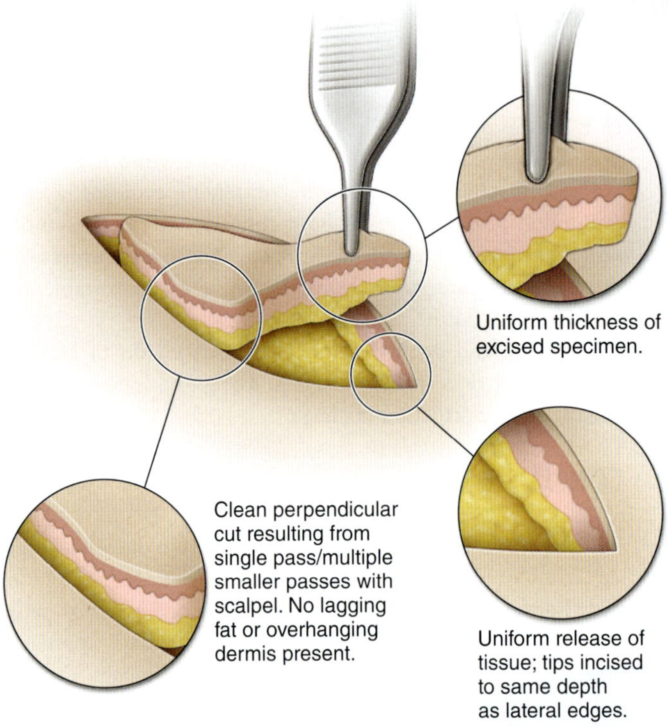

SUMMARY

- Linear closures involve direct side-to-side closure of the surgical wound.
- Layered linear closure remains the gold standard for wound closure given its predictable outcomes, reasonable cost to the patient and healthcare system, and low risk of complications.
- Even very large defects, including those on the face, can often be closed in a linear fashion, as long as aggressive undermining and dog-ear correction are performed.
- A significant advantage of linear closures is their predictability; since outstanding blood flow is maintained to the wound edge, these closures often result in fine-line nearly imperceptible scars when carefully designed and executed.

Beginner Tips

- Breaking down the excision and linear repair into its component parts helps conceptualize each requisite step.
- Never attempt to rush a step; most shortcuts result in the need for a far more time-consuming correction.

Pitfalls and Cautions

- Always carefully identify the source of any oozing and address it directly; judicious use of electrosurgical approaches will help reduce the amount of necrotic tissue left in a wound.
- Gentle tissue handling will result in improved outcomes, decreasing the risk of necrosis and infection.

Expert Tips

- Large defects on the face do not necessarily require flap repair.
- Linear closures have almost no risk of flap loss, and so are particularly useful approaches for closures in tobacco users.
- Using a rhombus or tangent-to-circle closure approach may result in smaller apical angles and less dog-ear formation.

Patient Education Points

- Explaining that any additional scar length will likely heal with a minimally visible line may go a long way toward patient reassurance.
- Always review the planned degree of eversion with the patient so that there is no confusion or worry in the immediate postoperative period regarding the ridged appearance of the wound.

Don't Forget!

- When deciding between a large linear closure and a flap, keep in mind that linear closures have less of a tendency to "burn bridges" for future repairs, an important consideration in the patient with florid skin cancers.
- If a wound closed with buried sutures alone results in significant gaping or overhanging dermis, do not attempt to solve this with superficial suture placement. Instead, remove the excess dermis and/or replace the deep sutures.

Billing Pearls

- As a general rule, extensive undermining, dog-ear correction, or other complex steps are needed to bill for a complex closure.
- No amount of undermining shifts a linear excision and repair to a bilateral advancement flap for billing purposes.

Layered Excision and Surgical Repairs

16

INTRODUCTION

Direct linear closure of surgical wounds is the primary technique used for defect closure in dermatologic surgery. Learning to perform an outstanding linear excision and repair will go a long way to making a budding clinician's career, as patients and providers alike place great value on well-executed excisions. Linear closure is favored for several reasons, including its ease of execution; reliable and predictable healing pattern; rapidity; and reproducibility. Even large or deep defects may be amenable to linear repairs, and indeed, this may represent the best option for many such wounds.[1-7] When feasible, layered linear closure remains the gold standard for wound closure given the predictable outcomes, reasonable cost to the patient and healthcare system, and low risk of complications. Fundamental linear closure techniques, including undermining, hemostasis, tissue handling, and suture placement, represent the bedrock of all surgical closures, from small punch biopsies to large flaps.

NOMENCLATURE

The term *elliptical excision* has been used historically to denote linear wound closures, although numerous authors have, over the years, pointed out that the basic shape used by most clinicians for closure design is not, in fact, an ellipse (**Figure 16-1**).[8-12] The term *fusiform excision* has therefore been proposed as an alternative, although it has yet to be universally adopted.

The rhombus, or tangent-to-circle, design is a geometrically efficient approach to linear wound closure. Note that *rhomboid*, however, does not mean rhombus-like, but rather refers to a specific geometric shape defined by Euclid as a parallelogram where adjacent sides are of unequal lengths. Therefore, these closures should not, from a Euclidean perspective, be referred to as rhomboid.

Most linear excisions are closed in a layered fashion, with repair of the dermis and/or fascia preceding epidermal approximation. Clinicians may refer to an *intermediate* closure and *complex* closure; these terms relate to the *billing* of closures using Common Procedural Terminology (CPT) code series. As a general rule, extensive undermining, dog-ear correction, or other ostensibly complex steps are needed to bill for a complex closure.

Some clinicians refer to undermined *flaps* of tissue that are *advanced* into the center of a wound in order to close a linear excision. While it is technically appropriate to refer to undermined sections of tissue as skin flaps, no degree of undermining shifts a linear excision and repair to a bilateral advancement flap for billing purposes, as the latter requires a true adjacent tissue transfer (for a detailed discussion of flap dynamics and advancement flaps, see Chapter 20; for a discussion of billing, see Chapter 8).

PREOPERATIVE EVALUATION

The preoperative consultation for most linear excisions and closures can safely take place on the day of surgery and includes a detailed medical and social history, with particular attention to the use of medications or supplements that may affect bleeding as well as tobacco use, which has a marked effect on the postoperative healing process. The details of the preoperative evaluation in general are addressed in Chapter 3.

Patients should understand that there is always more than one way to skin a cat; all surgical procedures present risk, and all surgical procedures have alternatives—including avoiding

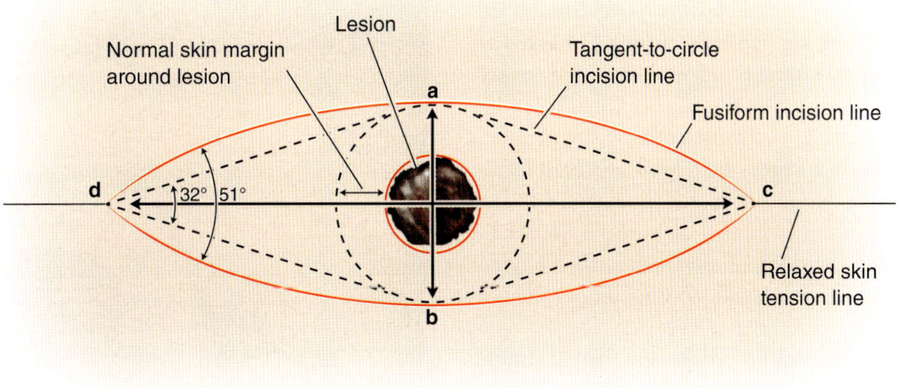

FIGURE 16-1 The rhombus (tangent-to-circle) closure inscribed within a fusiform design using a theoretical length-to-width ratio of 3.5:1.

surgery altogether. It is the balance of risk and benefit that must be addressed with each patient individually.

This individualized approach to patient consent and education should extend to the preoperative evaluation of the planned procedure as well. Thus, the planned surgical site should be carefully assessed visually and palpated, and the range of motion of the planned surgical site and surrounding tissues should be closely assessed. For example, when designing facial repairs, the clinician should sequentially have the patient move through the entire range of motion (frown, smile, grimace) in order to better gauge the relaxed skin tension lines (RSTLs) and the presence of any underlying fibrous attachments. In recent years, there has been a better understanding of the retaining ligaments in the cheek and beyond, which may have a significant impact on tissue mobility, particularly during larger repairs.[13]

On the hands, patients should similarly move through flexion and extension and should be asked to make a fist. Querying patients regarding occupational and leisure activities may also be particularly helpful, as a dorsal hand repair on a masseuse may be approached differently to that on a professional golfer. The potential for range-of-motion variation is also seen on the upper back, where baseline patient posture may affect the planned closure vector.

Linear closures near free margins should be carefully planned and assessed, and patients should understand potential risks, such as ectropion or eclabium, before the procedure is started. When assessing the potential for ectropion, the patient may be asked to gaze upward with their mouth wide open while in a semi-reclined position in order to better assess the potential for ectropion development.

As part of the informed consent process, the patient should understand that there will be a scar every time the skin is cut. The goal is not to avoid scarring altogether, which is impossible regardless of clinician or surgical technique; it is to create the least cosmetically obvious scar while definitively treating the underlying disease process. The assessment of scar quality has been the focus of renewed interest of late, particularly as this may be used as an outcome measure for quality-of-care assessments. The Scar Cosmesis Assessment and Rating (SCAR) scale is a recently developed validated scale that may be particularly helpful when determining the quality of postoperative scarring.[14,15]

The informed consent and consultation process, while unique to each patient's circumstances, should always move through the same steps. Thus, all patients are handed a mirror and asked to confirm the surgery site prior to marking, and then again asked to confirm the site verbally once the site has been marked. This approach is invaluable in engaging the patient as partner regarding biopsy site identification and may help limit potential liability exposure in cases where wrong-site surgery is alleged. In cases where the biopsy site location is equivocal, surgery should be delayed, and consultation should be undertaken with the referring physician (if applicable), or a small scouting biopsy may be performed.[16,17]

Prior to beginning the surgical procedure, the patient should be informed of the postoperative healing course. This includes a detailed explanation regarding limitations on physical activity, as well as an explanation regarding postoperative wound care. Furthermore, most patients (and many physicians) are not aware of the need to hyper-evert the wound edges postoperatively, and explaining that this is analogous to a subcutaneous splint that is present only temporarily until buried suture absorption is complete may be very helpful.[18]

LINEAR CLOSURE DESIGN AND GEOMETRY

The Apical Angle: Fusiform and Rhombus Closures

Classic descriptions of linear closure designs have highlighted the role of the apical angle as a determinant of dog-ear formation. The dogma of the 3:1 (or, more recently, 4:1) ellipse with 30-degree apical angles requires significant revision, particularly as geometrically even a 3:1 fusiform closure mathematically cannot yield 30-degree apical angles.[9,10,19]

Angulated (also known as tangent-to-circle and rhombus) closure designs, already advocated by Bennett in the 1980s, have also become more popular, as they permit narrow apical angles (in the neighborhood of 30 degrees) coupled with a relatively modest length-to-width ratio of approximately 3:1. Indeed, a 3:1 fusiform design results in a 74-degree apical angle, while a similar length-to-width ratio designed as a rhombus yields apical angles of only 37 degrees.

Another modification that blends the benefits of the rhombus design (narrower apical angles coupled with a shorter overall incision length) and the fusiform design (a gradual curving shape that is more amenable to closure without residual central gaping) is the inside rhombus–outside fusiform technique. Here, a rhombus design is first created and incised to the superficial dermis. At that point, lateral pressure on the incision (a technique that is useful in general to avoid overhanging dermis, as noted later) is used to turn the outside edges of the excision site into a fusiform shape while allowing the excised segment of skin to remain as a rhombus, albeit with overhanging dermis on its midsection (**Figures 16-2 and 16-3**).

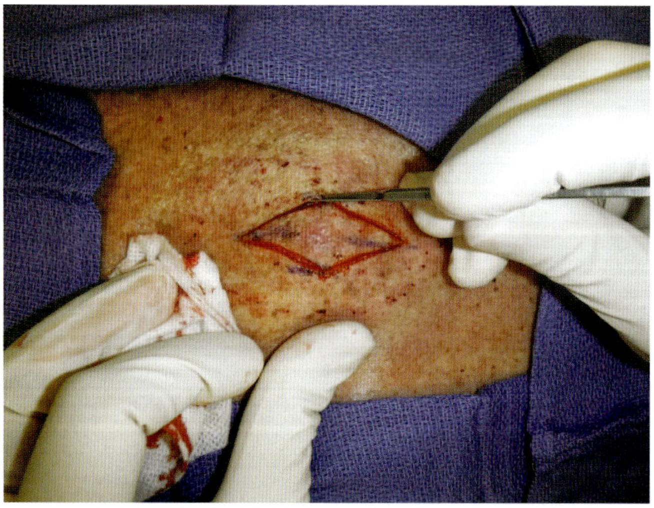

FIGURE 16-2 The inside rhombus–outside fusiform technique involves incising a rhombus shape initially and then aggressively pressing outward with the blade during subsequent passes.

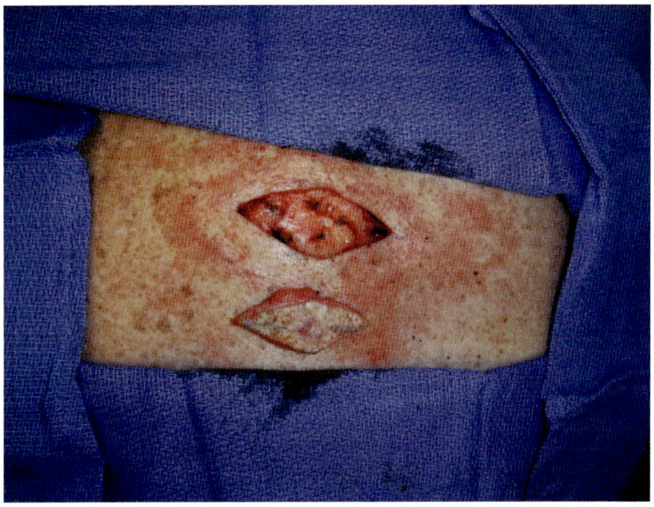

FIGURE 16-3 This leads to a defect that is shaped like a rhombus with narrow apical angles but a wound contour that appears more fusiform.

Topography

The three-dimensional topography of the wound should also be considered when designing a linear closure.[11] Indeed, restoring—or maintaining—the natural contours may be at least as important as repairing a wound with a thin scar.[20,21] For wounds over convex surfaces, designing a straight-line fusiform closure may lead to both short- and long-term undesirable outcomes. In the short term, dog-ear formation may be exaggerated over the extremes of convex surfaces, and such standing cones may not be resolved using standard dog-ear correction techniques. This is the origin of the "chasing the dog ear" phenomenon that may be seen classically when working on the forehead. In the long term, scar contraction occurs three dimensionally; when lateral scar contraction occurs over a convex surface, this may lead to a clinically apparent depressed scar.[11] Several approaches may be used to mitigate this risk, including the S-plasty.[22-25]

Cosmetic Subunits

Keeping a linear closure within a cosmetic subunit, and ideally along a cosmetic subunit boundary, may help lead to an ideal scar.[1,20] Even very large defects may be hidden very effectively as long as the suture line, however lengthy, remains along cosmetic subunit boundary lines (**Figures 16-4 to 16-6**). One of the central advantages of the linear closure design is that it results in a single fine line that is often effectively hidden. Flap repairs by their very nature result in angulated scars, and even with precise suturing techniques, these scars may remain visible, with pin-cushioning a possibility as well.[1] Angulated or geometric scars, once thought to be less obvious to the observer, may actually result in inferior cosmesis, and therefore, excisions performed with this goal in mind should probably best be avoided.

Tension Vectors

Understanding and planning for tension vectors parallel to RSTLs and perpendicular to free margins are important components

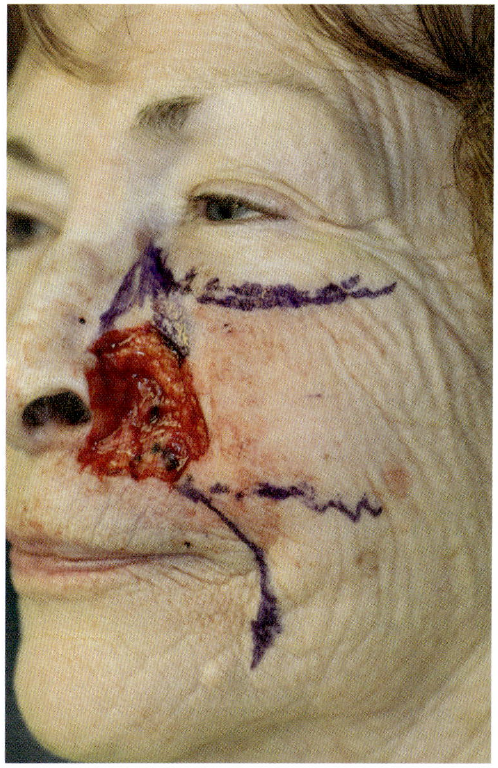

FIGURE 16-4 Moderately sized defect after Mohs micrographic surgery for basal cell carcinoma.

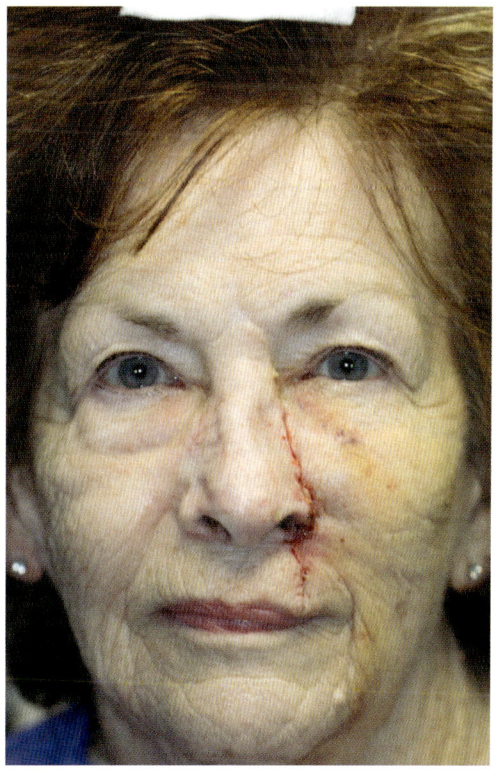

FIGURE 16-5 Largely linear repair respecting cosmetic subunit boundaries. Note the downward push on the lip caused by central axis lengthening.

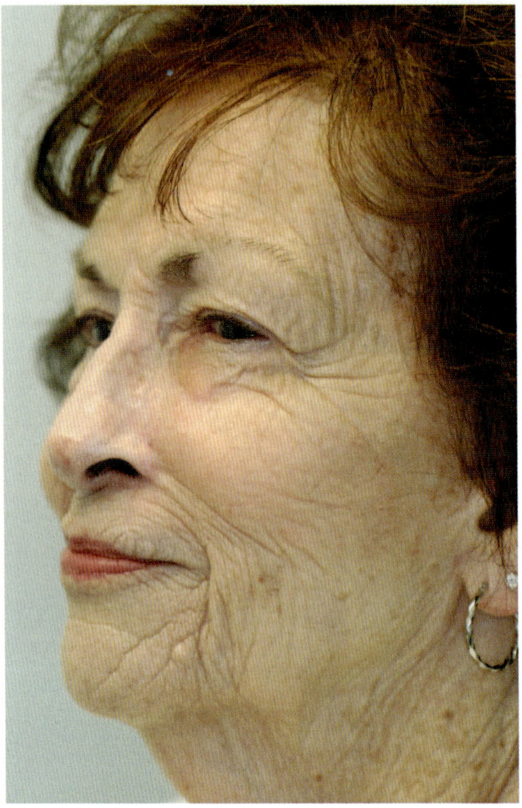

FIGURE 16-6 Six-month postoperative view showing a nearly undetectable scar and no residual push on the upper lip.

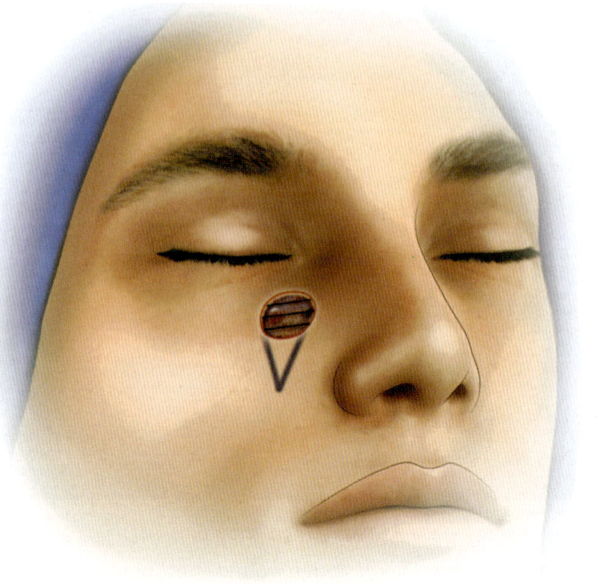

FIGURE 16-7 Orienting the tension vector of the sutures parallel to the free margin can permit closures without free-margin distortion.

of linear excisions and repairs. Preplanned ideal tension vectors are not uniformly reliable, even when designed by experienced clinicians.[26,27]

Moreover, the tension vector of the *suture line* is not necessarily the same as the tension vector of the *sutures*; since the tension vector of the sutures dictates the direction of tissue movement, this has important implications for reconstructive design (**Figure 16-7**). For example, repairs on the upper cheek or near the lower orbital rim are often closed in a linear or S-plasty fashion. To conform to RSTLs, portions of the excision may lay parallel to free margins such as the lower eyelid. By maintaining the tension vector across the sutures parallel to the free margin, an ectropion-free closure may be accomplished.

The RSTLs over extremities do not consistently conform to the angle of minimal tension under all circumstances, since range of motion has an impact on tension. For example, on the thigh, the true RSTL may be along the long axis with extension but along the transverse axis with flexion. The anticipated range of motion for the patient should therefore be addressed, and at times, using the average of the two angles—the mean RSTL—may be a helpful approach.

Moreover, conforming to the RSTL is not necessary or ideal in all cases. For repairs on the forearms, the RSTL would dictate closure along the long axis of the forearm. Yet given the convex surface of the forearm, this would also increase the risk of long-term dog-ear formation with scar contraction, necessitating a longer scar length. Transverse closures on the forearms may result in cosmetically more appealing closures given the ability to minimize the excision length. Conversely, for dorsal hand closures, the RSTL may run transversely, although closures are often best aligned along the long axis to minimize the long-term risk of lymphedema.

Free Margins

Free margins, such as the lips, eyelids, alar rims, and helical rims, are both more susceptible to distortion (given their lack of bony attachments) and more cosmetically obvious when distorted (given their prominence in facial cosmesis) than other areas on the face. Therefore, preserving the position of the free margins is of great importance. Free margins can be both pulled (as in a lower eyelid ectropion caused by downward pull on the lower lid) and pushed (as in an upper lip closure forcing a section of dog ear downward). Keep in mind the potential for central axis lengthening as a result of wound closure, as this "pushing" effect due to the differential between the length of the central axis (apex to apex) and the (longer) length of each of the outside wound edges means that postoperatively the length of the linear closure will be longer than anticipated; this may impact repairs around the lips, where tissue may be pushed, leading to an immediate postoperative puffiness that often resolves spontaneously.

Evaluation

A bright light and/or Wood's lamp is very helpful in adequately assessing clinical tumor margins. Side lighting and gently rubbing the lesion with an alcohol wipe and manipulating the skin are all helpful techniques.

Surrounding skin should be evaluated as well; this serves both to ensure that there is no local inflammation that may impede wound healing (eg, seborrheic dermatitis, angular cheilitis) and to assess whether the postexcision defect will impinge on other preexisting nevi skin lesions. For example, a banal nevus that was just lateral to a newly excised dysplastic nevus may appear directly adjacent to the scar line postoperatively. This should be noted and reviewed with the patient so that a focal area of pigmentation adjacent to the scar line is not confused with recurrence.

Scars elsewhere on the patient's body should be evaluated as well, if possible. This serves two purposes: first, it provides a baseline measure for the clinician regarding the patient's propensity to heal with hypertrophic or telangiectatic scarring. Second, it provides a reference point for patient education, so that the patient may be told what to expect in terms of healing relative to their existing scars. It may also be a significant motivator for encouraging adequate postoperative compliance.

Determining Excision Size

Clinicians perform linear excisions for many indications, including the treatment of nonmelanoma skin cancers, dysplastic nevi, banal or congenital nevi, cysts, and lipomas. For both melanoma and nonmelanoma skin cancer, various studies have examined appropriate surgical margins.[28-37]

With time and experience, clinicians may trend toward smaller excisions with tighter margins for most low-risk nonmelanoma skin cancers, although maintaining wide and deep margins for melanoma resection remains of critical importance to minimize the risk of potentially catastrophic recurrence.

Benign nevi may be excised en bloc or in segmental or staged fashion. Benign subcutaneous tumors may be excised via modestly sized access incisions and then dissected out subcutaneously to minimize the size of the postoperative scar.

LEARNING LINEAR REPAIRS

Several studies have evaluated techniques to both learn and assess surgical competency and technique.[38] Objectively assessing surgical skills is critical, as novice clinicians tend to significantly and consistently overestimate their competence.[39] Breaking down surgical excisions and repairs into their component parts, and focusing on particular quality metrics and checkpoints at each step, may be very helpful when learning these techniques.[40,41]

Of all skills, eversion is least often performed successfully by applicants to dermatologic surgery fellowship programs, suggesting that further focus on meticulous everting suturing techniques, including the set-back suture and buried vertical mattress suture, may be of significant didactic value.[42-44] While one study questioned the value of eversion per se as a contributor to postoperative cosmesis, it may represent a surrogate end point for meticulous wound edge approximation and tension reduction.[45]

OPERATIVE TECHNIQUE

The excision with linear repair may be broken down into several component parts.

Preparation

After the informed consent process and preoperative consultation are completed, the skin is prepped and infused with local anesthetic (see Chapter 9). A sterile skin prep is generally performed for dermatologic surgery excisions, although data have suggested that the use of sterile gloves for brief and straightforward procedures may not confer a reduced risk of postoperative wound infection.[46-48] Common surgical scrubs include chlorhexidine and povidone-iodine; the former confers the advantage of rapid onset of action even while wet,[49] although chlorhexidine should be kept out of the eyes and ears due to risks of keratitis and ototoxicity, respectively.[50]

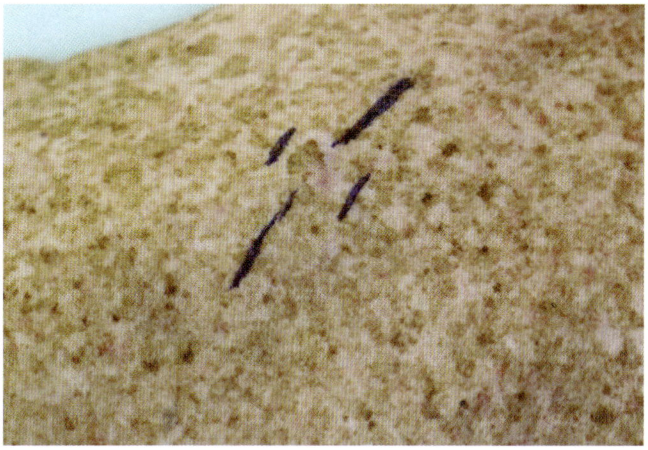

FIGURE 16-8 Minimal markings that outline the closure vector, closure extent, and margins around the lesion to be excised can be used. This provides key information to the assistant for local anesthesia infiltration while using a minimal amount of ink that may later need to be removed.

Marking

Skin marking is important when preparing for linear closures; many clinicians draw a fusiform (or rhombus) shape to delineate the planned excision. Another approach that minimizes the amount of tissue marking used is to draw only minimal markings that outline the closure vector, closure extent, and margins around the lesion to be excised (**Figure 16-8**).

Regardless of the planned defect shape, it may be useful to mark additional anatomic landmarks as well. On the face, cosmetic subunit boundaries may be marked prior to local anesthetic infiltration (**Figure 16-9**). On the extremities, particularly when more than one vector appears a priori appropriate, both vectors may be drawn out and prioritized (**Figure 16-10**). Finally, when working around tattoos or near large superficial vessels, pacemaker leads, or other structures that should be avoided, these may be marked as well in a clear and consistent manner (**Figure 16-11**).

Most clinicians use felt-tipped surgical marking pens given their ease of use and low cost; patients should be told that any residual ink may be removed with alcohol. Other options include gentian violet, specialized white tissue markers, and white eyeliner markers.

Local Anesthetic Infiltration

Local anesthesia revolutionized the field of surgery in the late 19th century.[51] Patients judge the quality of their clinician based largely on the painlessness of the procedure and the absence of long-term scarring. Particularly given its impact on patient

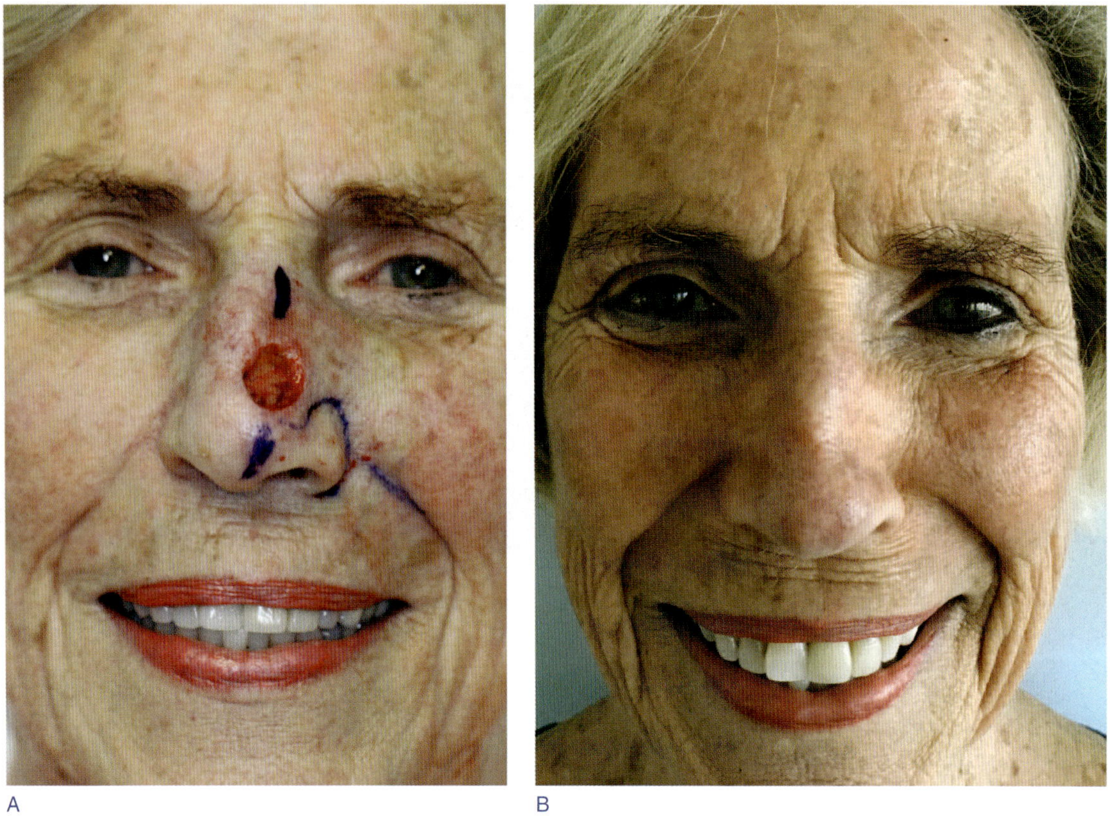

FIGURE 16-9 Cosmetic subunit boundaries may be marked prior to local anesthetic infiltration. **A.** Preoperative photograph. **B.** Postoperative photograph.

anxiety, adequate and comprehensive local anesthetic infiltration is a prerequisite for successful dermatologic surgery. For smaller cases, direct infiltration is effective. For larger surgical sites, a ring block, nerve block (if possible), or tumescent anesthesia may be considered. For a detailed discussion of local anesthetic infiltration, see Chapter 9.

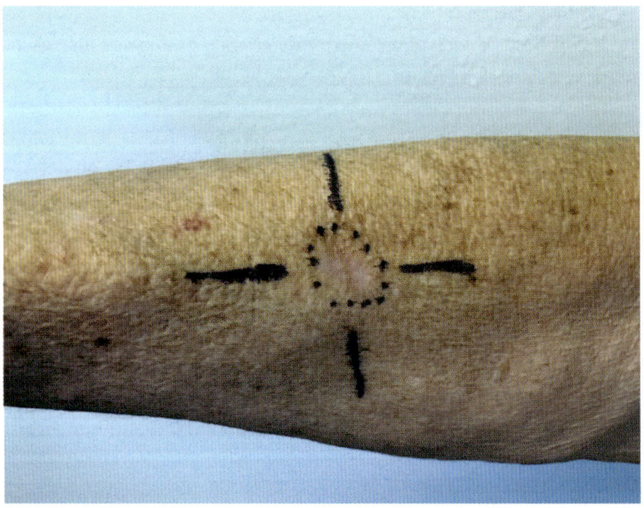

FIGURE 16-10 Multiple tension vectors may be drawn out if needed, and sufficient local anesthetic may be infused to use either vector. A circular excision may be performed, and the lowest tension vector can then be chosen.

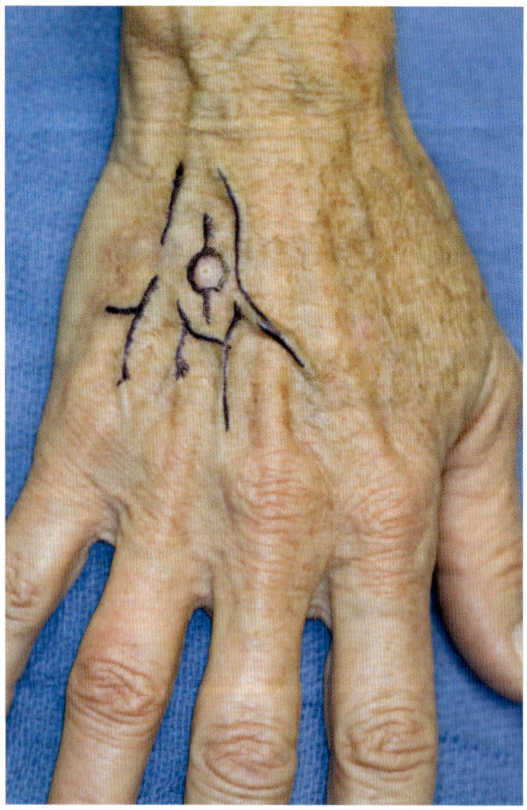

FIGURE 16-11 Marking structures to be avoided in a clear manner is a helpful preoperative step.

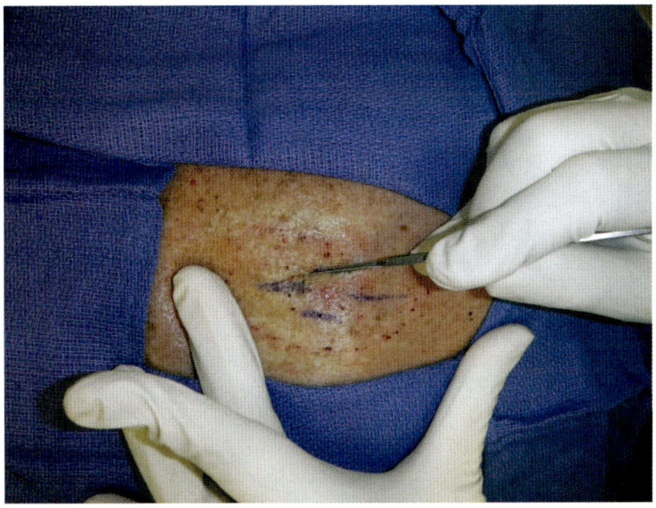

FIGURE 16-12 An incision is made along the marked axis with the blade held perpendicular to the skin or with a slight outward bevel.

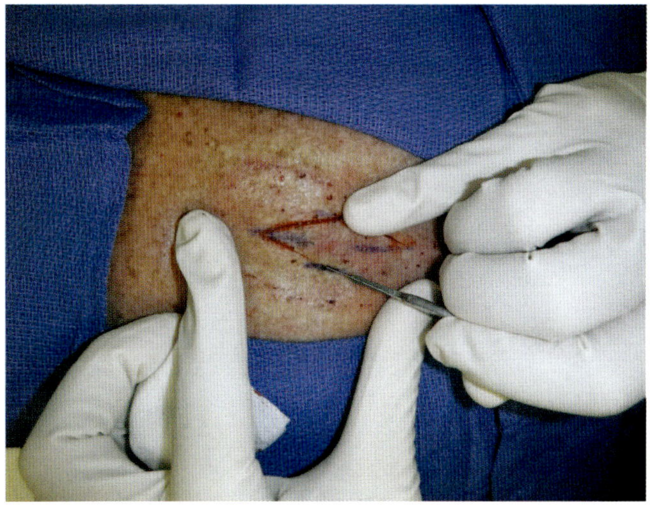

FIGURE 16-13 The incision is made to a uniform depth including the apices.

Incision

After sterile skin preparation and draping, the lesion is excised. The ideal scalpel entry angle for a fusiform excision has been classically described as 90 degrees to the skin[41]; others have suggested a 10-degree outward (reverse) bevel, while more recently it was suggested that a more dramatic reverse bevel may be desirable.[52,53] In practice, when working on facial skin or on the forearms, true perpendicular incision angles work well; on the back, particularly in younger patients with a robust dermis, a reverse bevel may be advantageous and minimize the need for removal of any residual overhanging dermis (**Figures 16-12 to 16-20**). This is particularly an issue because after the initial release of epidermis and superficial dermis, there is a tendency for the outside (nonincised) edges of the excision to spring laterally (**Figure 16-21**).[41] Stabilizing the surrounding skin during scalpel entry and during incision creation may help maintain a consistent angle.

Most standard descriptions call for the tip of the scalpel to be used initially, followed by the belly of the blade, which is ostensibly sharper than the tip. While common surgical folklore, this is more critical when using the larger #10 blade than when using the #15 blade that is typically used in dermatologic surgery. Similarly, references to holding the surgical blade like a violin bow are largely a result of translating general surgery techniques to dermatologic surgery. The violin bow technique is classically described when using a #10 blade, which is significantly larger than the #15 blade. Similarly, some textbooks historically advocated that a single pass of the scalpel should incise through epidermis and dermis and through to the subcutaneous fat; in practice, this is both unnecessary and difficult to achieve unless excessive force is used. Therefore, the surgical blade may be held like a pencil, and careful and consistent traction may be used to permit a smooth incision through the dermis, although multiple passes, particularly when working on the back, are perfectly acceptable.

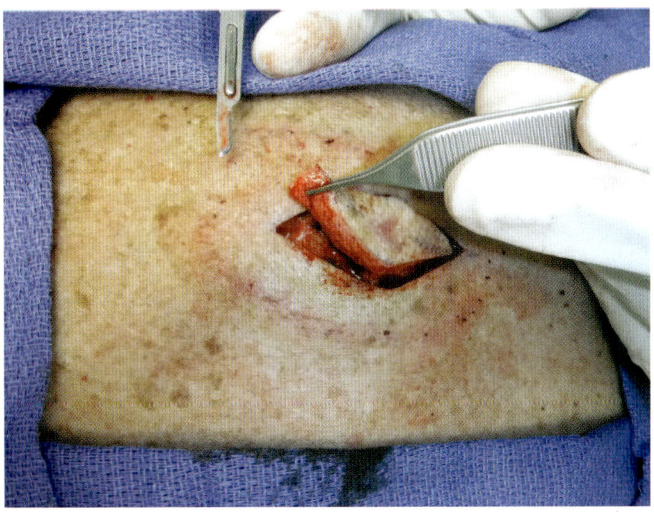

FIGURE 16-14 The specimen is incised at a uniform depth on its undersurface.

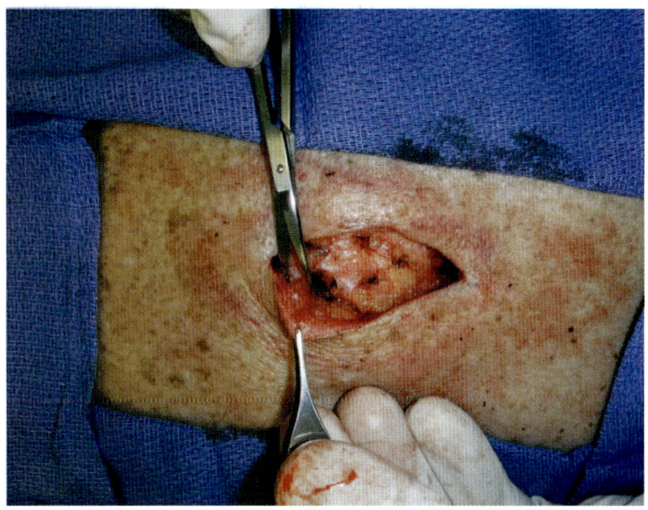

FIGURE 16-15 Sharp undermining is performed with surgical scissors or a scalpel.

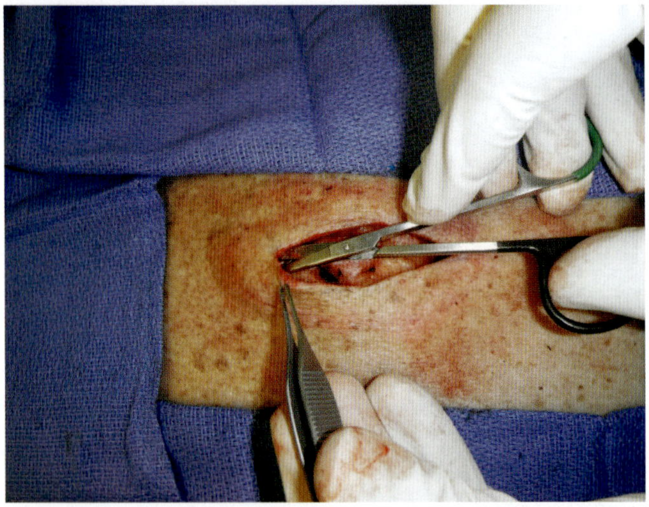

FIGURE 16-16 The apices are undermined extensively.

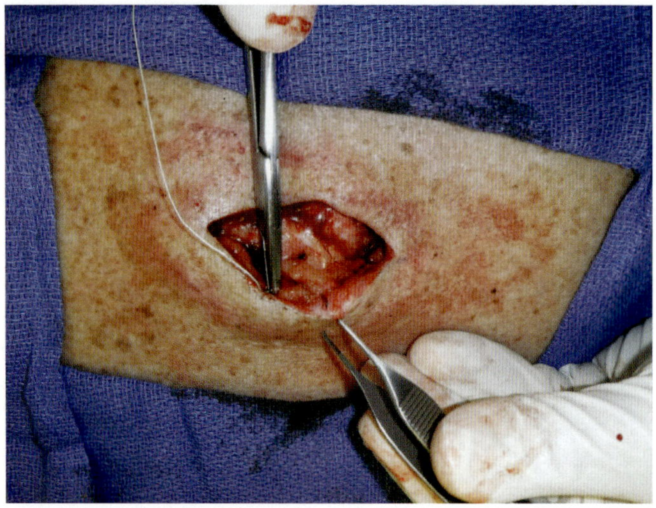

FIGURE 16-17 A fascial plication suture is placed to reduce tension and decrease the apical angle further.

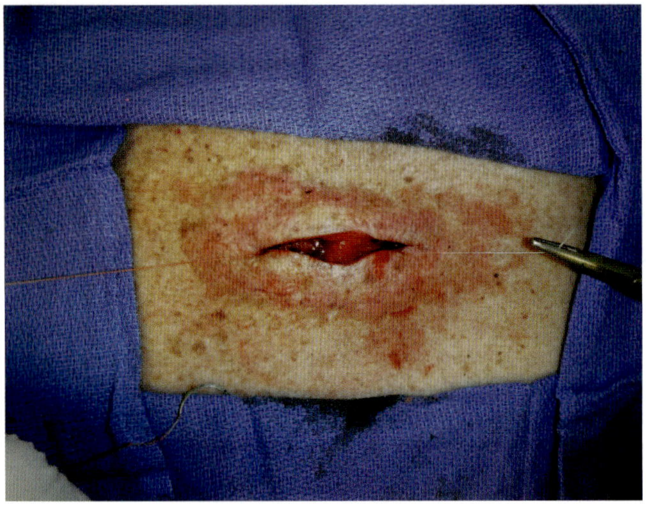

FIGURE 16-18 Tightening this suture leads to narrower apical angles.

Tissue Release

Uniform excision and tissue release is very helpful in elegantly excising tissue and preparing the nascent wound for reconstruction. The tendency to bevel the excision inward at the apices may result in the rowboat deformity, which increases the risk of dog-ear formation unless the excess tissue is separately removed prior to reconstruction. Therefore, excision to a uniform depth and with a uniform angle is desirable. A well-planned excision saves significant reconstructive time by obviating the need to trim overhanging dermis prior to wound closure.

Some authors have referred to the "lagging fat" phenomenon, where the epidermis and dermis tend to retract away from the center of the wound after tissue release, but deep fat—without lateral fibrous attachments—lags centrally and presents a physical impediment to wound closure.[41] In clinical practice, there is

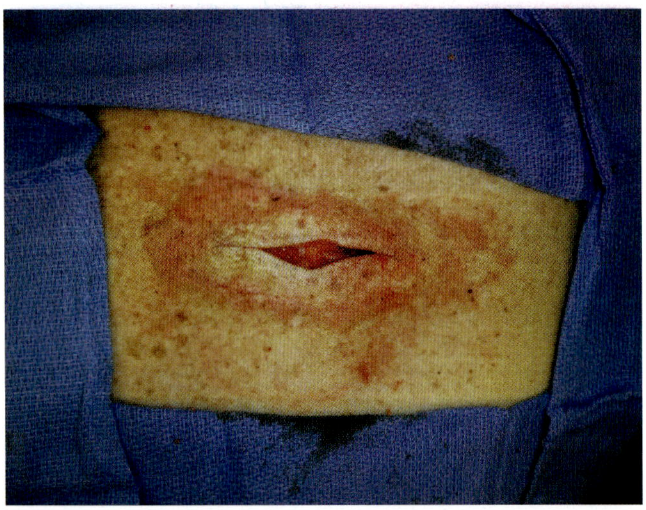

FIGURE 16-19 After a single fascial plication suture is placed, the bulk of the wound is closed and tension is reduced.

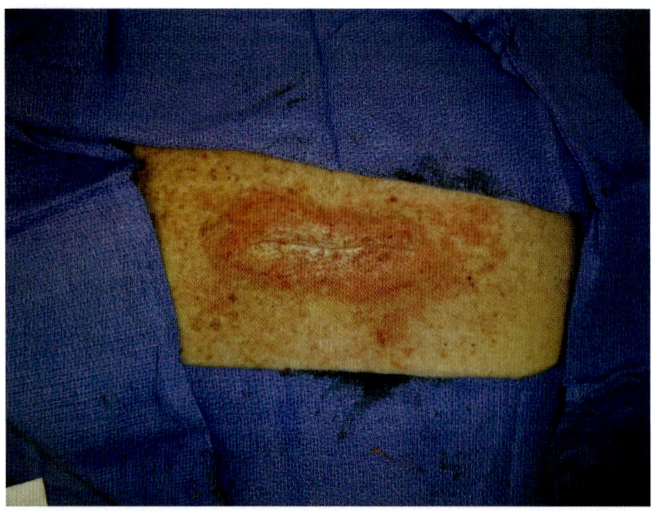

FIGURE 16-20 Set-back or buried vertical mattress sutures are then placed, allowing the wound edges to drape together under minimal tension.

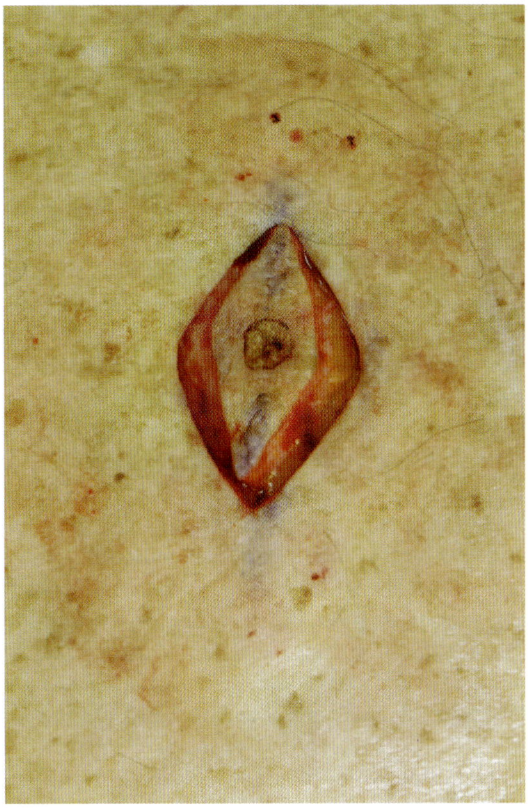

FIGURE 16-21 After incising and tissue release, there is a tendency for the lateral edges of the wound to spring back from the central defect.

often a significant lagging *dermis* phenomenon, where even with a 90-degree perpendicular incision a significant amount of reticular dermis may protrude centrally, particularly in areas with a more robust dermis such as the back. This may be obviated by either excising tissue with a reverse bevel or, after the fact, trimming the lagging dermis (**Figure 16-22**). Importantly, no degree of suturing technique–based correction can solve this physical problem

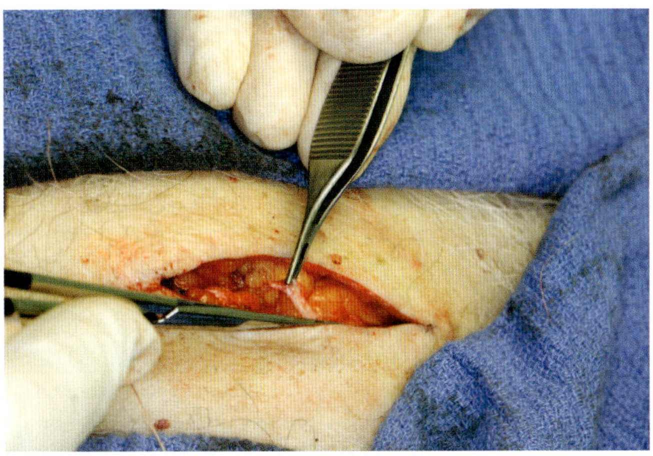

FIGURE 16-22 Trimming any lagging dermis is a critical step that must always take place if dermis is present medial to the epidermal edge.

definitively, and investing a few moments in assuring that the wound edges are uniform prior to closure is time well spent.

Undermining

Undermining serves several purposes. First, it permits closure of large (based on defect size) or tight (based on lack of elasticity, such as on the scalp and lower leg) defects under tension that would otherwise not close easily. Second, it reduces tension across moderately tense defects by recruiting adjacent skin for the closure. Third, it frees up underlying attachments that would otherwise lead to both lateral and downward pull, potentially leading to wound inversion.

It is important to undermine the apices as well as the lateral portions of the wound.[11] In fact, wide apical undermining may in some cases be *more* important than lateral undermining given its potential to partially mitigate dog-ear formation.

Disadvantages of undermining include its potential impact on blood supply, as wide undermining essentially creates a small local random pattern flap.[54] Undermining also increases intraoperative morbidity by creating a potential space for hematoma or seroma formation.

The plane of undermining has a profound effect on surgical outcomes, as it may affect the risk of bleeding (and the resulting need for more aggressive and time-consuming hemostatic measures), as well as the risk of nerve damage. Remaining in a uniform plane is important and may be aided by retracting back the skin with uniform pressure.

Novices often prefer to err on the side of remaining superficial and have a tendency to attempt all undermining at the level of the superficial fat, fearing an increased risk of bleeding or nerve compromise with deeper undermining. Understanding the vascular supply of various anatomic areas may be helpful, as overly superficial undermining may also increase the risk of damage to perforating vessels supplying the dermal plexus, decreasing vascular supply, and increasing the risk of necrosis. Deeper undermining may permit the reapproximation of deeper, well-vascularized structures rather than only the relatively thin dermis and epidermis. This phenomenon may be seen when performing a linear closure on the nose, where deep submuscular undermining affords a robust vascular supply to the advancing wound edge, while superficial subdermal undermining leads to a significant risk of postoperative necrosis.

When undermining, keep in mind that a scalpel and scissors work from opposite directions: the scalpel cuts from the distal point to the more proximal point, while scissors begin cutting proximally and extend the incision distally.

One recent study evaluated the relative merits of wide undermining and imbrication.[54] In this porcine study, both undermining and imbrication were studied to assess their effect on wound tension and perfusion. Not surprisingly, both techniques led to decreased tension across the surface of the wound, and both led to a marginal drop in wound perfusion, although imbrication was associated with a slightly more dramatic decrease in perfusion. Notably, the experimental wounds were undermined a full 4 cm, significantly beyond the point that most surgical wounds are undermined in dermatologic surgery.

When feasible, undermining should be minimized in patients on thrombolytic agents such as aspirin or in those with very ruddy skin who are prone to numerous small wound-edge bleeding vessels.

Pragmatically, undermining is best performed under direct visualization. Sharp dissection may lead to less tissue trauma as it avoids shearing forces that may be seen with blunt or spread undermining. While many clinicians prefer blunt-tipped surgical scissors, such as blepharoplasty scissors (for almost all cases) or Metzenbaum, facelift, or Mayo scissors (for larger cases), on a practical level, sharp undermining may also be performed with a scalpel or using electrocautery on either a pure cut or blend setting. Radiofrequency cutting devices, as well as newer cold plasma devices, may also be used. These confer the advantages of reduced thermal injury, although they are also associated with a significantly increased cost that makes them impractical for most linear excisions and repairs.

Hemostasis

Achieving adequate hemostasis prior to wound closure is an absolute requirement. Experience is very helpful in distinguishing between low-level wound-edge oozing that may resolve with suturing and pressure and true bleeding that should be addressed with aggressive hemostatic measures. There is a delicate balance between mitigating the risk of hematoma formation and overly dessicating wound edges that may impair healing over the long and short term. Larger vessels should be clamped and ligated, rather than treated with electrosurgical approaches, in order to minimize the risk of bleeding in the acute postoperative period. Bipolar forceps may be useful, although they are not necessary.

Bleeding should always be addressed under direct visualization, and skin hooks—usually used as a pair to tent up the overlying epidermis and dermis—may be very helpful for this purpose.

Suturing

Suturing techniques play a critical role in the efficiency of surgical reconstruction, and technique choice may also impact the design of linear closures. A detailed discussion of suturing techniques and their variations may be found in Chapter 10.

Historically, most linear closures relied on a bilayered closure approach, with sutures placed in the dermis for tension relief and transepidermally for wound edge approximation. This paradigm has shifted over the past few years, with the realization that recruiting deeper tissue planes may have a profound effect on wound strength and cosmesis.[55,56]

Fascial plication is one of the most useful techniques for linear closures, as it confers several advantages simultaneously.[55] First, it leads to significant tension reduction over the wound surface by shifting tension to the deep fascia. Second, it decreases the amount of undermining needed to permit effective closure, theoretically improving vascular supply to the undersurface of the advancing wound edges and reducing the risk of potential space formation that may increase the risk of hematoma formation. Finally, fascial plication has a significant effect on wound geometry, as a single fascial plication suture shifts a wound from a 3:1 fusiform shape to a 6:1 ratio and decreases the apical angles significantly.[55]

Fascial plication sutures need not be used for all linear closures. This technique is most appropriate for areas under significant tension or for large excisions where minimizing the postoperative wound length is desirable. On the face, recruiting the superficial muscular aponeurotic system (SMAS) may be very helpful. When designing the closure of a round defect, the fascial plication suture should be placed prior to removing the dog ears. The risks of fascial plication sutures include possible pain, a theoretically increased infection risk (since the fascial envelope has been pierced by suture), and a theoretical risk of vascular compromise through inadvertent pressure-induced ligation of perforating vessels. In practice, these complications are infrequent, although patients may experience transient pain during needle entry and immediately after the fascial plication suture is tied. If pain persists for more than 5 minutes, the suture should be removed.

Buried dermal sutures are the cornerstone of linear repairs. Two central suturing techniques are useful, the buried vertical mattress suture and the set-back dermal suture. The former yields significant wound edge eversion and epidermal approximation, while the latter is easier to execute. A randomized controlled trial has suggested that the set-back suture leads to cosmetically more appealing scarring than the buried vertical mattress suture.[42] Its ease of use is a significant advantage as well, particularly as effective wound edge eversion is one of the most challenging (and clinically critical) components of the linear excision and closure.[38]

Set-back dermal sutures result in marked wound edge eversion, although this can be adjusted based on how set back each bite is taken from the incised wound edge. For a detailed discussion of step-by-step suture placement, see Chapter 10.

Although many manuscripts and chapters addressing linear closures advocate the placement of a key suture in the center of the wound followed by closure using the rule of halves, in practice, this may be less desirable than starting at one edge of the wound—typically the edge most distant from the clinician—and moving proximally. The latter technique allows tension to be gradually relieved, minimizing the tension across any single suture. This permits tissue creep to gradually take place over the course of the closure.

The set-back or buried vertical mattress sutures may be placed closer together in the center of the wound, where tensile forces are greatest. After placement of a full row of buried sutures, the wound edges should be well everted and ideally drape together under no tension. With assiduous attention to detail, this layer of sutures may lead to ideal wound edge approximation, obviating the need for transepidermal sutures.

If transepidermal sutures are placed, they may be performed in a simple interrupted or running fashion. Ideally, there should be no tension across the wound surface after deep suture placement, and therefore, running sutures may be appropriate. Alternatively, some mild depth correction may be needed, and in such cases, depth-correcting simple interrupted suture can be used. Running horizontal mattress sutures, often with intermittent simple loops, may also be helpful for yielding excellent wound eversion and avoiding suture material crossing over the incised wound edge.[57,58] Running subcuticular sutures may be used as well, although in the context of well-placed buried sutures, they often confer only minimal advantage while introducing additional foreign body material across the wound.

Most clinicians use reverse-cutting needles; these confer several advantages and may theoretically decrease the risk of suture

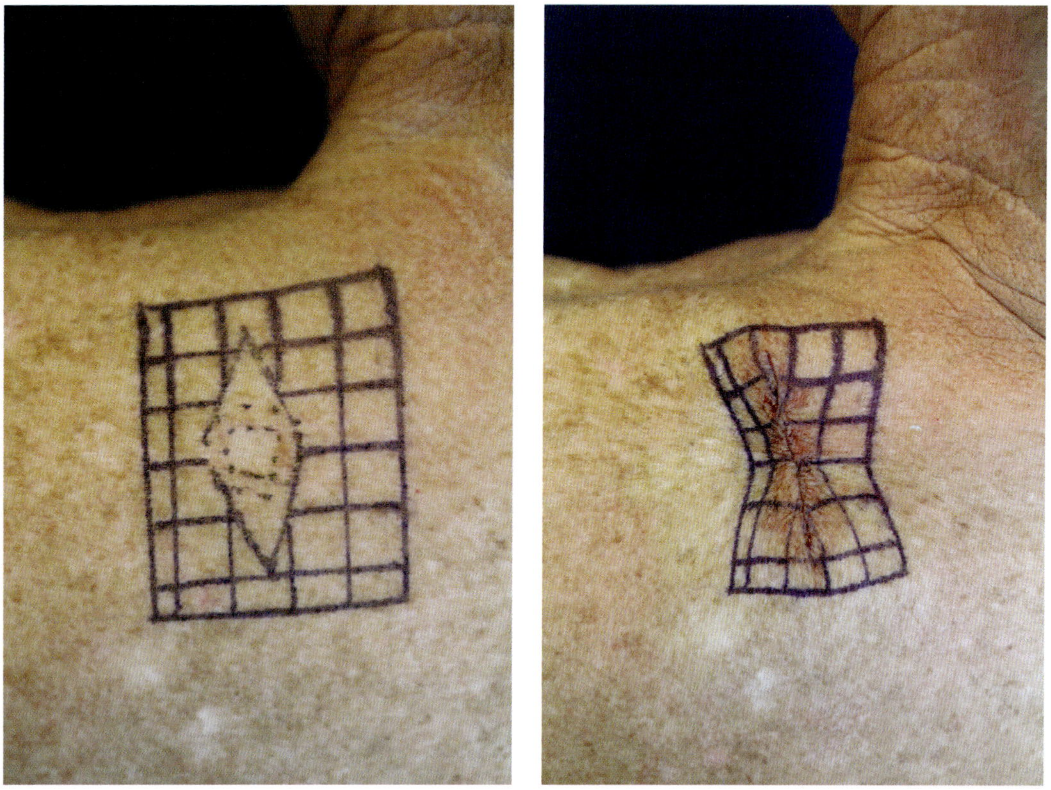

FIGURE 16-23 In this elliptical excision, the movement at the midpoint of the closure is pure advancement, although the apices rotate slightly as illustrated by the curvature of the lines. This rotational force contributes to tissue puckering and dog-ear formation.

material tear-through since the cut edges are on the opposite sides of the vector of maximal postoperative tension.

Dog-Ear Repair

The geometric property that contributes most significantly to the formation (or prevention) of dog ears is the length of the wound edges relative to wound width.[2] If one visualizes the long axis of the excision as the line that connects the apices, it becomes clear that the sides of the wound are invariably longer than this axis. As closure approaches the apices of the wound, the movement of the edges becomes more rotational, pivoting at the point of the apex and resulting in compression of the periapical skin (**Figure 16-23**). When this rotational movement and compression overcome the skin's elastic qualities, a dog ear forms.[1,3,5] Increasing the apical angle increases the rotational movement, subsequently increasing the risk of redundant tissue gathering at the apex.[3]

In addition to the length-to-width ratio, the edges of the fusiform excision should be symmetric to prevent large or unevenly positioned dog ears; if the arcs are unequal, excess tissue will be gathered on the longer side and not be uniformly positioned at the apex. Correction of an uneven dog ear such as this will not result in a linear closure, but will create a curved or angled scar (crescentic repair). This may be advantageous to the skillful clinician when trying to place a scar within natural skin lines or along favorable lines of tension.

Because each layer of skin is anchored to the structures beneath it, undermining is an essential method for augmenting the skin's functional pliability. As an ellipse is closed, the edges pull on the underlying tissue, compressing the tissue at the base of the wound and causing vertical displacement of the wound edges.[1,2] Undermining can release the wound edges from the anchored tissues beneath, mitigating the compression by allowing lateral dissipation of pressure as the skin is stretched.[2,5]

In addition to wound geometry and tissue elasticity, the contour of the surgical site may also affect the closure and formation of dog ears. Because the geometric principles of lines and angles differ between planar and curved surfaces,[6] the prudent clinician must account for the curvature of the skin when preparing an excision. Closure on a convex surface is more likely to produce dog ears, whereas concave surfaces are more forgiving.[1,2]

High-tension repairs, such as those on the lower leg, may also lead to changes that mimic true dog ears. When an ellipse is closed in an area under significant tension, such as the lower leg or scalp, the tension on the skin may cause central wound depression. This depression sometimes causes the tips of the ellipse to appear raised, simulating dog ears; however, this is illusionary due to the central depression. The tips are not truly redundant and generally resolve without intervention.

Small dog ears in cosmetically less sensitive areas can sometimes be addressed through the "rule of halves." This approach effectively divides a single noticeable region of puckering into multiple smaller puckered areas, each with a much smaller degree of excess, that ultimately become clinically insignificant. A suture is placed in the center of the area of concern (halving it), and

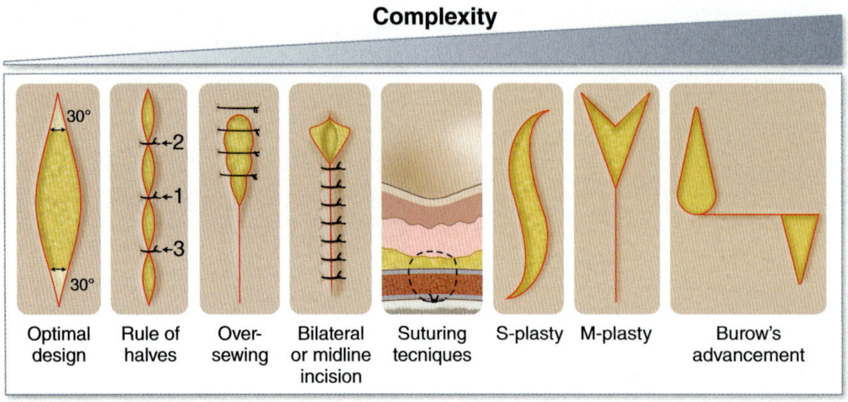

FIGURE 16-24 Techniques for dog-ear repair.

subsequent sutures progressively halve each remaining segment. Alternatively, particularly when working in areas with fairly thin skin, one can "oversew" the dog ear by suturing over it and effectively tacking it down to deeper structures. If these approaches are not sufficient, techniques that excise the excess tissue by lengthening the scar along the wound's long axis are generally among the simplest and most frequently used methods of dog-ear revision (**Figure 16-24**).

BILATERAL-INCISION EXTENSION TECHNIQUE

This approach is very straightforward and can be used in the majority of cases. This is the primary method of dog-ear removal for the authors of this chapter. With practice, this technique is an efficient and elegant way to repair dog-ear redundancies.

1. Using forceps or a skin hook, grasp the apex of the dog ear and pull lightly in an outward direction until just taut. This maneuver will produce a triangular shape to the cone of tissue, with its base aligned with the original wound incision.
2. With the skin tented, it is important to note the extent of the redundancy, as this will indicate how much wound extension is required. This is denoted by the tip of the cotton-tipped applicator in the figure (**Figure 16-25A**).
3. While lightly gripping the apex of the cone, drape the redundancy to one side. Then make an incision connecting the point of extension (step 2) with the surgical wound. Particular attention should be paid to creating an incision that aligns with the existing incision with little to no angle change (**Figure 16-25B**).
4. Elevate the redundancy and undermine the flap of skin. This can be accomplished with a scalpel or scissors (**Figure 16-25C**).
5. Once undermined, drape the redundant skin across the long axis of the original wound. Incise the remaining side of the redundancy along the long axis to release the tissue. Again, particular attention should be paid to creating an incision that aligns with the existing wound with little to no angle change (**Figure 16-25D**).
6. Finally, closure of the wound should continue with a standard linear closure technique (**Figure 16-25E**).

MIDLINE-INCISION EXTENSION TECHNIQUE

This technique has the same result as the bilateral-incision method, using a slightly different approach.

1. Using forceps or a skin hook, grasp the apex of the dog ear and pull lightly outward until just taut. This maneuver will produce a triangular shape to the cone of tissue, with its base aligned with the original wound incision.
2. With the skin tented, it is important to note the extent of the redundancy, as this will indicate how much wound extension is required, as is denoted by the tip of the cotton-tipped applicator (**Figure 16-26A**).
3. While lightly gripping the apex, incise the redundant tissue directly along the long axis of the wound with a scalpel or scissors, effectively bisecting the cone into two equal triangular flaps. If working with very thin skin, the clinician may find using scissors an easier approach (**Figure 16-26B**).
4. Undermine beneath the dog ear to release the flaps of skin (**Figure 16-26C**).
5. With forceps or a hook, grasp one of the flaps and drape it across the incision line (the long axis) (**Figure 16-26D**).
6. Remove this flap by excising it at its base along the incision line. Be careful not to impose excessive traction when pulling the flap across the wound, as this will result in excision of excess tissue (**Figure 16-26D**).
7. After the first triangular flap is removed, repeat the process with the opposite flap (**Figure 16-26E**).
8. Finally, closure of the wound should continue with a standard linear closure technique (**Figure 16-26F**).

M-PLASTY MODIFICATION

This technique may be employed when lengthening of the scar would yield a suboptimal result, commonly encountered when performing surgery around certain anatomic sites, such as the eye or lip, or when the resultant lengthened scar would cross a cosmetic junction. M-plasty is used to shorten the final scar length, and additionally removes less normal skin.[9]

1. Using forceps or a skin hook, grasp the apex of the cutaneous cone and pull lightly in an outward direction. This maneuver will produce a triangular shape to the cone, with its base aligned with the original wound incision.
2. With the skin tented, note the extent of the redundancy. It may be useful to outline the base of the cone. Mark a point on each side of the cone's base that is approximately two-thirds the length of the redundancy (**Figure 16-27A**).
3. Incise along the base of the redundancy, connecting one of the points to the existing wound. Repeat this step with the second point on the other side (**Figure 16-27B**). This will result in a flap of skin that resembles a rectangle, which is only attached along one of its long edges (**Figure 16-27C**). Note that the apex of the original wound now terminates at the midpoint of the flap's free edge.
4. Undermine flap of skin so it can be laid flat on the skin surface.
5. With scissors or a scalpel, excise a portion of the flap by cutting from the midpoint to the point previously marked in step 2. Then repeat on the other side (**Figures 16-27D and 16-27E**).
6. For good approximation of the tip of the M-plasty, a tip-stitch (half-buried horizontal mattress suture) is often used. Suturing of the remainder of the M-plasty is performed in a conventional fashion (**Figure 16-27F**).

VARIATIONS

S-Plasty

The S-plasty variation of the linear repair is useful for closures over convex surfaces. Given the tendency for linear closures to contract during wound healing, straight-line repairs may lead to scar contraction over convexities that is particularly visible as scar maturation occurs. By lengthening the overall scar length—and particularly extending the scar length over the convexities—the S-plasty may result in better long-term cosmesis for these repairs.

Some authors have advocated the S-plasty as a technique for all closures, arguing that the extended scar leading to decreased lateral contraction may ultimately provide a superior cosmetic results even in the absence of a convexity.[59] This theoretical benefit should be weighed against the desire for a straight-line linear repair. Some variations of the S-plasty use shortened or differentially angled arms to reduce the overall incision length or rely on suturing techniques to add curvature to an otherwise linear repair.[10]

S-PLASTY MODIFICATION

This technique permits redirection of the closure line of redundant tissue. This is particularly helpful on convex surfaces, such as the extremities, the chin, and the ear, which often require length-to-width ratios much greater than the standard 3:1 to reduce the apical angle for optimal closure. Redirection of the excision has two primary benefits: (1) it guides the suture line from the convex surface onto a flatter surface, thereby mitigating the risk of "chasing" the dog ear on the convexity and decreasing the required suture line length; and (2) as scars tend to depress on convex surfaces, S-plasty redirects the depressive forces onto a flat plane, thereby decreasing the formation of such central indentation.

To perform this procedure (**Figure 16-28**), the clinician will follow many of the same steps as the bilateral-incision technique. However, rather than bisecting the cone to a point aligned with the wound's axis, a different point is selected either to the right or left of it. The further right or left the clinician goes, the more dramatic the S-plasty. Curvilinear lines are created and the edges are undermined as needed. As one edge will be longer than the other, the rule of halves should be used when suturing to decrease the risk of forming another dog ear: the first suture approximates the midpoint of the long arc to the midpoint of the short arc, essentially halving the wound (**Figure 16-28D**); the second suture then approximates the midpoints of the subsequent arcs, and so on and so forth the strategy continues, successively halving the wound each time until closure is complete. The rule of halves allows the excess tissue of the longer wound edge to be evenly distributed along the entirety of the wound's closure, minimizing or eliminating the need for redundancy removal.

When orienting the S-plasty, the curved tips of the repair should follow the RSTLs as much as possible. All S-plasty repairs should be conceptually repaired using the rule of halves, which in practice requires that all sutures are placed perpendicular to the excision (**Figures 16-29 to 16-32**). If this is not done, a defect incised as an S-plasty may ultimately appear as a longer straight line.

Eccentric Parallelogram

The eccentric parallelogram has been advocated as an alternative to both the fusiform and rhombus repair.[10] This approach provides some geometrical advantages, although like the S-plasty, it results in a curved final scar. A variation of the eccentric parallelogram may also be performed using a triangle-square-triangle technique that may result in a straight-line closure.

Crescentic Excisions

Since a goal of all surgical repairs is to hide the postoperative scar as effectively as possible, some scars may be purposely curved for optimal cosmesis, such as those in the nasolabial and melolabial folds. When designing a crescentic excision, the curved side will dictate the final angle of the repair as long as suturing is performed using the rule of halves.

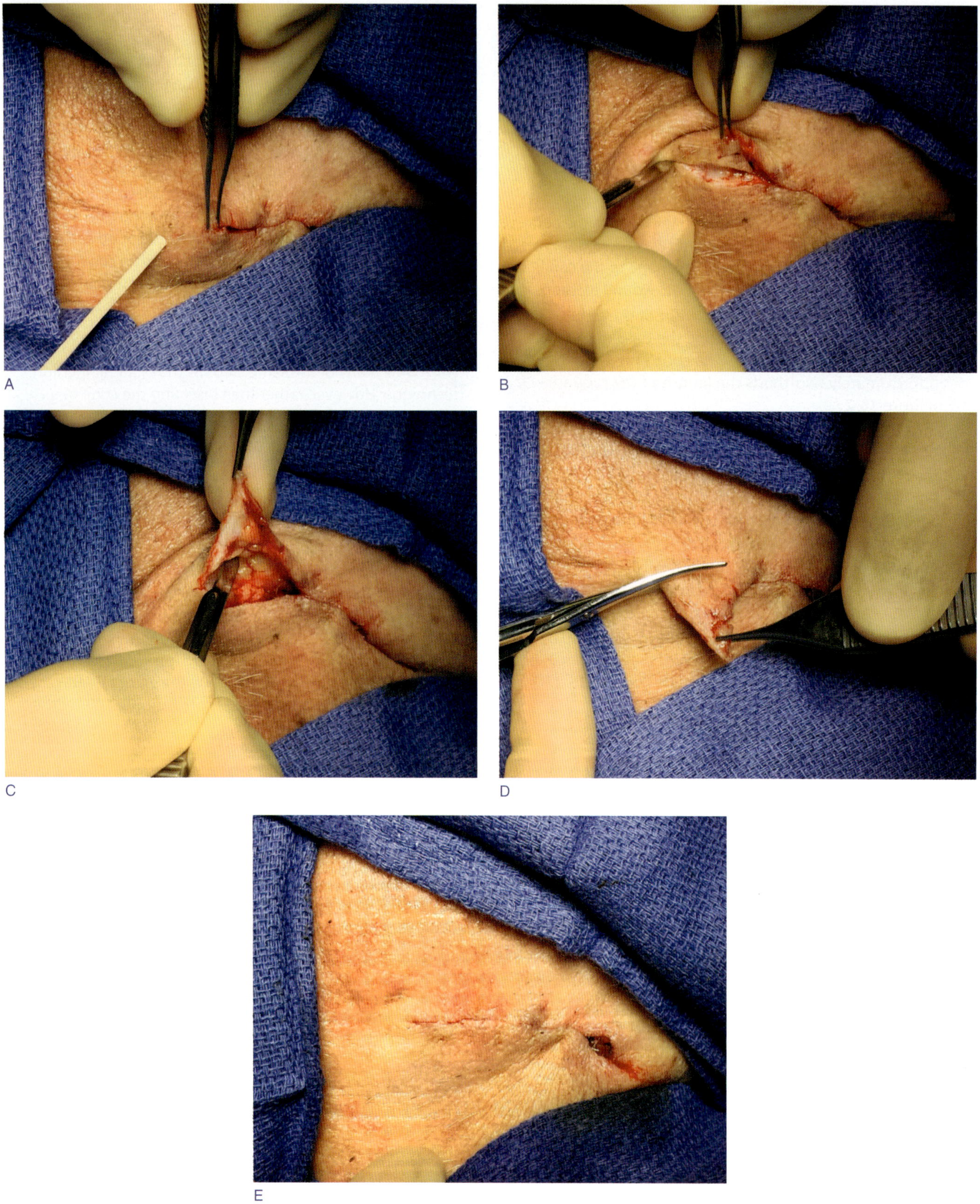

FIGURE 16-25 The bilateral-incision extension technique. First, (**A**) the dog ear is gently elevated with surgical forceps, and its extent is noted (here by the presence of the cotton-tipped applicator). Then, (**B**) the dog ear is gently pulled laterally, and an incision is made in line with the already existing excision line. This nascent flap of skin is then undermined (**C**). The dog ear is then pulled in the opposite direction (**D**), and another incision is made. This technique results in dog-ear removal and the extension of the original excision line (**E**).

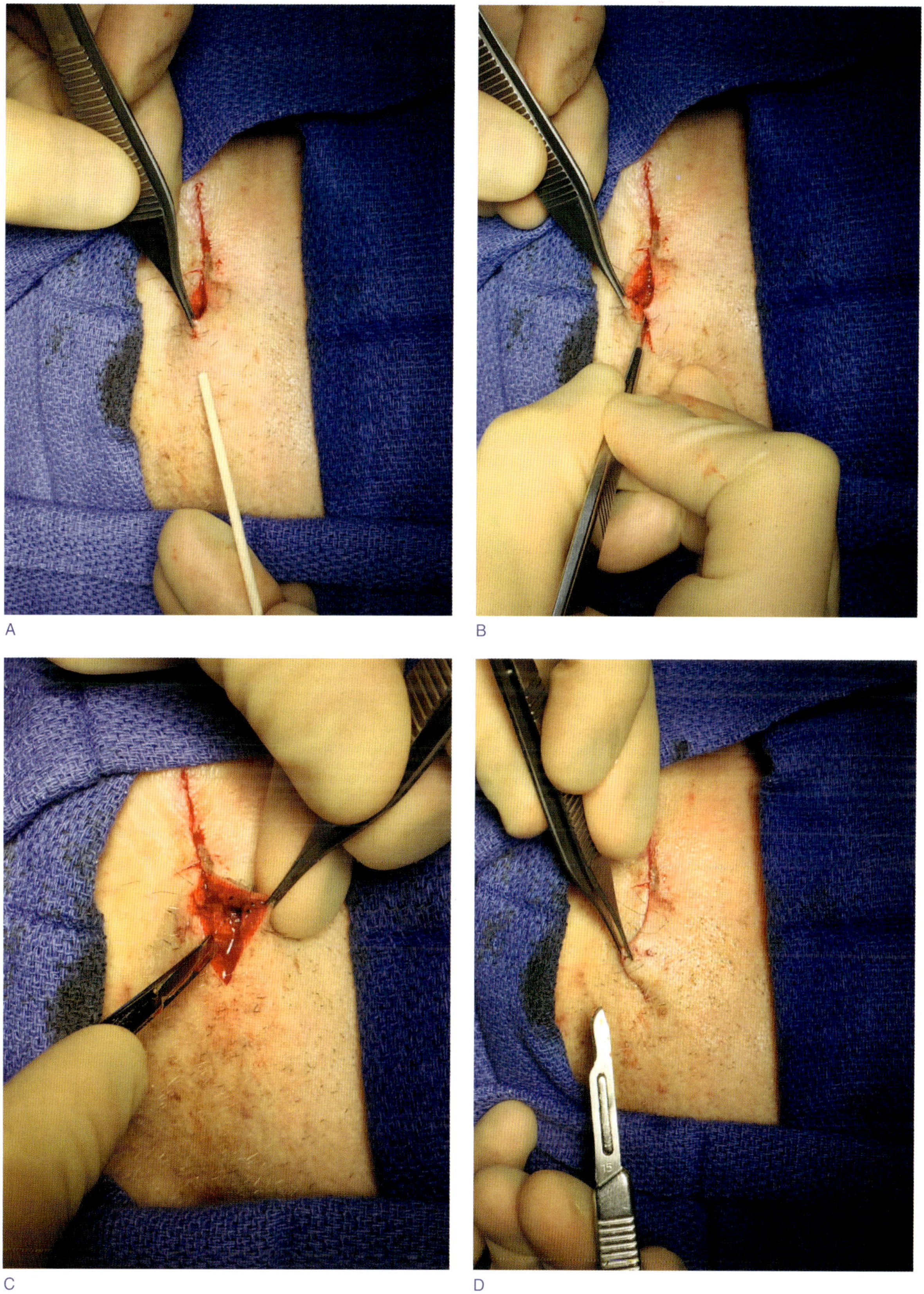

FIGURE 16-26 The midline-incision extension technique. First, (**A**) the dog ear is gently elevated with surgical forceps, and its extent is noted (here by the presence of the cotton-tipped applicator). Then, (**B**) the dog ear is gently pulled upward away from the skin, and an incision is made in the midline extending the already existing excision line. This area is then undermined bilaterally (**C**). The dog ear is then pulled gently laterally (**D**), and the half-triangle is removed in line with the original excision line. Finally, the dog ear is pulled in the opposite direction (**E**), and the process is repeated (**F**). This technique results in dog-ear removal and the extension of the original excision line (**G**).

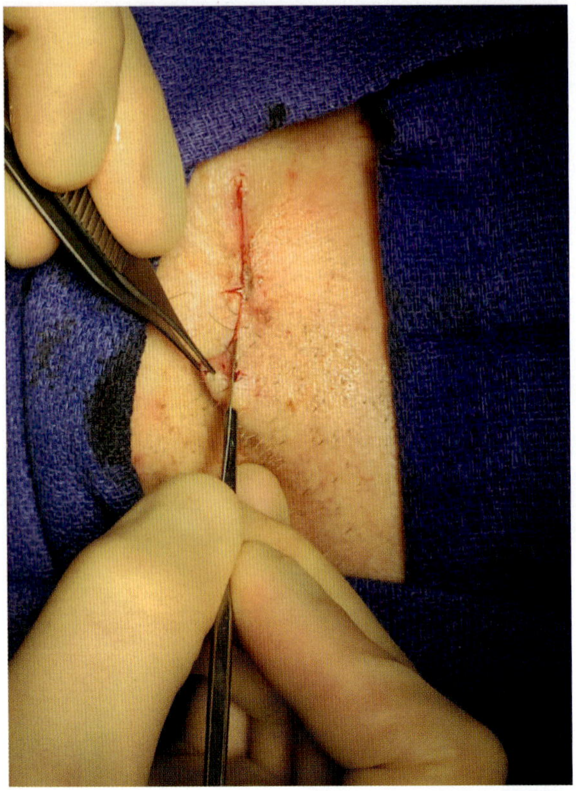

E

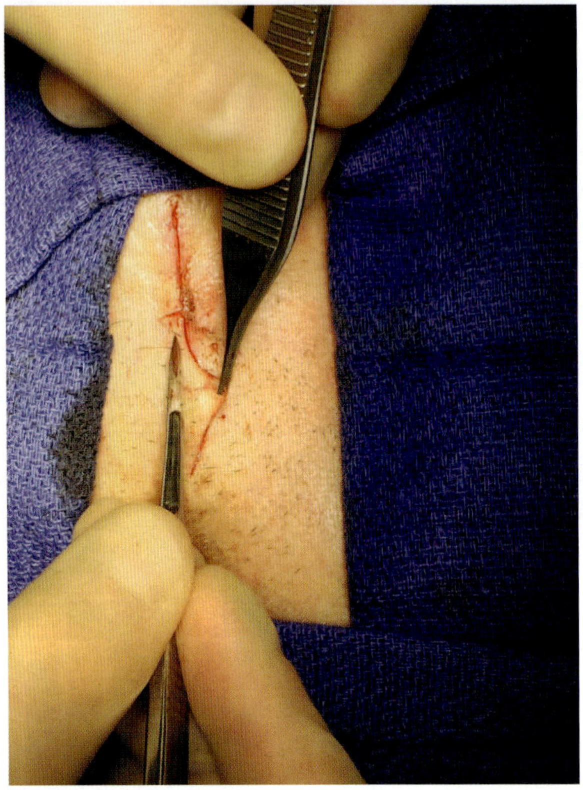

F

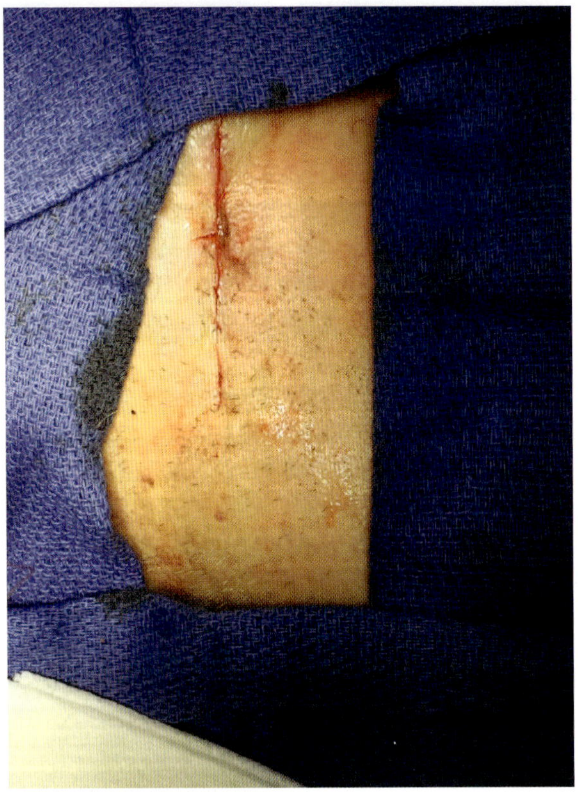

G

FIGURE 16-26 *(Continued)*

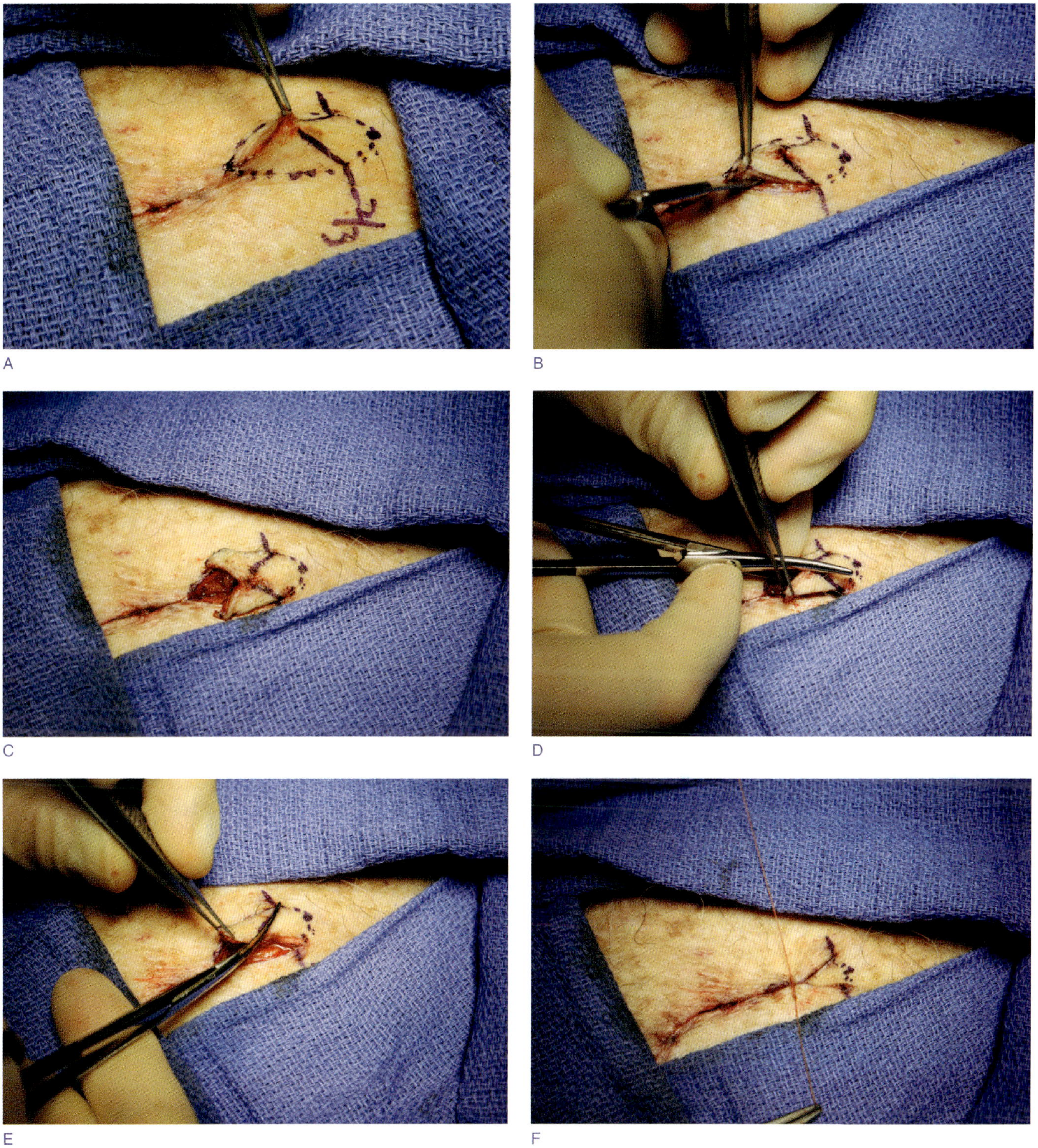

A B C D E F

FIGURE 16-27 The M-plasty technique. The extent of the raised dog ear is delineated (**A**), and a point two-thirds along the length of each cone's base is marked. Incise along the base of the redundancy, connecting one of the points to the existing wound (**B**). Repeat this step with the second point on the other side. This will result in a flap of skin that resembles a rectangle, which is only attached along one of its long edges (**C**). Next, excise a portion of the flap by cutting from the midpoint to the point previously marked (**D**) and repeat on the other side (**E**). A tip stitch (**F**) is often used to secure the tip of the M-plasty in place.

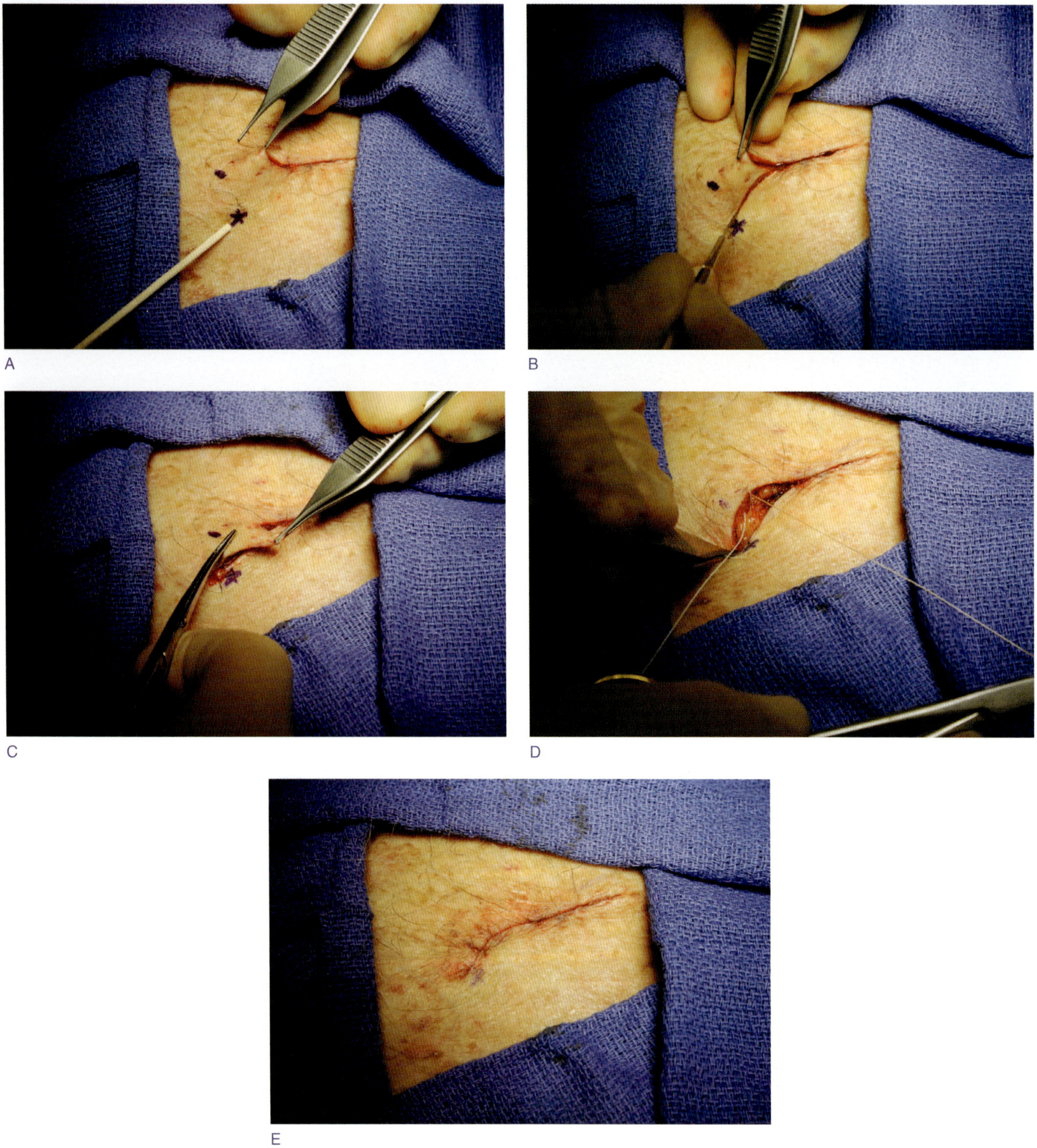

FIGURE 16-28 The S-plasty modification. In order to exaggerate the curve at the end of the closure, a target point (asterisk) is chosen outside of the standard dog-ear removal cone, lateral to the base of the standing cone (**A**). A curvilinear incision is made from the end of the existing excision line to the target point (**B**), and the dog ear is then draped laterally and removed (**C**). The first deep suture is placed in the center of the nascent dog-ear repair, using the rule of halves (**D**). Light tension pulling the new wound apex away from the center of the wound helps to better delineate the precise location of the center of the repair. The final result (**E**) is a curvilinear repair terminating at the target point.

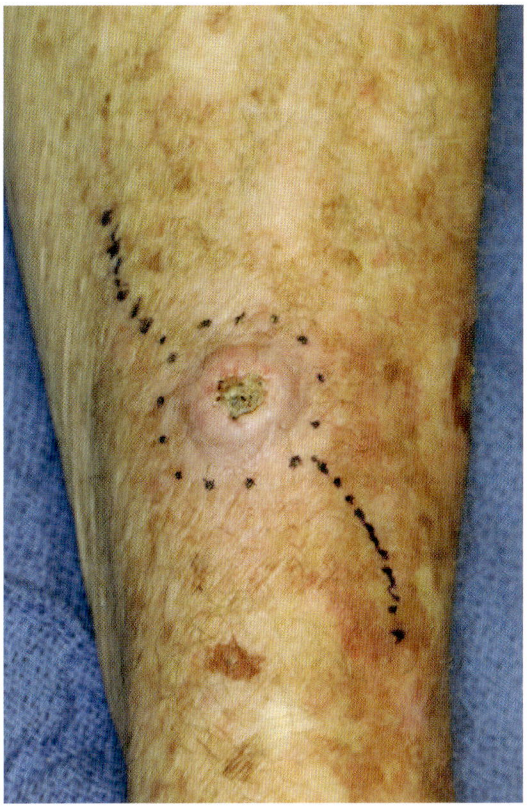

FIGURE 16-29 An S-plasty may be used when working over a convex surface, such as the forearm.

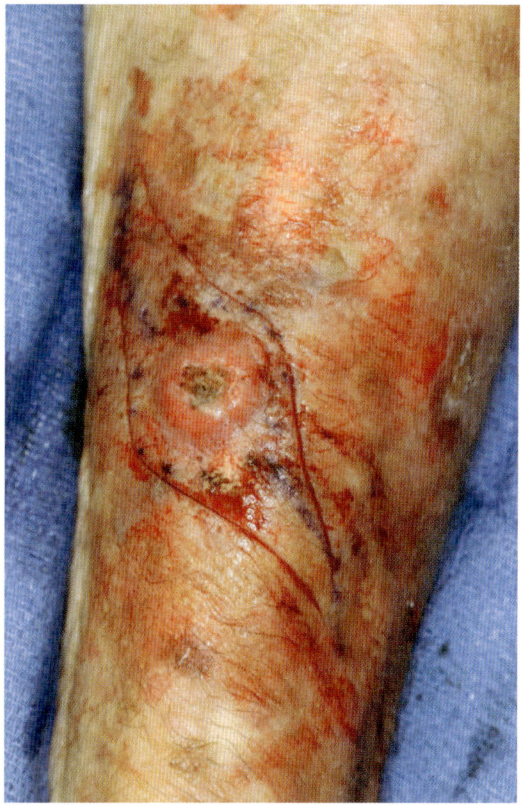

FIGURE 16-30 The S-plasty incision is made to a uniform depth.

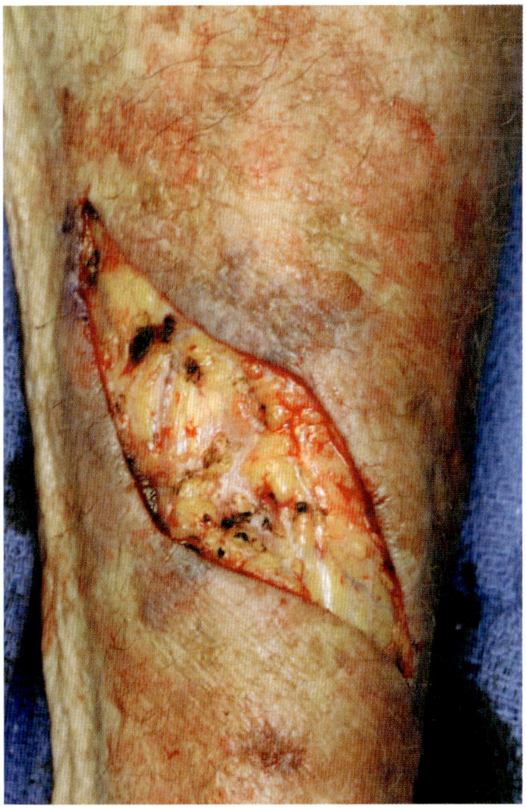

FIGURE 16-31 The excision is performed leaving an elongated S-shaped defect.

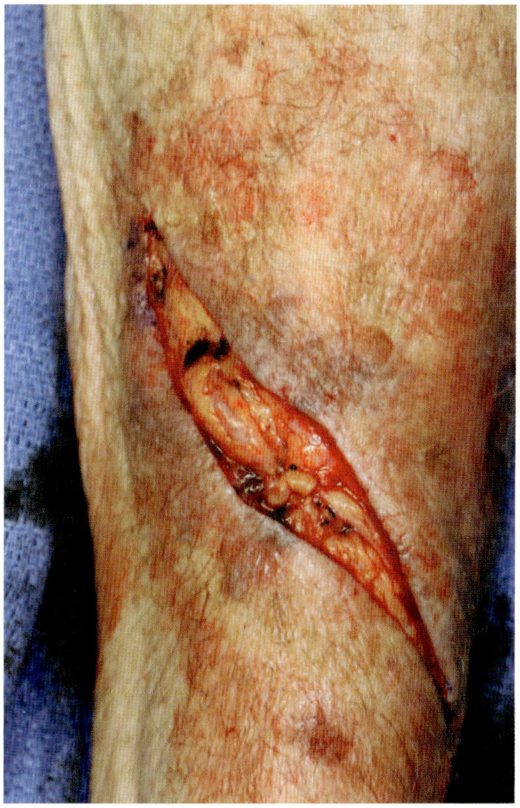

FIGURE 16-32 A fascial plication suture may be used to reduce tension and increase the apical angles.

Circular Defect with Dog-Ear Repair

Not all linear closures must begin as fusiform or rhombus shapes. Indeed, several studies have suggested that the round excision with ensuing dog-ear correction may yield a shorter postoperative scar than primarily designed fusiform closure. An additional advantage of this freestyle technique is that the ideal closure vector can be determined once the central defect has been created, which is a significant advantage because even experienced clinicians do not consistently select the ideal closure vector.[26,27,60]

This approach is particularly useful when performing a large excision, where the ideal vector of tissue closure is not a priori obvious. This approach also provides an easily oriented specimen for the laboratory. The excision is performed to conform to the native margins of the lesion being excised. It is carried to the appropriate depth, and a perpendicular incision is made circumferentially to minimize the risk of residual overhanging dermis. Once the excision is completed and the specimen is appropriately tagged, wide undermining may be performed and the different potential angles for closure are explored. A fascial plication suture along the appropriate axis may be useful prior to contemplating dog-ear removal, as this may limit the amount of additional tissue that needs to be excised. After dog-ear removal, the wound is then closed in a layered linear fashion.

Delayed Dog-Ear Repair

The tendency toward standing cone formation at the apices of a linear excision is a function of (1) tissue bunching and redundancy; (2) wound edema; and (3) a more pronounced central depression. As two of the three causes of immediate dog-ear appearance are only temporary, it may be preferable to err on the side of taking a smaller dog ear at the time of closure. This must be weighed against patient concerns in the immediate postoperative period regarding the appearance of the nascent dog ears, as some patients are less concerned regarding postoperative cosmesis and would prefer to have a shorter scar. Additionally, especially in areas such as the lower leg that are at high risk of dehiscence, creating the smallest possible wound is a clear advantage.

M-Plasty

M-plasty can be conceptualized as a small V-Y closure at one pole of an otherwise linear repair and is useful for reducing the length of a linear closure. This approach is classically used around the eyelids, where the M-plasty may be hidden along the rhytides, although it can be used in any situation where a standard dog-ear repair would approach free margins or adjacent cosmetic subunits. The net result of M-plasty formation is that the dog-ear length is reduced by approximately half.

Non-Undermined Repairs

While undermining is a standard technique to facilitate both lateral tissue movement and permit the placement of deeper buried sutures (eg, the set-back suture), it is neither necessary nor appropriate in all situations. As noted earlier, undermining itself leads to some vascular compromise, as has been demonstrated in a porcine model.

Markedly atrophic skin should almost never be undermined. This is not due to concern regarding skin tear or skiving, but rather because with atrophic skin the underlying fibrous attachments between the underside of the dermis and the deeper subcutaneous tissues provide the greatest purchase for buried sutures. A modified simple buried dermal suture is used in these cases, taking as large a bite as possible on each side, beginning on the undersurface of the deep subcutaneous tissue or even underlying fascia. Avoiding undermining may permit such wounds to be closed easily without resorting to adjuvant approaches such as suturing through tissue adhesive bolsters.[61,62]

Second, wounds in areas of very poor baseline perfusion, such as the lower legs, may sometimes be repaired without undermining. This serves two purposes: first, it obviates the risk of perfusion reduction secondary to undermining proper, and second, it creates a smaller subdermal defect in the event of dehiscence.

Partial Closure

Partial wound closure may be considered in areas where there is extreme wound tension across the central portion of the defect, such as those on the scalp and lower leg. In such cases, the poles of the wound may be approximated in a linear fashion, but a central area of wound gaping may remain. One option for these repairs is via a Burow's graft, taken from one of the poles of the wounds (see Chapter 20 for a detailed discussion of skin grafts), although permitting this small area to heal by secondary intention is appropriate as well. Adequate patient preparation is of course a prerequisite to this approach.

Another technique for partial closure is used when extreme tension across a wound does not permit direct side-to-side wound apposition at all.[63] While traditionally other repairs would be entertained, in select patients, partial linear closure allowing the remainder of the wound to heal by secondary intention may be appropriate. This can be conceptualized as a strategy to reduce the size of the defect that will heal by secondary intention. Such repairs may also be performed prior to skin graft placement.

At times, portions of an otherwise linear repair may be purposely left to heal by secondary intention. For example, when recreating the alar groove, the deepest part of the groove may be left to heal secondarily (or grafted) as an alternative to inverting suture placement.

Staged (Serial) Excision

When excising a large benign lesion, such as a congenital nevus, staged excisions may permit wound closure with a smaller ultimate repair size than would be needed otherwise. This approach combines several fundamental principles, including tissue creep, tissue stretch, and the ability to perform all but the final stage of the repair as purse-string closures to minimize the final scar length. Other approaches, including a torus (doughnut) approach to staged excisions, as well as a compressed design method using an X-shaped repair, have been described as well.[64]

Multidirectional Vector Excision

The multidirectional vector excision was proposed as a single-stage alternative to the staged excision for the removal of benign lesions. With this technique, multiple small triangular-shaped sections of the benign lesion are pulled with skin hooks in order to determine the optimal closure vector.[65] Future investigation is needed regarding this niche technique.

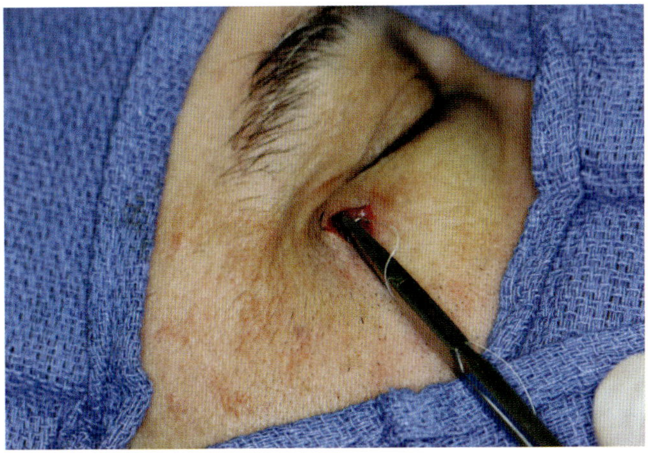

FIGURE 16-33 The first suture is placed with the goal of maintaining tension vectors parallel to the free margin.

SPECIAL ANATOMIC CONSIDERATIONS

Eyelids

Linear repairs on the upper eyelids may be performed as long as significant postoperative asymmetry is not anticipated. If this occurs, a modified blepharoplasty on the contralateral lid may be performed to restore symmetry. On the lower eyelid, excisions may be designed parallel to the lower lid as long as the tension vector across the sutures is perpendicular to this axis (**Figures 16-33 to 16-36**). If needed, a stress maneuver with open mouth and upward gaze should be performed prior to closure design. Keep in mind that Frost sutures (**Figure 16-37**) do not mitigate the risk of ectropion due to poorly designed repairs; they simply prevent this occurrence secondary to edema in the immediate postoperative period.

Nose

Linear repairs on the nose are possible even for fairly large defects, particularly those located in the midline.[1] This approach is predicated on a high length-to-width ratio closure in order to avoid the risk of dog-ear formation at the apices, which is particularly

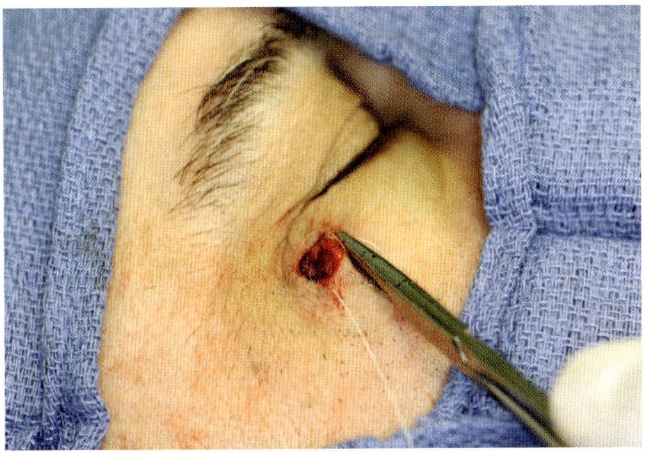

FIGURE 16-34 The second half of the suture is placed.

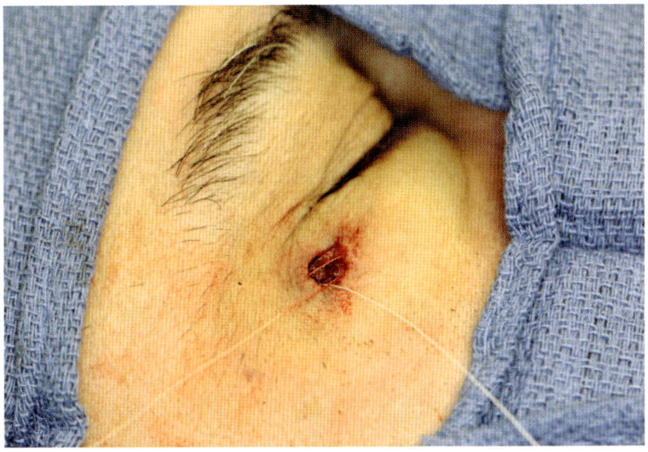

FIGURE 16-35 Note that the suture material is oriented horizontally so that there will be no vertical pull on the lower eyelid, reducing the risk of ectropion.

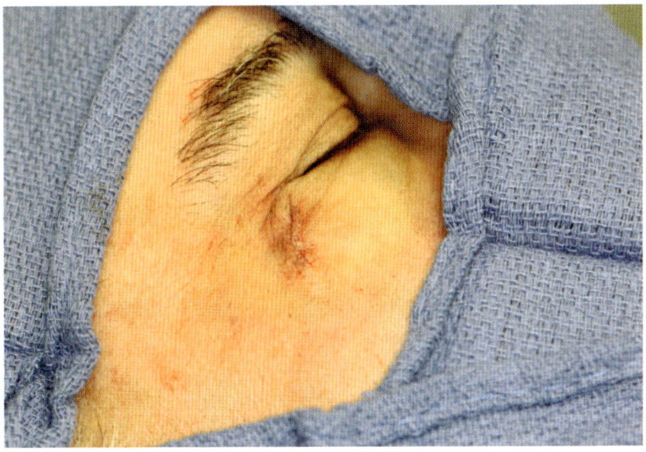

FIGURE 16-36 The wound is shown after the placement of an additional buried suture. Note the wound eversion without any evidence of ectropion.

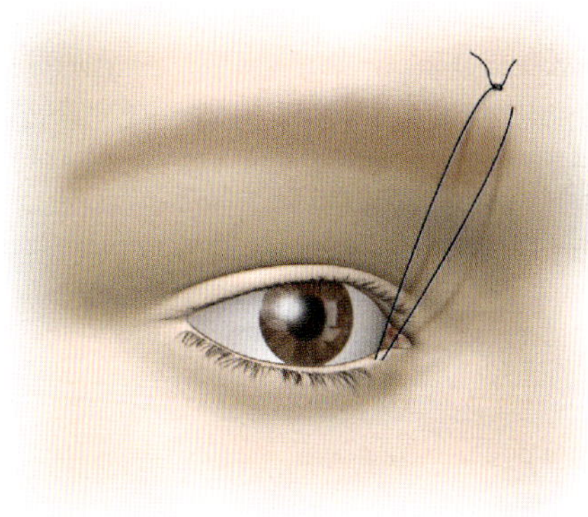

FIGURE 16-37 A Frost suture may be used to minimize ectropion secondary to postoperative edema in an otherwise well-designed repair.

noticeable on the nose. The depth of the excision and suture placement should be significant, as superficially placed sutures and superficial undermining on the nose increases the risk of dehiscence. Buried sutures should ideally include nasalis muscle in order to provide optimal cosmesis.

Patients should be informed that all nasal repairs should be conceptualized as multistaged, given the sebaceous nature of nasal skin. Postoperative dermabrasion is often useful, and if patients are told before the procedure that this may be needed, they will be more satisfied with the ultimate outcome.

Lips

Linear repairs on the lips often heal very well, as long as the white line and wet line are appropriately prioritized. Deep defects should be performed in a layered fashion, including repair of the orbicularis oris. While silk sutures have traditionally been advocated for the outer layer of lip closures, braided absorbable suture, such as polyglactin 910, is also very soft and may permit layered closure with a single suture packet.

Ears

Linear repairs on the ear are often possible and provide outstanding cosmesis. When orienting a repair along the helix, a high length-to-width ratio is helpful in maintaining the natural curvature of the ear. Percutaneous sutures may be helpful (see Chapter 10) when working with atrophic skin.

Cheeks

The cheeks are subject to significant tensile stress and often include significant convex components. Therefore, both S-plasty and crescentic approaches may be useful. Even large defects on the cheeks can often be closed in a linear fashion (**Figures 16-38 to 16-40**). Patients should go through their full range of facial movement before deciding on an optimal tissue vector. Occasionally, M-plasty may be useful when approaching free margins. Fascial plication and set-back sutures are useful for maintaining well-everted wound edges under minimal tension.

Forehead

The forehead is usually repaired in a linear fashion, although closure vectors are of particular importance given the potential impact of repairs on eyebrow positioning. Many small forehead defects are repaired along the rhytides in a transverse fashion, and small defects often result in only temporary eyebrow elevation. Large repairs are best performed in a layered vertical fashion, and with meticulous suturing technique and eversion, the resulting scar may be almost undetectable. On the temples, wounds should be repaired in a radial fashion, with special attention paid to the baseline rhytides and vectors of tissue laxity.

Scalp

Repairs on the scalp should take into account the inelastic nature of scalp skin. Linear repairs are often limited by this inelasticity, although with subgaleal undermining (and possibly galeal relaxing incisions), even fairly large defects may be closed in a linear fashion. There is considerable individual variation in scalp

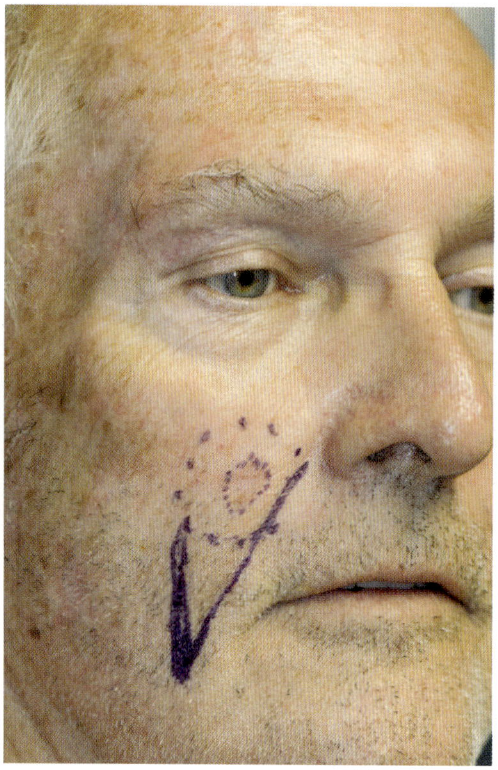

FIGURE 16-38 Lentigo maligna on the cheek can be easily closed in a linear fashion.

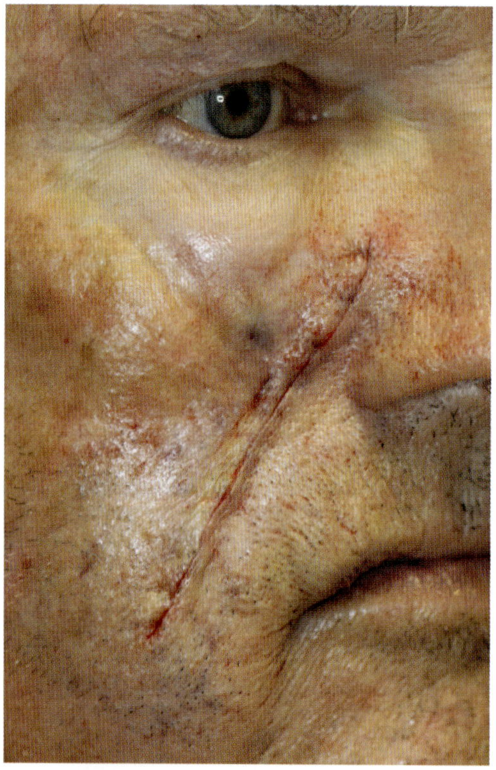

FIGURE 16-39 Wound appearance immediately after superficial muscular aponeurotic system (SMAS) plication and buried suture placement. Note the presence of overhanging dermis that will be removed prior to the completion of the repair.

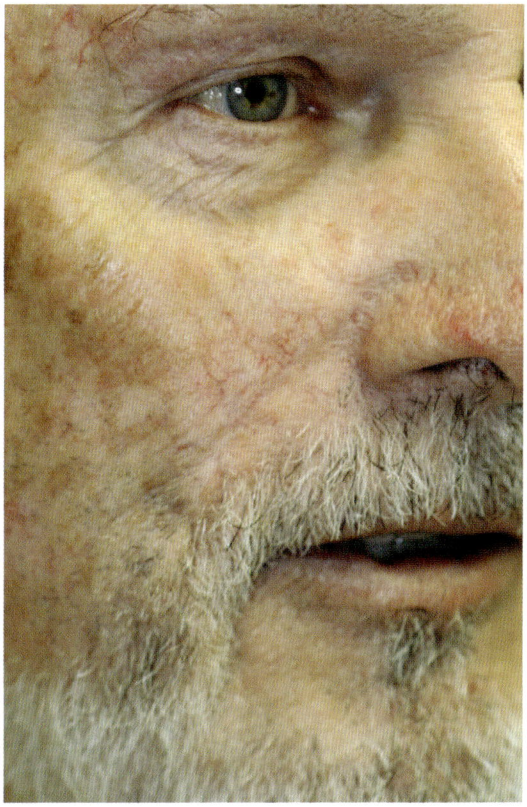

FIGURE 16-40 At 6-month follow-up, the wound has healed with barely visible scarring.

elasticity, and this should always be judged by attempting lateral compression on the scalp in multiple directions prior to closure. Although debatable, considerable tissue creep may be seen in some patients, suggesting a role for intraoperative tissue expansion using either temporary sutures or a towel clamp.

Hands and Feet

Linear repairs on the hand may be subject to significant tension as well as repetitive trauma from daily exposure as well as the insertion and removal of the hand from a pocket or purse. Most linear repairs on the hand are oriented along the long axis of the hand, although depending on the orientation of the defect as well as the patient's activity level, this axis may be individualized. Transversely oriented closures may increase the risk of postoperative lymphedema due to an increased risk of lymphatic transection. Exploring the full range of motion rather than relying on RSTLs alone is helpful. The loose areolar tissue just beneath the dermis provides an excellent plane for undermining. Use particular caution with transepidermal sutures to avoid inadvertently entering or ligating one of the many small superficial vessels of the dorsal hand.

COMPLICATIONS

As with any surgical procedure, bleeding, hematoma formation, dehiscence, and infection are the most common postprocedure complications seen with linear repairs.

Clinicians should make every effort to personally see every patient with a postoperative complication. This both serves to assuage the patient's concerns and helps the clinician with feedback regarding optimal technique. Additionally, the clinician is best qualified to assess whether some mild edema or erythema truly represents a complication or whether it is simply an expected part of the healing process.

Dog-ear formation is also frequently seen with linear closures, and a delicate balance between maintaining the natural curvature of the skin and not exaggerating the length of the wound must be maintained. Dog-ear correction should generally not be considered for at least the first few postoperative months, as significant wound flattening and maturation is expected within this period.

Most linear closures do not require surgical drains; for the rare patient with persistent pinpoint bleeding or a background bleeding diathesis, placement of a small Penrose, Jackson-Pratt, or wick drain could be considered, although in general, it is far better to achieve adequate and meticulous hemostasis prior to wound closure. A rapidly expanding hematoma necessitates evacuation in the context of surgical revision, where the wound should be anesthetized, prepped in a sterile fashion, opened, explored, and all sources of bleeding definitively addressed. Smaller or stable hematomas may be managed conservatively.

Mild wound dehiscence should be managed with sharp debridement. Usually, local anesthetic is not required because only devitalized tissue—and often only the overlying eschar—is debrided. Patients may be seen weekly if desired and should be advised to keep the wound bed moist with ointment application at least three times per day. It is vital to debride the advancing edges of the wound in order to maximize the chance of rapid healing. Patients should be told that postdebridement bleeding is not only expected but also desirable.

Active wound infections, while rare, should be cultured if possible, and empiric antibiotics may be started. True abscesses should be drained. Patients should understand that even wounds with significant postoperative complications may ultimately heal with outstanding cosmesis.

Repairs on sebaceous skin, such as the nose, may result in a scar that appears depressed relative to the surrounding skin. This may be approached with dermabrasion (or laser) postoperatively, although waiting 3 to 6 months may be prudent as the scar may improve significantly without intervention.

Persistent wound eversion, though rare, may be treated with intralesional triamcinolone injection, although this should not be considered until 6 months have passed.

POSTOPERATIVE MANAGEMENT

Even the best surgical repair can be undone by less-than-optimal postoperative care. Clear written instructions on wound care are of vital importance and should be reviewed verbally with the patient as well. For most linear repairs, only minimal postoperative management is required. For wounds closed without transepidermal sutures, a simple adhesive film dressing may be applied immediately postoperatively. This gas-permeable film will permit the wound to breathe while providing a moist environment for wound healing.

Patients should be warned that a small amount of blood or serous fluid drainage is expected and that this will typically become trapped beneath the film dressing. The film dressing may be left in place for the next 1 to 2 weeks, depending on patient and clinician preference. The advantage of this approach is that it requires no effort on the patient's part, which is particularly useful for difficult-to-reach wounds or for patients living alone. Leaving the dressing in place for more than 2 weeks may increase the risk of maceration.

For wounds closed with transepidermal sutures, film dressings remain an option, although often a nonstick dressing is simply cut to size and placed over the wound after application of a thin film of ointment.

A moderate-pressure dressing is applied postoperatively and left in place for approximately 24 hours. When placing a pressure dressing over adherent film, the gauze should extend beyond the edge of the film so that the adhesive tape holding the pressure dressing in place does not touch the film, as otherwise the film may be inadvertently removed at the time of the first dressing change.

Pressure should be sufficient to mitigate the risk of oozing but should not restrict blood flow to the wound. Additionally, downward and inward pressure should be exerted just lateral to the wound edges, resulting in a net effect of the wound edges being pressed together. Direct pressure over the surface of the sutured wound should be avoided, as this does not address potential space created laterally to the suture line and also serves as a distracting force against the sutures. This same principle should be emphasized to surgical assistants when they are asked to hold pressure on a partially sutured wound.

When needed, suture removal may be performed between postoperative days 3 and 10, depending on the anatomic site of the surgery and clinician preference. For patients who are unable to return for suture removal, options include avoiding transepidermal sutures or placing the transepidermal sutures using fast-absorbing gut or fast-absorbing synthetic sutures.

For wounds covered with an adhesive film, no care is needed. For those covered with a nonstick pad, the wound may be gently cleaned once or twice daily and a thin film of petrolatum should be placed over the suture line using a cotton-tipped applicator. For wounds in dependent areas, patients should be advised to keep their legs elevated as much as possible for several weeks postoperatively.

Patients often ask about using over-the-counter scar healing aids. Most have little or no evidence of efficacy, and in general, they should not be recommended. For patients with a history of true keloid formation, consideration may be given to intraoperative or immediate postoperative triamcinolone injection along the suture line, with repeat monthly treatments for maintenance, although risks, including delayed wound healing, atrophy, and telangiectasias, should be discussed with the patient. As noted earlier, patients should be told to expect dramatic wound eversion postoperatively and be reassured that this is only temporary.[18]

CONCLUSIONS

The linear closure is the most useful and broadly applicable closure technique in dermatologic surgery. One of the great advantages of linear closures is their predictability; since outstanding blood flow is maintained to the wound edge, these closures often result in fine-line, nearly imperceptible scars when carefully designed and executed. Attention to detail and customizing approaches for each individual patient and anatomic location serve to create closures that will ultimately be difficult to detect from a conversational distance.

REFERENCES

1. Soliman S, Hatef DA, Hollier LH Jr, Thornton JF. The rationale for direct linear closure of facial Mohs' defects. *Plast Reconstr Surg.* 2011;127(1):142-149.
2. Goldberg LH, Silapunt S, Alam M, Peterson SR, Jih MH, Kimyai-Asadi A. Surgical repair of temple defects after Mohs micrographic surgery. *J Am Acad Dermatol.* 2005;52(4):631-636.
3. Behroozan DS, Goldberg LH. Combined linear closure and Burow's graft for a dorsal nasal defect. *Dermatol Surg.* 2006;32(1):107-111.
4. Dang M, Greenbaum SS. Modified Burow's wedge flap for upper lateral lip defects. *Dermatol Surg.* 2000;26(5):497-498.
5. Whitaker DC, Goldstein GD. Lateral nose and perinasal defects: options in management following Mohs micrographic surgery for cutaneous carcinoma. *J Dermatol Surg Oncol.* 1988;14(2):177-183.
6. Wesley NO, Yu SS, Grekin RC, Neuhaus IM. Primary linear closure for large defects of the nasal supratip. *Dermatol Surg.* 2008;34(3):380-384; discussion 384-385.
7. Godek CP, Weinzweig J, Bartlett SP. Lip reconstruction following Mohs' surgery: the role for composite resection and primary closure. *Plast Reconstr Surg.* 2000;106(4):798-804.
8. Ling N, Martin A. Three suturing techniques for closing fusiform excisions. A randomised controlled study. *Australas J Dermatol.* 2016;57(4):271-277.
9. Etzkorn JR, Sobanko JF, Miller CJ. Free margin distortion with fusiform closures: the apical angle relationship. *Dermatol Surg.* 2014;40(12):1428-1432.
10. Goldberg LH, Alam M. Elliptical excisions: variations and the eccentric parallelogram. *Arch Dermatol.* 2004;140(2):176-180.
11. Zitelli JA. TIPS for a better ellipse. *J Am Acad Dermatol.* 1990;22(1):101-103.
12. Borges A-F, Alexander JE. Relaxed skin tension lines, Z-plasties on scars, and fusiform excision of lesions. *Br J Plast Surg.* 1962; 15:242-254.
13. Pepper JP, Baker SR. Local flaps: cheek and lip reconstruction. *JAMA Facial Plast Surg.* 2013;15(5):374-382.
14. Kantor J. Reliability and photographic equivalency of the Scar Cosmesis Assessment and Rating (SCAR) Scale, an outcome measure for postoperative scars. *JAMA Dermatol.* 2017;153(1):55-60.
15. Kantor J. The SCAR (Scar Cosmesis Assessment and Rating) scale: development and validation of a new outcome measure for postoperative scar assessment. *Br J Dermatol.* 2016;175(6):1394-1396.
16. Zhang J, Rosen A, Orenstein L, et al. Factors associated with biopsy site identification, postponement of surgery, and patient confidence in a dermatologic surgery practice. *J Am Acad Dermatol.* 2016;74(6):1185-1193.
17. Perlis CS, Campbell RM, Perlis RH, Malik M, Dufresne RG Jr. Incidence of and risk factors for medical malpractice lawsuits among Mohs surgeons. *Dermatol Surg.* 2006;32(1):79-83.

18. Kantor J. The subcutaneous splint: a helpful analogy to explain post-operative wound eversion. *JAMA Dermatol.* 2014;150(10):1122.
19. Moody BR, McCarthy JE, Sengelmann RD. The apical angle: a mathematical analysis of the ellipse. *Dermatol Surg.* 2001;27(1):61-63.
20. Sobanko JF. Optimizing design and execution of linear reconstructions on the face. *Dermatol Surg.* 2015;41(Suppl 10):S216-S228.
21. Toll EC, Loizou P, Davis CR, Porter GC, Pothier DD. Scars and satisfaction: do smaller scars improve patient-reported outcome? *Eur Arch Otorhinolaryngol.* 2012;269(1):309-313.
22. Liu H, Yu N, Shi J, Hu X, Lv X, Han Y. A new modified S-plasty for skin defect closure. *Aesthetic Plast Surg.* 2015;39(1):100-105.
23. Hafiji J, Salmon P, Hussain W. Modifying the S-plasty to optimize a curvilinear scar. *Clin Exp Dermatol.* 2012;37(2):199-200.
24. Kim P, Kim HJ. S-plasty: clinical applications for skin surgery. *Aust Fam Physician.* 2011;40(4):224-225.
25. Sebastian S, Bang RH, Padilla RS. A simple approach to the S-plasty in cutaneous surgery. *Dermatol Surg.* 2009;35(8):1277-1279.
26. Hudson-Peacock MJ, Lawrence CM. Comparison of wound closure by means of dog ear repair and elliptical excision. *J Am Acad Dermatol.* 1995;32(4):627-630.
27. Seo SH, Son SW, Kim IH. Round excisions lead to shorter scars and better scar positioning than traditional elliptical excisions. *Dermatology.* 2008;217(3):276-280.
28. Kauvar AN, Arpey CJ, Hruza G, Olbricht SM, Bennett R, Mahmoud BH. Consensus for nonmelanoma skin cancer treatment, part II: squamous cell carcinoma, including a cost analysis of treatment methods. *Dermatol Surg.* 2015;41(11):1214-1240.
29. Kauvar AN, Cronin T Jr, Roenigk R, Hruza G, Bennett R, American Society for Dermatologic Surgery. Consensus for nonmelanoma skin cancer treatment: basal cell carcinoma, including a cost analysis of treatment methods. *Dermatol Surg.* 2015;41(5):550-571.
30. Felton S, Taylor RS, Srivastava D. Excision margins for melanoma in situ on the head and neck. *Dermatol Surg.* 2016;42(3):327-334.
31. MacKenzie Ross AD, Haydu LE, Quinn MJ, et al. The association between excision margins and local recurrence in 11,290 thin (T1) primary cutaneous melanomas: a case-control study. *Ann Surg Oncol.* 2016;23(4):1082-1089.
32. Haydu LE, Stollman JT, Scolyer RA, et al. Minimum safe pathologic excision margins for primary cutaneous melanomas (1-2 mm in thickness): analysis of 2131 patients treated at a single center. *Ann Surg Oncol.* 2016;23(4):1071-1081.
33. Hayes AJ, Maynard L, Coombes G, et al. Wide versus narrow excision margins for high-risk, primary cutaneous melanomas: long-term follow-up of survival in a randomised trial. *Lancet Oncol.* 2016;17(2):184-192.
34. Akhtar S, Bhat W, Magdum A, Stanley PR. Surgical excision margins for melanoma in situ. *J Plast Reconstr Aesthet Surg.* 2014;67(3):320-323.
35. Duffy KL, Truong A, Bowen GM, et al. Adequacy of 5-mm surgical excision margins for non-lentiginous melanoma in situ. *J Am Acad Dermatol.* 2014;71(4):835-838.
36. Kunishige JH, Brodland DG, Zitelli JA. Margins for standard excision of melanoma in situ. *J Am Acad Dermatol.* 2013;69(1):164.
37. Newlands C, Currie R, Memon A, Whitaker S, Woolford T. Non-melanoma skin cancer: United Kingdom National Multidisciplinary Guidelines. *J Laryngol Otol.* 2016;130(S2):S125-S132.
38. Alam M, Nodzenski M, Yoo S, Poon E, Bolotin D. Objective structured assessment of technical skills in elliptical excision repair of senior dermatology residents: a multirater, blinded study of operating room video recordings. *JAMA Dermatol.* 2014;150(6):608-612.
39. Hu Y, Tiemann D, Michael Brunt L. Video self-assessment of basic suturing and knot tying skills by novice trainees. *J Surg Educ.* 2013;70(2):279-283.
40. Miller CJ, Antunes MB, Sobanko JF. Surgical technique for optimal outcomes: part II. Repairing tissue: suturing. *J Am Acad Dermatol.* 2015;72(3):389-402.
41. Miller CJ, Antunes MB, Sobanko JF. Surgical technique for optimal outcomes: Part I. Cutting tissue: incising, excising, and undermining. *J Am Acad Dermatol.* 2015;72(3):377-387.
42. Wang AS, Kleinerman R, Armstrong AW, et al. Set-back versus buried vertical mattress suturing: results of a randomized blinded trial. *J Am Acad Dermatol.* 2015;72(4):674-680.
43. Kantor J. The set-back buried dermal suture: an alternative to the buried vertical mattress for layered wound closure. *J Am Acad Dermatol.* 2010;62(2):351-353.
44. Zitelli JA, Moy RL. Buried vertical mattress suture. *J Dermatol Surg Oncol.* 1989;15(1):17-19.
45. Kappel S, Kleinerman R, King TH, et al. Does wound eversion improve cosmetic outcome? Results of a randomized, split-scar, comparative trial. *J Am Acad Dermatol.* 2015;72(4):668-673.
46. Mehta D, Chambers N, Adams B, Gloster H. Comparison of the prevalence of surgical site infection with use of sterile versus nonsterile gloves for resection and reconstruction during Mohs surgery. *Dermatol Surg.* 2014;40(3):234-239.
47. Xia Y, Cho S, Greenway HT, Zelac DE, Kelley B. Infection rates of wound repairs during Mohs micrographic surgery using sterile versus nonsterile gloves: a prospective randomized pilot study. *Dermatol Surg.* 2011;37(5):651-656.
48. Rogers HD, Desciak EB, Marcus RP, Wang S, MacKay-Wiggan J, Eliezri YD. Prospective study of wound infections in Mohs micrographic surgery using clean surgical technique in the absence of prophylactic antibiotics. *J Am Acad Dermatol.* 2010;63(5):842-851.
49. Dumville JC, McFarlane E, Edwards P, Lipp A, Holmes A. Preoperative skin antiseptics for preventing surgical wound infections after clean surgery. *Cochrane Database Syst Rev.* 2013;3:CD003949.
50. Steinsapir KD, Woodward JA. Chlorhexidine keratitis: safety of chlorhexidine as a facial antiseptic. *Dermatol Surg.* 2017;43(1):1-6.
51. Tetzlaff JE. The pharmacology of local anesthetics. *Anesthesiol Clin North America.* 2000;18(2):217-233, v.
52. Nantel-Battista M, Murray C. Dermatologic surgical pearls: enhancing the efficacy of the traditional elliptical excision. *J Cutan Med Surg.* 2015;19(3):287-290.
53. Breuninger H. Double butterfly suture for high tension: a broadly anchored, horizontal, buried interrupted suture. *Dermatol Surg.* 2000;26(3):215-218.
54. Krishnan NM, Brown BJ, Davison SP, et al. Reducing wound tension with undermining or imbrication: do they work? *Plast Reconstr Surg Glob Open.* 2016;4(7):e799.
55. Kantor J. The fascial plication suture: an adjunct to layered wound closure. *Arch Dermatol.* 2009;145(12):1454-1456.
56. Dzubow LM. The use of fascial plication to facilitate wound closure following microscopically controlled surgery. *J Dermatol Surg Oncol.* 1989;15(10):1063-1066.

57. Wang SQ, Goldberg LH. Surgical pearl: running horizontal mattress suture with intermittent simple loops. *J Am Acad Dermatol.* 2006;55(5):870-871.

58. Moody BR, McCarthy JE, Linder J, Hruza GJ. Enhanced cosmetic outcome with running horizontal mattress sutures. *Dermatol Surg.* 2005;31(10):1313-1316.

59. Paolo B, Stefania R, Massimiliano C, Stefano A, Andrea P, Giorgio L. Modified S-plasty: an alternative to the elliptical excision to reduce the length of suture. *Dermatol Surg.* 2003;29(4):394-398.

60. Tilleman TR. Direct closure of round skin defects: a four-step technique with multiple subcutaneous and cutaneous "figure-of-8" sutures alleviating dog-ears. *Plast Reconstr Surg.* 2004;114(7):1761-1767.

61. Tayebi B, Kaniszewska M, Mahoney AM, Tung R. A novel closure method for surgical defects in atrophic skin using cyanoacrylate adhesive and suture. *Dermatol Surg.* 2015;41(1):177-180.

62. Bain MA, Peterson EA, Murphy RX Jr. Dermabond bolster-assisted primary closure of atrophic skin. *Plast Reconstr Surg.* 2009;123(4):147e-149e.

63. Redondo P. Guitar-string sutures to reduce a large surgical defect prior to skin grafting or flap movement. *Dermatol Surg.* 2014;40(1):69-72.

64. Fife DJ, Alam M. Alternative techniques for reduction of scar length during staged excision. *J Am Acad Dermatol.* 2011;65(4):811-818.

65. Oh SI, Lee YH. Multidirectional vector excision leads to better outcomes than traditional elliptical excision of facial congenital melanocytic nevus. *Arch Plast Surg.* 2013;40(5):570-574.

Approach to Dysplastic Nevi

17

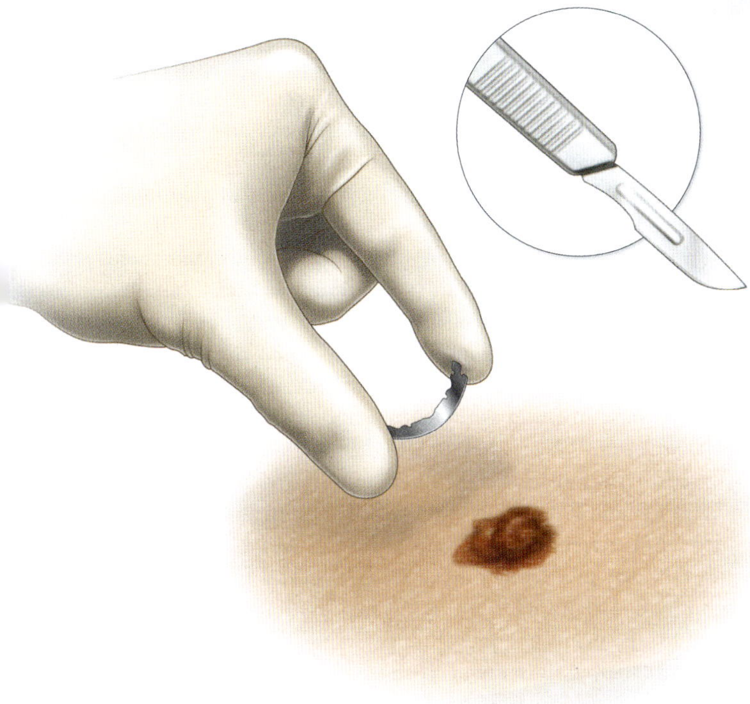

SUMMARY

- CAN and DN are clinicopathologic markers of patients at an increased risk for melanoma. Patients with CAN/DN should be screened regularly for melanoma.
- CAN are not obligate precursors to melanoma, and they do not have to be removed—they may be clinically monitored for change.
- The majority of melanomas are believed to arise de novo, and are not associated with a precursor nevus.

Beginner Tips

- A biopsy of a pigmented lesion is performed if there is a high level of suspicion for melanoma. Other reasons for biopsy may include irritation, cosmesis, or atypical lesions in areas difficult to self-monitor.
- An excisional biopsy is the preferred method to remove any lesion concerning for melanoma to provide the most accurate diagnosis and smallest risk of recurrence.

Pitfalls and Cautions

- While the morbidity of a biopsy should always be considered, there is no substitute for biopsy in cases where a true concern for evolving melanoma exists.
- Serial photography has no impact on the development of melanoma unless the clinician has a low threshold for biopsy for any evolving CAN.

Expert Tips

- Reexcisions need not always be performed in mildly and moderately DN with clear margins on the original biopsy.
- Mildly DN with positive histologic margins and no clinical residual pigmentation can be safely observed.

Patient Education Points

- Patients should be taught that all CAN do not evolve on to melanoma, and that they represent a marker of melanoma risk rather than a "precancer."
- Therefore, most CAN may be monitored clinically as long as there is no evolution and they appear similar to the patient's other CAN.

Don't Forget!

- Observation of moderately DN with positive histologic margins and no clinical residuum may be reasonable, but more data are needed.
- Severely DN with positive histologic margins should be reexcised.

Billing Pearls

- The decision of whether to code a shave as a biopsy or shave removal is based on the clinician's intent. Even a deep, broad scoop shave, if performed to *biopsy* the lesion in question, should be coded as a biopsy.

17 Approach to Dysplastic Nevi

INTRODUCTION

One of the greatest challenges to dermatologists and primary care clinicians alike is the management of complex pigmented lesions. Subtlety of diagnosis, slow evolution over time, and presentation in a broad array of demographic groups all add to the difficulty in appropriately assessing and managing these complex lesions. Most importantly, inadequate management or imprecise evaluation may result in tragic consequences, as melanoma represents the fifth most common cancer overall in the United States and is responsible for the majority of cancer deaths among women in the 25- to 30-year age group.[1] Moreover, the precipitous drop in 10-year survival as a result of delayed diagnosis—patients with lesions less than 1 mm thick have a survival rate of 88%, whereas those with melanomas 4 mm or greater in thickness with ulceration have a survival rate of 32%—means that early detection is critical and has the potential to save lives.[2]

Clinically atypical nevi (CAN)/dysplastic nevi (DN) are a subset of melanocytic nevi that clinically have an irregular, poorly defined border, asymmetric shape, and variegated pigmentation and are generally larger than 5 mm.[3] When biopsied, these lesions have certain histologic findings including disorganized melanocytic proliferations and associated atypical cells.[4] Although CAN/DN themselves are not obligate precursors to melanoma, they are clinicopathologic markers of patients with an increased risk for melanoma.[5,6] Some patients who have numerous CAN/DN can be challenging to follow clinically and may require surgical procedures for lesions suspicious for melanoma.

BACKGROUND

William Norris, a Scottish surgeon, reported the first case of cutaneous melanoma in 1820. He also observed high numbers of nevi on his patient and proposed that the two conditions may be related.[7] In the 1970s, CAN/DN were described among individuals from melanoma-prone families. In 1978, Clark et al[8] described CAN/DN as part of the "B-K mole syndrome" (named for two patients in the study) among patients from families affected by familial malignant melanoma. Around the same time, Lynch's group described four individuals in a melanoma-prone family and found three of them to have a larger number of CANs (>200).[9] In 1980, Elder et al[10] proposed the term *dysplastic nevus* for these morphologically atypical moles with irregular outlines and pigmentation that tended to occur more commonly on sun-protected areas when compared with common or banal nevi (CN) and had histologic evidence of dysplasia. The National Institutes of Health (NIH) held a consensus meeting to further define the histologic criteria for DN in 1992 and recommended the clinical term *atypical nevus* versus the pathologic term *nevus with architectural disorder*.[11]

PATHOPHYSIOLOGY

Several genetic alterations have been implicated in the development of DN. For example, mutations in a cell cycle regulator, $p16^{INK4a}$, appear to be involved in tumorigenesis and in DN.[12] Carriers of p16 mutations are more likely to have greater than 100 nevi, according to a study by Bishop et al[13] of five families with these mutations.[13] Other alterations in BRAF, NRAS, and mismatch repair enzymes are also present in DN, but these mutations can also be found in both melanoma and CN.[12,14-17] When gene expression patterns were examined by Scatolini et al[18] among CN, DN, and melanomas, it was noted that there are many similarities in gene expression between DN and CN including those involved with mitosis, apoptosis, and transcriptional regulation.[18] Nevertheless, DN demonstrate higher rates of Ki-67 positivity, a marker of proliferation, relative to CN. Levels of cyclin D1 and D3, which indicate cell division, are intermediate for DN between what is observed for CN and melanoma.[19,20] Thus, DN may proliferate more actively than CN but not as significantly as melanoma.[21] An autosomal dominant inheritance pattern for the nevus phenotype in melanoma-prone families has been postulated, with many of these families showing mutations at the CDKN2A locus.[22,23]

Ultraviolet exposure has also been postulated to lead to the development of DN. However, this is controversial, as some studies have failed to find a relationship between sun exposure and DN,[24] whereas another study found that CAN density was greatest on skin that was intermittently exposed to sun—so-called *traumatizing exposure*, or intense exposure that exceeds the natural resistance of the skin.[25] Finally, alterations in the host immune system may be related to the development of multiple DN ("eruptive DN"). This may occur in the context of immunosuppression for organ transplants, chemotherapy, systemic immunosuppression from HIV, and certain hematologic malignancies.[26-29]

CLINICAL FEATURES OF CLINICALLY ATYPICAL NEVI

The diagnosis of CAN is made clinically, and there are different sets of criteria to identify these nevi (**Table 17-1**).[30,31] In contrast to CN, CAN tend to be larger in diameter and may have some features of the ABCDs of melanoma (asymmetry, border irregularity, color variegation, enlarged diameter), which can make melanoma screening challenging in patients with numerous CAN. The criteria used by Tucker et al[30] are considered to be the most clinically relevant as they were used for one of the largest studies on melanoma risk and nevi. These consist of diameter ≥5 mm; presence of a macular component; and at least two of the following criteria: (1) variable pigmentation, (2) irregular and asymmetric outline, and (3) indistinct borders.[30] The Dutch Working Group proposed

TABLE 17-1 • Clinical Criteria for Diagnosing Atypical Nevi

Tucker et al[30]	≥5 mm in size, having a flat component At least two of the following three: 1. Variable pigmentation 2. Irregular and asymmetric outline 3. Having indistinct borders
Dutch Working Group[31]	1. ≥5 mm in diameter 2. Vague border 3. Asymmetric shape 4. Irregular pigmentation 5. Red hue

an alternative set of criteria for CAN also shown in **Table 17-1.**[31] Clinical examples of CAN are shown in **Figure 17-1**.

HISTOLOGIC FEATURES AND PATHOLOGIC REPORTING OF DYSPLASTIC NEVI

Histologically, DN have been described as having features distinct from CN. Clark et al[8] originally described DN as having both atypical cytology and architecture. These features included atypical melanocyte cytology, atypical melanocytic hyperplasia, papillary dermal fibroplasia, and a lymphocytic infiltrate. Other features of DN that have been described include elliptical nests with variability in shape and size that bridge adjacent rete ridges.[32] Epithelioid cell hyperplasia is another growth pattern seen in DN and is characterized by cells with large rounded nuclei and abundant pale cytoplasm.[33] Prominent

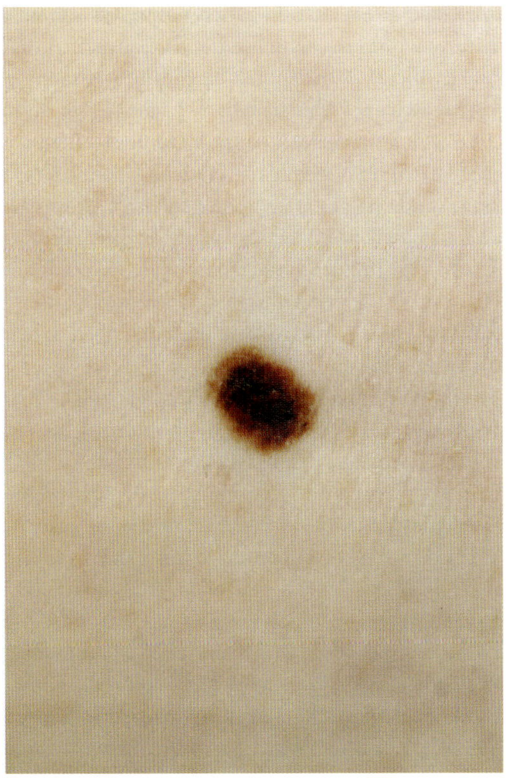

FIGURE 17-1 Clinically atypical nevus.

TABLE 17-2 • Criteria for the Histologic Diagnosis of Dysplastic Melanocytic Nevi from the World Health Organization Melanoma Program[33]

Major Criteria	Minor Criteria
1. Basilar proliferation of atypical nevomelanocytes (extending at least three ridges or "pegs" beyond any dermal nevocellular component) 2. Organization of this proliferation in a lentiginous or epithelioid cell pattern	1. Presence of lamellar fibrosis or concentric eosinophilic fibrosis 2. Neovascularization 3. Inflammatory response 4. Fusion of rete ridges

Both major criteria and two minor criteria are required for diagnosis.
Data from Bergman W, van Voorst Vader PC, Ruiter DJ: Dysplastic nevi and the risk of melanoma: a guideline for patient care. Nederlandse Melanoom Werkgroep van de Vereniging voor Integrale Kankercentra. Ned Tijdschr Geneeskd. *1997 Oct 18;141(42):2010-2014.*

vascularization in the papillary dermis can also be observed.[32] The World Health Organization has developed major and minor criteria for the histologic diagnosis, which was found to have an overall concordance of diagnosis for 141 specimens (including CN, DN, and melanoma) of 92% (**Table 17-2**).[33] Other groups such as the University of Pennsylvania, the European Organization for Research and Treatment of Cancer, and Duke University (**Table 17-3**) have also reported guidelines for reporting and grading DN.[34-36]

Pathologic reporting of DN is variable across institutions and practices, with some pathologists grading them on a scale ranging from mild, moderate, to severe dysplasia, and others preferring to report lesions as having low- or high-grade dysplasia. Given that these distinctions between lower and higher levels of dysplasia are based on degrees of histologic atypia interpreted by the dermatopathologist, it is important to note that variable interobserver concordance has been demonstrated, with the level of dermatopathologist experience potentially influencing the level of concordance.[5,37] One study did show that with a rigid set scoring system in place, the discrepancies among study dermatopathologists remained largely within one grade of the mean (55% of cases), whereas only 3% of cases differed by two or more grades.[38] DN can be heterogenous, meaning that atypical features may not be uniformly found across the lesion,[39] which can further nuance the grading of DN and lead to potential sampling error in partial incisional biopsies. The histologic features of a lesion have not been shown to correlate with the biologic behavior of the lesions.[40]

CLINICAL SIGNIFICANCE OF CAN/DN AND RISK OF TRANSFORMATION TO MELANOMA

CAN/DN can have both sporadic and familial origins and are associated with an increased risk for melanoma. CAN/DN have been described in the context of familial atypical mole and melanoma syndrome, where patients have a family history of melanoma along with greater than 50 nevi, at least one with atypical histologic features. These individuals have a significantly

TABLE 17-3 • Duke University Criteria for Grading of Dysplastic Nevi[36]

Architectural disorder	1. **Junctional component nested at both edges** (0: Yes, 1: No) 2. **Good overall symmetry** (0: Yes, 1: No) 3. **More than 5% nests cohesive** (0: Yes, 1: No) 4. **Suprabasal spread prominent or present at edge** (0: No, 1: Yes) 5. **More than 50% confluence of proliferation** (0: No, 1: Yes) 6. **Single-cell proliferation absent or focal** (0: Yes, 1: No) **Score key:** mild: 0-1; moderate: 2-3; severe: 4-6
Cytologic atypia	1. **Nuclei round or oval and euchromatic** (0: Yes, 1: No) 2. **Nuclei larger than those of basal-layer keratinocytes** (0: No, 1: Yes) 3. **Nucleoli prominent** (0: No, 1: Yes) 4. **Cell diameter more than twice that of basal keratinocytes** (0: No, 1: Yes) **Score key:** mild: 0-1; moderate: 2; severe: 3-4

Architectural disorder and cytologic atypia are scored separately by assigning a 0 or 1 for each criterion and summing.
Data from de Wit PE, van't Hof-Grootenboer B, Ruiter DJ, et al: Validity of the histopathological criteria used for diagnosing dysplastic naevi. An interobserver study by the pathology subgroup of the EORTC Malignant Melanoma Cooperative Group. Eur J Cancer. *1993;29A(6):831-839.*

increased risk of developing melanoma.[41] Nonfamilial CAN/DN as an isolated finding also confers an increased relative risk for developing melanoma of two- to eightfold.[11] A case-control study showed that 15% of patients with melanoma were diagnosed with CAN/DN, compared to only 2% of controls.[42] Another case-control study found that the presence of CAN (defined by irregular pigmentation and/or irregular border with a diameter of at least 5 mm) was significantly associated with the risk of melanoma among English and Australian patients.[43] Greater numbers of CAN appear to confer a greater risk for melanoma.[30] Moreover, a higher degree of atypia appears to correlate with an increased risk for melanoma: a history of mild, moderate, or severe atypia resulted in diagnosis of melanoma at a rate of 5.7%, 8.1%, and 19.7%, respectively, according to a study of 4481 patients.[44]

Although patients with CAN/DN are at increased risk for melanoma and need to be screened regularly, CAN are not obligate precursors to melanoma. CAN are not considered premalignant lesions or on a progression toward malignancy, unlike other models of dysplasia in cervical or colon cancer. Therefore, CAN be clinically followed to assess for stability, and biopsies may be reserved for changing lesions suspicious for melanoma or those that may be bothersome or difficult to self-monitor. Melanomas can arise from both CN and CAN/DN. Although there have been computed estimates of transformation rates of nevi to melanoma,[41] the true biological transformation rate of a CAN/DN into melanoma is not known. Several studies have demonstrated a comparable risk of developing melanoma among both DN and CN, suggesting that DN may not have an increased risk for malignant transformation and therefore do not need to be managed more aggressively.[45-48] Interestingly, in a study where histologically confirmed DN were transplanted into athymic mice, none were noted to transform into melanoma even following ultraviolet radiation.[49] Tucker et al[50] noted that among 844 individuals followed over a 25-year period, the majority of DN regressed or were stable. Most melanomas develop de novo, with only 20% to 40% of melanomas arising from precursor nevi.[51-53]

CLINICAL EVALUATION AND MANAGEMENT OF PATIENTS WITH CAN/DN

Because of their increased risk for melanoma, patients with CAN/DN need to be screened for melanoma on a regular basis. Given that the clinical features of CAN sometimes overlap with melanoma and some patients may have numerous CAN, the clinical examination can be challenging. Various clinical clues have been identified to help detect lesions concerning for malignancy. These include the ABCDEs (asymmetry, borders, color, diameter, and evolution) and the "ugly duckling sign," which uses the assumption that within an individual, most nevi tend to have similar phenotypic patterns, while a melanoma typically would stand apart in appearance.[54] The overall accuracy in clinically differentiating melanoma from CAN is estimated at 65% to 80%.[55-57]

Dermoscopy (epiluminescence microscopy) may increase the accuracy of clinical melanoma diagnosis and is an important diagnostic tool when caring for patients with CAN/DN.[58,59] Dermoscopy uses polarized light emitted from a handheld magnifying lens to visualize deeper pigmentation patterns as well as stromal and vascular structures within the skin. Studies have suggested that the use of dermoscopy increases melanoma diagnostic accuracy,[60] although training is necessary for this benefit.[61] There are six dermoscopic patterns into which the majority of DN can be classified: (1) reticular, (2) globular, (3) homogenous, (4) reticular globular, (5) reticular homogenous, and (6) globular homogenous.[62] Alternatively, DN can also be classified based on the pigment distribution into the following subtypes: uniform, multifocal hyper-/hypopigmentation, and central or eccentric hyper-/hypopigmentation. Various dermoscopy pattern analysis algorithms have been described to help distinguish melanoma from nevi.

Total-body photography (TBP) is another tool to help in the management of CAN/DN patients by monitoring for changes in nevi over time compared to a baseline set of images. TBP is especially useful for those with large numbers of nevi or those with more complex nevus patterns with a variety of colors, shapes, and sizes. Used in many pigmented lesion specialty clinics across the country, TBP encompasses a series of photographs in standardized positions to optimize viewing of nevi and dermoscopy images of individual nevi, which are used by clinicians at follow-up visits for patients over time. Through total-body baseline image comparison, new changes in pigmented lesions can more easily be detected. This method has been shown to allow clinicians to accurately detect melanoma in the earliest stages, while decreasing unnecessary biopsies and patient anxiety.[63-65] In one study published on TBP, biopsy rates of patients prior to care in a pigmented lesion clinic compared to rates after TBP in the clinic dropped significantly from 1.56 biopsies per year to less than 0.2 per year—a 3.8-fold reduction after TBP.[64] Skin self-photography has also been described as a reasonable approach for monitoring when professional photography services are unavailable.[66]

SURGICAL APPROACH

Deciding When and How to Biopsy

The decision to biopsy a pigmented lesion is based on the degree of clinical suspicion for melanoma, with the goal of detecting melanoma at its earliest, most curable stage, while also avoiding unnecessary biopsies of banal, stable CN and CAN.[2] Other scenarios in which clinicians consider biopsies include nevi that are irritated, cosmetically concerning, or in areas difficult to self-monitor. It is important in particular for patients with multiple CAN to be educated that CAN are not obligate precursors to melanoma, and the vast majority remain stable over one's lifetime. Careful self-monitoring and clinical monitoring by a clinician for suspicious changes can be recommended and may prevent the morbidity, downtime, and anxiety produced with numerous biopsies and excisions. Prophylactic excision of all a patient's nevi is both unnecessary and causes excessive morbidity to the patient. This strategy is also not effective at preventing melanoma, as melanomas may be more likely to arise de novo despite a patient having nevi.[21]

Prior to biopsy, the pigmented lesion should be examined to determine the best biopsy approach. Excisional biopsies are the preferred method for evaluating lesions that are suspicious for melanoma,[4] and the National Comprehensive Cancer Network (NCCN) and American Academy of Dermatology (AAD) guidelines recommend these biopsies be performed with a margin of 1 to 3 mm of normal skin beyond the area of clinical pigmentation.[67,68] This can be accomplished with a shave/scoop, punch, or fusiform excisional biopsy depending on the size and location of the lesion (**Table 17-4**).

The benefit of an excisional biopsy is that it produces the most complete specimen for histologic examination. This increases the likelihood of a correct diagnosis for pigmented lesions, in which the histologic diagnosis hinges on viewing the complete architecture of a lesion as well as the range of cytologic atypia.[4] Although a clinician may choose between a shave/scoop versus a punch/fusiform excision, a recent study demonstrated that the degree of clinical suspicion impacted this choice, with the majority of surveyed clinicians choosing a full-thickness punch or fusiform techniques for a lesion with a high degree of suspicion for melanoma, while the shave technique was used more frequently for lesions with a low degrees of suspicion.[69] Complete removal of a pigmented lesion also reduces the possibility of positive margins and recurrence. Recurrent nevi can appear clinically atypical and

TABLE 17-4 • Biopsy Techniques for Pigmented Lesions

	Technique	Benefits/Other Issues to Consider	Clinical Scenarios
Excisional biopsies	Shave/scoop excision	1. Complete assessment for accurate pathologic diagnosis assuming clinician did not transect peripheral or deep margins 2. Less invasive and fewer restrictions on patient activity given no need for sutures 3. Wound may take longer to heal by secondary intent	1. Lesions with higher suspicion for melanoma 2. Lesion in area of high tension or area difficult for primary closure (eg, mid back)
	Full-thickness (punch or fusiform excision)	1. Most complete control of peripheral and deep margins for accurate pathologic diagnosis. 2. Lower risk of clinical recurrence 3. Patient will have temporary restricted activity and sutures	1. Lesions with higher suspicion for melanoma 2. Primary closure is feasible
Partial incisional biopsies	Shave/scoop incisional biopsy	1. Fewer patient restrictions on patient activity given lack of sutures 2. Possibility of sampling error	1. Lesions with lower suspicion for melanoma; removal for irritation or cosmesis 2. Very large, suspicious macular lesion in which an excisional biopsy would be more complex
	Full-thickness (punch or elliptical) incisional biopsy	1. Patient may have temporary restricted activity and sutures 2. Can assess deeper components of lesion 3. Possibility of sampling error	1. Lesions with lower degree of suspicion for melanoma; removal for irritation or cosmesis 2. Very large, suspicious, papular or indurated lesion in which an excisional biopsy would be more complex

demonstrate histologic atypia that is nonmalignant (pseudomelanoma), histologically resembling superficial spreading melanoma, resulting in a misdiagnosis.[70]

There are certain clinical scenarios in which a partial incisional biopsy may be considered for pigmented lesions as well (**Table 17-4**). The AAD and NCCN guidelines support the use of partial incisional biopsy methods for certain anatomic areas (acral, cosmetically sensitive areas including the face) or for large lesions that would be difficult to fully excise.[71,72] In these cases, the most clinically atypical-appearing areas should be selected for biopsy.[4] However, in some instances, incisional biopsies can fail to diagnose a melanoma because sampling only part of a melanocytic lesion may not accurately reflect the biology of the entire lesion,[73] and studies have revealed that clinical atypia may not necessarily correlate with histologic atypia.[74] When partial incisional biopsy is used and obvious pigment remains, patients should be educated about monitoring for abnormal regrowth, and clinicians should continue to monitor the remaining pigmented lesion for the possibility of melanoma.

Punch Biopsy/Excision

Prior to performing a biopsy, the sites are typically cleaned with 70% isopropyl alcohol and anesthetized using lidocaine with epinephrine.[75] A punch biopsy relies on a metal cylinder with a sharp circular cutting edge to remove a full-thickness sample of skin, usually ranging in diameter from 2 to 8 mm. For pigmented lesions, the punch diameter should ideally extend at least 1 mm beyond the clinical pigment, with the goal of complete removal of the lesion. The clinician can score the skin around the pigmented lesion with light pressure to assess the correct-sized punch and map the best location for the punch to create clear clinical margins. The punch instrument is then rotated in a circular motion between the fingers until the instrument cuts through the dermis, meeting less resistance in the subcutaneous fat (**Figure 17-2**), at

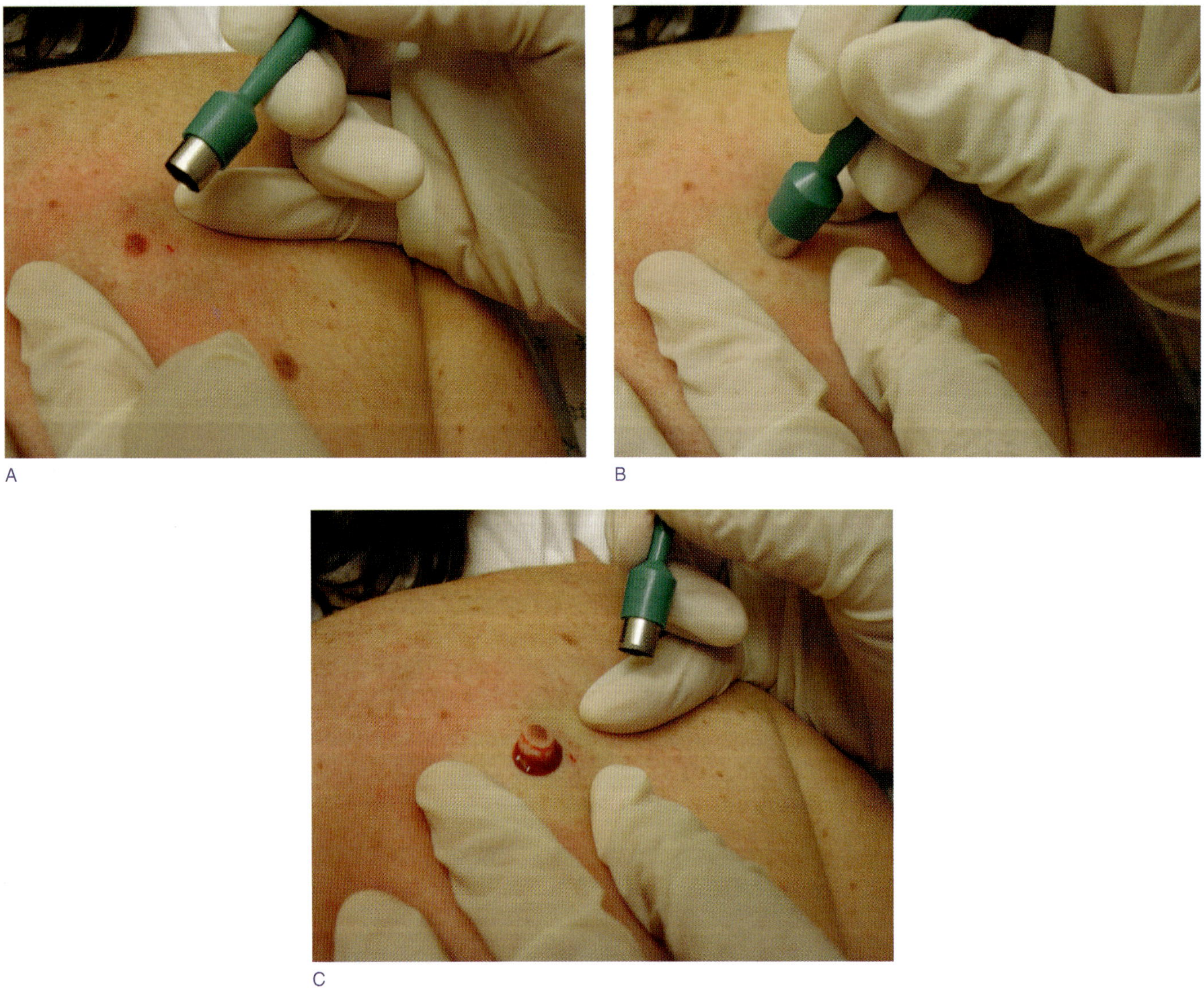

FIGURE 17-2 (**A**) Punch excisional biopsy technique (8-mm punch): Skin is held taut by hands and punch location is approximated to allow for margin of normal skin surrounding lesion. (**B**) Punch device is placed around lesion and rotated between fingers while applying pressure downward through the dermis until less resistance of the subcutaneous fat is felt. (**C**) The atypical pigmented lesion with surrounding 2 mm of normal skin is released by the punch technique, and the clinician cuts at the base of the tissue before placing sutures.

which time forceps are used to elevate the section and cut it away from the subcutaneous tissue.[75]

Hemostasis is achieved usually with one to three interrupted sutures; adhesive tape or a buried dermal suture can also be used for larger defects.[76] Nonabsorbable sutures are removed, in general, between 5 and 14 days after the procedure depending on anatomic site. Alternatively, if the punch is very small or the wound is very difficult to close primarily due to tension or other considerations, it may be appropriate to allow the wound to heal by secondary intention, in which case hemostasis can be achieved using gel foam if desired. Electrocautery, aluminum chloride, or other hemostatic agents are less desirable because these methods may impact wound healing.[77] Punch biopsy sites that heal by secondary intention may be appropriate for younger patients who can easily care for their biopsy site and may have outcomes comparable with 4-mm punch biopsies on the trunk or extremities that are closed with sutures. Older patients and those requiring larger punch biopsies may not be good candidates for healing through secondary intention because the outcomes are suboptimal in terms of postoperative pain, healing time, and scar formation. Adhesives are insufficient for closing punch biopsies because they do not bear adequate tension.[78]

An incisional punch biopsy by definition samples a portion of a larger lesion. For pigmented lesions, this may be considered in specific scenarios (**Table 17-4**). In general, although excisional biopsies are the preferred method of removal of lesions suspicious for melanoma, some pigmented lesions may be more difficult to remove in total due to size or sensitive anatomic area (such as on the face or feet), and clinicians may choose to sample a portion of these first. While not allowing a complete lateral architectural assessment of a lesion, the full depth of a lesion could be accurately assessed by punch biopsy and, therefore, is desirable for palpable or indurated suspicious lesions.

Shave/Saucerization Biopsy and Excision

Shave biopsies and excisions of pigmented lesions are rapid, commonly performed procedures that in certain clinical scenarios may result in comparable outcomes with punch biopsies or full-thickness skin excisions.[79,80] Generally, this procedure can be performed as a shave or saucerization using a sterile flexible razor blade. Clinicians may choose to use either a 15 blade with a handle, a split sterile flexible razor blade, or a DermaBlade. The skin is first anesthetized with an intradermal injection, which slightly elevates and tumesces the lesion and may make it easier to perform the biopsy. The nondominant hand is used to stabilize and hold the skin taught during the biopsy. Biopsies performed superficially may leave residual pigment either as a central dot or a peripheral rim.[80] This can be prevented by increasing the downward angle of the razor blade and lateral pressure. Another option for increasing the depth of the shave is to pinch the tissue beneath the nevus to create greater convexity of the area to be removed. Deeper shaves lead to more extensive wounds that may be associated with a depressed scar.[81] A 15 blade with handle may be used for saucerization of suspicious pigmented lesions in areas of higher tension such as the mid-back. In the saucerization technique, a 1- to 2-mm margin of normal skin around the lesion can be marked and scored by applying light pressure to the blade along the marking. This allows for control over the peripheral margins of the biopsy. Light, continuous pressure is then applied tangentially through the dermis to the scored areas to release the skin specimen. The removed specimen is convex on its undersurface[75,82] (**Figure 17-3**).

Larger shave excisions and saucerizations may take longer to heal than incisions repaired with sutures, and patients should be educated to continue wound care until the skin is healed completely. Patients who heal with hypertrophic scars or keloids may prefer punch or elliptical excisions. However, most patients consider the scars following shave biopsy to be acceptable and preferable to other methods such as more invasive excisions into the deep dermis or superficial subcutaneous layer[7,82] (**Figure 17-3**). The shave biopsy technique has been associated with a higher risk of recurrence of pigmented lesions.[83] In general, shave biopsies are more superficial than punch or elliptical excisions and are more likely to leave a positive deep margin, although clinician experience with the technique likely plays a role in how accurately a pigmented lesion is removed, and many pigmented lesions are effectively biopsied in this manner.

Although excisional biopsies of suspicious pigmented lesions are favored, certain scenarios may cause a clinician to favor a shave incisional biopsy of a pigmented lesion. These scenarios include larger diameter lesions difficult to remove in total; lesions in certain anatomic areas (acral and face); and lesions removed that are of lower clinical suspicion, such as those removed for irritation or cosmesis (**Table 17-4**). Limitations, such as sampling error and inability to assess deeper tissue, should be considered with shave incisional biopsies. As with any partial incisional biopsy, any clinical pigmented lesion remaining after the biopsy should be monitored for the possibility of melanoma.

Fusiform Excision

The fusiform or elliptical excision is a versatile technique that is a cornerstone of dermatologic surgery and the definitive removal of atypical pigmented lesions. The excision should ideally encompass at least a 2-mm margin of normal skin around a pigmented lesion, and the fusiform design results in a defect three to four times longer than the width of the planned excision[84] (**Figure 17-4**). The incision extends to the subcutis and should preferably be oriented such that the scar lies parallel to relaxed skin tension lesions. After surgical planning and orientation are established, the skin is marked with a surgical marker, cleaned, and prepped in a sterile fashion. Local anesthesia is administered. Once the incision lines are made to the subcutis, a uniform thickness of tissue is removed through the subcutaneous fat in the fusiform shape. After appropriate undermining and hemostasis are achieved, closure can be achieved by several methods with the goals to provide precise wound approximation and maximal wound eversion and reduce tension on the wound.[85] A layered closure is generally performed. For a complete discussion of linear excision and repairs, see Chapter 16.

Fusiform excisional biopsies with 2- to 3-mm clinical margins are an ideal way to achieve an excisional biopsy of suspicious pigmented lesions, as both peripheral and deep margins can be accurately controlled by the clinician. As the goal of the excisional biopsy is to remove the complete skin lesion for accurate

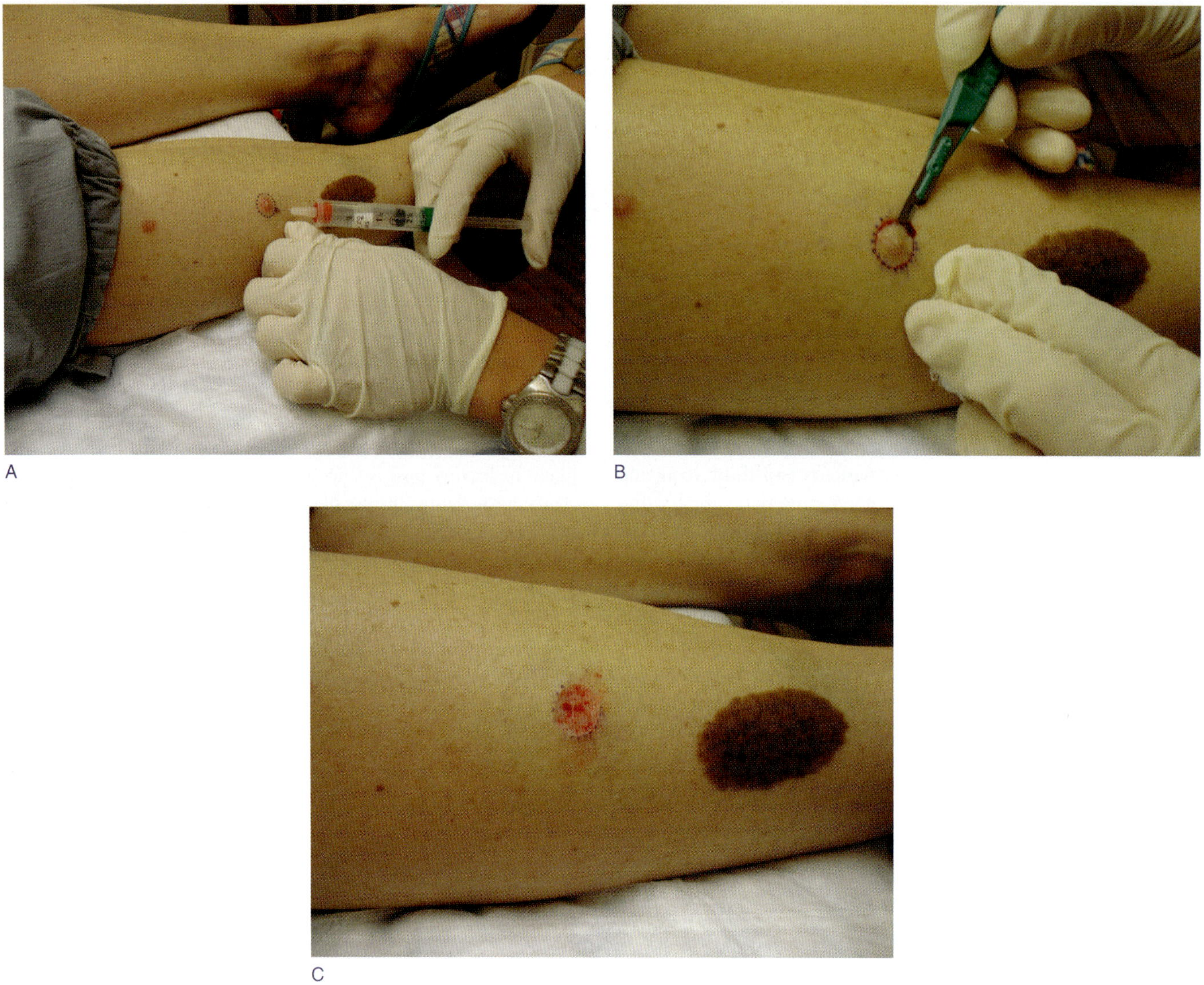

FIGURE 17-3 (**A**) Saucerization excisional biopsy technique: Lesion is marked with a surgical pen with 2- to 3-mm clinical margin of surrounding normal skin, cleaned, and anesthetized. (**B**) Marked lesion is scored around the margin, then blade is tangentially and continuously drawn through the dermis to scored areas. (**C**) Appearance of wound after removal of lesion.

diagnosis, margins beyond 2 to 3 mm are not necessarily needed at the time of initial removal. If the suspicious pigmented lesion is believed to represent melanoma, the possibility of a follow-up wide local excision with sentinel lymph node biopsy must be considered, and the clinician should be mindful of the orientation and size of the initial excision. This is important to allow for the greatest chance of closure of a second, wider excision and accurate sentinel lymph node mapping. Reexcisions of DN are also typically performed in a fusiform fashion to ensure complete removal of any residuum, with some clinicians favoring a 5-mm reexcision of severe DN via a fusiform excision.

Deciding When to Reexcise a DN

Despite the intent to perform an excisional biopsy of a pigmented lesion, histologically positive margins can be left behind. By definition, a histologically positive margin is expected in a partial incisional biopsy. The NIH consensus paper on DN from 1992 had no guidelines on reexcision of DN, and clinicians have had the challenge of determining when to recommend a reexcision after an initial biopsy of a DN.[11] The decision to perform reexcisions for DN have been variable geographically as there is a paucity of data to help understand the actual risk of transformation of melanoma from DN. In 2002, a survey of members of the AAD revealed that 67% of respondents preferred to reexcise DN with a positive histologic margin.[58] However, several recently published studies have examined the role of observation for DN with positive histologic margins.[86] In addition, studies by Goodson et al[83] and Hocker et al[87] also observed a combined total of 184 DN with positive histologic margins, and no melanomas eventuated from the biopsy sites with greater than 2 years and an average of 17.4 years of follow-up, respectively. Two additional studies examined a total of 219 reexcisions of DN with positive histologic margins to assess for presence of melanoma in the reexcision specimen.[88,89] While the study by Abello-Poblete et al[88] found no

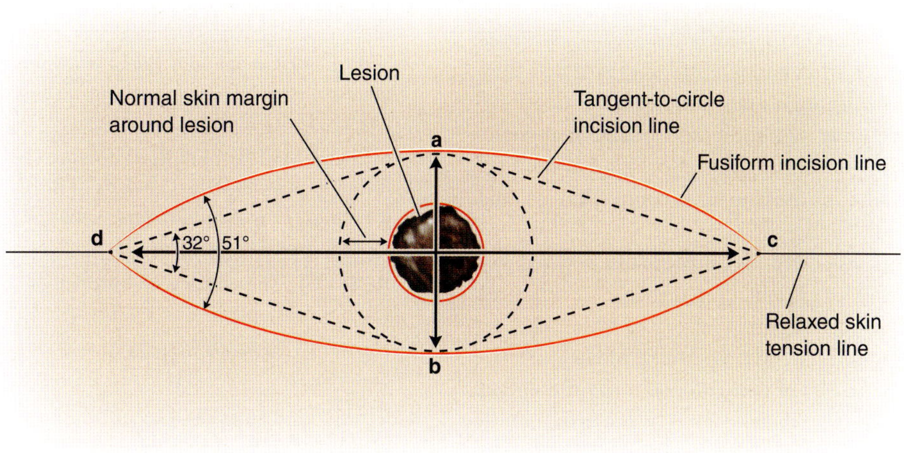

FIGURE 17-4 The fusiform excision.

melanomas within the reexcision of DN with positive histologic margins, the study by Reddy et al[89] found that 2 of 127 reexcisions (1.6%) revealed melanoma in situ arising from initial lesions biopsied and diagnosed as moderately to severely DN, and the authors suggested reexcisions for higher-grade DN with positive histologic margins. More recently, a study of 498 patients with mild or moderate DN with positive margins at biopsy demonstrated a very low rate of conversion to melanoma, with 2% of observed DN demonstrating conversion to melanoma versus 0.06% of reexcised DN.[90] Although this difference was not statistically significant, the study may not have been powered to detect such a small effect size, and therefore, careful consideration of reexcision should continue.

Recent studies have shown that over time, more clinicians choose clinical observation for lower grade DN with positive histologic margins. A 2009 survey of Chicago dermatologists revealed that although 79% of respondents observed mild DN with positive margins, 81% reexcised moderate DN with positive margins and 95% reexcised severe DN.[21] In a 2014 survey of New England dermatologists on management of DN with positive margins and no clinical residual pigment, 95% of respondents observed mild DN with positive histologic margins, while 39% observed moderate DN with positive margins, and 100% reexcised severe DN (**Table 17-5**).[69] Most dermatologists agree that severe DN with a positive margin should be reexcised because of the possibility that these lesions may overlap histologically with early melanoma.[58,69]

To highlight the clinical gap in recommendations for management of biopsied DN with positive margins, the Pigmented Lesion Subcommittee of the Melanoma Prevention Working Group published a consensus statement in 2015, and through the Delphi technique of consensus building, recommendations about management of DN with positive histologic margins were suggested by the authors.[2] Included in the recommendations was the consensus that DN with mild or moderate atypia and *clear* histologic margins do not need to be reexcised. Also, mild DN with positive histologic margins and no clinical residual pigmentation can be managed with observation. For moderate DN with positive histologic margins and no clinical residual pigmentation, the consensus statement recommended that clinical observation may be appropriate, although more data are needed. There was consensus that all severe DN with positive histologic margins should be reexcised to achieve a 2- to 5-mm clinically free margin.[91]

TABLE 17-5 • Results from a 2014 Survey of New England Dermatologists' Management of Dysplastic Nevi (DN) with Positive Histologic Margins and No Clinical Residual Pigment[69]

	Observe	Reexcise
Mild DN	95%	5%
Moderate DN	39%	61%
Moderate-severe DN	5%	95%
Severe DN	0%	100%

Data from Hocker TL, Alikhan A, Comfere NI, et al: Favorable long-term outcomes in patients with histologically dysplastic nevi that approach a specimen border. J Am Acad Dermatol. *2013 Apr;68(4):545-551.*

OTHER CLINICAL RECOMMENDATIONS FOR PATIENTS WITH CAN/DN

Patients with CAN/DN are at risk for melanoma and should be educated about the significance of their nevi as a risk marker—though not obligate precursor—for melanoma, reasons for biopsy, self-skin examinations, and sun protection. Monthly self-skin examinations can be recommended, and patients can be educated about concerning changes that should prompt clinical evaluation. The "ugly duckling" sign can be extremely helpful, particularly for patients with numerous CAN. This helps patients streamline their examination and recognize usual patterns of their nevi and to look for skin lesions that stand apart for any reason. Patients can be advised regarding wearing sun-protective clothing, minimizing sun exposure, and applying sunscreen with an SPF of 30 or higher to exposed skin. In terms of other screening recommendations, a survey of dermatologists found that few clinicians advised patients to be examined by an ophthalmologist to check for ocular melanocytic neoplasms (2.9%), whereas 11.5% reported usually referring patients and 45.5% stated they do so but infrequently.[58] Although many studies have identified a link between atypical mole syndrome and ocular malignant melanoma, a review article addressing this association also noted that there are several studies finding no such connection, so this relationship remains poorly defined.[92]

Timing of follow-up visits can be individualized based on number of nevi, complexity of examination, degree of clinical and histologic atypia, and personal or family history of melanoma. In one study, for a patient with DN and no personal history or family history of melanoma, 58.8% of dermatologists recommended follow-up every 12 months, whereas 32.8% preferred every 6 months.[58] All prior biopsy sites should be monitored for change and rebiopsied if changes are evident. Although recurrent pigmentation can occasionally be observed within a scar within the first several months after a biopsy, if new pigmentation extends beyond the scar or occurs after a longer delay after biopsy, this may be more concerning for melanoma, and the residual pigment should be rebiopsied.[91]

CONCLUSIONS

The evaluation and management of DN remain a considerable clinical challenge. Terminologic ambiguity, regional variation in management, and the clinical challenge of identifying those lesions at risk of evolution all contribute to the difficulties associated with DN evaluation and therapy. Clinically, any changing pigmented lesion in an adult likely merits biopsy or referral; those occurring in the context of a personal or family history of melanoma or associated with marked color or diameter change or the presence of underlying erythema merit particular concern. Educating patients on the importance of self-examinations and the utility of self-photography, as well as the simple act of offering a full skin examination to patients, may help mitigate the dramatic increase in melanoma seen over the past four decades.

From a procedural perspective, most DN are easily treated with a linear excision (see Chapter 16). Biopsy should always be performed with the goal of obtaining a representative, and ideally entire, sample of the lesion. The phrase "excisional biopsy" includes a number of approaches including deep or scoop shave biopsy, saucerization, punch biopsy, and fusiform excision. Ultimately, any procedural intervention should be performed in the context of an overall management approach that is tailored to the individual patient.

REFERENCES

1. Elston D. Practical advice regarding problematic pigmented lesions. *J Am Acad Dermatol.* 2012;67(1):148-155.
2. Balch CM, Buzaid AC, Soong SJ, et al. Final version of the American Joint Committee on Cancer staging system for cutaneous melanoma. *J Clin Oncol.* 2001;19(16):3635-3648.
3. Salopek TG. The dilemma of the dysplastic nevus. *Dermatol Clin.* 2002;20(4):617-628.
4. Kim CC, Swetter SM, Curiel-Lewandrowski C, et al. Addressing the knowledge gap in clinical recommendations for management and complete excision of clinically atypical nevi/dysplastic nevi: Pigmented Lesion Subcommittee consensus statement. *JAMA Dermatol.* 2015;151(2):212-218.
5. Piepkorn MW, Barnhill RL, Cannon-Albright LA, et al. A multiobserver, population-based analysis of histologic dysplasia in melanocytic nevi. *J Am Acad Dermatol.* 1994;30(5):707-714.
6. Steijlen PM, Bergman W, Hermans J, Scheffer E, Vloten WA, Ruiter DJ. The efficacy of histopathological criteria required for diagnosing dysplastic naevi. *Histopathology.* 1988;12(3):289-300.
7. Norris W. A case of fungoid disease. *Edinb Med Surg J.* 1820;16: 562-565.
8. Clark WH, Reimer RR, Greene M, Ainsworth AM, Mastrangelo MJ. Origin of familial malignant melanomas from heritable melanocytic lesions: the BK mole syndrome. *Arch Dermatol.* 1978;114(5):732-738.
9. Lynch HT, Frichot BC, Lynch JF. Familial atypical multiple mole-melanoma syndrome. *J Med Genet.* 1978;15(5):352-356.
10. Elder DE, Goldman LI, Goldman SC, Greene MH, Clark WH. Dysplastic nevus syndrome: a phenotypic association of sporadic cutaneous melanoma. *Cancer.* 1980;46(8):1787-1794.
11. Goldsmith LA, Askin FB, Chang AE, et al. Diagnosis and treatment of early melanoma: NIH Consensus Development Panel on Early Melanoma. *JAMA.* 1992;268(10):1314-1319.
12. Lee JY, Dong SM, Shin MS, et al. Genetic alterations of p16INK4a and p53 genes in sporadic dysplastic nevus. *Biochem Biophys Res Commun.* 1997;237(3):667-672.
13. Bishop JAN, Wachsmuth RC, Harland M, et al. Genotype/phenotype and penetrance studies in melanoma families with germline CDKN2A mutations. *J Invest Dermatol.* 2000;114(1):28-33.
14. Hussein MR, Roggero E, Sudilovsky EC, Tuthill RJ, Wood GS, Sudilovsky O. Alterations of mismatch repair protein expression in benign melanocytic nevi, melanocytic dysplastic nevi, and cutaneous malignant melanomas. *Am J Dermatopathol.* 2001;23(4):308-314.
15. Pollock PM, Harper UL, Hansen KS, et al. High frequency of BRAF mutations in nevi. *Nat Genet.* 2003;33(1):19-20.
16. Shpitz B, Klein E, Malinger P, et al. Altered expression of the DNA mismatch repair proteins hMLH1 and hMSH2 in cutaneous dysplastic nevi and malignant melanoma. *Int J Biol Markers.* 2004;20(1):65-68.
17. Uribe P, Wistuba II, Gonzalez S. Allelotyping, microsatellite instability, and BRAF mutation analyses in common and atypical melanocytic nevi and primary cutaneous melanomas. *Am J Dermatopathol.* 2009;31(4):354-363.
18. Scatolini M, Grand MM, Grosso E, et al. Altered molecular pathways in melanocytic lesions. *Int J Cancer.* 2010;126(8):1869-1881.
19. Alekseenko A, Wojas-Pelc A, Lis GJ, Furgał-Borzych A, Surówka G, Litwin JA. Cyclin D1 and D3 expression in melanocytic skin lesions. *Arch Dermatol Res.* 2010;302(7):545-550.
20. Lebe B, Pabuççuoglu U, Özer E. The significance of Ki-67 proliferative index and cyclin D1 expression of dysplastic nevi in the biologic spectrum of melanocytic lesions. *Appl Immunohistochem Mol Morphol.* 2007;15(2):160-164.
21. Duffy KL, Mann DJ, Petronic-Rosic V, Shea CR. Clinical decision making based on histopathologic grading and margin status of dysplastic nevi. *Arch Dermatol.* 2012;148(2):259-260.
22. Chin L. The genetics of malignant melanoma: lessons from mouse and man. *Nat Rev Cancer.* 2003;3(8):559-570.

23. Crijns MB, Vink J, Van Hees CLM, Bergman W, Vermeer BJ. Dysplastic nevi: occurrence in first-and second-degree relatives of patients with sporadic dysplastic nevus syndrome. *Arch Dermatol.* 1991;127(9):1346-1351.

24. Rampen FHJ, Fleuren BAM, de Boo TM, Lemmens W. Prevalence of common "acquired" nevocytic nevi and dysplastic nevi is not related to ultraviolet exposure. *J Am Acad Dermatol.* 1988;18(4):679-683.

25. Richard MA, Grob J-J, Gouvernet J, et al. Role of sun exposure on nevus: first study in age-sex phenotype-controlled populations. *Arch Dermatol.* 1993;129(10):1280-1285.

26. Reutter JC, Long EM, Morrell DS, Thomas NE, Groben PA. Eruptive post-chemotherapy in situ melanomas and dysplastic nevi. *Pediatr Dermatol.* 2007;24(2):135-137.

27. Richert S, Bloom EJ, Flynn K, Seraly MP. Widespread eruptive dermal and atypical melanocytic nevi in association with chronic myelocytic leukemia: case report and review of the literature. *J Am Acad Dermatol.* 1996;35(2):326-329.

28. Ulrich C, Christophers E, Sterry W, Meyer T, Stockfleth E. Skin diseases in organ transplant patients. *Hautarzt.* 2002;53(8): 524-533.

29. Duvic M, Lowe L, Rapini RP, Rodriguez S, Levy ML. Eruptive dysplastic nevi associated with human immunodeficiency virus infection. *Arch Dermatol.* 1989;125(3):397-401.

30. Tucker MA, Halpern A, Holly EA, et al. Clinically recognized dysplastic nevi: a central risk factor for cutaneous melanoma. *JAMA.* 1997;277(18):1439-1444.

31. Bergman W, van Voorst VPC, Ruiter DJ. [Dysplastic nevi and the risk of melanoma: a guideline for patient care. Nederlandse Melanoom Werkgroep van de Vereniging voor Integrale Kankercentra.]. *Ned Tijdschr Geneeskd.* 1997;141(42):2010-2014.

32. Elder DE. The dysplastic nevus. *Pathology.* 1985;17(2):291-297.

33. Clemente C, Cochran AJ, Elder DE, et al. Histopathologic diagnosis of dysplastic nevi: concordance among pathologists convened by the World Health Organization Melanoma Programme. *Hum Pathol.* 1991;22(4):313-319.

34. De Wit PEJ, Van't Hof-Grootenboer B, Ruiter DJ, et al. Validity of the histopathological criteria used for diagnosing dysplastic naevi: an interobserver study by the pathology subgroup of the EORTC Malignant Melanoma Cooperative Group. *Eur J Cancer.* 1993;29(6):831-839.

35. Elder DE, Murphy GF. *Melanocytic Tumors of the Skin.* Vol 2. Rockville, MD: American Registry of Pathology; 1991.

36. Shea CR, Vollmer RT, Prieto VG. Correlating architectural disorder and cytologic atypia in Clark (dysplastic) melanocytic nevi. *Hum Pathol.* 1999;30(5):500-505.

37. Duncan LM, Berwick M, Bruijn JA, Byers HR, Mihm MC, Barnhill RL. Histopathologic recognition and grading of dysplastic melanocytic nevi: an interobserver agreement study. *J Invest Dermatol.* 1993;100(3):S318-S321.

38. Weinstock MA, Barnhill RL, Rhodes AR, Brodsky GL. Reliability of the histopathologic diagnosis of melanocytic dysplasia. *Arch Dermatol.* 1997;133(8):953-958.

39. Barr RJ, Linden KG, Rubinstein G, Cantos KA. Analysis of heterogeneity of atypia within melanocytic nevi. *Arch Dermatol.* 2003;139(3):289-292.

40. Duffy K, Grossman D. The dysplastic nevus: from historical perspective to management in the modern era: part I. Historical, histologic, and clinical aspects. *J Am Acad Dermatol.* 2012;67(1): 1.e1-1.e16.

41. Mize DE, Bishop M, Resse E, Sluzevich J. Familial atypical multiple mole melanoma syndrome. 2009. https://www.ncbi.nlm.nih.gov/books/NBK7030/. Accessed February 19, 2020.

42. Newton JA, Bataille V, Griffiths K, et al. How common is the atypical mole syndrome phenotype in apparently sporadic melanoma? *J Am Acad Dermatol.* 1993;29(6):989-996.

43. Bataille V, Grulich A, Sasieni P, et al. The association between naevi and melanoma in populations with different levels of sun exposure: a joint case-control study of melanoma in the UK and Australia. *Br J Cancer.* 1998;77(3):505.

44. Arumi-Uria M, McNutt NS, Finnerty B. Grading of atypia in nevi: correlation with melanoma risk. *Modern Pathol.* 2003;16(8):764-771.

45. Goodson AG, Florell SR, Boucher KM, Grossman D. A decade of melanomas: identification of factors associated with delayed detection in an academic group practice. *Dermatol Surg.* 2011;37(11): 1620-1630.

46. Lucas CR, Sanders LL, Murray JC, Myers SA, Hall RP, Grichnik JM. Early melanoma detection: nonuniform dermoscopic features and growth. *J Am Acad Dermatol.* 2003;48(5):663-671.

47. Sagebiel RW. Melanocytic nevi in histologic association with primary cutaneous melanoma of superficial spreading and nodular types: effect of tumor thickness. *J Invest Dermatol.* 1993;100(3):322-325.

48. Skender-Kalnenas TM, English DR, Heenan PJ. Benign melanocytic lesions: risk markers or precursors of cutaneous melanoma? *J Am Acad Dermatol.* 1995;33(6):1000-1007.

49. Meyer LJ, Schmidt LA, Goldgar DE, Piepkorn MW. Survival and histopathologic characteristics of human melanocytic nevi transplanted to athymic (nude) mice. *Am J Dermatopathol.* 1995;17(4):368-373.

50. Tucker MA, Fraser MC, Goldstein AM, et al. A natural history of melanomas and dysplastic nevi: an atlas of lesions in melanoma-prone families. *Dermatol Nurs.* 2003;15(3):237-250.

51. Crucioli V, Stilwell J. The histogenesis of malignant melanoma in relation to pre-existing pigmented lesions. *J Cutan Pathol.* 1982;9(6):396-404.

52. Gruber SB, Barnhill RL, Stenn KS, Roush GC. Nevomelanocytic proliferations in association with cutaneous malignant melanoma: a multivariate analysis. *J Am Acad Dermatol.* 1989;21(4):773-780.

53. Marks R, Dorevitch AP, Mason G. Do all melanomas come from "moles"? A study of the histological association between melanocytic naevi and melanoma. *Australas J Dermatol.* 1990;31(2):77-80.

54. Gachon J, Beaulieu P, Sei JF, et al. First prospective study of the recognition process of melanoma in dermatological practice. *Arch Dermatol.* 2005;141(4):434-438.

55. Miller M, Ackerman AB. How accurate are dermatologists in the diagnosis of melanoma? Degree of accuracy and implications. *Arch Dermatol.* 1992;128(4):559-560.

56. Wolf IH, Smolle J, Soyer HP, Kerl H. Sensitivity in the clinical diag nosis of malignant melanoma. *Melanoma Res.* 1998;8(5):425-429.

57. Grin CM, Kopf AW, Welkovich B, Bart RS, Levenstein MJ. Accuracy in the clinical diagnosis of malignant melanoma. *Arch Dermatol.* 1990;126(6):763-766.

58. Tripp JM, Kopf AW, Marghoob AA, Bart RS. Management of dysplastic nevi: a survey of fellows of the American Academy of Dermatology. *J Am Acad Dermatol.* 2002;46(5):674-682.

59. Binder M, Schwarz M, Winkler A, et al. Epiluminescence microscopy: a useful tool for the diagnosis of pigmented skin lesions for formally trained dermatologists. *Arch Dermatol.* 1995;131(3):286-291.
60. Mayer J. Systematic review of the diagnostic accuracy of dermatoscopy in detecting malignant melanoma. *Med J Aust.* 1997;167(4):206-210.
61. Binder M, Puespoeck-Schwarz M, Steiner A, et al. Epiluminescence microscopy of small pigmented skin lesions: short-term formal training improves the diagnostic performance of dermatologists. *J Am Acad Dermatol.* 1997;36(2):197-202.
62. Hofmann-Wellenhof R, Blum A, Wolf IH, et al. Dermoscopic classification of atypical melanocytic nevi (Clark nevi). *Arch Dermatol.* 2001;137(12):1575-1580.
63. Del Mar CB, Green AC. Aid to diagnosis of melanoma in primary medical care. *BMJ.* 1995;310(6978):492-495.
64. Truong A, Strazzulla L, March J, et al. Reduction in nevus biopsies in patients monitored by total body photography. *J Am Acad Dermatol.* 2016;75(1):135-143.e5.
65. Moye MS, King SMC, Rice ZP, et al. Effects of total-body digital photography on cancer worry in patients with atypical mole syndrome. *JAMA Dermatol.* 2015;151(2):137-143.
66. Kantor J. Skin self-photography for dysplastic nevus monitoring is associated with a decrease in the number of biopsies at follow-up: a retrospective analytical study. *J Am Acad Dermatol.* 2015;73(4):704-705.
67. Bichakjian CK, Halpern AC, Johnson TM, et al. Guidelines of care for the management of primary cutaneous melanoma. *J Am Acad Dermatol.* 2011;65(5):1032-1047.
68. Coit DG, Thompson JA, Algazi A, et al. Melanoma, version 2.2016 clinical practice guidelines in oncology. *J Natl Compr Cancer Netw.* 2016;14(4):450-473
69. Tong LX, Wu PA, Kim CC. Degree of clinical concern and dysplasia affect biopsy technique and management of dysplastic nevi with positive biopsy margins: results from a survey of New England dermatologists. *J Am Acad Dermatol.* 2016;74(2):389-391.e382.
70. Kornberg R, Ackerman AB. Pseudomelanoma: recurrent melanocytic nevus following partial surgical removal. *Arch Dermatol.* 1975;111(12):1588-1590.
71. National Comprehensive Cancer Network. Clinical practice guidelines in oncology: melanoma. https://www.nccn.org/professionals/physician_gls/default.aspx. Accessed February 19, 2020.
72. Sober AJ, Chuang T-Y, Duvic M, et al. Guidelines of care for primary cutaneous melanoma. *J Am Acad Dermatol.* 2001;45(4):579-586.
73. Witheiler DD, Cockerell CJ. Sensitivity of diagnosis of malignant melanoma: a clinicopathologic study with a critical assessment of biopsy techniques. *Exp Dermatol.* 1992;1(4):170-175.
74. Annessi G, Cattaruzza MS, Abeni D, et al. Correlation between clinical atypia and histologic dysplasia in acquired melanocytic nevi. *J Am Acad Dermatol.* 2001;45(1):77-85.
75. Bart RS, Kopf AW. Techniques of biopsy of cutaneous neoplasms. *J Dermatol Surg Oncol.* 1979;5(12):979-987.
76. Collins SC, Whalen JD. Surgical pearl: percutaneous buried vertical mattress for the closure of narrow wounds. *J Am Acad Dermatol.* 1999;41(6):1025-1026.
77. Bush JA, Ferguson MWJ, Mason T, McGrouther DA. Skin tension or skin compression? Small circular wounds are likely to shrink, not gape. *J Plast Reconstruct Aesthet Surg.* 2008;61(5):529-534.
78. Christenson LJ, Phillips PK, Weaver AL, Otley CC. Primary closure vs second-intention treatment of skin punch biopsy sites: a randomized trial. *Arch Dermatol.* 2005;141(9):1093-1099.
79. Harrison PV. Good results after shave excision of benign moles. *Dermatol Surg.* 1985;11(7):668.
80. Hudson-Peacock MJ, Bishop J, Lawrence C. Shave excision of benign papular naevocytic naevi. *Br J Plast Surg.* 1995;48(5):318-322.
81. Gambichler T, Senger E, Rapp S, Alamouti D, Altmeyer P, Hoffmann K. Deep shave excision of macular melanocytic nevi with the razor blade biopsy technique. *Dermatol Surg.* 2000; 26(7):662-666.
82. Robinson JK, Anderson ER. Skin structure and surgical anatomy. In: *Surgery of the Skin: Procedural Dermatology.* Philadelphia, PA: Elsevier Mosby; 2005:3-23.
83. Goodson AG, Florell SR, Boucher KM, Grossman D. Low rates of clinical recurrence after biopsy of benign to moderately dysplastic melanocytic nevi. *J Am Acad Dermatol.* 2010;62(4):591-596.
84. Bennett RG. *Fundamentals of Cutaneous Surgery.* Philadelphia, PA: CV Mosby Company; 1988.
85. Moy RL, Waldman B, Hein DW. A review of sutures and suturing techniques. *J Dermatol Surg Oncol.* 1992;18(9):785-795.
86. Kmetz EC, Sanders H, Fisher G, Lang PG, Maize JC Sr. The role of observation in the management of atypical nevi. *South Med J.* 2009;102(1):45-48.
87. Hocker TL, Alikhan A, Comfere NI, Peters MS. Favorable long-term outcomes in patients with histologically dysplastic nevi that approach a specimen border. *J Am Acad Dermatol.* 2013;68(4):545-551.
88. Abello-Poblete MV, Correa-Selm LM, Giambrone D, Victor F, Rao BK. Histologic outcomes of excised moderate and severe dysplastic nevi. *Dermatol Surg.* 2014;40(1):40-45.
89. Reddy KK, Farber MJ, Bhawan J, Geronemus RG, Rogers GS. Atypical (dysplastic) nevi: outcomes of surgical excision and association with melanoma. *JAMA Dermatol.* 2013;149(8):928-934.
90. Fleming NH, Egbert BM, Kim J, Swetter SM. Reexamining the threshold for reexcision of histologically transected dysplastic nevi. *JAMA Dermatol.* 2016;152(12):1327-1334.
91. Blum A, Hofmann-Wellenhof R, Marghoob AA, et al. Recurrent melanocytic nevi and melanomas in dermoscopy: results of a multicenter study of the International Dermoscopy Society. *JAMA Dermatol.* 2014;150(2):138-145.
92. Hurst EA, Harbour JW, Cornelius LA. Ocular melanoma: a review and the relationship to cutaneous melanoma. *Arch Dermatol.* 2003;139(8):1067-1073.

Approach to Cysts and Lipomas

18

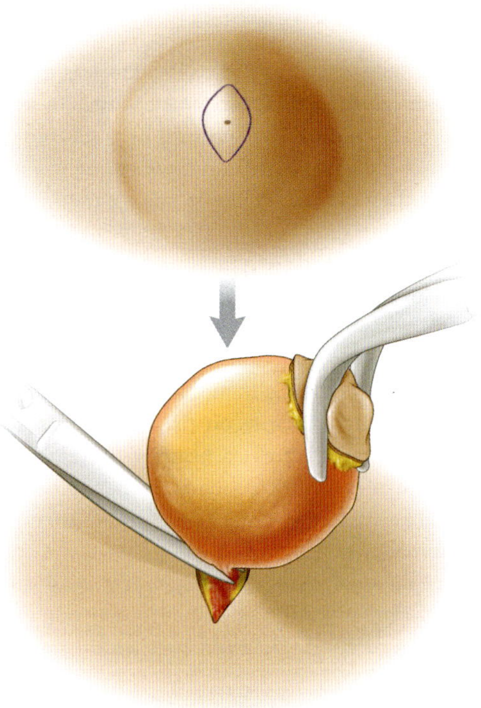

SUMMARY

- Cysts are a frequent patient complaint, and removal may be motivated by tenderness, functional compromise, or aesthetic concern.
- Most cysts respond well to excisional approaches, ranging from small punch excisions to large elliptical approaches.

Beginner Tips

- Never attempt to excise an actively infected cyst; instead, consider I&D or a course of antibiotic therapy prior to attempting aggressive surgical intervention.
- Cysts that have been previously treated, infected, or manipulated will be more recalcitrant to treatment and may require sharp dissection or full excision.

Pitfalls and Cautions

- Even expert diagnosticians may be fooled by cyst mimickers; therefore, all suspect cystic nodules should be removed, and every cyst should be sent for histopathology.
- Excising large cysts overlying nerve danger zones may entail a risk of permanent nerve damage; this should be explained to patients as part of the informed consent process.

Expert Tips

- With experience, cysts may be delicately dissected en bloc from a small incision site.
- Dead space minimization is vital for postoperative success, and may be accomplished via fascial plication sutures or percutaneous suture placement.

Patient Education Points

- Patients should always be told that they are trading the cyst for a scar; if they are at all hesitant, defer the procedure.
- Even with complete excision, cysts may recur; patients should be warned that this is a possibility before starting surgery.

Don't Forget!

- Though minimal access incisions may be tempting, this must be weighed against the undesirable smell associated with cyst rupture which may be disturbing to the patient.
- Careful removal of all cyst contents and the entirety of the cyst wall will help mitigate the risk of recurrence or postoperative complications.

Billing Pearls

- Depending on clinical practice, most excised cysts are removed for symptomatic reasons, and are therefore billed with a benign series excision code (11400 series) coupled with a repair code (12000 and 13000 series).
- Be sure to document the rationale for the medical necessity of cyst excision if it is to be billed to insurance.
- Cysts removed purely for cosmetic reasons should not be billed to insurance.

18 Approach to Cysts and Lipomas

INTRODUCTION

Cysts and lipomas are frequently encountered, as patients frequently present with a growing, irritated, or infected cystic nodule; while patients often present due to symptomatic concerns, they also occasionally seek treatment for aesthetic reasons as well. Most epidermal inclusion and pilar cysts can be identified clinically by their appearance and anatomic location, although excised nodules should always be evaluated histopathologically, as other skin and soft tissue tumors—everything from metastases to Merkel cell carcinoma—can clinically mimic epidermal cysts.

EPIDEMIOLOGY

Many patients and nonclinicians refer to epidermal inclusion and pilar cysts colloquially as *sebaceous* cysts. This terminology should probably be avoided, as the only truly sebaceous cyst is a steatocystoma, which is encountered only infrequently and is sometimes associated with pachyonychia congenita type 2 and steatocystoma multiplex.[1,2] Epidermal cysts are synonymous with infundibular cysts or epidermal inclusion cysts, as they are all derived from the follicular infundibulum. These are sometimes divided into primary and secondary lesions, caused by follicular disruption or traumatic transformation, respectively.

Epidermal cysts are the most common type of cyst and frequently occur on the face or upper trunk.[3] When epidermal cysts occur on the scalp, they are sometimes clinically confused with pilar or trichilemmal cysts. Pilar (trichilemmal) cysts differ histologically from epidermal cysts and occur almost exclusively on the scalp.[3] Milia, smaller variants of epidermal cysts, arise most frequently on the face in adults, although they may also be induced by secondary phenomena such as blistering, trauma, topical corticosteroid atrophy, laser resurfacing, and deep chemical peels.[4,5]

Lipomas are common soft tissue tumors and may occur both above and below the muscle. Submuscular lipomas may be challenging to remove and may entail more risk of damaging delicate neurovascular bundles, although localization is not always obvious preoperatively.

Surgical excision is the mainstay of treatment for epidermal and pilar cysts, although other surgical modalities may be explored as well. When multiple cysts are present, underlying syndromes, such as basal cell nevus syndrome and Gardner syndrome,[6,7] may be considered. Multiple milia can be found in the setting of oral-facial-digital syndrome, hereditary hypotrichosis, and Rombo and Bazex syndromes.[5] Similarly, multiple familial lipomatosis may sometimes be seen as well, particularly in those complaining of a history of multiple lipomas. Therefore, a complete history and physical examination are encouraged.

CLINICAL PRESENTATION

Epidermal inclusion cysts present as soft subcutaneous nodules, sometimes with a visible punctum (or puncta), and an associated yellow-white hue (**Figures 18-1 and 18-2**). These contain macerated keratin, and cyst contents are most frequently white or yellow, although they can be brown or gray-colored as well. Cyst size and location are variable, but they are most frequently found on the face and trunk and are typically a few centimeters in size, depending on location. Primary milia are usually 1- to 3-mm white papules, most commonly occurring around the eyelids and central face (**Figure 18-3**).

Clinically, pilar cysts are indistinguishable from epidermal cysts, although they occur primarily on the scalp and may be more firm to palpation. This increased firmness corresponds to the thick wall of the pilar cyst, which also makes them more resistant to rupture. Unlike epidermal cysts, a punctum is usually not seen with trichilemmal cysts[8] (**Figure 18-4**).

Compared to epidermal cysts, steatocystomas tend to be smaller, softer acneiform lesions (usually <1 cm) occurring on the chest and axillae[2] (**Figure 18-5**). Dermoid cysts appear similar to

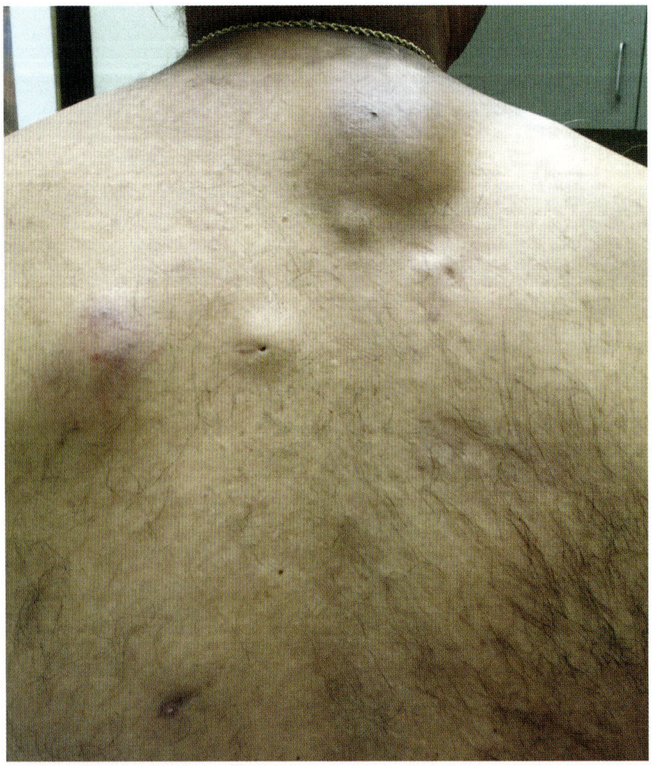

FIGURE 18-1 Epidermal inclusion cysts present as soft subcutaneous nodules, sometimes with a visible punctum (or puncta), and an associated yellow-white hue.

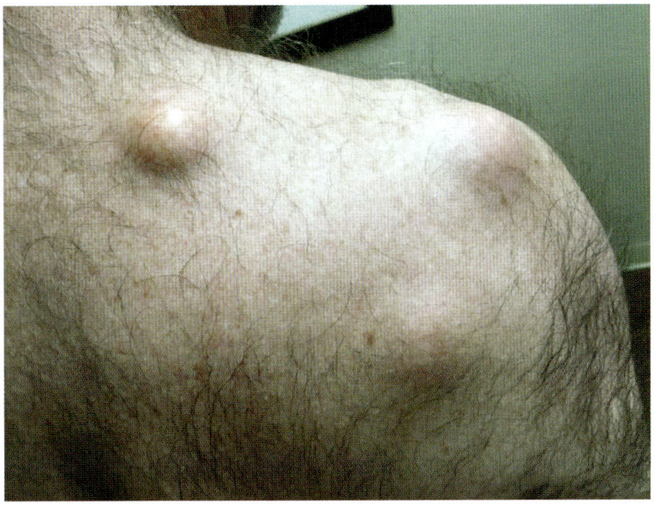

FIGURE 18-2 Epidermal inclusion cysts may become fairly large and are in variable proximity to the skin surface.

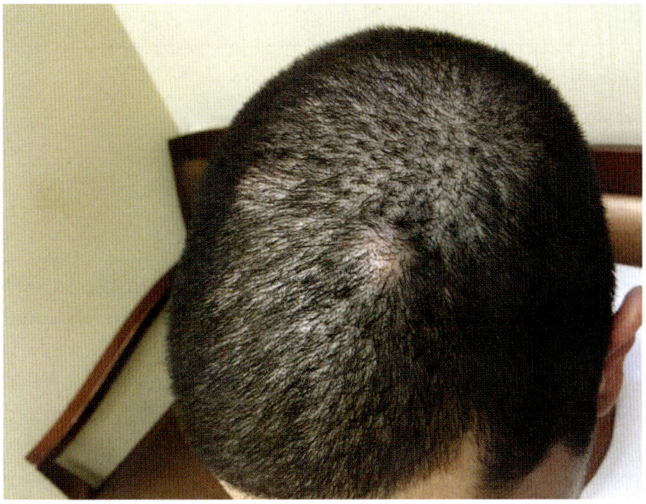

FIGURE 18-4 Unlike epidermal cysts, a punctum is usually not seen with trichilemmal (pilar) cysts.

epidermal cysts but typically occur in infants and are located along embryonic fusion planes.[3,9] Inflamed variants of each of these subtypes can occur and will appear erythematous, warm, and tender due to the inflammatory reaction to the ruptured cyst wall and contents. Other common mimickers of epidermal cysts include lipomas, juvenile xanthogranulomas, and reactive lymph nodes.

Lipomas are classically more rubbery feeling, although the clinical distinction between a cyst and lipoma may be challenging even for experienced clinicians in the absence of a visible punctum.

PATIENT EVALUATION AND SELECTION

Preoperative consultation is required to ensure adequate patient preparation and selection. This begins with a focused history, including prior excision, incision and drainage, or recurrent inflammation; this is helpful as there is increased risk of scar formation and recurrence because it may be more challenging to remove the cyst in its entirety.

Not all cysts are best served by immediate excision; inflamed cysts are better approached with intralesional corticosteroids or incision and drainage, as inflammation is an indication that the cyst wall has already ruptured. Inflammation causes local warmth, erythema, and pain from an acute foreign body reaction to the ruptured cyst contents. Occasionally, ruptured cysts become secondarily infected, requiring oral antibiotic therapy. In such cases, surgical excision should be delayed until frank infection has been cleared and the inflammation has markedly abated. A detailed conversation including the risks, benefits, and alternatives of surgery will not only permit the patient to better grasp the procedure, but may also help to mitigate the risk of adverse outcomes by encouraging improved compliance with postoperative

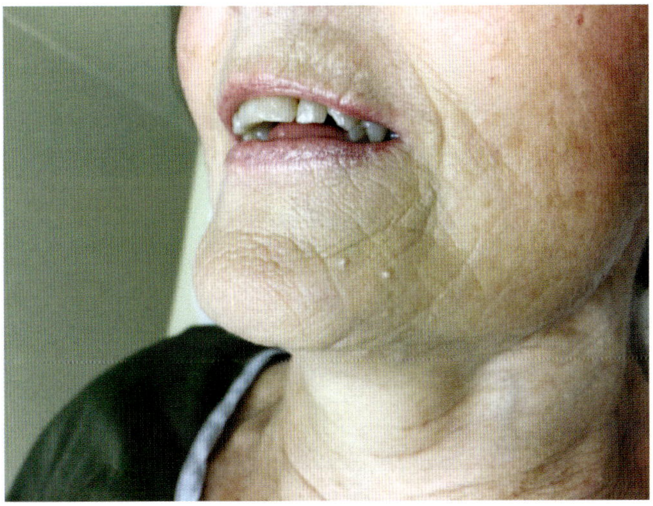

FIGURE 18-3 Primary milia are usually 1- to 3-mm white papules, most commonly occurring around the eyelids and central face.

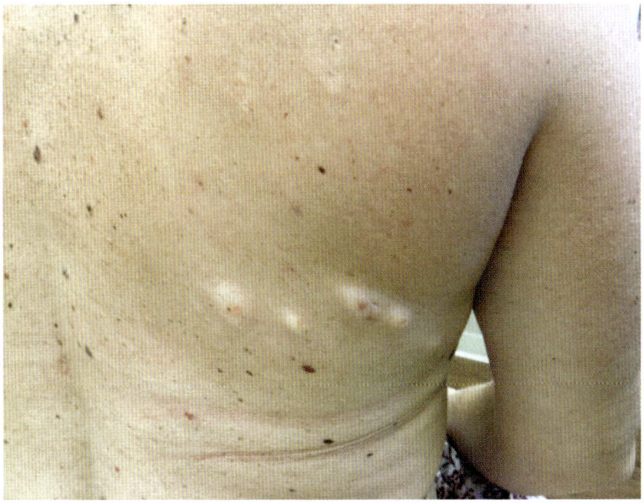

FIGURE 18-5 Compared to epidermal cysts, steatocystomas tend to be smaller, softer acneiform lesions (usually <1 cm) occurring on the chest and axillae.

instructions. Patients should always be advised regarding the risks of cyst excision, including the potential for recurrence, infection, and scarring.

PREOPERATIVE CONSIDERATIONS

Motivation

Cysts are removed for both aesthetic and symptomatic reasons, although there may be significant overlap between these motivations. Enlarging cysts may become increasingly tender, and cysts overlying bony structures or pressure points are particularly prone to tenderness. Cysts that have been inflamed or infected may cause significant pain, distress, and scarring. Aesthetically, patients sometimes feel that the cyst is noticeable, and it may become a source of embarrassment. Most patients presenting for cyst removal overtly state that they would prefer a scar to the cyst.

Anatomic Location

Location is an important consideration, particularly as cyst excision is often not truly medically required. Accordingly, the patient must be well informed and have reasonable expectations regarding the resulting scar. For example, if the patient has a cyst excised on the forehead or zygoma, the patient must understand that a scar will replace this cyst, and on these convex areas, a scar may be particularly evident. Cysts removed from thicker-skinned areas (eg, the back and flank), as well as the extremities, may require longer and larger excisions, because thinner-skinned areas are more flexible and malleable, allowing much of the cyst and contents to be squeezed out successfully from a smaller incision. Finally, cysts overlying anatomic danger zones shoulder always be approached with caution, especially as they may extend deeper than anticipated; thus, cysts on the preauricular area or over Erb's point should be dissected carefully, and patients should be warned preoperatively regarding the risk of permanent nerve damage.

Lesion History and Current State

Important considerations include the length of time that the cyst has been present, whether it has ever been irritated or inflamed, whether it has been otherwise traumatized or partially removed, and whether excision has been previously attempted.

General Preoperative Considerations

In addition to a problem-focused physical examination and explanation of any proposed procedure, general history should include medical, surgical, and social history and a review of current medications and allergies. Medical conditions may impact outcomes in dermatologic surgery, and these should be reviewed carefully, particularly if the patient has a history of hypertension, diabetes, smoking, alcohol use, or other cardiovascular disease.

SURGICAL APPROACHES

Instruments

A standard dermatologic surgery instrument tray (see Chapter 4) may be used. Some clinicians favor a serrated jaw forceps with no teeth for grasping the delicate cyst wall, as teeth may increase the risk of cyst wall puncture. Alternatively, hemostats may be used as well. A curette is sometimes useful when the cyst wall is adherent to surrounding tissue and when en bloc resection is not planned, as it permits the clinician to scrape the cyst contents from adjacent tissue with minimal damage to normal tissue.

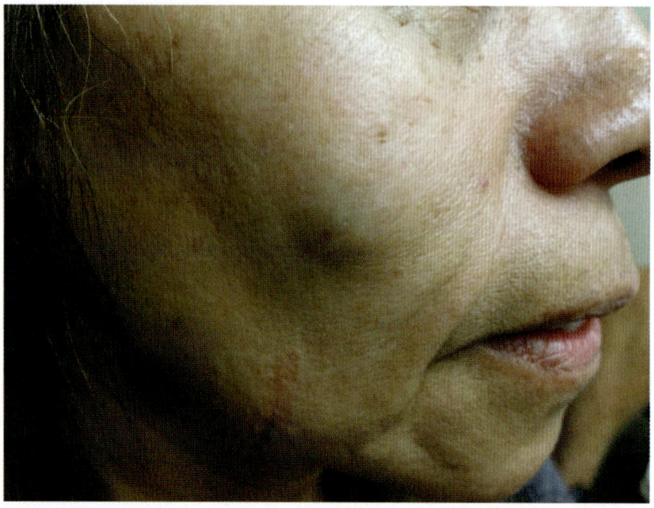

FIGURE 18-6 A moderately sized cyst is seen on the right cheek.

Preoperative Preparation and Anesthesia

A surgical marking pen is used to mark the punctum and the palpable margins of the cyst prior to local anesthetic infiltration, as local anesthesia may distort the cyst boundaries (**Figures 18-6 and 18-7**).

Tegaderm, a transparent film dressing, may be applied overlying the cyst immediately after marking and prior to local anesthetic infiltration. This may serve to mitigate the risk of cyst contents or local anesthetic agent backsplash contaminating the injector.

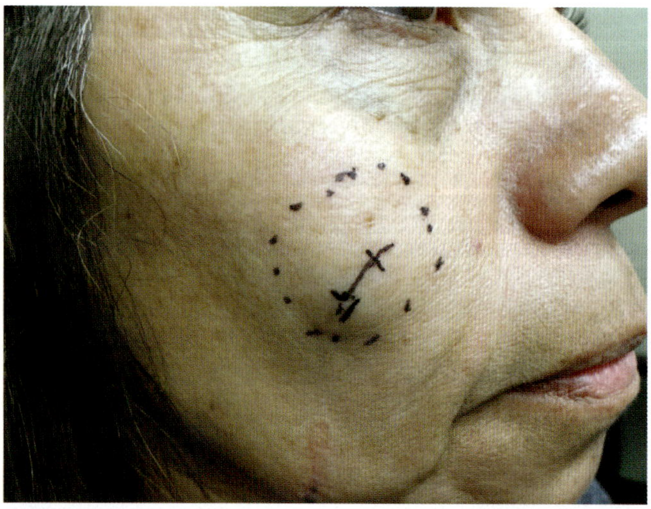

FIGURE 18-7 A surgical marking pen is used to mark the punctum and the palpable margins of the cyst prior to local anesthetic infiltration, as local anesthesia may distort the cyst boundaries.

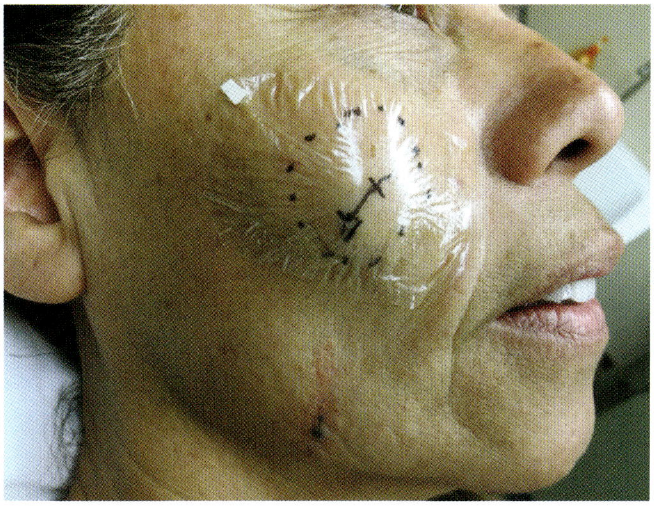

FIGURE 18-8 Tegaderm, a transparent film dressing, may be applied overlying the cyst immediately after marking and prior to local anesthetic infiltration. This may serve to mitigate the risk of cyst contents or local anesthetic agent backsplash contaminating the injector. The film is removed after local anesthesia infiltration, and the area is cleaned and sterilized per standard protocol.

The film is removed after local anesthesia infiltration, and the area is cleaned and sterilized per standard protocol[10] (**Figure 18-8**).

Injection of a local anesthetic agent may help to dissect the cyst from the surrounding tissue. If considerable fibrosis or scar tissue exists, little separation of the cyst from the surrounding tissue will occur. Care should always be taken not to inject directly into the cyst cavity, which may lead to cyst distention and possible rupture. Additional anesthetic can be infiltrated more deeply beneath the cyst as dissection and removal progresses, if necessary. Warning patient preoperatively that local anesthetic infiltration deep to the cyst may be incomplete may be worthwhile. Additionally, local anesthetic effect may be impeded in the acidic context of an infected cyst, although such cysts should generally not be approached surgically until the bulk of infection has been cleared through either incision and drainage or systemic antibiotic therapy.

Surgical Technique for Epidermal Cysts

There are many surgical approaches to epidermal cyst removal. Whichever approach is used in removal, extraction of all components is important, as residual cyst wall and cyst contents will increase the chances of recurrence and infections. The punctum or dilated pore in the skin overlying the lesion should be identified whenever possible, as the cyst adheres to skin at the site of the pore. In complete surgical excisions, the planned incision lines, oriented along relaxed skin tension lines, should include the epidermal pore if possible, and the goal is to create as small and/or imperceptible a scar as possible.

Slit Incision with Dissection: After a single incision line is marked over the cyst, including the punctum centrally, a shallow incision is made along the marked line (**Figure 18-9**). As with traditional elliptical excision, care must be taken not to incise too deeply and inadvertently incise into the cyst. Beveling the scalpel blade outward (a reverse bevel) may decrease the chance of cyst wall rupture. If the punctum is large, it may be removed. Once the cyst wall has been identified, grasp the epidermal edge with a skin hook and dissect the cyst wall free from the surrounding skin and subcutaneous tissue with iris or small gradle scissors. Firmly grasp the cyst with a tissue forceps or hemostat and deliver it through the incision if possible. If the cyst is too large for the incision size, it may be decompressed by making a small incision in the wall and, with gentle lateral pressure, expressing some of the keratinous contents through the incision. The partially collapsed cyst sac may then be delivered more easily through the incision. Be careful to ensure complete removal of cyst wall and the cyst contents to prevent recurrence. Lengthening the incision may be necessary. Although partially expressing the cyst contents is possible, en bloc cyst removal after dissection obviates patient concerns regarding the malodorous cyst contents and mitigates the risk of leaving residual keratinous debris in the excision site postoperatively. Layered wound closure should be completed as for traditional elliptical excision, taking care to reduce dead space.

Minimal or Punch Incision with Expression: Squeezing the capsule and contents through a minimal incision is another option for cyst removal (**Figure 18-10**).[11] Under local anesthesia, a stab incision is made in the center of the cyst using a #11 blade or trephine. When a punctum is visible, it should be included in the incision. Gentle lateral pressure is applied, expressing some of the cyst contents through the incision. The opening is extended using a hemostat, and the contents are gently expressed. A small curette may then be used to remove the remaining keratinous debris and to free the cyst wall from the surrounding tissue. Once visualized, the cyst wall is then grasped with the hemostat and removed. The cyst wall should be entirely removed, leaving no residue. Cyst contents may contaminate the wound during this procedure, and gentle irrigation should therefore be performed along with probing the wound with a curette to remove any residual keratinous fragments prior to closure.[12] Skin hooks work well to retract the wound edges and thoroughly inspect the margins of the wound for any residual cyst wall.

Alternatively, substituting a biopsy punch for a scalpel has been described as another minimally invasive method for cyst removal.[13-15] The punch hole may allow for better visualization and easier removal of the cyst wall as compared to a small linear incision, which often needs to be extended in order to remove the cyst completely, resulting in a longer scar. The biopsy punch is inserted perpendicular to the surface of the skin, preferably over a visibly enlarged punctum, until it penetrates the wall of the cyst. The overlying skin is then removed with iris or gradle scissors, and the contents of the cyst are squeezed through the hole until no further material can be extruded. At this point, the remaining cyst wall should be removed as described earlier. Usually, with appropriately chosen cysts, simple pressure is enough to dislodge the wall from the surrounding stroma, although it is sometimes necessary to dissect the wall away from the adjacent connective tissue with surgical scissors.

The resulting defect from incision or punch can be either sutured closed or allowed to heal by secondary intention. Warm compresses may be used for several days following surgery if the latter method is chosen. Healing by secondary intention is an

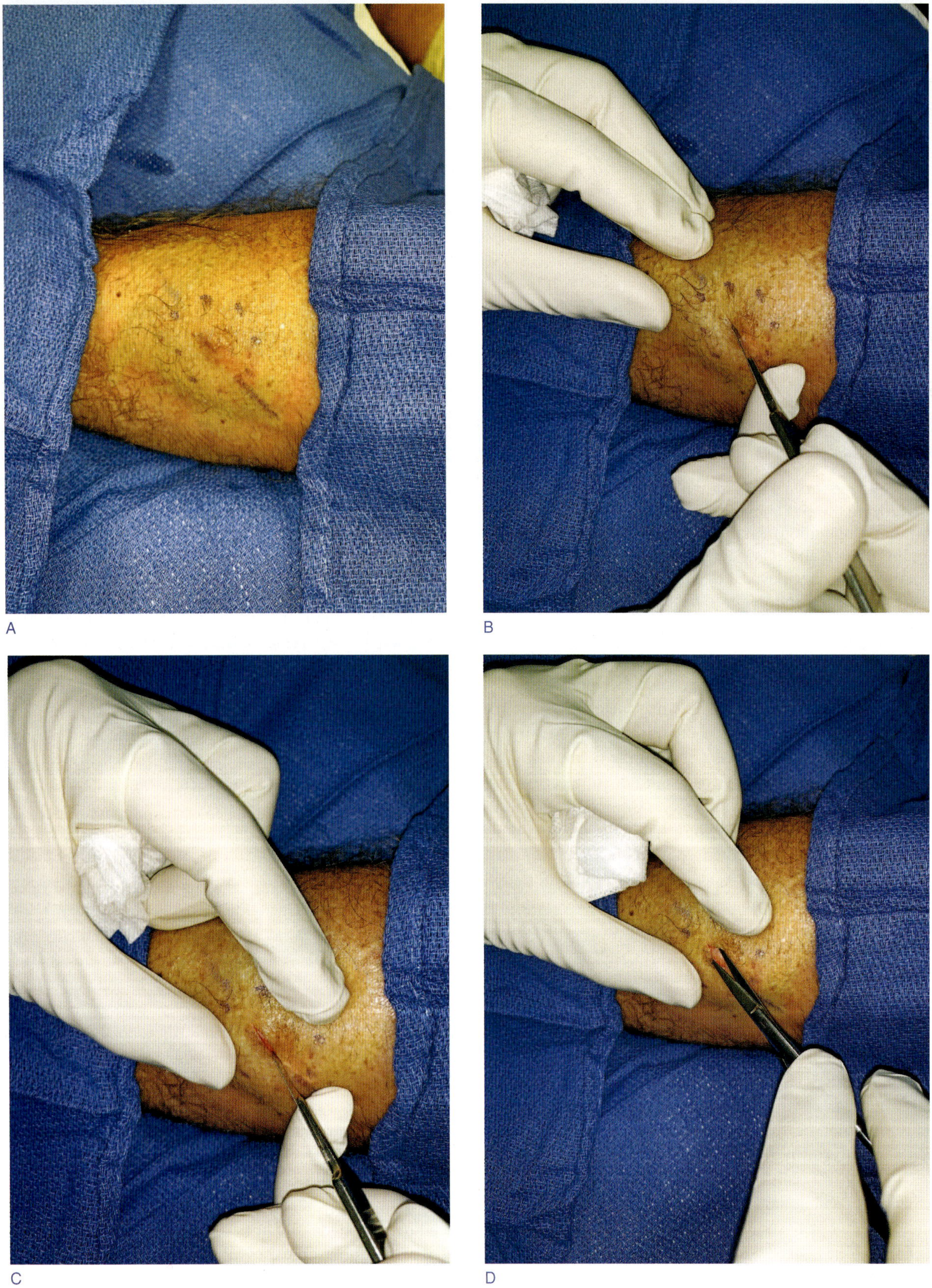

FIGURE 18-9 Cyst excision step by step.

a. Preoperative view of a subcutaneous nodule. No punctum was visible, and it was not clear if the lesion represented a cyst, lipoma, or other nodule.

b. A superficial incision is made.

c. The cyst wall is visible just deep to the incision.

d. Iris scissors are used to gently free up the lateral portion of the wall superficially adherent to the underlying dermis.

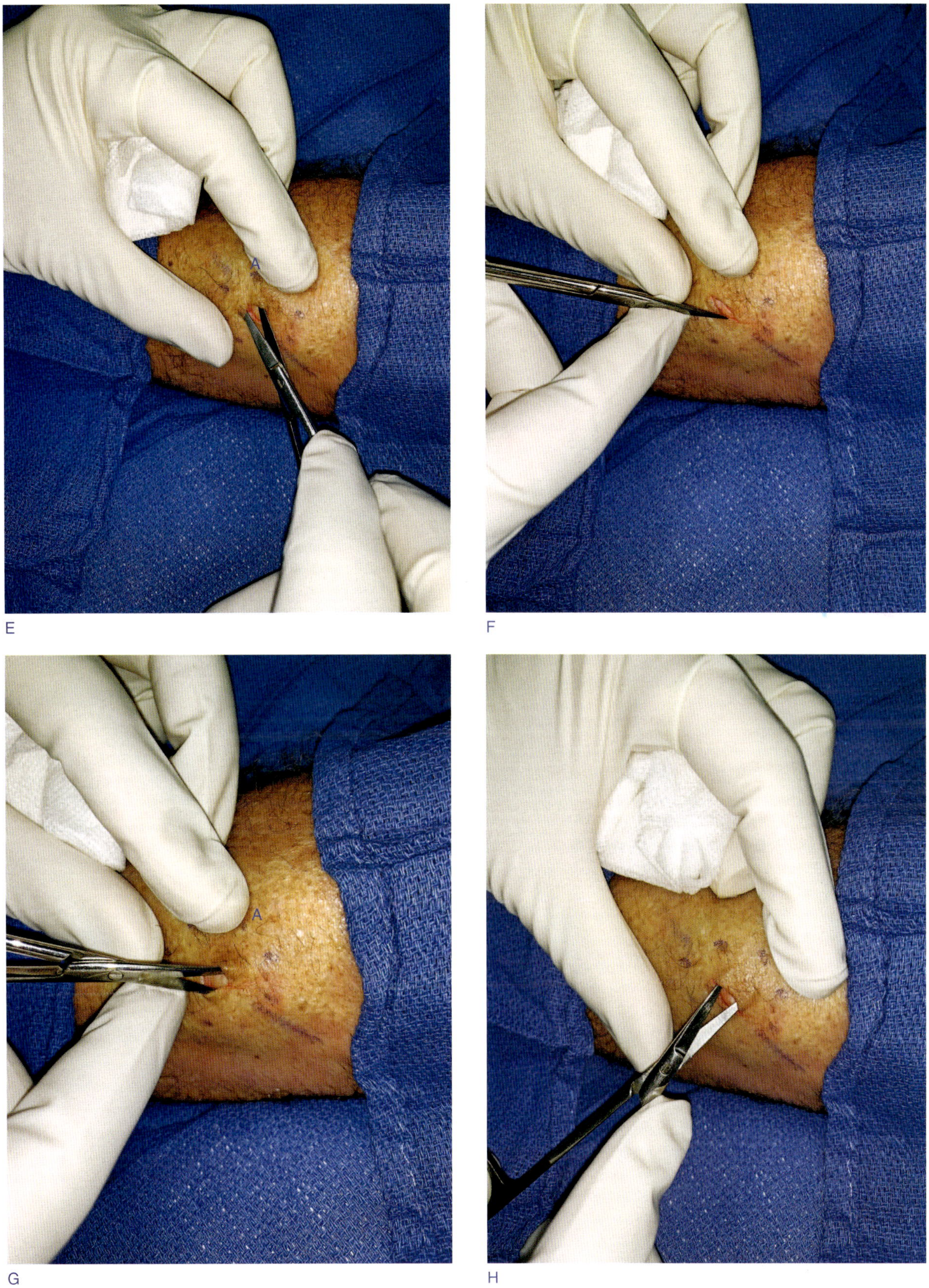

FIGURE 18-9 *(Continued)*

e. A spreading motion is used.
f. This is continued at the opposite pole.
g. Again, a spreading motion is used.
h. The lateral portion of the cyst is freed up as well. Note the very superficial plane from the visible blades of the scissors beneath the skin.

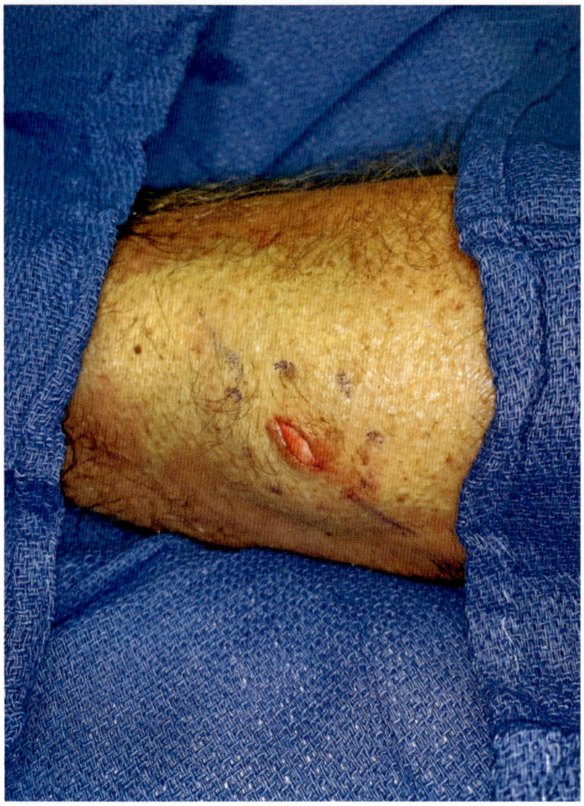

I

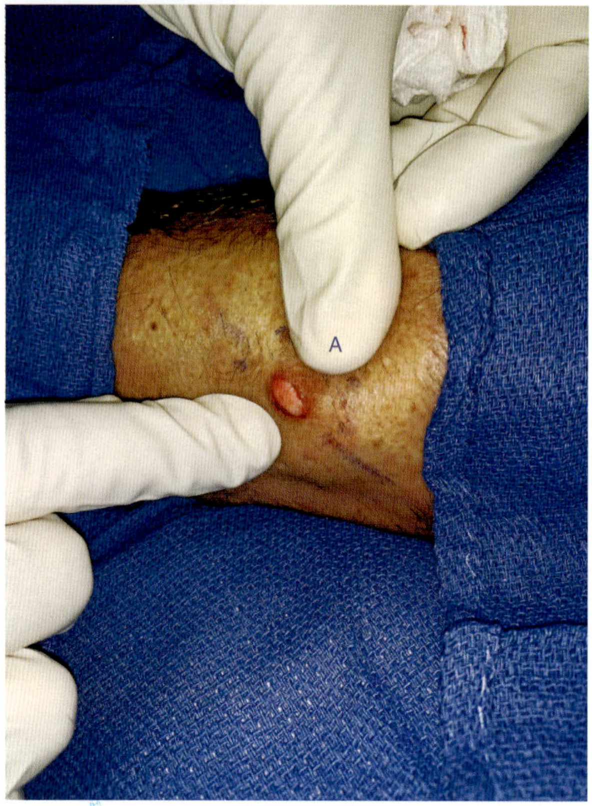

J

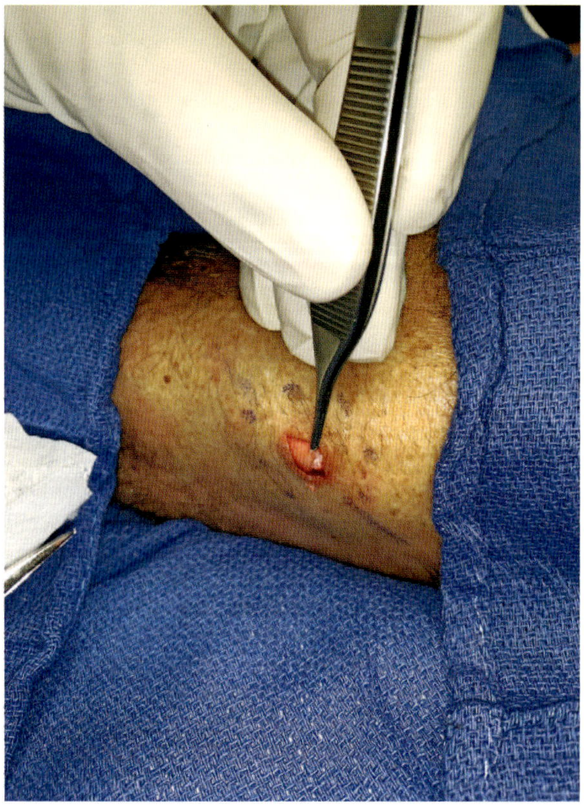

K

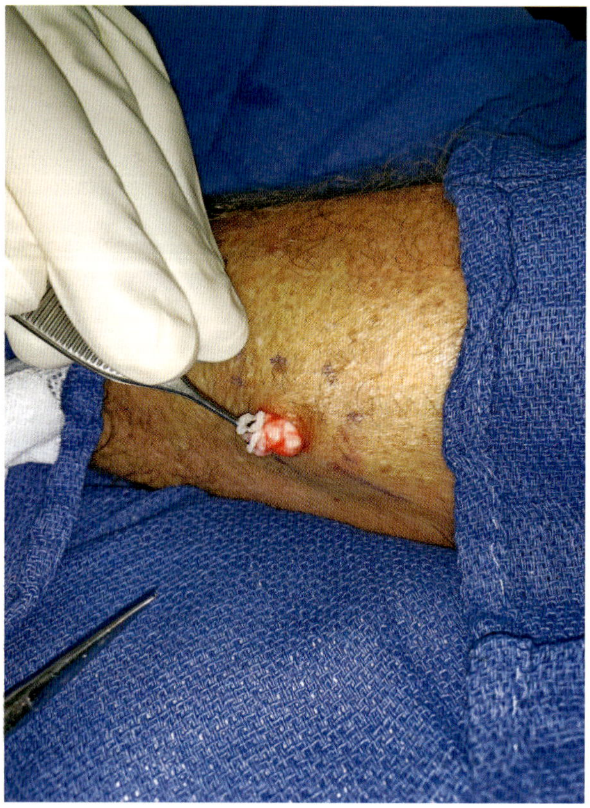

L

FIGURE 18-9 (*Continued*)

i. The cyst's appearance after being freed.
j. Gentle lateral pressure is applied.
k. Forceps are used to help deliver the cyst. Note the nascent tear in the cyst wall.
l. Some contents are extruded through the tear, although the cyst remains en bloc.

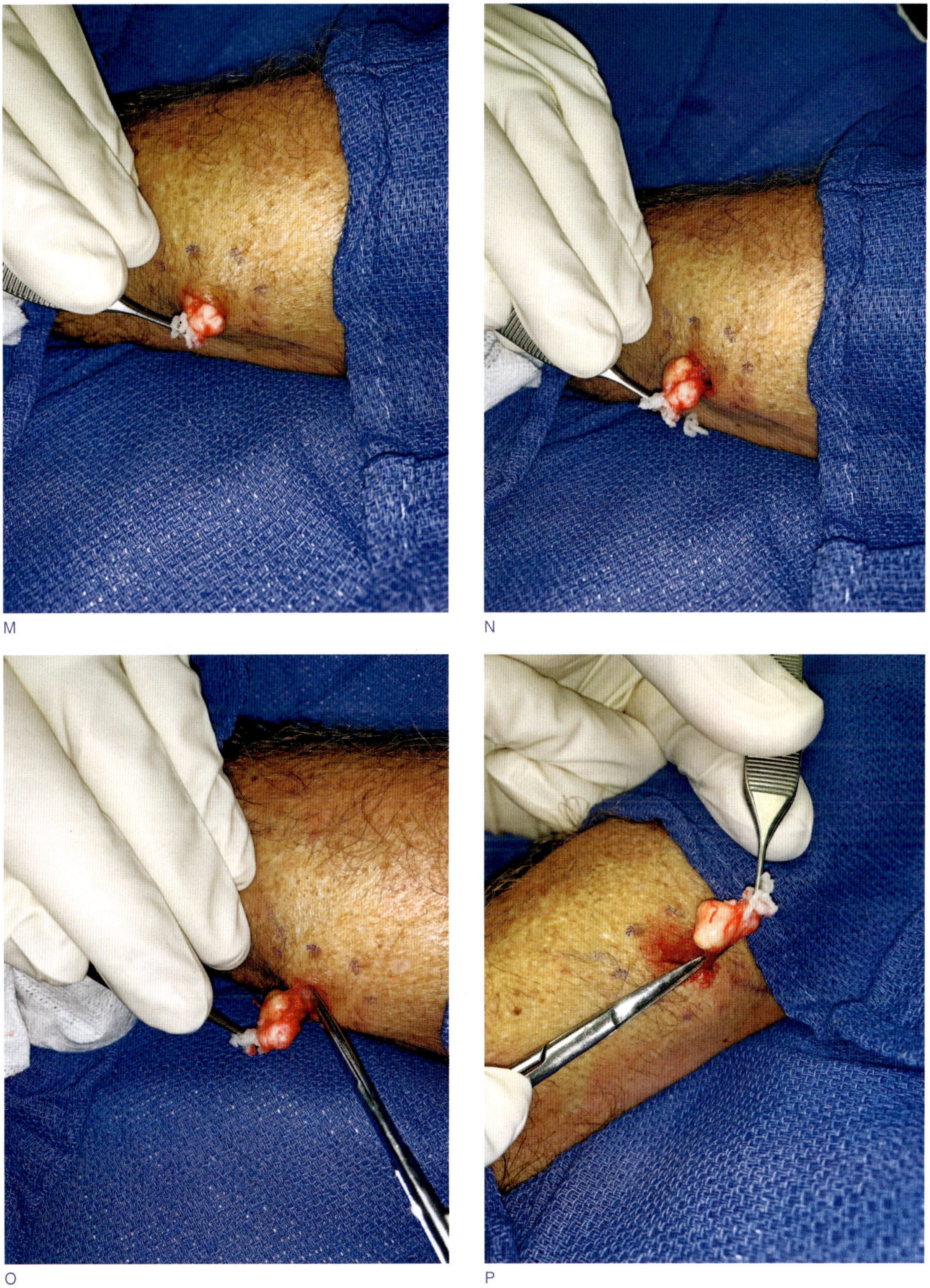

FIGURE 18-9 (*Continued*)
m. It is pulled very gently through the incision.
n. The deep fibrous attachments are now visible.
o. These attachments are cut using the iris scissors.
p. The cyst is pulled in the opposite direction to sever the remaining attachments.

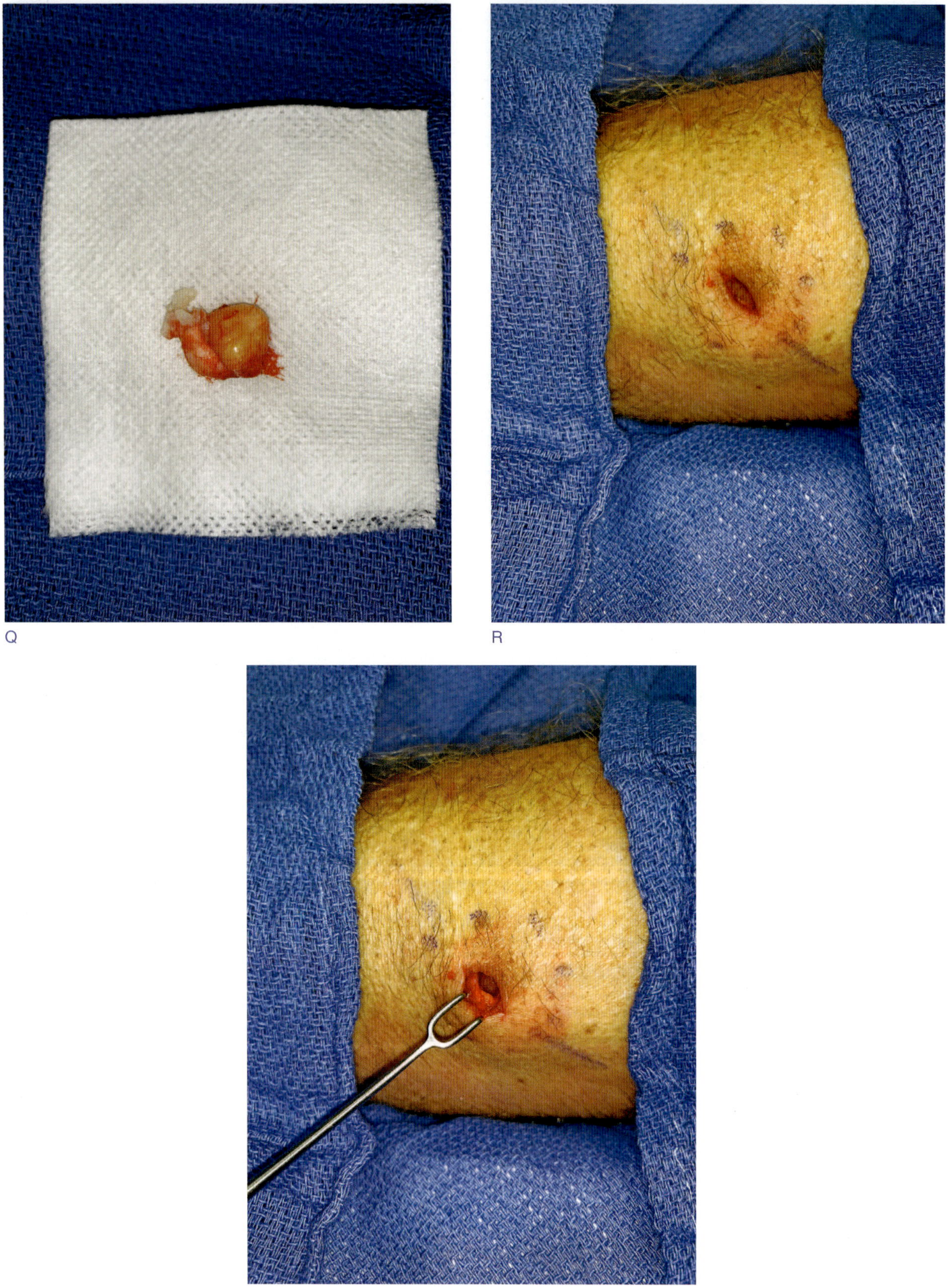

Q R S

FIGURE 18-9 *(Continued)*

q. The cyst's appearance after removal. Note that despite the tear, it is removed en bloc as a single unit.
r. The defect's appearance once the cyst has been removed.
s. This should be explored for residual extruded material or secondary ("daughter") cysts.

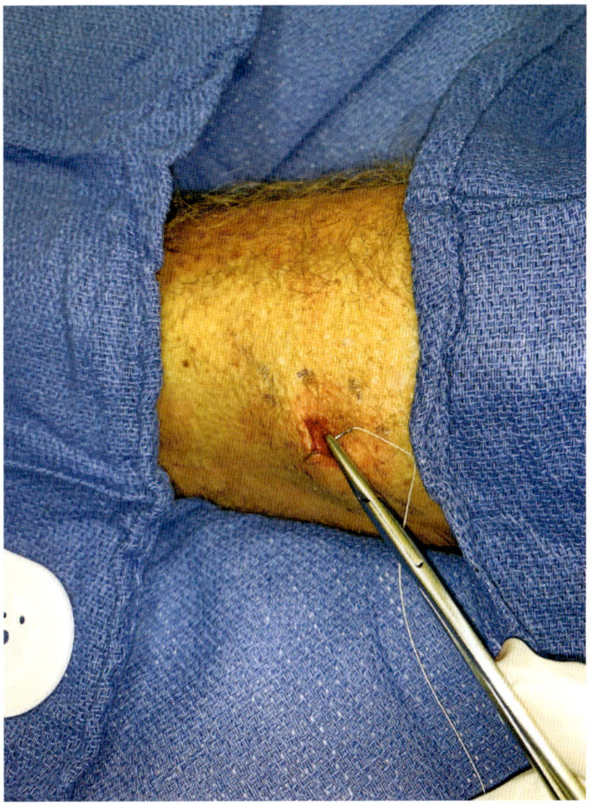

T

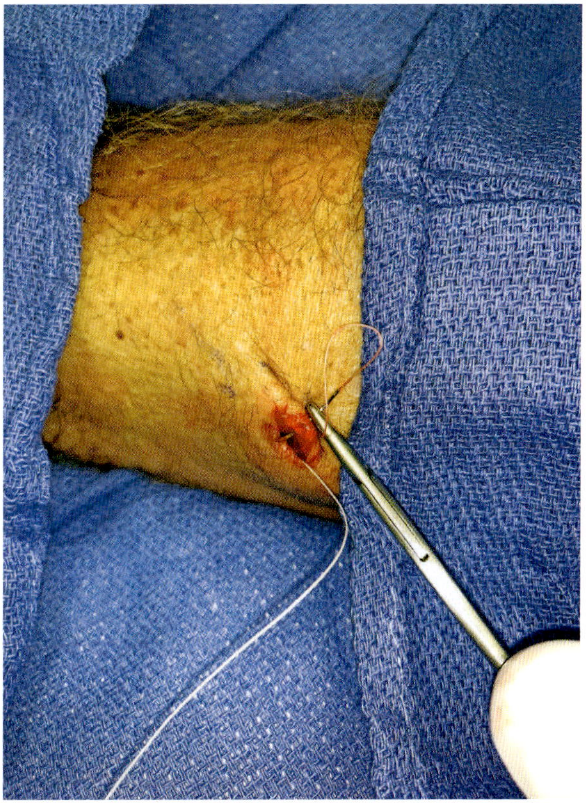

U

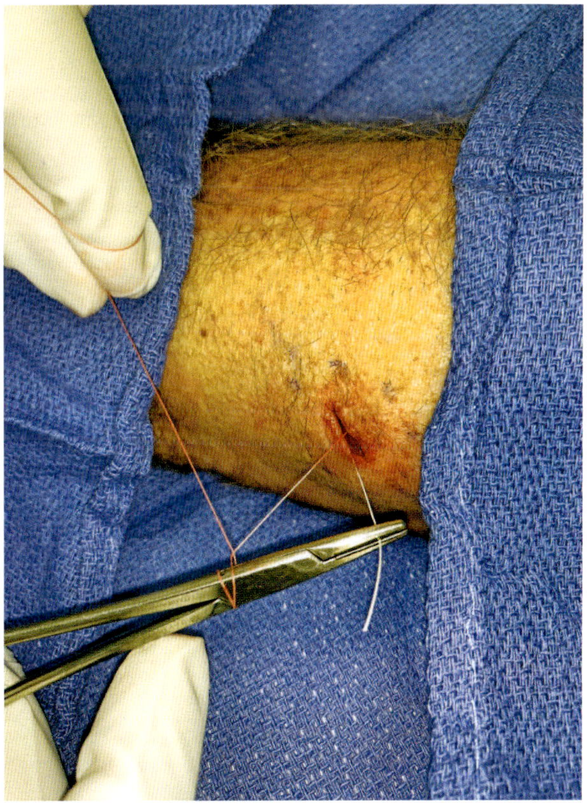

V

FIGURE 18-9 (*Continued*)

t. A buried vertical mattress suture is placed.
u. The suture's second bite is placed.
v. The wound's appearance prior to tying.

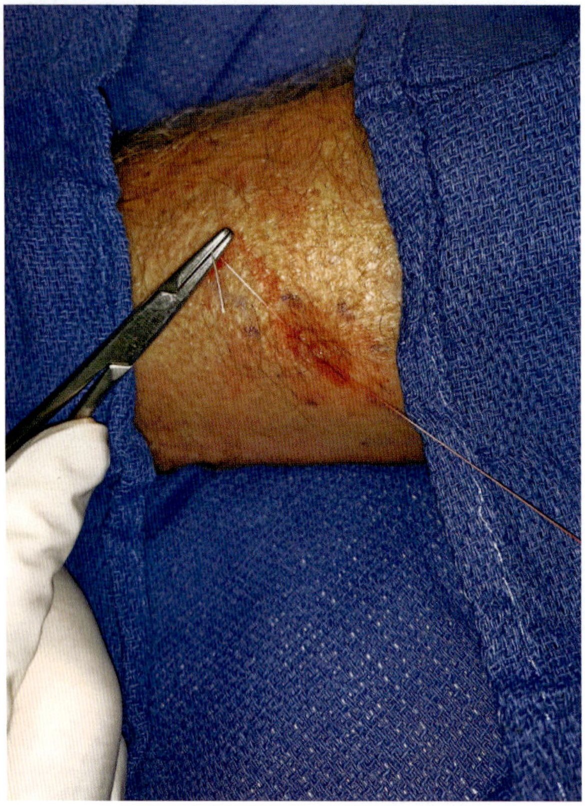
W

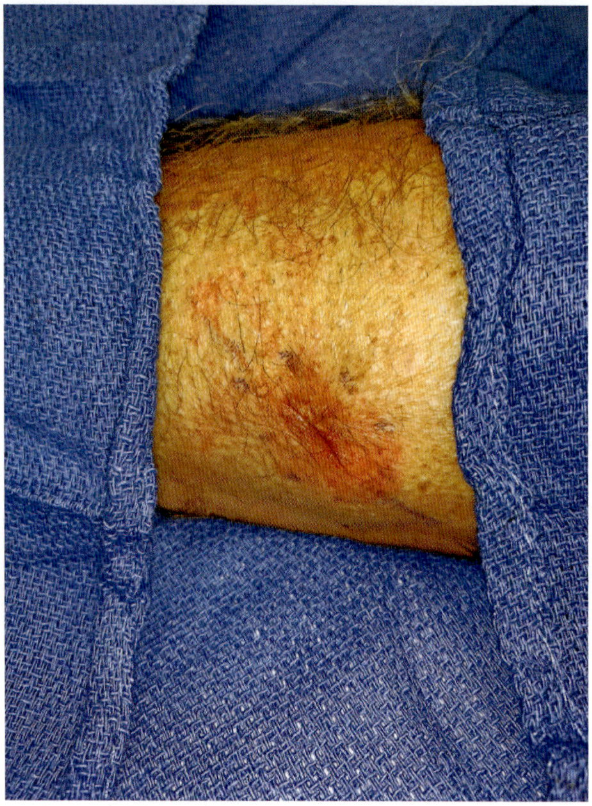
X

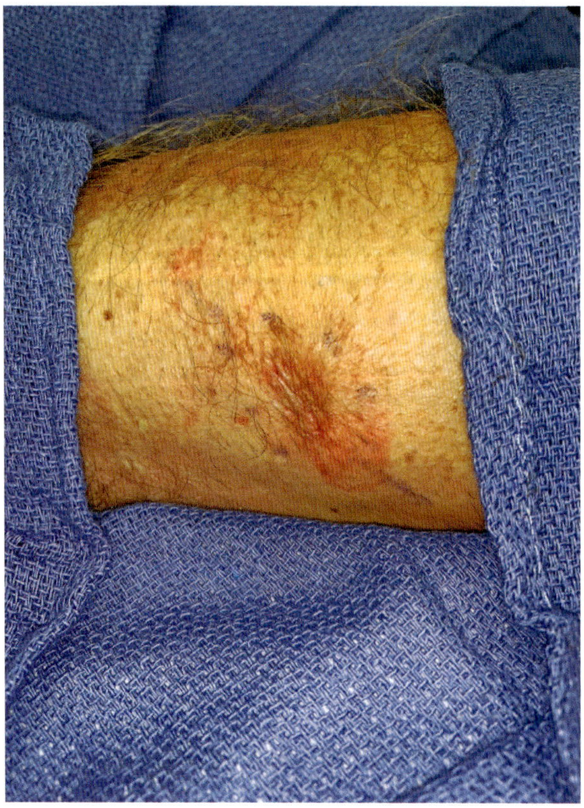
Y

FIGURE 18-9 (*Continued*)
w. Tying the suture. Note the excellent wound edge approximation with a single suture.
x. Appearance after one suture.
y. Appearance after a second buried suture is placed. Note the wound edge eversion.

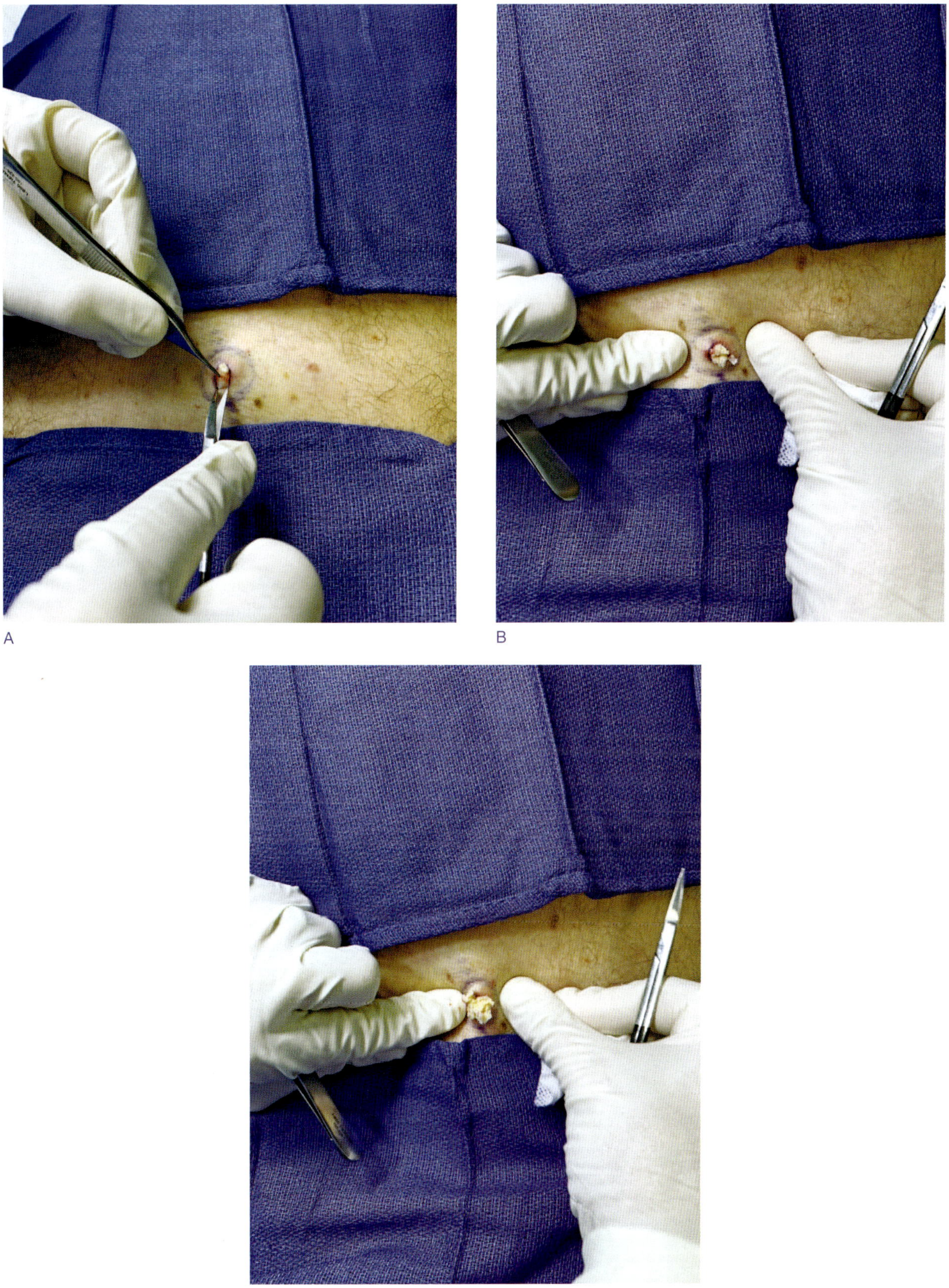

A B C

FIGURE 18-10 Sometimes a minimal slit excision is converted to an incision with expression when the cyst wall is very friable.

a. Dissection showing a cyst with some contents being extruded.
b. The friable cyst is gently squeezed.
c. The cyst contents are squeezed out. The cavity can then be evacuated further with forceps or a curette as needed. This approach is most useful for cysts with very thin and friable walls when a minimal slit dissection approach fails. An alternative approach would be converting this to a wide excision.

acceptable option if the defect is very small (2-3 mm), if it is in a cosmetically unimportant area, or if there is any doubt that the entire cyst wall and its contents have been removed. The benefits of secondary intention healing should be weighed against the risk of the wound healing as a dilated pore or depressed scar.

Wide Excision with Layered Closure: This is a reliable technique to prevent recurrence,[16] saving the patient further procedures, time, and expense. It is often indicated for larger cysts or those with previous inflammation, infection, or drainage suspected of having considerable surrounding fibrosis and scarring. The central disadvantage of this method is a longer scar and increased wound tension due to the removal of a fusiform ellipse of tissue.

After an ellipse is marked over the cyst, including the punctum centrally, and injection of local anesthetic around the cyst is complete, a shallow incision is made along the marked lines. As some cysts are quite superficial, care must be taken not to incise too deeply initially and inadvertently incise into the cyst. If the cyst has not previously been treated, the cyst wall may be visualized. Once the skin incision is made to the level of the cyst wall, the skin away from the ellipse can be carefully undermined to separate it from the cyst wall. A skin hook and iris or small gradle scissors work well for this approach. This process may be assisted by traction on the ellipse and underlying cyst using a hemostat, finely serrated tissue forceps, or stay sutures. The angles of the ellipse should be released to complete full cyst dissection. Often the cyst can be removed in its entirety without rupture. En bloc surgical excision may also remove considerable fibrosis or scar if present. This method also provides a large and well-oriented specimen for pathologic evaluation, which is useful when malignancy is suspected.[11,16]

Dead space closure is used to mitigate the risk of hematoma or seroma formation, as well as the risk of a dimpled or depressed scar. Layered closure with fascial plication sutures may be particularly helpful in this regard, and a layered closure is very helpful.

Previously manipulated (excised, incised and drained, or infected) cysts may be multiloculated, with significant surrounding scar tissue and adhesions. Such cysts are challenging to remove through a small incision and have an increased chance of recurrence. Therefore, wide en bloc excision is preferred in these cases to ensure complete removal.

Incision/Extraction of Milia

Milia can usually be removed easily by nicking the overlying skin with a #11 blade or lancet and removing the lesion with gentle lateral pressure using a comedone extractor. Alternatively, these lesions can also be removed by making a small incision using the tip of a sterile disposable needle and using the needle to enucleate the cyst. Larger lesions, particularly those around the eyes, may require a slightly longer incision with removal of the sac using fine forceps. They usually heal well by second intention or the placement of a few superficial sutures for larger lesions. New lesions are likely to occur, although treated lesions usually do not recur.

Surgical Technique for Pilar Cysts (Scalp)

Slit excision is a technique commonly used to remove these types of cysts on the scalp. Many patients avoid removing these because they fear that the surrounding area will be shaved. In general, shaving or clipping the hair is unnecessary beyond the small area overlying the portion of the scalp that may be excised completely. This is enormously appreciated by patients, and serves to make removal a very quick procedure that is gratifying for both the patient and clinician.

The area is first cleaned with chlorhexidine, pushing the hair in all directions away from the cyst. When dried, this assists in keeping the hair back away from the site of cyst removal. Additionally, ointment can be applied to the surrounding area, further helping to keep back the hair. Sterile hair clips and/or cloth tape may also be used in preventing hair from interfering with the procedure. Keeping hair from interfering with the procedure will not only make it easier, but also hair that is drawn into the wound at the time of closure can become a nidus for infection or later cyst formation and should be avoided. The surgical incision is started superficially, with the goal of visualizing the cyst without puncturing the wall. Once the wall is visualized, and after careful undermining laterally, gently applied lateral pressure alone often permits the cyst to easily emerge fully intact. This is the ideal scenario, as it ensures that the entire cyst has been removed and there will be little chance of recurrence. This approach results in no tension on the wound edges, although buried sutures may be helpful for dead space minimization.

Pilar cysts enlarge over time, leading to redundant skin development, particularly overlying larger cysts. This redundant tissue will often need to be removed at the time of closure. Large pilar cysts may include distorted hair shafts, decreased hair growth, or even complete alopecia over the central portion of the cyst, and this alopecic skin may be trimmed and removed at the time of closure. Percutaneous suturing approaches (see Chapter 10) may be helpful to reduce dead space when working in narrow scalp wounds.

Due to the vascularity of the scalp, postoperative bleeding is a risk, and careful intraoperative hemostasis coupled with dead space minimization and a pressure dressing application are helpful. Pressure dressings should ideally remain in place for 24 hours and can be secured with a tie-over ponytail using the patient's own surrounding hair (**Figure 18-11**).

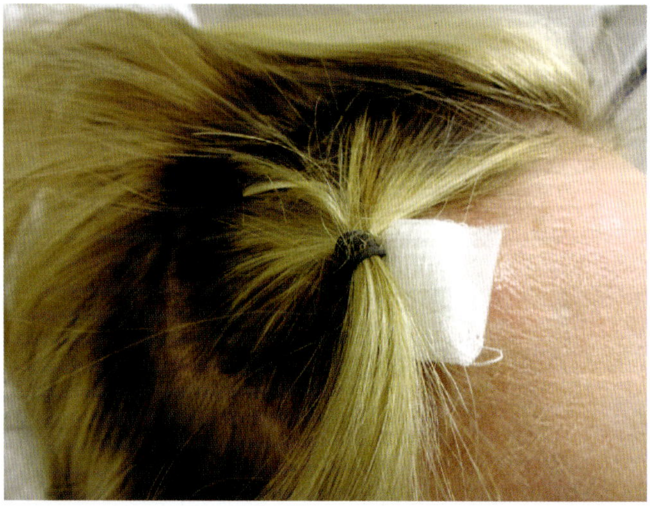

FIGURE 18-11 Pressure dressings should ideally remain in place for 24 hours and can be secured with a tie-over ponytail using the patient's own surrounding hair.

NONSURGICAL MANAGEMENT

Occasionally, patients present with the goal of decreasing cyst inflammation but prefer to avoid surgical management. In such cases, intralesional and perilesional corticosteroid injection may be helpful, although patients should be warned that this addresses only the underlying inflammation and that the cyst proper is unlikely to resolve. Similarly, incision and drainage may be used for inflamed epidermal cysts when excision would not otherwise be recommended (see Chapter 14). These approaches may be combined with the anti-inflammatory effects of nonsteroidal anti-inflammatory drugs and periodic application of warm compresses to encourage drainage and decrease pain. If infection is also suspected, prescribing an oral antibiotic to rapidly reduce the associated erythema and pain should be considered.

COMPLICATIONS

Rupture and Liquefaction

Epidermal cysts typically have a thin wall that can tear easily during removal and rupture the cyst, and larger cysts often have thinner walls. If a cyst has previously been inflamed, the contents may be liquefied due to previous inflammation. Pilar cysts have a thicker cyst wall, making them more resistant to rupture, and they more commonly extrude easily with gentle pressure.

Secondary Infection

Cysts are frequently mislabeled as infected rather than simply inflamed and irritated, especially as inflammation creates a vigorous foreign body inflammatory response leading to erythema, edema, and tenderness, simulating an abscess. Incision and drainage will often relieve the pressure and pain immediately; cultures are usually negative, and antibiotics are infrequently needed. For patients who are reluctant to undergo an intermediate procedure, antibiotic therapy may lead to significant reduction in erythema and edema, and the patient may then return in 2 weeks for a standard excision of the cyst.

Recurrence

If an epidermal cyst is not removed in its entirety, there is a chance of recurrence; this is possible even when the cyst wall is removed in its entirety, as tiny daughter cysts may exist adjacent to a larger cyst. Previously removed or manipulated cysts are at increased risk of recurrence. Patients should be informed of this risk before the procedure, particularly if the cyst has a history of manipulation, infection, or previous excision.

Scarring and Adhesions

When a cyst has been previously manipulated, inflamed, or partially excised, the potential for scarring, adhesions, and multiloculated cyst formation is increased. These characteristics make the cyst more difficult to completely identify intraoperatively and may necessitate a wider excision.

Histology/Misdiagnosis

Solid tumors may masquerade as a typical epidermal cyst. Proliferating pilar tumors often mimic pilar cysts, and even though they are usually benign, malignant transformation with local invasion and metastasis has been described.[17] If a solid tumor is suspected during minimal excision, it should be removed en bloc and sent for pathologic evaluation. Regardless of technique used and degree of clinical suspicion, all cysts that are removed surgically should be sent for histopathology.

CONCLUSIONS

Primary care clinicians are frequently called upon to remove cysts, which present a common patient complaint. Proper patient selection and preoperative management may be invaluable in selecting the ideal candidates for surgical intervention. Several fundamental techniques are available to the clinician, from small punch excisions of simple cysts to wide elliptical excisions of previously inflamed or manipulated cystic masses. Additionally, the differential diagnosis of subcutaneous cystic nodules remains broad, and malignant mimickers must be always considered. Clinicians should be particularly alert to rapidly growing cystic masses, which may be a harbinger of malignancy and should always be removed.

REFERENCES

1. Takeshita T, Takeshita H, Irie K. Eruptive vellus hair cyst and epidermal cyst in a patient with pachyonychia congenita. *J Dermatol.* 2000;27(10):655-657.
2. Cho S, Chang SE, Choi JH, et al. Clinical and Histologic features of 64 cases of steatocystoma multiplex. *J Dermatol.* 2002;29(3):152-156.
3. Al-Khateeb TH, Al-Masri NM, Al-Zoubi F. Cutaneous cysts of the head and neck. *J Oral Maxillofac Surg.* 2009;67(1):52-57.
4. Iacobelli D, Hashimoto K, Kato I, Ito M, Suzuki Y. Clobetasol-induced milia. *J Am Acad Dermatol.* 1989;21(2 Pt 1):215-217.
5. Berk DR, Bayliss SJ. Milia: a review and classification. *J Am Acad Dermatol.* 2008;59(6):1050-1063.
6. Ogata K, Ikeda M, Miyoshi K, et al. Naevoid basal cell carcinoma syndrome with a palmar epidermal cyst, milia and maxillary cysts. *Br J Dermatol.* 2001;145(3):508-509.
7. Leppard B, Bussey HJ. Epidermal cysts, polyposis coli and Gardner's syndrome. *Br J Surg.* 1975;62(5):387-393.
8. Leppard BJ, Sanderson KV, Wells RS. Hereditary trichilemmal cysts. Hereditary pilar cysts. *Clin Exp Dermatol.* 1977;2(1):23-32.
9. Eldesouky MA, Elbakary MA. Orbital dermoid cyst: classification and its impact on surgical management. *Semin Opthalmol.* 2018;33(2):170-174.
10. Kantor J, Dehbozorgi S, Lee S. Temporary application of transparent adhesive film dressing for the prevention of splash-back during local anesthetic administration in dermatologic surgery. *J Am Acad Dermatol.* 2017;77(1):e15-e16.
11. Zuber TJ. Minimal excision technique for epidermal (sebaceous) cysts. *Am Fam Phys.* 2002;65:1409-1412, 1417-1418, 1420.
12. Krull EA. The "little" curet (surgical gems). *J Dermatol Surg Oncol.* 1978;4:656-657.

13. Lee H, Yang C, Chen C, et al. Comparison of the surgical outcomes of punch incision and elliptical excision in treating epidermal inclusion cysts: a prospective, randomized study. *Dermatol Surg.* 2006;32:520-525.

14. Mehrabi D, Leonhardt JM, Brodell RT. Removal of keratinous cysts with the punch incision technique: analysis of surgical outcomes. *Dermatol Surg.* 2002;28:673-677.

15. Lieblich LM, Geronemus RG, Gibbs RC. Use of a biopsy punch for removal of epithelial cysts. *J Dermatol Surg Oncol.* 1982;8:1059-1062.

16. Suliman MT. Excision of epidermal (sebaceous) cyst: description of the operative technique. *Plast Reconstr Surg.* 2005;116(7):2042-2043.

17. Weiss J, Heime M, Grimmel M, Jung EG. Malignant proliferating trichilemmal cyst. *J Am Acad Dermatol.* 1995;32(5 Pt2):870-873.

Approach to Nonmelanoma Skin Cancer

19

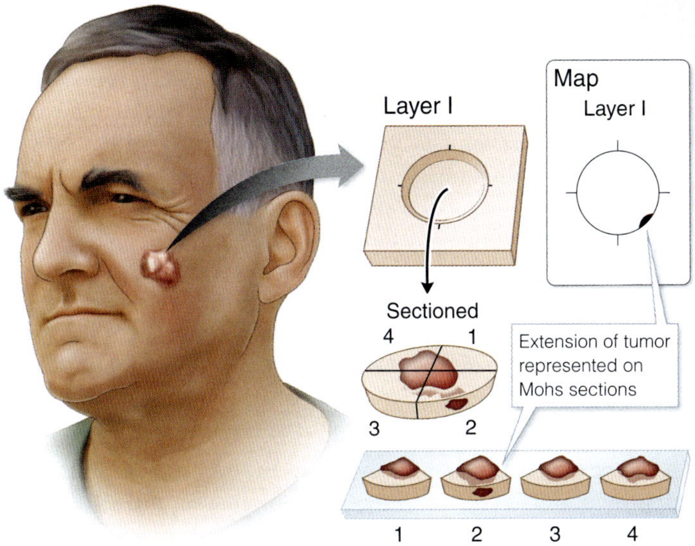

SUMMARY

- Nonmelanoma skin cancers are extraordinarily common, accounting for approximately 3 million new cases per year in the United States alone.
- Multiple treatment options are available, ranging from EDC to excision to Mohs surgery.
- Treatment decisions should be guided by both patient and tumor characteristics, and should always be individually tailored.

Beginner Tips

- Common treatment options for NMSC include EDC, excision, and Mohs micrographic surgery.
- The cost and ease of simple options such as EDC should always be weighed against both the increased healing time and decreased efficacy of these approaches when compared with excision or Mohs.

Pitfalls and Cautions

- Simple approaches such as cryotherapy and EDC should not be used on tumors at significant risk of recurrence.
- Appropriate tumor and patient selection for medical management or treatment with cryotherapy or EDC is critical; for example, some BCCs demonstrate both superficial and nodular growth patterns.

Expert Tips

- High-risk tumors may benefit from management in a multidisciplinary fashion.
- Adjuvant radiation therapy may be useful for select tumors at very high risk of recurrence.

Patient Education Points

- Full informed consent includes a discussion of both the ease of a particular procedure and the length and complexity of the healing process.
- Remind patients that even with very low rates of recurrence or complications, those numbers are not zero. Patients may otherwise fail to appreciate that a 98% chance of tumor clearance without complications means that, for a clinician who treats 100 patients per month, 2 patients monthly may have these undesirable outcomes.

Don't Forget!

- Select patients and tumors may benefit from primary medical management with topical or intralesional therapies.
- All surgical therapies entail risk, but this should be weighed against their effectiveness, rapid healing, and low recurrence rates.
- LN_2 treatment for NMSC is fundamentally different from AK treatment; intensity and depth of freeze must be significantly greater in order to lead to tumor destruction, and this will likely lead to significant surrounding tissue damage and hypopigmentation.

Billing Pearls

- Documentation is critical, and medical necessity is the ultimate arbiter of appropriateness.
- Some patients have poor (or no) prescription medication coverage; for them, medical management is generally not desirable.

19 Approach to Nonmelanoma Skin Cancer

INTRODUCTION

One of the most frequent reasons that patients present to a primary care office for an excision or destructive treatment is for the treatment of nonmelanoma skin cancer (NMSC). Indeed, as a group, these cancers represent the most common malignancy in the United States, with over 3 million cases annually.[1] NMSC is more common than all other malignancies combined, and its incidence continues to increase[2]; this burden has translated into a significant year-on-year increase in disease-related spending.[3] As the incidence of NMSC continues to increase, there are significant public health, patient safety, and cost implications, making it imperative that clinicians be able to effectively treat NMSC. Understanding broadly the options available to treat these common malignancies is therefore of significant value to the primary care clinician.

MANAGEMENT OPTIONS

Basal cell carcinoma (BCC) and squamous cell carcinoma (SCC) are by far the two most commonly diagnosed NMSCs, with BCC outnumbering SCC. Additional forms of NMSC include Merkel cell carcinoma and dermatofibrosarcoma protuberans. Despite histologic differences, surgical treatment modalities for BCC and SCC are essentially the same. Other forms of NMSC are treated almost exclusively with excisional surgery or Mohs micrographic surgery.

Although NMSC is the most commonly diagnosed malignancy, these cancers account for less than 0.1% of all cancer deaths.[4] Most cases of BCC and SCC have a relatively indolent course, and if detected early, there are many treatment modalities available that readily achieve cure. Both surgical and nonsurgical options are available for the treatment of NMSC.

In recent years, there have been significant advances in nonsurgical therapy for NMSC. Still, surgical treatment remains a well-tolerated and effective approach to clinical cure and generally remains the standard of care. The most common surgical approaches to treatment of BCC and SCC include electrodessication and curettage (EDC), cryosurgery, excision, or Mohs micrographic surgery (MMS). Treatment choice depends on lesion location, patient age, patient health status, and risks for recurrence. Prior to deciding on a surgical treatment, a biopsy should be obtained in order to histologically examine the tissue to confirm the presence of malignancy. Sampling to the base of the lesion is helpful to guide treatment by stratifying the degree of risk associated with the biopsied lesion, although deep biopsy must be weighed against the risk of aesthetic and functional compromise. Once pathology is confirmed, the clinician must decide the best treatment modality based on both patient (age, site, immune status) and tumor (histologic subtype and degree of invasion) characteristics.

Surgery is the most commonly used treatment approach for NMSC. MMS has become the gold standard for treating NMSCs that are recurrent, complex, or on anatomic locations that benefit from tissue sparing. Other surgical and medical modalities are also effective for less complex lesions. A 27-year review of BCCs treated at NYU Skin and Cancer that compared the efficacy of treatment with EDC, surgical treatment, and radiation therapy revealed that each of these methods has a very high cure rate at 5 years.[5] Regardless of what approach the clinician deems appropriate, the goal of therapy is to remove the tumor, achieve a high cure rate, preserve the maximal amount of normal surrounding tissue, and maintain an acceptable aesthetic and functional outcome.[6]

Electrodessication and Curettage

EDC is one of the most commonly employed surgical techniques to destroy NMSC. This approach involves removal of diseased tissue with a curette followed by application of a controlled electrical current to destroy the surrounding tissue. When considering EDC as a treatment modality for NMSC, it is important to assess lesion depth, size, and location. Nodular and superficial BCC and SCC in situ without deep follicular involvement may be treated with EDC, although anatomic location and patient characteristics must be considered as well.

The clinician can distinguish between malignancy and normal dermis based on the degree of tissue friability noted during curettage, as most NMSCs are less cohesive and more friable than normal skin.[7] Two techniques for curettage are frequently employed. First, the *pen technique* may be used, during which the clinician holds the curette like a pencil in the dominant hand while stabilizing the lesion with the nondominant hand. Alternatively, the *potato peeler technique* is encouraged for larger tumors and is accomplished by using the thumb to brace the tissue and create tension while the other four fingers are used to peel the lesion from the dermis.[8] Whichever method is chosen, curettage is performed vigorously until pinpoint bleeding occurs and a firm, normal-appearing dermis is observed. There is a learning curve to distinguish the feel of NMSC versus normal tissue, although this is probably most reliable on the taut skin of the trunk and extremities and less reliable on the face.[9]

Following curettage, the lesion is treated with electrodessication, applying high-voltage electricity to the tissue to invoke superficial tissue destruction. Electrodessication of the wound is performed to thoroughly destroy any remaining viable tumor tissue at the base of the wound. The char effect of electrodessication may lead to higher cure rates; three cycles of EDC have been proposed as the optimal treatment approach,[10] although this has not been definitively demonstrated.[11] Generally, a higher cure rate is achieved when an additional margin of healthy skin beyond the visually apparent lesion is treated,[12] although the exact margin has yet to be determined.[13] The cosmetic result of

EDC is site dependent, with the best results being on the trunk and extremities.

There is a large discrepancy in reported cure rates of NMSC treated with EDC. Several studies have assessed residual cancer following EDC and demonstrated residual malignancy in 8% to 12% of truncal lesions and 30% to 47% of facial lesions.[9,14] Another study compared different treatment modalities by stratifying anatomic sites as low, moderate, and high risk for recurrence.[5,15] Low recurrence risk locations included the neck, trunk, and extremities, with a 5-year recurrence of 8.6%. Moderate-risk locations included the scalp, forehead, and temples, and had a recurrence rate of 12.9% at 5 years. The nose, eyelids, chin, jaw, and ear were deemed high risk with a 17.5% risk of recurrence. Additionally, this study noted that recurrence risk was correlated with the size of the lesion treated with EDC, with the highest cure rates seen with lesions less than 1 cm in diameter. Other estimates show 5-year cure rates associated with EDC to be above 90%, and even higher when selecting low-risk lesions,[11,16] although well-designed randomized controlled trials are lacking.

The use of biopsy to confirm NMSC depth and morphology may help optimize EDC usage. Deeply invasive SCC and micronodular or infiltrative (morpheaform) BCC are not amenable to EDC and should be treated with excision or MMS. Additionally, recurrent NMSC at sites previously treated with EDC are best treated with MMS due to the presence of scar tissue and potential for skip areas and multifocal recurrence.[17] Other relative contraindications to EDC include patients who readily form keloids. Moreover, patients with unshielded implanted electrical devices may benefit from electrocautery (thermal cautery) rather than electrodessication.

EDC cure rate is both lesion and clinician dependent, and therefore, it is important to recognize the limitations of EDC so that clinicians provide and incorporate not only the least costly, but also the most curative, method.

Cryosurgery

Cryosurgery is a minimally invasive ablative technique that uses a cryogen to destroy tissue by rapidly freezing followed by a slow, prolonged thaw. Cryosurgery is a simple, fast, and inexpensive approach to NMSC management and is most appropriate for treating small discrete primary lesions such as superficial BCC and SCC in situ. Cryosurgery is particularly beneficial in patients with multiple NMSCs, as multiple lesions may be treated in a short period of time during a single office visit. This approach may be used safely in patients with complex medical conditions, although the ease of the procedure must be weighed against a possible extensive healing process. Moreover, cryosurgery does not provide any specimen for pathologic examination. Treatment should include a 2- to 5-mm margin of normal-appearing tissue to ensure adequate treatment.

The magnitude of destruction is a function of temperature, application pressure, and exposure time. Destruction of malignant cells requires temperatures between –40°C and –60°C. Liquid nitrogen (LN2) is the most commonly used cryogen in dermatologic surgery as its low temperature (–195.8°C) ensures the possibility of tissue destruction. The molecular basis for cryosurgery is multifactorial in nature (**Table 19-1**), involving direct cell injury during the initial freeze and mechanical destruction and crystallization of the cell wall leading to membrane instability and cell lysis.[18] During the thaw portion of treatment, vascular injury occurs. Intense vasoconstriction during the freeze cycle changes vessel wall permeability, and when blood flow resumes during the thaw, compensatory hyperperfusion leads to free radical damage and membrane oxidation with ensuing ischemia.[19] These mechanisms of injury lead to apoptosis even in regions where the temperature was not sufficiently low to lead to direct cell necrosis; additionally, an intense T-cell immunologic response occurs, further inhibiting tumor growth.[20-22]

TABLE 19-1 • Molecular Basis of Cryosurgery

	Mechanism	Time of Cycle
Direct injury	Ice crystal formation and cellular water movement	Freeze phase
Vascular injury	Circulatory collapse, free radical injury, and membrane oxidation lead to ischemic necrosis	Thaw phase
Apoptosis	Programmed cell death in response to injury	2-8 hours after rewarming
Immunologic response	T-cell response	Late

The cryogen delivery unit must accurately and reproducibly achieve temperatures capable of eliciting cell death at the deep and lateral margins of the lesion. There are four central cryogen delivery techniques for cryosurgery to the skin[23]:

- Open spray: LN2 is delivered through the open end of the cryogen delivery unit. Spray tips are available with different apertures to allow for treatment of different-sized lesions. Larger nozzles freeze more quickly, leading to a greater but less precise area of destruction.
- Confined spray cones: This variant of the open spray technique uses a circumscribed cone on a plastic plate to concentrate the spray on a specific area. This also reduces inadvertent tissue destruction or splashing of LN2.
- Chamber or closed cone: A metal cylinder with an open rubber covered base is firmly applied to the target tissue to help achieve a deep freeze.
- Closed system or probe: Cryoprobes are metal devices used to make direct contact for cryosurgery. This allows for direct contact and delivery of LN2 through the probe. It is ideal for lesions in hard to reach areas with a flat surface.

Once the proper delivery device is chosen, the area is frozen by delivering LN2 to the affected area in a controlled manner. It is then allowed to thaw for 60 to 120 seconds to return to the original skin temperature. Since much of the vascular injury occurs during the reperfusion of the thaw cycle, it is imperative to allow complete thawing before repeating the freeze-thaw cycles.

The optimal number of freeze-thaw cycles to adequately treat NMSC has not been determined. For very superficial NMSC, one cycle may be appropriate, although at least two cycles should be performed for thicker lesions. Studies suggest that the second freeze-thaw cycle increases the extent of original necrosis by 80%, significantly decreasing the risk of partial or inadequate treatment.[24]

Cryosurgery is typically reserved for BCC, well-differentiated SCC, and SCC in situ. Cure rates for cryosurgery at 5 years after procedure have been reported as 93% and 96% for low-risk BCC and SCC, respectively, although like EDC, it has not been rigorously studied in a randomized controlled trial setting.[25-27] Its advantages include ease, speed, and low cost. Disadvantages are similar to EDC and include prolonged healing duration (which may last 4-6 weeks), pain and edema at the site, postoperative bullae formation, and associated hypopigmentation. Future use of optical coherence tomography and confocal microscopy[28,29] may augment the reliability of cryosurgery, which may then be used as an adjuvant approach to minimize tumor recurrence.

Excision

Surgical excision is a mainstay of treatment for NMSC due to both the potential for rapid healing and the ability to examine tissue histologically to ensure complete tumor removal. Although EDC or cryosurgery may be appropriate for treatment of some NMSCs, surgical excision has both a higher cure rate and improved cosmesis over those options. Still, unlike MMS, where 100% of the margin is examined histologically, standard pathologic review of a surgical excision specimen examines only a portion of the tumor margin. Tumors that are well defined are ideal for surgical excision, as the clinician can assess clinical margins and confidently remove all of the tumor based on visual appearance alone.

Surgical technique for excision varies, although most lesions are excised with a fusiform ellipse with the long axis oriented along the relaxed skin tension lines. The length-to-width ratio of the ellipse should measure between 3:1 and 4:1, and the angles at the edges of the ellipse should be approximately 30 degrees to mitigate the risk of dog-ear formation. After the lesion is excised, the skin is undermined and a layered closure is performed. See Chapter 16 for a detailed discussion of linear closure approaches.

The goal of surgical excision is to completely remove the tumor while minimizing the removal and destruction of normal skin. Typically, surgical excision of NMSC requires that a margin of healthy skin surrounding the tumor be removed due to the risk of subclinical tumor extension.[30] When performing surgical excision for NMSC, obtaining adequate surgical margins reduces the risk of positive histologic margins and the subsequent need for reexcision.[31] In areas where there is limited excess skin and tissue preservation is vital, the limitations of excisional surgery must be recognized. In some circumstances, taking smaller surgical margins or referring for MMS may be more appropriate than simple surgical excision.

There are very few well-designed, qualitative, prospective studies examining appropriate surgical margins for NMSC. Although some advocate a 4-mm margin,[32] there is little evidence to support this, and individual practice varies.

BCC Margins: Features of the BCC that must be considered before determining surgical margins are how well defined the tumor is, tumor diameter and histologic subtype, anatomic location, and any prior treatments the patient has undergone.[33] Ill-defined tumors may be poor excisional candidates because an accurate assessment of the clinical margin is often not possible. It may be difficult to determine the degree of subclinical spread for larger tumors, and such lesions may be more appropriately treated with MMS. Although 4-mm margins are generally more than adequate for BCC, some circumstances require larger margins, and some tumors have very extensive subclinical spread.[32] Larger and recurrent tumors may require a larger margin of up to 10 mm.[33] Very aggressive histologic subtypes of BCC (morpheaform and sclerosing) are not appropriate for surgical excision because of their tendency to demonstrate aggressive subclinical spread. Facial lesions and recurrent lesions anywhere on the body are generally considered high risk and thus may be more appropriate for MMS.

SCC Margins: As with BCC, increased size, more invasive histologic subtypes, and higher-risk anatomic locations are less conducive to surgical excision. One additional parameter that should be considered is vertical depth of invasion.[33] As SCC invades deeper within the tissue, the surgical margins needed to clear the tumor also increase. It is generally accepted that a 4-mm margin is adequate when excising a low-risk SCC, whereas a 6-mm margin is adequate for higher-risk SCC.[34] These numbers are based on a study that progressively excised 1-mm margins until cure was achieved and found that 95% of low-risk SCCs were cured at a 4-mm margin and 95% of high-risk SCCs were cured at 6 mm.[35] Others have argued that these margins may not be appropriate and have suggested margins anywhere between 2 and 15 mm.[33]

In general, surgical excision has a very high cure rate for NMSC. Most tumors are adequately excised, but because there is no immediate histologic confirmation of negative margins, there is a risk for incomplete excision. One study showed that the cumulative 5-year recurrence risk with excision was 4.8% for BCC.[36] When stratified, the risk was lower on the trunk, neck, and extremities and slightly higher for excisions taking place on the head, with recurrence rates being highest for larger (>10 mm) lesions on the head. Studies evaluating cure rate of surgical excision of SCC suggest recurrence rates of 8% and 23% for primary and recurrent SCC, respectively.[37] The clinician must decide whether wide local excision or MMS is most appropriate in the setting of tumor recurrence or incomplete excision, especially as data regarding BCC demonstrated that recurrent tumors treated with MMS have a 5.4% recurrence rate compared to a 17.4% recurrence rate when treated with reexcision.[37] Still, given their sometimes indolent nature and propensity to affect the elderly, it is important to consider either approach, as well as watchful waiting, when deciding on management strategies for recurrent BCC in elderly patients. When considering recurrent SCC, MMS has similarly improved outcomes over standard reexcision.

Although guidelines for excision of NMSC have been set forth by the National Comprehensive Cancer Network, better-defined recommendations that take into account important tumor and patient characteristics need to be established. It is important to take into account patient's history, tumor history and histology, anatomic location, and tumor size in order to achieve optimal outcomes for surgical excision of NMSC.

Mohs Micrographic Surgery

MMS involves tangential removal of tissue and immediate processing with frozen section histology in order to ensure that 100% of the tumor margin has been histologically examined and excised. It has the distinct advantage of ensuring almost complete histologic removal of the tumor in real time and provides the least possible damage to adjacent normal tissues. Many studies have demonstrated both the safety and efficacy of MMS in treatment of NMSC. The strength of the technique is that it has the lowest documented recurrence rate of any surgical treatment method and maximizes tissue sparing.[37-39]

MMS is the treatment of choice for skin cancers on functionally or cosmetically sensitive areas, although it may be used anywhere the body. In general, MMS is indicated for NMSC in high-risk locations. It is also appropriate for larger tumors, incompletely excised tumors, tumors with aggressive histologic subtypes or indistinct clinical borders, and tumors in cosmetically or functionally sensitive areas.

The fresh frozen tissue technique[40] is performed by tangentially excising the tumor with a small amount of normal surrounding tissue. Orienting marks are made on the specimen and the corresponding site on the patient. The surgical specimen is then flattened in a manner that allows the three-dimensional margin to be cut in a two-dimensional plane and rapidly frozen. This allows the entire margin to be viewed in a microscopic section. The tissue is cut using a cryostat, and the margin is mounted on one or more slides and then stained and examined by the Mohs surgeon. Typically, a hematoxylin and eosin stain is used when examining NMSC, although other special stains exist that are specific to different types of tumors. Positive margins are marked on an operative map, and additional tissue can then be removed to ensure the greatest possible tissue sparing. Processing of the tissue, histologic examination, and reexcision are repeated in stages until a negative margin is obtained.

Assuming that 100% of the epidermis and deep margin are visualized, once there are no positive margins, complete removal of the tumor has been achieved.[41] The resulting defect from the excision can be repaired, allowed to heal by secondary intention, reconstructed, or referred to a colleague for reconstruction. Occasionally during the course of MMS, tumors will be encountered that are unresectable. This typically will not be apparent until many stages are performed or in cases of perineural invasion. When surgical margins cannot be obtained or complete resection cannot be achieved, it is helpful to map out the positive margins so that future surgery or radiotherapy can be targeted most accurately.

Indications for MMS have evolved as the technique has become more widely adopted and more actively sought out by patients. Appropriate use guidelines were developed by performing a thorough review of all available literature from 1940 to 2011 to help guide clinicians in determining when MMS is medically necessary.[42] A rating system was developed to guide clinical decision making and ensure rational use of MMS depending on patient characteristics, type of NMSC, tumor characteristics, and clinical scenario.

MMS has been very well studied for the treatment of NMSC and has the highest cure rate of all treatment modalities for BCC and SCC. A review of the Australian Mohs database showed 5-year recurrence rates of primary BCC and SCC to be 1.4% and 2.6%, respectively.[38] Additionally, it found the 5-year recurrence rates of recurrent BCC and SCC treated with MMS to be 4% and 5.9%, respectively.[38,43] Other large retrospective studies have shown that MMS has lower recurrence rates than any other treatment modality in both SCC and BCC, likely because all of the tissue margins are examined.[37] Although MMS may be more costly than excision or EDC, several studies have highlighted its cost effectiveness, particularly because it can be performed in the office, the surgeon also acts as the pathologist, and it has an extremely high cure rate.[44]

OPERATIVE CONSIDERATIONS

All surgical approaches have risks, including but not limited to bleeding, infection, risk of hypertrophic scar development, dyspigmentation, poor cosmetic outcome, and risk of incomplete treatment. These risks must be discussed with the NMSC patient in order to ensure that the patient is part of the informed consent process prior to deciding whether to undergo surgical management.

A detailed medical history should be obtained by the clinician to ensure a thorough understanding of the patient's comorbidities and overall immune status.[45] Additionally, the skin should be cleaned preoperatively in enlarging concentric circles beginning at the excision site and extending outward beyond the area covered by the sterile drape.[46] Bacteremia rates during cutaneous surgery have been documented to range from 0.7% to 7%, which is similar to spontaneous bacteremia rates in healthy adults.[47,48] The American Academy of Dermatology has recently reviewed and published a statement on the use of prophylactic antibiotics in dermatologic surgery, stating that it is unnecessary for cutaneous surgery unless mucosal skin is involved, the operative site is inflamed or infected, or the patient is high risk.[49] In these situations, a single dose of antibiotics should be administered 1 hour prior to surgery. Despite proper precautionary measures, wound infections will occur in approximately 2% of cases.[50] If this occurs, sutures should be removed and the patient should be started empirically on antibiotics such as a first-generation cephalosporin until culture and sensitivity results from the wound are obtained.[46]

The risk of postoperative bleeding is generally low for dermatologic surgery. In order to minimize bleeding complications, all medications and supplements should be disclosed to the clinician preoperatively.[51] Patients taking aspirin are more susceptible to bleeding complications. There have been several published studies regarding the cessation of anticoagulants prior to dermatologic surgery, and in general, the risk of postoperative bleeding after dermatologic surgery is much less than the risk of thromboembolic events. Therefore, medically necessary anticoagulants should not be routinely discontinued prior to surgery.[52]

MEDICAL THERAPY FOR NMSC

Although EDC, excision, and MMS are the cornerstones of NMSC management, select, largely superficial tumors may be managed noninvasively as well. Options include topical

5-fluorouracil and imiquimod for superficial BCC and SCC in situ, as well as photodynamic therapy. Topical 5-fluorouracil is typically applied twice daily for 6 weeks, with typical side effects including erythema, local irritation, and crusting. Imiquimod is typically applied daily five times weekly for 6 weeks and has a similar side effect profile to 5-fluorouracil.[53] Although these approaches may be useful in select tumors and patients, the inconvenience of multiple applications coupled with sometimes vigorous local tissue reaction and their modest complete clearance rate make these second-line options for NMSC management.

Intralesional approaches represent another treatment modality for NMSC, although like medical therapies, they have not been studied extensively. Intralesional 5-fluorouracil, methotrexate, and bleomycin have all been explored and have demonstrated variable success in managing NMSC.[53]

Advanced or unresectable BCC may also be treated using vismodegib, a novel hedgehog pathway inhibitor. Given the significant cost and—more importantly—side effect profile associated with this treatment, it should be reserved for select cases that are not amenable to surgical management.

RADIATION THERAPY FOR NMSC

Radiation has been used for decades to treat NMSC, although generally its use has been limited by considerations of cost and convenience. Recently, superficial radiation therapy and electronic brachytherapy have again come into vogue, and their use by clinicians in the United States has been increasing. Limitations of these approaches include a paucity of data regarding cure and recurrence rates as well as cost and availability. Radiation therapy may also be used as an adjuvant approach for select high-risk NMSC.

CONCLUSIONS

There are many surgical and nonsurgical techniques available to successfully treat NMSC. No multicenter studies are available to directly compare different surgical approaches for NMSC, although single-center studies comparing the recurrence rates of EDC, cryosurgery, surgical excision, and MMS have generally shown that MMS has the lowest recurrence rate (**Tables 19-2 and 19-3**).[37,54] Generally, clinician comfort with each of these modalities as well as tumor size, clinical and histologic characteristics, patient age, anatomic location, and recurrence status will help to guide the clinician in choosing the most appropriate treatment.

TABLE 19-2 • Estimated Cumulative Recurrence Rates for Primary Basal Cell Carcinoma by Treatment Modality

Treatment	Cumulative 5-Year Recurrence Rate
Cryosurgery	1.0%-16.5%
Curettage and electrodessication	2.0%-26%
Surgical excision	1.7%-10.1%
Mohs surgery	0.7%-1.7%

Data from Metterle L, Russell JS, Patel NS: An overview of the medical management of nonmelanoma skin cancer. Curr Probl Cancer. *2015 Jul-Aug;39(4):226-236.*

TABLE 19-3 • Estimated Cumulative Recurrence Rates for Primary Squamous Cell Carcinoma by Treatment Modality

Treatment	Cumulative 5-Year Recurrence Rate
Cryosurgery	Not available at 5 years, 3.2% in short term
Curettage and electrodessication	3.7%
Surgical excision	8.1%
Mohs surgery	3.1%

Data from Rowe DE, Carroll RJ, Day CL Jr: Prognostic factors for local recurrence, metastasis, and survival rates in squamous cell carcinoma of the skin, ear, and lip. Implications for treatment modality selection, J Am Acad Dermatol. *1992 Jun;26(6):976-990.*

Although other options for NMSC management, such as medical therapies and radiation therapy, are becoming increasingly common, surgical treatments will likely continue to represent the primary approach to NMSC because they achieve high cure rates and have minimal side effects, reasonable cost, and acceptable cosmetic outcomes.

REFERENCES

1. Rogers HW, Weinstock MA, Harris AR, et al. Incidence estimate of nonmelanoma skin in the United States, 2006. *JAMA Dermatol.* 2010;146(3):283-287.
2. Lomas A, Leonardi-Bee J, Bath-Hextall F. A systematic review of the worldwide incidence of nonmelanoma skin cancer. *Br J Dermatol.* 2012;166(5):1069-1080.
3. Rogers HW, Weinstock MA, Feldman SR, Coldiron BM. Incidence estimate of nonmelanoma skin cancer (keratinocyte carcinomas) in the US population, 2012. *JAMA Dermatol.* 2015;151(10):1081-1086.
4. American Cancer Society. *Cancer Facts and Figures 2006.* Atlanta, GA: American Cancer Society; 2006.
5. Silverman M, Kopf A, et al. Recurrence rates of treated basal cell carcinomas. Part 1: overview. *J Dermatol Surg Oncol.* 1991;17(9):713-718.
6. Neville JA, Welch E, Lefell DJ. Management of nonmelanoma skin cancer in 2007. *Nat Clin Pract Oncol.* 2007;4:462-469.
7. Sturm HM, Leider M. An editorial on curettage. *J Dermatol Surg Oncol.* 1979;5:532-533.
8. Adam JE. The technic of curettage surgery. *J Am Acad Dermatol.* 1986;15:697-702.
9. Salasche SJ. Curettage and electrodessication in the treatment of midfacial basal cell epithelioma. *J Am Acd Dermatol.* 1983;8:496-503.
10. Kopf W, Bart RS, Schrager D, et al. Curettage-electrodessication treatment of basal cell carcinomas. *Arch Dermatol.* 1977;113:439-443.
11. Sheridan AT, Dawber RPR. Curettage, electrosurgery and skin cancer. *Australas J Dermatol.* 2000;41:19-30.
12. Knox JM, Lyles TW, Shaprio EM, et al. Curettage and electrodessication in the treatment of skin cancer. *Arch Dermatol.* 1960;82:197-203.

13. Whelan CS, Deckers PJ. Electrocoagulation and curettage for carcinoma involving the skin of the face, nose, eyelids, and ears. *Cancer.* 1973;31:159-164.
14. Suhge d'Aubermont PC, Bennett PG. Failure of curettage and electrodessication for removal of basal cell carcinoma. *Arch Dermatol.* 1984;120:1456-1460.
15. Silverman M, Kopf A, et al. Recurrence rates of treated basal cell carcinomas. Part 2: curettage-electrodessication. *J Dermatol Surg Oncol.* 1991;17(9):720-726.
16. Peikert JM. Prospective trial of curettage and cryosurgery in the management of non-facial, superficial, and minimally invasive basal and squamous cell carcinoma. *Int J Dermatol.* 2011;50: 1135-1138.
17. Rowe DE, Carroll RJ, Day CL Jr. Mohs surgery is the treatment of choice for recurrent (previously treated) basal cell carcinoma. *J Dermatol Surg Oncol.* 1989;15(4):424-431.
18. Baust JG, Gage AAA. The molecular basis of cryosurgery. *BJU Int.* 2005;95(9):1187-1191.
19. Gage AA, Baust JG. Mechanisms of tissue injury in cryosurgery. *Cryobiology.* 1998;47:171-186.
20. Hollister WR, Mathew AJ, Baust JG, et al. Effects of freezing on cell viability and mechanisms of cell death in human prostate cancer cell line. *Mol Urol.* 1998;2:13-18.
21. Gage AA, Baust JM, Baust JG. Experimental cryosurgery investigations in vivo. *Cryobiology.* 2009;59:229-243.
22. Joosten JJA, van Muijen JNP, Wobbes T, et al. In vivo destruction of tumor tissue by cryoablation can induce inhibition of secondary tumor growth: an experimental study. *Cryobiology.* 2001;42(1):49-58.
23. Zouboulis CC. Principles of cutaneous cryosurgery: an update. *Dermatology.* 1999;2:111-117.
24. Gage AA, Baust JG. Cryosurgery for tumors. *J Am Coll Surg.* 2007;205(2):342-356.
25. Kuflik EG. The five-year cure rate achieved by cryosurgery for skin cancer. *J Am Acad Dermatol.* 1991;24:1002-1004.
26. Kuflik EG. Cryosurgery for skin cancer: 30 year experience and cure rates. *Dermatol Surg.* 2004;30-297-300.
27. Zacarian SA. Cryosurgery of cutaneous carcinomas. An 18-year study of 3,022 patients with 4,228 carcinomas. *J Am Acad Dermatol.* 1983;9:947-956.
28. Morgensen M, Thrane L, Jørgensen TM, et al. OCT imaging of skin cancer. *J Biophotonics.* 2009;2(6-7):442-451.
29. Karen JK, Gareau DS, Dusza SW, et al. Detection of basal cell carcinomas in Mohs excisions with fluorescence confocal mosaicking microscopy. *Br J Dermatol.* 2009;160:1242-1250.
30. Bennett RG. The meaning and significance of tissue margins. *Adv Dermatol.* 1989;4:343-357.
31. Lane JE, Kent DE. Surgical margins in the treatment of nonmelanoma skin cancer and Mohs micrographic surgery. *Curr Surg.* 2005;62:518-526.
32. Wolf DJ, Zitelli JA. Surgical margins for basal cell carcinoma. *Arch Dermatol.* 1987;123(3):340-344.
33. Huang CC, Boyce SM. Surgical margins of excision for basal cell carcinoma and squamous cell carcinoma. *Semin Cutan Med Surg.* 2004;23:167-173.
34. Thomas DJ, King AR, Peat BG. Excision margins for nonmelanotic skin cancer. *Plastic Reconstr Surg.* 2003;112(1):57-63.
35. Broadland DG, Zitelli JA. Mechanisms of metastasis. *J Am Acad Dermatol.* 1992;27(1):1-8.
36. Silverman M, Kopf A, Bart RS, et al. Recurrence rates of treated basal cell carcinomas. Part 3: surgical excision. *J Dermatol Surg Oncol.* 1992;18(6):471-476.
37. Rowe DE, Carroll RJ, Day CL Jr. Prognostic factors for local recurrence, metastasis, and survival rates in squamous cell carcinoma of the skin, ear, and lip. Implications for treatment modality selection. *J Am Acad Dermatol.* 1992;26(6):976-990.
38. Leibovitch I, Huilgol SC, Selva D, et al. Basal cell carcinoma treated with Mohs surgery in Australia II. Outcome at 5-year follow up. *J Am Acad Dermatol.* 2005;53(3):452-457.
39. Rowe DE, Carroll RJ, Day CL Jr. Long-term recurrence rates in preciously untreated (primary) basal cell carcinoma: implications for patient follow-up. *J Dermatol Surg Oncol.* 1989;15(3):315-328.
40. Brodland DG, Amonette R, Hanke CW, et al. The history and evolution of Mohs micrographic surgery. *Dermatol Surg.* 2000;26(4): 303-307.
41. Drake LA. Guidelines of cure for Mohs micrographic surgery. *J Am Acad Dermatol.* 1995;33:271.
42. Connolly SM, Baker DR, Coldiron BM, et al. AAD/ACMS/ASDAA/ASMS 2012 appropriate use criteria for Mohs micrographic surgery: a report of the American Academy of Dermatology, American College of Mohs Surgery, American Society for Dermatologic Surgery Association, and the American Society for Mohs Surgery. *J Am Acad Dermatol.* 2012;67(4):531-550.
43. Leibovitch I, Huilgol SC, Selva D, et al. Cutaneous squamous cell carcinoma treated with Mohs micrographic surgery in Australia I. Experience over 10 years. *J Am Acad Dermatol.* 2005;53(2):253-260.
44. Coo J, Zitelli J. Mohs micrographic surgery: a cost analysis. *J Am Acad Dermatol.* 1995;39:698-703.
45. Chan BCY, Patel DC. Perioperative management and the rate of adverse events in dermatologic procedures performed by dermatologists in New Zealand. *Australas J Dermatol.* 2009;50:171-175.
46. Hurst EA, Grekin RC, Yu SS, et al. Infectious complications and antibiotic use in dermatologic surgery. *Semin Cutan Med Surg.* 2007;26:47-53.
47. Carmichael AJ, Flanagan PG, Holt PJ, et al. The occurrence of bacteremia in skin surgery. *Br J Dermatol.* 1996;134:120-122.
48. Halpern AC, Leyden JJ, Dzubow LM, et al. The incidence of bacteremia in skin surgery of the head and neck. *J Am Acad Dermatol.* 1998;19:112-116.
49. Wright TI, Baddour LM, Berbari EF, et al. Antiobiotic prophylaxis in dermatologic surgery: advisory statement 2008. *J Am Acad Dermatol.* 2008;59:464-473.
50. Futoryan T, Grande D. Postoperative wound infection rates in dermatologic surgery. *Dermatol Surg.* 1995;21(6):509-514.
51. Dinehart SM, Henry L. Dietary supplements: altered coagulation and effects on bruising. *Dermatol Surg.* 2005;31:819-826.
52. Otley CC. Continuation of medically necessary aspirin and warfarin during cutaneous surgery. *Mayo Clin Proc.* 2003;78(11):1392-1396.
53. Metterle L, Russell JS, Patel NS. An overview of the medical management of nommelanoma skin cancer. *Curr Probl Cancer.* 2015;39(4):226-236.
54. Thissen MRTM, Neumann MHA, Schouten LJ. A systematic review of treatment modalities for primary basal cell carcinomas. *Arch Dermatol.* 1999;135(10):1177-1183.

20 Flaps and Advanced Techniques

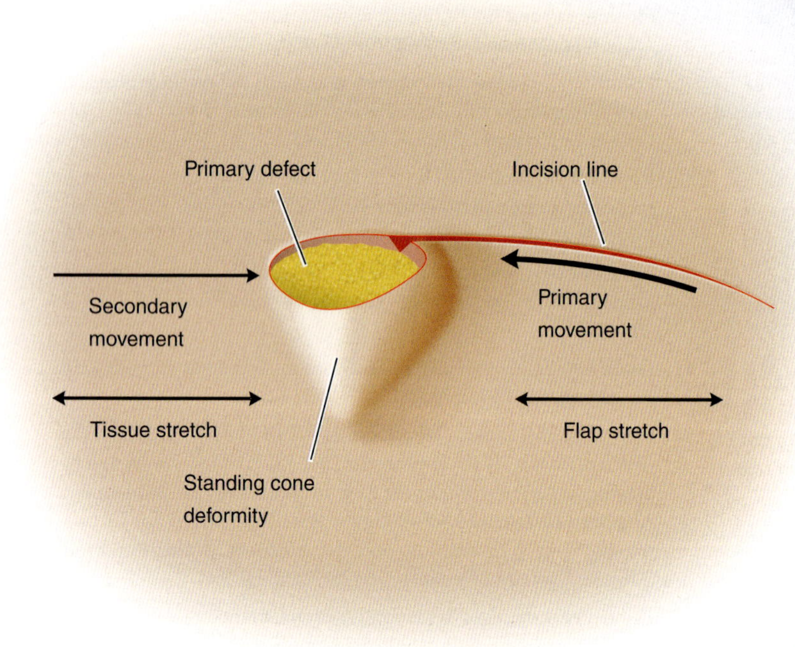

SUMMARY

- Understanding flap dynamics is a prerequisite for the performance of any flap procedures.
- Advancement flaps can be conceptualized as geometric variations of linear repairs with dog-ear redistribution.
- Rotation flaps recruit tissue through rotational movement around a pivot point, and rely on tissue laxity adjacent to the defect.
- The ability of transposition flaps to push tissue into the defect by redirecting tension vectors perpendicular to the primary closure direction, coupled with their ability to close a defect using a smaller total surface area than sliding flaps (and the possible added benefit of a broken-up repair line), make these flaps particularly useful for larger defects.

Beginner Tips

- Understanding flap dynamics is predicated on an appreciation of the forces that oppose tissue movement.
- Undermining mitigates most deep restraint, while horizontal restraint is addressed by using a sufficiently lengthy incision that recruits lax skin.

Pitfalls and Cautions

- Failing to account for pivotal restraint is one of the most common flap design challenges. Appropriately oversizing rotation flaps and widely undermining the pivot point may go a long way to mitigating this problem.
- Once relocated to the primary defect, flaps should be under minimal tension.

Expert Tips

- Horizontal, deep, and pivotal restraints must all be addressed for optimal flap outcomes.
- Obstructive restraint can be addressed prior to flap movement.
- On the face, the robust blood supply means that even random pattern flaps may behave more like axial flaps in terms of viability.

Patient Education Points

- Patients should be warned prior to flap closure that they will have an incision stretching well beyond the initially visible defect.
- Explaining that the additional scar length will likely heal with a minimally visible line may go a long way toward patient reassurance.

Don't Forget!

- Undermining beyond 1 to 2 cm from the incision line may be counterproductive and lead to an increased risk of tissue ischemia.
- Flap length:width ratios should ideally not be significantly greater than 3:1, at least when working in poorly perfused areas such as the legs. On the face, there is often a forgiving and robust blood supply.

Billing Pearls

- Flap repair codes (140XX series) include the excision component, so it is not appropriate to bill both an excision and a flap repair code simultaneously.
- When coding a flap, medical necessity is the ultimate arbiter of appropriateness.

Flaps and Advanced Techniques 20

INTRODUCTION

Linear closures are the preferred technique to approach most defects given their reliability, predictability, and low rate of dehiscence or infection. At times, however, repairs performed by clinicians in the primary care or emergency room setting may necessitate more complex closures such as random pattern flaps.

These advanced techniques assume a higher level of familiarity with tissue movement, anatomy, and surgical technique than linear approaches to closure, but concomitantly permit the effective closure of even substantially sized (or awkwardly located) defects.

FLAP TYPES

Flap repairs may be classified in many ways, although when discussing their use for the repair of superficial skin defects, it is straightforward to subdivide them into two categories, sliding or lifting, based on the overall tissue movement required (**Table 20-1**). The predominant movement in sliding flaps is direct translational movement of the flap into the primary defect. This creates a secondary defect, which typically has unequal wound-edge lengths and is often closed with the assistance of removal of standing cone deformities. The key, tension-bearing sutures are placed to close the primary defect. Both advancement and rotation flaps represent examples of sliding flap repairs.[1,2]

Lifting flap repairs involve initial upward movement of the flap across a bridge of normal tissue to close the primary defect. As opposed to sliding flaps, the key tension-bearing sutures are used to close the secondary defect. Transposition flap repairs are examples of commonly performed lifting flap repairs.[1,2]

All flaps must move from the donor site into the recipient site; this movement can be accomplished in various ways, depending on flap type. Irrespective of flap type, movement is maximized through minimization of restraint. The key principles of closure must always be followed (**Table 20-2**).

TABLE 20-1 • Sliding and Lifting Flaps

	Sliding	Lifting
Flap types	Advancement, rotation	Transposition
Movement	Direct translational movement	Lifting over bridge of normal tissue
Key suture placement	Primary defect	Secondary defect

ADVANCEMENT FLAPS

Advancement flaps may be conceptualized as modified linear closures, with one or both apical standing cones (dog ears) moved laterally to facilitate aesthetic or functional closure. When a free margin, such as the eyelid or lip, or a cosmetic subunit junction would be violated by a linear closure, advancement flaps may be used to direct the standing cones away from these natural boundaries (**Figure 20-1**). Additionally, advancement flaps often camouflage scars by placing incision lines along natural creases or cosmetic subunit junctions.

Types of Advancement Flaps

Advancement flap may be categorized based on the number and locations of standing cones that are displaced due to tissue advancement. Thus, with two standing cones on the sides of the defect and (in a simplified example) two directions to move the standing cones, four potential basic advancement flap designs are available. Additionally, the crescentic advancement flap is a frequently used approach in dermatologic surgery as well.

Burow's Wedge Flap (O-to-L): The O-to-L advancement flap, also known as a unilateral Burow's wedge flap, is perhaps the most common variant of advancement flap used by clinicians. Here, one standing cone is moved laterally along the base of the flap. Common locations for this flap are the cutaneous lip, the nasal sidewall, the forehead, the suprabrow, the temple, the lower eyelid, and the mid cheek. A step-by-step approach to this flap technique is demonstrated in **Figure 20-2**.

A-to-T Flap: A frequently used technique, also known as an O-T advancement flap, the A-to-T advancement flap splits one standing cone into two smaller cones along the base of the flap (**Figure 20-3**). Often, the standing cone is at least partially sewn out by a "rule of halves" suturing technique that may obviate the need for large displaced dog ears. This approach is frequently used on the forehead and lips.

Unilateral Advancement Flap (O-to-U): This classic unilateral advancement flap is often used for eyebrow defects, eyelid defects, and forehead defects. The principal disadvantage of this advancement flap design is that the advancing edge of the flap may be

TABLE 20-2 • Closure Hierarchy

I	Preserve function
II	Avoid free-margin distortion
III	Place incisions within cosmetic subunit boundaries
IV	Situate incisions in relaxed skin tension lines

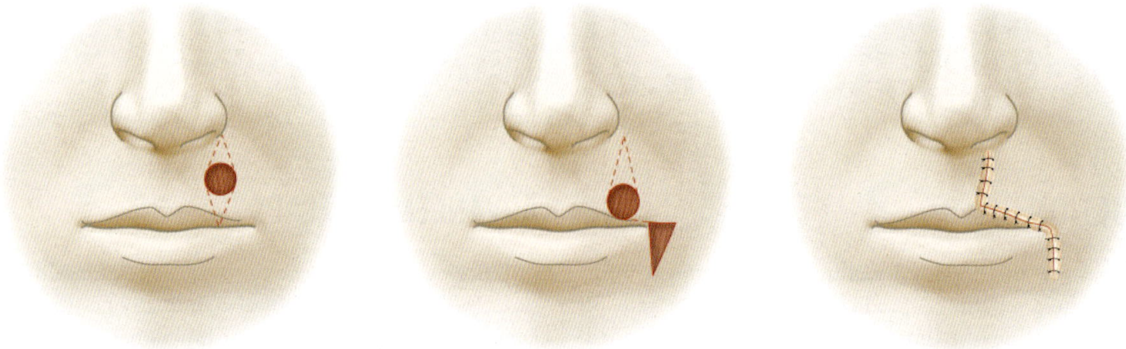

FIGURE 20-1 Advancement flaps allow for displacement of standing cones when they may infringe on free margins or cosmetic subunit junctions.

quite distant from the vascular pedicle, depending on the degree of undermining. However, if the vascular supply is robust, successful results can be achieved even with high length-to-width ratios.

A common variation of this approach is the helical rim advancement flap (**Figures 20-4 and 20-5**). This technique is useful for even fairly large defects on the helix given the robust blood supply available to this flap.[3]

Bilateral Advancement Flap (O-to-H): The bilateral advancement flap, also known as an H-plasty, is formed by creating two opposing O-to-U unilateral advancement flaps. The result is an H-shaped scar that is ideally masked within relaxed skin tension lines or along cosmetic subunit junctions. Prior to making incisions for the second pedicle of the flap, it may be prudent to completely undermine and mobilize the first pedicle to assess if the second arm is absolutely necessary. The two arms of the flap may be sized differently depending on the degree and location of required tissue movement.

Crescentic Advancement Flap: The crescentic advancement flap is a simple, yet powerful, variation of a unilateral advancement flap. Traditionally used along the alar crease and nasofacial sulcus, this technique is frequently employed for modestly sized nasal sidewall defects. This permits the clinician to effectively hide incision lines in cosmetic subunit boundaries, and—importantly—as the curved crescents of tissue lengthen, this approach may obviate the need for dog-ear removal as well (**Figure 20-6**).

Complications

Lower Eyelid Edema: Edema of the lower eyelid is frequently seen after advancement flaps are performed on the eyelids and upper cheeks. Warning patients of this eventuality may help mitigate anxiety and distress in the postoperative period, especially as this process generally resolves spontaneously over a period of months.

Disruption of Cosmetic Subunit Junctions: A cheek-to-nose flap may bridge the concavity of the nasofacial sulcus as the wound contracts, unless flap length is adjusted accordingly and tacking sutures are used to recreate the concavity. While this may be corrected with a secondary procedure, it is far better to appropriately design the flap de novo and use an appropriate-sized flap with tacking sutures, saving the patient the significant morbidity and cost associated with a secondary procedure.

On the lip, advancement flaps that require excision of the superior standing cone along the base of the nose may ablate the apical triangle and divert the nasolabial fold toward the lateral ala.[4,5] If there is no alternative to preserve the apical triangle, patients should be counseled preoperatively that the nasolabial fold may appear to dive into the nasal sill as opposed to continuing seamlessly onto the nasal sidewall. The natural course of the nasolabial fold can be restored with a Z-plasty.

Displacement of Free Margins: Whenever an advancement flap is adjacent to a free margin, the clinician must be careful to keep from pulling or pushing the margin out of position. To avoid pulling on a free margin, the primary tension vector for closure should be parallel to the free margin. Pushing may occur when the opposing sides of the advancement flap that come into apposition are significantly longer than the length of the original tissue that is being resurfaced, similar to the phenomenon that occurs with fusiform linear closures.[6]

ROTATION FLAPS

Rotation flaps recruit tissue via rotational movement around a pivot point. Inherent in this design is the formation of a broad pedicle and a desirable length-to-width ratio. Rotation flaps differ from primary repairs or advancement flaps by the orientation of tension vectors. In primary repairs or advancement flaps, the tension vectors generally are directed perpendicular to the long axis across the wound, whereas in a rotation flap, the tension vectors can be dispersed variably across the arcuate path of the flap.

As with the design of any flap, it must first be determined which tissue reservoir will be recruited. A rotation flap is, by definition, a sliding flap. The tissue reservoir must be immediately adjacent to the defined surgical defect. When choosing a tissue reservoir, cosmetic subunits and potential distortion of free margins must be taken into consideration. Once the most

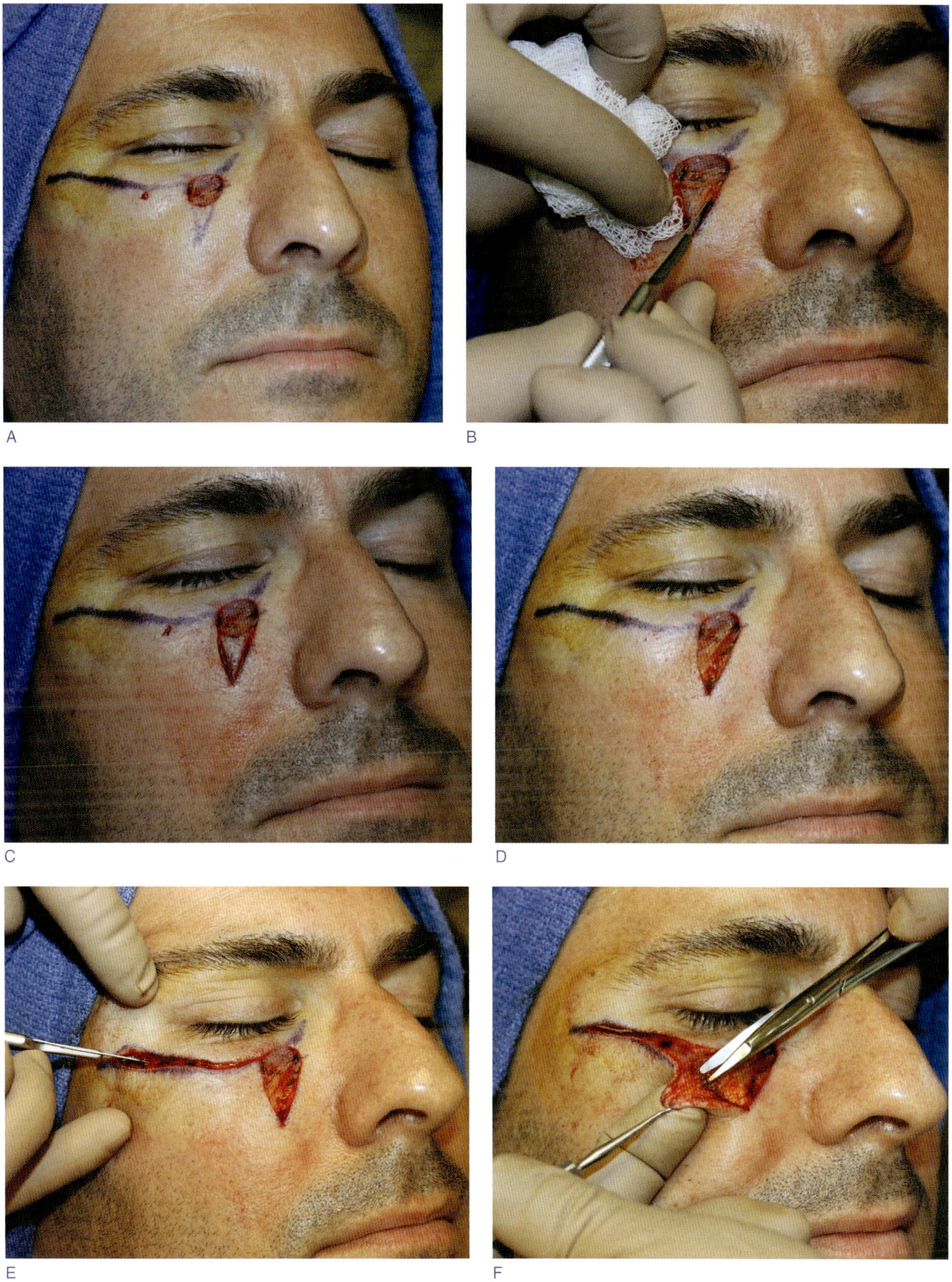

FIGURE 20-2 Advancement flap design (**A**). The inferior standing cone was removed (**B, C, D**). Then the incision along the junction of the cheek and eyelid was performed (**E**), and the flap was undermined above the superficial muscular aponeurotic system (SMAS) (**F**). The skin around the defect was undermined.

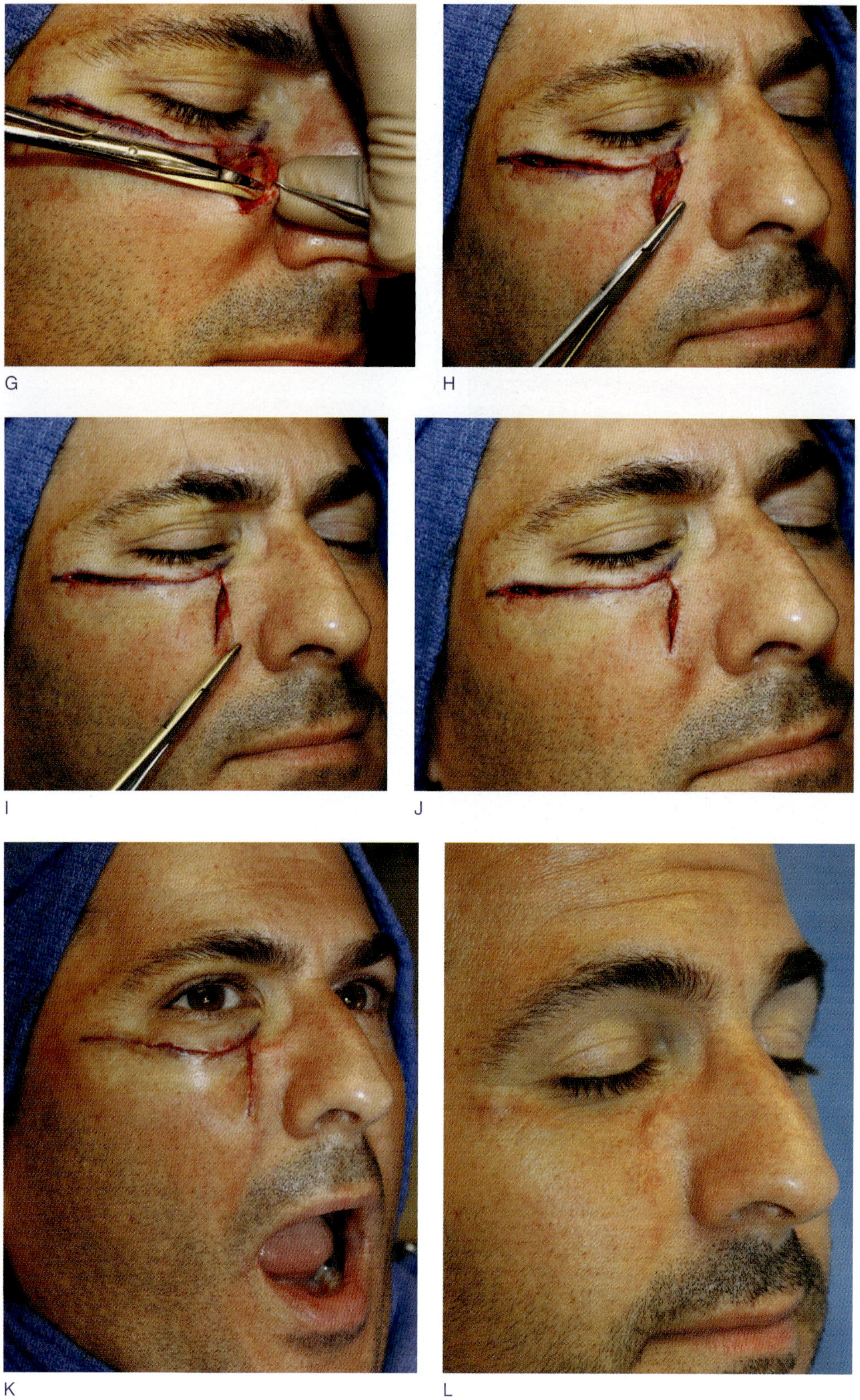

FIGURE 20-2 (*Continued*) (**G**). The first key suture was placed at the point of the highest tension (**H, I, J**). The remainder of the deep (**K**) and superficial sutures are placed, and the patient is instructed to open his mouth widely, open his eyes, and look up to place the lower lid under maximal stress and assess for ectropion (**K**). Six-week follow-up image is shown (**L**).

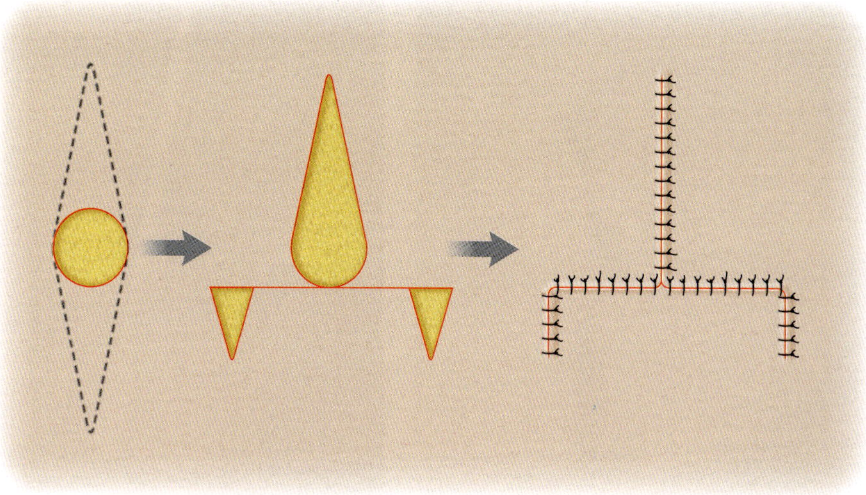

FIGURE 20-3 O-to-T flap design. Bidirectional primary tissue movement and one standing cone displaced.

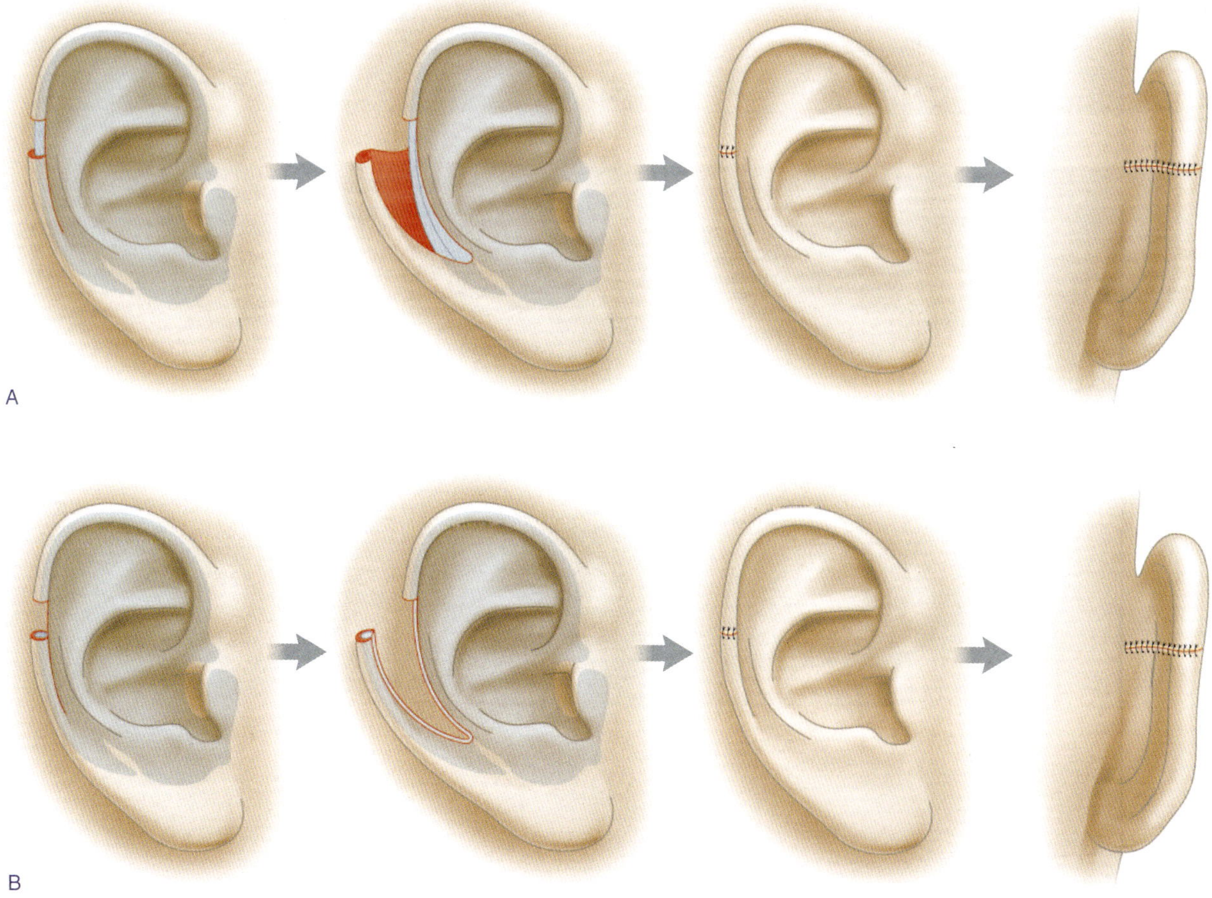

FIGURE 20-4 Schematic of helical rim advancement. **A.** A typical helical rim advancement flap. An incision is created along the anterior surface of the ear and carried into the lobule where a medial standing tissue cone is removed. The tissue is reflected off the cartilage and maintained on a posterior pedicle. The flap is advanced and the helical rim is approximated with eversion. A standing tissue cone is removed on the posterior surface of the ear. **B.** A chondrocutaneous advancement flap. Incision is carried out through cartilage and the flap is advanced and rotated into place. The inclusion of cartilage may be of greater benefit when the defect is higher on the helix or when more cartilage has been lost in the operative wound.

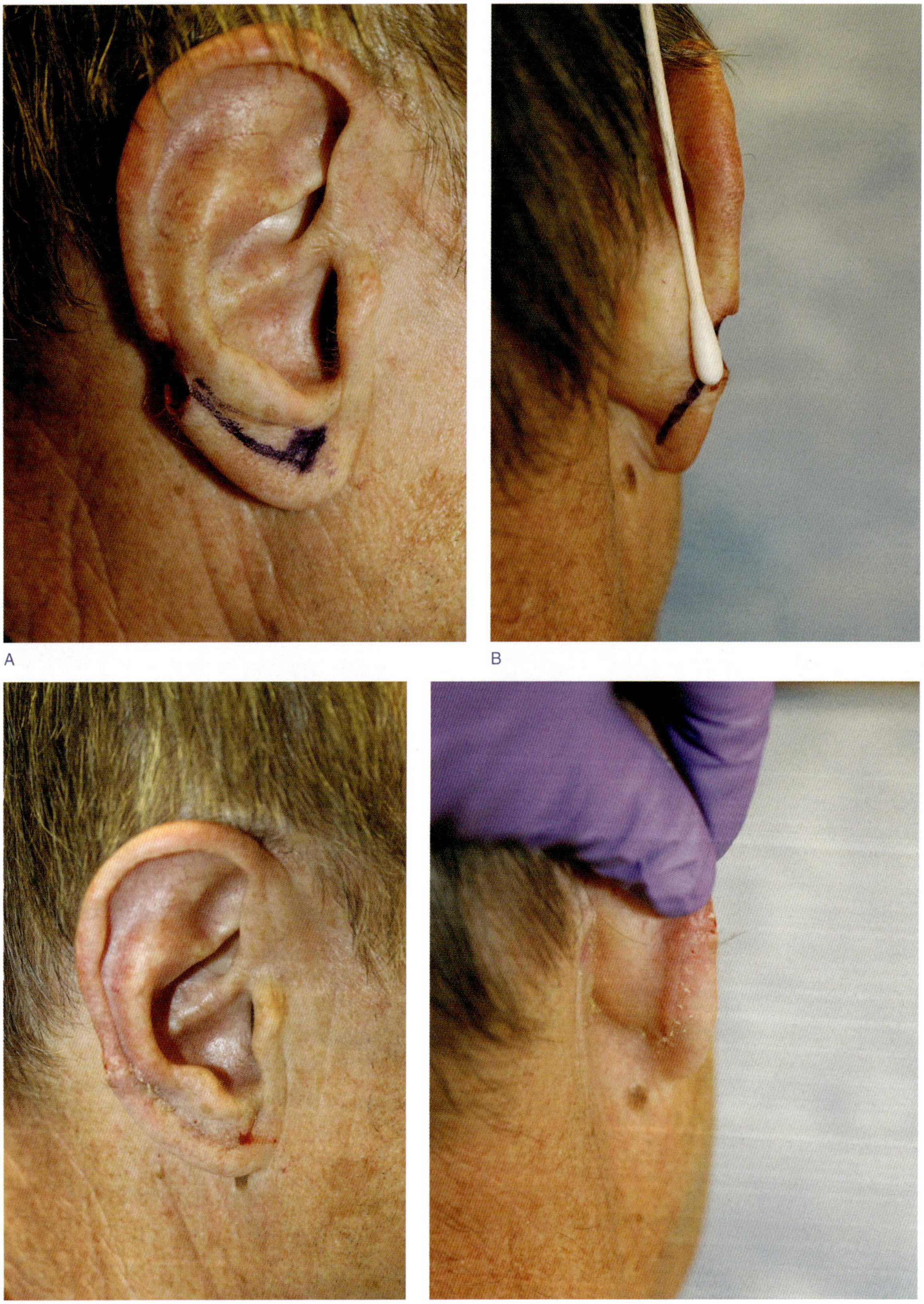

A B C D

FIGURE 20-5 Defect and advancement flap design (**A, B**) with full-thickness incision planned through the helical rim for reconstruction. The 4-week postoperative result is shown (**C, D**).

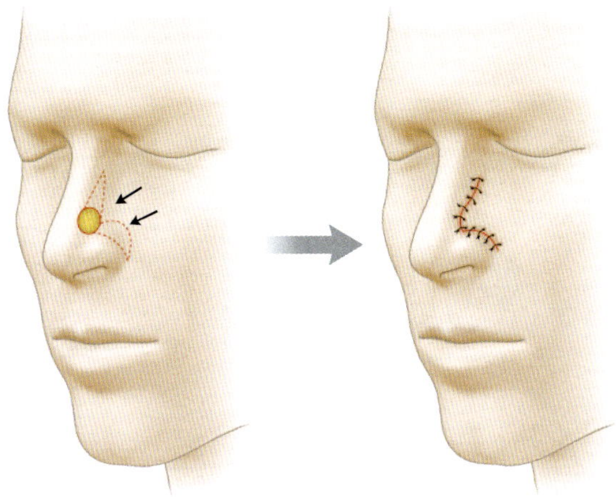

FIGURE 20-6 A crescentic advancement flap is designed to close an operative wound adjacent to the nasal ala with the upper and lower limbs of the advancement falling along the nasofacial sulcus, alar crease, and nasolabial fold. The design is simple in appearance but deceptively complex. As the flap advances, the shorter crescentic limbs stretch out to meet their destination and dog ears are not produced. Crescentic modification of a bilateral advancement flap may avoid the need for the removal of standing tissue cones.

appropriate reservoir has been identified, a curvilinear arc is extended from the wound around a central pivot point. Ideally, this arcuate incision may lie within a relaxed skin tension line, although this is not always possible. After the flap is incised, the flap and primary and secondary defects are all widely undermined. The flap can then be rotated inward to fill the primary defect (**Figure 20-7**).

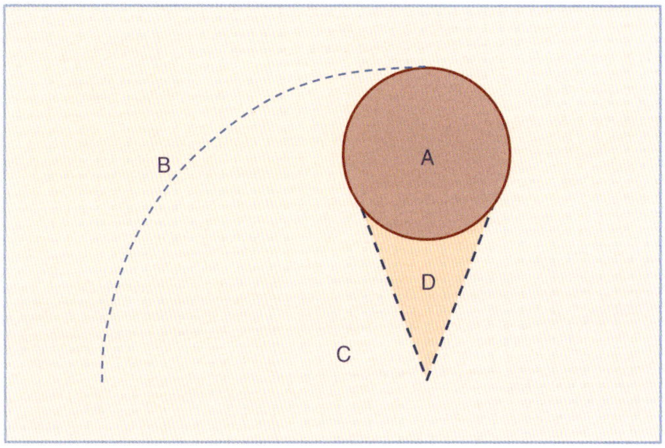

FIGURE 20-7 Rotation flap geometry. (**A**) The primary surgical defect is denoted by the red circle. After determination of the tissue recruitment area, a sweeping curvilinear arc is carried away from the primary defect with a tangential start point (**B**) around a central pivot point (**C**). Tissue redundancy can be anticipated adjacent to the pivot (**D**), and often is removed preemptively as a standing cone.

A critical consideration in flap design is sizing of the flap. All rotation flaps are subject to rotational shortening and pivotal restraint; as the flap tip rotates inward to fill the primary defect, the arc length of the flap decreases. The arc of rotation for a standard rotation flap classically begins tangentially to the defect. With the forces of pivotal restraint, the flap tip is shortened upon rotation into the defect, and the tip must be advanced upward to completely fill the gap. As a result, tension is transferred to the flap tip, already the area most susceptible to necrosis. To combat this design flaw, a vertical offset or "step-up" of the take-off point of the flap can be used,[7] extending the length of the leading edge of the flap past the surgical defect (**Figure 20-8**). This approach

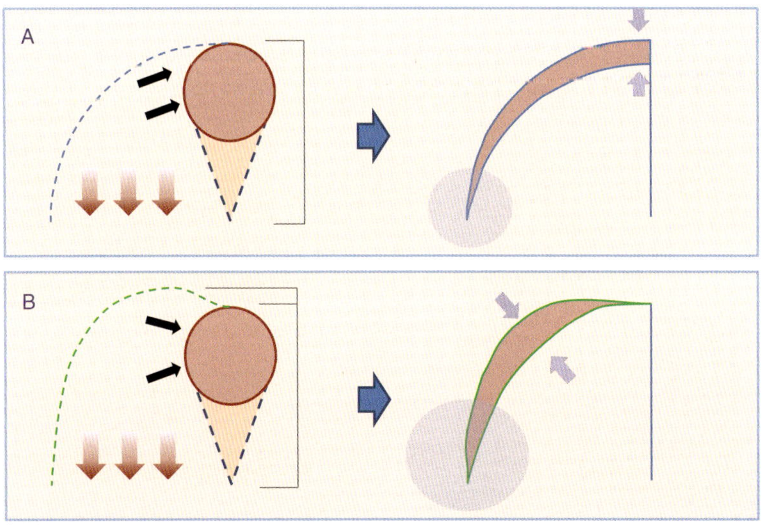

FIGURE 20-8 Rotational shortening. (**A**) Rotation flap designed with "traditional" tangential takeoff angle. Pivotal restraint effectively shortens the flap tip as it moves through the arc of rotation, and places additional tension on the tip once the flap movement is complete. (**B**) Oversized rotation flap design overcomes rotational shortening but creates a larger secondary defect and potentially creates more tissue redundancy. Black arrows, primary flap movement; red arrows, vector of pivotal restraint; purple arrows, the greatest area of tension on secondary defect; purple circles, potential tissue redundancy.

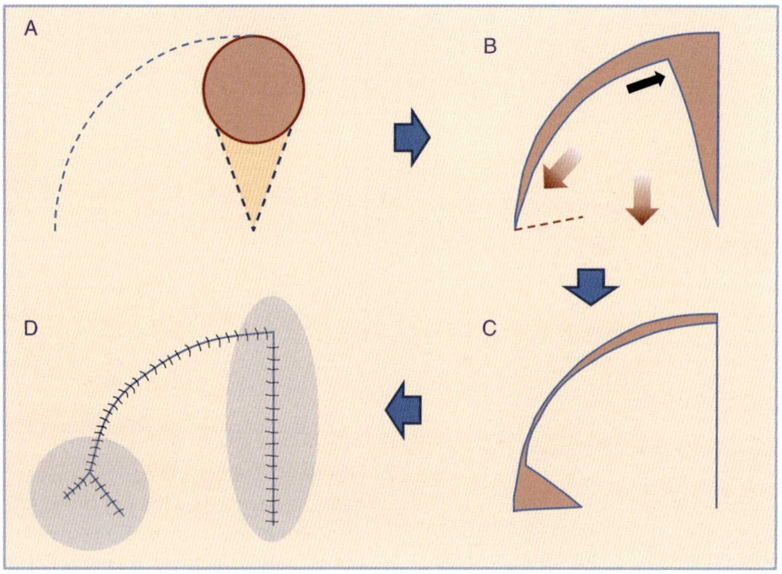

FIGURE 20-9 Backcut modification. (**A**) A standard rotation flap is designed, but occasionally excess laxity is needed to complete the rotation. (**B**) A backcut is designed and incised. (**C**) This allows the completion of the rotation arc. (**D**) Final closure—the secondary defect of the backcut is closed in a V-Y fashion. Black arrow, primary flap movement; red arrows, tissue restraint vectors; purple circles, tension on final closure.

allows the rotation flap to fill the defect under minimal tension on the flap tip, although increasing the length of the leading edge of the flap will result in a larger secondary defect, which may be undesirable depending on the cosmetic subunit.

The use of a backcut can further reduce pivotal restraint and assist in rotating the flap into place (**Figure 20-9**). However, careful attention must be paid to the length of a backcut that is used, as a backcut inherently reduces the width of the pedicle and may compromise flap perfusion.

Rotation flaps are often used to close large defects on the head and neck (**Figure 20-10**), many of which are unlikely to be encountered in primary care practice. Smaller rotation flaps, however, have a role in select straightforward closures that would benefit from shifting tension vectors or suture lines, or those perhaps used more frequently in response to trauma such as the O-to-Z double rotation flap that is often used for scalp defects (**Figure 20-11**). Moreover, traumatic injuries to the lip (as well as excisions) can occasionally be repaired with rotation flaps as well (**Figures 20-12 and 20-13**).

Complications and Management

Rotation flaps are susceptible to many of the same pitfalls that affect other types of flaps, including bleeding, dehiscence, and infection. Bulky pressure dressings may help in preventing bleeding in the postoperative period.

Should persistent bleeding continue beneath the flap during the postoperative period, a true hematoma may develop. Within the first 24 to 48 hours following surgery, hematomas should be

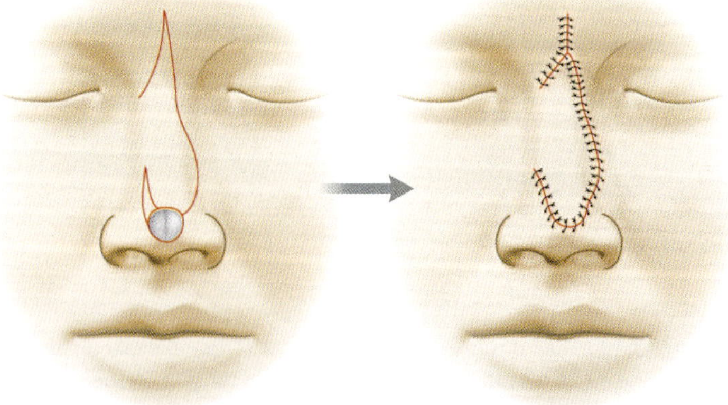

FIGURE 20-10 The dorsal nasal rotation flap. Note the use of a large backcut in the glabellar area to better mobilize the flap.

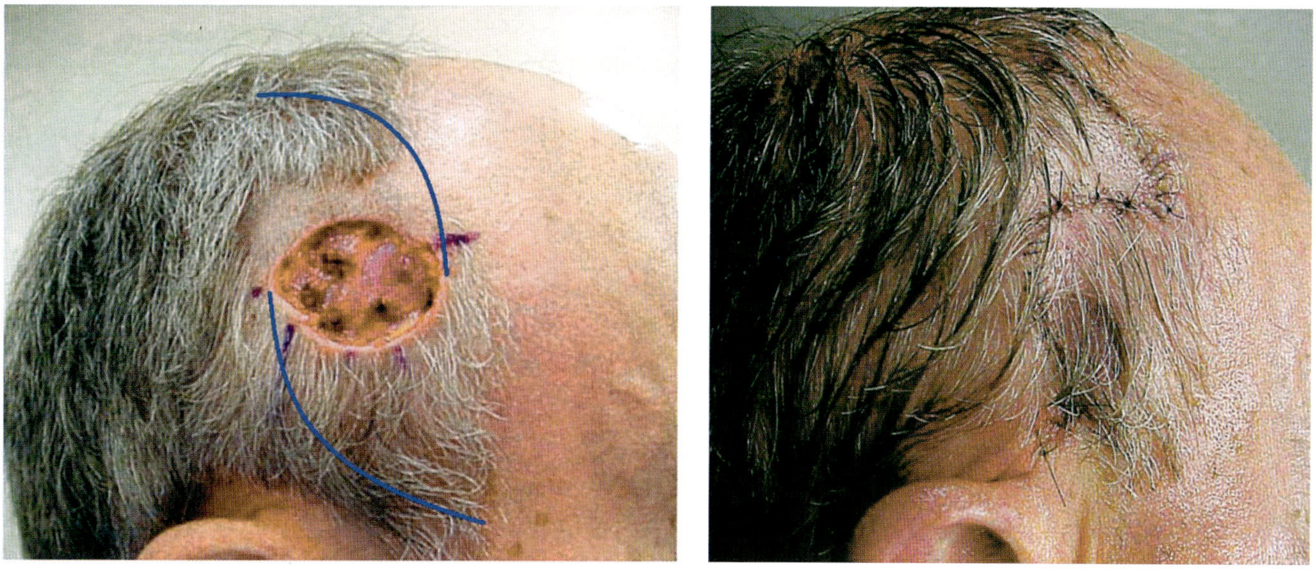

A B

FIGURE 20-11 O-to-Z rotation flap of the scalp—large defects of the scalp can be closed with opposing rotation flaps in a "Z" orientation. Repair shown with good results and minimal distortion of surrounding free margins.

evacuated to ensure the greatest chance for flap survival. If the hematoma is not yet organized, attempts can be made to remove the blood with a syringe and 18-gauge needle. However, it is likely that the sutures will need to be removed and the hematoma physically evacuated while also irrigating the wound. This offers the opportunity to visualize and address the source of bleeding, a critical step if the hematoma seems to be increasing in size. Outside of the first 2 days postoperatively, hematomas are more likely to be organized and less amenable to evacuation. Hematomas also significantly increase the risk of wound infections that may adversely affect flap viability. Thus, regardless of the time following surgery, the presence of a hematoma is an indication for prophylactic antibiotics, as hematomas serve as a nidus of infection.

Complications that are unique to rotation flaps derive from the design and tissue movement of these flaps. When unaccounted for, rotational shortening can produce excessive tension on the leading edge of the flap. This may result in dehiscence of the wound or flap ischemia and necrosis along this edge. Unnecessarily high tension due to rotational shortening may be combated by increasing the length of the leading edge of the rotation flap beyond the defect and wide undermining.

Lastly, rotation flaps may also be complicated by altering the position of free margins. The long arcuate incisions often created

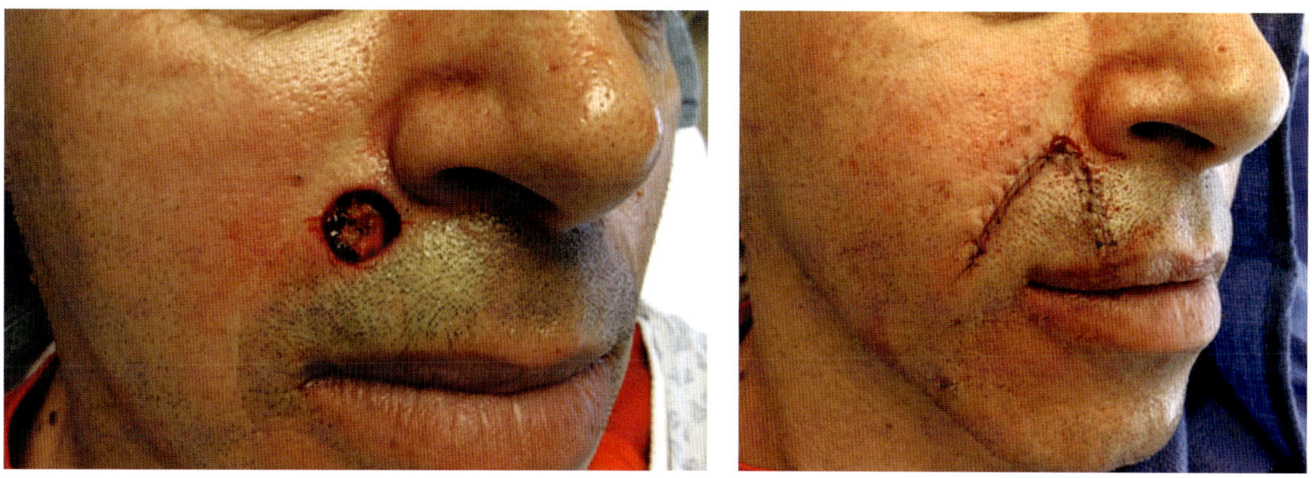

A B

FIGURE 20-12 Defect of the right upper cutaneous lip–nasolabial fold repaired with a rotation flap. (**A**) Preoperative appearance. (**B**) Postoperative appearance.

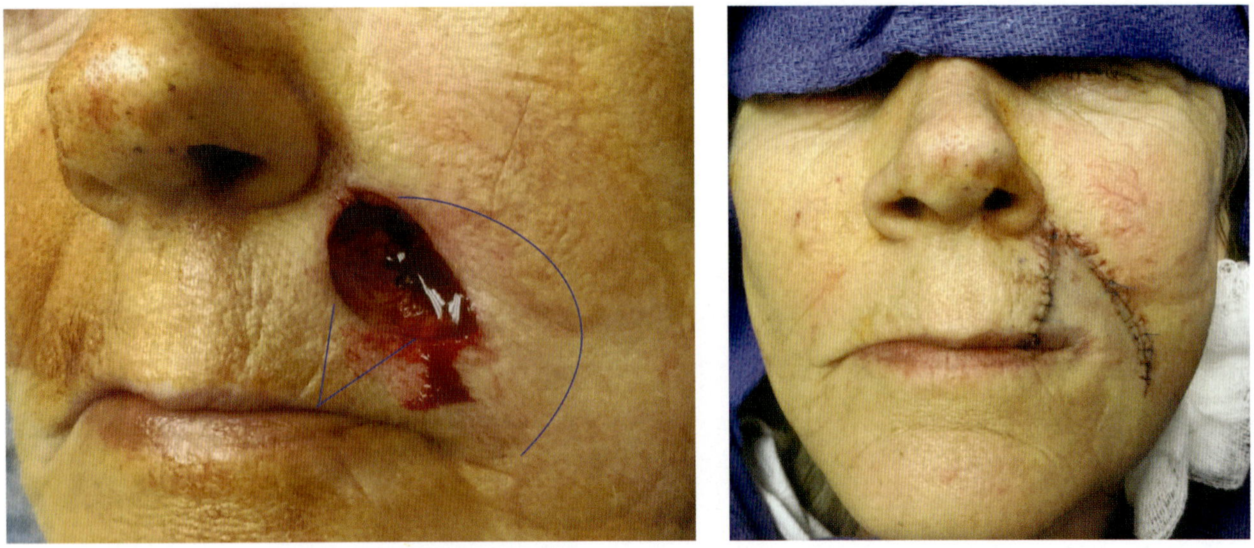

A B

FIGURE 20-13 Rotation flap of the lateral upper cutaneous lip ("Hatchet flap"). Note the rotation flap is designed such that the rotational arm of the flap recreates the nasolabial folds and the standing cone lines within the vertical perioral furrows.

by these flaps result in long secondary defects. It is important to be cognizant of the course of these secondary defects, especially when in close proximity to free margins. To varying degrees, there will always be secondary movement of the surrounding tissue to close the secondary defect. While it is true that increasing the length of the arc of rotation will decrease tension across the secondary defect, this must be weighed against extending the secondary defect to an anatomic location where a given amount of secondary tissue movement is unacceptable.

TRANSPOSITION FLAPS

Transposition flaps are often useful when tension at the primary defect precludes side-to-side closure or the use of sliding flaps, such as advancement or rotation flaps. To transpose means to switch positions, which aptly describes the flap's essence, as the position of the main tension vector is changed from the primary defect to a more ample adjacent tissue reservoir, and the elevated flap is transposed into the primary defect under little to no tension. Common transposition flaps include the rhombic (single-lobed), bilobed, and trilobed flaps, although the latter two flaps in particular involve a significant rotational component.

Pinching or squeezing together the primary wound edges is a simple strategy to guide flap selection. If pinching easily approximates the wound edges, then side-to-side closure or a sliding advancement or rotation flap will usually be possible (**Figure 20-14**). The pinch test can identify a suitable donor site for a transposition flap (**Figure 20-15**). If the skin immediately adjacent to the wound pinches easily and without anatomic distortion, a single-lobed rhombic flap may be possible. If the skin adjacent to the primary wound is too tight, then the pinch test may identify a sufficiently lax tissue reservoir more remote from the primary wound. A bilobed or trilobed flap may be necessary to reach a distant reservoir.

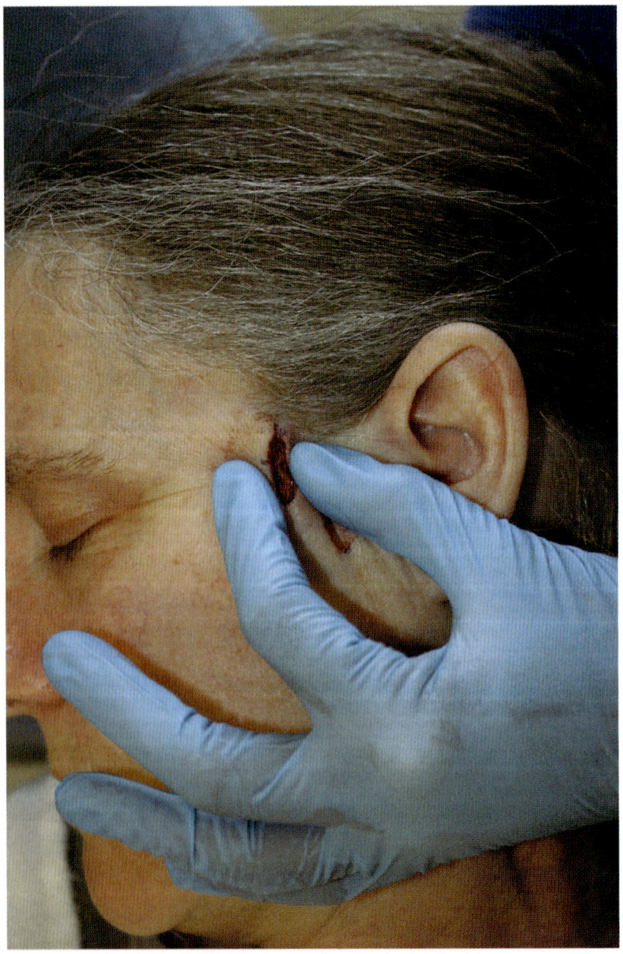

FIGURE 20-14 Pinching the primary wound edges guides flap selection. A linear closure or sliding flap is usually possible if the wound edges are easily approximated. If pinching the wound edges causes excessive tension or free-margin distortion, a transposition flap may be useful to transfer tension to and recruit tissue from an adjacent reservoir.

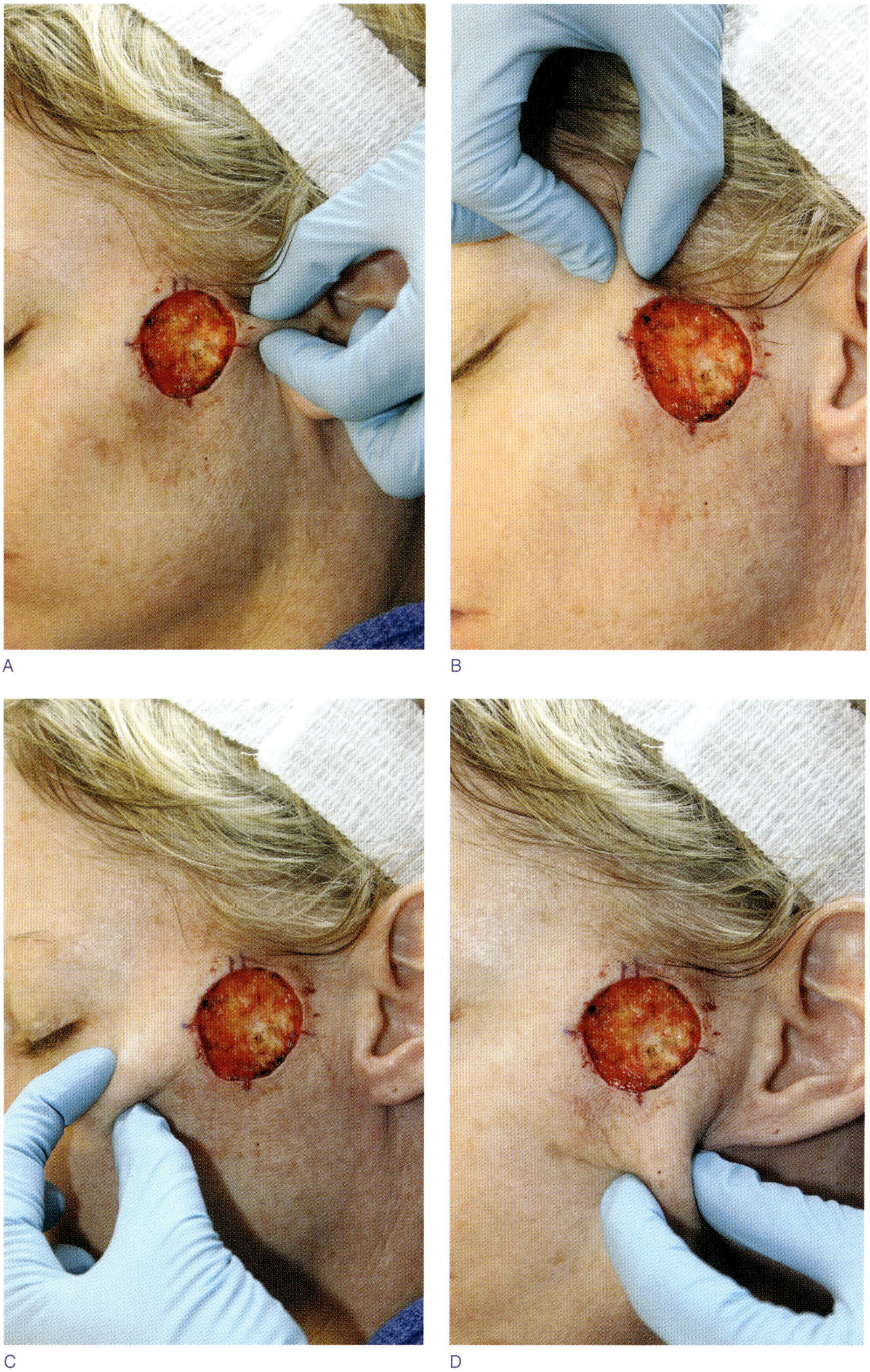

FIGURE 20-15 A suitable tissue reservoir for a transposition flap is identified using the pinch test. For this defect on the preauricular cheek, tissue reservoirs located posteriorly (**A**) and superiorly (**B**) lack sufficient volume, laxity, and vascularity. The anterior tissue reservoir (**C**), while ample, may lead to anatomic distortion. An inferior donor site (**D**) pinches easily without anatomic distortion and would be ideal. In order to reach this donor site, one or more lobes may be needed.

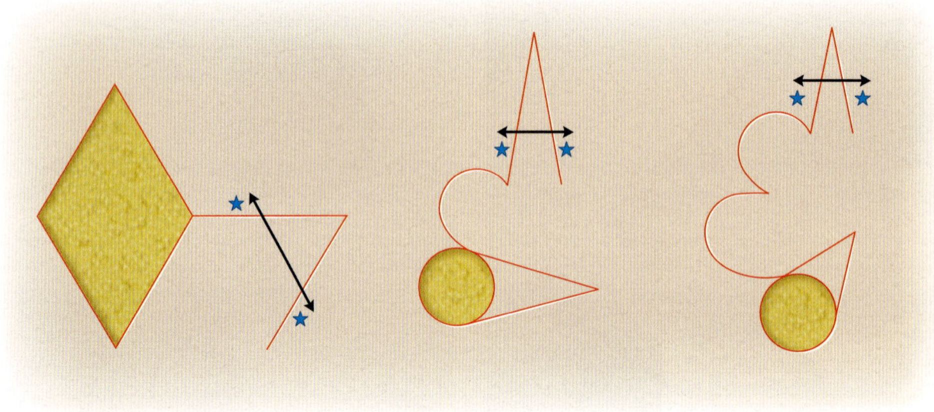

FIGURE 20-16 Transposition flaps displace tension from the primary defect to the final donor site (*stars* denote key stitch and *arrows* demonstrate direction of tension vector).

In general, tension is transferred from the primary defect to the terminal donor site or lobe (ie, the secondary lobe of a bilobed flap and the tertiary lobe of a trilobed flap; **Figure 20-16**). The fixed base at the pedicle tethers the flap and serves as a pivot point as the flap is rotated toward the primary defect. As the arc of rotation increases, pivotal restraint increasingly restricts and shortens the flap length.[7] If the shortened flap does not have enough surface area to cover the defect, the consequent secondary motion of the recipient tissue will increase tension at the primary defect and may compromise the blood supply of the distal flap, as with a rotation flap (**Figure 20-17**). The most commonly used transposition flaps are single-lobed (rhombic) and bilobed flaps, although other variations are possible as well.

Transposition Flap Types

Rhombic Flaps: The donor site of single-lobed transposition flaps is immediately adjacent to the defect. This proximity magnifies the importance of donor site selection and flap design. Among many important considerations are determining the appropriate takeoff angle (**Figure 20-18**) as well as ensuring equal widths for the flap and defect and tapering the flap endpoint appropriately (**Figure 20-19**).

Bilobed Flaps: When there is not enough tissue immediately adjacent to the wound to allow closure with a single-lobed flap, additional lobes may be added to access a suitable tissue reservoir. A classic example is the use of bilobed and trilobed flaps to close distal nasal defects (**Figure 20-20**), although these approaches are useful in other areas as well, such as hand repairs (**Figure 20-21**).

Complications

Pin-cushioning, or trapdoor deformity, may occur with transposition flaps. Several etiologies have been suggested, such as excessive flap thickness, inadequate undermining, and circumferential wound contraction. Strategies to minimize pin-cushioning include appropriately sizing the flap, careful suturing

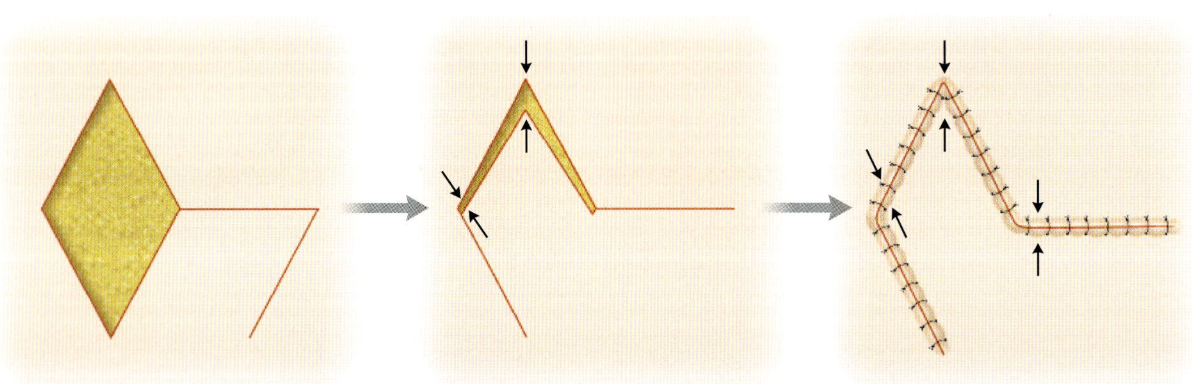

FIGURE 20-17 If the flap design does not take into account the consequences of pivotal restraint and the recipient site is unable to provide secondary motion, excess tension may compromise blood supply to the distal edges of the flap.

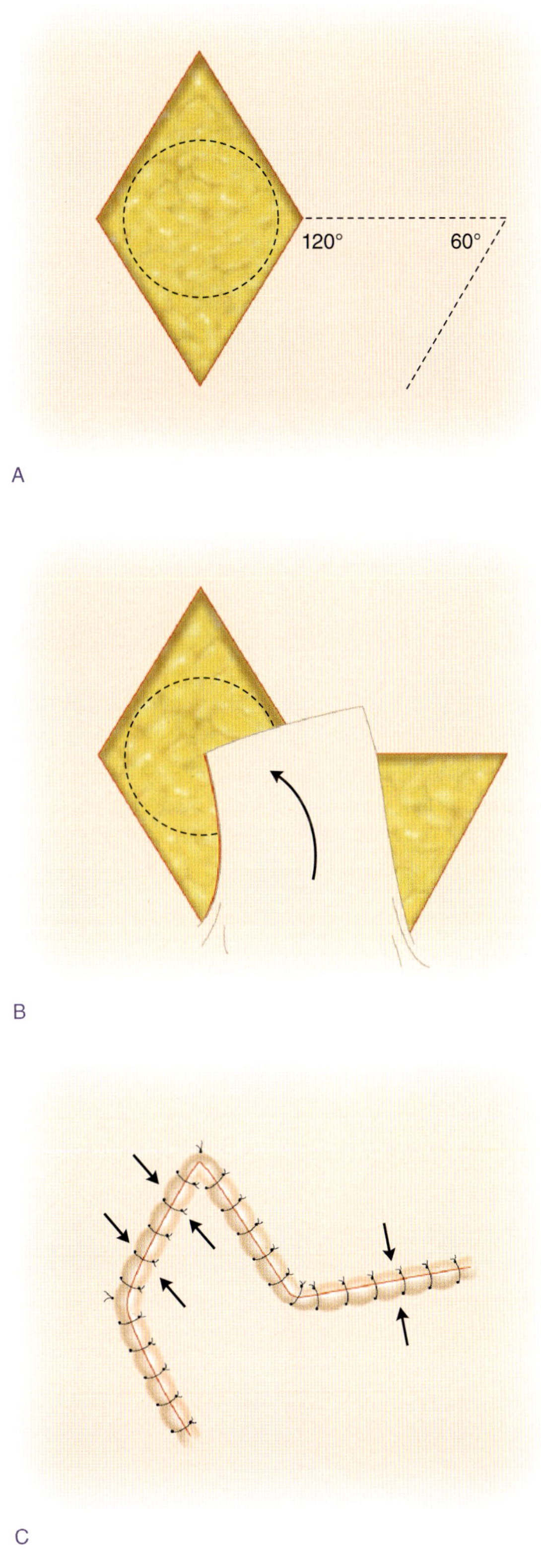

FIGURE 20-18 The takeoff angle between the first limb of the rhombic flap and primary defect is usually 90 degrees. There is no sharing of tension since the primary key stitch and secondary key stitch are nearly perpendicular. Acute takeoff angles result in competing tension vectors caused by closure of the primary and secondary defects. As a result, greater secondary motion is required at the primary defect.

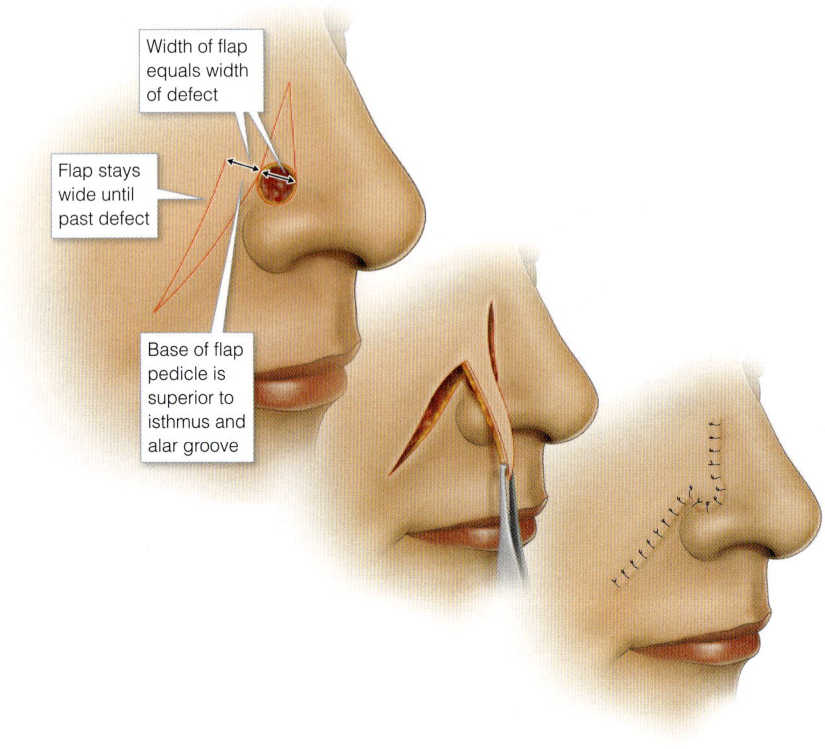

FIGURE 20-19 Design characteristics of the nasolabial transposition flap include equal widths of the flap and defect, maintaining the width of the flap until past the defect, and tapering the flap arms to an angle of 30 degrees or less.

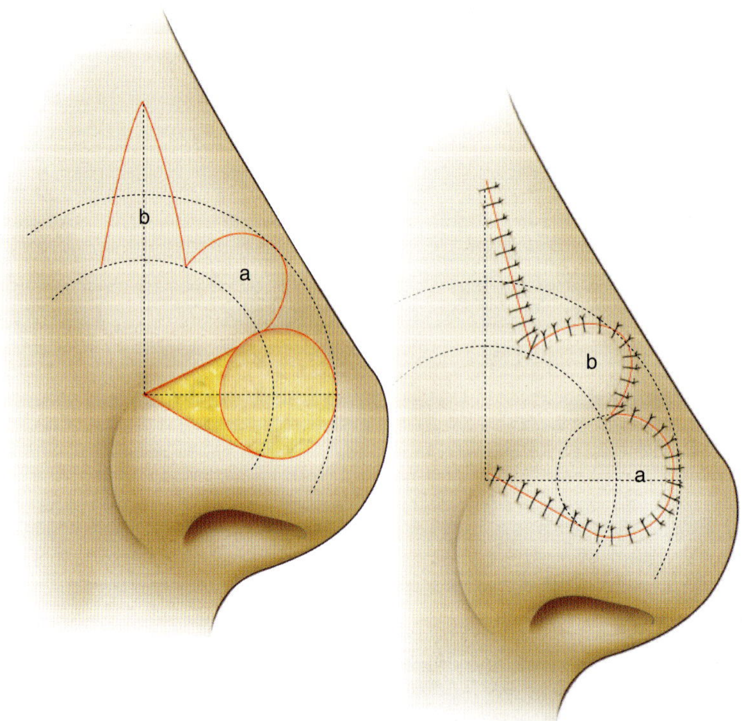

FIGURE 20-20 Zitelli modifications of the bilobed flap. Decreased angle of tissue transfer and incorporation of a Burow's triangle reduces standing cone deformity. The apex serves as a focal point for the design. Each donor lobe is designed around one arc through the center of the defect, and another arc through the distal end of the defect.

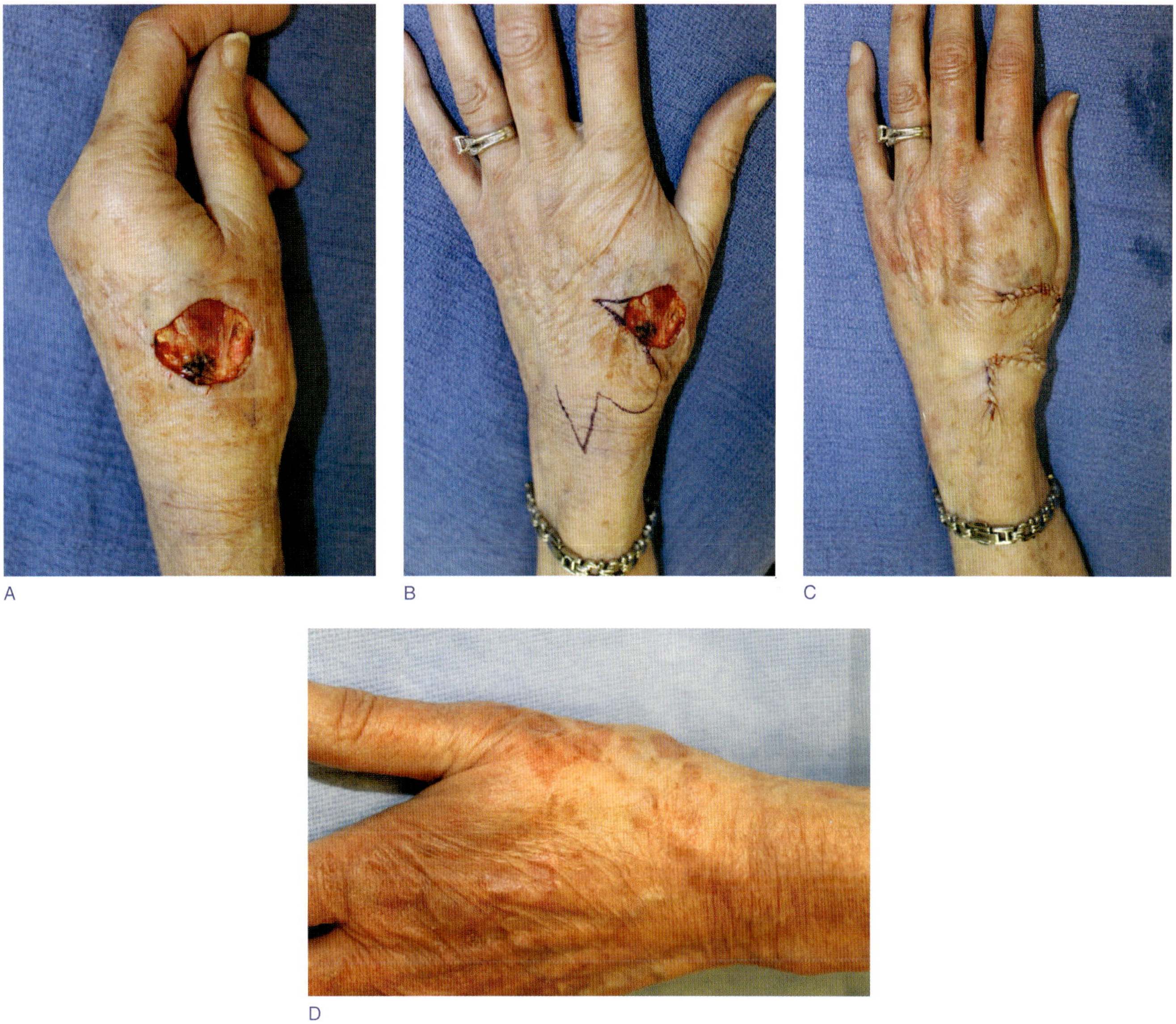

FIGURE 20-21 Defect on the radial dorsal hand repaired with a bilobed flap. (**A**) Mohs defect. (**B**) Flap design. Note the more favorable location of the tertiary defect which facilitates closure. (**C**) Immediate postoperative appearance. (**D**) Long-term follow-up.

of all anatomic layers, circumferentially undermining the primary defect, and closing any dead space under the flap. Contact inhibition of the pin-cushioning effect may be accomplished by ensuring that the undersurface of the flap is sutured to the defect; a flap that is kept in contact with the wound bed may have a decreased tendency to pin cushion. These buried quilting or basting sutures do not need to be tacked to deeper immobile structures, as is performed with suspension sutures, since the goal is to maintain contact of the flap base with the underlying defect, not to recreate a natural sulcus. The vascular supply to the flap should never be compromised, however, by overly zealous attempts at contact inhibition. If intralesional corticosteroids do not resolve pin-cushioning, surgical thinning may be necessary.

The curved lines that result from most transposition flaps require meticulous suturing, as they rarely fall along cosmetic subunit junctions or relaxed skin tension lines. This attention to detail is particularly critical for successful execution of flaps on sebaceous skin, such as the distal nose.

CONCLUSIONS

Flap repairs, while used much less frequently than linear closures, are an important and valuable addition to the clinician's armamentarium. It is important to understand the fundamental principles of tissue movement, as well as the possible risks associated with each approach, before embarking on any form of flap closure. These advanced techniques often draw on a blend of experience, skill, and anatomic finesse, and therefore, investing significant effort in understanding tissue movement—and suturing techniques—will pay dividends many times over.

REFERENCES

1. Johnson TM, Swanson N, Baker SR. Concepts of sliding and lifting tissue movement in flap reconstruction. *Dermatol Surg.* 2000;26:274-278.
2. Chilukuri S, Leffell DJ. Basic principles in flap reconstruction. In: Rohrer TE, Cook J, Nguyen TH, Mellette JR, eds. *Flaps and Grafts in Dermatologic Surgery*. Philadelphia, PA: Saunders; 2007:15-29.
3. Zilinsky I, Cotofana S, Hammer N, et al. The arterial blood supply of the helical rim and the earlobe-based advancement flap (ELBAF): a new strategy for reconstructions of helical rim defects. *J Plast Reconstr Aesthet Surg.* 2015;68(1):56-62.
4. Wang SQ, Behroozan DS, Goldberg LH. Perialar crescentic advancement flap for upper cutaneous lip defects. *Dermatol Surg.* 2005;31(11 Pt 1):1445-1447.
5. Johnson-Jahangir H, Stevenson M, Ratner D. Modified flap design for symmetric reconstruction of the apical triangle of the upper lip. *Dermatol Surg.* 2012;38(6):905-911.
6. Etzkorn JR, Sobanko JF, Miller CJ. Free margin distortion with fusiform closures: the apical angle relationship. *Dermatol Surg.* 2014;40(12):1428-1432.
7. Dzubow LM. The dynamics of flap movement: effect of pivotal restraint on flap rotation and transposition. *J Dermatol Surg Oncol.* 1987;13(12):1348-1353.

Nail Procedures

21

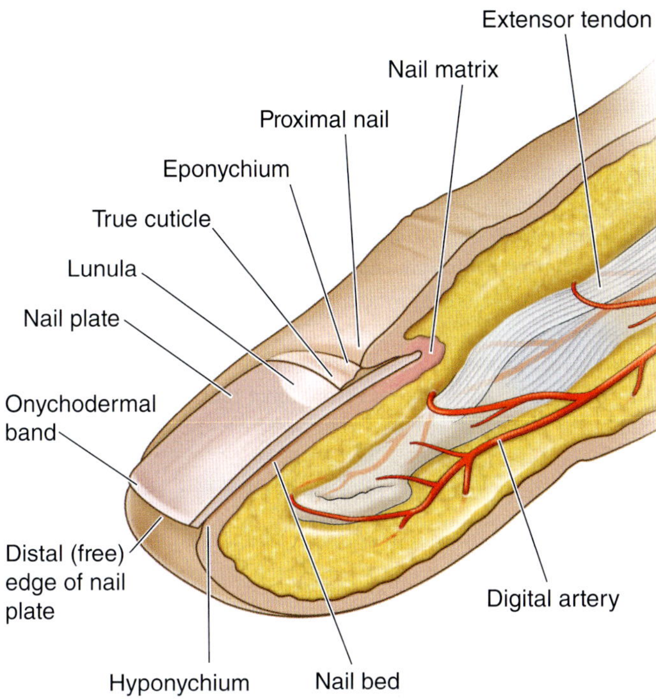

SUMMARY

- Nail procedures are is frequently performed for diagnostic and reconstructive purposes.
- A detailed understanding of nail anatomy and the implications of damage to specific areas of nail anatomy are a prerequisite for performing nail surgery.
- Visualization of the nail unit is required for surgical intervention; therefore, tourniquets are used for many nail procedures.

Beginner Tips

- Ensure that the dermatopathology laboratory has experience with handling nail specimens.
- Examination of the free edge of the nail allows the clinician to determine whether the disorder originates in the proximal matrix (if the pathology is on the outer surface of the nail plate) or in the distal matrix (if the pathology is on the inner surface of the nail plate).
- A 15-minute dilute chlorhexidine soak may help limit the risk of infection.

Pitfalls and Cautions

- A rare complication of the transthecal block is injury to the flexor tendon that can result in scar or trigger finger.
- For moderate bleeding, oxidized cellulose or calcium alginate dressings work nicely; for severe postoperative bleeding, injection of some anesthetic (0.5 mL) in a wing block fashion will act as a volumetric tourniquet (anesthetic tamponade of the nail unit) until clotting occurs.
- Postoperative dysesthesia after nail surgery is common.

Expert Tips

- The distal digital (wing) block is faster and safer than a proximal block.
- The main indication for matrix biopsy is longitudinal melanonychia.
- Because the proximal nail matrix gives rise to the upper part of the nail plate, biopsies in this area are more likely to induce surface dystrophy or nail scarring.
- Tangential shave biopsy is highly effective for wide pigmented lesions of the matrix.

Patient Education Points

- Describing the anatomy of the nail unit, the usual rate of nail growth and the patient's specific surgery prepares the patient for a postoperative course that meets their expectations. Preoperative discussion should also include a discussion of risks including pain, infection, bleeding, scar, nerve damage, nondiagnostic biopsy, and permanent nail dystrophy.
- If surgery is to be performed on a toenail, the patient should be advised to bring footwear with adequate space to accommodate the postoperative dressing and a driver to escort them home safely. Elevation of the surgically manipulated limb is mandatory in order to limit postoperative pain and edema.

Don't Forget!

- When possible, a partial nail avulsion is preferred to complete nail avulsion.
- Matrixectomy is faster, easier, and more comfortable when performed in a chemical, rather than surgical, fashion.
- Nail bed biopsies should be oriented longitudinally; matrix biopsies should be oriented transversely.

Billing Pearls

- Nail biopsy is coded using 1175.
- Avulsion is coded using 11730.
- Graft repair is coded using 11762.
- Lateral wedge resection is coded using 11765.
- Excision for onychocryptosis or onychogryphosis is coded using 11750.

21 Nail Procedures

INTRODUCTION

The nail unit is a complex anatomic structure that is important for both form and function. The nail plate serves as protection for the tip of the digit. It also provides counterpressure to nail unit soft tissues, thereby providing sensory feedback during movement. Moreover, the aesthetic value of the nail unit is highlighted by the popularization of manicures and nail art.

Disorders of the nail unit require diagnostic or therapeutic surgery. When nail procedures are performed, it is critical to restore the nail unit as close to its natural form as possible. Accomplishing this requires knowledge of nail anatomy and the variety of available surgical approaches.

To ensure an accurate diagnosis, the surgical specimen should ideally be evaluated by a dermatopathologist familiar with normal and abnormal histopathology of the nail apparatus and experienced in disorders of the nail unit. This is of particular importance when evaluating melanocytic neoplasms whose histologic and immunohistochemical nuances have features unique to this anatomic location.

ANATOMY

The nail unit is composed of nail plate, nail matrix, nail bed, hyponychium, nail folds, nerves, and blood vessels (**Figures 21-1 and 21-2**). The latter derive from branches of the common volar digital arteries that have arterial anastomoses over the dorsal surface of the distal phalanx (**Figure 21-3**). Innervation to the nail unit is supplied by sensory nerves that travel along the lateral aspects of the digits in close proximity to the aforementioned arteries. The perionychium (tissues surrounding the nail plate) is supplied by the common volar digital nerves, which branch dorsally distal to the distal interphalangeal joint.[1] Venous drainage of the perionychium coalesces laterally and dorsally, drains in a random fashion over the dorsum of the digit, and progresses toward anastomoses at the level of the distal interphalangeal joint. Lymphatics of the nail unit parallel the venous drainage, and are most dense at the hyponychium.

A comprehensive physical examination is critical in localizing the origin of nail unit pathology. The proximal nail matrix gives rise to the outer surface of the nail plate, whereas the distal nail matrix produces the undersurface of the nail plate.

Examination of the free edge of the nail allows the clinician to determine whether the disorder originates in the proximal or distal matrix (**Figure 21-4**).

After examination of the digit and identification of the source of nail pathology, the clinician may discuss with the patient the various surgical approaches that are relevant for the pathology.

PREOPERATIVE EVALUATION

A thorough preoperative discussion with the patient is one of the most important elements of successful nail surgery. The discussion should include preparation by the patient for surgery as well as anticipated postoperative care. Describing the anatomy of the nail unit, the usual rate of nail growth, and the patient's specific surgery prepares the patient for a postoperative course that meets their expectations. Preoperative discussion should also include a discussion of risks of any nail surgery including pain, infection,

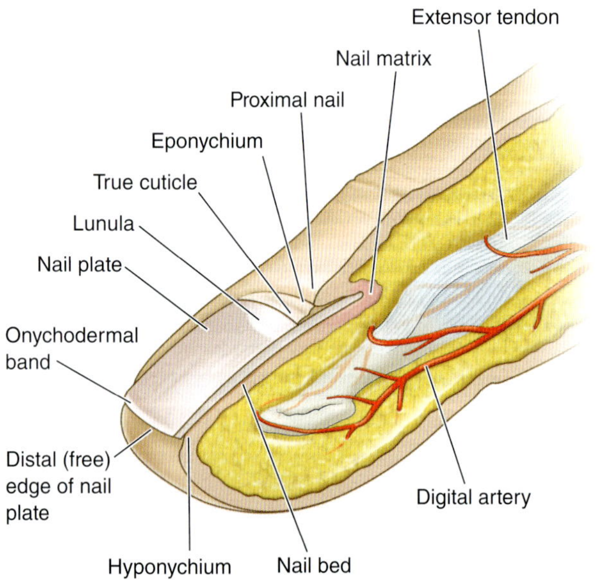

FIGURE 21-1 Distal digit anatomy.

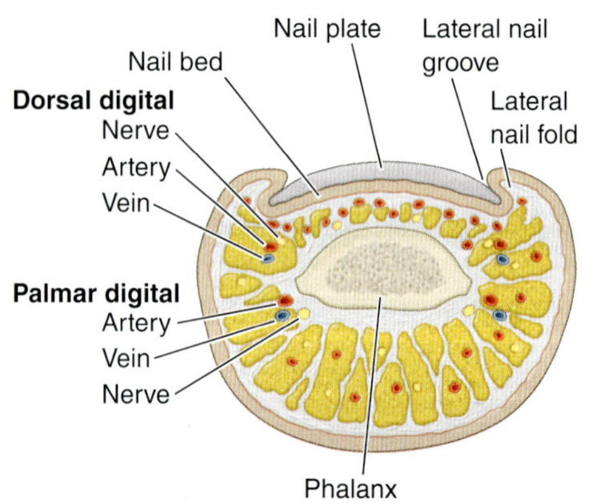

FIGURE 21-2 Transverse section of anatomy through the distal digit.

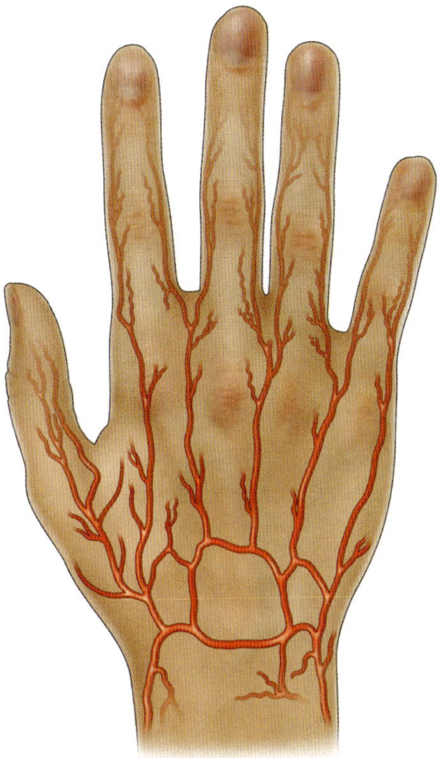

FIGURE 21-3 Dorsal hand arterial supply.

bleeding, scar, nerve damage, nondiagnostic biopsy, and permanent nail dystrophy. The actual rate of these complications varies by surgical approach and the expertise of the clinician.

The preoperative plan takes into account any peripheral vascular compromise that might be encountered in associated conditions such as Raynaud phenomenon, peripheral vascular disease, and diabetes. Smoking cessation is known to improve the microvasculature, leading to reduced ischemic injury and improved wound healing.[2,3] Any medically necessary anticoagulants are continued, as the risk of stopping anticoagulation outweighs the surgical benefits.[4,5]

As with all surgeries, the patient should be asked if they have any allergies or adverse reactions to anesthetics, wound care materials, and/or pain medications planned for use in their surgery. Rarely, patients may benefit from oral anxiolytics.[6] If surgery is to be performed on a toenail, the patient should be advised to bring footwear with adequate space to accommodate the postoperative dressing and a driver to escort them home safely. Elevation of the surgically manipulated limb is mandatory in order to limit postoperative pain and edema.

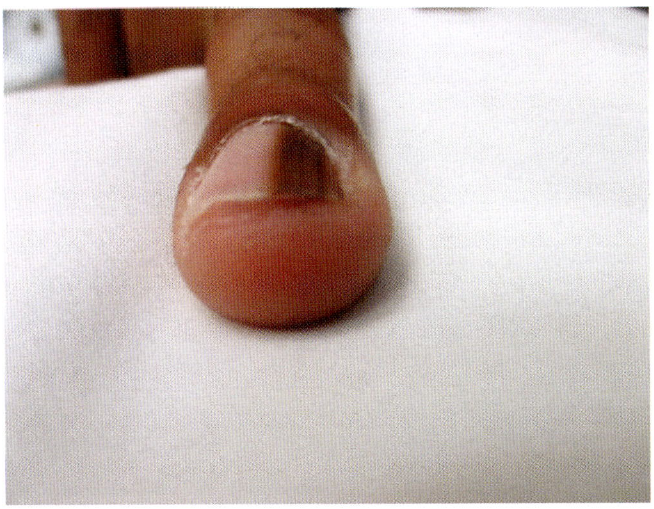

FIGURE 21-4 Examination of the free margin. Pigment can be seen on the surface of the nail plate, which indicates that the lesion of interest is located in the proximal matrix.

ANESTHESIA

Adequate anesthesia is the first procedural step of surgery. Although lidocaine with epinephrine is safe, it is generally unnecessary because nail surgery is often performed with a tourniquet.

The injection site is cleansed and prepped. One technique used in nail surgery to attempt to reduce the bacterial burden, as well as soften the nail plate, is a dilute chlorhexidine soak for 5 to 15 minutes. Distractive measures during injection such as concurrent vibration help limit the pain of injection.[7] After anesthesia, nail surgery is performed under aseptic conditions using sterile gloves and drapes.

If surgery is to be performed on a finger, an arm board can be useful for both patient comfort and as a stable work surface for the clinician.

Distal Digital Block

The most commonly used approach to anesthetizing digits for nail surgery is the distal digital ("wing") block. Its advantages are a quick onset of anesthesia, the use of smaller volumes of anesthetic, and a tumescent effect providing hemostasis. Lidocaine 1% to 2% buffered and ropivacaine 0.25% are appropriate choices for this indication. A 0.5-mL dose of anesthetic is injected into a point 5 mm proximal and lateral to the junction of the proximal and lateral nail fold on each side of the digit such that a total of approximately 1 mL of anesthesia is used. If a clinician chooses to use epinephrine in their anesthetic, there should be minimal risk of intra-arterial injection due to the small caliber of arterioles in this anatomic location. If using lidocaine, then the addition of bupivacaine 0.25% to 0.5% will prolong anesthesia for up to 8 to 12 hours.

Proximal Digital Block

Because the injection sites are far from the nail unit, a proximal digital block is an optimal approach when performing surgery on a painful distal nail, such as in the context of acute paronychia. It is of slower onset, and up to 20 minutes may be needed before complete numbing of the distal tip of the digit takes place. Unlike the distal digital block, it carries a potential risk for damage to the neurovascular bundles.[8]

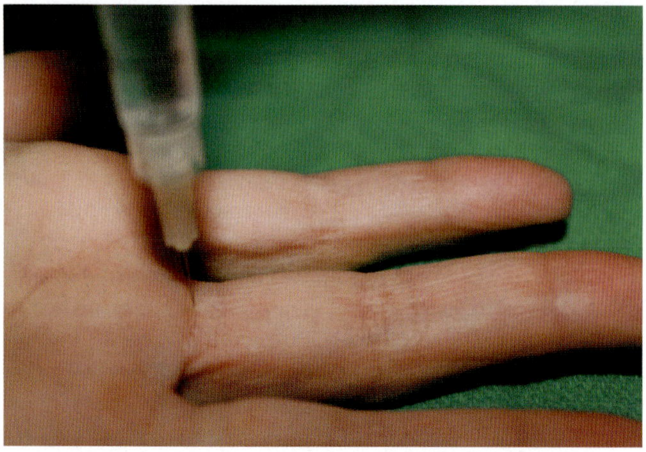

FIGURE 21-5 Transthecal block. This proximal digital block can only be used for digits 2, 3, and 4 of the hands. It has the advantage of quicker onset of action as compared to proximal blocks laterally performed.

Approximately 1 mL of anesthetic is injected laterally at the level of the metacarpophalangeal or metatarsophalangeal joints into each of the radial and ulnar (or the tibial and fibular) sides of the digit. Care should be taken to draw back on the syringe before injection to avoid injecting into an arteriole of the common digital artery (**Figure 21-3**).

Transthecal Block

This procedure is a useful approach for surgery of fingers 2, 3, and 4.[2,9] Due to anatomic variation, this approach is not advised for surgery on any other digit.

Its advantages are its fast onset (2-5 minutes) and the absence of risk to neurovascular bundles, as the needle is inserted on the palmar aspect of the digit (**Figure 21-5**). A rare complication is injury to the flexor tendon that can result in scar or trigger finger.

SURGICAL INSTRUMENTS

Nail surgery requires a few specific instruments, including a freer elevator and a nail splitter (English anvil nail splitter) (**Figure 21-6**).

A bloodless field is necessary for adequate visualization during surgery and for phenolization of the matrix. To accomplish this, a tourniquet is often required. The tourniquet may be a Penrose drain secured with a sturdy hemostat or a sterile glove with a small hole snipped in the fingertip of the glove finger to be operated on and rolled back to the base of the digit, achieving a full exsanguination of the finger or toe (**Figure 21-7**). Debate exists as to a safe duration for use of a tourniquet, with the goal always being to keep it in place for as little time as necessary for adequate visualization. Surgical loupes that provide magnification of 2.5 to 4.2 times can also aid in visualization during the procedure.[10]

The surgical specimen must be submitted to dermatopathology review in a condition adequate for interpretation. One useful approach for submission of small specimens, including those obtained during tangential excision, is to place the specimen on filter paper (ideally with a nail template) in a cassette padded with sponges that is then placed in the formalin container.[11]

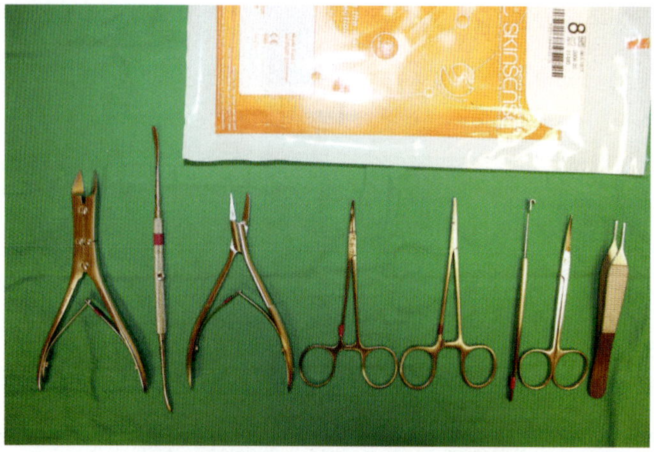

FIGURE 21-6 Surgical tray for nail surgery. **From left to right:** Dual-action nail nippers, freer elevator, English anvil nail splitter, curved hemostat, mosquito, skin hook, iris scissors, forceps.

NAIL PROCEDURES

Nail Bed

When the source of pathology based on physical examination findings is noted to be in the nail bed, a nail bed biopsy is indicated. If an incision is necessary, align it along the longitudinal axis of the digit to limit the risk of scarring and postoperative nail deformities, including split nail.

Punch Biopsy of the Nail Bed (Figure 21-8): A 3- to 4-mm punch biopsy of the bed will heal via secondary intention with very little risk of scarring.

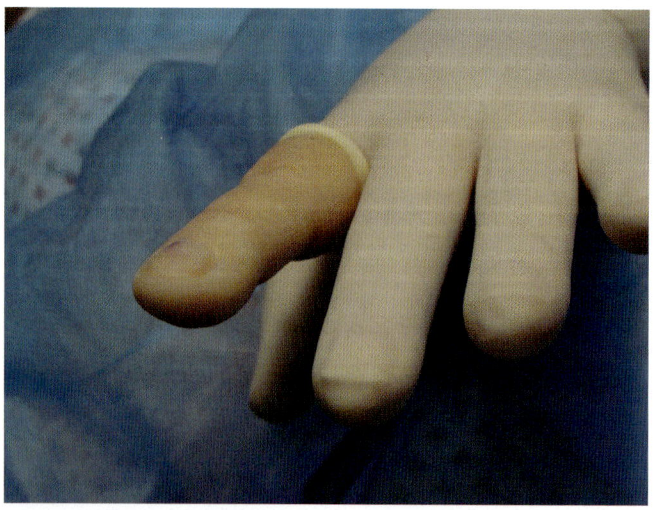

FIGURE 21-7 Glove tourniquet. A sterile surgical glove can be used as a tourniquet by rolling back the glove finger on the affected digit.

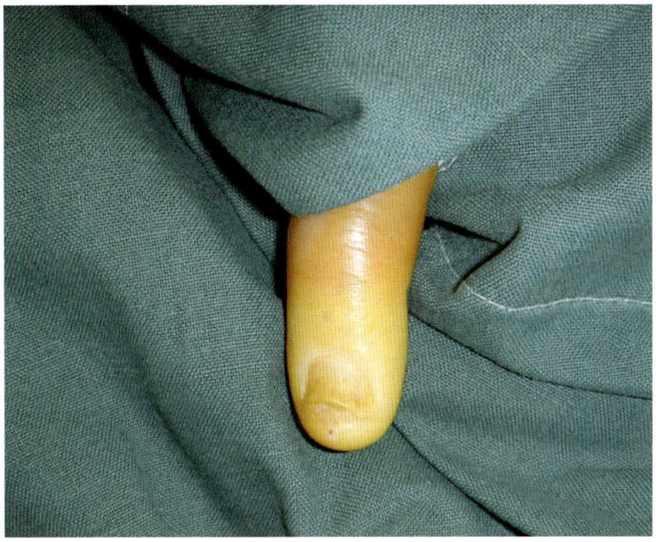

A

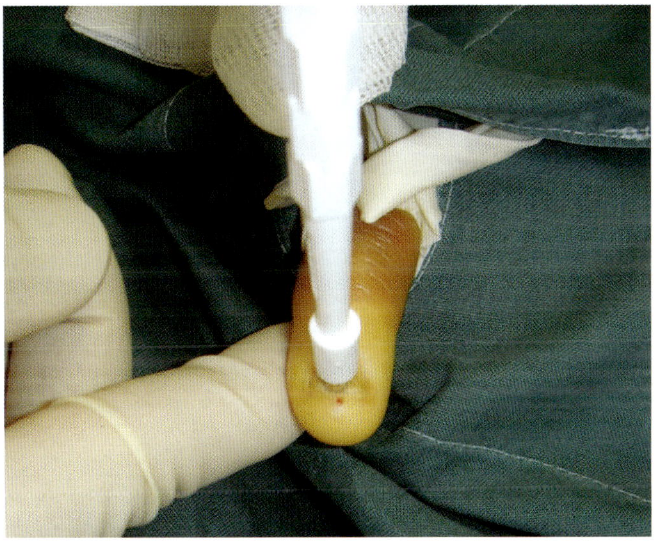

B

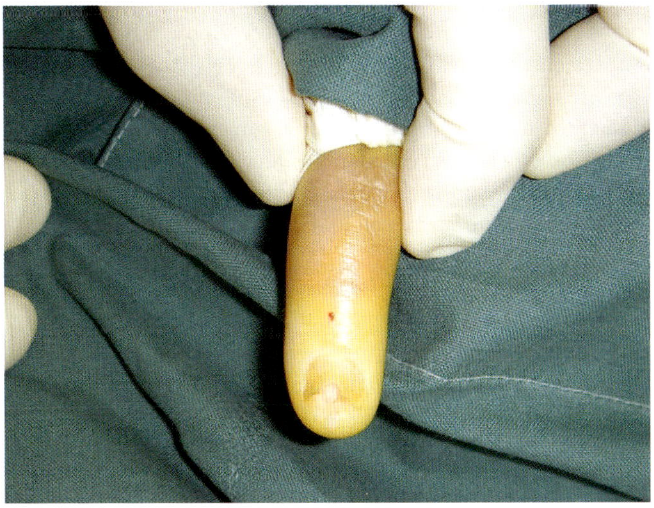

C

FIGURE 21-8 (**A-C**) Nail bed punch biopsy.

A common indication for this procedure is the differential diagnosis of subungual hyperkeratosis that may result from nail psoriasis or lichen planus. Squamous cell carcinoma of the bed is also a common indication. The punch tool is inserted to the bone using a twisting motion. A narrow-tipped scissors such as iris scissors is used to snip the base of the specimen off the periosteum. This can be best be achieved by inserting the scissor tips perpendicular to the nail bed surface down to periosteum with the curvature facing upward, then opening the tips and turning the open scissor tips along the base of the biopsy specimen. The biopsy specimen then can be snipped free from the periosteum. If possible, harvest the specimen with the scissors, as using forceps may crush the delicate specimen. Always check that the punch tool is free of tissue prior to discarding.

Nail Bed Incisions: The nail bed is incised to remove a nail bed tumor (eg, squamous cell carcinoma, onychopapilloma) or to reach a deep tumor (eg, glomus tumor of the nail bed or subungual exostosis). After a partial or a lateral plate avulsion, the area of the involved nail bed is fully exposed. Any incision on the bed should be aligned along the longitudinal axis of the digit to limit the risk of scarring and postoperative nail deformity.

The elliptical excision is carried with a #15 blade and should be no wider than 4 mm to limit the risks of onycholysis (**Figure 21-9**). The nail bed adheres strongly to the bony phalanx and is therefore relatively immobile. Reapproximation of tissue edges requires wide undermining of the lateral edges of the wound with the blade. Undermining should be carried out at the level of periosteum, skimming the bone. For larger defects, longitudinal releasing incisions parallel to the lateral edge of the ellipse, associated with lateral undermining, are often required. High tension across the sutures is not recommended, as the fragile nail bed may tear off. Part of the defect may be left to heal by secondary intention. Suturing is performed with 5-0 absorbable suture. The plate is always put back in place (although some lateral trimming may be necessary) and secured to the lateral nail folds.

Matrix

When the source of pathology is in the nail matrix, then a nail matrix biopsy is indicated. The main indication for matrix biopsy is longitudinal melanonychia. This should be performed as an excisional biopsy to ensure complete examination of the pigmented lesion by the pathologist. Complete visualization of the matrix area is mandatory. This is perfectly achieved with a proximal partial nail avulsion completed with a reclination of the proximal fold.

In some cases, the matrix is incised to reach a submatricial tumor. Incisions on the matrix should preferably be aligned along the transverse axis of the digit to limit postoperative nail deformity, especially split nail.

The origin of pigmented streaks causing longitudinal melanonychia can be localized by dermoscopy of the free margin of the nail plate (**Figure 21-10**).[12] As the distal nail matrix gives rise to the undersurface of the nail plate, biopsies in this area have a low risk of scarring. Because the proximal nail matrix gives rise

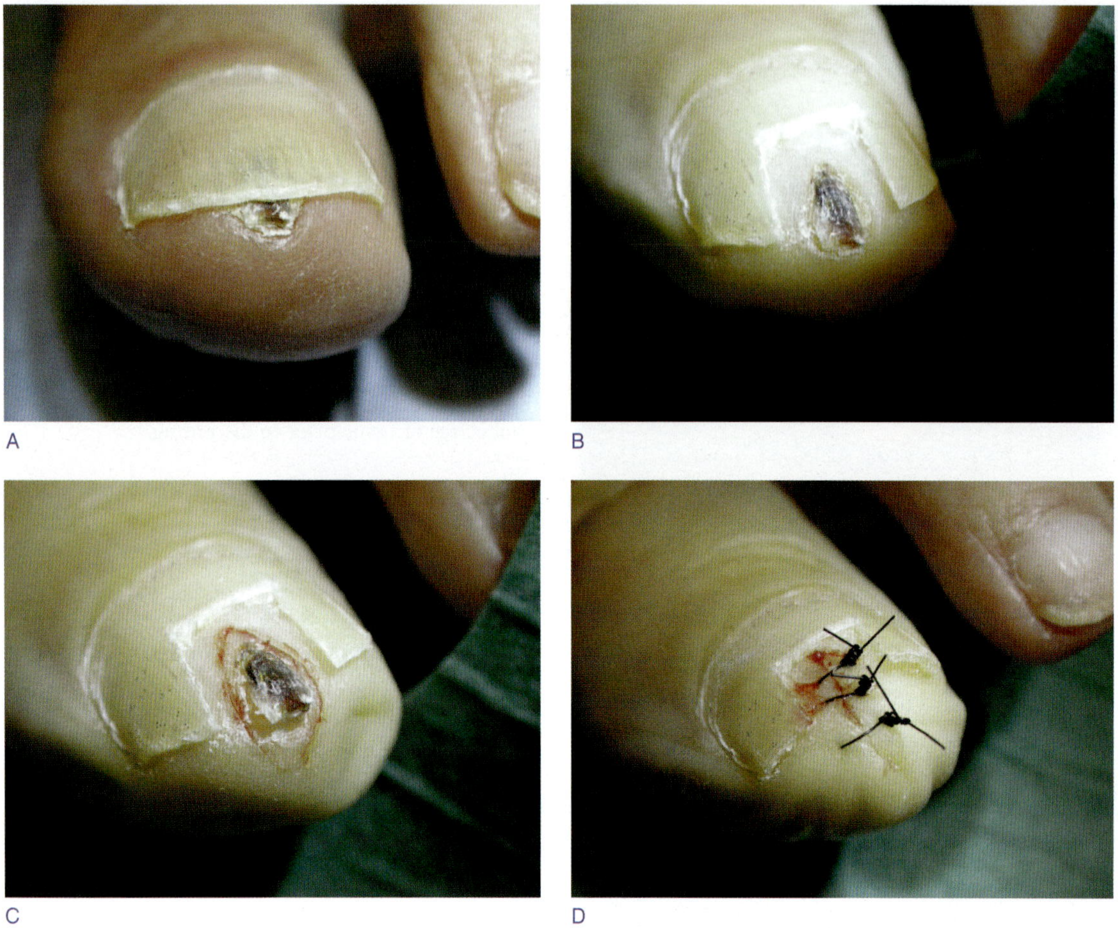

FIGURE 21-9 Excision of nail bed. (**A**) Onychoclavus of distal nail bed. (**B**) Nail plate removal to expose onychoclavus. (**C**) Appearance of nail bed after excision of onychoclavus. (**D**) Sutured defect after excision of onychoclavus.

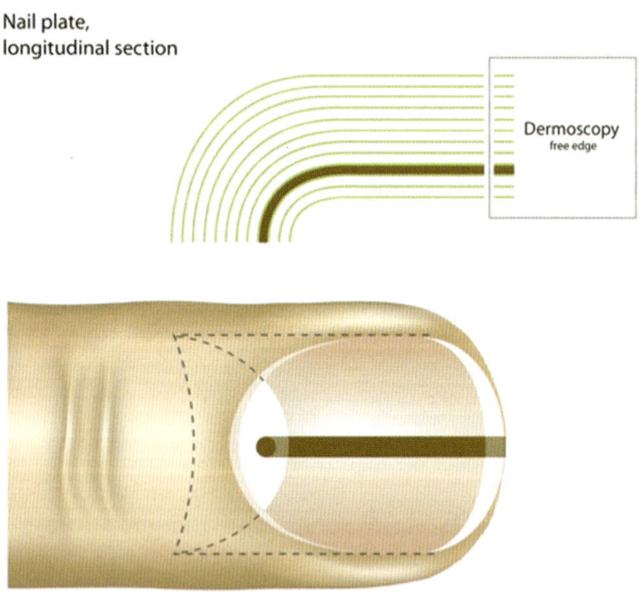

FIGURE 21-10 Diagram of origin of pigment. The origin of melanonychia can be localized by dermoscopy of the free margin of the nail plate.

to the upper part of the nail plate, biopsies in this area are more likely to induce surface dystrophy or nail scarring.

Punch Biopsy[13]*:* This procedure is a very simple and easy option for pigmented lesions of the distal matrix less than 3 mm in diameter. After a proximal nail avulsion exposing the entire matrix, the pigmented macule is removed with a punch technique down to the periosteum and harvested in the same fashion as described for nail bed punch biopsies (**Figure 21-11A-D**). The plate is replaced and secured to the lateral nail fold (**Figure 21-11E**).

Tangential Shave Biopsy: Tangential shave biopsy of the matrix is an extremely useful technique and is widely regarded by many as the preferred method for removal of wide (>4 mm) macular pigmented lesions of the matrix, including the proximal matrix. This technique, while technically demanding, provides outstanding results in skilled hands and allows adequate diagnosis in all cases. Its main drawback is a recurrence of the pigmentation in about 75% of cases.[14] Removal of a thin layer of matrix may result in a thinner nail and, very rarely, nail dystrophy.

After partial nail avulsion to expose the matrix, a shallow incision is carried out around the pigmented zone, with extra

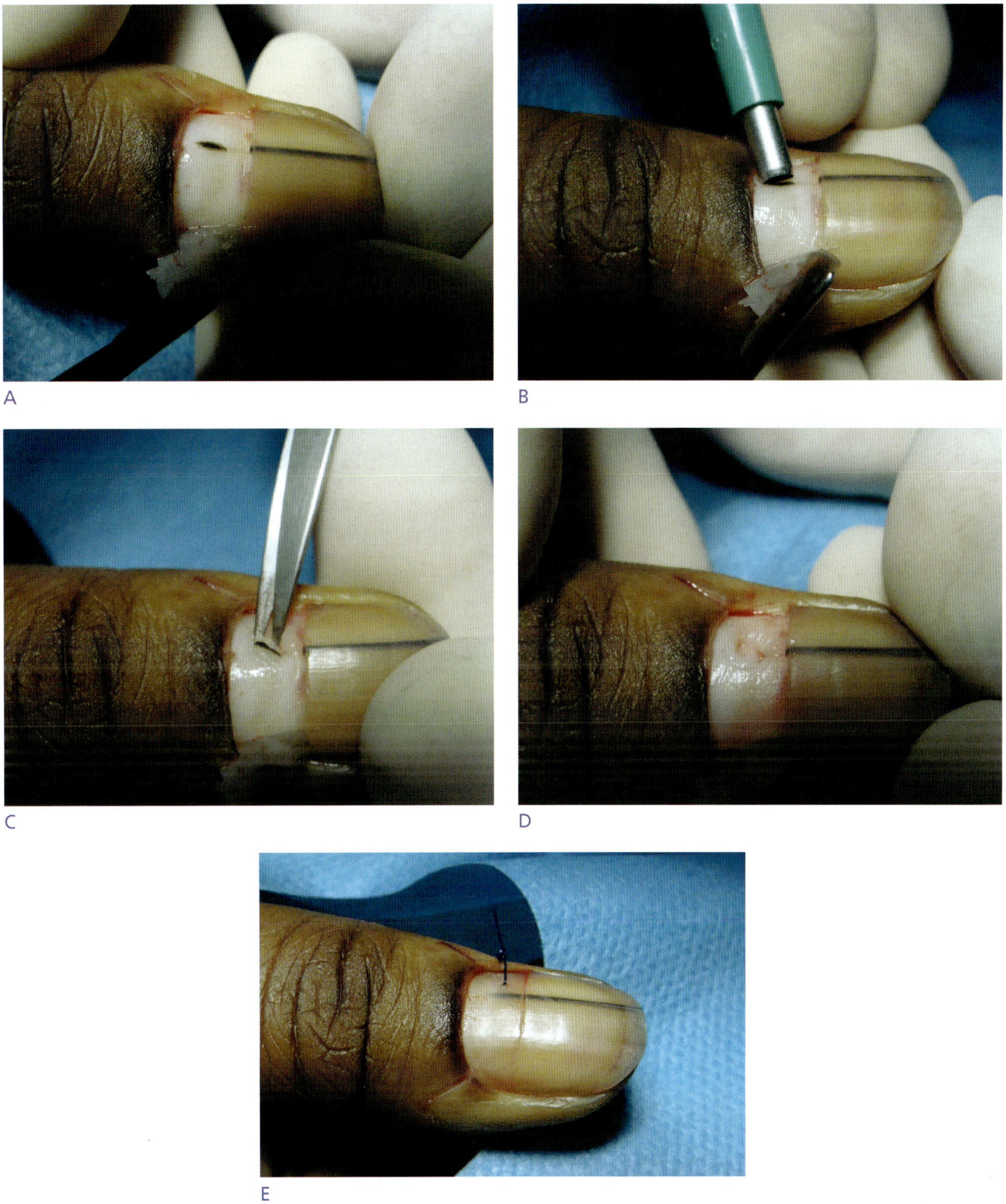

FIGURE 21-11 (**A**) Proximal avulsion exposes matrix and pigmented macule. (**B**) Punching the macule. (**C**) Harvesting the specimen with scissors. (**D**) Defect in the matrix left for secondary intention healing. (**E**) Nail plate replaced and sutured to the lateral nail fold.

margins. The scalpel is then held horizontally, and the lesion is removed from the deep dermis using a gentle sawing motion. The specimen should not be thicker than 0.5 mm. The avulsed nail is replaced and secured to the lateral fold.

Lateral Longitudinal Excision (En Bloc Excision): For laterally located longitudinal melanonychia or other tumors (eg, squamous cell carcinoma in situ), lateral longitudinal excisions are indicated. The patient must be informed that this type of biopsy will narrow the nail permanently due to partial amputation of the lateral horn of the matrix.

The specimen should not exceed 3 mm in width in order to avoid postoperative lateral deviation. The incision begins halfway between the cuticle and the crease of the distal interphalangeal joint and runs distally through the proximal nail fold and the nail plate/nail bed, until the hyponychium is reached. A second incision performed in the lateral nail fold parallels the first and joins it at the tip of the finger. Proximally, the incision takes on a laterally curved direction that extends about 5 mm laterally in order to remove the lateral horn of the matrix (**Figure 21-12A**).[15] This is especially important when performing a biopsy of the great toenail. The specimen is then carefully detached from the bone with fine scissors. At the proximal tip of the biopsy, the matrix must be preserved, and particular care should be taken to avoid raising the scissors too soon and foreshortening the specimen. The defect is reapproximated with horizontal mattress stiches in order to re-create a lateral nail fold (**Figure 21-12B**). This type of excision allows the study of the whole nail apparatus: proximal nail fold, matrix, nail bed, nail plate, and hyponychium. The laboratory and dermatopathologist should be experienced with handling such specimens and section them longitudinally to allow visualization of the architecture of the pigmented lesion.

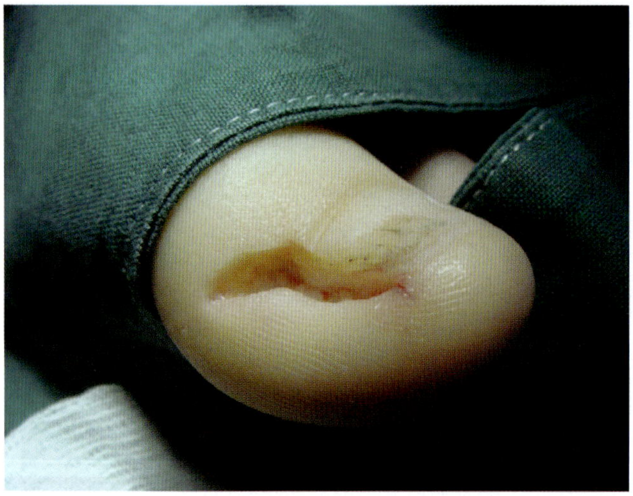

A

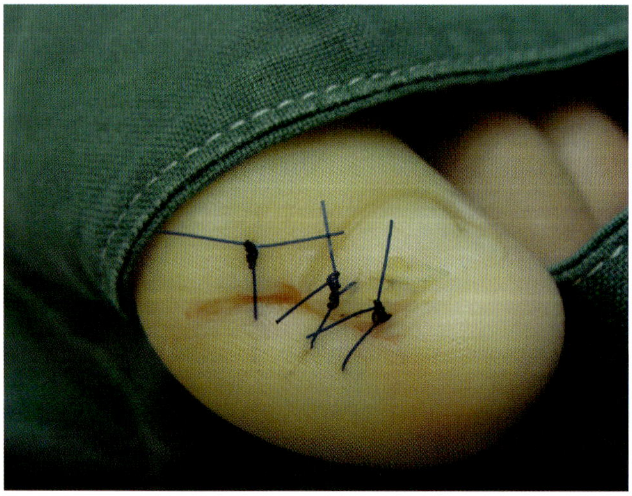

B

FIGURE 21-12 (**A**) Lateral longitudinal biopsy: used for diagnosis of lichen planus in a child. Note the lazy S incision that curves proximally to be sure to remove the lateral horn of the matrix. (**B**) Lateral longitudinal biopsy: suturing perfectly reapproximates the edges of the excision.

Matrix Excisions: Sometimes, the pigmented macule may present as a narrow longitudinal patch. This may be removed using a longitudinal ellipse with minimal margins. The edges of the incision are widely undermined and reapproximated with 5-0 or 6-0 absorbable sutures. The nail is laid back in place and sutured to the lateral nail fold. If the proximal nail matrix is not involved, the risk of dystrophic sequelae is very unlikely. Another removal option is the tangential excision.

Other indications for matrix excisions are submatricial tumors, such as a glomus tumor, superficial acral fibromyxoma, and pseudomyxoid cyst. Incisions are carried out in transverse or curvilinear fashion with a #15 blade in the distal matrix, a few millimeters behind the junction of the nail matrix and nail bed. Closure with 5-0 or 6-0 absorbable suture should be performed delicately under minimal tension.

POSTOPERATIVE CONSIDERATIONS

Surgical planning includes anticipation of and preparation for postoperative considerations. Patients leave the clinic with a padded bandage in place. An in-office dressing change at 48 hours postoperatively should be offered, and although some patients appreciate this, most patients choose instead to change the dressing at home. Written instructions are provided.

Pain management is an important concern after surgery. It is important to stress to patients that elevation of the surgical site and following activity restrictions are important parts of pain prevention. For punch and tangential biopsies and phenolization, acetaminophen for the first 48 hours is adequate. Total nail avulsion is painful, and for the first 48 hours, narcotic pain medication may be prescribed. For lateral longitudinal excisions, flaps, and grafts, narcotics are almost always needed. It is not unusual for patients to only need analgesics for the first 24 hours after a light and limited nail surgery.

COMPLICATIONS[16]

All surgical procedures have risks.[16] These include pain, bleeding, infection, scarring, dysesthesia, implantation cysts, necrosis, recurrence, and nondiagnostic biopsy. Careful surgical planning and thorough patient education limit the complications of nail surgery. Patients undergoing nail surgery should be informed of the risks of nerve damage and permanent nail dystrophy.

Postoperative pain is minimized with replacement of the nail plate after surgery, with instructions for the patient to keep the digit elevated and limit activity for 48 hours after surgery, and by anticipating pain with adequate analgesics.

Bleeding is the most common complication of nail surgery and occurs when the tourniquet is removed. Anticoagulants and antiplatelet agents should not be interrupted prior to nail surgery, as the risks from stopping those drugs outweigh the potential benefit.

For moderate bleeding, oxidized cellulose or calcium alginate dressings work nicely; for severe postoperative bleeding, injection of some anesthetic (0.5 mL) in a wing block fashion will act as a volumetric tourniquet (anesthetic tamponade of the nail unit) until clotting occurs. Electrocoagulation should not be used. Subungual hematoma is a rare complication of nail surgery because the nail plate should be laid back over the nail bed/matrix rather than tightly fixing it in place.

Nail infections rarely occur after nail surgery because surgery is performed in a sterile environment and digits are well vascularized. Daily wound care further limits postoperative infection. Most infections result from poor homecare and/or lack of hygiene.

Necrosis is an unpredictable complication. It may occur after accidental extended use of a tourniquet, from the use of lidocaine with epinephrine in patients with impaired blood supply of the limbs, from overly tight stitches, or from excess volume infiltration of local anesthetic.

Postoperative dysesthesia after nail surgery is common. In one study, a sensory disturbance was observed in about half of all patients, without any relationship to the extent of the surgery undertaken.[17] There is no clear explanation for this phenomenon.

Implantation cysts were reported as being the most common complication after full-thickness grafts following complete nail unit excision.[18]

Complex regional pain syndrome is a poorly understood, idiosyncratic, dreaded, and thankfully very rare complication of nail surgery. Pain is severe and out of proportion to the surgical intervention and may spread up the limb. Associated signs include textural changes of the skin (atrophic), altered adnexae (altered sweating, loss of hair in affected areas), stiffness, and reduced range of motion of nearby joints. Recovery may be partial or complete and is aided by early intervention in consultation with a neurologist.

CONCLUSION

Nail surgery is often a part of the diagnosis and management of nail disorders. Knowledge of nail anatomy and physiology is a prerequisite to successful nail surgery. By targeting the source of pathology with the least invasive surgical approach, the clinician obtains diagnostic material for dermatopathology while limiting the risk of postoperative complications.

REFERENCES

1. Zook EG, Van Beek AL, Russell RC, Beatty ME. Anatomy and physiology of the perionychium: a review of the literature and anatomic study. *J Hand Surg Am*. 1980;5(6):528-536.
2. Haneke E. Nail surgery. *Clin Dermatol*. 2013;31(5):516-525.
3. Haneke E. Nail surgery. *J Cutan Aesthet Surg*. 2011;4(3):163-164.
4. Wolfe SW, Pederson WC, Hotchkiss RN, Kozin SH, Cohen MS. *Green's Operative Hand Surgery*. Philadelphia, PA: Elsevier; 2017.
5. Alcalay J, Alcalay R. Controversies in perioperative management of blood thinners in dermatologic surgery: continue or discontinue? *Dermatol Surg*. 2004;30(8):1091-1094.
6. Richert B. Basic nail surgery. *Dermatol Clin*. 2006;24(3):313-322.
7. Jellinek NJ. Nail surgery: practical tips and treatment options. *Dermatol Ther*. 2007;20(1):68-74.
8. Flarity-Reed K. Methods of digital block. *J Emerg Nurs*. 2002; 28:351-354.
9. Kim JE, Ahn HS, Cheon MS, Lee KJ, Cho BK, Park HJ. Proximal nail fold-lunula double punch technique: a less invasive method for sampling nail matrix without nail avulsion. *Indian J Dermatol Venereol Leprol*. 2011;77(3):346-348.
10. Abimelec P, Dumontier C, Nail B. Nail surgery. In: Scher RK, Daniel CR III, eds. *Nails: Therapy, Diagnosis, Surgery.* 3rd ed. New York, NY: Elsevier; 2005:276-291.
11. Reinig E, Rich P, Thompson CT. How to submit a nail specimen. *Dermatol Clin*. 2015;33(2):303-307.
12. Braun RP, Baran R, La Gal FA, et al. Diagnosis and management of nail pigmentations. *J Am Acad Derm*. 2007:56(5):835-847.
13. Jellinek N. Nail matrix biopsy of longitudinal melanonychia: diagnostic algorithm including the matrix shave biopsy. *J Am Acad Dermatol*. 2007;56(5):803-810.
14. Richert B, Theunis A, Norrenberg S, André J. Tangential excision of pigmented nail matrix lesions responsible for longitudinal melanonychia: evaluation of the technique on a series of 30 patients. *J Am Acad Dermatol*. 2013;69(1):96-104.
15. De Berker DA, Baran R. Acquired malalignment: a complication of lateral longitudinal biopsy. *Acta Derm Venereol*. 1998;78(6):468-470.
16. Moossavi M, Scher RK. Complications of nail surgery: a review of the literature. *Dermatol Surg*. 2001;27(3):225-228.
17. Walsh ML, Shipley DV, de Berker DA. Survey of patients' experiences after nail surgery. *Clin Exp Dermatol*. 2009;34(5):e154-e156.
18. Lazar A, Abimelec P, Dumontier C. Full thickness skin graft for nail unit reconstruction. *J Hand Surg*. 2005;30:194-198.

22 Managing Surgical Complications

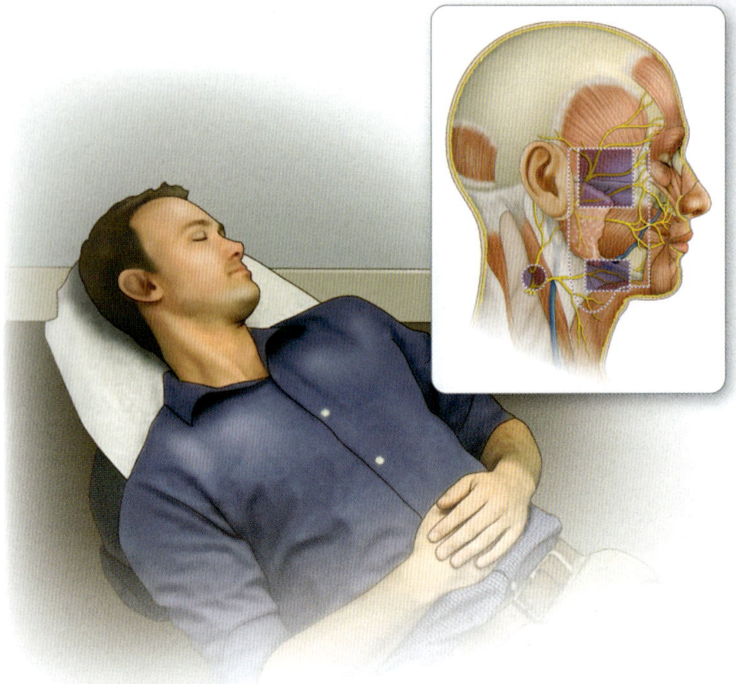

SUMMARY

- The rate of complications remains under 1%, and the rate of serious complications is vanishingly rare.
- The risk of bleeding is the greatest in the first 24 hours postoperatively and is most frequent in the first 6 hours.
- Prophylactic antibiotics are only indicated in specific circumstances (surgery on the mucosa or infected skin) to prevent joint infection, endocarditis, and surgical site infection.

Beginner Tips

- Be able to recognize signs and symptoms of vasovagal reaction, epinephrine reaction, anesthetic overdose, and anaphylaxis.
- To avoid a delayed suture reaction, or spitting suture, place absorbable sutures deep in the dermis, cut sutures at the knot, and close wounds with minimal tension.

Pitfalls and Cautions

- Poor closure design can lead to tension on an anatomic free margin and subsequent cosmetic and functional impairment. The clinician should design closures that place tension perpendicular to the free margins.

Expert Tips

- Digital blocks with lidocaine with epinephrine are considered safe, though the clinician should avoid using more than 2 to 4 mL of anesthesia per digit, as the mass effect of the anesthetic volume added can lead to nerve and artery compression.

Patient Education Points

- Taking time to actively consent patients and inform them of possible complications may lead to a significant improvement in patient satisfaction.

Don't Forget!

- The nerves at the greatest risk for injury during cutaneous surgery are the temporal and marginal mandibular branches of the facial nerve and the spinal accessory nerve. Know the anatomical danger zones of these nerves, but also appreciate that nerve location cannot be precisely identified by anatomic location due to extensive individual variability.

Billing Pearls

- Clinicians should be familiar with global periods; most complications treated within the global period of a given procedure cannot, by definition, be billed for separately.
- Weigh the value of charging patients for revision procedures against the goodwill fostered by performing these procedures as a courtesy.

Managing Surgical Complications 22

INTRODUCTION

The safety and efficacy of dermatologic surgical procedures have been supported by multiple clinical studies.[1] A prospective study following 2370 surgical procedures over a 1-year period found a total of 56 surgical complications in 51 patients. Bacterial wound infections occurred in 13 cases (0.5%), and bleeding complications occurred in 5 cases (0.2%).[2] A prospective multicenter study examined the intraoperative and postoperative adverse events at 23 centers. Among 20,821 Mohs surgery procedures, there were 149 adverse events (0.72%), including 4 serious events (0.02%), and no deaths were reported. Of the adverse events, 61.1% were infections, 20.1% were wound dehiscence or partial- or full-depth necrosis, and 15.4% were related to bleeding or hematomas.[3]

Noninvasive to minimally invasive cosmetic dermatologic procedures are also associated with a low rate of adverse events.[4] A multicenter, prospective cohort study of procedures performed using laser and energy devices, injectable neurotoxins, and soft-tissue augmentation materials (20,399 total procedures) reported only 48 adverse events (0.24%) and no serious adverse events.[5]

Overall, the risk of minor adverse events in dermatologic procedures is low, and severe complications such as hospitalization and death almost never occur. Nonetheless, complications still arise, and clinicians must be able to successfully prevent, diagnose, and manage these complications.

PREOPERATIVE CONSIDERATIONS

The preoperative risk for surgical complications is a function of patient factors, including medical comorbidities, medications and behaviors, and the procedure being performed. The degree of preoperative assessment should be dictated in part by the extent of the procedure. Dermatologic procedures such as cryotherapy and shave biopsies are low risk, whereas flaps, grafts, Mohs micrographic surgery (MMS), and large excisions are considered higher risk. Patient risk factors may impact the clinician's choice of surgical modality or the type of surgical reconstruction performed. Prior to the procedure, the patient should be counseled in detail on the expected postoperative course, including activity limitations, wound care, pain control, and medication management.

A thorough preoperative evaluation includes a medical history and physical examination. Diabetes, hypertension, liver failure, renal failure, immunosuppression, inherited bleeding disorders, inflammatory skin conditions, and prior radiation therapy are examples of conditions that can complicate dermatologic surgery.[6] A thorough list of medications and supplements should be collected; many medications may impact intraoperative and postoperative bleeding. The clinician should also assess and quantify the patient's smoking and alcohol consumption. Alcohol use and smoking may increase the risk of complications, and even minor decreases in consumption can improve postoperative results.[6] Identifying patients with implantable electrical cardiac devices or other implantable electric devices can guide the safe use of electrosurgery.[7] Allergies, particularly medication reactions and prior reactions to latex or other medical materials, should be obtained. Vital signs may be obtained on the day of surgery as part of the physical examination. While there is a range of blood pressures within which clinicians comfortably operate, one comprehensive review suggests that for patients with a systolic pressure of 180 mm Hg or lower and a diastolic pressure of 100 mm Hg or lower and no other medical contraindications, cutaneous surgery may proceed.[8] Higher blood pressures often warrant surgical deferment. Many clinicians rely on patient-reported history to ascertain whether a history of uncontrolled hypertension exists. Surgery should be avoided on areas of active infection or inflammation.

INTRAOPERATIVE COMPLICATIONS

Anxiety

Anxiety in dermatologic surgery results from multiple potential factors, including concern about the risks of the procedure, separation from loved ones, unfamiliar environment, loss of control, reliance on strangers, needle phobia, cosmetic concerns, and anticipation of intraoperative and postoperative pain.[9,10] Increased levels of anxiety may have a negative impact on the patient's surgical course. The release of epinephrine into the bloodstream causes blood vessel constriction, increased heart rate, increased blood pressure and temperature, flushing, and sweating.[11] These physiologic changes may result in increased intraoperative and postoperative bleeding. Anxiety has also been shown to increase postoperative pain in dermatologic surgery; Chen et al[12] demonstrated that higher preoperative scores on two validated questionnaires, the Pain Catastrophizing Scale and Pain Anxiety Symptoms Scale, correlate with increased pain after MMS. Anxiety can also decrease patient satisfaction.[13] To minimize patient anxiety, it is key to manage patient expectations and provide clear explanations before, during, and after surgical procedures.

Before surgery, patient anxiety can be decreased by a phone call discussing the diagnosis and what to expect on the day of the surgery, as well as reading written material or searching the internet for information regarding the procedure.[13] Calls from providers, as opposed to nurses or other team members, have also been shown to be effective in reducing patient anxiety.[13] Listening to music has been demonstrated to reduce anxiety in patients undergoing dermatologic surgery, especially those undergoing surgery for the first time.[14] Eating throughout the day, watching TV, bringing a guest, and engaging in small talk with the clinician and staff during the procedure have also been shown to subjectively decrease patients' anxiety.[13] Other potential relaxation strategies include slower breathing, biofeedback, progressive muscular relaxation, guided imagery, hypnosis, and meditation.[15]

Some patients may require a preoperative oral anxiolytic such as diazepam, alprazolam, or midazolam. During MMS, midazolam has been shown to offer the benefit of amnesia, reduced alertness, and reduced blood pressure with no clinically significant adverse effects.[16] In patients requiring an anxiolytic, informed consent should be obtained before medication administration. The patient should be accompanied to their surgical appointment and should be instructed not to operate a vehicle the day of the surgery.[17] The most notable side effects of benzodiazepine use include drowsiness and respiratory depression, which require intra- and postoperative patient monitoring. It is important to note that less than 1% of individuals taking a benzodiazepine may paradoxically experience agitation, restlessness, hyperactivity, and combativeness and may require flumazenil for reversal of the medication.[18]

Reaction to Anesthesia

Pain: Given that the majority of dermatologic surgeries are performed with the patient awake, intraoperative pain management is a key concern. For instance, while MMS is typically well tolerated, significant intraoperative pain is one of the risk factors for aborting a case prior to achieving clear surgical margins.[19] Injectable local anesthesia (LA), most commonly lidocaine, is used for intraoperative pain management in dermatologic surgery. For a full discussion of LA in dermatologic surgery, see Chapter 9.

LA injection can be painful due to needle sticks, tissue distension, and burning associated with the anesthetic itself.[20] Several techniques can help minimize discomfort during the administration of LA. First, buffering lidocaine with sodium bicarbonate in a 10:1 ratio can decrease injection site pain by alkalinizing the solution toward a more physiologic range.[21] By increasing the pH, there is a 10-fold reduction in hydrogen ion concentration, which decreases local irritation and causes a much more rapid disbursement of the anesthetic, resulting in near-instantaneous nerve blockade.[22,23] Second, various injection techniques can be used for pain minimization. These include using a small-bore needle (most commonly a 30-gauge), injecting slowly, topical skin cooling prior to injection, using warmed anesthesia, providing distraction stimuli with pinching or vibration, injecting perpendicularly to the skin initially, using as few needle sticks as possible, and ensuring adequate depth and width of the anesthetic.[24-28]

The use of topical anesthetics prior to LA injection can minimize both patient anxiety and pain. Topical anesthetics may decrease the pain of the needle placement but will not impact the pain due to anesthetic infiltration. Patients should be provided instructions on safe use of the topical medication and apply the topical anesthetic under occlusion 30 to 60 minutes before arriving for their procedure.[29]

Topical anesthetics exist in many different preparations and vehicles for delivery. There are numerous commercially available, US Food and Drug Administration (FDA)–approved topical anesthetics for use in dermatology including:

1. Eutectic mixture of local anesthetics (EMLA; Astra Pharmaceuticals, Westborough, MA), which is an oil-in-water emulsion of 2.5% lidocaine and 2.5% prilocaine.
2. Topical lidocaine products, such as Topicaine (ESBA Laboratories, Jupiter, FL), Lidoderm (Endo Pharmaceuticals, Chadds Ford, PA), and LMX (Ferndale Laboratories, Ferndale, MI).
3. Topical S-Caine peel marketed as Pliaglis (Galderma Laboratories, Fort Worth, TX), which is a eutectic mixture of 7% lidocaine and 7% tetracaine in a cream base, and topical S-Caine patch marketed as Synera (Zars Inc, Salt Lake City, UT), which is a eutectic mixture of 70 mg of lidocaine and 70 mg of tetracaine under a patented heating element that enhances delivery of the anesthetic.

All topical anesthetics have associated risks of cardiotoxicity and central nervous system toxicity, which are heightened with prolonged application, the use of inappropriately high concentrations, and application to a large surface area. The prilocaine portion of EMLA can induce methemoglobinemia by oxidizing iron in red blood cells from the ferrous to the ferric state, impairing hemoglobin transport of oxygen.[29] Very young patients or patients with glucose-6-phosphate dehydrogenase deficiencies are more susceptible to methemoglobinemia.

Non–FDA-approved, pharmaceutically compounded topical anesthetics should be used with caution. These products typically contain higher concentrations of the compounded anesthetic mixtures than their FDA-approved counterparts and lack appropriate warnings or directions for use. These factors increase both the risk of adverse events and provider liability. Practitioners may wish to limit the use of topical anesthetics to those approved by the FDA, or at least those prepared by reputable compounding pharmacies.[29]

Local Reactions: Tenderness, bruising, and edema are commonly seen after LA infiltration. Edema is often more pronounced in the thinner skin of the periorbital area or the oral mucosa and vermillion lip (**Figure 22-1**). Transient motor nerve paralysis can be seen if there is anesthetic involvement of large myelinated nerve fibers. This paralysis may persist several hours after sensory nerves have returned to normal function, and patients should be counseled on this potential outcome prior to the procedure.[30]

Allergy/Anaphylaxis: A rare but important side effect of LAs is allergic reaction. These reactions involve either type I (immediate) or type IV (delayed type) hypersensitivity. Most true allergic reactions to LAs are type IV reactions, also known as contact allergy. A retrospective chart review of 1819 patients found that type IV hypersensitivity to LAs has been increasing, with benzocaine (45%), lidocaine (32%), and dibucaine (23%) being the most common allergens.[31] This phenomenon is thought to be due to an increased number of over-the-counter products containing lidocaine, resulting in unnecessary exposure and sensitization. Type IV hypersensitivity results in a local eczematous dermatitis, characterized by erythematous papules and/or vesicles that may progress to plaques and bullae; anaphylaxis is not a risk.[31,32]

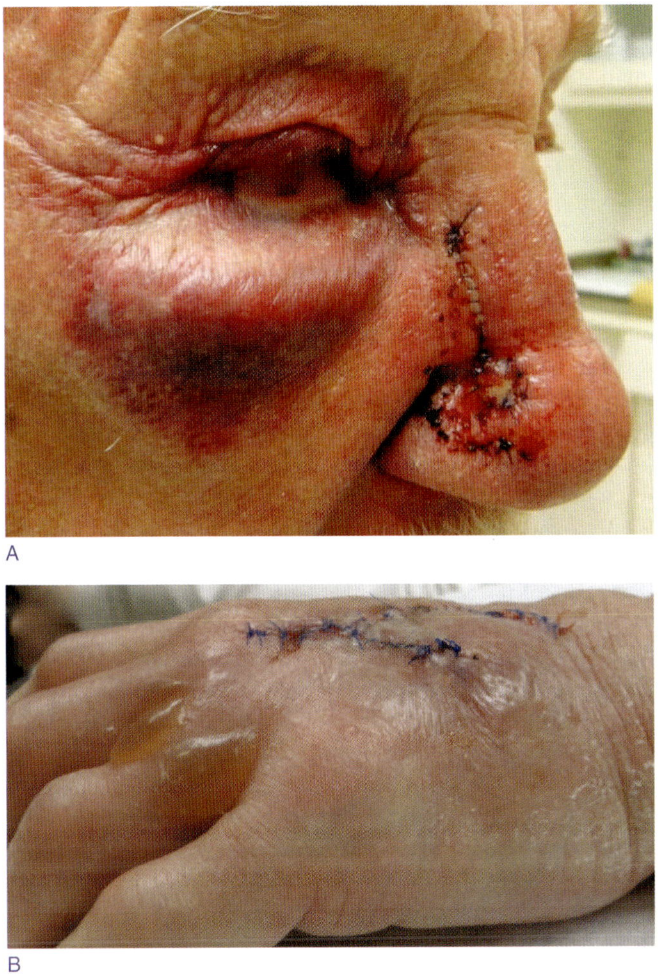

FIGURE 22-1 (**A**) Periorbital bruising and edema after Burow's graft closure on nose. (**B**) Edema bullae on the hand after rotation flap closure. Reconstruction on the hand often leads to extensive swelling; this can be minimized by wrapping the hand, including the fingers and thumb to the distal interphalangeal joints, to the mid-forearm with a self-adherent wrap.

The time course of type IV hypersensitivity is most commonly at least 48 hours after exposure.

In contrast, type I reactions are immunoglobulin E (IgE) mediated and occur minutes to hours after exposure to an antigen. Local manifestations of type I hypersensitivity are isolated urticaria or angioedema without laryngeal involvement. Systemic manifestations, or anaphylaxis, include bronchospasm and peripheral vasodilation, presenting as tachycardia and hypotension (**Table 22-1**). Overall, the rate of true IgE-mediated allergy to LAs in very high-risk populations (patients reporting an LA allergy) has been found to be around 1%.[32] Thus, the prevalence of IgE-mediated LA allergy in the general population is presumably significantly lower. While latex, found in surgical gloves, was previously one of the most common causes of anaphylaxis in the medical setting, widespread efforts to reduce latex exposure and sensitization have resulted in a marked decrease in the number of reactions.[33] Reports of anaphylaxis due to antibiotics, dyes, and chlorhexidine have been increasing in frequency.[33]

There are two classes of commercially available LAs: amides and esters. True type I allergy to amide anesthetics, including lidocaine and bupivacaine, is exceedingly rare. Most true LA allergies have been reported with ester anesthetics, including procaine, tetracaine, and benzocaine. The ester anesthetics more commonly elicit an allergic reaction because they are *p*-aminobenzoic acid (PABA) derivatives. There is no cross-reactivity between amide and ester anesthetics, but the preservative methylparaben, used as a stabilizer in multiple-dose vials of lidocaine, is structurally related to PABA. Thus, PABA and other preservatives, including sodium metabisulfite, are likely the most common cause of a reported allergy to amide LAs.[34-36] Single-dose vials of lidocaine are available without preservatives.

If a history of type I LA allergy is documented, patients can be referred to an allergy specialist for evaluation. If an LA allergy is reported but considered low risk based on patient history, an intradermal or subcutaneous challenge can be performed in the office. This assessment is performed by injecting into the skin a 2- to 3-mm superficial bleb of a 1:1000 dilution of an LA (without epinephrine) from the opposite class as the suspected allergen. In addition, a positive control (0.10 mg/mL of histamine base) and negative control (normal saline) should be injected for comparison. The wheal and flare reaction should be evaluated at 15 to 20 minutes, and if the longest diameter of the wheal is at least 3 mm greater than the negative control, the test is considered positive. If the result of the 1:1000 dilution is negative, an increased concentration of 1:100 should also be tested before deeming the test negative. If negative, a subcutaneous challenge can then be performed with an undiluted concentration of LA.[32]

It is important to be able to differentiate an anaphylactic reaction to LA from the much more common vasovagal and epinephrine reactions, which are frequently interpreted by patients as an "allergy" to LA. When a patient has systemic symptoms after administration of an LA, a set of vitals should be taken, as well as a thorough review of systems.

With true anaphylaxis, tachycardia is coupled with hypotension. The patient may have bronchospasm, urticaria, angioedema, or other systemic symptoms such as nausea, vomiting, and

TABLE 22-1 • Distinguishing Reactions to Local Anesthetics in Dermatologic Surgery

	Anaphylaxis	Epinephrine Sensitivity	Vasovagal Reaction
Signs	Tachycardia + hypotension	Tachycardia + hypertension	Bradycardia + hypotension
Management	IM epinephrine 0.3-0.5 mg every 5 minutes.	No treatment. Nonselective β-blocker if needed.	Trendelenburg position. Atropine 0.4 mg SC if needed.

IM, intramuscular; SC, subcutaneously.

diarrhea. Intramuscular epinephrine should immediately be given for anaphylaxis, and the threshold for administration should be low. Treatment with antihistamines or steroids is inappropriate in cases of suspected anaphylaxis. The recommended dosing for an adult is 0.3 to 0.5 mg (this typically equals the same volume: 0.3-0.5 mL of a 1 mg/mL solution) of a 1:1000 solution delivered intramuscularly. This injection may be repeated every 5 minutes as needed. For a child, the recommended dosing is 0.01 mg/kg up to the adult dose of 0.5 mg. Commercially available autoinjectors deliver a preset dose of epinephrine. Clinicians should have epinephrine solution or epinephrine autoinjectors readily available to treat suspected anaphylaxis.

If the patient is having a benign reaction to epinephrine, tachycardia with hypertension is expected. The most commonly used concentrations of epinephrine in dermatologic surgery are 1:100,000 and 1:200,000 for LA and 1:1,000,000 to 1.5:1,000,000 for tumescent anesthesia.[37] Even the low concentrations of epinephrine in these formulations can cause systemic effects, such as palpitations, flushing, and a feeling of panic. Epinephrine effects typically resolve spontaneously and usually do not require treatment. If needed, the recommended treatment is a nonselective β-blocker.[32] Patients can interpret the epinephrine response as anxiety or a cardiac complication, so it is important to provide reassurance as to the benign and temporary nature of this reaction. Epinephrine should be avoided in patients who have a medical history of uncontrolled hyperthyroidism or pheochromocytoma.[32] Local infiltration with epinephrine has been used safely for dermatologic procedures in patients with stable cardiovascular diseases including hypertension, ischemic heart disease, arrhythmia, coronary artery disease, and heart transplantation. If there is any concern about a patient's ability to safely undergo a procedure due to cardiovascular disease, the patient's cardiologist should be consulted.[37]

In a vasovagal reaction, bradycardia and hypotension are typically seen. This will be the most commonly encountered scenario in clinical practice. Vasovagal reaction is due to activation of the vagus nerve in response to anxiety, fear of needles, or pain on injection and results in heightened parasympathetic tone.[38] The patient will likely describe sweating, nausea, and hyperventilation.[32] Patients may feel like they are about to lose consciousness (presyncope) or may lose consciousness (syncope). Patients who experience syncope may lose bladder control and have rhythmic movements that can mimic a grand mal seizure.[39] One study revealed that young patients are more likely to experience presyncope compared with older patients and that young males are most prone to develop true syncope.[40] If the patient is having a vasovagal response, reassurance, placing a cool towel on the forehead, and placing the patient in Trendelenburg can alleviate the symptoms. For vasovagal reactions not responding to these measures, atropine 0.4 mg delivered subcutaneously can be considered.[32] Given the risk of vasovagal reactions, it is helpful to always infiltrate LA with the patient in a supine position.

Overdose: Life-threatening systemic toxicity can potentially occur when LAs exceed their maximum dosage or when excretion is impaired. Lidocaine has a maximum, weight-based dose of 4.5 mg/kg without epinephrine and 7.0 mg/kg with epinephrine.[37] Lidocaine toxicity is rare in dermatologic surgery; a 2010 study demonstrated that perioperative peak lidocaine levels during MMS do not result in serum levels approaching toxic limits, even when relatively high total lidocaine doses (up to 50 mL) are used.[41] Despite this finding, toxicity has been reported as a complication of dermatologic surgery, and it is important for clinicians to be aware of the signs, symptoms, and management of LA toxicity.[42,43] Inadvertent intravascular administration of local anesthetic may cause systemic toxicity more commonly than gross excess of infiltrated anesthetic.[42,43]

Overdose of lidocaine results in central nervous system toxicity and cardiovascular toxicity due to decreased cardiomyocyte contractility (**Table 22-2**). Initial signs and symptoms of lidocaine overdose occur at blood concentrations of 1 to 6 μg/mL and include perioral and digital numbness or tingling, restlessness, and lightheadedness. The patient may be increasingly talkative and describe a metallic taste in their mouth. At a concentration of 6 to 9 μg/mL, the patient may experience nausea, vomiting, twitching, tremors, blurred vision, tinnitus, and confusion. While the patient may still have a normal pulse and blood pressure, consider treating with benzodiazepines or barbiturates and ensure the airway is patent. At a blood concentration of 9 to 12 μg/mL, seizures may occur. Anticonvulsants may be used prophylactically in this situation. Additionally, initial manifestations of cardiovascular compromise may be seen, with the patient having lower than normal pulse and blood pressure. At a blood concentration of greater than 12 μg/mL, the patient is at risk of coma and cardiopulmonary arrest.[44]

Bupivacaine has a maximum, weight-based dose of 2.5 mg/kg without epinephrine and 3.0 mg/kg with epinephrine.[37] Of the nonlidocaine LAs, bupivacaine exhibits the smallest therapeutic range. Acutely elevated plasma levels may result in ventricular tachyarrhythmias and asystole, even before central nervous system symptoms develop.[44] If there is any concern for LA overdose of any type, anesthesia administration should be stopped and vital signs obtained. Clinicians should have a low threshold for a transfer to a higher level of care in these cases, given the potential morbidity and mortality of anesthetic toxicity.

Digital Anesthesia: There is a historically entrenched belief that epinephrine can cause tissue ischemia and necrosis due to vasoconstriction of end arteries via α-1 receptors, particularly of the digits.[45] In recent years, research and reviews have invalidated

TABLE 22-2 • Signs of Lidocaine Toxicity

Blood Level	Clinical Signs
1-6 μg/mL	Perioral/digital paresthesias, restlessness, lightheadedness
6-9 μg/mL	Nausea, vomiting, twitching, tremors, blurred vision, tinnitus, confusion
9-12 μg/mL	Seizures
>12 μg/mL	Coma, cardiopulmonary arrest

this doctrine, and current evidence demonstrates that LA with epinephrine is safe for use in all clinical locations, including the digits. One study demonstrated no digital necrosis using 0.5% lidocaine with epinephrine 1:200,000 for digital anesthesia in 63 cases, including patients with peripheral vascular disease, hypertension, and diabetes mellitus.[46] Another study examined patients who accidentally injected themselves with an epinephrine pen used for anaphylaxis. No cases of digital gangrene were noted, and the epinephrine concentrations used in epinephrine autoinjectors are much higher than those used in LA for cutaneous surgery.[47] Phentolamine is a reversible nonselective α-adrenergic antagonist recommended for epinephrine-induced digital vasospasm, although its use after dermatologic surgery has not been reported.[48-51]

Digital blocks can be safely performed with LA with epinephrine. The clinician should avoid using more than 2 to 4 mL of anesthesia per digit, as the mass effect of the LA volume can potentially lead to nerve and artery compression. Circumferential ring blocks should also be avoided for this same reason.[52] It is important to note that tubular dressings, rather than epinephrine or large volumes of LA, are the most common cause of iatrogenic digital ischemia and necrosis due to a tourniquet effect.[53-56]

Intraoperative Bleeding

Clinicians must consider therapeutic antithrombotic medications, herbal supplements, inherited hemorrhagic disorders, and other comorbidities that may place a patient at higher risk of intra- and postprocedural bleeding (**Table 22-3**).[7] Many patients, particularly those undergoing treatment for skin cancer, will have medical conditions that require therapy with anticoagulant and antiplatelet agents. Anticoagulants inhibit thrombin generation and fibrin formation and include vitamin K antagonists (warfarin), indirect thrombin inhibitors (unfractionated and low-molecular-weight heparins), direct thrombin inhibitors (dabigatran, argatroban, bivalirudin, and lepirudin), and factor Xa inhibitors (rivaroxaban, apixaban, edoxaban, and fondaparinux). Antiplatelet drugs block platelet activation and aggregation and include aspirin and clopidogrel. Both classes of medications may increase a patient's risk of intraoperative and postoperative bleeding and should be noted prior to the procedure.[57,58]

Individuals on dual antithrombotic therapy are at the highest risk for procedure-related bleeding. A 2011 prospective study of 1911 patients demonstrated that patients taking both warfarin and clopidogrel had a 40 times greater risk of bleeding complications compared to other subjects.[59] In their retrospective study of 760 patients undergoing skin surgery, another group found a significantly higher rate of bleeding complications in patients taking two or more antithrombotic medications at the time of the procedure.[60] In addition to prescription medications, herbal supplements, including ginseng, gingko, vitamin E, fish oil, garlic, dong quai, and others, may potentiate bleeding risks.[61-64] Inherited hemorrhagic disorders, including von Willebrand disease, hemophilia, and clotting factor deficiencies, should also be identified prior to a dermatologic procedure. These inherited conditions should be managed in conjunction with the patient's hematologist, given the potential need for premedication or infusions prior to the procedure. Other patient comorbidities, such as uremia, liver disease, excessive alcohol consumption, vitamin K deficiency, immune thrombocytopenia, and bone marrow failure, may further impair thrombosis.[7]

For patients with increased bleeding risk, pertinent preoperative laboratory data such as prothrombin time, international normalized ratio (INR), and platelet count may be reviewed. Studies suggest that it is safe to proceed with dermatologic surgery if the

TABLE 22-3 • Risk Factors for Increased Intraoperative Bleeding

Medications	Supplements	Genetic Diseases	Other Patient Factors
Aspirin	Ginseng	von Willebrand disease	Uremia
Clopidogrel	Gingko	Hemophilia A/B (factor VIII and IX deficiency)	Liver disease
Nonsteroidal anti-inflammatory drugs	Vitamin E	Other clotting factor deficiencies	Hepatosplenomegaly
Warfarin	Fish oil		Excessive alcohol use
Heparin	Garlic		Myeloproliferative diseases/bone marrow failure
Dabigatran	Dong quai (*Angelica sinensis*)		Vitamin K deficiency
Argatroban	Feverfew		Immune thrombocytopenia
Bivalirudin	Licorice		
Lepirudin	Bilberry		
Rivaroxaban	German chamomile		
Apixaban	Red clover		
Edoxaban	Poplar		
Fondaparinux	Meadowsweet		
	Willow bark		
	Tamarind		
	Danshen		
	Alfalfa		
	Goldenseal		
	Green tea		

INR is less than 3.5 within 1 week of the operation.[65,66] A platelet count below 50,000 is widely considered a relative contraindication to an invasive procedure. It is recommended to discontinue elective acetylsalicylic acid and/or nonsteroidal anti-inflammatory drugs (NSAIDs) 7 to 10 days before surgery.[66] In 2012, the American College of Chest Physicians recommended continuing warfarin or aspirin perioperatively and optimizing local hemostasis during minor dermatologic procedures.[67] The current consensus is that individuals should *not* stop any medically necessary anticoagulants or antiplatelet medications prior to dermatologic surgery, as the risk of catastrophic thrombotic complications exceeds the risk of bleeding.[58,65] There may be instances in which reduction or cessation of anticoagulation is warranted. In such cases, the decision is best made on an individual basis, with active involvement of the prescribing provider.[68] A 2015 randomized, double-blind, placebo-controlled study demonstrated that when patients with atrial fibrillation stopped warfarin therapy prior to an elective procedure, forgoing bridging anticoagulation with low-molecular-weight heparin was noninferior to bridging for the prevention of arterial thromboembolism and resulted in a decreased risk of major bleeding.[69] This study indicates that there may be circumstances in which anticoagulation may be stopped without increased risk to the patient.

Consideration of closure type should also be made when operating on patients with an elevated bleeding risk. Of all closure types, flaps, grafts, and partial repairs have the highest risk of bleeding.[59] Undermining is important in surgical reconstruction but should be performed only to the degree necessary to ensure adequate tissue movement. Wide and deep undermining can cause damage to large vessels and result in extensive dead space beneath the closure, thus increasing the risk of bleeding and hematoma formation.[7] Drain placement may be appropriate in patients who have a large postoperative wound cavity and/or a baseline bleeding propensity. Drains may be passive or active; passive drains rely on gravity to evacuate fluid, while active drains are attached to a vacuum device. In dermatologic surgery, the drain used most frequently is a passive Penrose drain. The Penrose drain may exit a wound through the inferior aspect of the suture line or from a small opening near the incision. Active drains like Jackson-Pratt or Hemovacs are closed systems that connect to a reservoir and have the advantage of removing bleeding through negative pressure. Drains should be removed within 24 to 48 hours to minimize the risk of infection (**Figure 22-2**).

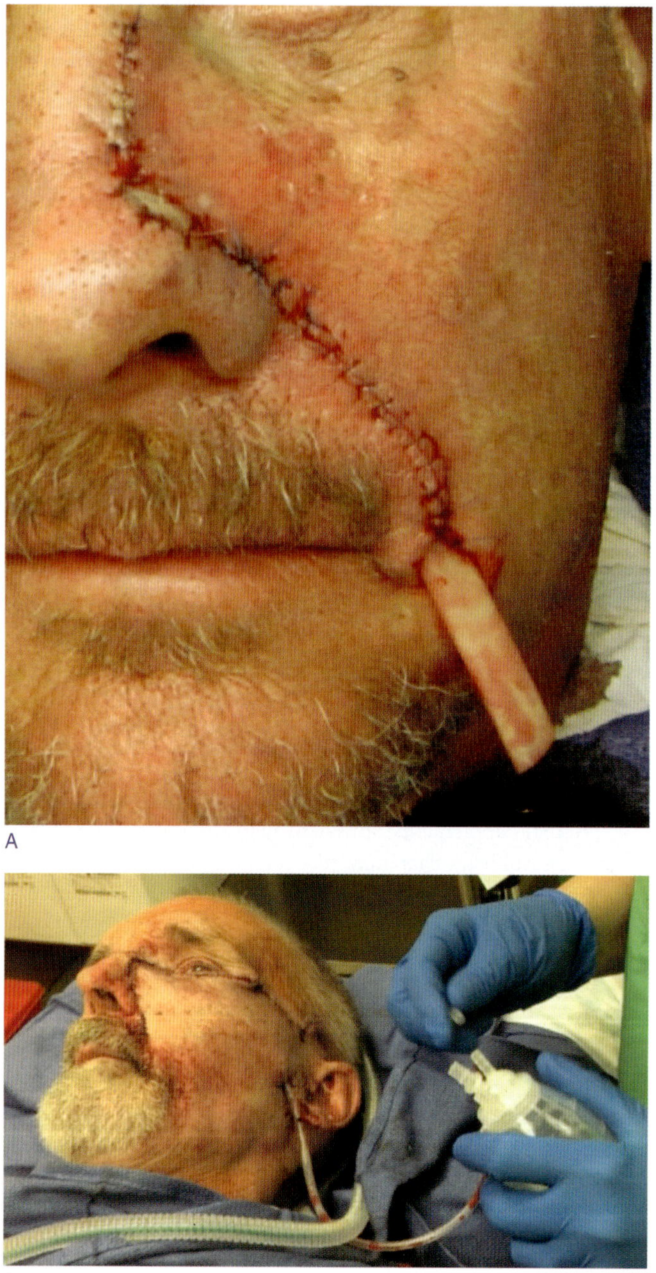

A

B

FIGURE 22-2 (**A**) Penrose drain placed in a large flap closure. This passive drain needs to be placed at the most inferior aspect of the wound. (**B**) Jackson-Pratt drain placed in a large flap closure.

Management of Uncontrolled Bleeding Intraoperatively: Direct pressure over a bleeding vessel for 15 to 20 minutes can tamponade active bleeding, thus allowing physiologic hemostasis to take place. This method is simple and effective, although it prolongs operative time and thus is infrequently used.[7] In the postoperative period, pressure dressings at the surgical site left in place for 48 hours can reduce the risk of bleeding after the procedure.

Epinephrine is often added to local anesthetics. In addition to improving the duration of action of the anesthetic, epinephrine provides transient vasoconstriction. A recent triple-blind, randomized controlled trial found that the time to maximal cutaneous vasoconstriction with lidocaine containing epinephrine 1:1000 is 25.9 minutes.[70] One caveat is that some patients may be excessively sensitive to the vasoconstrictive effects of the epinephrine, resulting in an intraoperative pseudo-hemostasis that manifests postoperatively with an increased risk of bleeding or hematoma formation. If this is suspected, meticulous hemostasis of all visible bleeding should take place.[7]

Suturing techniques may also aid in achieving hemostasis. Occasionally, transection of a larger vessel (>2 mm in diameter) leads to brisk bleeding not amenable to electrosurgery. Suture ligation offers a secure and long-lasting method of hemostasis for these vessels. After identifying the bleeding vessel, both ends of the transected vessel should be clamped with curved hemostats, and each end of the vessel can be directly ligated. Alternatively, in cases where the vessel cannot be directly sutured, a figure-of-eight suture or horizontal mattress suture may be placed around the bleeding area leading to compression and hemostasis.[7]

Topical hemostatic agents are also commonly used to control intraoperative bleeding. These may be categorized as physical hemostatic agents, chemical hemostatic agents, biologic scaffold hemostatic agents, and biologically active hemostatic agents.[71] Physical hemostatic agents function to tamponade blood vessels. Chemical hemostatic agents are caustic and lead to local tissue injury and subsequent thrombus formation. Biologic scaffold hemostatic agents provide a meshwork for platelet aggregation. Biologically active hemostatic agents are purified proteins in the coagulation pathway.[7] These materials are listed in **Table 22-4**. For intraoperative bleeding that will not respond to electrosurgery alone, the most frequently used topical agents are absorbable gelatin (Gelfoam), oxidized cellulose (Surgicel), bovine thrombin (Thrombin-JMI), and recombinant thrombin (Recothrom).

Electrosurgery is the most commonly used method of hemostasis in cutaneous surgery (Chapter 13). This leads to thermal damage, protein coagulation, and subsequent sealing of bleeding vessels. Electrosurgery includes electrodessication, electrofulguration, electrosection, and electrocoagulation. Another method of hemostasis, electrocautery, does not use electricity but rather direct heat to coagulate bleeding vessels. Electrosurgery and electrocautery are key components of dermatologic surgery but, when used in excess, can result in delayed wound healing and poor cosmesis due to thermal tissue damage and injury to the surrounding lymphovasculature.[7]

Complications Associated with Electrosurgery

Cardiac Implantable Electronic Devices: In North America alone, there are more than 250,000 new cardiac devices implanted each year.[72] Because older patients are at higher risk for both skin cancers and cardiac conditions requiring implantable electronic devices (IEDs), understanding the potential implications of electrosurgery is prudent.[73] Electromagnetic interference (EMI) from electrosurgical devices is relatively rare, as electrosurgery in office-based settings generates relatively low electromagnetic fields. In 2000, a survey of 166 Mohs surgeons revealed a low rate of complications due to electrosurgery (0.8 cases in 100 years of surgical practice) with no significant morbidity or mortality.[74] Complications included skipped beats (eight patients), reprogramming of a pacemaker (six patients), firing of an implanted cardioverter-defibrillator (ICD; four patients), asystole (three patients), bradycardia (two patients), depleted battery life of a pacemaker (one patient), and an unspecified tachyarrhythmia (one patient). Bipolar forceps were not associated with any complications.

Cardiac pacemakers are electronic devices consisting of a pulse generator and leads, which provide electrical stimulation to cause cardiac contraction if the intrinsic heart rhythm is absent or slowed.[75] In general, pacemaker patients are classified as *dependent* or *independent*. Pacemaker-dependent patients have inadequate or even absent intrinsic rhythm and, therefore, can suffer significant symptoms or even cardiac arrest after cessation of pacing.[76] As a result, patients who are pacemaker dependent are at higher risk of complications from EMI during electrosurgery. ICDs can detect and terminate life-threatening tachyarrhythmias via high-energy shocks and pace bradyarrhythmias. If EMI is erroneously identified as a life-threatening arrhythmia, a shock may be delivered or the ICD may respond by inhibiting cardioversion or pacing.[77] ICDs are more sensitive to EMI than pacemakers. Additionally, with poorly grounded or nonisolated electrosurgery, an implantable cardiac device can work as an indifferent plate and cause myocardial burn or arrhythmia because the delivered energy is localized to a small area.[74] Safeguards against EMI are under continuous development and include insulated coatings to limit the distance current must flow between electrodes and protective algorithms and filters that limit nonphysiologic interference.[72,78] As a result of the protective circuitry of modern pacemakers, complications from EMI are currently quite rare.[72]

As office-based monopolar electrosurgical units such as hyfrecators are low powered compared to their hospital operating room counterparts, a grounding pad is not consistently required.[78] Without a grounding pad, current disperses throughout the body and results in relatively safe means of obtaining hemostasis in most patients. However, since the current travels to a distant site, there is a potential risk of EMI with cardiac IEDs. In bipolar electrosurgery, current travels through a two-electrode instrument from one electrode, through tissue, to a second adjacent electrode, completing an electrical circuit. A grounding pad is not required, and electrical energy capable of interfering with an IED is minimized.[78] A recent in vitro study observed that monopolar electrosurgical units did not interfere with defibrillators and affected pacemakers only when used in close proximity to the device.[79] It was concluded that these devices are safe to use in patients with defibrillators at any distance and within 2 inches of pacemakers. However, conservative guidelines advise that electrosurgery should be avoided within 15 cm of a cardiac device without consultation from an electrophysiologist.[78] The safest forms of cautery in patients with cardiac IEDs is electrocautery (heat cautery) and electrosurgery with bipolar forceps (**Figure 22-3**).

A magnet placed over a pacemaker will switch most demand pacemakers to an asynchronous mode.[72,80] In this mode, the heart is paced at a fixed rate regardless of the patient's underlying rhythm.[78] This method has been used to protect patients from the inhibition of the pacemaker by EMI. When the magnet is removed, the device should revert to previous programmed pacing. Rare case reports of pacemaker malfunction have been associated with magnet use.[35,77] For ICDs, tachycardia detections can be disabled by magnet application without having an effect on pace mode or rate. Most ICDs will revert to prior arrhythmia detection upon removal of the magnet. An important feature unique to ICDs is that magnet response will not affect ICD antibradycardia pacing functions.[80] Unlike pacemakers, the pacemaker function of an ICD will not be rendered asynchronous. Thus, if a patient is dependent on the intrinsic antibradycardia pacing of their ICD, they will be potentially vulnerable to bradyarrhythmias from electrosurgery-induced EMI inhibiting the pacing function.[80] Clinicians should obtain direction from

TABLE 22-4 • Topical Hemostatic Agents

Agent	Mechanism of Action	Advantages	Disadvantages	Formulations	Notes
Physical hemostatic agents					
Bone wax (beeswax)	Physical tamponade to bleeding	Easy to apply	Nonresorbable, development of foreign body, granulomas	Paste	Most commonly used for bleeding vessels on the calvarium
Acrylates	Rapid polymerization to block bleeding	Nonreactive	Moderately expensive, can adhere to mucous membranes	Solution	Acetone can dissolve excess. Often used for closure of small cutaneous surgical wounds
Chemical hemostatic agents					
Aluminum chloride	Protein precipitation, thrombus formation	No risk of tattoo, low cost	Tissue irritation	Solution	Flammable even without an alcohol base
Monsel's solution (ferric subsulfate)	Protein precipitation, thrombus formation	Skin or mucosal application, ease of use	Can lead to permanent tattooing effect, tissue reaction	Solution	May interfere with tissue staining in Mohs surgery
Zinc paste	Caustic agent, thrombus formation	Theoretical tumor destruction effect	Painful to apply, extensive tissue destruction	Paste	Used in early Mohs surgery tissue fixation in vivo
Silver nitrate	Silver ions bind and precipitate tissue proteins	Low cost, ease of use	Tattoo risk, theoretical risk of argyria with large area application	Solution	Commonly used to treat hypergranulation tissue
Biologic scaffold hemostatic agents					
Gelatin	Meshwork to promote clot formation	Nonreactive, resorbable, low cost	Infection risks; swelling can lead to nerve or vascular compression	Foam, powders	Can be combined with thrombin
Cellulose	Meshwork to promote clot formation	Low risk of infection, resorbable	Not for graft bed or near perichondrium	Mesh, gauze, sponge	
Microfibrillar collagen	Meshwork to promote clot formation	May be removed once hemostasis achieved	Easily adheres to wet surfaces, allergic reactions	Fibrils	Bovine source
Biologically active hemostatic agents					
Thrombin	Converts fibrinogen to fibrin	Nonreactive	Risk of disseminated intravascular clotting if introduced to large-bore vessel; expensive	Solution, powder	Works best with biologic scaffold hemostatic agent
Fibrin glue	Direct coagulation	Nonreactive	Expensive	Solution	Prepared from patient's cryoprecipitate obtained from homologous donor, or synthetic

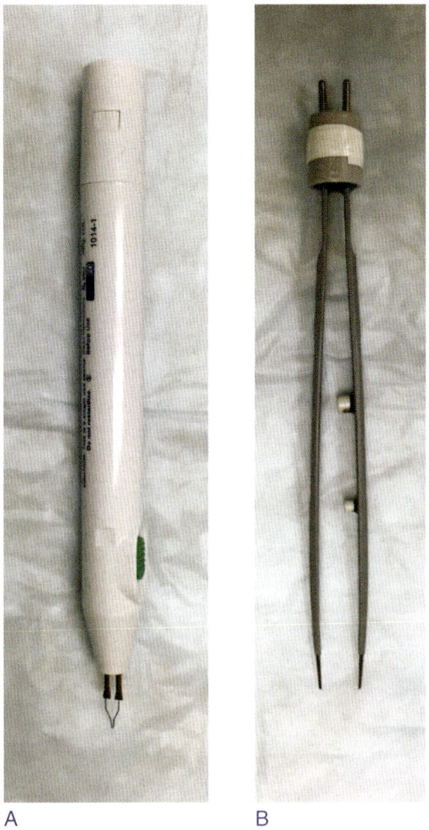

FIGURE 22-3 (**A**) Electrocautery and (**B**) bipolar forceps. These two methods of cautery are the safest in patients with implantable electrical cardiac devices.

a cardiologist or the patient's pacemaker/ICD clinic prior to the use of magnets due to the low but potentially significant risks.

Noncardiac Implanted Electrical Devices: Noncardiac IEDs include deep brain stimulators, spinal cord stimulators, vagal and phrenic nerve stimulators, gastric stimulators, and cochlear implants. These IEDs can also develop complications related to EMI.[78] To limit the risk of EMI, many of these devices can be turned off with an external remote control. However, some devices cannot be inactivated due to functional or medical reasons. Electrosurgery can lead to electrode heating and tissue injury around the stimulator, as well as paresthesias and electrical shocks, even if the device is deactivated.[72] As with cardiac devices, the risk is greatest with monopolar electrosurgical devices. If a noncardiac IED cannot be deactivated or the clinician is working close to the electrodes, the physician managing the device should be consulted.

Burns and Fires: Approximately 50 to 100 surgical fires occur in the United States each year, with the majority involving either electrosurgery or laser devices.[81,82] Of these cases, one to two per year result in death.[82,83] In dermatology specifically, electrosurgical pencil tips for coagulation are a common ignition source.[82] Dermatologists also routinely use flammable and combustible chemicals, such as surgical dressings, drapes, and certain cleansers (eg, isopropyl alcohol).[17] Petrolatum has not been found to be flammable and can be safely used in a surgical field.[84] Supplemental oxygen has been found to be a contributing factor in 74% of all surgical fires.[81] Because 90% of surgical fires are caused by monopolar electrosurgical units and laser devices, bipolar electrosurgery is the preferred method of coagulation by the Emergency Care Research Institute as a means to prevent surgical fires in situations where oxygen supplementation is required.[81] In the majority of dermatologic surgery procedures, patients' oxygen can be turned off while using electrosurgery without adverse effects. All surgical personnel should be trained in fire safety procedures, including initiating a "Code Red" and knowing the location of fire extinguishers and fire alarms.

Burns can also be a major complication secondary to electrosurgery.[82] In one survey of otolaryngologists, 324 complications from electrosurgical instruments were reported out of 99,664 cases performed in 1 year. These complications included 219 unanticipated direct burns, 48 burns secondary to current flow through a metallic retractor or instrument, 13 grounding pad burns, and 11 fires.[85] Grounding pad burns typically occur due to a pad with dry gel, an improperly sized pad, moisture under the pad, or improperly positioning the pad. Single-use grounding pads should be placed on clean, dry skin overlying a well-perfused large muscle ipsilateral and close to the surgical site.[82]

POSTOPERATIVE COMPLICATIONS

Pain

Postoperative pain is common: the majority of healthy patients who undergo MMS experience mild to moderate postprocedure pain.[86] A study of 433 MMS cases demonstrated that postoperative pain was greatest on the day of surgery and associated most strongly with flap repairs, age less than 66 years, greater number of lesions treated, and the use of narcotics for pain relief.[87] Longer lasting LAs, particularly 0.5% bupivacaine, can be injected into the surgical site to achieve extended postoperative anesthesia. Bupivacaine has an anesthesia onset of greater than 5 minutes and duration of 4 to 6 hours, compared to lidocaine, which works in less than 2 minutes and lasts 1 to 2 hours. It is important to note that bupivacaine injected without preanesthesia with lidocaine may be painful.[88] Nerve blocks can be used as an alternative to, or in addition to, infiltrative anesthesia for procedures on the face, hands, feet, and digits. Nerve blocks have the benefit of decreasing tissue swelling/distortion, prolonging anesthesia, and reducing postoperative discomfort for the patient.[37] For a detailed discussion of nerve block options, see Chapter 9.

Management of postoperative pain with analgesics is an important consideration in dermatologic surgery. Studies have shown that a preventive, single dose of acetaminophen of 1 g or less, ibuprofen 400 mg, diclofenac 50 mg, or etoricoxib 120 mg immediately after surgery reduces postoperative pain and opioid use.[89,90] Options for postoperative pain control include cold analgesia with ice or gel cold packs at the surgical site, acetaminophen, NSAIDs, opioids, and combination therapy.[91] Acetaminophen remains the mainstay of pain management for minor dermatologic procedures. Doses of 500 mg to 1 g provide significant improvement in mild to moderate pain over 4 to 6 hours, up to a maximal daily dose of 3 g.[92] At high doses of acetaminophen, rare side effects include liver failure and Stevens-Johnson syndrome. Because of risks of bleeding and hepatorenal syndrome, acetaminophen at a maximum daily dose of 2 g/d is the preferred analgesic in patients with advanced liver disease.[93] NSAIDs, such as ibuprofen, ketorolac, naproxen, celecoxib, and etoricoxib, are also commonly used to treat mild postoperative pain. Risks include impairment of renal perfusion, exacerbations of preexisting renal dysfunction, weakening of gastric mucosa resulting in bleeding or perforation, worsening of underlying conditions such as hypertension, and induction of life-threatening hepatorenal syndrome in patients with cirrhosis.[91]

A common concern in dermatologic surgery is the effect of NSAIDs on hemostasis in the perioperative period. While it has been shown that NSAIDs do indeed increase bleeding time, the elevations are mostly within the normal range and last only hours.[94] A case series found that, in individuals taking aspirin or NSAIDs after cutaneous surgery, postoperative bleeding could not be attributed to either medication.[95] Research in the field of otolaryngology has demonstrated that the postoperative use of ibuprofen does not cause greater bleeding complications compared to acetaminophen.[96] Thus, the use of NSAIDs after dermatologic procedures likely confers a low risk for bleeding complications. A 2011 randomized controlled trial showed that the combination of acetaminophen 1000 mg and ibuprofen 400 mg offers superior pain control compared with acetaminophen alone when given immediately after surgery and every 4 hours thereafter for four or fewer doses after MMS.[97]

Despite these favorable outcomes, some patients may still require opioid analgesics to control postoperative pain. Opioids are considered second-line therapy due to their adverse effect profile including nausea, constipation, and respiratory distress. Another potential risk of using opioids for acute pain management is that regular use for as little as 1 week can result in dependence and withdrawal.[91] Either manufactured or a-la-carte combination regimens including both an opioid (codeine, hydrocodone, or oxycodone) and nonopioid (acetaminophen, ibuprofen, or aspirin) analgesic are commonly used.

Hematoma

Hematomas are postoperative bleeding complications that occur if bleeding continues within a closed wound. Hematomas are problematic because they provide a substrate for bacterial growth, leading to infections; prevent wound healing; and increase wound tension, leading to possible dehiscence.[6] Despite optimal perioperative patient management, meticulous surgical technique, and attentive hemostasis, hemorrhagic complications may still occur after dermatologic surgery procedures.[98] The risk of bleeding is greatest in first 24 hours and is most frequent in the first 6 hours.[99] If a hematoma is suspected, the patient should place immediate firm pressure with ice as a first step.[98] Any bleeding that does not resolve with pressure within 1 hour or any rapidly expanding, painful subcutaneous mass should be evaluated on a more urgent basis.

Rapidly expanding hematomas indicate that there is an active bleed. They typically manifest as an enlarging, ecchymotic, fluctuant to firm mass with acute, throbbing pain (**Figure 22-4**). For a rapidly expanding hematoma, the surgical closure must be partially or full opened, and the sources of bleeding identified and stopped.[99] Once hemostasis is obtained, the wound can be

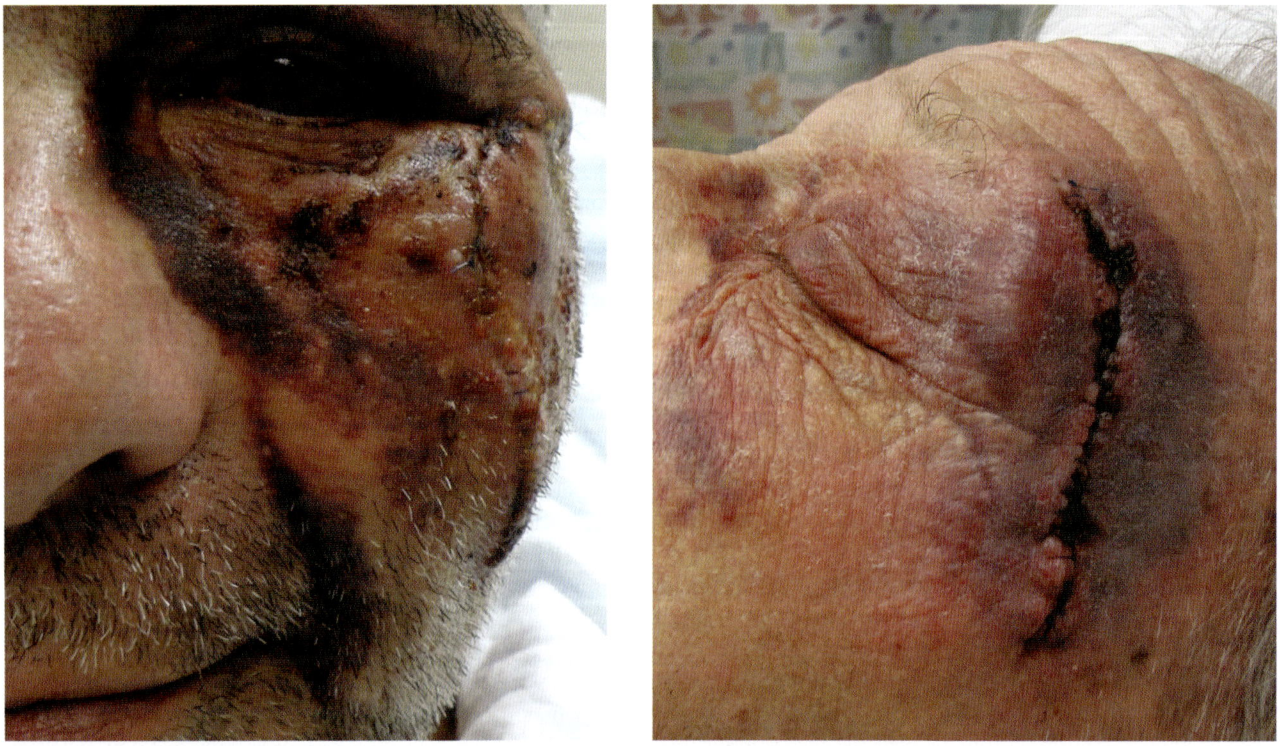

A B

FIGURE 22-4 (**A**) Large hematoma of the cheek after rotation flap closure. (**B**) Stable late hematoma of the temple after primary closure.

resutured. After postoperative bleeding is controlled, a pressure dressing should be left in place for a full 48 hours, and placement of a drain may be considered.[6]

Nonexpanding hematomas, or stable hematomas, also commonly develop within the first 48 hours. These hematomas tend to be small and do not compromise tissue viability. No immediate surgical intervention is necessary. Within 2 to 10 days, the hematoma tends to organize into a fibrotic clot, and after 14 days, the hematoma becomes fluctuant and eventually resorbs. Organized hematomas can be treated by incising with a #11 blade along the suture line or 1 cm away from the suture line, with subsequent expression of the contents. Fluctuant hematomas can be aspirated with a large-bore needle. For small hematomas, no intervention may be necessary,[99] although even small hematomas can contribute to delayed wound healing and tissue fibrosis.

Wound Dehiscence

Wound dehiscence is defined as separation of the epidermal and/or dermal edges of a wound (**Figure 22-5**). The most vulnerable period for dehiscence is just after suture removal,[99] although wound dehiscence occurs in less than 1% of surgical cases. Anatomic location, but not type of closure, was significantly associated with wound dehiscence (**Figure 22-6**). Surgery on the chest in particular has a significantly increased risk of dehiscence when compared to other anatomic sites.[59] Causes of wound dehiscence include high wound tension, infection, necrosis, residual tumor, suture reaction, trauma to the wound and poor wound healing secondary to anemia, hypoalbuminemia, diabetes mellitus, renal failure, and steroid use.

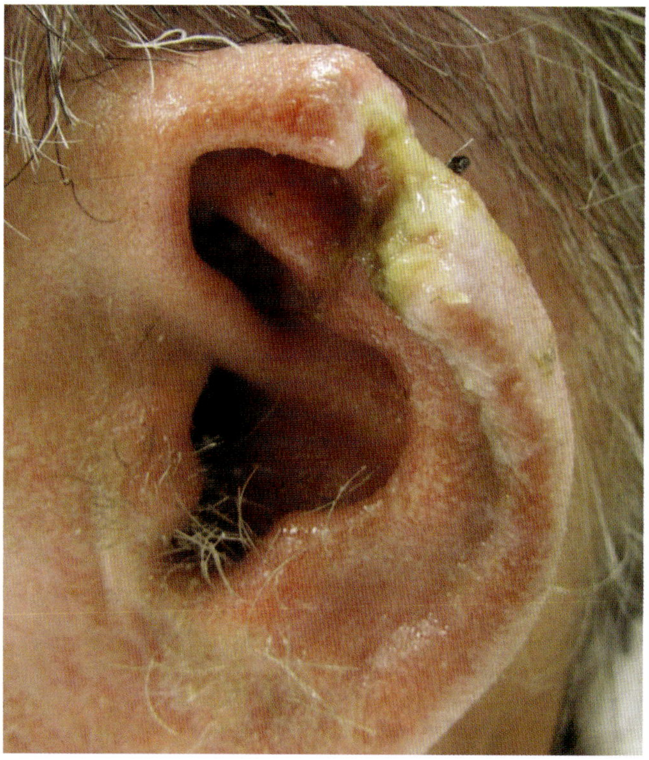

FIGURE 22-6 Dehiscence of wedge reconstruction on ear.

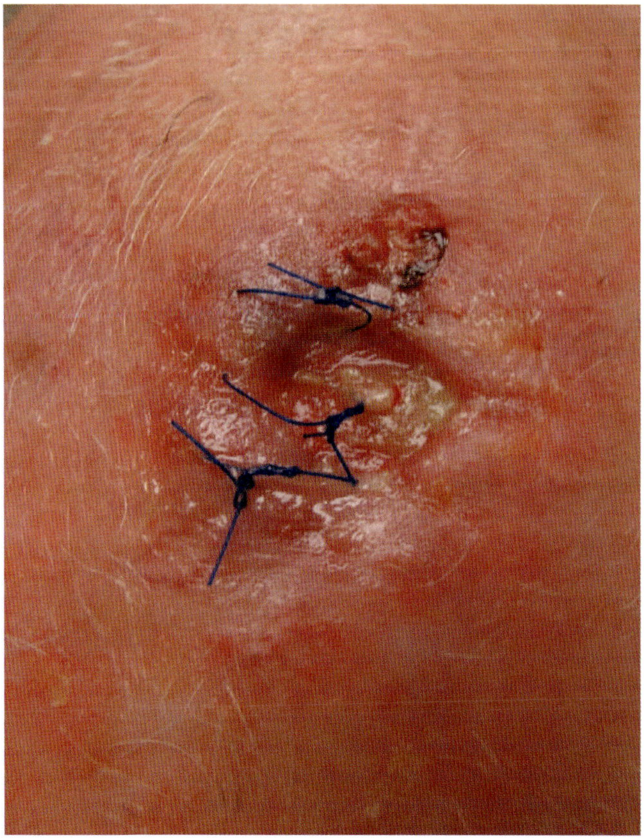

FIGURE 22-5 Wound dehiscence—epidermal and dermal separation of primary closure.

Whenever possible, wound dehiscence should aim to be prevented with proper surgical technique and detailed patient education. Removing wound tension through appropriate suturing techniques, closure design, and adequate undermining is key. Infections should be prevented and treated, and every effort should be made to remove residual tumor. The patient should be notified that the tensile strength of a surgical incision is only 10% at 2 weeks postoperatively.[99] Appropriate wound care instructions should be provided to the patient, including the use of moist occlusion, gentle wound cleansing, and appropriate dressing material use. Patients should also be advised to limit certain activities or exercises that place undue tension on the wound.

The wound may be re-sutured in cases of early dehiscence due to premature suture removal or trauma without infection.[99] The clinician should remove any devitalized tissue. The sutures should be removed and the wound explored if there is suspicion for hematoma. If the wound is infected or at a high risk for an infection, healing by second intention is preferred.

Skin Necrosis

Tissue ischemia is a result of decreased vascular perfusion that does not allow for adequate tissue perfusion. Ischemia can eventually result in tissue necrosis or death.[99] Black, densely adherent eschar represents tissue necrosis (**Figure 22-7**).[6] Skin necrosis is

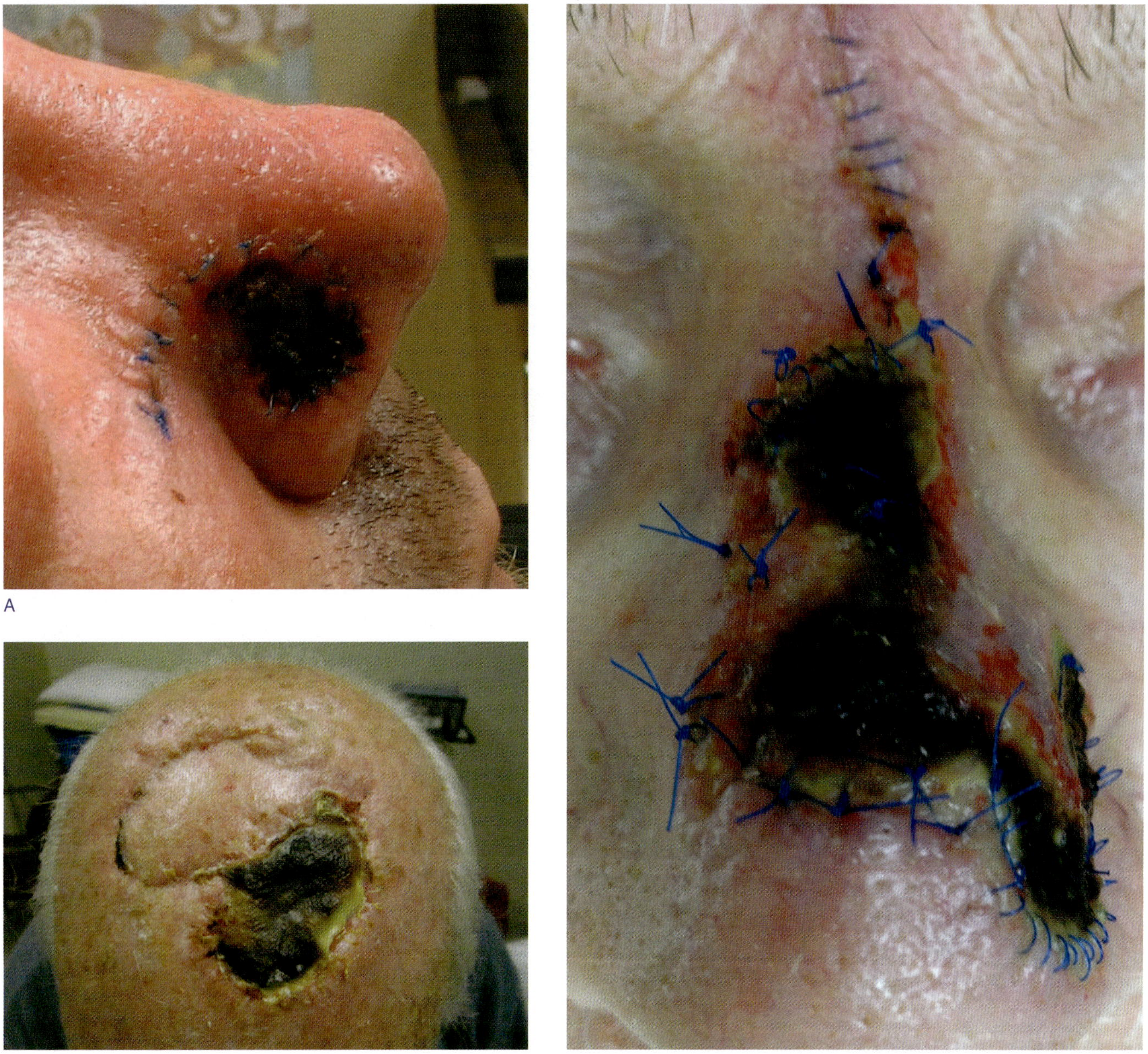

A B C

FIGURE 22-7 (**A**) Impending necrosis of rotation flap. (**B**) Tissue necrosis of full-thickness skin graft. (**C**) Tissue necrosis of transposition flap.

a rare complication seen in cutaneous surgery. Necrosis is often seen as a result of patient risk factors, anatomic risk factors, poor closure design (eg, excessive tension), postoperative bleeding, or wound infection. Patient risk factors include anticoagulant use, hepatic or renal insufficiency, excessive alcohol consumption, and smoking (heavy smokers develop necrosis three times more frequently than never smokers).[100,101] Tobacco use decreases cutaneous blood flow via nicotine (causes vasoconstriction) and carbon monoxide (impairs cutaneous oxygenation). It is recommended that patients decrease their smoking to less than one pack per day for 2 days prior to surgery and for 1 week postoperatively to minimize complications.[6]

Proper surgical technique also plays a major role in preventing ischemia and necrosis. Delicate tissue handling is important. The clinician should aim to avoid macerating tissue edges; this can be achieved by using skin hooks or toothed forceps rather than serrated forceps.[6,99] When undermining, the clinician should avoid disrupting the dermal plexus by undermining at the appropriate depth.[102] Strangulation of tissue with sutures can also lead to tissue ischemia. Elastic sutures may have a lower risk of necrosis because the suture material can expand with tissue edema.[103] The tip stitch, or half buried mattress suture, minimizes compression on the subdermal vessels in order to minimize ischemic necrosis of vulnerable flap tips.[104] Mattress sutures, in contrast, may increase the risk of necrosis. Finally, prevention of hematoma, as noted earlier, may also prevent tissue ischemia and necrosis.

From the standpoint of closure design, high-tension closures should be avoided in order to minimize the risk of tissue ischemia.[105]

Techniques to minimize closure tension include appropriate undermining, using plication sutures and/or dermal and subcutaneous sutures to decrease tension on the epidermal edge,[106] and using relaxation incisions or Z-plasties. Flaps and grafts have an increased risk of tissue ischemia compared to primary closures.[105] In flaps, the vascularity is based only on the pedicle supplying the tissue. The length of the pedicle correlates with the risk of flap necrosis. One study examining dermatologic surgery complications prospectively found that 4 (1.7%) of 241 flap repair patients had evidence of partial flap necrosis; no complete flap necrosis occurred. The authors also found no significant association between anatomic site and flap necrosis. Graft necrosis tends to occur more frequently. In the same study, partial graft necrosis occurred in 13 (8.6%) of 152 patients. Average graft loss was 50% of the total graft area.[59]

The first signs of ischemia and necrosis may be seen intraoperatively. In the event of arterial insufficiency, the tissue tends to be dusky or pale and cool to the touch. If venous congestion is present, the tissue is typically dark purple and bleeds readily if pricked. In both of these settings, the clinician should redesign or modify the closure to maximize blood flow. In the postoperative period, arterial ischemia can be reversed by early intervention, as the tissue is capable of surviving up to 13 hours. In venous congestion, the tissue progresses to necrosis much more rapidly. Serial pinpricks can be performed in the postoperative period to mitigate venous congestion. Postoperatively, tissue necrosis appears as a dusky eschar with tissue sloughing. Nonviable tissue should not be debrided given the risk of damaging underlying viable tissue. The wound should be kept moist and occluded, and patients should be counseled on the expected clinical course, including tissue sloughing and odor. Once the necrotic tissue has completely sloughed off, healing by second intention or surgical intervention can be considered. No surgical closure should be attempted with devitalized tissue still present in the wound bed.

Infection

Wounds can be classified (class I-IV) according to the site and status of the wound preoperatively (**Table 22-5**).[107] While there are differing definitions of localized surgical skin infections, the Centers for Disease Control and Prevention state that a superficial surgical site infection (SSI) can be diagnosed if it involves skin, subcutaneous tissues, or muscle above the fascial layer at the incision site, occurs within 30 days of surgery, and at least one of the following is present:

- Purulent discharge from the incisional wound is present.
- Organisms are isolated on culture of aseptically obtained wound fluid or tissue.
- One or more of the following is present: pain, tenderness, localized swelling, redness, or heat.
- The clinician deliberately reopens the wound (unless culture of the incision is negative).
- The treating doctor diagnoses a superficial incisional SSI.[107-109]

The overall rate of infection is very low in dermatologic surgery, ranging from 0.7% to 3.5%.[59,110,111] A wound infection develops when sufficient pathogenic bacteria contaminating the wound overcome the local tissue defenses and host response.[112] Postoperative surgical wound infections may have a significant effect on the outcome of a dermatologic surgical procedure, including the final cosmetic appearance of the wound.[113] Higher-risk procedures include those below the knee or in the groin area, wedge excisions of the lip and ear, flaps on the nose, and all skin grafts.[107,111,112,114]

Intrinsic factors that place a patient at higher risk of infection include coincident remote site infections or colonization, cigarette smoking, diabetes, systemic immunosuppression, obesity, extremes of age, and poor nutritional status.[107] The most common bacteria found in wound infections (in order of decreasing frequency) are *Staphylococcus aureus, Staphylococcus epidermidis, Enterococcus* species, *Escherichia coli,* and *Pseudomonas aeruginosa.*[108] It is commonly thought that *P aeruginosa* is the main pathogenic organisms in infections of the ear after dermatologic surgery; however, it has been shown that *S aureus* is actually the most common bacteria cultured from SSIs on the ear.[115] *Enterococcus* and *E coli*, as well as other gram-negative bacteria, are commonly cultured from groin and lower extremity infections.[107,108] Most bacterial SSIs are a result of the presence of bacteria on the patients' skin or mucosa.[116] Other potential sources of bacterial contamination include colonized surgical personnel, surgical suite fomites, adhesive dressings, and contaminated disinfectant solutions.[117]

Signs and symptoms of wound infection usually develop within 4 to 8 days postoperatively and are characterized by pain,

TABLE 22-5 • Wound Classification Based on 1985 Centers for Disease Control and Prevention Classification of Wounds[107]

Class	Skin Condition	Body Location/Surgical Technique	Antibacterial Recommendations
I	Clean	Sterile procedure	No prophylaxis
II	Clean contaminated	Oral cavity, nasal mucosa, perineum, axilla; sterile procedure	Prophylaxis only if immunocompromised
III	Contaminated	Traumatic wounds, nonpurulent inflammation; nonsterile procedure	Therapeutic antibacterials
IV	Infected	Gross contamination, devitalized tissue, foreign body contamination	Therapeutic antibacterials

erythema, tenderness, and purulent discharge (**Figure 22-8**). Cellulitis occurs when the infection spreads into the surrounding skin and soft tissue beyond the incision and manifests as swelling, warmth, expanding redness, and pain. Infection is a clinical diagnosis based on the patient's signs and symptoms. Wound cultures may guide treatment, but a positive culture does not necessarily indicate active infection. Normal skin flora may be seen in wound cultures, and chronic wounds (>6 weeks) will almost universally be contaminated with bacteria.

Severe Infections: Special considerations must be made when treating methicillin-resistant *S aureus* (MRSA). MRSA can be hospital or community acquired; hospital-associated strains often exhibit multiple antibiotic resistance, while community-associated strains are often only resistant to methicillin.[118] To diagnose MRSA, bacterial culture with antibiotic sensitivity should be obtained. MRSA should be suspected if SSI persists despite empiric antibiotic treatment. Treatment includes surgical drainage when an abscess is present and an appropriate antibiotic regimen consisting of either trimethoprim/sulfamethoxazole double-strength twice daily for 7 to 10 days, clindamycin 300 mg orally four times daily for 7 to 10 days, or doxycycline 100 mg twice daily for 7 to 10 days.[117] Culture sensitivities and clinical response will subsequently determine whether alternative or additional antibiotic agents are necessary. The rates and antibiotic sensitivities of MRSA vary by region.

Necrotizing fasciitis occurs when pathogens extend beyond the skin and subcutis and involve the superficial fascia. The infection is usually polymicrobial, although *Streptococcus pyogenes* has been implicated in many cases.[119,120] While early necrotizing fasciitis can

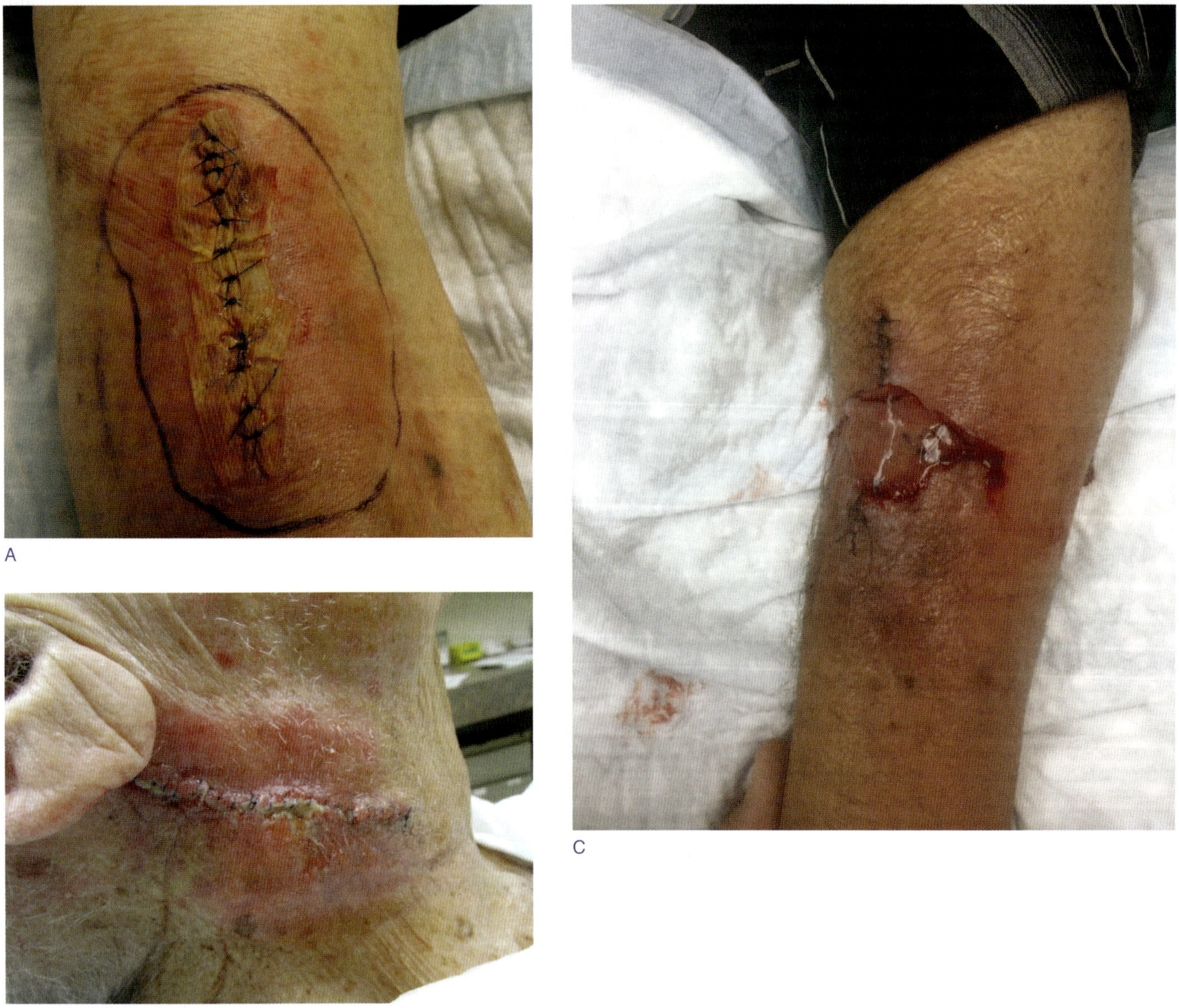

FIGURE 22-8 (**A**) Superficial surgical site infection of primary closure on arm. (**B**) Surgical site infection of primary closure on the infra-auricular with underlying abscess. (**C**) Expressing pus from an abscess on the arm.

be difficult to distinguish from cellulitis, red-flag symptoms include exquisite pain, violaceous bullae, eschar, necrosis, and decreased sensation.[121] Necrotizing fasciitis is exceedingly rare following dermatologic surgery but has been reported after excision of a melanoma.[122] Inpatient management with surgical debridement, broad-spectrum antibiotics, and hemodynamic support is required.[117]

Very rarely, staphylococcal wound toxic shock syndrome can cause early fever and systemic signs following a surgical procedure.[123,124] In these cases, the wound is often benign in appearance. Erythroderma tends to occur early with subsequent desquamation. Fever, hypotension, abnormal hepatic and renal blood studies, and diarrhea are early systemic findings. The incision should be opened and cultured and the patient should begin antistaphylococcal treatment.[125]

Infection Prevention: Many techniques exist to prevent infection in dermatologic surgery. Patient hygiene should be encouraged. Based on data from the general surgery literature, patients are often advised to shower before dermatologic surgery, despite a lack of data showing a clear benefit in cutaneous procedures.[126] A large systematic review recently illustrated no evidence of benefit for preoperative showering or bathing with chlorhexidine over other wash products.[127] If possible, surgery on areas of active infection or active inflammatory skin disease should be avoided. When it is necessary to remove hair, the existing evidence suggests that clippers are associated with fewer SSIs than shaving with razors.[128,129]

Antiseptic agents are an initial line of defense against SSIs. The widely accepted technique for cleansing the skin prior to cutaneous surgery is to scrub with antiseptic in concentric expanding circles until a wide region is cleansed around the surgical site. This technique minimizes the chance of spreading pathogens from the periphery into the procedure site and provides a sterile zone around the site where surgical instruments may contact without becoming contaminated.[117]

Commonly used surgical antiseptics include isopropyl alcohol 70%, povidone-iodine, and chlorhexidine gluconate with or without alcohol. Isopropyl alcohol acts by denaturing microbial proteins and has a rapid onset. However, isopropyl alcohol is flammable and can irritate the skin.[108] Povidone-iodine acts through oxidation and substitution by free iodine. It has a broad spectrum of antimicrobial activity and a rapid onset of action, typically within minutes, but must be left on the skin to have sustained activity.[109] Povidone-iodine is inactivated by blood and sputum, can cause a contact allergy, and has been known to cause hypothyroidism in neonates when there is chronic maternal use.[108] Chlorhexidine gluconate disrupts cell membranes and has excellent gram-positive coverage and good gram-negative and viral coverage but poor mycobacterial and fungal coverage.[108,109] Chlorhexidine binds to the stratum corneum and maintains antimicrobial activity for longer than 6 hours even when wiped off. Chlorhexidine can cause keratitis and cochlear damage in the setting of a ruptured tympanic membrane, so use around the eye and ears should be performed with caution.[108,109]

Some research supports the efficacy of intraincisional antibiotics (nafcillin or clindamycin) to prevent postoperative wound infections when compared with placebo. The benefits of intraincisional antibiotic prophylaxis include immediate delivery to the surgical site, ease of use, enhanced compliance, and low cost compared with other routes of delivery.[113] The limitations of this technique include the risk of patient allergy and theoretically increased bacterial resistance. Postoperative topical antibiotic preparations have not been found to differ from petrolatum ointment in healing time or infection rate for clean surgical wounds.[130] Allergic contact dermatitis is a well-documented adverse effect of topical antibacterial agents. For this reason, topical antibacterial preparations are not commonly indicated for routine use after dermatologic surgery procedures.

A few controversies exist in infection prevention techniques in dermatologic surgery. First, although many clinicians wear sterile gloves for dermatologic procedures such as excisions and MMS, a 2010 study suggested that a clean, nonsterile technique is adequate for achieving an exceedingly low SSI rate.[131] More recent studies also demonstrated no difference in infection rate when sterile versus nonsterile gloves are used during MMS resection and reconstruction, with the use of nonsterile gloves resulting in significant cost savings.[132,133]

Second, a common practice is to use one sterile set of instruments for tumor removal and a different sterile set for the repair during MMS. One recent study suggested that using a single set of sterile surgical instruments for both removal and repair stages of MMS maintains SSI rates within an acceptable range and leads to cost savings.[134] However, further investigation is needed before this technique is broadly adopted, given concerns for SSI and potential issues of tumor spread from using a single set of instruments during MMS. Moreover, many clinicians use a minimalist instrument set for the performance of MMS (blade and forceps), while reconstructive surgical sets are generally much more involved. Thus, in practice, it is not clear whether using the same instrument set would result in any significant cost or time savings.

Antibiotic Prophylaxis

Indiscriminate oral antibiotic prophylaxis is discouraged in cutaneous surgery, in light of the risk of possible adverse effects, antibiotic cost, and the potential for contributing to the development of antibiotic-resistant bacteria.[107] Antibiotics are associated with numerous adverse side effects ranging from mild gastrointestinal upset to serious cutaneous reactions such as toxic epidermal necrolysis, acute hepatitis, nephrotoxicity, and *Clostridium difficile* colitis.[108] Not only is the incidence of community-acquired MRSA on the rise, but also antimicrobial resistance to viridans group streptococci, one of the major causes of infective endocarditis, is also increasingly reported in the literature.[108,135]

An advisory statement published in 2008 provided an update on the indications for antibiotic prophylaxis in dermatologic surgery for the prevention of SSI, infective endocarditis (IE), and hematogenous total joint infection (HTJI).[114] This statement incorporated recommendations from the 2007 American Heart Association (AHA) guidelines for endocarditis prophylaxis, as well as the 1997 and 2003 American Dental Association (ADA) and American Academy of Orthopaedic Surgeons (AAOS) advisory statements regarding prophylactic antibiotics in preventing HTJI following dental procedures.[136-138]

TABLE 22-6 • Cardiac Conditions for Which Antibiotic Prophylaxis Is Recommended to Prevent Infective Endocarditis in Surgery Involving the Oral Mucosa or Infected Skin

Prosthetic cardiac valve or prosthetic material used for cardiac valve repair

Previous infective endocarditis

Congenital heart disease (CHD) from the following:

- Unrepaired cyanotic CHD, including palliative shunts and conduits
- Completely repaired congenital heart defect with prosthetic material or device, whether placed by surgery or by catheter intervention, during the first 6 months after the procedure
- Repaired CHD with residual defects at the site or adjacent to the site of a prosthetic patch or prosthetic device (which inhibit endothelialization)

Cardiac transplantation recipients who develop cardiac valvulopathy

If a dermatologic procedure involves the oral mucosa or infected skin (class II), patients with certain cardiac conditions (**Table 22-6**) or joint conditions should receive prophylactic antibiotics to prevent IE and HTJI, respectively. High-risk indications for HTJI include a history of total joint replacement within the preceding 2 years, previous prosthetic joint infections, and certain comorbidities with a history of joint replacement at any point in time.[114] High-risk comorbidities include insulin-dependent (type 1) diabetes, malignancy, immunosuppression, HIV, malnourishment, and hemophilia. Finally, antibacterial prophylaxis may be warranted for high-risk cardiac and whole-joint prosthesis patients undergoing dermatologic surgery in sites that are associated with higher rates of infection (below the knee, in the groin, flaps on the ear and nose, wedge excisions, or grafts). These high-risk dermatologic surgery patients may also receive preoperative antibiotic prophylaxis to prevent SSI, but no guidelines exist delineating if and when this is warranted.[107]

A suggested antibiotic prophylaxis regimen for dermatologic surgical procedures that breach oral mucosa or involve infected skin of high-risk patients is shown in **Table 22-7**.[114] The same 2008 advisory statement suggested antibiotic prophylaxis regimens for patients at increased risk of SSIs (**Table 22-8**).[114] Finally, in the setting of endocarditis prophylaxis, the AHA advises that an antibiotic should be given 60 minutes prior to a procedure but may be given up to 2 hours after the procedure if it is inadvertently not given before the procedure.[135] The ADA and AAOS recommended antibiotics to be administered 60 minutes prior to the procedure.[114]

Treatment: Once an SSI is diagnosed, wound culture should be obtained and the patient should be started on empiric antibiotics

TABLE 22-7 • Suggested Antibiotic Prophylaxis Regimens for Dermatologic Surgical Procedures That Breach the Oral Mucosa or Involve Infected Skin in Patients at High Risk for Infective Endocarditis or Hematogenous Total Joint Infection

Surgical Site	Medication Restrictions	Agent	Adult Dose
Nonoral	No PCN allergy	Cephalexin OR Dicloxacillin	2 g PO 2 g PO
Nonoral	Patient with PCN allergy	Clindamycin OR Azithromycin/clarithromycin	600 mg PO 500 mg PO
Nonoral	Patient unable to take PO medication	Cefazolin/ceftriaxone	1 g IM/IV
Nonoral	Patient unable to take PO medication and has PCN allergy	Clindamycin	600 mg IM/IV
Nonoral (skin infected and pathogen known)	No PCN allergy	Antibiotic specific for pathogen	
Oral (breach of oral mucosa)	No PCN allergy	Amoxicillin	2 g PO
Oral	Patient has PCN allergy	Clindamycin OR Azithromycin/clarithromycin	600 mg PO 500 mg PO
Oral	Patient unable to take PO medication	Cefazolin/ceftriaxone OR Ampicillin	1 g IM/IV 2 g IM/IV
Oral	Patient unable to take PO medication and has PCN allergy	Clindamycin	600 mg IM/IV

IM, intramuscular; IV, intravenous; PCN, penicillin; PO, by mouth.

TABLE 22-8 • Suggested Antibiotic Prophylaxis Regimens for Patients at Increased Risk of Surgical Site Infection

Surgical Site	Medication Restrictions	Agent	Adult Dose
Wedge excision of lip or ear; flaps on nose; all grafts	No PCN allergy	Cephalexin OR Dicloxacillin	2 g PO 2 g PO
Lesions in groin and lower extremities	No PCN allergy	Cephalexin OR TMP-SMX-DS OR Levofloxacin	2 g PO 1 tablet PO 500 mg PO
Wedge excision of lip or ear; flaps on nose; all grafts	Patient with PCN allergy	Clindamycin OR Azithromycin/clarithromycin	600 mg PO 500 mg PO
Lesions in groin and lower extremities	Patient with PCN allergy	TMP-SMX-DS OR Levofloxacin	1 tablet PO 500 mg PO
Wedge excision of lip or ear; flaps on nose; all grafts	Patient unable to take PO medications	Cefazolin/ceftriaxone	1 g IM/IV
Lesions in groin and lower extremities	Patient unable to take PO medications	Ceftriaxone	1-2 g IV
Wedge excision of lip or ear; flaps on nose; all grafts	Patient unable to take PO medications; has PCN allergy	Clindamycin	600 mg IM/IV
Lesions in groin and lower extremities	Patient unable to take PO medications; has PCN allergy	Clindamycin and gentamicin	600 mg/2 mg/kg IV

IM, intramuscular; IV, intravenous; PCN, penicillin; PO, by mouth; TMP-SMX-DS, trimethoprim-sulfamethoxazole, double strength.

based on the most likely causal organism. A 7-day course of oral antibiotics is sufficient treatment for most SSIs. In the majority of cases, empiric treatment with an antibiotic that has activity against *S aureus* is effective. This treatment includes either a first-generation cephalosporin, such as cephalexin 250 to 500 mg orally three or four times daily, or a penicillinase-resistant penicillin, such as dicloxacillin 250 to 500 mg orally twice, three times, or four times daily.[117] Antibiotic therapy should be modified, if necessary, based on culture and sensitivity results. If an abscess is present, it should be drained in a sterile setting under LA. Some or all sutures may need to be removed to permit adequate drainage. The wound then may either be packed with sterile gauze or allowed to remain open to drain. The patient should be seen for close follow-up to ensure resolution of the infection and to monitor for future complications.

Nerve Damage

Sensory Nerves: Cutaneous nerves are commonly transected during dermatologic surgery. As a result, patients frequently experience paresthesias at the procedure site. Given that most areas on the skin have diffuse sensory innervation and sensory nerves often regenerate, there are rarely significant permanent deficits from cutaneous surgery. Patients should be counseled preoperatively about risk of paresthesias at the surgical site and that normal sensation usually returns within 18 months. Occasionally, complete sensation never returns. Areas most prone to sensory nerve injury and appreciable deficits are the digits, forehead, and scalp. In particular, procedures that require deep tissue removal or dissection risk permanent damage to the branches of the trigeminal nerve on the face, with subsequent sensory loss.

Motor Nerves: Injury to motor nerves can result in more severe consequences than damage to sensory nerves. Although rare, damage to motor nerves can cause significant functional impairment. While many of the muscles of the head and neck have significant redundancy in innervation, there are specific motor nerve "danger zones" that are most at risk during dermatologic surgery. Overall, the risk of motor nerve damage in dermatologic surgery is very low, but patients need to be counseled preoperatively when operating in high-risk locations. Clinicians also need to be aware that significant individual variability exists in the anatomic course of nerves. Additionally, patients with tissue atrophy, such as seen with normal aging or HIV lipoatrophy, will have motor nerves coursing in a more superficial plane. If motor nerve damage occurs, it may be temporary (neuropraxia) or permanent. It is prudent to consult with the appropriate specialty (generally neurology or otolaryngology) early to optimize management after motor nerve damage. The nerves at greatest risk for injury during cutaneous surgery are the temporal and marginal mandibular branches of the facial nerve and the spinal accessory nerve.[44]

The temporal branch of the facial nerve is the most commonly injured nerve in facial surgery. When damaged, it will lead to ipsilateral brow ptosis secondary to paralysis of the frontalis muscle (**Figure 22-9**).[139] The nerve branches off the facial nerve trunk within the parotid gland and courses superficially across the zygomatic arch within the innominate fascia (a plane deep to the superficial muscular aponeurotic system and superficial temporal fascia) and crosses the temple with little overlying subcutaneous fat.[140] If nerve damage is permanent, this complication can be addressed with a direct or indirect brow lift. Over time, patients may develop a compensatory brow elevation on the contralateral side of injury.[139]

The marginal mandibular branch of the facial nerve traverses the mandible near the facial artery and vein, covered only by skin and thin platysma muscle. While the nerve is normally located approximately 1 to 2 cm below the mandible, in individuals with lax or atrophic tissues (as seen with aging), the branches can be as low as 3 to 4 cm below the mandible.[141] This nerve innervates the lip depressors, and damage presents clinically as asymmetric facial expressions and mouth function compromise. This asymmetry and lip imbalance are readily noticeable during opening of the mouth (**Figure 22-10**).[142] The marginal mandibular nerve is at risk during liposuction of the jowls and neck dissections, as well as after deoxycholic acid injections for submental fat.[143,144] The buccal and zygomatic branches are deeper, with more collateral innervation, and are at less risk of damage when compared to the other branches of the facial nerve.

Finally, damage to the spinal accessory nerve results in a winged scapula due to trapezius muscle palsy. This palsy results in dropping of the shoulder girdle inferiorly and laterally along with flaring of the wing of the scapula and loss of abduction of the arm.[44] The spinal accessory nerve exits behind the sternocleidomastoid (SCM) muscle at the junction of the upper and middle third of the SCM, then courses across the posterior triangle of the neck. It primarily innervates the trapezius and partially innervates the SCM. Inadvertent transection can occur during procedures in the posterior triangle of the neck, including radical neck dissection, lymph node dissection, and extensive cyst or tumor resection.

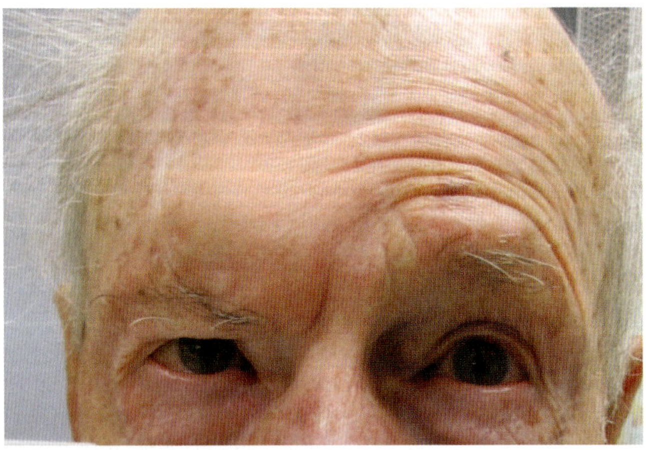

FIGURE 22-9 Injury to the temporal branch of the facial nerve resulting in the inability to raise the right brow due to frontalis muscle paralysis.

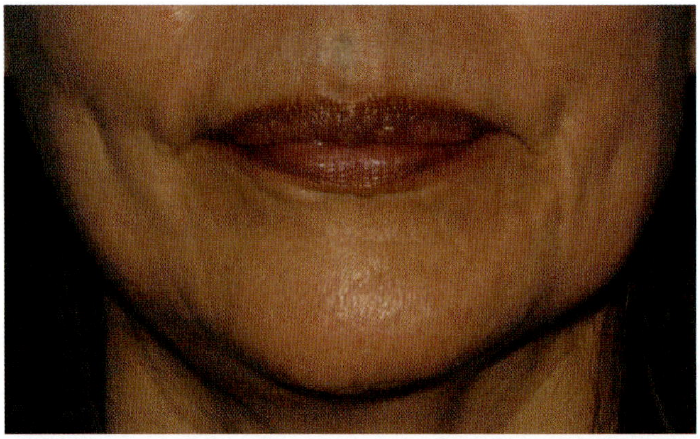

A

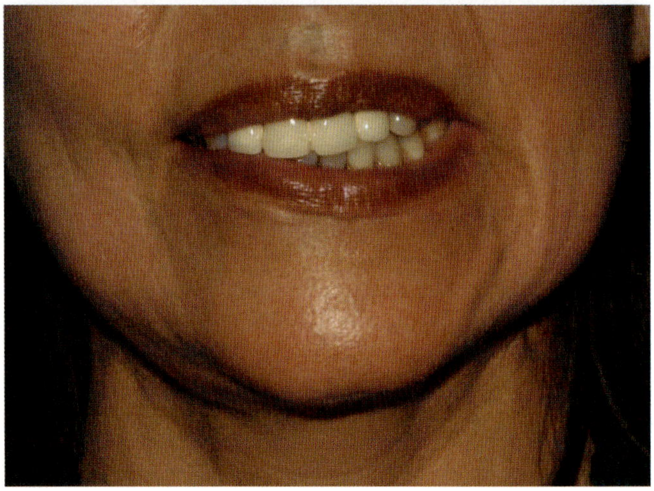

B

FIGURE 22-10 Marginal mandibular nerve paralysis after neck dissection, with injury on the right side: (**A**) at rest; (**B**) smiling showing compensation on the left side.

Suture Reaction

All sutures elicit some degree of inflammatory response when embedded in tissue, but the response is variable. Several factors contribute to tissue reactivity including suture material, configuration, caliber, and absorbability. The degree of inflammatory response to biologic sutures (eg, fast, chromic, or plain gut or silk) is much higher than that seen with synthetic sutures (eg, nylon or polypropylene).[145] Additionally, monofilament configurations of suture are thought to lead to less reactivity when compared to a multifilament configuration. Immediate postoperative suture reaction is characterized by erythema and tenderness of the skin. When suture reaction develops later in the postoperative course, it often presents as a "spitting suture," where there is residual suture material in the skin and/or an inflammatory foreign body reaction (**Figure 22-11**). Spitting sutures tend to occur 1 to 4 months postoperatively and present as a focal, aseptic pustule at the site of a buried suture. One study examined 140 patients and found that suture reaction was significantly less with poliglecaprone-25 (3.1%) as compared to polyglactin-910 (11.4%).[146] Surgical techniques that can help prevent spitting sutures include

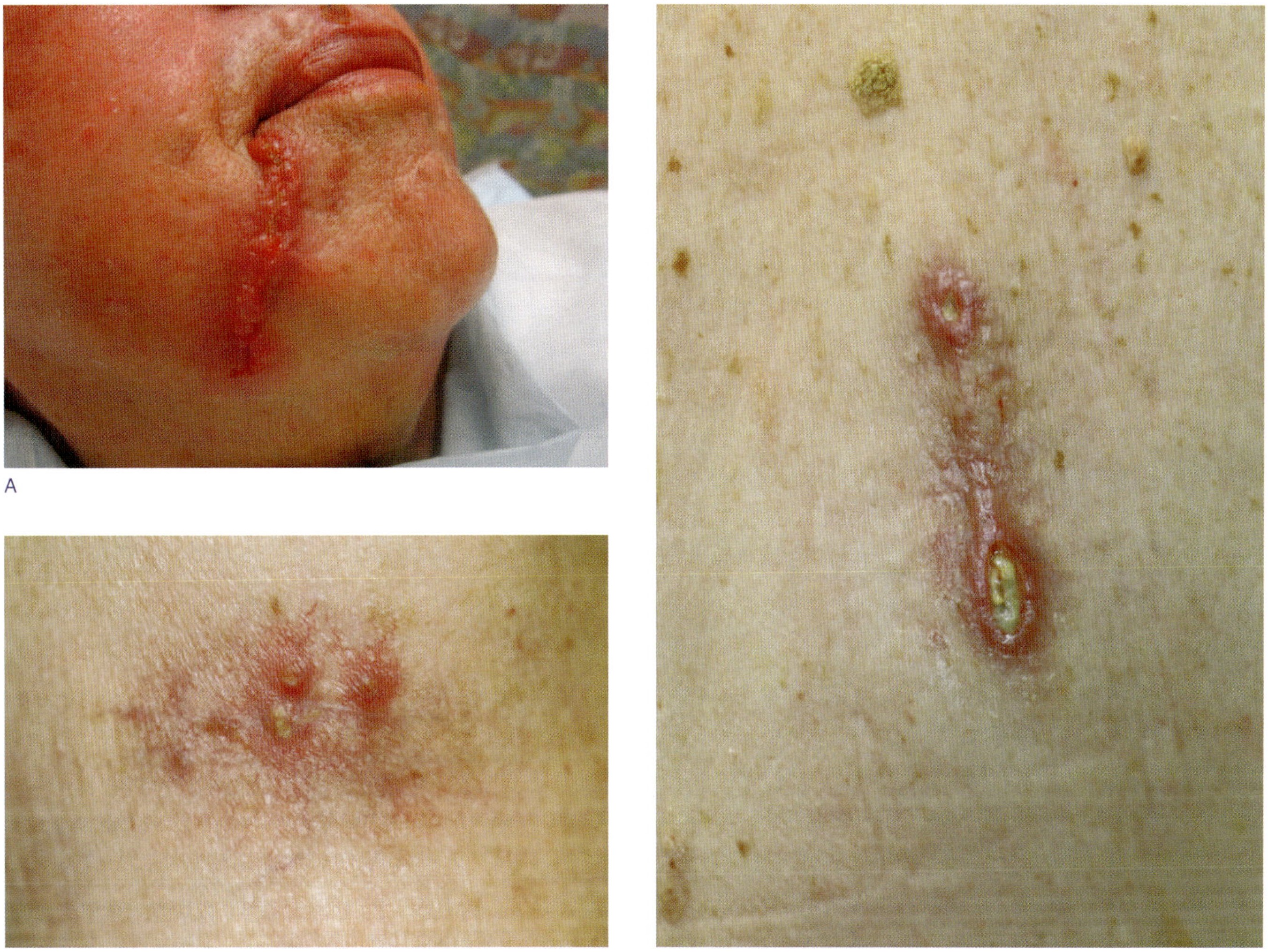

A B C

FIGURE 22-11 (**A**) Immediate suture reaction presenting as erythema and edema at 1 week postoperative. (**B**) Late suture reaction to deep sutures presenting as sterile pustules along the closure line at 6 weeks postoperative. (**C**) Late suture reaction presenting as small ulceration along suture line.

placing absorbable sutures deep in the dermis, using the set-back suture technique, cutting sutures at the knot, and closing wounds with minimal tension.[146-148] To treat a spitting suture, the site can be nicked with an 11 blade and the purulence expressed and residual suture removed.

Contact Dermatitis

Allergic contact dermatitis (ACD) represents a type IV hypersensitivity reaction and ranges in presentation from mildly pruritic erythema to intensely pruritic vesicular, bullous, or indurated plaques. The presence of erythema and induration around a postoperative surgical site may initially raise concern for SSI, but the clinical appearance of a contact dermatitis differs from infection. Contact dermatitis often occurs away from the wound edges, may have an angulated appearance, lacks purulence and tenderness, and is frequently itchy (**Figure 22-12**). ACD may be caused by any material in dermatologic surgery, including surgical antiseptics and wound dressings. Antiseptics used to prepare the surgical site are common causes of contact dermatitis. Most commonly, this is seen with povidone-iodine, but a similar reaction has also be reported to chlorhexidine.[149] Postoperatively, fixatives (eg, benzoin and Mastisol), dressings (eg, colophony), and antibiotics (eg, bacitracin and neomycin) are potential sources of ACD. If a patient has a history of ACD, it is recommended that white petrolatum be used instead of any potential allergy-inducing products.[149] Contact dermatitis will frequently resolve spontaneously once the implicated agent is removed from the skin. However, in cases of severe reactions that present with blistering or severe pruritus, topical or even systemic steroids may be helpful.

Abnormal Wound Healing and Scarring

Excessive Granulation Tissue: Excessive granulation tissue is considered a type of abnormal wound healing and is often seen in wounds healing by second intention.[150] Associated factors include wound site, prolonged inflammation, an imbalance in matrix metalloproteinases, and excessive angiogenesis. While a

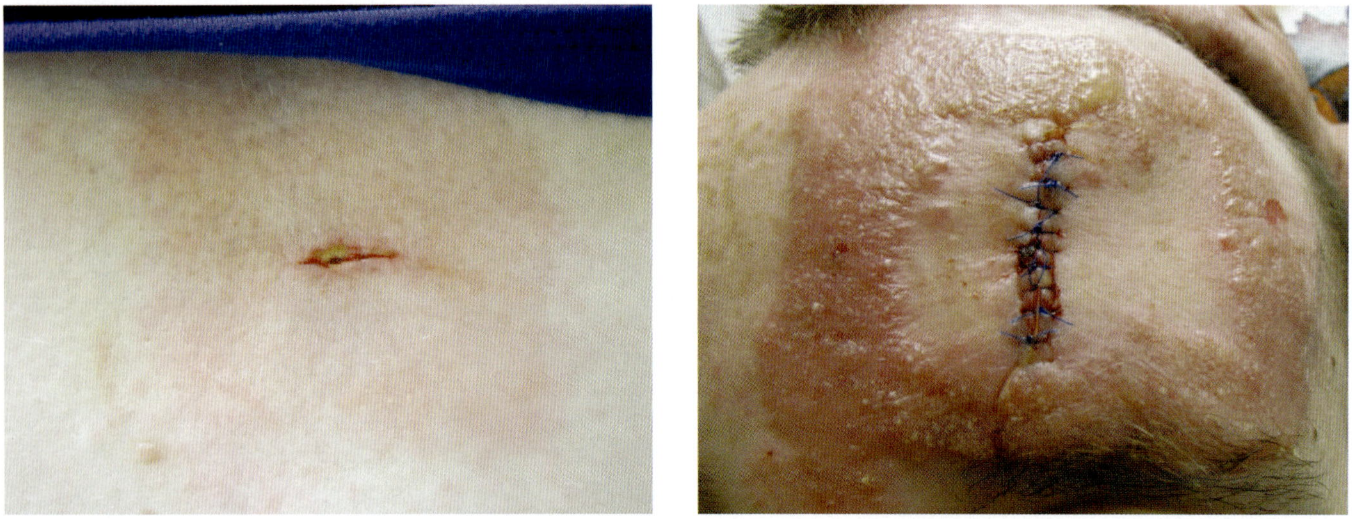

A B

FIGURE 22-12 Contact dermatitis presenting as angulated erythema corresponding to the location of adhesives. (**A**) Mild erythema and itching. (**B**) Severe reaction with blisters and edema.

modest amount of granulation tissue is considered favorable in wound healing by second intention, too much granulation tissue inhibits wound healing by preventing fibroblast proliferation. Granulation tissue appears beefy red and friable and may extend above the level of normal skin. Management of excessive granulation tissue includes destruction with silver nitrate, laser ablation, cautery, curettage, or shave removal of the tissue. Medium- to high-potency topical corticosteroids have also been used with success.[150,151]

Scarring: Scarring after skin cancer surgery can profoundly affect psychosocial functioning, especially when scars are located on the head and neck.[152] For many patients, the success of a surgical procedure is often tied to the aesthetic appearance of the final scar. Surgical scars tend to have a variable presentation and may have multiple features that must be addressed for optimal scar reduction. Scars may be characterized by abnormal erythema or pigmentation, firmness, visibility, contour irregularity, and other negative factors. Additionally, the position, location, age of the scar, and skin type of the patient should be considered. For many surgical scars, time will resolve many of the adverse features. Laser therapy with multiple different energy modalities has been shown to improve scar features.[153,154] Dermabrasion is another method for treating surgical scars and is particularly useful on sebaceous nasal skin.[155] Surgical scar revision may be attempted if the scar is not exhibiting favorable characteristics long term. Multiple techniques may be used, including scar excision with linear closure, Z-plasty, W-plasty, and geometric broken line closure.[155]

Hypertrophic/Keloid Scars. Hypertrophic scars and keloids are two forms of abnormal wound healing characterized by local fibroblast proliferation and excessive collagen production in response to cutaneous injury. Hypertrophic scars tend to remain confined to the scar line, whereas keloids extend beyond the margin of the scar. Hypertrophic scars often arise earlier than keloids, usually within 4 weeks postoperatively. Keloids may develop months to a year after trauma or surgery.[156] Hypertrophic scars can regress without intervention, whereas keloids do not, and indeed frequently recur after surgical removal. Keloids are more common on the chest and back of darker skinned patients and are often also seen at the sites of wounds healing by second intention.[157] In contrast, spread scars tend to be more atrophic, with thin, fragile tissue centrally. Spread scars occur in areas under high tension, areas with high use (shoulders, chest, back), and in the context of infection or dehiscence.

The first-line treatment for hypertrophic scars and keloids is intralesional steroid injections.[158] While this approach is considered largely effective, it may be associated with cutaneous atrophy, pigmentary alteration, and telangiectasias.[159] Reexcision with the addition of pressure therapy, postoperative radiation, and intralesional steroid injections has also been performed with success for keloids,[160,161] and one study has demonstrated an effective combination of reexcision and closure with the set-back suture coupled with postoperative radiation.[162] Finally, silicone gel sheeting, 585- or 595-nm pulsed dye laser, cryotherapy, intralesional 5-fluorouracil (5-FU), interferon alfa-2b injections, fractional nonablative lasers, and ablative laser treatment may also be of benefit for keloids.[163-168]

Suture Track Marks. Track marks are often seen when epidermal sutures are left in place longer than necessary or are placed too tightly (**Figure 22-13**).[104] Postoperative edema tends to exacerbate track marks due to increased tension on epidermal sutures. To prevent track marks, sutures should be removed as early as possible, wound tension should be maximally decreased by performing adequate undermining, buried dermal or subcutaneous sutures should be used for tension reduction, and sutures of appropriate size should be used for a given anatomic location. A recent randomized controlled trial found the set-back suture to be superior to the buried vertical mattress suture for postoperative

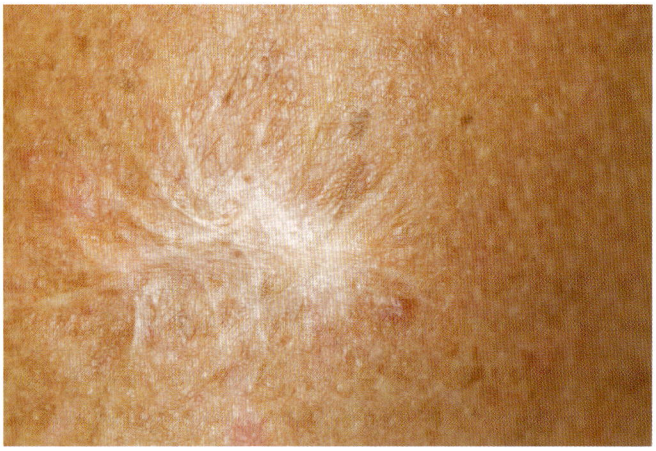

FIGURE 22-13 Spread surgical scar.

scar cosmesis.[148] Tissue adhesives or adhesive strips may also be used in place of epidermal sutures in order to prevent track marks as long as dermal sutures have been placed to reduce tension.[169]

Trapdoor Phenomenon: The trapdoor phenomenon, or pin-cushioning, is a contour irregularity due to scar elevation above the surrounding skin surface. This abnormal scarring is most frequently seen in flaps on the nose and upper cutaneous lip (**Figure 22-14**). Irregular flap contour may be due to several factors, including lymphatic or venous obstruction, postoperative ischemia, resolving hematoma, scar hypertrophy, excessive subcutaneous fat or flap tissue, and scar contracture. The deformity typically appears within 3 weeks to 6 months after surgery and can be prevented with optimal flap design, wide undermining of the recipient site, squaring of the corners (versus circular trimming), appropriately thinning the flap, and the judicious use of dermal sutures to reapproximate muscle and dermis. Potential treatments include surgical revision by lifting and thinning of the flap, intralesional steroid injection, and dermabrasion. Over time, improvement may be seen without intervention.[170,171]

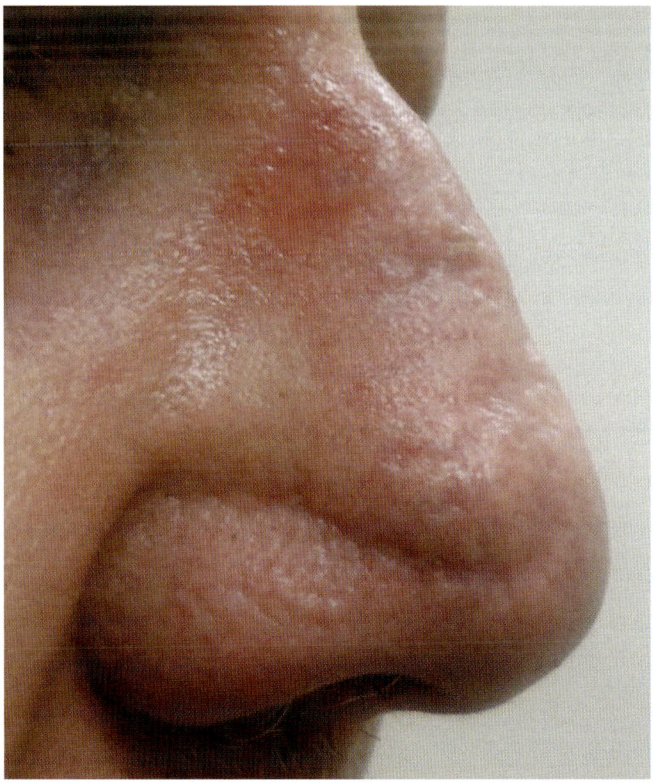

FIGURE 22-14 Pin-cushioning or trapdoor deformity of transposition flap on the nose.

Free Margin Retraction: Free margins are anatomic areas where the skin surface remains unattached to the surrounding tissue. Common free margins on the face are the eyelid, helical rim of the ear, alar rim of the nose, and the vermilion lip. Because they offer little resistance to tension created by surgical reconstruction or scar contracture, free margins are vulnerable to distortion (**Figure 22-15**).

Disruption of these natural contours is both aesthetically displeasing and functionally significant. Ectropion may result in difficulty closing the eyelids with subsequent dry eyes and corneal irritation, alar rim retraction can cause nasal valve obstruction, and eclabium can lead to challenges when creating a tight oral seal.

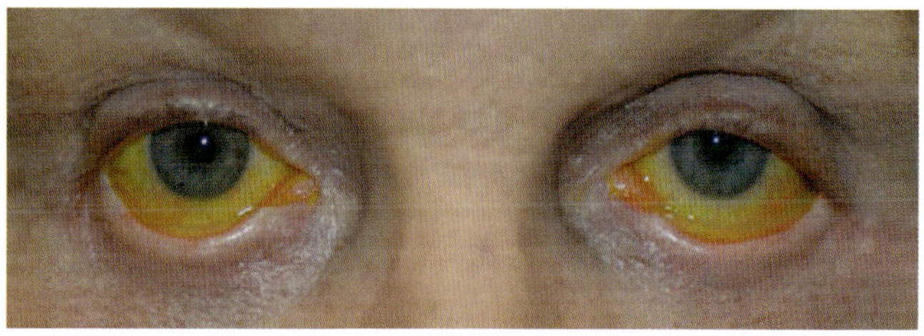

A

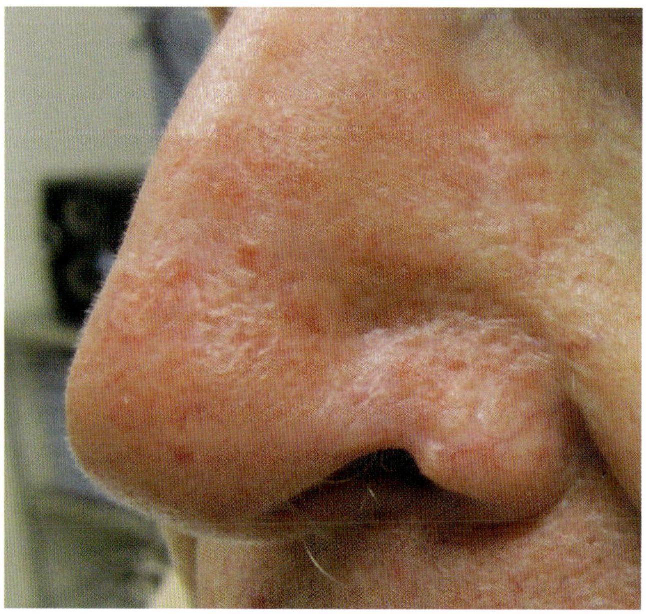

B

FIGURE 22-15 Contracture of a free margin resulting in (**A**) ectropion after lower blepharoplasty and (**B**) alar retraction after interpolated flap necrosis.

To prevent these complications, surgical closures must be designed to minimize tension on the free margin; this is often achieved by orienting closure tension vectors perpendicular to the free margins to avoid "pulling" the free margin out of position.[172] Cartilage grafts may be used to prevent alar rim retraction, and Frost sutures may be used to prevent ectropion in the immediate postoperative period, although they cannot compensate for poorly designed closures.[173] Caution should be used when using second intention healing or when placing skin grafts in locations near a free margin, as clinically significant contraction may occur. Treatment of free margin retraction includes intralesional steroids and scar revision.

SEVERE POSTOPERATIVE RISKS OF DERMATOLOGIC SURGERY

The incidence of catastrophic complications in dermatologic surgery is exceedingly low, but providers should be aware of potential emergent situations so that early detection may mitigate adverse outcomes. Such emergent scenarios include anaphylaxis from type I immune hypersensitivity reactions, cardiac arrhythmias from electrosurgery, and local anesthetic/lidocaine toxicity.[44]

Life-threatening air embolism resulting from the removal of large scalp tumors has been reported in the dermatologic surgery literature.[174,175] Positioning the patient flat during surgery, so as to minimize a pressure gradient, and using airtight dressings between MMS stages helps to prevent this complication.[43] If faced with a potential air embolism, the clinician should immediately refer the patient to a higher level of care, due to the risk of permanent neurologic insult.

Venous thromboembolism, including deep vein thrombosis and pulmonary embolism, is another reported complication after MMS.[176,177] Most cases of deep vein thrombosis and pulmonary embolism after dermatologic surgery have occurred in patients with underlying hypercoagulability who have discontinued anticoagulation perioperatively. Treatment includes anticoagulation, inferior vena cava filters, thrombolysis, and compression stockings.[43]

RISKS TO THE CLINICIAN AND OTHER HEALTH CARE PERSONNEL

Surgical Smoke

Surgical smoke or plume is the gaseous by-product produced by the destruction of human tissue by electrosurgery or other procedures.[178] It is estimated that a Mohs surgeon who performs 1000 cases per year receives approximately 50 hours of continuous smoke exposure per year.[179] Surgical smoke and plume generated by electrosurgery and lasers has been demonstrated to harbor live viruses and bacteria in addition to hazardous chemicals. As a result, the potential exists for infection, carcinogenesis, and pulmonary damage from surgical smoke exposure.[180] Surgeons' exposure to smoke is more concentrated than for other perioperative personnel because they are closest to the tissue destruction. The use of standard surgical masks offers little to no protection against inhalation of surgical smoke. The best protection for surgical personnel is the use of smoke evacuator units during electrosurgery. Integrated cautery and smoke evacuator units are convenient and easy to use, decrease the need for extra staff, and improve patient comfort by aiding in removal the unpleasant odor of surgical smoke.

Sharps Injuries

The Centers for Disease Control and Prevention estimate that more than 380,000 sharps exposures occur annually.[181] Sharps injuries pose an occupational hazard to dermatologists because of the large number of procedures they perform. A 2013 cross-sectional survey of practicing dermatologists and trainees revealed that 85.1% of 336 responders had experienced a needle-stick injury during their career. Importantly, 64% of respondents experienced a sharps injury that they did not report.[182] The most frequently cited reason for not reporting an injury was the belief that the patient was a low risk for a hematologically spread infectious disease. A similar 2016 survey of dermatology residents showed that, of 351 responders, 76% had a sharps injury during training and 34% went unreported.[183] Given the risk of communicable diseases such as hepatitis B virus, hepatitis C virus, and HIV, it is important to promptly report injuries to occupational health services so that appropriate baseline and follow-up testing can be informed and prophylactic medication administered. Improving the ease of access to reporting systems, ensuring anonymity, and encouraging ongoing sharps safety training may increase the prevalence of reporting.[182] In addition, continued efforts to decrease the stigma associated with medical errors are essential.

To prevent sharps injuries in clinicians and other team members, several preoperative, intraoperative and postoperative techniques can be employed.[184] Preoperatively, one should wear protective devices (gloves, masks, protective eyewear, and protective footwear). Intraoperatively, it is important to practice safe handling and transferring of sharp instruments, minimize the use of sharps, and protect from backsplash injuries. When treating patients with known infectious hepatitis or HIV, the use of blunt skin hooks, safety scalpels, safety syringes, smoke evacuators, a separate ink supply during MMS, or 24-hour formalin fixation resulted in no exposures in 188 surveyed Mohs surgeons.[185] Postoperative measures that should be taken include the proper disposal of used sharps.

CONCLUSIONS

The rate of surgical complications in dermatologic procedures is very low, and the rate of serious surgical complications remains vanishingly rare. Adhering to standard safety recommendations may increase the level of safety for clinicians and their patients, and developing protocols for management of surgical complications may help mitigate the severity of these problems when they arise. Critically, patients must be educated preoperatively regarding the risks associated with a given procedure, as managing patient expectations regarding the baseline risk of undesirable outcomes may help foster a team approach to care and management.

REFERENCES

1. American Society for Dermatologic Surgery. ASDS Consumer Survey on Dermatologic Procedures. 2014. https://www.asds.net/Portals/0/PDF/consumer-survey-2014-infographic.pdf. Accessed February 24, 2020.
2. Elliott TG, Thom GA, Litterick KA. Office based dermatological surgery and Mohs surgery: a prospective audit of surgical procedures and complications in a procedural dermatology practice. *Australas J Dermatol.* 2012;53(4):264-271.
3. Alam M, Ibrahim O, Nodzenski M, et al. Adverse events associated with Mohs micrographic surgery: multicenter prospective cohort study of 20,821 cases at 23 centers. *JAMA Dermatol.* 2013;149(12):1378-1385.
4. Newlove T, Cook J. Safety of staged interpolation flaps after Mohs micrographic surgery in an outpatient setting: a single-center experience. *Dermatol Surg.* 2013;39(11):1671-1682.
5. Alam M, Kakar R, Nodzenski M, et al. Multicenter prospective cohort study of the incidence of adverse events associated with cosmetic dermatologic procedures: lasers, energy devices, and injectable neurotoxins and fillers. *JAMA Dermatol.* 2015;151(3):271-277.
6. Delaney A, Diamantis S, Marks VJ. Complications of tissue ischemia in dermatologic surgery. *Dermatol Ther.* 2011;24(6):551-557.
7. Chen DL, Carlson EO, Fathi R, Brown MR. Undermining and hemostasis. *Dermatol Surg.* 2015;41(Suppl 10):S201-S215.
8. Bunick CG, Aasi SZ. Hemorrhagic complications in dermatologic surgery. *Dermatol Ther.* 2011;24(6):537-550.
9. Gillen E, Biley F, Allen D. Effects of music listening on adult patients' pre-procedural state anxiety in hospital. *Int J Evid Based Healthc.* 2008;6(1):24-49.
10. Mitchell M. Patient anxiety and modern elective surgery: a literature review. *J Clin Nurs.* 2003;12(6):806-815.
11. Vaughn F, Wichowski H, Bosworth G. Does preoperative anxiety level predict postoperative pain? *AORN J.* 2007;85(3):589-604.
12. Chen AF, Landy DC, Kumetz E, Smith G, Weiss E, Saleeby ER. Prediction of postoperative pain after Mohs micrographic surgery with 2 validated pain anxiety scales. *Dermatol Surg.* 2015;41(1):40-47.
13. Locke MC, Wilkerson EC, Mistur RL, Nisar M, Love WE. 2015 arte poster competition first place winner: assessing the correlation between patient anxiety and satisfaction for Mohs surgery. *J Drugs Dermatol.* 2015;14(9):1070-1072.
14. Vachiramon V, Sobanko JF, Rattanaumpawan P, Miller CJ. Music reduces patient anxiety during Mohs surgery: an open-label randomized controlled trial. *Dermatol Surg.* 2013;39(2):298-305.
15. Shenefelt PD. Relaxation strategies for patients during dermatologic surgery. *J Drugs Dermatol.* 2010;9(7):795-799.
16. Ravitskiy L, Phillips PK, Roenigk RK, et al. The use of oral midazolam for perioperative anxiolysis of healthy patients undergoing Mohs surgery: conclusions from randomized controlled and prospective studies. *J Am Acad Dermatol.* 2011;64(2):310-322.
17. Robinson JK. *Surgery of the Skin: Procedural Dermatology.* Philadelphia, PA: Elsevier Mosby; 2014.
18. Heller M, Hayes CM, Krejci NC. Paradoxical reaction to midazolam reversed with flumazenil in a patient undergoing tumescent liposuction. *Dermatol Surg.* 2009;35(7):1144-1146.
19. Zbar RI. Identifying and managing those patients at risk for aborted mohs micrographic surgery. *Ann Plast Surg.* 2012;68(1):67-71.
20. Nimigan AS, Gan BS. Pain and efficacy rating of a microprocessor-controlled metered injection system for local anaesthesia in minor hand surgery. *Pain Res Treat.* 2011;2011:362396.
21. Matsumoto AH, Reifsnyder AC, Hartwell GD, Angle JF, Selby JB, Tegtmeyer CJ. Reducing the discomfort of lidocaine administration through pH buffering. *J Vasc Interv Radiol.* 1994;5(1):171-175.
22. Bancroft JW, Benenati JF, Becker GJ, Katzen BT, Zemel G. Neutralized lidocaine: use in pain reduction in local anesthesia. *J Vasc Interv Radiol.* 1992;3(1):107-109.
23. Christoph RA, Buchanan L, Begalla K, Schwartz S. Pain reduction in local anesthetic administration through pH buffering. *Ann Emerg Med.* 1988;17(2):117-120.
24. Hogan ME, vanderVaart S, Perampaladas K, Machado M, Einarson TR, Taddio A. Systematic review and meta-analysis of the effect of warming local anesthetics on injection pain. *Ann Emerg Med.* 2011;58(1):86-98.e81.
25. Zilinsky I, Bar-Meir E, Zaslansky R, Mendes D, Winkler E, Orenstein A. Ten commandments for minimal pain during administration of local anesthetics. *J Drugs Dermatol.* 2005;4(2):212-216.
26. Fosko SW, Gibney MD, Harrison B. Repetitive pinching of the skin during lidocaine infiltration reduces patient discomfort. *J Am Acad Dermatol.* 1998;39(1):74-78.
27. Al-Qarqaz F, Al-Aboosi M, Al-Shiyab D, Al Dabbagh Z. Using cold air for reducing needle-injection pain. *Int J Dermatol.* 2012;51(7):848-852.
28. Scarfone RJ, Jasani M, Gracely EJ. Pain of local anesthetics: rate of administration and buffering. *Ann Emerg Med.* 1998;31(1):36-40.
29. Sobanko JF, Miller CJ, Alster TS. Topical anesthetics for dermatologic procedures: a review. *Dermatol Surg.* 2012;38(5):709-721.
30. Hruza GJ. Anesthesia. *Dermatology.* 3rd ed. Philadelphia, PA: Elsevier Saunders; 2012.
31. To D, Kossintseva I, de Gannes G. Lidocaine contact allergy is becoming more prevalent. *Dermatol Surg.* 2014;40(12):1367-1372.
32. Fathi R, Serota M, Brown M. Identifying and managing local anesthetic allergy in dermatologic surgery. *Dermatol Surg.* 2016;42(2):147-156.
33. Mertes PM, Volcheck GW, Garvey LH, et al. Epidemiology of perioperative anaphylaxis. *Presse Med.* 2016;45(9):758-767.
34. Nagel JE, Fuscaldo JT, Fireman P. Paraben allergy. *JAMA.* 1977;237(15):1594-1595.
35. Fader DJ, Johnson TM. Medical issues and emergencies in the dermatology office. *J Am Acad Dermatol.* 1997;36(1):1-16; quiz 16-18.
36. Dooms-Goossens A, de Alam AG, Degreef H, Kochuyt A. Local anesthetic intolerance due to metabisulfite. *Contact Dermatitis.* 1989;20(2):124-126.
37. Kouba DJ, LoPiccolo MC, Alam M, et al. Guidelines for the use of local anesthesia in office-based dermatologic surgery. *J Am Acad Dermatol.* 2016;74(6):1201-1219.
38. Tetzlaff JE. The pharmacology of local anesthetics. *Anesthesiol Clin North Am.* 2000;18(2):217-233.
39. Asadi-Pooya AA, Nikseresht A, Yaghoubi E. Vasovagal syncope treated as epilepsy for 16 years. *Iran J Med Sci.* 2011;36(1):60-62.

40. Shalom A, Westreich M, Hadad E, Friedman T. Complications of minor skin surgery performed under local anesthesia. *Dermatol Surg.* 2008;34(8):1077-1079.
41. Alam M, Ricci D, Havey J, Rademaker A, Witherspoon J, West DP. Safety of peak serum lidocaine concentration after Mohs micrographic surgery: a prospective cohort study. *J Am Acad Dermatol.* 2010;63(1):87-92.
42. Auroy Y, Narchi P, Messiah A, Litt L, Rouvier B, Samii K. Serious complications related to regional anesthesia: results of a prospective survey in France. *Anesthesiology.* 1997;87(3):479-486.
43. Minkis K, Whittington A, Alam M. Dermatologic surgery emergencies: complications caused by occlusion and blood pressure. *J Am Acad Dermatol.* 2016;75(2):243-262.
44. Minkis K, Whittington A, Alam M. Dermatologic surgery emergencies: complications caused by systemic reactions, high-energy systems, and trauma. *J Am Acad Dermatol.* 2016;75(2):265-284.
45. Denkler K. A comprehensive review of epinephrine in the finger: to do or not to do. *Plast Reconstr Surg.* 2001;108(1):114-124.
46. Firoz B, Davis N, Goldberg LH. Local anesthesia using buffered 0.5% lidocaine with 1:200,000 epinephrine for tumors of the digits treated with Mohs micrographic surgery. *J Am Acad Dermatol.* 2009;61(4):639-643.
47. Fitzcharles-Bowe C, Denkler K, Lalonde D. Finger injection with high-dose (1:1,000) epinephrine: does it cause finger necrosis and should it be treated? *Hand (N Y).* 2007;2(1):5-11.
48. Markovchick V, Burkhart KK. The reversal of the ischemic effects of epinephrine on a finger with local injections of phentolamine. *J Emerg Med.* 1991;9(5):323-324.
49. Khairalla E. Epinephrine-induced digital ischemia relieved by phentolamine. *Plast Reconstr Surg.* 2001;108(6):1831-1832.
50. Hardy SJ, Agostini DE. Accidental epinephrine auto-injector-induced digital ischemia reversed by phentolamine digital block. *J Am Osteopath Assoc.* 1995;95(6):377-378.
51. Bodkin RP, Acquisto NM, Gunyan H, Wiegand TJ. Two cases of accidental injection of epinephrine into a digit treated with subcutaneous phentolamine injections. *Case Rep Emerg Med.* 2013;2013:586207.
52. Krunic AL, Wang LC, Soltani K, Weitzul S, Taylor RS. Digital anesthesia with epinephrine: an old myth revisited. *J Am Acad Dermatol.* 2004;51(5):755-759.
53. Giandoni MB, Vinson RP, Grabski WJ. Ischemic complications of tubular gauze dressings. *Dermatol Surg.* 1995;21(8):716-718.
54. Corre KA, Arnold A. Iatrogenic digital compromise with tubular dressings. *West J Emerg Med.* 2009;10(3):190-192.
55. Spruiell MD, Messina MJ, Mitchell JJ, Scott FA. A deadly digital dressing: a case of surgical decompression for finger ischemia due to circumferential finger dressing. *J Emerg Med.* 2014;46(5):655-658.
56. Norris RL, Gilbert GH. Digital necrosis necessitating amputation after tube gauze dressing application in the ED. *Am J Emerg Med.* 2006;24(5):618-621.
57. Stewart LC, Langtry JA. Clopidogrel: mechanisms of action and review of the evidence relating to use during skin surgery procedures. *Clin Exp Dermatol.* 2010;35(4):341-345.
58. Callahan S, Goldsberry A, Kim G, Yoo S. The management of antithrombotic medication in skin surgery. *Dermatol Surg.* 2012;38(9):1417-1426.
59. Bordeaux JS, Martires KJ, Goldberg D, Pattee SF, Fu P, Maloney ME. Prospective evaluation of dermatologic surgery complications including patients on multiple antiplatelet and anticoagulant medications. *J Am Acad Dermatol.* 2011;65(3):576-583.
60. Shimizu I, Jellinek NJ, Dufresne RG, Li T, Devarajan K, Perlis C. Multiple antithrombotic agents increase the risk of postoperative hemorrhage in dermatologic surgery. *J Am Acad Dermatol.* 2008;58(5):810-816.
61. Dinehart SM, Henry L. Dietary supplements: altered coagulation and effects on bruising. *Dermatol Surg.* 2005;31(7 Pt 2):819-826; discussion 826.
62. Cupp MJ. Herbal remedies: adverse effects and drug interactions. *Am Fam Physician.* 1999;59(5):1239-1245.
63. Chang LK, Whitaker DC. The impact of herbal medicines on dermatologic surgery. *Dermatol Surg.* 2001;27(8):759-763.
64. Collins SC, Dufresne RG. Dietary supplements in the setting of Mohs surgery. *Dermatol Surg.* 2002;28(6):447-452.
65. Ah-Weng A, Natarajan S, Velangi S, Langtry JA. Preoperative monitoring of warfarin in cutaneous surgery. *Br J Dermatol.* 2003;149(2):386-389.
66. Henley J, Brewer JD. Newer hemostatic agents used in the practice of dermatologic surgery. *Dermatol Res Pract.* 2013;2013:279-289.
67. Douketis JD, Spyropoulos AC, Spencer FA, et al. Perioperative management of antithrombotic therapy: Antithrombotic Therapy and Prevention of Thrombosis, 9th ed: American College of Chest Physicians Evidence-Based Clinical Practice Guidelines. *Chest.* 2012;141(2 Suppl):e326S-350S.
68. O'Neill JL, Taheri A, Solomon JA, Pearce DJ. Postoperative hemorrhage risk after outpatient dermatologic surgery procedures. *Dermatol Surg.* 2014;40(1):74-76.
69. Douketis JD, Spyropoulos AC, Kaatz S, et al. Perioperative bridging anticoagulation in patients with atrial fibrillation. *N Engl J Med.* 2015;373(9):823-833.
70. McKee DE, Lalonde DH, Thoma A, Glennie DL, Hayward JE. Optimal time delay between epinephrine injection and incision to minimize bleeding. *Plast Reconstr Surg.* 2013;131(4):811-814.
71. Palm MD, Altman JS. Topical hemostatic agents: a review. *Dermatol Surg.* 2008;34(4):431-445.
72. Howe N, Cherpelis B. Obtaining rapid and effective hemostasis: part II. Electrosurgery in patients with implantable cardiac devices. *J Am Acad Dermatol.* 2013;69(5):677.e671-679.
73. Matzke TJ, Christenson LJ, Christenson SD, Atanashova N, Otley CC. Pacemakers and implantable cardiac defibrillators in dermatologic surgery. *Dermatol Surg.* 2006;32(9):1155-1162; discussion 1162.
74. El-Gamal HM, Dufresne RG, Saddler K. Electrosurgery, pacemakers and ICDs: a survey of precautions and complications experienced by cutaneous surgeons. *Dermatol Surg.* 2001;27(4):385-390.
75. Chapas AM, Lee D, Rogers GS. Excision of malignant melanoma overlying a pacemaker. *Dermatol Surg.* 2005;31(1):112-114.
76. Crawford MH. *Cardiology.* 3rd ed. Philadelphia, PA: Mosby/Elsevier; 2010.
77. Dawes JC, Mahabir RC, Hillier K, Cassidy M, de Haas W, Gillis AM. Electrosurgery in patients with pacemakers/implanted cardioverter defibrillators. *Ann Plast Surg.* 2006;57(1):33-36.

78. Voutsalath MA, Bichakjian CK, Pelosi F, Blum D, Johnson TM, Farrehi PM. Electrosurgery and implantable electronic devices: review and implications for office-based procedures. *Dermatol Surg.* 2011;37(7):889-899.

79. Weyer C, Siegle RJ, Eng GG. Investigation of hyfrecators and their in vitro interference with implantable cardiac devices. *Dermatol Surg.* 2012;38(11):1843-1848.

80. Crossley GH, Poole JE, Rozner MA, et al. The Heart Rhythm Society (HRS)/American Society of Anesthesiologists (ASA) Expert Consensus Statement on the perioperative management of patients with implantable defibrillators, pacemakers and arrhythmia monitors: facilities and patient management this document was developed as a joint project with the American Society of Anesthesiologists (ASA), and in collaboration with the American Heart Association (AHA), and the Society of Thoracic Surgeons (STS). *Heart Rhythm.* 2011;8(7):1114-1154.

81. Arefiev K, Warycha M, Whiting D, Alam M. Flammability of topical preparations and surgical dressings in cutaneous and laser surgery: a controlled simulation study. *J Am Acad Dermatol.* 2012;67(4):700-705.

82. Poore SO, Sillah NM, Mahajan AY, Gutowski KA. Patient safety in the operating room: II. Intraoperative and postoperative. *Plast Reconstr Surg.* 2012;130(5):1048-1058.

83. Kaye AD, Kolinsky D, Urman RD. Management of a fire in the operating room. *J Anesth.* 2014;28(2):279-287.

84. Winslow E, Jacobson A. Dispelling the petroleum jelly myth. *Am J Nursing.* 1998;98(11):16.

85. Smith TL, Smith JM. Electrosurgery in otolaryngology-head and neck surgery: principles, advances, and complications. *Laryngoscope.* 2001;111(5):769-780.

86. Limthongkul B, Samie F, Humphreys TR. Assessment of postoperative pain after Mohs micrographic surgery. *Dermatol Surg.* 2013;39(6):857-863.

87. Firoz BF, Goldberg LH, Arnon O, Mamelak AJ. An analysis of pain and analgesia after Mohs micrographic surgery. *J Am Acad Dermatol.* 2010;63(1):79-86.

88. Morris R, McKay W, Mushlin P. Comparison of pain associated with intradermal and subcutaneous infiltration with various local anesthetic solutions. *Anesth Analg.* 1987;66(11):1180-1182.

89. De Oliveira GS, Castro-Alves LJ, McCarthy RJ. Single-dose systemic acetaminophen to prevent postoperative pain: a meta-analysis of randomized controlled trials. *Clin J Pain.* 2015;31(1):86-93.

90. Moore RA, Derry S, McQuay HJ, Wiffen PJ. Single dose oral analgesics for acute postoperative pain in adults. *Cochrane Database Syst Rev.* 2011;9:CD008659.

91. Glass JS, Hardy CL, Meeks NM, Carroll BT. Acute pain management in dermatology: risk assessment and treatment. *J Am Acad Dermatol.* 2015;73(4):543-560; quiz 561-562.

92. Toms L, McQuay HJ, Derry S, Moore RA. Single dose oral paracetamol (acetaminophen) for postoperative pain in adults. *Cochrane Database Syst Rev.* 2008;4:CD004602.

93. Imani F, Motavaf M, Safari S, Alavian SM. The therapeutic use of analgesics in patients with liver cirrhosis: a literature review and evidence-based recommendations. *Hepat Mon.* 2014;14(10):e23539.

94. McIntyre BA, Philp RB, Inwood MJ. Effect of ibuprofen on platelet function in normal subjects and hemophiliac patients. *Clin Pharmacol Ther.* 1978;24(5):616-621.

95. Lawrence C, Sakuntabhai A, Tiling-Grosse S. Effect of aspirin and nonsteroidal antiinflammatory drug therapy on bleeding complications in dermatologic surgical patients. *J Am Acad Dermatol.* 1994;31(6):988-992.

96. Chen T, Adamson PA. Comparison of ibuprofen and acetaminophen with codeine following cosmetic facial surgery. *J Otolaryngol Head Neck Surg.* 2009;38(5):580-586.

97. Sniezek PJ, Brodland DG, Zitelli JA. A randomized controlled trial comparing acetaminophen, acetaminophen and ibuprofen, and acetaminophen and codeine for postoperative pain relief after Mohs surgery and cutaneous reconstruction. *Dermatol Surg.* 2011;37(7):1007-1013.

98. Hurst EA, Yu SS, Grekin RC, Neuhaus IM. Bleeding complications in dermatologic surgery. *Semin Cutan Med Surg.* 2007;26(1):40-46.

99. Salasche SJ. Acute surgical complications: cause, prevention, and treatment. *J Am Acad Dermatol.* 1986;15(6):1163-1185.

100. Tønnesen H, Nielsen PR, Lauritzen JB, Møller AM. Smoking and alcohol intervention before surgery: evidence for best practice. *Br J Anaesth.* 2009;102(3):297-306.

101. Goldminz D, Bennett RG. Cigarette smoking and flap and full-thickness graft necrosis. *Arch Dermatol.* 1991;127(7):1012-1015.

102. Boyer JD, Zitelli JA, Brodland DG. Undermining in cutaneous surgery. *Dermatol Surg.* 2001;27(1):75-78.

103. Bennett RG. Selection of wound closure materials. *J Am Acad Dermatol.* 1988;18(4 Pt 1):619-637.

104. Moy RL, Waldman B, Hein DW. A review of sutures and suturing techniques. *J Dermatol Surg Oncol.* 1992;18(9):785-795.

105. Salasche SJ, Grabski WJ. Complications of flaps. *J Dermatol Surg Oncol.* 1991;17(2):132-140.

106. Kantor J. The fascial plication suture: an adjunct to layered wound closure. *Arch Dermatol.* 2009;145(12):1454-1456.

107. Rosengren H, Dixon A. Antibacterial prophylaxis in dermatologic surgery: an evidence-based review. *Am J Clin Dermatol.* 2010;11(1):35-44.

108. Rossi AM, Mariwalla K. Prophylactic and empiric use of antibiotics in dermatologic surgery: a review of the literature and practical considerations. *Dermatol Surg.* 2012;38(12):1898-1921.

109. Shurman DL, Benedetto AV. Antimicrobials in dermatologic surgery: facts and controversies. *Clin Dermatol.* 2010;28(5):505-510.

110. Chan BC, Patel DC. Perioperative management and the associated rate of adverse events in dermatological procedures performed by dermatologists in New Zealand. *Australas J Dermatol.* 2009;50(1):23-28.

111. Maragh SL, Brown MD. Prospective evaluation of surgical site infection rate among patients with Mohs micrographic surgery without the use of prophylactic antibiotics. *J Am Acad Dermatol.* 2008;59(2):275-278.

112. Futoryan T, Grande D. Postoperative wound infection rates in dermatologic surgery. *Dermatol Surg.* 1995;21(6):509-514.

113. Huether MJ, Griego RD, Brodland DG, Zitelli JA. Clindamycin for intraincisional antibiotic prophylaxis in dermatologic surgery. *Arch Dermatol.* 2002;138(9):1145-1148.

114. Wright TI, Baddour LM, Berbari EF, et al. Antibiotic prophylaxis in dermatologic surgery: advisory statement 2008. *J Am Acad Dermatol.* 2008;59(3):464-473.

115. Mailler-Savage EA, Neal KW Jr, Godsey T, Adams BB, Gloster HM Jr. Is levofloxacin necessary to prevent postoperative infections of auricular second-intention wounds? *Dermatol Surg.* 2008;34(1):26-30; discussion 30-31.

116. Altemeier WA, Culbertson WR, Hummel RP. Surgical considerations of endogenous infections: sources, types, and methods of control. *Surg Clin North Am.* 1968;48(1):227-240.

117. Wood LD, Warner NM, Billingsley EM. Infectious complications of dermatologic procedures. *Dermatol Ther.* 2011;24(6):558-570.

118. Baba T, Takeuchi F, Kuroda M, et al. Genome and virulence determinants of high virulence community-acquired MRSA. *Lancet.* 2002;359(9320):1819-1827.

119. García-Casares E, Mateo Soria L, García-Melchor E, et al. Necrotizing fasciitis and myositis caused by streptococcal flesh-eating bacteria. *J Clin Rheumatol.* 2010;16(8):382-384.

120. Abolnik IZ, Sexton DJ. Necrotizing fasciitis and myositis caused by group A streptococci. Epidemiology, diagnosis, and treatment of "flesh-eating bacteria." *N C Med J.* 1994;55(10):464-466.

121. Bisno AL, Stevens DL. Streptococcal infections of skin and soft tissues. *N Engl J Med.* 1996;334(4):240-245.

122. Gibbon KL, Bewley AP. Acquired streptococcal necrotizing fasciitis following excision of malignant melanoma. *Br J Dermatol.* 1999;141(4):717-719.

123. Huntley AC, Tanabe JL. Toxic shock syndrome as a complication of dermatologic surgery. *J Am Acad Dermatol.* 1987;16(1 Pt 2): 227-229.

124. Bosley AR, Bluett NH, Sowden G. Toxic shock syndrome after elective minor dermatological surgery. *BMJ.* 1993;306(6874):386-387.

125. Stevens DL, Bisno AL, Chambers HF, et al. Practice guidelines for the diagnosis and management of skin and soft tissue infections: 2014 update by the infectious diseases society of America. *Clin Infect Dis.* 2014;59(2):147-159.

126. Dizer B, Hatipoglu S, Kaymakcioglu N, et al. The effect of nurse-performed preoperative skin preparation on postoperative surgical site infections in abdominal surgery. *J Clin Nurs.* 2009;18(23):3325-3332.

127. Webster J, Osborne S. Preoperative bathing or showering with skin antiseptics to prevent surgical site infection. *Cochrane Database Syst Rev.* 2015;2:CD004985.

128. Tanner J, Norrie P, Melen K. Preoperative hair removal to reduce surgical site infection. *Cochrane Database Syst Rev.* 2011;11:CD004122.

129. Moro ML, Carrieri MP, Tozzi AE, Lana S, Greco D. Risk factors for surgical wound infections in clean surgery: a multicenter study. Italian PRINOS Study Group. *Ann Ital Chir.* 1996;67(1):13-19.

130. Smack DP, Harrington AC, Dunn C, et al. Infection and allergy incidence in ambulatory surgery patients using white petrolatum vs bacitracin ointment. A randomized controlled trial. *JAMA.* 1996;276(12):972-977.

131. Rogers HD, Desciak EB, Marcus RP, Wang S, MacKay-Wiggan J, Eliezri YD. Prospective study of wound infections in Mohs micrographic surgery using clean surgical technique in the absence of prophylactic antibiotics. *J Am Acad Dermatol.* 2010;63(5):842-851.

132. Mehta D, Chambers N, Adams B, Gloster H. Comparison of the prevalence of surgical site infection with use of sterile versus nonsterile gloves for resection and reconstruction during Mohs surgery. *Dermatol Surg.* 2014;40(3):234-239.

133. Xia Y, Cho S, Greenway HT, Zelac DE, Kelley B. Infection rates of wound repairs during Mohs micrographic surgery using sterile versus nonsterile gloves: a prospective randomized pilot study. *Dermatol Surg.* 2011;37(5):651-656.

134. Nasseri E. Prospective study of wound infections in Mohs micrographic surgery using a single set of instruments. *Dermatol Surg.* 2015;41(9):1008-1012.

135. Moorhead C, Torres A. I PREVENT bacterial resistance. an update on the use of antibiotics in dermatologic surgery. *Dermatol Surg.* 2009;35(10):1532-1538.

136. American Dental Association, American Academy of Orthopaedic Surgeons. Advisory statement. Antibiotic prophylaxis for dental patients with total joint replacements. *J Am Dent Assoc.* 1997;128(7):1004-1008.

137. American Dental Association, American Academy of Orthopaedic Surgeons. Antibiotic prophylaxis for dental patients with total joint replacements. *J Am Dent Assoc.* 2003;134(7):895-899.

138. Wilson W, Taubert KA, Gewitz M, et al. Prevention of infective endocarditis: guidelines from the American Heart Association: a guideline from the American Heart Association Rheumatic Fever, Endocarditis, and Kawasaki Disease Committee, Council on Cardiovascular Disease in the Young, and the Council on Clinical Cardiology, Council on Cardiovascular Surgery and Anesthesia, and the Quality of Care and Outcomes Research Interdisciplinary Working Group. *Circulation.* 2007;116(15):1736-1754.

139. Hendi A. Temporal nerve neuropraxia and contralateral compensatory brow elevation. *Dermatol Surg.* 2007;33(1):114-116.

140. Agarwal CA, Mendenhall SD, Foreman KB, Owsley JQ. The course of the frontal branch of the facial nerve in relation to fascial planes: an anatomic study. *Plast Reconstr Surg.* 2010;125(2):532-537.

141. Baker DC, Conley J. Avoiding facial nerve injuries in rhytidectomy. Anatomical variations and pitfalls. *Plast Reconstr Surg.* 1979;64(6):781-795.

142. Arden RL, Sinha PK. Vertical suture plication of the orbicularis oris muscle: a simple procedure for the correction of unilateral marginal mandibular nerve paralysis. *Facial Plast Surg.* 1998;14(2):173-177.

143. Ramírez OM. Advanced considerations determining procedure selection in cervicoplasty. Part one: anatomy and aesthetics. *Clin Plast Surg.* 2008;35(4):679-690, viii.

144. Humphrey S, Sykes J, Kantor J, et al. ATX-101 for reduction of submental fat: a phase III randomized controlled trial. *J Am Acad Dermatol.* 2016;75(4):788-797.e787.

145. Regula CG, Yag-Howard C. Suture products and techniques: what to use, where, and why. *Dermatol Surg.* 2015;41(Suppl 10): S187-S200.

146. Regan T, Lawrence N. Comparison of poliglecaprone-25 and polyglactin-910 in cutaneous surgery. *Dermatol Surg.* 2013;39(9):1340-1344.

147. Kantor J. The set-back buried dermal suture: an alternative to the buried vertical mattress for layered wound closure. *J Am Acad Dermatol.* 2010;62(2):351-353.

148. Wang AS, Kleinerman R, Armstrong AW, et al. Set-back versus buried vertical mattress suturing: results of a randomized blinded trial. *J Am Acad Dermatol.* 2015;72(4):674-680.

149. Butler L, Mowad C. Allergic contact dermatitis in dermatologic surgery: review of common allergens. *Dermatitis.* 2013;24(5): 215-221.

150. McShane DB, Bellet JS. Treatment of hypergranulation tissue with high potency topical corticosteroids in children. *Pediatr Dermatol.* 2012;29(5):675-678.

151. Mandrea E. Topical diflorasone ointment for treatment of recalcitrant, excessive granulation tissue. *Dermatol Surg.* 1998;24(12):1409-1410.

152. Sobanko JF, Sarwer DB, Zvargulis Z, Miller CJ. Importance of physical appearance in patients with skin cancer. *Dermatol Surg.* 2015;41(2):183-188.

153. Alster TS. Improvement of erythematous and hypertrophic scars by the 585-nm flashlamp-pumped pulsed dye laser. *Ann Plast Surg.* 1994;32(2):186-190.

154. Dierickx C, Goldman MP, Fitzpatrick RE. Laser treatment of erythematous/hypertrophic and pigmented scars in 26 patients. *Plast Reconstr Surg.* 1995;95(1):84-90; discussion 91-92.

155. Thomas JR, Somenek M. Scar revision review. *Arch Facial Plast Surg.* 2012;14(3):162-174.

156. Murray JC. Keloids and hypertrophic scars. *Clin Dermatol.* 1994;12(1):27-37.

157. Sidgwick GP, McGeorge D, Bayat A. A comprehensive evidence-based review on the role of topicals and dressings in the management of skin scarring. *Arch Dermatol Res.* 2015;307(6):461-477.

158. Hayashi T, Furukawa H, Oyama A, et al. A new uniform protocol of combined corticosteroid injections and ointment application reduces recurrence rates after surgical keloid/hypertrophic scar excision. *Dermatol Surg.* 2012;38(6):893-897.

159. Balaraman B, Geddes ER, Friedman PM. Best reconstructive techniques: improving the final scar. *Dermatol Surg.* 2015;41(Suppl 10):S265-S275.

160. Park TH, Seo SW, Kim JK, Chang CH. Outcomes of surgical excision with pressure therapy using magnets and identification of risk factors for recurrent keloids. *Plast Reconstr Surg.* 2011;128(2):431-439.

161. Yamawaki S, Naitoh M, Ishiko T, Muneuchi G, Suzuki S. Keloids can be forced into remission with surgical excision and radiation, followed by adjuvant therapy. *Ann Plast Surg.* 2011;67(4):402-406.

162. Wang LZ, Ding JP, Yang MY, Chen B. Forty-five cases of chest keloids treated with subcutaneous super-tension-reduction suture combined with postoperative electron-beam irradiation. *Dermatol Surg.* 2014;40(12):1378-1384.

163. Gladsjo JA, Jiang SI. Treatment of surgical scars using a 595-nm pulsed dye laser using purpuric and nonpurpuric parameters: a comparative study. *Dermatol Surg.* 2014;40(2):118-126.

164. Ren Y, Zhou X, Wei Z, Lin W, Fan B, Feng S. Efficacy and safety of triamcinolone acetonide alone and in combination with 5-fluorouracil for treating hypertrophic scars and keloids: a systematic review and meta-analysis. *Int Wound J.* 2017;14(3):480-487.

165. van Drooge AM, Vrijman C, van der Veen W, Wolkerstorfer A. A randomized controlled pilot study on ablative fractional CO2 laser for consecutive patients presenting with various scar types. *Dermatol Surg.* 2015;41(3):371-377.

166. Berman B, Flores F. Comparison of a silicone gel-filled cushion and silicon gel sheeting for the treatment of hypertrophic or keloid scars. *Dermatol Surg.* 1999;25(6):484-486.

167. Berman B, Flores F. Recurrence rates of excised keloids treated with postoperative triamcinolone acetonide injections or interferon alfa-2b injections. *J Am Acad Dermatol.* 1997;37(5 Pt 1):755-757.

168. Rusciani L, Paradisi A, Alfano C, Chiummariello S, Rusciani A. Cryotherapy in the treatment of keloids. *J Drugs Dermatol.* 2006;5(7):591-595.

169. Yang S, Ozog D. Comparison of traditional superficial cutaneous sutures versus adhesive strips in layered dermatologic closures on the back: a prospective, randomized, split-scar study. *Dermatol Surg.* 2015;41(11):1257-1263.

170. Kaufman AJ, Kiene KL, Moy RL. Role of tissue undermining in the trapdoor effect of transposition flaps. *J Dermatol Surg Oncol.* 1993;19(2):128-132.

171. Koranda FC, Webster RC. Trapdoor effect in nasolabial flaps. Causes and corrections. *Arch Otolaryngol.* 1985;111(7):421-424.

172. Etzkorn JR, Sobanko JF, Miller CJ. Free margin distortion with fusiform closures: the apical angle relationship. *Dermatol Surg.* 2014;40(12):1428-1432.

173. Guyuron B. Alar rim deformities. *Plast Reconstr Surg.* 2001;107(3):856-863.

174. Goldman G, Altmayer S, Sambandan P, Cook JL. Development of cerebral air emboli during mohs micrographic surgery. *Dermatol Surg.* 2009;35(9):1414-1421.

175. Kantor J. Risk of cerebral air emboli associated with calvarial fenestration. *Dermatol Surg.* 2016;42(7):907-908.

176. Sukal SA, Geronemus RG. Deep venous thrombosis following Mohs micrographic surgery: case report. *Dermatol Surg.* 2008;34(3):414-417.

177. Alam M, Goldberg LH. Serious adverse vascular events associated with perioperative interruption of antiplatelet and anticoagulant therapy. *Dermatol Surg.* 2002;28(11):992-998; discussion 998.

178. Bigony L. Risks associated with exposure to surgical smoke plume: a review of the literature. *AORN J.* 2007;86(6):1013-1020; quiz 1021-1024.

179. Oganesyan G, Eimpunth S, Kim SS, Jiang SI. Surgical smoke in dermatologic surgery. *Dermatol Surg.* 2014;40(12):1373-1377.

180. Bell ML, Zanobetti A, Dominici F. Evidence on vulnerability and susceptibility to health risks associated with short-term exposure to particulate matter: a systematic review and meta-analysis. *Am J Epidemiol.* 2013;178(6):865-876.

181. Phillips EK, Conaway MR, Jagger JC. Percutaneous injuries before and after the Needlestick Safety and Prevention Act. *N Engl J Med.* 2012;366(7):670-671.

182. Donnelly AF, Chang YH, Nemeth-Ochoa SA. Sharps injuries and reporting practices of U.S. dermatologists. *Dermatol Surg.* 2013;39(12):1813-1821.

183. Nambudiri VE, Qureshi AA, Vleugels RA. Sharps injuries among US dermatology trainees: a cross-sectional study. *J Am Acad Dermatol.* 2016;74(4):756-758.

184. Alghamdi KM, Alkhodair RA. Practical techniques to enhance the safety of health care workers in office-based surgery. *J Cutan Med Surg.* 2011;15(1):48-54.

185. LoPiccolo MC, Balle MR, Kouba DJ. Safety precautions in Mohs micrographic surgery for patients with known blood-borne infections: a survey-based study. *Dermatol Surg.* 2012;38(7 Pt 1):1059-1065.

PART III

Cosmetic Procedures

The Cosmetic Consultation

23

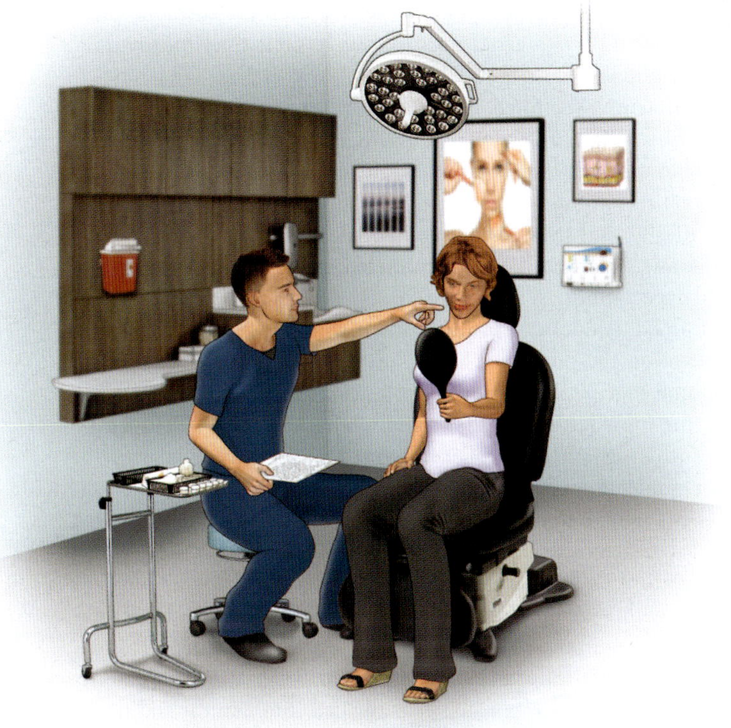

SUMMARY

- The demand for cosmetic procedures, both invasive and noninvasive, is increasing dramatically.
- A thorough consultation is invaluable for patient education and comfort.
- Patients vary widely in their desires and expectations, and the consultation is the ideal time to tease out a patient's individual preferences.

Beginner Tips

- The interaction with the front desk sets the stage for everything that follows.
- Etiquette for a clinician's office staff must be similar to that seen in high-level hotels or retail stores.

Pitfalls and Cautions

- Patient expectations must be set by the clinician with both clinical and financial boundaries: the patient who expects to pay for one syringe of a filler but requires at least six syringes to attain the desired result will not be satisfied.
- Body dysmorphic disorder is the most common psychiatric condition seen in patients seeking cosmetic procedures.

Expert Tips

- A cosmetic interest questionnaire that lists problems and procedures the patient wants to discuss helps to streamline the consultation.
- Use a variant of responsive listening—repeating back to the patient what he or she expressed to the nurse or assistant in the preliminary interview.

Patient Education Points

- Be clear that nonsurgical procedures can provide excellent, but still not surgical, results.
- A clinician must say "no" to any treatment they believe is medically or aesthetically inadvisable.

Don't Forget!

- The appearance of the reception area is particularly important when treating cosmetic patients.
- The public generally does not understand that surgery may be less expensive than the combination of nonsurgical procedures necessary to produce desirable results.

Billing Pearls

- Do not automatically write off procedure fees or offer reimbursement without checking with your malpractice carrier; returning money to a patient prior to discussion with your carrier could negate your insurance coverage if the incident is litigated.

23 The Cosmetic Consultation

INTRODUCTION

Every interaction between a clinician's office and the patient represents both opportunity and risk. Opportunities for the clinician include solidifying the practice and provider's credentials and expertise, establishing rapport and trust, and highlighting the possible benefits for the patient. At the same time, risks include discouraging the patient from seeing the provider through less-than-stellar customer service, portraying the practice in an unprofessional light, and giving off an air of unavailability and aloofness that will likely result in a cancelled appointment—or frustrated new patient. Therefore, spending extra time training the office staff in best practices for patient management, and particularly for new patient management, often pays significant dividends.[1-3]

PATIENT INTERACTIONS

The first contact a prospective patient has with the office is with office staff, whether by phone, online, or in person. That interaction will set the stage for everything else that follows. Phone calls and emails must be answered promptly. The volume of phone calls received by medical offices has increased up to 50% over the past decade as patients seek help managing approvals for prescriptions (which may be needed even for cosmetic procedures) and try to avoid doctor visits by soliciting information by telephone.[4]

Any employee hired for direct patient contact on the phone must be polite, professional, and friendly, and have the ability to remain calm. Etiquette for clinician's office staff must be similar to that seen in high-level hotels or retail stores (**Table 23-1**).[5]

Ideally, staff speaking with potential patients should be knowledgeable regarding the services offered, the clinicians, and financial expectations. When new procedures are added, staff must be informed: it does not inspire patient confidence if the first staff person on the phone has never heard of the procedure. Do not assume that patients know the clinician's qualifications: talking up the provider during that initial phone call can make the difference in whether the caller becomes a patient. Many offices do not quote procedure prices by phone. However, the incoming patient must be informed of consult cost, the scope of the visit, and whether there is a possibility of additional fees if procedures are performed on that day. Callers must have the opportunity to speak with someone in detail about upcoming procedures, especially if they may be performed on the date of the consult. Some practices cross-train all employees to have that discussion. At other times, staff responsibility is divided into clinical and nonclinical groups, and therefore, excellent communication between them is critical.

TABLE 23-1 • Phone Etiquette

Basic Phone Etiquette When Scheduling the Cosmetic Consult

1. Never let the phone ring more than 3 times before picking up.
2. When answering, speak clearly and smile. Smiling while on the phone helps keep your tone positive.
3. Identify yourself and the office and ask for the name of the caller, like: "Hello, Dr. Jones Cosmetics. This is Jane. To whom am I speaking?"
4. Repeat the caller's name and ask the reason for the call: "Hello, Mrs. Smith. How may I help you today?" Be sure to take notes with the patient's name and contact information while speaking in case the call is lost.
5. If the call cannot be taken immediately, do not place the caller on hold before asking and receiving permission to do so. "Mrs. Smith, I apologize that I am on another line. May I put you on hold briefly?"
6. If you know it will be a long wait on hold, instead offer to call the patient back. "Mrs. Smith, I don't want to keep you waiting. May I take your information and get back to you?" And return the call as promised.
7. If the caller asks a question for which you do not have the answer, be honest. "Mrs. Smith, I apologize that I can't answer that question for you, but I will have our cosmetic coordinator return your call. She can explain everything." Or "I will ask the doctor as soon as she is between patients and get back to you."
8. When transferring phone calls to other staff members, be sure to share the name of the patient so they too can start with the patient's name. "Mrs. Smith, this is Kathy, Dr. Jones's nurse. Jane said you had some questions for me before setting up your appointment."
9. Always get the best number (and an alternate) and the best time to have a call returned to the caller, especially if a manager or another team member must return the call.
10. Always thank the caller for his or her time and patience.
11. When possible, let the caller hang up first, and if using a receiver, hang up the phone gently.

THE OFFICE

When new patients arrive for a cosmetic consult, they should feel welcomed. The area for patient check-in should be clearly marked and situated so the patient sees the receptionist's smiling face on initial entry. If the receptionist is not yet ready to take care of a patient, or if there will be a delay before seeing the clinician, a smile, apology, and the offer of a beverage or snack while waiting are generally appreciated. If the wait will be significant, staff should be instructed to call patients before they arrive; this conveys to patients that the office values their time.

The appearance of the reception area is particularly important when treating cosmetic patients, as it is a reflection of the clinician's aesthetic. At the most basic level, it should be clean and uncluttered with enough personal space for the patient to check in with a sense of privacy. A smooth and organized flow from reception to waiting room or rest room and then examination or procedure room adds to the new patient's foundation of trust for the office.

Office décor should reflect the clinician's brand, location, and patient base. A beautiful cosmetic office in Arizona may have a southwestern theme with muted tones and stone; one in New Orleans, crystal and glass; and in New York, ultramodern spare white and oak. An office catering primarily to men might choose to include sports-themed memorabilia. Millennials may prefer a high-tech environment. Walking into the office may also give a sense of the clinician and can incorporate their hobbies or interests, whether by displaying photos of travel, Hollywood memorabilia, or midcentury furniture.

The color palette is also important. Studies in the fields of design, marketing, and branding have revealed strong connections between color and emotional and even physical reactions, an effect termed *chromodynamics*. Colors are considered cool or warm based on their respective association with water and sky (blues) or the sun (reds). Red, yellow, and orange are "high arousal" colors and may raise blood pressure. Blues, greens, and violets are "low arousal" colors that tend to calm and relax. Particular colors are associated with psychological characteristics and traits, such as red for both war and love, green for nature and healing, and blue for stability and trust.[6] Color combinations can trigger responses based on where the reflected light hits the retina. Color fatigue is a pulsating or vibrating effect caused by conflicting signals coming from the optic nerve when seeing adjacent bright complementary colors.[6]

New patients are often excited and anxious. The choice of color for your office entry, reception, and waiting areas can act in one of three ways: active, passive, or neutral. The stimulatory effect of a red waiting room would not be ideal. Pale yellow used as an accent may be soothing and make the occupant feel happy, but too much has been shown to make people more likely to feel frustrated and lose their temper. Blues may reduce blood pressure, although some pale blues may appear chilly or impersonal.[7]

Research has shown that the average time spent in any doctor's waiting room is 21 minutes.[8] An uncomfortable space will make the wait seem longer. Chairs or couches should be easy to get in and out of without assistance, and there should be surfaces on which to put a beverage. A cosmetic practice may make the patient feel more cared for by having a beverage or snack area. Information about procedures offered and products sold can be accessible but not cluttered. Depending on the patient population and personal preferences of the clinician, offices may also provide up-to-date popular magazines, interesting coffee table books, computer monitors with educational information, or television monitors.[9]

THE CONSULT

Preparation

The past medical history and list of medications are as important for a cosmetic consult as for any medical visit.[10] Whether patients fill out these forms online via a patient portal or in the office, the nurse or medical assistant must review details with the patient to make sure it is complete. The medication list must include both prescriptions and over-the-counter medications, vitamins, and supplements. Allergies and sensitivities must be noted where they will be visible on each visit. The clinician must be aware of the patient's general health, past procedures, or underlying conditions. Patients are generally unaware of the anticoagulant effect of fish oil and baby aspirin, but it can be significant when using injectables.[11] Patients with history of herpes simplex virus may require antiviral prophylaxis for facial or genital procedures. A predisposition to keloid formation is a relative contraindication to injecting poly-l-lactic acid and to some surgical procedures or may require preplanning postprocedure interventions. Radiofrequency or ultrasound heating should not be used over an untreated hernia and might also be problematic over surgical mesh from a herniorrhaphy. Staff must be aware of procedure-specific concerns and highlight them in the patient record.

Equally important is a detailed history of past cosmetic procedures. Patients frequently forget (or decline) to include cosmetic procedures in their surgical history. Rhinoplasty, even if done 30 years earlier, can have implications on vascular anatomy and, therefore, on safe filler injection. Seeing how a patient healed after rhytidectomy or abdominoplasty is informative. Staff must question patients about prior treatment with botulinum toxin, filling agents, lasers, other energy-based devices, suture or thread lifts, chemical peels, noninvasive fat reduction, and cosmetic surgery. In addition to eliciting approximate dates the procedures were done, questions should include product used, provider of the service or procedure, and patient satisfaction. Most patients do not know the exact filler or toxin injected, but if injection was done by a reputable clinician, it is a reasonable assumption that it was US Food and Drug Administration (FDA) approved, and if needed, records can be obtained. The distinction is medically important when planning future treatment: injecting filler over some permanent fillers not available in the United States can ignite an inflammatory, nodular, or infectious reaction. Moreover, for those with excess or inappropriately placed filler, knowing it if it is a hyaluronic acid gel determines whether hyaluronidase injection will be helpful. Finding out whether the patient was happy with the results—and why—helps the clinician determine if realistic expectations can be achieved. The patient's current skincare regimen and experience with retinoids, hydroquinone, or other common ingredients also should be documented in order to maximize results and to provide postprocedure instructions.

A cosmetic interest questionnaire that lists problems and procedures the patient wants to discuss helps to streamline the consultation (**Figure 23-1**). If appropriate, it allows the nurse, medical assistant, or cosmetic coordinator doing the initial patient interview to begin to review potential procedures offered in the office. An associated question is: "Why now?" Is the cosmetic improvement being sought to prepare for an upcoming event like a wedding, to recover from a serious life event like a divorce, or to feel better after an illness like cancer? This facilitates a smoother visit once the patient is brought in the room.

After review of the medical and cosmetic history and patient's cosmetic interests, the patient should be prepared for the clinician. That may include the patient removing facial makeup, pulling hair away from the face, or changing into an examination gown. Some offices take photos at this time, whereas others wait until immediately before the procedure. These preparations save time for the clinician who can now focus on the patient.

PATIENT NAME____ DATE_______________________

Are there other conditions/services we provide that interest you? [YES] [NO].

If NO, end here IF YES, please CIRCLE all that apply:

I AM INTERESTED IN FINDING OUT MORE ABOUT TREATMENT OPTIONS FOR:

Skin discoloration	Facial lines, wrinkles	Facial sagging	Looking "old" and/or "tired"
Dull looking skin	Dark circles under eyes	Drooping brows or eyelids	Sagging skin body
Blotchy skin	Undereye "bags" or puffiness	Sunken cheeks and/or temples	Unwanted fat
Uneven skin tone	Frown lines between brows	Jowels, jaw drooping	Loss of contour abdomen, hips, thighs, buttocks
Large pores	Forehead lines	Turkey neck	Excessive sweating
Rough skin texture	Nasolabial folds or "parentheses"	Thin lips	Stretch marks
Skin discoloration	Lip lines	Unwanted "moles"	Acne scars
Age spots/brown spots	Marionette lines	Hands "look old"	Surgical or traumatic scars
Red spots/spider veins	Nose shape	Unwanted hair	Keloid scars
Face and/or neck redness	Neck and/or chest lines/wrinkles	Leg veins	Unwanted tattoos

I AM INTERESTED IN FINDING OUT MORE ABOUT THE FOLLOWING TREATMENT(S):

Skin products/skin regimen	Botox, Dysport, Xeomin for lines and wrinkles	Fraxel laser for photoaging (wrinkles, discoloration)
VBeam lasers for red spots and spider vessels	Fine line orwrinkle treatment with fillers	Fraxel laser for scars or stretch marks
QsNd:YAG lasers for brown spots	Facial contour restoration with fillers	Thermage tissue tightening
IPL (photofacial) for red and brown spots	Lower lid tear trough correction with fillers	Coolsculpting or Kybella noninvasive fat reduction
Clear & brilliant for pores, fine lines, dull skin	Lip restoration with fillers	Sclerotherapy for leg veins
Microdermabrasion or chemical peels	Laser hair removal	Cosmetic mole removal

WHEN LOOKING AT MYSELF IN THE MIRROR, COMPARED TO MY TRUE AGE, I BELIEVE I LOOK:

Younger than my age	--------------------------	My age	--------------------------	Older than my age
1	2	3	4	5

FIGURE 23-1 The cosmetic questionnaire.

Evaluation

A successful consult—one that converts an interested consumer into a patient—rests on the rapport between the clinician and patient. Before entering the examination room, clinician and staff should put cell phones on silent to minimize distraction. If the clinician knows she will be interrupted for an expected phone call, explain and apologize to the patient in advance. Even if there is only one clinician in the office, the clinician should introduce herself to the patient on entering. Older studies suggested that patients prefer to be called by their last name, but this may have changed, along with the transformation of "doctor" and "patient" to "healthcare provider" and "consumer," respectively.[12] A safe standard is to refer to the patient by last name until she or he says otherwise. Taking the time to sit down during the consultation rather than standing has been shown to have a positive effect on the doctor-patient relationship.[13]

The single most important factor in establishing a good relationship with the patient is to listen. Despite the inclination to get the answers via rapid fire questions, speak slowly, use open-ended questions, and let the patient speak. If time is of the essence, use a variant of responsive listening—repeating back to the patient what he or she expressed to the nurse or assistant in the preliminary interview; for example, "My nurse Tina and I reviewed your conversation. My understanding is that you are most concerned about your jowls." This defines the clinician's assistants as part of the team and lets the patient know that the team has heard their concerns.[14] After reviewing the history, hand the patient a hand mirror and ask for him or her to point out major concerns. This keeps the focus on what the concern is, rather than on one specific treatment option about which that the patient may have heard.[10,15]

After reviewing the pertinent history and establishing the patient's concerns, it is time for the clinician evaluation. For most noninvasive cosmetic dermatology procedures, it is best to examine the patient sitting upright or standing in order to see the effect of gravity. Look at the patient from multiple angles and gently palpate, pull, and pinch tissue as needed and ask the patient to make expressions. Include additional physical examination as appropriate for the specific procedures being considered. Document pertinent negatives, such as the absence of thyromegaly or umbilical hernia during a consult for submental or abdominal fat reduction, respectively.

Recommendations

The clinician's recommendations should be based on the patient's physical, social, and economic concerns. Sometimes the answer is straightforward, such as treating facial telangiectasias with a series of vascular laser or intense pulsed light treatments. More often, achieving the requested results noninvasively will require a combination of procedures to volumize, relax, resurface, tighten, or lift. If you think referral for surgery is appropriate, find out if it is a consideration, and if not, why not. Be clear that nonsurgical procedures can provide excellent, but still not surgical, results. The public generally does not understand that surgery may be less expensive than the combination of nonsurgical procedures necessary to produce results. Patient expectations must be set by the clinician with both clinical and financial boundaries. A patient who expects to pay for one syringe of a filler but requires at least six syringes to get to the desired result will not be satisfied.

Today, most patients arrive for consultation after having already researched procedures on individual clinician, specialty, academy, industry, informational, and community websites. While educational, these sites also provide opinion boards for dissatisfied patients. The clinician bears the burden not only of explaining their own recommendations, but of dispelling common myths. Be prepared to explain what you expect the procedure will achieve for that particular patient, how it is performed, the number of times it must be performed and at what interval, the expected degree of discomfort, down time and posttreatment care expected, and risks involved. If multiple procedures are being considered, explain why one is recommended or why the patient might prefer one over the other. If there are multiple procedures, design a reasonable plan that balances the patient's priorities with what you as the expert think will make the most significant improvement in appearance within the patient's health, time, and budget constraints. In addition, be prepared if asked to let the patient know how many of each of those procedure you have done: Is it your bread and butter everyday type, or is it something new that you have just started but in which you feel quite comfortable, and why?[16] Finally, be clear that every procedure has benefits and risks and that there are no guarantees of outcome.

The time required for adequate explanation may be more than the clinician has available during a busy schedule. Engaging assistants who regularly work with you and know your thought process to begin the consultation during their preliminary patient interview provides a frame of reference for understanding. When in the room with the patient, be present, face the patient, and show that you are actively listening and remembering.[14] The clinician and staff should use similar language that is easily understandable to a layperson and provides a consistent message. Use of visual paper or digital educational resources developed by the doctor, specialty association, and/or industry may be helpful. After the clinician provides specific recommendations, he or she can leave the room (without appearing to rush out) in order for the staff to review the details.

THE DIFFICULT PATIENT

Most successful aesthetic clinicians gain personal and job satisfaction from knowing they have many appreciative, long-time patients who refer family and friends, thereby increasing the circle of happiness. However, patients, like doctors, are as diverse as the world population. Especially in the field of aesthetics, personality, appearance, communication skills, and appearance can attract or repel a prospective patient regardless of clinical skills. Thus, no clinician is going to be the perfect fit for everyone. Conversely, there are times when the patient is not the perfect fit for the clinician. A clinician must say "no" to any treatment they believe is medically or aesthetically inadvisable. The clinician will be held responsible for any complication, and a bad aesthetic result, even if it is what the patient wants, is the worst advertisement for your practice.

During the consultation, the clinician and staff can screen patients by noting the patient's verbal and nonverbal cues. These may suggest the patient will not be satisfied with the clinician, office, or procedure. There are also patients who must be approached carefully because of mental illness. One study found that up to 47.7% of patients seeking cosmetic surgery in a Japanese plastic surgery center between 1980 and 1997 met the criteria for a mental disorder.[17] Not all mental disease is a contraindication for cosmetic procedures, and there are many patients without diagnosable mental illness who should be treated only with extreme caution. What follows are four common categories of "difficult" patients seen in aesthetic practice and guidelines for how to manage them.

Body Dysmorphic Patients

Body dysmorphic disorder (BDD) is the most common psychiatric condition seen in patients seeking cosmetic procedures.[12] *The Diagnostic and Statistical Manual of Mental Disorders*, fifth edition (DSM-V) defines BDD as "distress due to a perceived physical anomaly."[18] In a literature review, it was estimated that 6% to 15% of patients presenting for treatment in a surgical dermatology practice suffer from body dysmorphia.[19] Another article noted that BDD occurs in 2.4% of the US population and makes up 2% to 7% of patients in cosmetic surgery practices and 9% to 15% in dermatology practices.[20] Although cosmetic practices generally see more female than male patients, body dysmorphia is equally common in both men and women in outpatient mental health settings.[19,20] Any area of the body may be the focus of concern, although the most common BDD complaints involve the skin (eg, scarring), hair, and nose.[20] Because these patient concerns are "perceived" rather than real, it is not surprising that few patients are satisfied with any treatment: one study reported 75% of BDD patients being dissatisfied with their results.[21]

The easiest way to screen for BDD during the consultation is to have the patient point out concerns while looking in a mirror. Confirm that you see what the patient sees. Unfortunately, some patients have a more subtle presentation of BDD. The issue may not become apparent until follow-up to a procedure while reviewing before and after photos. Whenever it becomes clear that a patient is not able to see what the clinician and staff see, it is time to discontinue additional treatment. Tell the patient that unfortunately you are not seeing what she sees, and as such, you are unable to change it. Suggest that another aesthetic clinician may serve her better. An official discharge from the practice is usually not necessary, just your empathetic acknowledgement that you wish you could help but you cannot, although check with your malpractice carrier regarding the advisability of discharging the patient from the practice.[20]

The Overly Anxious Patient

The overly anxious patient is generally benign but may be the most time-consuming and emotionally draining type of patient. This patient repeats the same questions before every decision, despite similar repeated detailed answers given by the clinician and staff. Some excessively anxious patients just require reassurance. However, informed consent requires that the patient has had all of her questions answered. Determining whether the patient wants the clinician to make the decision for her or whether she is not ready for the procedure can sometimes be difficult. If unsure, suggest that the patient return another day after thinking about it further. Both clinician and staff should be prepared for frequent calls before and after any procedure. Most important, despite the frustration of having to repeat the same information, everyone must treat the patient with kindness and seriousness.[22]

The Haggler Patient

The increased competition for patient dollars has given rise to the commoditization of aesthetic procedures. Advertised specials by "syringe" or "cycle" and bundled procedure deals promoted through online sites give rise to "doctor shoppers"—patients who choose an office based on the price rather than the clinician. Although there are certainly patients who initially find a clinician through a discount and remain because of the results, most doctor shoppers switch providers based on the latest deal. Since they usually insist on getting prices before coming in for a consult, refusing to publish your procedure prices is an effective screening tool.

The more difficult are the patients who routinely "haggle" over price. While clinician offices can set their own prices for services not covered by third-party payors and certainly can give a discount or free services, ethics and practicality require reasonably standardized pricing. Some people feel entitled to a deal, while others complain that they cannot afford the doctor's prices and should receive a discount. To those patients, say with kindness that you understand that cosmetic procedures are a luxury item and your staff will be happy to help figure out if there is a plan that fits their budget. Other patients do not value the clinician's time. Explain that the cost is based on the clinician's years of training and experience, as well as the cost of product that is used. The patient who values the clinician, staff, and office will generally understand at this point.[23,24]

The Angry Patient

This category of patients is generally the most difficult. Anger due to an understandable reason, such as a clerical error or the clinician running significantly late, must be respected in order to salvage the doctor-patient relationship. The clinician and/or involved staff should apologize and reassure the patient that the office considers the patient their priority and will address those concerns. A token gift, such as a cosmeceutical, may drive home the clinician's sincerity.

Unfortunately, the patient who is irrationally angry is harder to manage. This patient wants to create a scene and may become abusive to the office staff even before seeing the clinician. In this case, the first priority is to move the patient calmly and smoothly from the public to a private area, such as an examination room, office manager's office, or even the staff break room if no other room is available.[24] Ideally, if a procedure has already been done, staff should take photos to document results. As quickly as possible, the clinician accompanied by a staff member should be with the patient and listen. The patient must have the opportunity to vent without interruption. Instead of becoming defensive, the physician should practice responsive listening. A technique of summarizing what was said by the other person, responsive listening shows that person you were listening and confirms to both parties that you understand. Striking a balance of calm strength and empathy without condescension is not easy when listening to someone degrade you and your office. Do not take it personally. And be very careful with your apology: remember that saying you are sorry that your office was not able to make the patient happy may help defuse the situation without being a legal admission of guilt. It may be easiest to write off your consult fee in this situation. Do not automatically write off procedure fees or offer reimbursement without checking with your malpractice carrier. Returning money to a patient prior to discussion with your carrier can negate your insurance coverage if the incident turns into a legal case. Finally, be sure the patient is led out of the office expeditiously. If it would be helpful to document further clinical results, suggest the patient return before or after normal patient office hours. If it is necessary to discharge the patient from your practice, your carrier should be able to provide you with a template letter that includes the reason, referral information to a local medical society (so the patient can find another clinician), and a records release form. Depending on your state, you will likely need to offer to see the patient for follow-up or emergencies related to any procedure done for a reasonable period of time (usually 30 days).[25,26]

CONCLUSION

A successful encounter between clinician and patient involves the interplay of various factors beyond procedural recommendations. The office setting, staff communication skills, and perceived attention from the clinician combine to create a successful cosmetic consult that launches a long-term clinician-patient relationship.

REFERENCES

1. American Society of Surgical Dermatology. ASDS survey: twice as many considering cosmetic procedures. https://www.asds.net/_Media.aspx?id=9576&terms=asds%20survey%202016. Accessed February 27, 2017.
2. The American Society for Aesthetic Plastic Surgery. American Society for Aesthetic Plastic Surgery reports more than $13.5 billion spent for the first time ever. Statistics, surveys, and trends 2016. http://www.surgery.org/media/news-releases/american-society-for-aesthetic-plastic-surgery-reports-more-than-135-billion-spent-for-the-first-time-ever. Accessed December 20, 2016.
3. Quora. Who said: "You never get a second chance to make a first impression!"? https://www.quora.com/Who-said-You-never-get-a-second-chance-to-make-a-first-impression. Accessed February 27, 2017.
4. Wieczner J. The doctor won't take your call. Market Watch. http://www.marketwatch.com/story/the-doctor-wont-take-your-call-2013-07-16. Accessed January 19, 2017.
5. Angeles S. Customer service 101: phone etiquette for small businesses. Business News Daily. May 20, 2014. http://www.businessnewsdaily.com/6444-call-center-phone-etiquette.html/. Accessed January 19, 2017.
6. Przybyla D. The psychology and meaning of colors. ColorPsychology.org. http://www.colorpsychology.org. Accessed January 19, 2017.
7. Pantone. Color psychology: how does color affect us. https://www.pantone.com/color-psychology-how-does-color-affect-us. Accessed December 20, 2016.
8. Vitals. How long will you wait at your next doctor's appointment? http://www.vitals.com/about/wait-time. Accessed February 27, 2017.
9. Mihai. Room color and how it affects your mood. Freshome. http://freshome.com/room-color-and-how-it-affects-your-mood/. Accessed January 18, 2017.
10. Werschler P, Calkin J, Lamb D, Mauricio T, Narurkar V, Rich P. Aesthetic dermatologic treatments: consensus from the experts. *J Clin Aesthet Dermatol.* 2015;8(10):S2-S7.
11. Doctors Health Press. Stop taking herbs before surgery. April 20, 2006. http://www.doctorshealthpress.com/heart-health-articles/stop-taking-herbs-before-surgery. Accessed February 27, 2017.
12. Gillette R, Filak A, Thorne C. First name or last name: which do patients prefer? *J Am Board Fam Pract.* 1992;5:517-522.
13. Swayden KJ, Anderson K, Connelly L, Moran J, McMahon J, Arnold P. Effect of sitting vs standing on perception of provider time at bedside: a pilot study. *Patient Educ Couns.* 2012;86(2):166-171.
14. Larsen B. Six listening techniques that can change everything. Standard Examiner. October 22, 2014. http://www.standard.net/Success-Strategies/2014/10/22/6-listening-techniques-that-can-change-everything. Accessed February 26, 2017.
15. Hilton L. The "art" of the cosmetic consult. *Dermatology Times.* November 10, 2016. http://dermatologytimes.modernmedicine.com/dermatology-times/news/art-cosmetic-consult. Accessed February 26, 2017.
16. American Board Cosmetic Surgery. What to ask a cosmetic surgeon: 5 essential questions to ask at your cosmetic surgery consult. September 29, 2014. http://www.americanboardcosmeticsurgery.org/5-essential-questions-for-cosmetic-surgery-consult/. Accessed February 26, 2017.
17. Ishigook J, Iwao M, Suzuki M. Dermographic features of patients seeking cosmetic surgery. *Psychiatry Clin Neurosci.* 1998;52:283-287.
18. American Psychiatric Association. *Diagnostic and Statistical Manual of Mental Disorders.* 5th ed. Washington, DC: American Psychiatric Association; 2013.
19. Malick F, Howard J, Koo J. Understanding the psychology of the cosmetic patients. *Dermatol Ther.* 2008;21:47-53.
20. Medscape. Never-ending cosmetic surgeries—the patient with body dysmorphic disorder: an expert interview with Eva Ritvo, MD. July 20, 2010. http://www.medscape.com/viewarticle/725216. Accessed February 27, 2017.
21. Wilson JB, Erpey CJ. Body dysmorphic disorder: suggestions for detection and treatment in a surgical dermatology practice. *Dermatol Surg.* 2004;30:1391-1399.
22. GP Online. Consultation skills: consultations with anxious patients. December 3, 2008. http://www.gponline.com/consultation-skills-consultations-anxious-patients/article/866068. Accessed February 27, 2017.

23. Sacopulos M. Video: how to handle hagglers and other tough patients. Modern Aesthetics. http://modernaesthetics.com/tv/?f=how-to-deal-with-hagglers-and-other-tough-patients. Accessed February 27, 2017.

24. Waldorf H. Video: the difficult patient part 2. Modern Aesthetics. http://modernaesthetics.com/tv/?f=the-difficult-patient-part-2. Accessed February 27, 2017.

25. Waldorf H. Video: the difficult patient. Modern Aesthetics. http://modernaesthetics.com/tv/?f=the-difficult-patient. Accessed February 27, 2017.

26. HPSO. Handling the angry patient. http://www.hpso.com/risk-education/individuals/articles/Handling-the-Angry-Patient#. Accessed February 27, 2017.

24 Botulinum Toxin

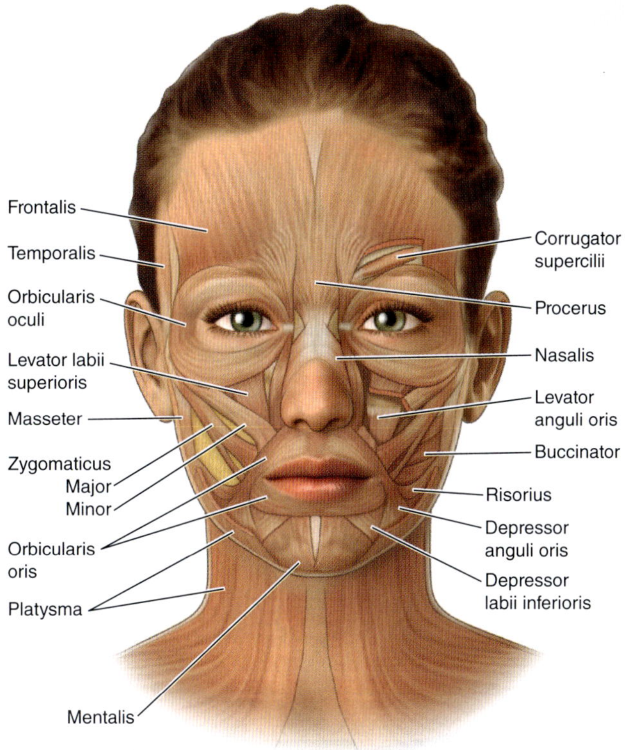

SUMMARY

- The most popular dermatologic uses of BTX include the reduction of facial rhytides, facial contouring, and treatment of focal hyperhidrosis. It is commonly used for the following areas of the face:
  - Upper face
    - Glabellar lines
    - Lateral canthal lines
    - Horizontal forehead lines
    - Bunny lines
    - Infraorbital region
  - Lower face
    - Nasal tip droop
    - Nasal flare
    - Perioral rhytides
    - Depressor anguli oris
    - Hypertrophic masseters
    - Excessive gum show
    - Wrinkled chin

Beginner Tips

- Expert consensus guidelines recommend that a vial of BTX can be refrigerated or refrozen for at least 4 weeks before injection without significant risk for contamination or decreased effectiveness, and that a single vial can be used to treat multiple patients, assuming appropriate handling.
- Using preservative-containing sterile normal saline for reconstitution significantly reduces subsequent injection pain and is therefore recommended.

Pitfalls and Cautions

- Cultural and ethnic norms should also be taken into account when tailoring individual treatments, as desires and expectations can vary significantly between these diverse populations.
- Inferolateral extension of lateral canthal lines down toward and across the zygoma should not be "chased" with BTX due to the risk of facial asymmetry.

Expert Tips

- Variations in muscular patterns in the upper face are well established, and studies have demonstrated that targeted individualized treatment delivers superior outcomes.
- Due to the interrelationship between the facial musculature, it is useful to conceptualize the upper and lower face as global treatment regions rather than focus on a specific area such as the glabella or lateral canthus. This mindset promotes the goal of achieving a harmonious, balanced, natural, and aesthetically pleasing outcome.

Patient Education Points

- Important areas to consider include: establishment of realistic goals, assessment of desired treatment area, understanding of expectations and potential side effects, written informed consent, and photographic documentation.
- Photographic documentation is highly recommended for both pre- and posttreatment status.

Don't Forget!

- Simple mechanical distraction administered by an assistant tapping on the patient's shoulder or forehead during injections is a highly effective and efficient way to decrease injection pain.
- Brow ptosis is especially common in those with smaller foreheads, naturally low brows, minimal frontalis bulk, or with a tendency to overutilize the frontalis muscle for brow elevation during facial expressions.

24 Botulinum Toxin

INTRODUCTION

Botulinum toxin (BTX) has revolutionized the practice of aesthetic medicine. When appropriately injected, its safety, efficacy, reproducibility, and overall satisfaction are exceptional.

Although the toxin itself was isolated in the 1940s, early work with BTX for medical purposes began in the 1970s and 1980s with the pioneering research of Alan Scott on strabismus and blepharospasm. Experiments in monkeys[1] laid the groundwork for successful clinical trials in humans.[2,3] In 1989, BTX received US Food and Drug Administration (FDA) approval for blepharospasm and nystagmus.

In parallel with the above efforts, the ophthalmologist-dermatologist, wife-husband team of Jean and Alastair Carruthers made an unexpected discovery: a subject being treated for blepharospasm in a clinical trial reported that BTX therapy also seemed to give her an untroubled, unworried appearance.[4] Seizing upon this observation, the Carruthers explored the potential of BTX therapy for aesthetic concerns and published their initial work in 1992.[5] This report spawned the ensuing decades of research and refinement of the dermatologic uses for BTX. In the present day, BTX therapy forms a cornerstone in the clinician's armamentarium for facial rejuvenation and beyond.

Types of BTX

In the United States, there are currently three BTX type A preparations that are FDA approved for dermatologic use: onobotulinumtoxin (ONA; Botox Aesthetic, Allergan), abobotulinumtoxin (ABO; Dysport Aesthetic, Galderma), and incobotulinumtoxin (INCO; Xeomin, Merz), as well as one BTX type B preparation that is FDA approved for cervical dystonia (rimabotulinumtoxin, Myobloc, Elan Corp, Dublin, Ireland). Other BTX preparations are available in different regions of the world. Types of BTX are summarized in **Table 24-1**.

BTX: Structure and Function

Seven different serotypes of BTX exist and are labeled A, B, C_1, D, E, F, and G. All serotypes exhibit a similar molecular structure. The toxin is produced as an inactive 150-kDa single-chain protein that undergoes tissue proteolysis to form a 100-kDa heavy chain and a 50-kDa light chain, which serves as a zinc-dependent protease. This di-chain complex is held together by a disulfide bond. The active molecule has a variety of different effects including inhibition of the presynaptic neuromuscular junction, alteration of fibroblast function, and modification of skin mechanical properties.

Neuromodulation

The most well-known function of BTX is its inhibition of acetylcholine (Ach) release at the presynaptic neuromuscular junction. This mechanism of action involves three discrete stages: binding, internalization, and prevention of neurotransmitter release.[6] Both the 50-kDa and 100-kDa active components have unique roles in these stages. Binding of the presynaptic receptor is triggered by the 100-kDa heavy chain, which then induces receptor-mediated endocytosis for internalization of the molecule. Once internalized, the 50-kDa light chain cleaves proteins that facilitate the docking of Ach at the presynaptic membrane, thus inhibiting its release. BTX serotypes A, C, and E cleave synaptosome-associated protein-25 (SNAP-25), and serotypes B, D, F, and G cleave vesicle-associated membrane protein (VAMP).

This presynaptic inhibition is temporary. Reversal occurs in two phases, explaining the gradual loss of clinical efficacy.[7,8] First, de novo nerve terminals sprout from the existing parent terminal

TABLE 24-1 • Botulinum Toxins Approved by the US Food and Drug Administration (FDA)

	Botox	Dysport	Xeomin	Myobloc
Generic name	OnabotulinumtoxinA	AbobotulinumtoxinA	IncobotulinumtoxinA	RimabotulinumtoxinB
Active substance	Botulinum toxin type A	Botulinum toxin type A	Botulinum toxin type A	Botulinum toxin type B
FDA indication	Blepharospasm, cervical dystonia, hyperhidrosis, temporary correction of glabellar and lateral canthal hyperdynamic rhytides	Cervical dystonia, temporary correction of glabellar hyperdynamic rhytides, upper and lower limb spasticity	Cervical dystonia, temporary correction of glabellar hyperdynamic rhytides, blepharospasm, upper limb spasticity	Cervical dystonia
Mechanism of action	SNAP-25	SNAP-25	SNAP-25	VAMP
Total antigen load	5 ng/100 units	5 ng/100 units	0.6 ng/100 units	100 ng/10,000 units

axon during the first 28 days after BTX exposure, leading to the establishment of a nascent neuromuscular junction. Following this first phase, the parent terminal axon gradually synthesizes new SNAP-25 proteins with simultaneous regression and elimination of the new sprouts. This second phase takes place over the next 3 months, which explains why the effects of BTX tend to dissipate around this time frame.

Hyperhidrosis

Although the mechanism of action of BTX in the setting of focal hyperhidrosis has not been fully elucidated, it is likely analogous to its action at the neuromuscular junction. Focal hyperhidrosis is caused in part by an overactivity of the postganglionic sympathetic sudomotor C fibers innervating the eccrine sweat glands.[9,10] These sudomotor terminals contain Ach as well as other co-transmitters such as vasoactive intestinal peptide (VIP) and calcitonin gene-related peptide (CGRP). By blocking Ach transmission, BTX therapy inhibits eccrine overstimulation and therefore alleviates hyperhidrosis.[11,12] As with the neuromuscular junction, chemodenervation with subsequent neural sprouting and reinnervation explain the clinical efficacy and impermanence of this treatment, although the timing of these events may follow a more prolonged course.[13]

Dermal Remodeling

Aside from the effects of muscular paralysis and sweat gland denervation, BTX therapy has also been observed to promote a global antiaging effect and to have a potentially positive impact on scar tissue remodeling. In vitro studies have shed some light onto these phenomena. When normal human fibroblasts were cultured in the presence of BTX, upregulation of collagen-1 and collagen-3 protein expression measured by enzyme-linked immunosorbent assay (ELISA) was detected in a dose-dependent fashion. Concurrently, downregulation of matrix metalloproteinases (MMP)-1 and -3 was also observed.[14,15] These cellular effects likely contribute to alterations in skin mechanical properties such as elasticity and pliability following BTX treatment.[16-18] Fibroblasts derived from hypertrophic scars, however, may respond differently to BTX than normal, nonscar fibroblasts. In this specific cell population, BTX has an inhibitory effect, which may account for its utility in facilitating scar remodeling.[19,20] It is important to note that the above data are largely preliminary, and conflicting evidence exists. Further research into these pathways is required.

The Immunology of BTX

Neutralizing antibodies against BTX can decrease or abolish clinical efficacy of the treatment. The development of these antibodies correlates with total antigen load, defined as the combined amount of neurotoxin product, complexing proteins, and residual proteins. A higher total antigen load increases the risk of antibody development. For example, ONA was originally formulated with a total antigen load of 25 ng per 100 units, which was subsequently reduced to 5 ng per 100 units. Patients treated with the original formulation (prior to 1998) were six times more likely to have neutralizing antibodies than those who received the newer formulation.[21] Of the three FDA-approved BTX type A formulations currently available, INCO has the lowest total antigen load at 0.44 ng per 100 units.[22] However, due to the small total antigen loads in all current formulations, the clinical relevance of this distinction is unknown.

CLINICAL APPLICATION OF BTX THERAPY

Successful BTX therapy depends on appropriate knowledge of anatomy and medication effects, preparation of product, and injection technique.

Product Preparation

Reconstitution and storage of the product play an important role in achieving maximal safety and efficacy. Original recommendations from the manufacturer, as well as Centers for Disease Control and Prevention (CDC) guidelines, suggested that BTX be used within 4 hours of reconstitution and that each vial should only be used to treat a single patient. However, multiple clinical studies have since established that refrigerated storage after reconstitution for periods of weeks does not decrease efficacy,[23-26] freeze-thawing of reconstituted BTX is allowable,[27] mechanical agitation does not damage the active molecule,[28] use of a single vial for multiple patients with appropriate precautions does not increase infectious risk,[29] and prolonged storage of reconstituted product under appropriate conditions does not lead to detectable microbial growth.[30] Expert consensus guidelines therefore recommend that a vial of BTX can be refrigerated or refrozen for at least 4 weeks before injection without significant risk for contamination or decreased effectiveness and that a single vial can be used to treat multiple patients, assuming appropriate handling.[31,32] Other important considerations regarding the preparation of BTX include the reconstitution medium and different reconstitution techniques for different commercial preparations. Using preservative-containing sterile normal saline for reconstitution significantly reduces subsequent injection pain and is therefore recommended.[33,34] Particular attention needs to be paid to INCO vials, which require both swirling and inversion of the vial in order to dissolve all of the product within.[35] INCO is also unique among current FDA-approved BTX-A preparations in that room temperature storage (25°C) for 1 week appears to have no impact on treatment efficacy.[36] Volume of dilution in clinical practice ranges from 1 to 10 mL per vial, with 2.5 to 3 mL being most commonly employed.[37] Variations in dilution do not impact efficacy as long as absolute number of units remains equivalent,[38] although injection of smaller volumes promotes more precise technique.[39]

Preoperative Assessment

Prior to initiating BTX treatment, the patient must be thoroughly assessed for contraindications and educated in terms of goals and expectations. Contraindications to BTX include the following:

1. Known hypersensitivity to BTX or any of the components in the formulation
2. Active infection at the injection site

3. Neuromuscular diseases such as myasthenia gravis, Eaton-Lambert syndrome, or amyotrophic lateral sclerosis, which may increase risk of generalized muscle weakness, diplopia, ptosis, dysphonia, dysarthria, severe dysphagia, and respiratory symptoms
4. Pregnancy and lactation (pregnancy category C)

Patient education remains one of the most crucial steps to the success of any dermatologic surgical procedure. First-time BTX patients may arrive with a variety of preconceptions, and it is the responsibility of the clinician to provide safe and appropriate guidance toward achieving individual goals. Important areas to consider include establishment of realistic goals, assessment of desired treatment area, understanding of expectations and potential side effects, written informed consent, and photographic documentation.

First, priority should be given to developing trust and rapport with the patient and a thorough understanding of their treatment goals. At this stage, it is important to identify patients who may have an element of body dysmorphism, as this syndrome has a small but significant prevalence in cosmetic offices.[40] Treatment of patients with unrealistic goals should be avoided.

Next, a careful evaluation of the treatment area should be conducted with the patient being an active participant in the examination. One effective technique is to have the patient look into a handheld mirror while explaining the difference and interrelation between dynamic and static rhytides. It is important for the patient to understand that improvements in dynamic rhytides will likely be swift and sure, but static lines will often require multiple treatments over a more prolonged time course. By actively engaging the patient in this assessment and conversation, the clinician can also highlight the long-term benefits of BTX therapy in the treatment of facial rhytides.[41] In almost all cases of BTX treatment, clinical effects will be temporary, and repeated treatment sessions will be required to maintain or achieve a certain aesthetic goal. This remains an important concept to explain during patient education. Simple side effects such as bruising and swelling should always be mentioned, whereas discussion of other complications should be guided in a focused manner in keeping with the patient's baseline clinical status and the specific type of BTX treatment being administered. The clinician should always leave ample time for answering patient questions and concerns.

Once the patient has been thoroughly educated and a treatment plan agreed upon, written informed consent should always be obtained. Photographic documentation is highly recommended for both pre- and posttreatment status and can be obtained either by standard digital photography or dedicated imaging devices. In the case of facial rhytid treatment, it is often useful to schedule a 2-week follow-up appointment, at which time minor touch ups (if required) can be administered. This can also help to avoid unnecessary patient anxiety during the immediate postoperative period when the treatment begins taking effect. After treatment, patients should be counseled to avoid lying down, manipulating the area, or undergoing strenuous physical activity for a period of 4 hours. In-office ice packs can be offered to decrease swelling.

Treatment

The most popular dermatologic uses of BTX include the reduction of facial rhytides, facial contouring, and treatment of focal hyperhidrosis. However, BTX can also have pleasing effects on the neck and chest, scars and wounds, preexisting or iatrogenic facial palsies and asymmetries, body contouring, and skin boosting.

Injection Technique: The patient is seated upright or slightly tilted for comfort in an examination chair with an elevated head rest. Prior to injection, the skin should be cleansed with an antiseptic agent such as 70% alcohol or 4% chlorhexidine gluconate. The treatment area should be identified and muscular patterns may be marked with a skin marker. Each patient potentially presents with subtle anatomic differences, and these should guide the clinician in delivering optimally tailored treatment regimens. Variations in muscular patterns in the upper face are well established,[42,43] and studies have demonstrated that targeted individualized treatment delivers superior outcomes.[44] Some injectors advocate the use of real-time imaging aids to identify and avoid vasculature while injecting so as to minimize the possibility of bruising, although there is no evidence to suggest an impact on outcomes.[45] Additionally, ultrasound examination may be helpful to guide injections directly into muscle bellies.[46] For the majority of patients, these adjunctive techniques are unnecessary for successful treatment.

Several techniques may be used to decrease injection pain, including application of ice pack just prior to injection, cold air prior to and during injection, mechanical distraction, or topical anesthesia. Simple mechanical distraction administered by an assistant tapping on the patient's shoulder or forehead during injections is a highly effective and efficient way to decrease injection pain. In general, BTX should be delivered intramuscularly, although due to diffusion, perimuscular or subcutaneous placement of medication may sometimes be acceptable.[47,48] For most facial applications, the optimal needle for injection is a 32-gauge 0.3-mL insulin syringe (Becton, Dickinson and Company, Franklin Lanes, NJ), although other needles may be used as well.

Due to the interrelationship between the facial musculature, it is useful to conceptualize the upper and lower face as global treatment regions rather than focus on a specific area such as the glabella or lateral canthus. This mindset promotes the goal of achieving a harmonious, balanced, natural, and aesthetically pleasing outcome.

Upper Face: Treatment of the upper face includes the glabella, the lateral canthus, the forehead, the infraorbit, and the bunny lines.

Glabellar Frown Lines: The glabellar frown lines form secondary to hyperactivity of the procerus, corrugator supercilii, and depressor supercilii muscles. Treatment in this area can relax these wrinkles and relieve a habitually angry or displeased expression. Three to five injection points should be used depending on the patient's presenting muscular pattern (**Figure 24-1**). One study demonstrated no additional benefit

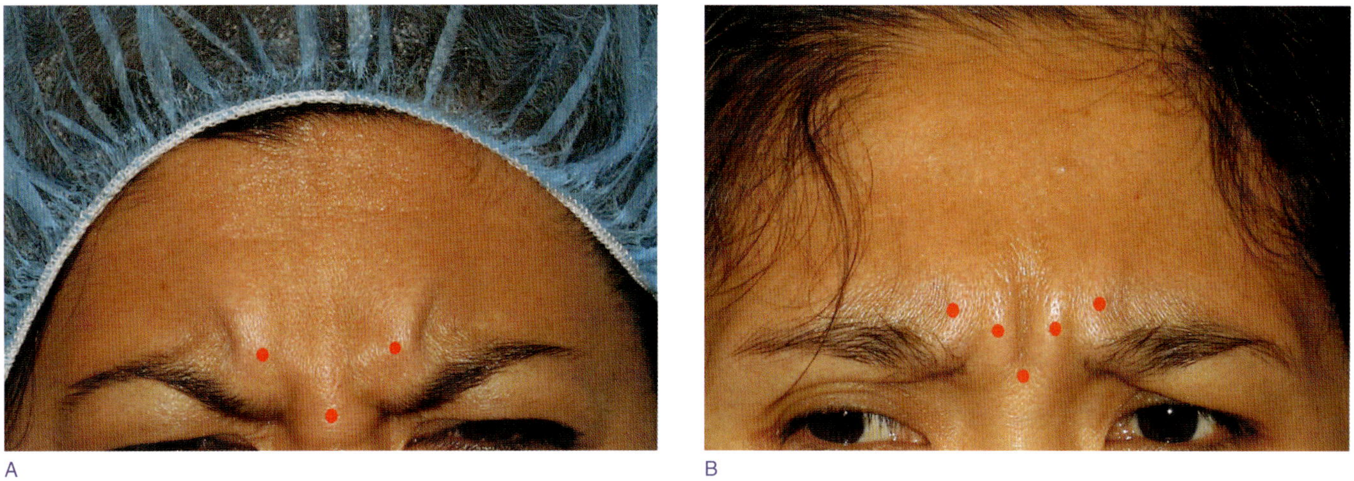

FIGURE 24-1 Patterns of glabellar injection. By analyzing the patient's anatomical predisposition, the appropriate number of injection points can be determined. (**A**) Three injection points. (**B**) Five injection points.

to five injection points over three.[49] In order to limit complications such as ptosis, injections should be placed medial to the mid-pupillary line and 1 cm above the eyebrow. A typical starting dose for the majority of patients is 20 units of ONA,[50] 50 units of ABO,[51] or 20 units of INCO.[52] Use of lesser amounts of medication has been correlated with reduced effect duration and patient satisfaction.[53-56] However, the most important guiding principle for treatment dosage remains the clinical assessment of what is required to achieve a certain aesthetic goal (**Figure 24-2**).

There are several considerations when treating glabellar frown lines. Men tend to require higher dosages due to increased muscular activity.[57] Race does not have an impact on treatment efficacy.[58-60] Isolated treatment of glabellar frown lines can lead to dramatic, and sometimes unwanted, changes in eyebrow position,[61] which can be balanced with treatment of the forehead and/or lateral canthus. The long-term benefits of repeated glabellar frown line treatments at regular intervals include reduction of static rhytides and improvement in skin texture and quality.[62-64]

Lateral Canthal Lines: Excessive lateral canthal lines (sometimes referred to as "crow's feet") can give the impression of an aged and tired appearance. They are secondary to hyperactivity of the orbicularis oculi muscle and typically present as a fan-shaped pattern radiating from the lateral canthal region.[42] Treatment with BTX in this area should be delivered in one to five injection points that are placed superficially 1 to 1.5 cm lateral to the orbital rim (**Figure 24-3**). Given the heterogeneity canthal line patterns, injections should be customized

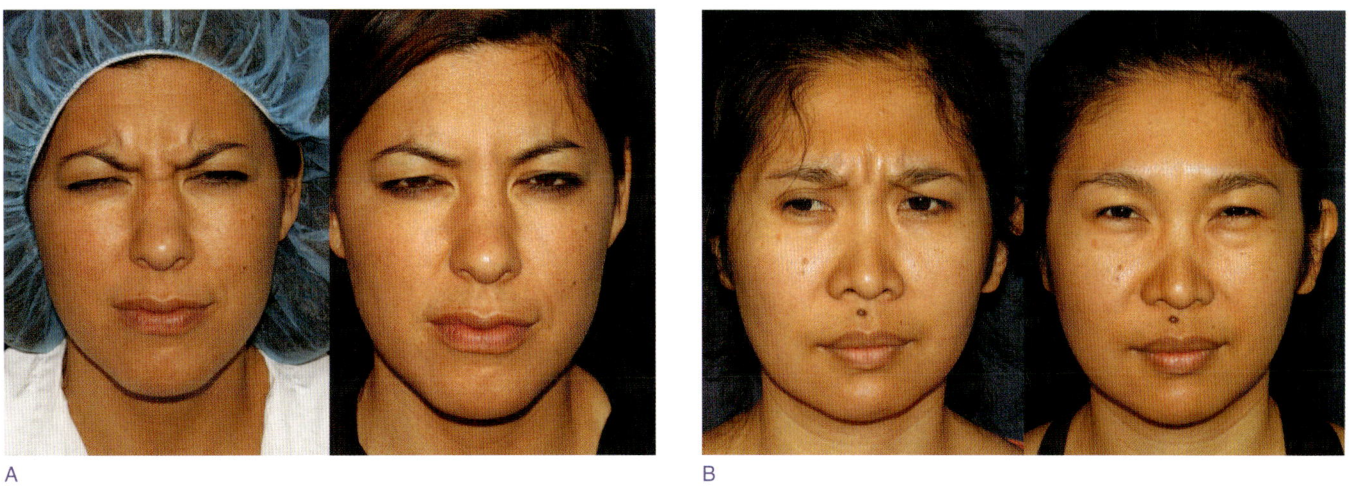

FIGURE 24-2 Before and after glabellar treatment. Note reduction of habitually angry expression. (**A**) Three injection points. (**B**) Five injection points.

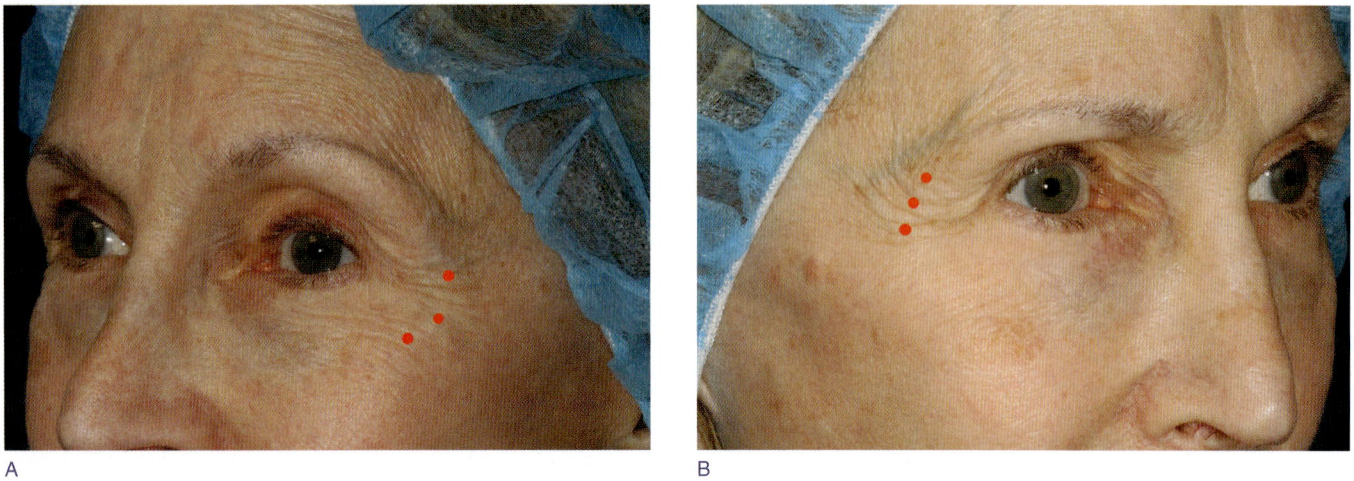

FIGURE 24-3 Patterns of lateral canthal lines. Different patterns can present in the same individual. (**A**) Downward fan pattern. (**B**) Upward fan pattern.

for each patient (**Figure 24-4**). Once again, treatment dosage should be determined clinically, but a typical starting point to each side is 12 units of ONA,[65,66] 36 units of ABO,[67,68] or 12 units of INCO.[69,70] Much lower dosages may be effective as well. In this area, minimizing injection points can help to reduce pain and side effects while maintaining equivalent efficacy.[68] As with glabellar frown lines, repeated and regular BTX treatment in the lateral canthal region confers long-term benefits.[64] One important consideration in this area is that many patients present with significant inferolateral extension of lateral canthal lines down toward and across the zygoma. These rhytides should not be "chased" with BTX due to risk of denervation of the zygomaticus muscle and resultant facial asymmetry (**Figure 24-5**).

Horizontal Forehead Lines: Horizontal creasing along the forehead is a cause of concern for many patients presenting to cosmetic clinics. This phenomenon is caused by hyperactivity of the frontalis muscle. Treatment with BTX in this area is typically delivered over four to eight injection points with small doses ranging from 2 to 8 units of ONA, 5 to 20 units of ABO, or 2 to 8 units of INCO (**Figure 24-6**).[71] The goal of treatment is to soften existing wrinkles while avoiding freezing of all expressiveness or induction of brow ptosis. The most feared complication of isolated frontalis treatment is brow ptosis. In order to avoid this complication, careful assessment of the patient is required. Some patients will present with smaller foreheads, naturally low brows, or minimal frontalis bulk or exhibit the tendency to overuse the frontalis muscle for brow elevation when making facial expressions. These features must be noted prior to treatment and should lead the clinician to consider lowering treatment dosage or placing injection points higher on the forehead approaching the hairline. Another way to minimize risk of brow ptosis is to simultaneously treat the glabellar region in order to balance the muscles of the upper face. In the majority of cases, this is the most reliable way to achieve a beautiful outcome.[72] Simultaneous treatment of the glabellar region serves to prevent brow ptosis as well as relax central horizontal forehead lines, and in general, even patients who request treatment of the forehead alone should have the glabella treated as well (**Figure 24-7**).

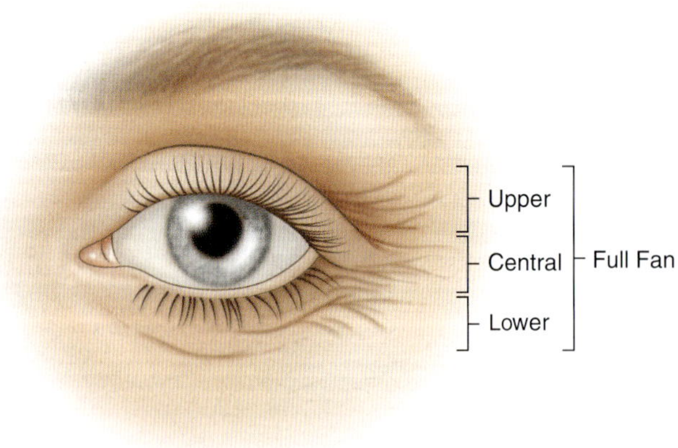

FIGURE 24-4 Four patterns have been described for crow's feet; full, upper, lower, and central fan.

Bunny Lines and Infraorbit: Hyperactivity of the upper nasalis muscle produces a horizontal or fan-shaped pattern of rhytides at the radix of the nose, sometimes referred to as "bunny lines." This concern can be addressed with 2 to 3 units of ONA (or equivalent ABO or INCO) injected in two injection points in the superior nasalis muscle.[73] Caution should be taken to maintain the injection points at least 1 cm above the nasolabial fold to minimize the risk of affecting lip elevators, which may result in unwanted lip ptosis.

The immediate infraorbital region can be treated with BTX with the aim of targeting the pretarsal portion of the orbicularis oculi muscle. Hypertrophy of this muscle can be associated with a decrease in the size of the palpebral aperture. Two units of ONA placed 2 to 3 mm inferior to the lower eyelid margin

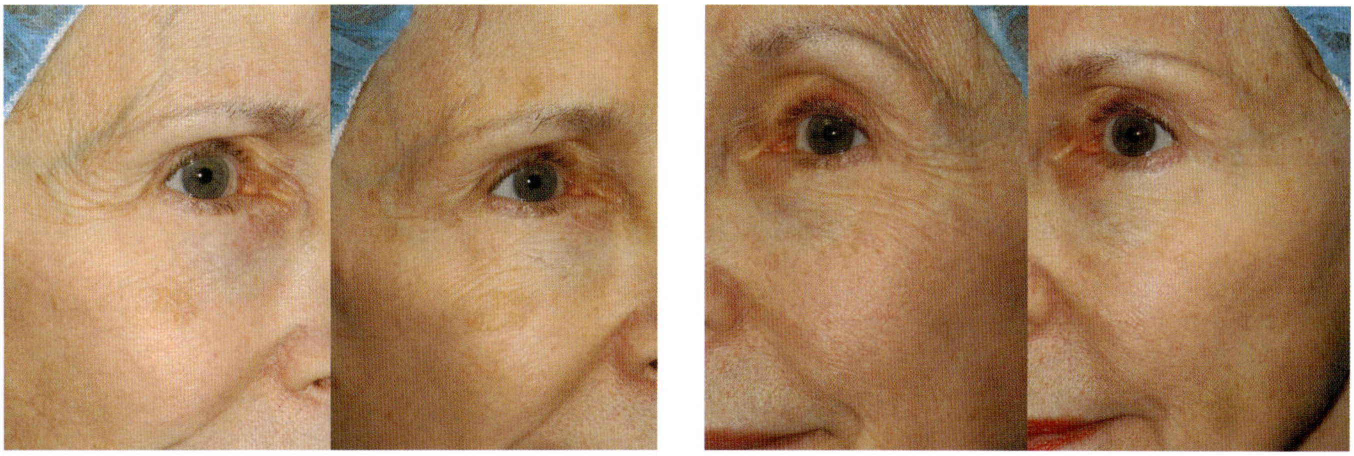

A B

FIGURE 24-5 Before and after lateral canthal line treatment. Note the relaxation of lateral canthal lines producing a natural, worry-free, and more youthful expression.

along the mid-pupillary line are typically sufficient to relax infraorbital wrinkling and subtly increase the palpebral aperture (**Figure 24-8**).[74,75]

Lower Face: Common concerns in the lower face that are amenable to BTX therapy include excessive nasal flare, nasal tip droop, perioral rhytides, upper gum show, hypertrophic masseters, depressed oral commissures, and wrinkled chin.[76] These advanced techniques are off-label and are associated with some risk, and therefore, they should only be approached by experienced injectors.

Nasal Tip Droop: A plunging nasal tip can be due to an overactive depressor septi muscle and can give the impression of a shortened upper lip, especially while smiling. For patients who are not candidates for rhinoplasty, BTX represents a simple alternative to improve this issue. Two to 10 units of ONA should be delivered at the columella-labial angle for this purpose.[77,78]

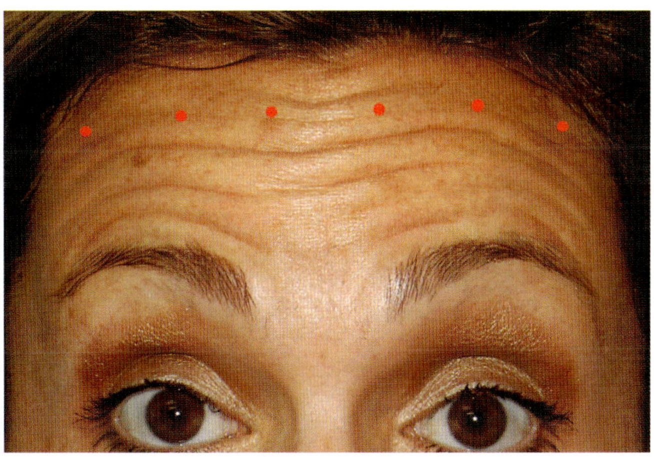

FIGURE 24-6 Frontalis injection. A small number of units should be placed high into the frontalis in order to minimize the chance of inducing brow ptosis.

Perioral Rhytides: The orbicularis oris is a circular muscle that extends circumferentially around the oral aperture and is primarily responsible for the development of hyperdynamic vertical perioral rhytides. Treatment of this muscle with judicious amounts of neuromodulator can achieve temporary improvement of these lines. An early, uncontrolled, open-label trial[79] studied 18 patients who had received between 7 and 18 units of ONA to the perioral region. Effacement of perioral wrinkles and enhanced lip eversion and fullness were observed. More recently, a randomized, double-blind trial demonstrated that a dose of 7.5 units of ONA distributed in several injection points perioally was sufficient to achieve the desired clinical effect.[80] Often, total dosages ranging between 4 and 6 units of ONA (or equivalent neuromodulator) are used. One-unit aliquots are delivered over four injection points along the superior vermilion border, and two injection points are used along the lower vermilion border, staying 1 cm medial to the oral commissure to avoid unwanted spread into muscles inserting into the modiolus (**Figure 24-9**). Prior to moving forward with treatment, patients are warned that they may have difficulty pursing their lips, pronouncing their "p's," drinking out of straws, and playing a wind instrument. A minimal amount of units is used initially since a second treatment, if necessary, can be performed a week after the first injection session and is preferable to overtreating with resultant excessive muscle paralysis in a single treatment session.

Upper Gum Show: Excessive gingival display when smiling is a result of hyperactivity of the levator labii superioris alaeque nasi muscle, which originates from the upper frontal process of the maxilla and inserts into the skin of the lateral part of the nostril and upper lip. This slender muscle can be targeted by BTX injected just lateral and inferior to the nasal ala bilaterally

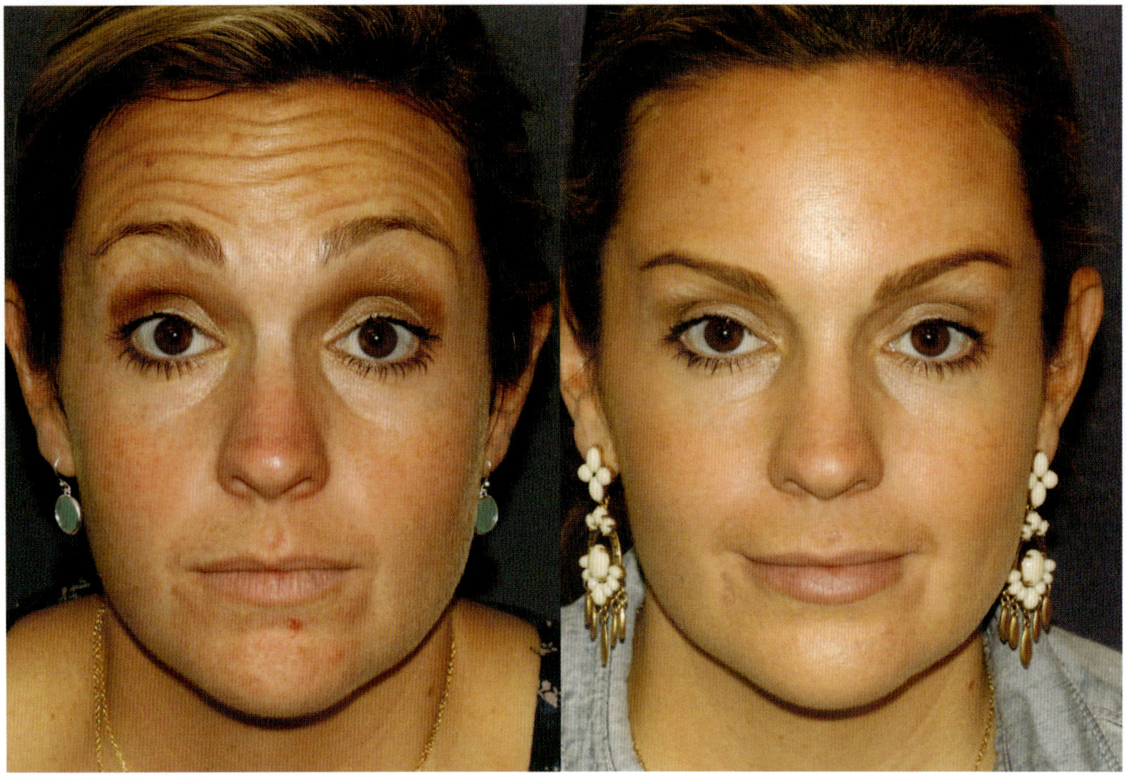

FIGURE 24-7 Reduction of horizontal forehead lines. Concomitant treatment of glabella and frontalis is recommended to achieve the optimal cosmetic result.

(**Figure 24-10**). Two to 3 units of ONA per injection site are all that is required (**Figure 24-11**).[81]

Masseters: Masseteric hypertrophy conveys the impression of heaviness and squaring of the lower face. Genetic predisposition and mastication habits contribute to the development of this feature that is often considered aesthetically displeasing, especially in women because it can masculinize the face. A significant body of evidence supports the use of BTX in the reduction of unwanted masseteric hypertrophy. All commercially available type A BTXs have been used successfully for this purpose.[70,82,83] Anatomic considerations should be taken into account when selecting the appropriate injection points for neuromodulator contouring of the masseters.[84] Misplaced injections can result in disturbance of

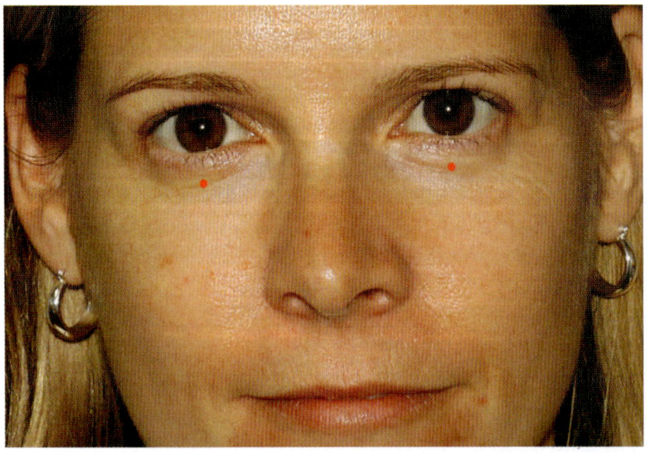

FIGURE 24-8 Infraorbital injection. The purpose of this placement is to relax the pretarsal orbicularis oculi, reducing fine lines and leading to a subtly increased palpebral aperture.

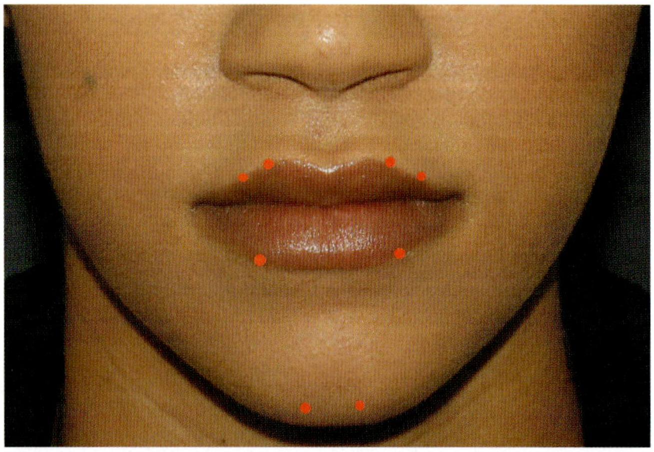

FIGURE 24-9 Orbicularis oris and mentalis injection.

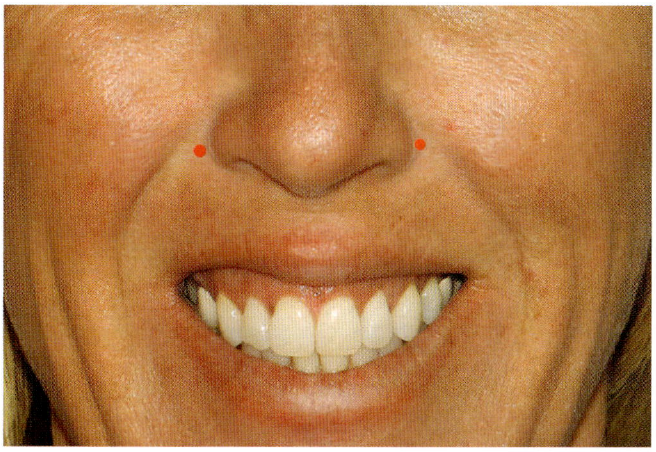

FIGURE 24-10 Reduction of excessive upper gum show is achieved by targeting the levator labii superioris alaeque nasi muscle.

the risorius muscle and resultant facial asymmetry. Injection of neuromodulators deep and directly into the belly of the masseter muscle may diminish the risk of unwanted diffusion. The following technique can be used to optimize safety and efficacy of treatment in this area. First, palpate the point of maximal muscle hypertrophy upon clenching along the mandibular border and mark this as the primary injection point. Next, administer two adjunctive injections approximately 1 cm superolateral and 1 cm superomedial, in the shape of an inverted triangle, keeping the superomedial injection point 1 cm posterior to the medial border of the masseter. By remaining inferior and lateral along the muscle, the risk of adversely affecting the zygomaticus major and risorius muscles is decreased. A total of 20 to 30 units of ONA may be injected into each muscle initially, depending on the degree of hypertrophy. Utilization of multiple injection points as opposed to single injection minimizes the risk of imbalanced muscle atrophy (**Figure 24-12**). A follow-up visit is scheduled 4 weeks after injection for additional slimming of the muscle if necessary to achieve the desired facial contour (**Figure 24-13**).

Downturned Oral Commissures: The depressor anguli oris (DAO) originates at the outer surface of the mandible posterior to the oblique line and inserts into the modiolus at the angle of the mouth. It is innervated by the mandibular branch of the facial nerve and serves primarily to depress the oral commissure. A hyperactive DAO contributes to the accentuation of the melomental fold (marionette line) and creates an impression of disapproval and sadness. It can also lend an appearance of an aged lower face. Chemodenervation of the DAO via application of ONA can improve this appearance and create the impression of a more youthful and vibrant outlook. However, placement and dosage of medication must be carefully considered. The modiolus is an insertion point for several key muscles of facial expression, including the zygomaticus major, risorius, levator anguli oris, orbicularis oris, DAO, and depressor labii inferioris (DLI). As such, misplacement of neuromodulator in this area has the

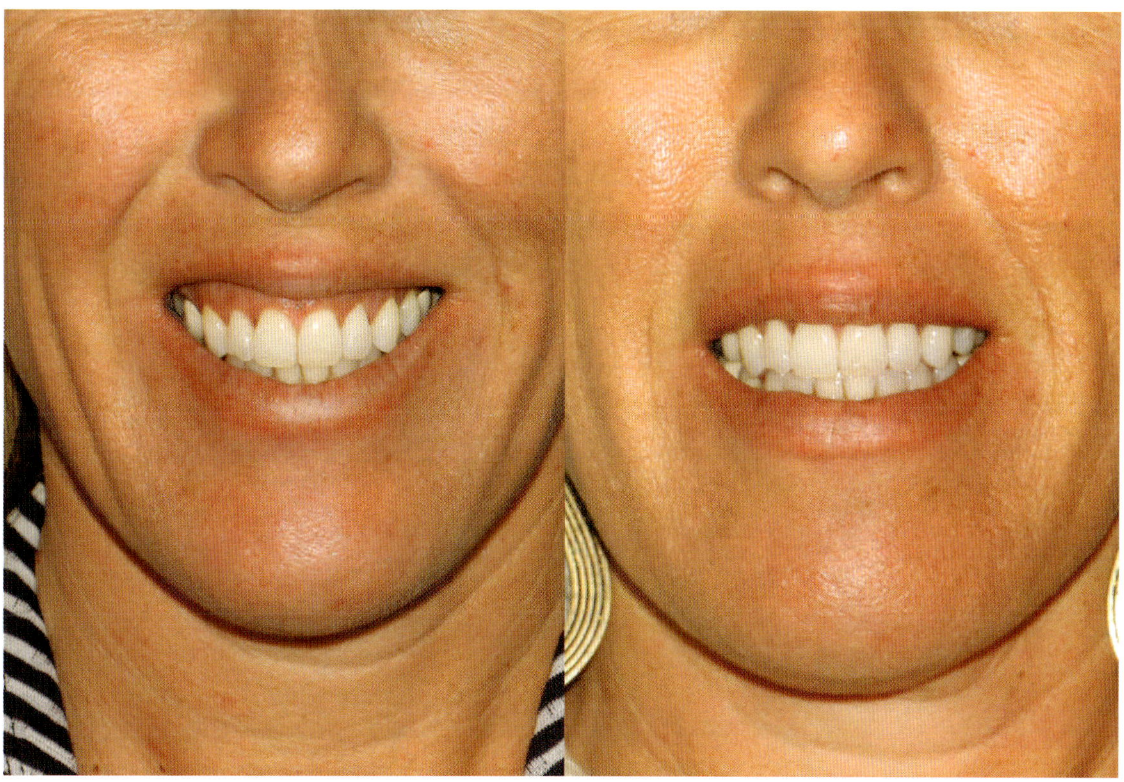

FIGURE 24-11 Before and after reduction of excessive upper gum show. Also note the concomitant elimination of the infranasal crease.

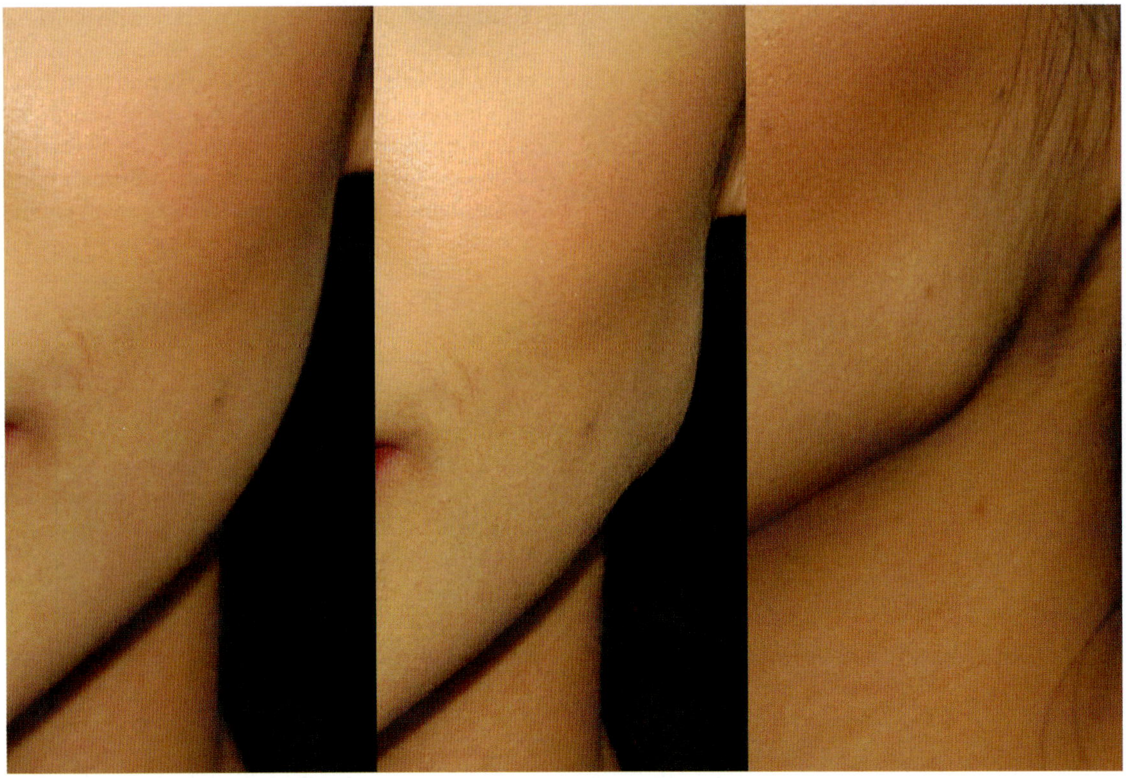

FIGURE 24-12 Imbalanced atrophy of the masseter muscle. This patient was treated with a single injection point into the masseter muscle and developed excessive atrophy at that point while simultaneously developing relatively abnormal hyperactivity in untreated areas. Left panel: At rest. Middle panel: Clenching the jaw. Right panel: Clenching the jaw at 45-degree angle photograph.

potential to negatively alter expressivity, phonation, and facial symmetry. Recent anatomic studies have shed light on the appropriate location for safe injection of neuromodulator targeting the DAO.[84] Prior to injection, to avoid treatment of the DLI when injecting along its insertion on the mandible, patients are asked to pull down the corners of their mouths to aid in the location of the DAO. Following this landmark identification, 4 units of ONA are injected into the DAO on each side along the mandibular border staying 1 cm lateral to the oral commissure.[85] In this fashion, the fan-shaped belly of the DAO

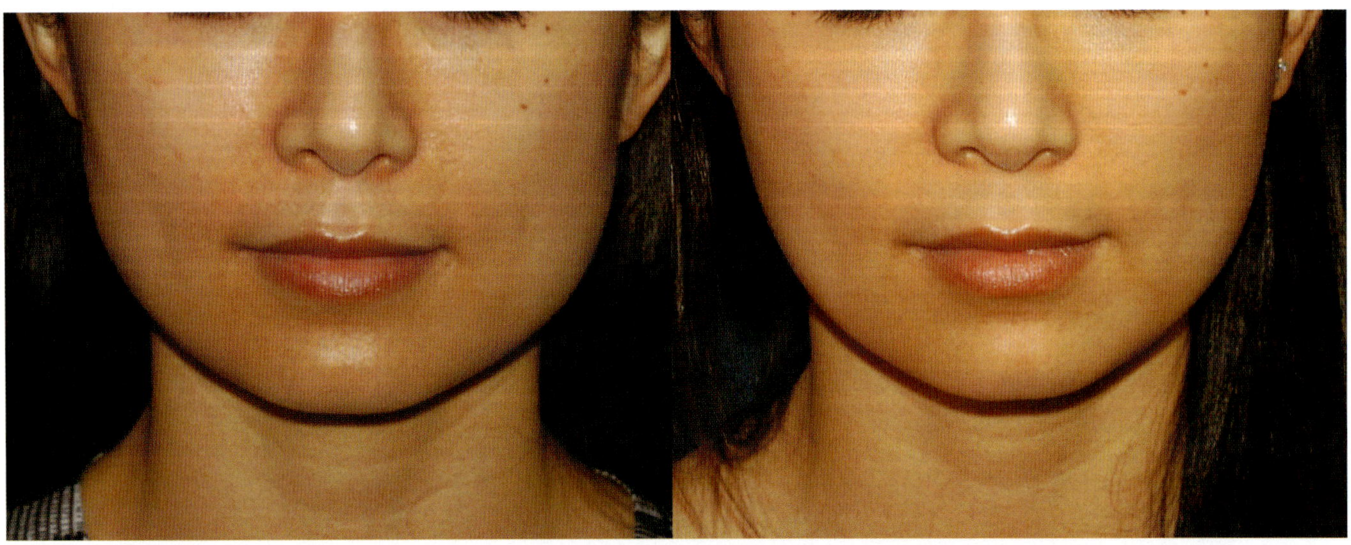

FIGURE 24-13 Before and after masseter muscle reduction. Note the slimming of the lower face contour, a subtle but pleasing aesthetic effect.

is most accurately targeted while minimizing the possibility of medication diffusion affecting adjacent musculature.

Chin Wrinkling: The mentalis muscle is the primary evertor of the lower lip and also serves to elevate the skin of the chin. Its fibers intermingle with the orbicularis oris and DLI.[86] A hyperdynamic mentalis muscle can create unwanted wrinkling and creasing with a peau d'orange appearance. Appreciation of this effect is best noticed when the patient is performing facial expressions. Correction of this phenomenon can be achieved with the injection of either 4 units of ONA directly into the insertion point of both bellies of the mentalis muscle centrally on the mandible or 2 units of ONA into each belly of the muscle, staying close to the midline to avoid spread to the DLI (**Figure 24-9**). It is also important to place injections deep to avoid the more superficial DLI.

Neck and Chest: Excessive platysmal banding is an increasingly common problem with aging. The vertical banding is a result of platysmal muscle hypertrophy. Treatment of this area should be performed in a series of injection points delivered superficially. Injections begin at the jawline and proceed inferiorly along the band with approximately 2-cm spacing. Each injection point should deliver 5 to 10 units of ONA, and the maximum dose per side should not exceed 50 units (**Figure 24-14**).[78,87]

Décolleté wrinkles have also been shown to respond to BTX therapy. In this setting, a V-shaped pattern of injection points following the distribution of "necklace lines" should be used. Each injection is delivered at a depth of 4 mm with 5 to 10 units of ONA per injection site. The total dosage typically ranges between 75 and 120 units.[78,87] Interestingly, flushing of the chest may also respond and improve with this treatment.[88]

OTHER APPLICATIONS

Other uses of BTX therapy that may present to an aesthetic clinic include migraine treatment,[89,90] hyperhidrosis,[91-93] body contouring,[94,95] scar revision,[96] correction of spasmodic facial deformities,[97] enhancing wound healing,[98] and mesotherapy.[88,99]

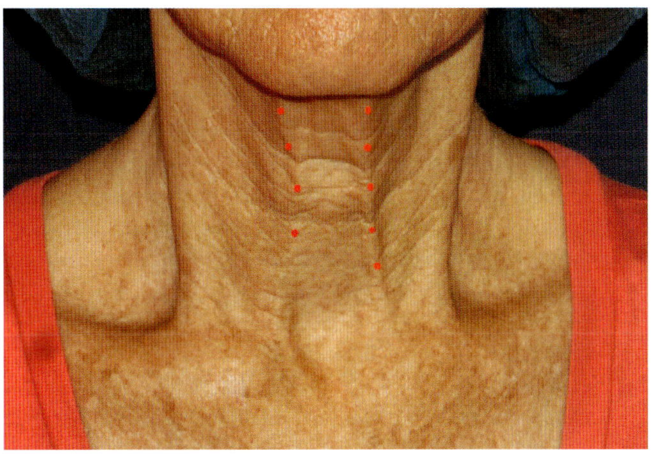

FIGURE 24-14 Platysmal band injection. Once again, treatment should be tailored to match each individual's unique anatomic variations.

SPECIAL CONSIDERATIONS

The above recommendations serve as a template for the aesthetic application of BTX therapy. However, the most critical guideline to bear in mind is to always tailor each treatment to the individual anatomic, personal, and cultural preferences of each patient. Appreciation should be given to both gender and ethnic differences. Men tend to have heavier musculature and therefore usually require a higher dosage in order to achieve the same efficacy and longevity. The male aesthetic is also different, especially where it concerns brow shape and jawline. These considerations should be discussed with the patient prior to treatment so that the correct expectations can be set and the necessary adjustments in injection technique can be applied.

Cultural and ethnic norms should also be taken into account when tailoring individual treatments, as desires and expectations can vary significantly between these diverse populations.[100] Asian patients tend to desire a subtler brow arch or no arch at all, and so alterations in glabellar and frontalis injections may be required. Additionally, these patients also place higher importance and benefit more from infraorbit and masseter treatment.[101,102] Other ethnic preferences that have been studied include Hispanic,[103] Russian,[104] Indian,[105] African,[106] and Middle Eastern.[107] Once again, the duty of the clinician is to explore these nuances with each patient in order to deliver an optimized treatment regimen.

OUTCOMES AND COMPLICATIONS

In the overwhelming majority of cases, if used properly, aesthetic application of BTX is exceedingly safe, effective, and a rewarding experience for both injector and patient. However, as with any cosmetic procedure, appropriate establishment of expectations as well as ability to manage complications are paramount. To avoid dissatisfaction, patients need to be counseled on the differences between the immediate short-term benefits of a single treatment and the long-term benefits of continued maintenance therapy. A recent meta-analysis of clinical trials reported that the most common complications of upper face BTX include headache, eyelid ptosis, and heavy eyelids or brow ptosis.[108] Other complications include "Spock" brow (excessive brow arch), undesired alteration of facial expression, redistribution of muscular bulk in the case of incorrect masseter injection (**Figure 24-12**), and difficulty with head elevation after overtreatment of platysmal banding. For the most part, these complications can be addressed with judicial balancing treatments with additional neuromodulator. In the case of overinjection, time and supportive measures will reassure the patient that the effect is temporary. Eyelid ptosis can be treated with apraclonidine eyedrops until natural improvement occurs.[109]

CONCLUSIONS

BTX remains one of the cornerstones of aesthetic and antiaging medicine. While some patients desire BTX alone, newer trends include a combination approach with neuromodulators, soft-tissue fillers, and energy-based devices for the ultimate outcome.[110] In almost every circumstance, the appropriate use of BTX therapy can enhance an aesthetic treatment regimen, leading to better patient outcomes and satisfaction.

REFERENCES

1. Scott A, Rosenbaum A, Collins C. Pharmacologic weakening of extraocular muscles. *Invest Ophthalmol.* 1973;12(12):924-927.
2. Scott A, Kennedy R, Stubbs H. Botulinum A toxin injection as a treatment for blepharospasm. *Arch Ophthalmol.* 1985;103(3):347-350.
3. Scott A. Botulinum toxin injection into extraocular muscles as an alternative to strabismus surgery. *Ophthalmology.* 1980;87(10): 1044-1049.
4. Carruthers A. History of the clinical use of botulinum toxin A and B. *Clin Dermatol.* 2003;21(6):469-472.
5. Carruthers J, Carruthers J. Treatment of glabellar frown lines with *C. botulinum*-A exotoxin. *J Dermatol Surg Oncol.* 1992;18(1): 17-21.
6. Lam S. The basic science of botulinum toxin. *Facial Plast Surg Clin North Am.* 2003;11(4):431-438.
7. de Paiva A, Meunier FA, Molgó J, Aoki KR, Dolly JO. Functional repair of motor endplates after botulinum neurotoxin type A poisoning: biphasic switch of synaptic activity between nerve sprouts and their parent terminals. *Proc Natl Acad Sci U S A.* 1999;96(6):3200-3205.
8. Alderson K, Holds J, Anderson R. Botulinum-induced alteration of nerve-muscle interactions in the human orbicularis oculi following treatment for blepharospasm. *Neurology.* 1991;41(11): 1800-1805.
9. Iwase S, Ikeda T, Kitazawa H, Hakusui S, Sugenoya J, Mano T. Altered response in cutaneous sympathetic outflow to mental and thermal stimuli in primary palmoplantar hyperhidrosis. *J Auton Nerv Syst.* 1997;64(2-3):65-73
10. Manca D, Valls-Sole J, Callejas M. Excitability recovery curve of the sympathetic skin response in healthy volunteers and patients with palmar hyperhidrosis. *Clin Neurophysiol.* 2000;111(10):1767-1770.
11. Weinberg T, Solish N, Murray C. Botulinum neurotoxin treatment of palmar and plantar hyperhidrosis. *Dermatol Clin.* 2014;32(4):505-515.
12. Doft M, Hardy K, Ascherman J. Treatment of hyperhidrosis with botulinum toxin. *Aesthet Surg J.* 2012;32(2):238-244.
13. Swartling C, Naver H, Pihl-Lundin I, Hagforsen E, Vahlquist A. Sweat gland morphology and periglandular innervation in essential palmar hyperhidrosis before and after treatment with intradermal botulinum toxin. *J Am Acad Dermatol.* 2004;51(5): 739-745.
14. Permatasari F, Hu YY, Zhang JA, Zhou BR, Luo D. Antiphotoaging potential of botulinum toxin type A in UVB-induced premature senescence of human dermal fibroblasts in vitro through decreasing senescence-related proteins. *J Photochem Photobiol B.* 2014;133:115-123.
15. Oh S, Lee Y, Seo YJ, et al. The potential effect of botulinum toxin type A on human dermal fibroblasts: an in vitro study. *Dermatol Surg.* 2012;38(10):1689-1694.
16. Min P, Zhang Z, Grassetti L. Alteration of skin mechanical properties in patients undergoing botulinum toxin type A injections of forehead rhytides. *Aesthetic Plast Surg.* 2016;40(3):410-420.
17. Bonaparte J, Ellis D. Alterations in the elasticity, pliability, and viscoelastic properties of facial skin after injection of onabotulinum toxin A. *JAMA Facial Plast Surg.* 2015;17(4):256-263.
18. Bonaparte J, Ellis D. Skin biomechanical changes after injection of onabotulinum toxin A: prospective assessment of elasticity and pliability. *Otolaryngol Head Neck Surg.* 2014;150(6):949-955.
19. Chen M, Yan T, Ma K, et al. Botulinum toxin type A inhibits alpha-smooth muscle actin and myosin II expression in fibroblasts derived from scar contracture. *Ann Plast Surg.* 2016;77(3):e46-e49.
20. Jeong H, Lee BH, Sung HM, et al. Effect of botulinum toxin type A on differentiation of fibroblasts derived from scar tissue. *Plast Reconstr Surg.* 2015;136(2):171e-178e.
21. Jankovic J, Vuong K, Ahsan J. Comparison of efficacy and immunogenicity of original versus current botulinum toxin in cervical dystonia. *Neurology.* 2003;60(7):1186-1188.
22. Lorenc Z, Kenkel JM, Fagien S, et al. IncobotulinumtoxinA (Xeomin): background, mechanism of action, and manufacturing. *Aesthet Surg J.* 2013;33(Suppl 1):S18-S22.
23. Lizarralde M, Gutierrez S, Venegas A. Clinical efficacy of botulinum toxin type A reconstituted and refrigerated 1 week before its application in external canthus dynamic lines. *Dermatol Surg.* 2007;33(11):1328-1333; discussion 1333.
24. Hui J, Lee W. Efficacy of fresh versus refrigerated botulinum toxin in the treatment of lateral periorbital rhytids. *Ophthal Plast Reconstr Surg.* 2007;23(6):433-438.
25. Jabor M, Kaushik R, Shayani P, et al. Efficacy of reconstituted and stored botulinum toxin type A: an electrophysiologic and visual study in the auricular muscle of the rabbit. *Plast Reconstr Surg.* 2003;111(7):2419-2426; discussion 2427-2431.
26. Yang G, Chiu R, Gillman G. Questioning the need to use Botox within 4 hours of reconstitution: a study of fresh vs 2-week-old Botox. *Arch Facial Plast Surg.* 2008;10(4):273-279.
27. Parsa A, Lye K, Parsa F. Reconstituted botulinum type A neurotoxin: clinical efficacy after long-term freezing before use. *Aesthetic Plast Surg.* 2007;31(2):188-191; discussion 192-193.
28. Shome D, Nair AG, Kapoor R, Jain V. Botulinum toxin A: is it really that fragile a molecule? *Dermatol Surg.* 2010;36(Suppl 4):2106-2110.
29. Alam M, Yoo SS, Wrone DA, White LE, Kim JY. Sterility assessment of multiple use botulinum A exotoxin vials: a prospective simulation. *J Am Acad Dermatol.* 2006;55(2):272-275.
30. Osaki T, Osaki MH, Osaki TH, Sant'Anna AE, Yu MC, Hofling-Lima AL. Absence of bacterial or fungal growth in vials of reconstituted botulinum toxin type A after storage. *Aesthet Surg J.* 2015;35(2):189-193.
31. Alam M, Bolotin D, Carruthers J, et al. Consensus statement regarding storage and reuse of previously reconstituted neuromodulators. *Dermatol Surg.* 2015;41(3):321-326.
32. Liu A, Carruthers A, Cohen JL, et al. Recommendations and current practices for the reconstitution and storage of botulinum toxin type A. *J Am Acad Dermatol.* 2012;67(3):373-378.
33. Alam M, Dover J, Arndt K. Pain associated with injection of botulinum A exotoxin reconstituted using isotonic sodium chloride with and without preservative: a double-blind, randomized controlled trial. *Arch Dermatol.* 2002;138(4):510-514.
34. Allen S, Goldenberg N. Pain difference associated with injection of abobotulinumtoxinA reconstituted with preserved saline and

preservative-free saline: a prospective, randomized, side-by-side, double-blind study. *Dermatol Surg.* 2012;38(6):867-870.

35. Carey W. Incorrect reconstitution of incobotulinumtoxinA leads to loss of neurotoxin. *J Drugs Dermatol.* 2014;13(6):735-738.
36. Soares D, Dejoseph LM, Zuliani GF, Liebertz DJ, Patel VS. Impact of postreconstitution room temperature storage on the efficacy of incobotulinumtoxinA treatment of dynamic lateral canthus lines. *Dermatol Surg.* 2015;41(6):712-717.
37. Klein A. Dilution and storage of botulinum toxin. *Dermatol Surg.* 1998;24(11):1179-1180.
38. Carruthers A, Carruthers J, Cohen J. Dilution volume of botulinum toxin type A for the treatment of glabellar rhytides: does it matter? *Dermatol Surg.* 2007;33(1 Spec No.):S97-S104.
39. Carruthers A, Carruthers J. Botulinum toxin type A. *J Am Acad Dermatol.* 2005;53(2):284-290.
40. Wilson J, Arpey C. Body dysmorphic disorder: suggestions for detection and treatment in a surgical dermatology practice. *Dermatol Surg.* 2004;30(11):1391-1399.
41. Rivkin A, Binder W. Long-term effects of onabotulinum toxin A on facial lines: a 19-year experience of identical twins. *Dermatol Surg.* 2015;41(Suppl 1):S64-S66.
42. Kane M, Cox SE, Jones D, Lei X, Gallagher CJ. Heterogeneity of crow's feet line patterns in clinical trial subjects. *Dermatol Surg.* 2015;41(4):447-456.
43. Kim H, Kim C, Cho H, Hwang JY, Kim YS. A study on glabellar wrinkle patterns in Koreans. *J Eur Acad Dermatol Venereol.* 2014;28(10):1332-1339.
44. Guerrrerosantos J, Carlos Eduardo PG, Mateos Arriola J, et al. Effectiveness of botulinum toxin (type-A) administered by the fixed-site dosing approach versus the muscle area identification. *Aesthetic Plast Surg.* 2015;39(2):243-251.
45. Lowe N, Halliday D. Vein imaging laser reduces bruising in bruise-prone botulinum toxin injected patients. *J Cosmet Laser Ther.* 2016;18(3):162-164.
46. Quezada-Gaon N, Wortsman X, Peñaloza O, Carrasco JE. Comparison of clinical marking and ultrasound-guided injection of Botulinum type A toxin into the masseter muscles for treating bruxism and its cosmetic effects. *J Cosmet Dermatol.* 2016;15(3):238-244.
47. Gordin E, Luginbuhl AL, Ortlip T, Heffelfinger RN, Krein H. Subcutaneous vs intramuscular botulinum toxin: split-face randomized study. *JAMA Facial Plast Surg.* 2014;16(3):193-198.
48. Campos J, Oliveira LB, Queiroz TO, Santos KP, Freitas FM. Comparison between intramuscular and perimuscular injections of botulinum toxin type A. *Aesthetic Plast Surg.* 2006;30(6):700-703; discussion 704.
49. Rzany B, Ascher B, Fratila A, Monheit GD, Talarico S, Sterry W. Efficacy and safety of 3- and 5-injection patterns (30 and 50 U) of botulinum toxin A (Dysport) for the treatment of wrinkles in the glabella and the central forehead region. *Arch Dermatol.* 2006;142(3):320-326.
50. Carruthers J, Lowe NJ, Menter MA, et al. A multicenter, double-blind, randomized, placebo-controlled study of the efficacy and safety of botulinum toxin type A in the treatment of glabellar lines. *J Am Acad Dermatol.* 2002;46(6):840-849.
51. Monheit G, Carruthers A, Brandt F, Rand R. A randomized, double-blind, placebo-controlled study of botulinum toxin type A for the treatment of glabellar lines: determination of optimal dose. *Dermatol Surg.* 2007;33(1 Spec No.):S51-S59.
52. Carruthers A, Carruthers J, Coleman WP 3rd, et al. Multicenter, randomized, phase III study of a single dose of incobotulinumtoxinA, free from complexing proteins, in the treatment of glabellar frown lines. *Dermatol Surg.* 2013;39(4):551-558.
53. Mangano A, Albertin A, La Colla L. A double-blind, randomized, placebo-controlled, two-dose comparative study of botulinum toxin type A for treating glabellar lines in Japanese subjects: what if sample size and statistical tests mattered? *Aesthetic Plast Surg.* 2009;33(5):788.
54. Kawashima M, Harii K. An open-label, randomized, 64-week study repeating 10- and 20-U doses of botulinum toxin type A for treatment of glabellar lines in Japanese subjects. *Int J Dermatol.* 2009;48(7):768-776.
55. Carruthers A, Carruthers J. A single-center, dosecomparison, pilot study of botulinum neurotoxin type A in female patients with upper facial rhytids: safety and efficacy. *J Am Acad Dermatol.* 2009;60(6):972-979.
56. Carruthers A, Carruthers J. A single-center dosecomparison study of botulinum neurotoxin type A in females with upper facial rhytids: assessing patients' perception of treatment outcomes. *J Drugs Dermatol.* 2009;8(10):924-929.
57. Carruthers A, Carruthers J. Prospective, double-blind, randomized, parallel-group, dose-ranging study of botulinum toxin type A in men with glabellar rhytids. *Dermatol Surg.* 2005;31(10):1297-1303.
58. Banegas R, Farache F, Rancati A, et al. The South American Glabellar Experience Study (SAGE): a multicenter retrospective analysis of real-world treatment patterns following the introduction of incobotulinumtoxinA in Argentina. *Aesthet Surg J.* 2013;33(7):1039-1045.
59. Taylor S, Callender VD, Albright CD, Coleman J, et al. AbobotulinumtoxinA for reduction of glabellar lines in patients with skin of color: post hoc analysis of pooled clinical trial data. *Dermatol Surg.* 2012;38(11):1804-1811.
60. Wu Y, Zhao G, Li H, et al. Botulinum toxin type A for the treatment of glabellar lines in Chinese: a double-blind, randomized, placebo-controlled study. *Dermatol Surg.* 2010;36(1):102-108.
61. Carruthers A, Carruthers J. Eyebrow height after botulinum toxin type A to the glabella. *Dermatol Surg.* 2007;33(1 Spec No.):S26-S31.
62. Carruthers A, Carruthers J, Lei X, Pogoda JM, Eadie N, Brin MF. OnabotulinumtoxinA treatment of mild glabellar lines in repose. *Dermatol Surg.* 2010;36(Suppl 4):2168-2171.
63. Dailey R, Philip A, Tardie G. Long-term treatment of glabellar rhytides using onabotulinumtoxinA. *Dermatol Surg.* 2011;37(7):918-928.
64. Carruthers J, Rivkin A, Donofrio L, et al. A multicenter, randomized, double-blind, placebo-controlled study to evaluate the efficacy and safety of repeated onabotulinumtoxinA treatments in subjects with crow's feet lines and glabellar lines. *Dermatol Surg.* 2015;41(6):702-711.
65. Carruthers A, Bruce S, de Coninck A, et al. Efficacy and safety of onabotulinumtoxinA for the treatment of crow's feet lines: a multicenter, randomized, controlled trial. *Dermatol Surg.* 2014;40(11):1181-1190.

66. Lowe N, Ascher B, Heckmann M, Kumar C, Fraczek S, Eadie N; Botox Facial Aesthetics Study Team. Double-blind, randomized, placebo-controlled, doseresponse study of the safety and efficacy of botulinum toxin type A in subjects with crow's feet. *Dermatol Surg.* 2005;31(3):257-262.

67. Kassir R, Kolluru A, Kassir M. Triple-blind, prospective, internally controlled comparative study between abobotulinumtoxinA and onabotulinumtoxinA for the treatment of facial rhytids. *Dermatol Ther (Heidelb).* 2013;3(2):179-189.

68. Fabi S, Sundaram H, Guiha I, Goldman MP. A two-center, open-label, randomized, split-face study to assess the efficacy and safety of one versus three intradermal injection sites of abobotulinumtoxinA in the treatment of lateral periocular rhytides. *J Drugs Dermatol.* 2013;12(8):932-937.

69. Kerscher M, Rzany B, Prager W, Turnbull C, Trevidic P, Inglefield C. Efficacy and safety of incobotulinumtoxinA in the treatment of upper facial lines: results from a randomized, double-blind, placebo-controlled, phase III study. *Dermatol Surg.* 2015;41(10):1149-1157.

70. Lee J, Park JH, Lee SK, et al. Efficacy and safety of incobotulinum toxin A in periocular rhytides and masseteric hypertrophy: side-by-side comparison with onabotulinum toxin A. *J Dermatolog Treat.* 2014;25(4):326-330.

71. Monheit G. Neurotoxins: current concepts in cosmetic use on the face and neck-upper face (glabella, forehead, and crow's feet). *Plast Reconstr Surg.* 2015;136(Suppl 5):S72-S75.

72. Solish N, Rivers JK, Humphrey S, et al. Efficacy and safety of onabotulinumtoxinA treatment of forehead lines: a multicenter, randomized, dose-ranging controlled trial. *Dermatol Surg.* 2016;42(3):410-419.

73. Tamura B, Odo MY, Chang B, Cucé LC, Flynn TC. Treatment of nasal wrinkles with botulinum toxin. *Dermatol Surg.* 2005;31(3):271-275.

74. Flynn T, Carruthers JA, Carruthers JA, Clark RE 2nd. Botulinum A toxin (BOTOX) in the lower eyelid: dose-finding study. *Dermatol Surg.* 2003;29(9):943-950; discussion 950-951.

75. Flynn T, Carruthers J, Carruthers J. Botulinum-A toxin treatment of the lower eyelid improves infraorbital rhytides and widens the eye. *Dermatol Surg.* 2001;27(8):703-708.

76. Wu D, Fabi S, Goldman M. Neurotoxins: current concepts in cosmetic use on the face and neck-lower face. *Plast Reconstr Surg.* 2015;136(Suppl 5):S76-S79.

77. Cigna E, Sorvillo V, Stefanizzi G, Fino P, Tarallo M. The use of botulinum toxin in the treatment of plunging nose: cosmetic results and a functional serendipity. *Clin Ter.* 2013;164(2):e107-e113.

78. Ascher B, Talarico S, Cassuto D, et al. International consensus recommendations on the aesthetic usage of botulinum toxin type A (Speywood Unit)-Part II: wrinkles on the middle and lower face, neck and chest. *J Eur Acad Dermatol Venereol.* 2010;24(11):1285-1295.

79. Semchyshyn N, Sengelmann R. Botulinum toxin A treatment of perioral rhytides. *Dermatol Surg.* 2003;29(5):490-495; discussion 495.

80. Cohen J, Dayan SH, Cox SE, Yalamanchili R, Tardie G. OnabotulinumtoxinA dose-ranging study for hyperdynamic perioral lines. *Dermatol Surg.* 2012;38(9):1497-1505.

81. Suber J, Dinh TP, Prince MD, Smith PD. OnabotulinumtoxinA for the treatment of a "gummy smile." *Aesthet Surg J.* 2014;34(3):432-437.

82. Lee S, Wee SH, Kim HJ, et al. Abobotulinum toxin A and onabotulinum toxin A for masseteric hypertrophy: a split-face study in 25 Korean patients. *J Dermatol Treat.* 2013;24(2):133-136.

83. Lee D, Jin SP, Cho S, et al. RimabotulinumtoxinB versus onabotulinumtoxinA in the treatment of masseter hypertrophy: a 24-week double-blind randomized split-face study. *Dermatology.* 2013;226(3):227-232.

84. Bae J, Choi DY, Lee JG, Seo KK, Tansatit T, Kim HJ. The risorius muscle: anatomic considerations with reference to botulinum neurotoxin injection for masseteric hypertrophy. *Dermatol Surg.* 2014;40(12):1334-1339.

85. Carruthers J, Carruthers A. Aesthetic botulinum A toxin in the mid and lower face and neck. *Dermatol Surg.* 2003;29(5):468-476.

86. Hur M, Kim HJ, Choi BY, Hu KS, Kim HJ, Lee KS. Morphology of the mentalis muscle and its relationship with the orbicularis oris and incisivus labii inferioris muscles. *J Craniofac Surg.* 2013;24(2):602-604.

87. Levy P. Neurotoxins: current concepts in cosmetic use on the face and neck-jawline contouring/platysma bands/necklace lines. *Plast Reconstr Surg.* 2015;136(Suppl 5):S80-S83.

88. Geddoa E, Matar H, Paes T. The use of botulinum toxin-A in the management of neck and anterior chest wall flushing: Pilot study. *Int J Dermatol.* 2013;52(12):1547-1550.

89. Binder W, Blitzer A. Treatment of migraine headache with botulinum toxin type A. *Facial Plast Surg Clin North Am.* 2003;11(4):465-475.

90. Silberstein S. Clinical results of botulinum toxin type A treatment of migraine headache. *Aesthet Surg J.* 2002;22(1):91-93.

91. Goldman A. Treatment of axillary and palmar hyperhidrosis with botulinum toxin. *Aesthetic Plast Surg.* 2000;24(4):280-282.

92. Shelley W, Talanin N, Shelley E. Botulinum toxin therapy for palmar hyperhidrosis. *J Am Acad Dermatol.* 1998;38(2 Pt 1):227-229.

93. Glogau R. Botulinum A neurotoxin for axillary hyperhidrosis. No sweat Botox. *Dermatol Surg.* 1998;24(8):817-819.

94. Lee HJ, Lee DW, Park YH, Cha MK, Kim HS, Ha SJ. Botulinum toxin a for aesthetic contouring of enlarged medial gastrocnemius muscle. *Dermatol Surg.* 2004;30(6):867-871; discussion 871.

95. Han K, Joo YH, Moon SE, Kim KH. Botulinum toxin A treatment for contouring of the lower leg. *J Dermatol Treat.* 2006;17(4):250-254.

96. Freshwater M. Botulinum toxin for scars: can it work, does it work, is it worth it? *J Plast Reconstr Aesthet Surg.* 2013;66(3):e92-e93.

97. Chundury R, D'Angelo AS, Couch SM, Holds JB. Subjective and objective measures in the treatment of hemifacial spasm with onabotulinumtoxinA. *Ophthal Plast Reconstr Surg.* 2016;32(2):133-137.

98. Ziade M, Domergue S, Batifol D, et al. Use of botulinum toxin type A to improve treatment of facial wounds: a prospective randomised study. *J Plast Reconstr Aesthet Surg.* 2013;66(2):209-214.

99. Eshghi G, Khezrian L, Alirezaei P. Botulinum toxin A in treatment of facial flushing. *Acta Med Iran.* 2016;54(7):454-457.

100. Wimalawansa S, McKnight A, Bullocks J. Socioeconomic impact of ethnic cosmetic surgery: trends and potential financial impact the African American, Asian American, Latin American, and Middle Eastern communities have on cosmetic surgery. *Semin Plast Surg.* 2009;23(3):159-162.

101. Wu W, Liew S, Chan HH, et al. Consensus on current injectable treatment strategies in the Asian face. *Aesthetic Plast Surg.* 2016;40(2):202-214.

102. Liew S, Wu WT, Chan HH, et al. Consensus on changing trends, attitudes, and concepts of Asian beauty. *Aesthetic Plast Surg.* 2016;40(2):193-201.

103. Cobo R, Garcia C. Aesthetic surgery for the Mestizo/Hispanic patient: special considerations. *Facial Plast Surg.* 2010;26(2):164-173.

104. Yutskovskaya Y, Gubanova E, Khrustaleva I, et al. IncobotulinumtoxinA in aesthetics: Russian multidisciplinary expert consensus recommendations. *Clin Cosmet Investig Dermatol.* 2015;8: 297-306.

105. Shetty R. Outer circle versus inner circle: Special considerations while rejuvenating an Indian face using fillers. *J Cutan Aesthet Surg.* 2015;8(3):169-172.

106. Brissett A, Naylor M. The aging African-American face. *Facial Plast Surg.* 2010;26(2):154-163.

107. Farahvash M, Arad S. Clostridium botulinum type A toxin for the treatment of upper face animation lines: an Iranian experience. *J Cosmet Dermatol.* 2007;6(3):152-158.

108. Jia Z, Lu H, Yang X, et al. Adverse events of botulinum toxin type A in facial rejuvenation: a systematic review and meta-analysis. *Aesthetic Plast Surg.* 2016;40(5):769-777.

109. Scheinfeld N. The use of apraclonidine eyedrops to treat ptosis after the administration of botulinum toxin to the upper face. *Dermatol Online J.* 2005;11(1):9.

110. Carruthers J, Burgess C, Day D, et al. Consensus recommendations for combined aesthetic interventions in the face using botulinum toxin, fillers, and energy-based devices. *Dermatol Surg.* 2016;42(5):586-597.

25 Fillers

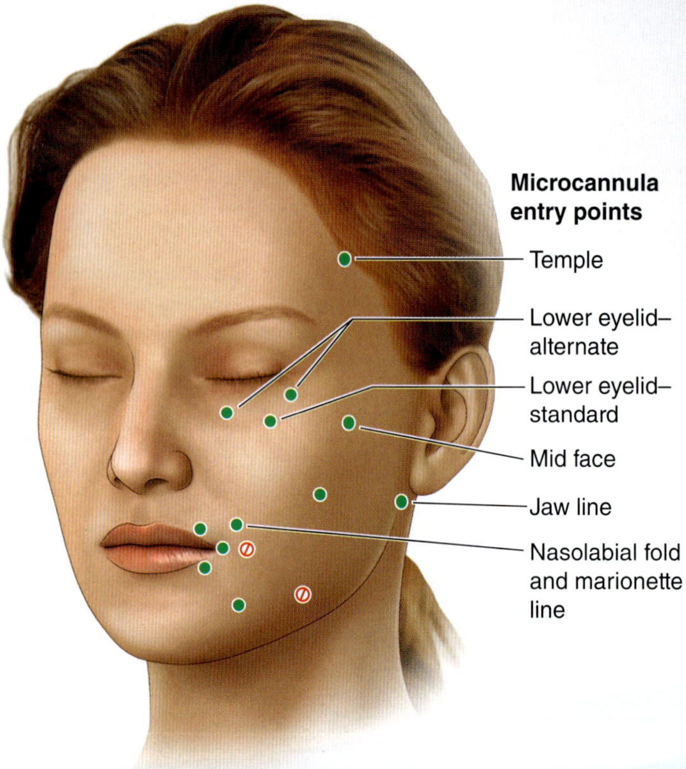

SUMMARY

- *Serial puncture technique*: Small aliquots of filler are injected close together so that they integrate continuously along a rhytid or fold. Postinjection massage further facilitates this blending.
- *Linear threading technique*: The full length of the needle is introduced dermally or subcutaneously, and filler is injected linearly either retrograde (as the needle is withdrawn) or anterograde (as the needle is inserted), which creates a plane of blunt dissection.
- *Cross-hatching or radial injection technique*: Regularly spaced, linear threads created by injecting in more than one direction to form a grid pattern.
- *Fanning technique*: The needle is inserted at a single site then passed multiple times in different directions without fully withdrawing the tip from the skin.
- *Depot injection techniques*: Boluses of filler are injected along the periosteum, usually to correct volume deficiency in the temporal, zygomatic cheek, and chin areas. Postprocedural massage helps prevent nodularity and smooth contour irregularities.

Beginner Tips

- Injection of commercially available hyaluronidase degrades hyaluronic acid filler if it is misplaced (i.e., too superficially), overinjected, or if it produces inflammatory reactions or occludes vasculature.
- Differences in formulation and manufacturing techniques help impart the unique characteristics of each filler.

Expert Tips

- Because of its ability to decrease edema and, consequently, external vessel compression, some recommend hyaluronidase injection irrespective of filler type.
- Sculptra is essentially pulverized polyglactin 910 and can be prepared with as much as 8 to 11 mL of sterile water in >24 hours.
- Calcium hydroxyapatite is radiopaque, though it does not obscure radiographic findings.

Don't Forget!

- Persistent papulonodules are more likely with Sculptra, Bellafill/Artefill, and silicone than other agents.
- Both hypersensitivity and infection with or without biofilm can contribute to the formation of delayed nodules.
- For fat grafts, massage and vigorous dynamic facial movement should be avoided postprocedure.

Pitfalls and Cautions

- Superficial HA can cause a temporary bluish tint due to the Tyndall effect.
- If intralesional hyaluronidase is ineffective or nodules occur in the setting of non-HA augmentation, other reported medical therapies include oral antibiotics (antimicrobial and anti-inflammatory effects); topical, intralesional, or systemic corticosteroids; intralesional 5-fluorouracil; oral immunosuppressants such as cyclosporine; lasers; or combination therapies.

Patient Education Points

- All injectable fillers entail risk; while the risk of serious adverse events is low, it is not inconsequential.
- Patients should have realistic expectations regarding potential outcomes and the need for repeated treatments. Many of the commercially touted before-and-after photos reflect patients treated with large volumes of filler; given the cost, many patients attempt treatment with significantly less volume and should be warned that their results may be less dramatic.
- Though rare, potentially irreversible vascular complications are the most dreaded and serious adverse events following soft tissue augmentation, and patients should understand this possibility and alert the clinician immediately in the event of any symptoms.

Fillers

25

INTRODUCTION

The use of fillers and injectable implants for facial rejuvenation is one of the most important forms of minimally invasive correction and represents a key class of interventions for the aging face. These interventions can be largely grouped into the four "R's": redrape (surgical procedures that pull, lift, or tighten); resurface (chemical peels, dermabrasion, ablative or nonablative lasers); relax (chemodenervation with neuromodulatory agents); and replace or recontour (injection of filler agents for soft-tissue augmentation). The last has become increasingly popular, as the number of safe, effective dermal filling agents has increased and as the public's demand for minimally invasive approaches has grown. It is helpful to keep in mind the various etiologies of facial volume loss when contemplating augmentation (**Table 25-1**).

Approval by the US Food and Drug Administration (FDA) of the first hyaluronic acid (HA) filler, Restylane, in 2003 marked the beginning of a new period in injectable agents for facial rejuvenation. HA fillers quickly supplanted all other products. Current FDA-approved formulations fall into three families: Restylane/Perlane (now marketed as Restylane Lyft), Juvederm/Juvederm Voluma, and Belotero. Hyalorm, derived from rooster coombs; Captique, a plant-based HA; Elevess; and Prevelle Silk are other approved agents no longer sold in the United States.[1,2] The FDA has also approved two longer-acting agents (poly-L-lactic acid [Sculptra] and calcium hydroxylapatite [Radiesse]), as well as one permanent filler, polymethylmethacrylate (Bellafill, formerly marketed as Artefill).[3] Different products are placed at different depths in order to exert an ideal cosmetic effect; notably, in recent years, there has been a strong push away from using fillers simply to fill in grooves (as with the first generation of fillers) and toward a three-dimensional understanding of the potential benefit of accomplishing superficial—and particularly deep—volumizing through precise placement of filler material (**Table 25-2**).

TABLE 25-1 • Causes of Facial Volume Loss

	Skin	Fat	Bone
Age of onset	20 years	40 years	50 years; later in males
Effect	Pore size, tired look	Gaunt, aged	Gaunt, aged
Approach to repair	Superficial fillers	Deep fillers	Deep fillers

TABLE 25-2 • Typical Products in a Hyaluronic Acid Filler Family Designed for LayeredImplantation, and Their Usual Implantation Depths[a]

Product Type	Usual Implantation Depth
Deep volumizer	Supraperiosteal and subcutaneous
Midlevel volumizer	Subcutaneous and sometimes intradermal; submucosal to lips; supraperiosteal to nasojugal folds
Superficial volumizer	Intradermal and superficial subcutis; submucosal to lips; supraperiosteal to nasojugal folds
Additional specialty products	Lips, submucosal, nasojugal folds, supraperiosteal, and subcutaneous

Data from Sundaram H: Igniting discovery, dialogue, and global innovation through international collaboration. J Drugs Dermatol. *2014 Apr;13(4):386-388.*

GENERAL INJECTION TECHNIQUE

Consultation

Major goals of the initial consultation are baseline evaluation, understanding of relevant medical history, and patient education. The clinician must evaluate the type, location, depth, and diameter of the deficit, as well as the quality of surrounding tissue, which may alter the final appearance of augmentation. Appreciating the etiology of cutaneous defects will help select the most appropriate therapeutic modality and tailor the treatment plan accordingly. Distinction should be made between static and dynamic rhytides (the latter are usually more amenable to chemodenervation) and between changes as a result of chronologic age compared to solar damage (**Table 25-3**). Patients should be evaluated in a seated or gravity-dependent position with ample lighting streaming from an acute angle that highlights subtleties. This careful positioning allows for better selection of filler product and injection technique. Standardized, before-and-after photography is strongly recommended to track change over time and help explain procedures.

Appropriate patient selection is key in ensuring good outcomes and involves taking a detailed past medical history. **Table 25-4** outlines some helpful medical information to determine which patients are candidates for soft-tissue augmentation and which products may be most suitable for them. A history of prior allergic reaction to the filler material or its constituents (ie, amide anesthetics such as lidocaine or, for some HA fillers,

TABLE 25-3 • Etiology of Cutaneous Defects and Deficits

Etiology	Description
Chronologic age	Gravity-related tissue dissent and sagging Loss of subcutaneous fat Bone resorption
Photodamage	Pigmentary alterations (eg, solar lentigines, melasma) Rhytides from decreased extracellular matrix turnover and degradation Neoplasia
Scarring	Acne Varicella, zoster Surgery Trauma Other
Inflammation	Infection-related lipoatrophy or wasting (eg, HIV) Collagen vascular disease (eg, linear morphea, Parry-Romberg disease, lupus, other)
Other	Congenital lipoatrophy Medication side effects (eg, antiviral therapy) Exercise-induced lipoatrophy and gravity-related changes Nutritional deficiencies Idiopathic lipoatrophy

HIV, human immunodeficiency virus.

TABLE 25-4 • Preprocedure Evaluation and Consultation Considerations

Patient goals and expectations	Defect(s) of concern Expected outcomes Expected duration of correction Acceptable recuperation time/downtime
Medical history	Past medical history (eg, infectious disease, collagen vascular disease, granulomatous disease, scarring condition including propensity for keloids) History and location of herpes simplex viral infection Past facial surgery (eg, facelifts, reconstruction) Past rejuvenation procedures (eg, injections, implants) History of hypersensitivity reaction to filler products or their constituents Medications, particularly anticoagulant and antiplatelet agents Current or anticipated pregnancy/lactation
Defect assessment	Anatomic location Type (eg, superficial, medium, or deep folds and wrinkles; volume loss; localized or global lipoatrophy) Volume of product necessary for correction Quality of adjacent skin Benefits, risks, alternative or complementary treatments

gram-positive bacterial proteins) is a major contraindication. Intervention should be postponed for infections or inflammation in the treatment area. Care should be taken in those with bleeding disorders, and all nonessential anticoagulation and/or antiplatelet medications may be held to limit the risk of ecchymosis. If taken for primary prevention only, patients may discontinue aspirin 10 to 14 days and nonsteroidal anti-inflammatory drugs (NSAIDs) 5 to 7 days before the procedure. There are many other over-the-counter supplements that may increase bleeding and bruising, such as omega-3 fatty acids/fish oil, garlic, ginseng, gingko biloba, St. John's wort, and high-dose vitamin E, so these too should be temporarily stopped.[1,3]

Patient education is another critical component of the consultation. Clinicians should inquire about subjective deficits and teach about the relevant anatomy contributing to these "problem" areas. There should be a frank discussion about the indications, benefits, limitations, risks, and alternatives of soft-tissue augmentation, including surgery, resurfacing, neuromodulation, and no intervention. The anticipated duration of results; need for repeat treatments in the future; estimated financial costs; and postprocedural recovery should be emphasized. In the end, overall success and satisfaction rely on setting and achieving clear, realistic expectations.[1,3]

Sex Differences

Hormonal differences contribute to the development of male facial features.[4] Overall, men have a squarer facial appearance attributable to flat, concave, and more angular features. Women have rounder, softer features leading to a more triangular face (**Table 25-5**).[5]

Gender differences also vary based on location on the face. Upper facial features include the brow, the nose, supraorbital ridge, and associated muscles. Men have a straight brow that sits lower on the face, whereas women have an arched brow that sits higher on the face. The nose is slightly longer, and the fat compartments

TABLE 25-5 • Key Sex Differences in Men and Women

	Female	Male
Temples	Convex	Flat
Lips	Pronounced-augment. Inject vermilion border	Thin-replace at most. Inject vermilion body
Zygoma	Superior augmentation	Inferior augmentation

above the brows are very small in men. Men also have a more prominent supraorbital ridge, resulting in the appearance of deep-set eyes.[4] The corrugator is stronger in men and extends more laterally, while the frontalis muscle is larger and stronger.[5]

Overall, the midface is wider in men than women. Although the zygomatic arch is more prominent in men, the midface is flatter, with more lateral cheek projection and less anterior cheek projection. This is likely a function of women's relatively increased superficial fat compartments in the midface and cheeks. Men also have a more pronounced, angular jawline in the lower face while the chin is prominent, leading to a squarer facial appearance. Women generally have a softer jawline, creating a more triangular face.[5]

Men do not generally seek the oval face shape that women often pursue. Men enjoy some benefits in regard to aging of the face. Compared to women, the male facial skeleton retains its shape much longer with age.[6] Special attention should be paid to key focus areas including the cheekbones, chin, and jawline.

The midface ages more slowly in men, and as the cheekbones recede, the male cheek tends to move inferiorly and medially.[4] When placing facial filler in the male cheek, it is important to avoid feminization. Practically, this means aiming to restore the cheek rather than augment it. The position of the male cheek apex is more medial and inferior relative to females. Facial fillers should be placed lower along the zygomatic arch and with less volume relative to female patients. Adding volume to the anterior compartment of the cheek should be avoided (**Figure 25-1**).

Men often appreciate augmentation of the chin when necessary. A strong chin is a defining feature of the male face. Although both genders exhibit retrograde movement of the chin, the lateral aspect of the mandible moves inward in women but outward in men. Adding volume can enhance projection of a recessed chin in men.

Treatment of lips in male patients is often not desired or accepted. Males have thinner lips in general, and this becomes more pronounced with age. If attempted, the focus of fillers in male lips should be restoration rather than augmentation. Filler placement should be concentrated at the vermillion body and not at the vermillion border.

Special attention should be paid toward sexual dimorphism in the temple and the zygoma. The temple is an important area for volumization in order to address aging. However, the youthful appearance of females derives from round and slightly convex temples. In contrast, males prefer straight and flat temples. Similarly, the focus of the zygoma in females is the superior aspect, while in men the focus is slightly inferior.

Facial structure is not limited to gender influences only, but includes ethnic differences as well. Ethnicity therefore changes the goals of treatment and the method by which those goals are achieved. Asians, blacks, and Latinos tend to appear younger longer due to less skin aging and sagging compared to Caucasians.[7-9] As previously discussed, the skin, fat, and craniofacial skeleton are the major foci for these differences.

Preprocedure

After thorough evaluation and discussion, written consent should be obtained and the skin sterilized with isopropyl alcohol, chlorhexidine, or equivalent agent.[10] Clean technique from start to finish helps prevent contamination and seeding of the implant. This should be adhered to when handling, mixing, and injecting the filler and prepping the skin as well. Gloves should be changed after contact with the oral mucosa.

Anesthesia to decrease discomfort from injections is another component of many treatment protocols. Some newer agents (ie, Restylane, Perlane, Juvederm, Bellafill/Artefill) come premixed with lidocaine, while others require clinicians to compound their own off-label (**Table 25-6**). Cryoanesthesia with ice or commercial devices and topical anesthetic preparations, such

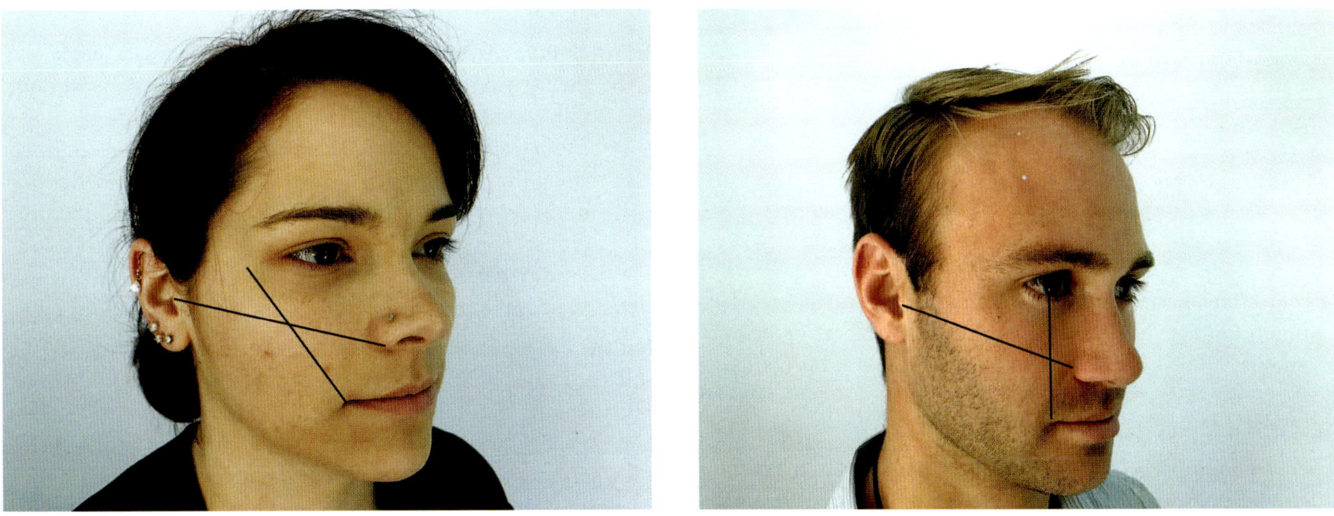

A B

FIGURE 25-1 Using Hinderer's lines to determine the point of maximal zygomatic projection. In a female (**A**), the first of Hinderer's lines is drawn from the lateral canthus to the oral commissure and the second from the tragus to the alar lobule. In a male (**B**), the first line is a vertical line drawn directly down from the lateral iris to the lateral oral commissure, and the second from the tragus to the alar lobule. This corresponds to the apex of a male cheek being inferomedial to a female's.

TABLE 25-6 • Food and Drug Administration–Approved Soft-Tissue Fillers in the United States (US)

No Longer Available in US[a]	Available in US
Bovine-derived collagen ■ Zyderm I, Zyderm II, Zyplast	Nonanimal stabilized hyaluronic acid ■ Restylane/Restylane-L[b], Perlane/Perlane-L[b] ■ Juvederm Ultra/Juvederm Ultra XC[b], Juvederm Ultra Plus/Juvederm Ultra Plus XC[b] ■ Belotero Balance ■ Juvederm Voluma XC
Porcine-derived collagen ■ Evolence	Synthetic[c] ■ Poly-L-lactic acid (Sculptra/Scupltra Aesthetic) ■ Calcium hydroxyapatite (Radiesse) ■ Polymethylmethacrylate (Bellafill/Artefill)
Noncadaveric human collagen ■ CosmoDerm 1, CosmoDerm 2, CosmoPlast Cadaveric human collagen ■ Dermalogen, Cymetra Avian-derived hyaluronic acid ■ Hylaform, Hylaform Plus Nonanimal stabilized hyaluronic acid ■ Captique, Elevess, Prevells Silk Autologous fibroblast therapy ■ Autologen, Fibrel, Isolagen	Autologous ■ Autologous fat ■ Autologous fibroblast therapy (Azficel-T/laViv)

[a]*Production suspended because of voluntary manufacturer discontinuation or decreased demand in favor of other products.*
[b]*Contains lidocaine.*
[c]*Silicone injected off-label for soft-tissue augmentation.*
Reproduced with permission from the U.S. Food & Drug Administration. www.fda.gov.

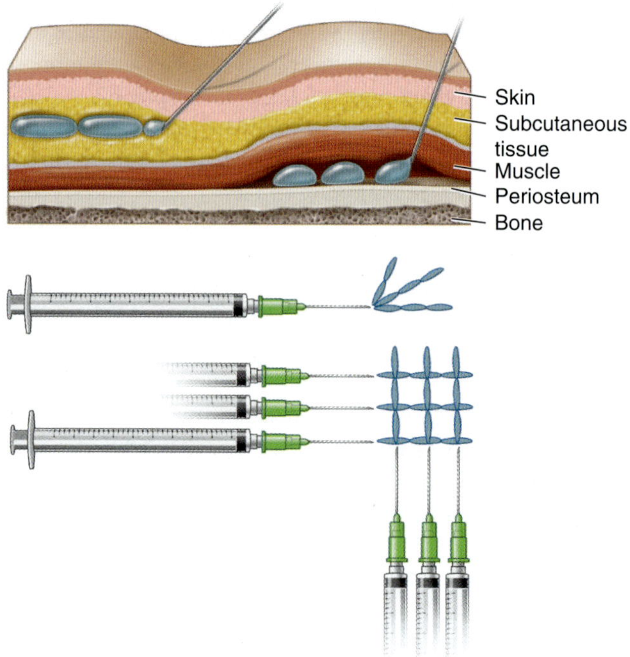

FIGURE 25-2 Soft-tissue filler injection technique options using a sharp needle include serial puncture with microdroplets, linear retrograde and anterograde threading, fanning, and cross-hatching.

as benzocaine, lidocaine, prilocaine, and/or tetracaine, are other common adjunctive methods. Less often, nerve blocks or regional anesthesia can be used to limit pain associated with injections.

Injection Techniques

There are multiple acceptable injection techniques, and selecting the most appropriate is often a question of provider preference and experience. Some anatomic locations and fillers are more amenable to particular techniques (**Figure 25-2**).[10]

- *Serial puncture technique.* Small aliquots of filler are injected close together so that they integrate continuously along a rhytid or fold. Postinjection massage further facilitates this blending.
- *Linear threading technique.* The full length of the needle is introduced dermally or subcutaneously, and filler is injected linearly either retrograde (as the needle is withdrawn) or anterograde (as the needle is inserted), which creates a plane of blunt dissection.
- *Cross-hatching or radial injection technique.* Regularly spaced, linear threads are created by injecting in more than one direction to form a grid pattern.
- *Fanning technique.* The needle is inserted at a single site then passed multiple times in different directions without fully withdrawing the tip from the skin.
- *Depot injection techniques.* Boluses of filler are injected along the periosteum, usually to correct volume deficiency in the temporal, zygomatic cheek, and chin areas. Postprocedural massage helps prevent nodularity and smooth contour irregularities.

Historically, augmentation focused on directly filling folds, but there is now an emphasis on facial volumizing to replace the soft tissue and bone loss that occurs with age or photodamage. Furthermore, this volumizing effect indirectly smooths wrinkles and fine lines, and understanding the facial fat pads can be helpful when considering this approach (**Figure 25-3**).[11]

Blunt-tipped cannulas may be less likely to puncture vessels and may reduce the risk of intravascular injection, bruising, discomfort, and number of injection sites; however, there is a learning curve with cannulas, so that precise product placement may be suboptimal initially. In addition, previous facial surgery, scarring, or tissue augmentation may contribute to tissue fibrosis,

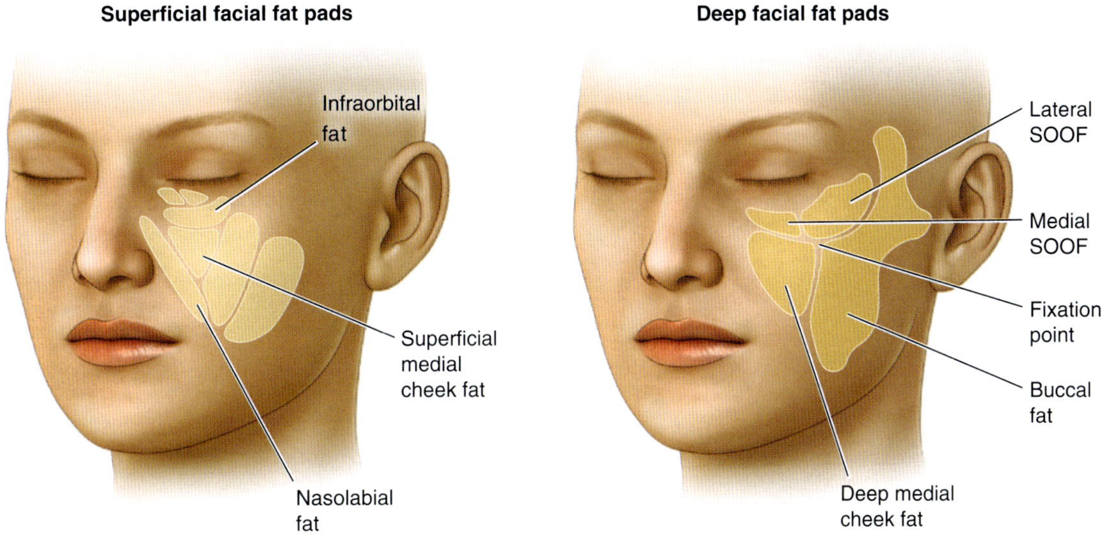

FIGURE 25-3 Knowledge of the facial fat pads is essential for successful filler placement. SOOF, suborbicularis oculi fat.

making use of a cannula more challenging.[12,13] Combined use of sharp needle injections and blunt microcannulas, depending on the site and treatment goals, may be used to achieve a balance of safety and efficacy. A consensus panel has advocated for different blunt cannula sizes (**Table 25-7**) and entry points (**Figure 25-4**) for different facial regions.[13]

Pertinent Vascular Anatomy

In addition to knowledge of multiple injection techniques, expert practitioners should have a detailed grasp of relevant vascular anatomy in an attempt to avoid devastating adverse events. This has been investigated in detail in the past,[14] and some of the most high-risk and frequently discussed regions are addressed in **Figure 25-5**.

The majority of facial blood supply comes from branches of the external carotid artery, which anastomose with divisions off the internal carotid artery at the nose. The facial artery is the most studied and frequently compromised branch of the external carotid. It extends along the mandible up toward the medial canthus under the platysma, zygomaticus major, and lip elevator muscles to terminate in the angular artery that runs along the lateral nose. These landmarks are general guidelines, however, and the path is tortuous with substantial individual variation,[15,16] so

TABLE 25-7 • Preferred Blunt Microcannulas for Specific Areas and Products

Area	Microcannula Diameter and Length	Preferred Filler Product(s)
Lower eyelid	27- or 25-gauge, 38 mm	HA
Upper eyelid and around eyebrow	27- or 25-gauge, 38 mm or longer	HA
Midface	25- or 22-gauge, 38 mm or longer	HA, CaHA, or PLLA
Temple	25- or 22-gauge, 38 mm or longer	HA, PLLA, or CaHA
Lower face	25- or 22-gauge, 38 mm or longer	HA, CaHA, or PLLA
Lips	27- or 25-gauge, 38 mm	HA
Hand (dorsum)	25- or 22-gauge, 38 mm or longer	CaHA or HA
Décolletage	25-gauge, 38 mm	HA

CaHA, calcium hydroxylapatite; HA, hyaluronic acid; PLLA, poly-L-lactic acid.

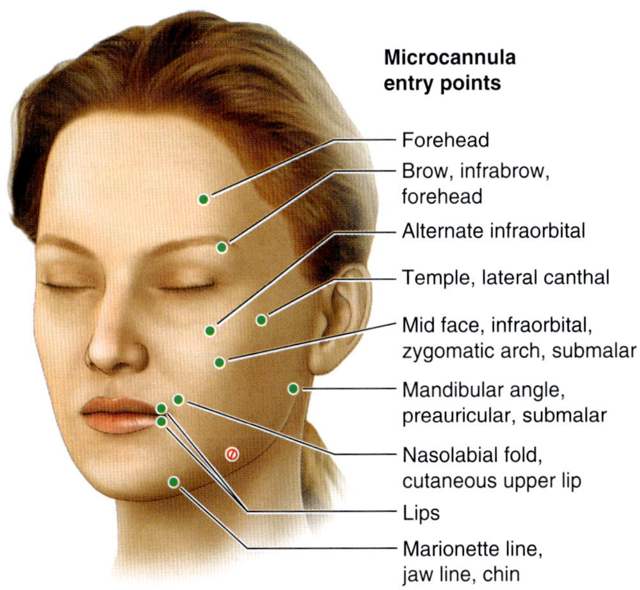

FIGURE 25-4 Select microcannula entry point suggestions.

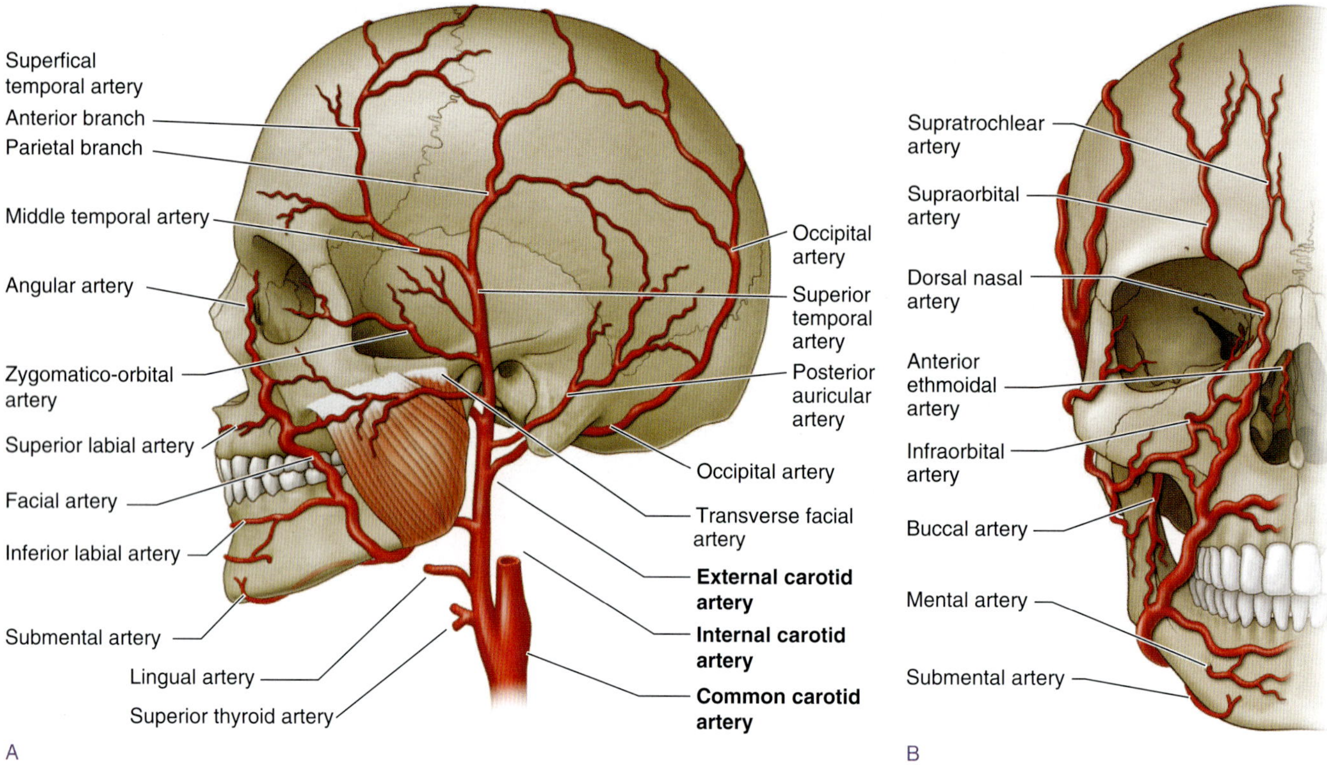

FIGURE 25-5 Anastomoses of the internal and external carotid circulations.

care must be taken when injecting at the medial cheek and along the nasal sidewall because there is a higher risk of arterial occlusion. Blunt tip cannulas that do not pierce vessel walls as easily as needles may be safer in these regions, although this has yet to be definitively established.

The angular artery supplies the nasal sidewall before joining with the dorsal nasal artery, one of two divisions of the ophthalmic artery, at the root of the nose. The latter continues down the nose, irrigating its root and dorsum, before anastomosing with the lateral nasal artery, a branch of the facial artery. There have been reports of retrograde emboli and blindness due to these interconnection, and again, care must be taken to inject small aliquots under low pressure periosteally and perichondrally along the nose.

Similarly, anastomoses between the cutaneous and ophthalmic circulation in the upper face may lead to blindness and even cerebrovascular deficits. Both the supraorbital and supratrochlear arteries branch off the internal carotid near the glabella. The supraorbital emerges from the supraorbital notch just medial to the mid-pupillary line, whereas the supratrochlear lies beneath the medial-most glabellar rhytid. They run along bone for approximately 1 cm, then pierce the frontalis muscle and branch superficially. Hence, injections at the medial portion of the upper face should only be performed with cannula or superficially in the dermis, while those in the mid to upper portion of the forehead should be periosteal deep to the level of the vasculature. As with the dorsal nose, complications occur from direct injection into or compression of the vessels or retrograde emboli into the ophthalmic and then terminal retinal arteries off the internal carotid.

INJECTABLE SOFT-TISSUE FILLER MATERIALS

Filler Selection

The number of available filler materials for soft-tissue augmentation and rejuvenation continues to increase.[2] They can be categorized based on different qualities: derivation (autologous, xenograft, allograft, synthetic, semi-synthetic); depth of cutaneous injection (dermal, subcutaneous); reversibility (reversible and nonreversible); and longevity (temporary and permanent). **Table 25-8** compares selected FDA-approved agents. Knowledge of these different properties allows for appropriate placement at the appropriate anatomic location.

Hyaluronic Acid Derivatives

Since their first approval in 2003, HA derivatives have become the most common filler used for rejuvenation (87% of all soft-tissue filler procedures).[17] HA, also called hyaluronan, is an endogenous glycosaminoglycan, contributing to the extracellular matrix and conserved among mammals and tissue types. It serves many biologic functions, regulating tissue remodeling and cell migration. HA's anionic structure readily binds water to form a gel, which is particularly important for hydration, lubrication, and volumization of connective tissue. Because of its hygroscopic property, the amount of dermal HA dictates tissue

INJECTION TECHNIQUE PEARLS

Anatomic Region	
Forehead	*Glabella* • Supraorbital and supratrochlear arteries run periosteally medial to mid iris; *avoid* deep injections. • Inject intradermally along etched-in lines using a 32-gauge, ½-inch needle tenting up on skin. • If deeper injections necessary, use cannula inserted lateral to mid-pupillary line perpendicular to vessels. *Mid to superior forehead* • Arteries perforate the frontalis muscle superficially 1 cm above the glabella. • Inject periosteal depots (≤0.1 mL) deep to the vessels for volume deficits. • Inject intradermally along etched-in lines using a 32-gauge, ½-inch needle tenting up on skin.
Temples	• Inject periosteally at the point 1 cm up along temporal fusion line and 1 cm inferolateral. • Place finger along hairline to prevent product from spreading posteriorly.
Midface and naso-jugal folds (tear troughs)	*Lateral midface* • Relatively avascular lateral to the mid-pupillary line. • Inject periosteal depots (≤0.1 mL) using a 30- or 32-gauge, ½-inch needle for lift and volumization. • Products of choice have high G′ or high cohesivity: Juvederm Voluma, Restylane Lyft, calcium hydroxyapatite. *Medial midface and nasojugal folds* • Infraorbital artery emerges from its foramen 5 to 8 mm below the orbital rim in the mid-iris to mid-pupil region. • Facial artery transitioning to angular artery runs at the medial cheek and along the nasal sidewall. • *High-risk* vascular territory because of tortuous and variable path. • Inject tear troughs in the suborbicularis oculi fat (SOOF) using cannula.
Nasolabial folds	*Nasolabial creases* • Facial artery runs tortuously and variably. • Inject in a linear retrograde technique along the fold using a cannula with an inferior insertion point. *Piriform fossa* • Inject a periosteal depot in direction of contralateral commissure.
Jawline and mandible	• Facial artery traverses the mandible 1 cm anterior to the border of the masseter muscle and runs deeply. • Inject subcutaneously between the bone and subdermal layers above the level of vasculature except for at the gonial angle where injections may be deep periosteal. • Insert cannula superficially over artery and thread filler linearly along mandibular ramus. • Products of choice are calcium hydroxyapatite and highly elastic hyaluronic acid (Juvederm Voluma, Restylane Lyft).
Chin	• Inject periosteal depots (≤0.1 mL) anteriorly or inferiorly to mandibular symphysis to augment projection and height, respectively.
Lips and perioral	• Inject in a linear retrograde technique along vermillion border using a 30-gauge, ½- or 1-inch needle. • Subsequent augmentation into at the philtral columns, wet-dry, or pillows as necessary. • Inject depot deep to modiolus muscle at the oral commissure. • Ideal vertical height ratio of upper to lower lip: 1:1.6 in Caucasian patients and 1:1 in African or Asian patients. • Particulate (ie, poly-L-lactic acid, calcium hydroxylapatite) and permanent (ie, polymethylmethacrylate) fillers contraindicated due to nodule formation.

viscoelasticity; therefore, as the concentration of HA decreases with age, so does the skin's ability to retain water and maintain contour.[18,19]

HA is a linear mucopolysaccharide with long repeating disaccharide chains of D-glucuronic acid and N-acetylglucosamine. The longer the chains, the higher the molecular weight. Hyaluronidase cleaves high-molecular-weight hyaluronan into oligosaccharides, while β-N-glucuronidase and β-N-acetylhexosaminidase degrade these smaller cleaved sugars. This degradation occurs continually under normal circumstances,

TABLE 25-8 • Important Properties of Soft-Tissue Fillers

Filler Trade Name	Major Materials	FDA Indication(s)[a]	Availability	Longevity	Skin Testing	Reversible	Unique Features
Zyderm I/II, Zyplast	Bovine-derived collagen (98% purified type I in phosphate-buffered saline, 0.3% lidocaine)	Dermal injection for soft-tissue contour irregularities	No longer in United States (US)	3-6 months	Yes	No	▪ Zyplast cross-linked with glutaraldehyde—less immunogenic and longer lasting ▪ Lip augmentation most common application ▪ Hypersensitivity 3%
Evolence	Porcine-derived collagen (type I collagen crosslinked with ribose sugar)	Dermal injection for moderate to severe facial wrinkles and folds such as nasolabial folds	No longer in US	Up to 1 year	No	No	▪ Less immunogenic than bovine collagen ▪ Avoid lip enhancement; risk of nodule formation
CosmoDerm 1/2, CosmoPlast	Human bioengineered collagen (single human fibroblast cell line, tested for disease)	Papillary dermal injection for soft-tissue contour deficiencies such as wrinkles, acne scars	No longer in US	3-6 months	No	No	▪ Similar properties to bovine collagen except no risk of hypersensitivity
Fascian	Cadaveric fascia lata	Marketed in accordance with Tissue Reference Group (TRG) criteria rather than as a device, no prescribed indications Grafts applicable to subdermal correction at any anatomic location	No longer in US	Up to 8 months	No	No	▪ Highly biocompatible ▪ Requires large-bore needle for pretunneling or subcision ▪ Trace amounts of polymyxin sulfate, bacitracin, gentamycin; avoid if history of allergy ▪ Substantial postprocedural edema
Restylane/ Restylane-L/ Restylane Silk Perlane/ Perlane-L	Bacterial-derived hyaluronic acid	Dermal injection for (1) Moderate to severe to facial wrinkles and folds (2) Lip augmentation in adults (Restylane-L and Silk only)	Yes	6-9 months	No	Yes	▪ Highly biocompatible ▪ Rare risk of hypersensitivity ▪ Room temperature storage, biodegradable, long shelf life ▪ Reversible with off-label hyaluronidase (Vitrase, Hylenex) degradation
Belotero Balance	Bacterial-derived hyaluronic acid	Dermal injection for moderate to severe wrinkles and folds	Yes	6-9 months	No	Yes	See Restylane

Juvederm Ultra/ Juvederm Ultra XC Juvederm Ultra Plus/ Juvederm Ultra Plus XC	Bacterial-derived hyaluronic acid	Dermal injection for moderate to severe facial wrinkles and folds					See Restylane
Juvederm Voluma XC	Bacterial-derived hyaluronic acid	Subcutaneous or supraperiosteal injection for age-related volume loss in the midface in adults over 21 years	Yes	Up to 24 months	No	No	▪ Higher risk of delayed nodularity compared to other hyaluronic acid derivatives
Hylaform, Hylaform Plus	Hyaluronic acid from rooster combs	Dermal injection for moderate to deep wrinkles and folds	No	6-9 months	No	Yes	See Restylane
Fibrel, Autologen, Isolagen, Azficel-T (laViv)	Autologous fibroblasts; cutaneous punch biopsy shipped to manufacturer where fibroblasts isolated and expanded in vitro	(1) Depressed scars that distend with manual stretching of the borders (2) Moderate to severe nasolabial fold wrinkles in adults	Only azficel-T (laViv)	Uncertain, phase III trial with benefit at 6 months	No; autologous	No	▪ Limited product yield at high cost ▪ Requires two procedures (punch biopsy from which fibroblasts harvested)
Autologous fat	Suspension of aspirated autologous adipocytes	None	Yes	Variable, potentially permanent	No	No	▪ Potential indications include correction of (1) Wrinkles and folds (2) Atrophic scars (3) Stable, inflammation-induced, facial atrophy (ie, linear morphea, Parry-Romberg syndrome) (4) HIV-related lipoatrophy (5) Volume loss at the dorsal hands ▪ Highly biocompatible even at large volumes ▪ Variable graft ($\leq$50%) ▪ Efficacy depends on technique ▪ Need for two procedures ▪ Substantial postprocedural edema

(Continued)

TABLE 25-8 • Important Properties of Soft-Tissue Fillers (Continued)

Filler Trade Name	Major Materials	FDA Indication(s)[a]	Availability	Longevity	Skin Testing	Reversible	Unique Features
Radiesse	Calcium hydroxyapatite	Subdermal injection for (1) HIV-associated lipoatrophy (2) Moderate to severe facial wrinkles and folds (eg, nasolabial folds) (3) Volume loss at the dorsal hands	Yes	12 months clinically, up to 20 months histologically	No	No	▪ Highly biocompatible ▪ Lip augmentation contraindicated (granulomas) ▪ Migration and beading around mouth from frequent movement
Sculptra, Sculptra Aesthetic	Poly-L-lactic acid	Subdermal injection for (1) HIV-associated lipoatrophy (2) Shallow to deep nasolabial fold contour deficiencies and other facial wrinkles	Yes	Variable and cumulative over time, up to 18-24 months	No	No	▪ Highly biocompatible ▪ Higher risk of papulonodules ▪ Postprocedural massage recommended (rule of 5s: 5 minutes, 5 times per day, for 5 days)
Bellafill/ Artefill, Artecoll, Arteplast	Polymethylmethacrylate spheres in 3.5 bovine collagen, 0.3% lidocaine	Correction at the nasolabial folds	Only Bellafill/ Artefill	Permanent	Yes	No	▪ Risk of delayed-onset nodules, granulomas
Silikon 1000, AdatoSil 5000	Liquid injectable silicone	Licensed for ophthalmic indications	Yes; off-label	Permanent	No	No	▪ Lowest risk complications with microdroplet technique, low total volumes, pure product ▪ Correction of HIV-associated lipoatrophy

[a]*Reproduced with permission from the U.S. Food & Drug Administration. www.fda.gov.*

and unmodified HA persists in vivo for only 12 to 24 hours. Crosslinking the polysaccharide side chains increases tissue stability and ensures a more acceptable tissue residence time of manufactured products.[18] HA in all the currently FDA-approved fillers is isolated from streptococcal bacteria and chemically crosslinked using 1,4-buanediol diglycidyl ether (BDDE).

Differences in formulation and manufacturing techniques help impart the unique characteristics of each filler. For the Restylane/Perlane family, sieving HA through mesh produces identically shaped and sized particles that are suspended in phosphate-buffered saline at a concentration of 20 mg/mL. One milliliter of Restylane contains 100,000 particles, whereas Perlane/Restylane Lyft particles are larger, with only 10,000/mL, making the latter more suitable for deeper folds. In contrast, Juvederm products use a proprietary manufacturing technology, termed Hylacross, to generate particles of variable shapes and sizes that bind together as a homogenous gel with a concentration of 24 mg of HA per milliliter. Juvederm Ultra (Juvederm 24HV) is less crosslinked than Ultra Plus (Juvederm 30 HV). Both the concentration of HA and degree of crosslinking impact product stiffness and longevity. Juvederm Voluma XC consists of 20 mg/mL HA produced via Vycross technology. While most fillers contain only higher molecular weight particles, Voluma is a 9:1 mix of high- to low-molecular-weight HA. The short polysaccharide chains in the lower weight molecules allow for formation of more crosslinks and provide a greater lifting capacity.[20] The third family of Belotero products undergoes two sequential rounds of crosslinking to form a nonparticulate gel comprised of 22.5 mg/mL of HA with different density zones.[21] All of the above agents, except for Belotero, are available prepackaged with lidocaine anesthesia.

Restylane, Juvederm, and Belotero all gained initial FDA approval for the treatment of moderate to severe facial wrinkles, such as at the nasolabial folds (**Table 25-9**), based on data from 6-month, multicenter, blinded, randomized, controlled, split-faced, phase III trials comparing the HA agent in question to Zyplast bovine collagen.[22-24] Each was found to better correct facial folds at 6 months than the Zyplast control and to be safe in all skin types (**Figure 25-6**). It appears that subsequent treatments after 6 months require less volume to achieve optimal effect, with results lasting up to 1 to 2 years.[24-26] Restylane and Juvederm family fillers treat facial folds (ie, nasolabial folds) by injecting into the superficial subdermal plane. Deposition too superficially may produce an uneven contour and bluish tint because of irregular light scattering (Tyndall effect). Owing to its nonparticulate composition, Belotero better integrates into the dermis so that discoloration is less likely,[27] a property making Belotero appropriate for treatment of etched lines such as those seen periorally (**Figure 25-7**). Restylane-L and Restylane Silk later received FDA approval for lip augmentation in patients aged 21 years and older; both showed improvement over no treatment at 8 weeks.[28,29] Juvederm and Belotero are used off-label for this indication.[30]

Juvederm Voluma XC was the first product to seek FDA approval for deep injection at the midface to counteract age-related volume loss (**Figure 25-8**). It should be placed at the deep subcutaneous and/or periosteal planes rather than in the lip, glabella, or intradermally. In the pivotal phase III randomized, controlled, single-blind trial, patients saw improvement in moderate to severe volume deficits of the cheeks at 6 months versus no treatment (**Figures 25-9 and 25-10**). These results persisted at 24 months in nearly half of patients, a longer duration than that achieved with other HA fillers on the market.[31,32]

TABLE 25-9 • Off-Label Indications for Soft Tissue Fillers

Indication	Examples
Nondynamic rhytides and folds	Glabellar and forehead lines Nasojugal folds (medial tear trough) Prejowl sulcus Marionette lines Mental crease
Volume deficits	Hollow temples Sunken cheeks Tear trough deformities Hanging ear lobes Atrophic dorsal hands
Structural prominences	Lateral eyebrow elevation Nasal bridge and tip Malar/zygoma Chin Jawline contouring
Distensible and depressed scars	Acne Trauma Surgery Varicella
Perioral	Lip augmentation Vertical lip lines Vermilion and philtrum flattening Oral commissures

Adverse reactions to HA fillers are rare, occurring in less than 2% of patients.[33] Unlike other materials, HA is "reversible," so treatment-related complications can often be mitigated. Injection of commercially available hyaluronidase (Vitrase or Hyalanex) degrades the filler if it is misplaced (eg, too superficially) or overinjected or it produces inflammatory reactions or occludes vasculature.

Poly-L-Lactic Acid

Sculptra, a synthetic polymer of poly-L-lactic acid, provides subtle but buildable rejuvenation that persists for up to 18 to 24 months by upregulating endogenous neocollagenesis. It typically requires multiple treatments to obtain desired results. Sold as a freeze-dried powder that can be stored at room temperature, Sculptra is essentially pulverized polyglactin 910 (Vicryl) suture material and must be reconstituted with sterile water or saline into a suspension for injection.

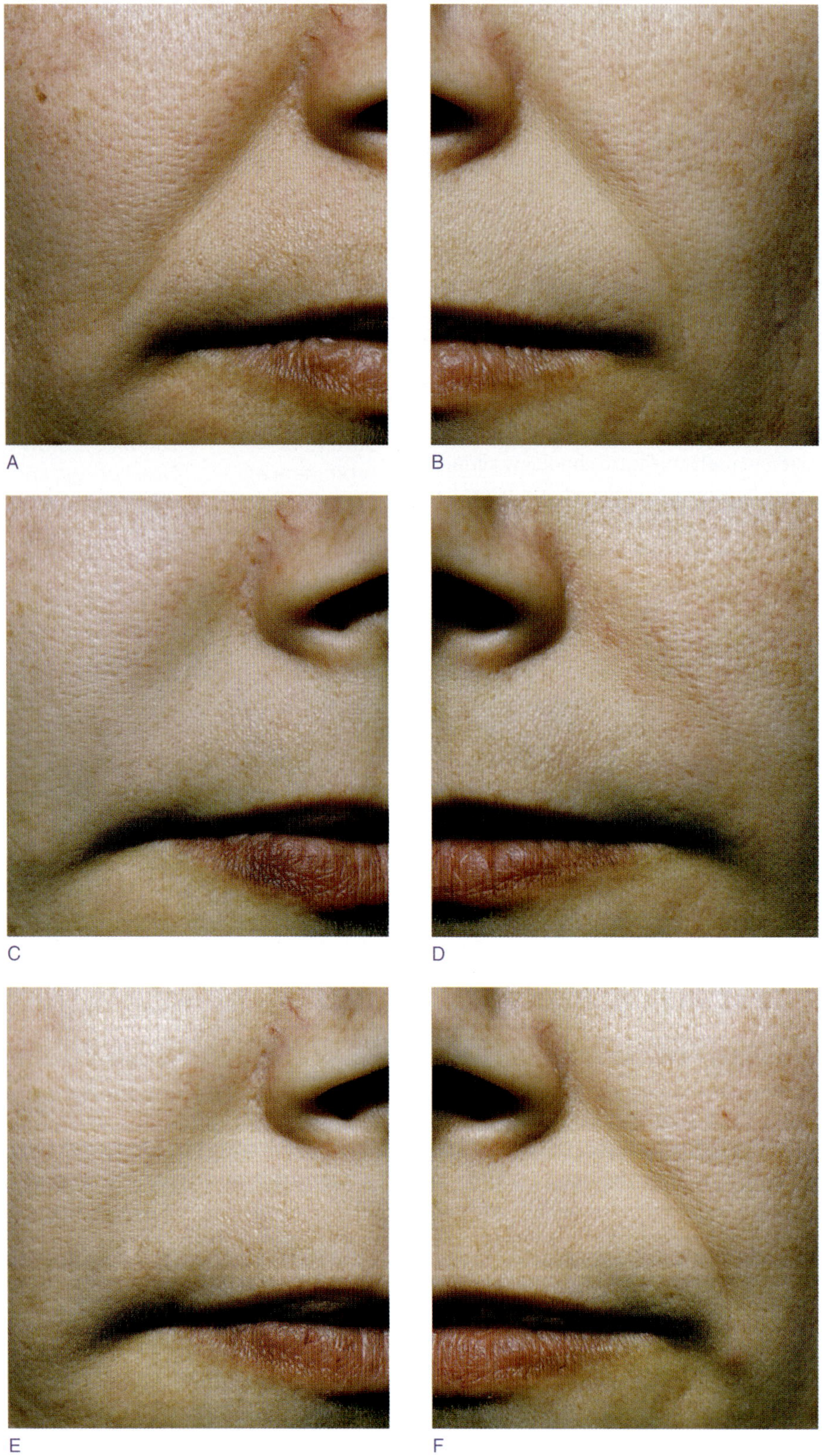

FIGURE 25-6 Treatment of nasolabial folds with Juvederm Ultra versus Zyplast at baseline (**A and B**), 2 weeks (**C and D**), and 24 weeks (**E and F**).

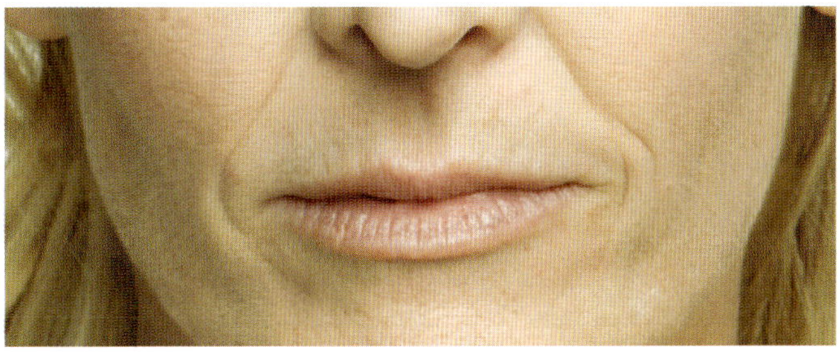

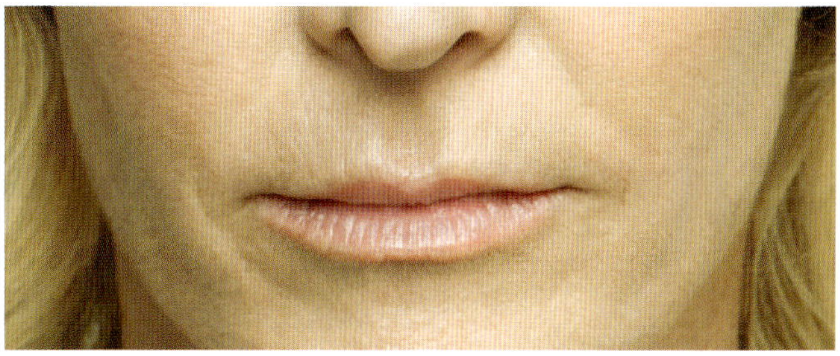

A B

FIGURE 25-7 Belotero correction of perioral rhytides at baseline (**A**) and 2 weeks (**B**).

First developed and marketed in Europe as New-Fill, Sculptra gained FDA approval for treatment of HIV-related facial lipoatrophy in 2004. In 2009, the FDA approved Sculptra Aesthetic for shallow to deep wrinkles, including the nasolabial folds, in immunocompetent patients. Panfacial injections are an off-label option in patients with limited volume loss. Sculptra is typically injected with 25- or 26-gauge needles serially or as depots into the subcutaneous plane. More superficial deposition increases the risk of visible nodules. After injection, immediate correction is the result of edema and solvent from the solution, which dissipates. Persistent augmentation takes longer to appear and requires three or more treatment sessions, spaced every 3 to 6 weeks.[34]

Preparation and storage practices vary among practitioners. Current packaging suggests reconstituting each vial with 4 mL of sterile water and 1 mL of lidocaine just 2 hours before use. However, the resultant 5 mL of solution is thick and can clog syringes or more readily form papulonodules, so most clinicians prepare their mixture with as much as 8 to 11 mL of sterile water at greater than 24 hours.[33] Agitating the vial and/or syringe also helps maintain particles in solution. Nonetheless, frequent needles changes or back aspiration may be needed if the product precipitates.

Although not unique to this filler, formation of delayed-onset papules, nodules, or granulomatous reactions at the site of injection is an important adverse effect after Sculptra (**Figure 25-11**). In the phase III extension study, these complications occurred in 17.8% (20/116 patients) of treated sites compared to 12.8% (15/117 patients) of control sites and appeared months later, often persisting for more than a year.[35] Reconstituting the solution farther in advance, diluting with larger volumes, injecting into the subcutis rather than the dermis, administering smaller aliquots, and massaging treatment sites postprocedurally are strategies used to prevent papulonodule formation. In fact, massaging should continue at home in accordance with the "Rule of 5's": 5 minutes, 5 times per day, for 5 days. No controlled studies to date have determined whether this technique truly limits the development of delayed reactions.

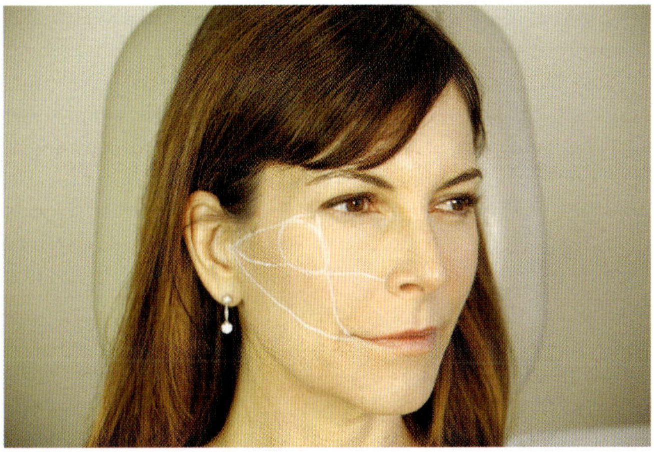

FIGURE 25-8 Analyzing the mid-face. Lines extend from the tragus to the lateral canthus, ala, and oral commissure and from the lateral canthus to oral commissure. In women, maximal light reflection falls in the uppermost quadrant of these intersecting lines.

Calcium Hydroxyapatite

Calcium hydroxyapatite has been marketed in the United States under the name Radiesse since 2006. It is a semi-solid suspension of 25- to 45-µm calcium hydroxyapatite microspheres in a gel carrier of sterile water, glycerin, and sodium carboxymethylcellulose. The primary mineral component of these spheres is the same as the calcium phosphate in bone and teeth, so the filler is biocompatible with low risk of allergic reaction. Mechanistically, new collagen forms over the calcium hydroxyapatite framework and replaces the carrier solution. These effects have been documented histologically for nearly 20 months, although clinical results beyond 12 months are less clear.[11]

On-label applications of Radiesse include correction of (1) moderate to severe facial folds and wrinkles such as the nasolabial folds, (2) lipoatrophy associated with HIV, and (3) volume loss of the dorsal hands, an often overlooked area that shares the same photo- and age-related volume changes as the face.[33,36,37] Facial revolumizing in immunocompetent patients is an off-label indication[11,38] (**Figure 25-12**); Radiesse should be injected at the dermal-subcutaneous junction or over periosteum. Results are immediate, with correction persisting for about 12 months. It should not be used for lip augmentation due to the risk of granuloma formation and should be used with care around the mouth, where constant contraction of the orbicularis oris during phonation may lead to migration and beading of the filler.[38] Because of substantial pain and throbbing after injection, the FDA allows for premixing of Radiesse with 2% lidocaine before treatment.

Of note, patients should understand that while Radiesse is radio-opaque and may be visible on radiographs, computed

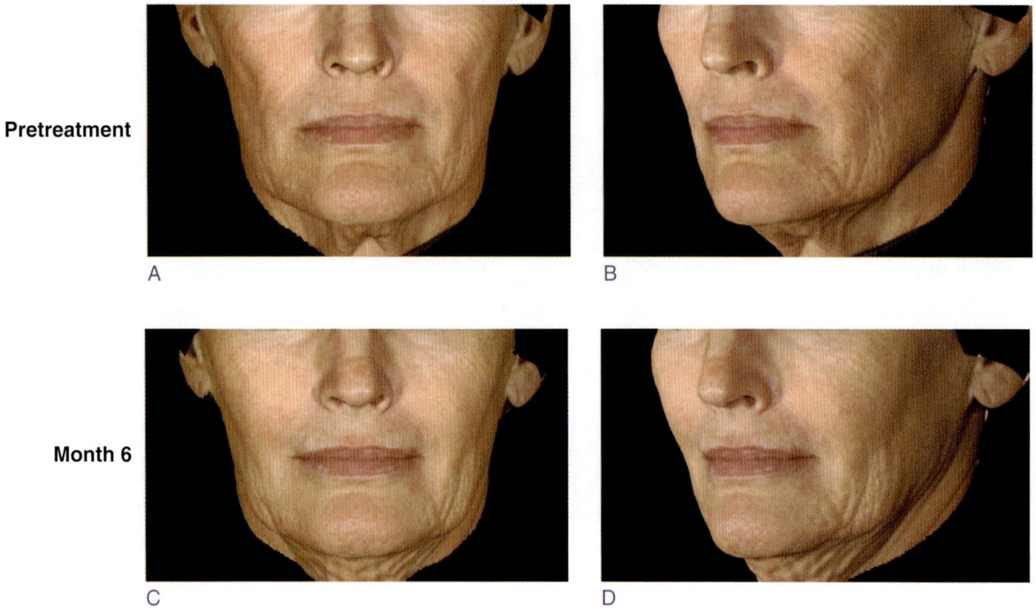

FIGURE 25-9 Three-dimensional midfacial volume restoration with Juvederm Voluma XC at baseline and 6 months.

tomography scans, and mammograms, the filler has not been shown to limit interpretation or obscure findings.[39]

Polymethylmethacrylate

Bellafill, formerly marketed as Artefill in the United States, is a solution of polymethylmethacrylate (PMMA) beads in 3.5% bovine collagen and 0.3% lidocaine with sterile water, phosphate buffer, and sodium chloride. The 30- to 50-µm microspheres are nonabsorbable and inert, made of the same compound as acrylic glass (trade names Plexiglass, Lucite, and Perspex) or as in orthopedic bone cement and intraocular lens implants for cataract surgery. The collagen in Bellafill/Artefill acts as a fluid carrier that degrades over 1 to 3 months and leaves intact beads, which become encapsulated in endogenous collagen.[33,40]

In 2006, Bellafill/Artefill became the first and only FDA-approved permanent filler available for correction of the nasolabial folds.[41] In 2015, it gained an indication for treatment of moderate to severe, distensible, atrophic acne scars in those over age 21 years. Skin testing for hypersensitivity reaction to the bovine collagen component is necessary before augmentation.

Unlike its predecessors Arteplast and Artecoll, Bellafill/Artefill has a lower rate of inflammatory adverse reactions, because the PMMA particles are more spherical, smooth, and uniformly sized. The manufacturer eliminated smaller microspheres measuring less than 20 µm, which are readily phagocytosed and cause granulomas.

A 5-year follow-up analysis of patients on the Bellafill/Artefill FDA pivotal nasolabial folds trial found that most were satisfied or very satisfied (95% and 83%, respectively) with their long-term results. Only 2% reported delayed adverse events, including irregular contour or granuloma formation, most of which were treatable.[42] Seventy-seven percent of participants in the acne scarring phase III trial reported improvement at 6 months compared to 44% of controls; these results persisted for up to 1 year of follow-up. There were no delayed granulomas noted in the latter study. The authors do not recommend injecting this product off-label in large quantities for volumizing, where there is a greater incidence of severe, recurrent subcutaneous inflammation and induration.[43]

Autologous Fibroblasts

The FDA licensed Azficel-T (laViv) in 2011 as a biologic product for the correction of moderate to severe nasolabial folds. Preparation of the material requires isolation and culture of autologous fibroblasts from punch biopsies of posterior auricular skin. These specimens are sent to the manufacturer who grows the cells in vitro until there is 1.2 mL of suspension containing 18 million patient-specific fibroblasts in Dulbecco's Modified Eagle Medium (DMEM). In the pivotal phase III trial, there was a statistically significant improvement in the appearance of nasolabial folds at 6 months versus placebo. Efficacy beyond that length of time is less well established.[44]

Drawbacks of Azficel-T compared to other fillers include requisite skin biopsies, producing secondary defects and scars; delay between time of specimen collection and fibroblast injection; unclear duration of correction; limited yield based on volume and quality of biopsy tissue sent; and high cost. Hence, several other products (ie, Autologen, Fibrel, Isolagen) derived from autologous fibroblasts are no longer sold in the United States.

Fat Transfer

Some consider autologous fat the optimal filler, since it is relatively abundant, highly biocompatible, able to provide natural-appearing volumetric correction, and potentially permanent, although rates of graft survival are variable.[45] The concept of fat transfer is not new. However, older en bloc techniques required

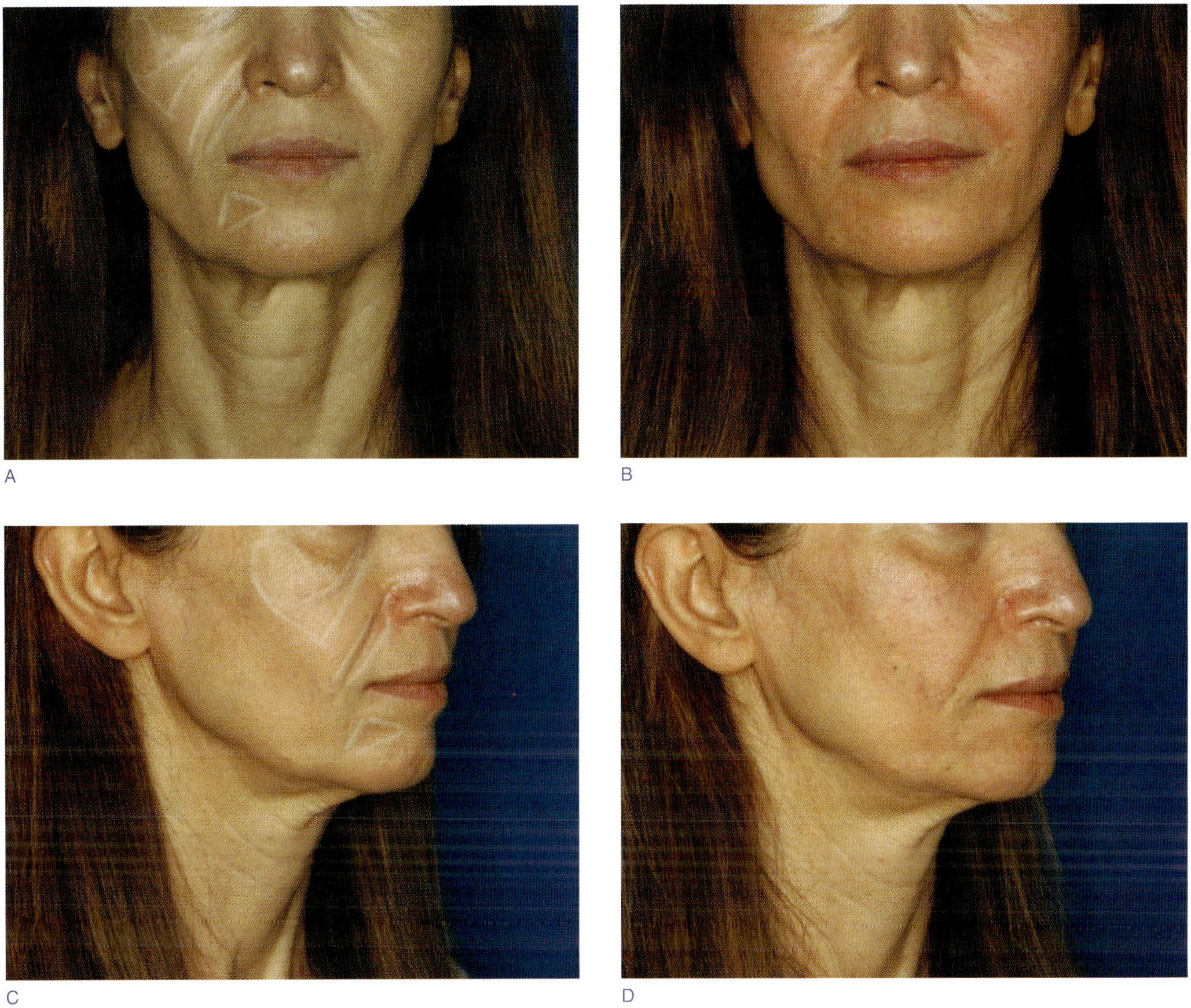

FIGURE 25-10 Midfacial volume restoration with 2 mL of Juvederm Voluma XC and 1 mL of Juvederm Ultra Plus. Baseline (**A and C**) and after (**B and D**).

excision of a solid section of tissue with subsequent implantation in larger segments, a process that left not only a new donor-site defect but also possible graft-site incisional scars. The advent and popularity of liposuction in the 1980s made lipotransfer more feasible. Aspirated fat could be reinjected through small-bore cannulas or needles with minimal scarring.[46,47]

Deficits at the nasolabial folds, cheeks, marionette lines, lips, and infraorbital region, as well as atrophic scars (ie, those from acne) and areas of stable, subcutaneous, facial atrophy (ie, from linear morphea or Parry-Romberg syndrome), may all be improved with autologous fat transfer. Correction of HIV-related lipoatrophy and rejuvenation of the dorsal hands are other documented indications. Lipotransfer is unable to treat fine lines or small, superficial scars that require dermal placement of filler.[48-50]

There are multiple modalities for harvesting, processing, and injecting fat.[51,52] No studies to date have established an optimal donor site, and any region of excess adipose may be reasonable. Common sites are readily accessible, insensitive to weight loss via diet and exercise, and associated with low morbidity: periumbilical, lumbar back, trochanteric buttocks and/or medial thigh, and medial knee or arm.[53] Common harvesting practices involve premedicating patients with anxiolytic and/or narcotic drugs as needed; infiltrating the subcutaneous space at the donor site with tumescent anesthesia, consisting of saline admixed with small amounts of lidocaine with epinephrine; and making small incisions. A traditional aspiration cannula or 14-gauge, single-holed microcannula attached to a hypodermic Luer-Lok syringe can be used to harvest the fat. Graft survival is directly related to graft trauma, and care must be taken to maintain suction at less than

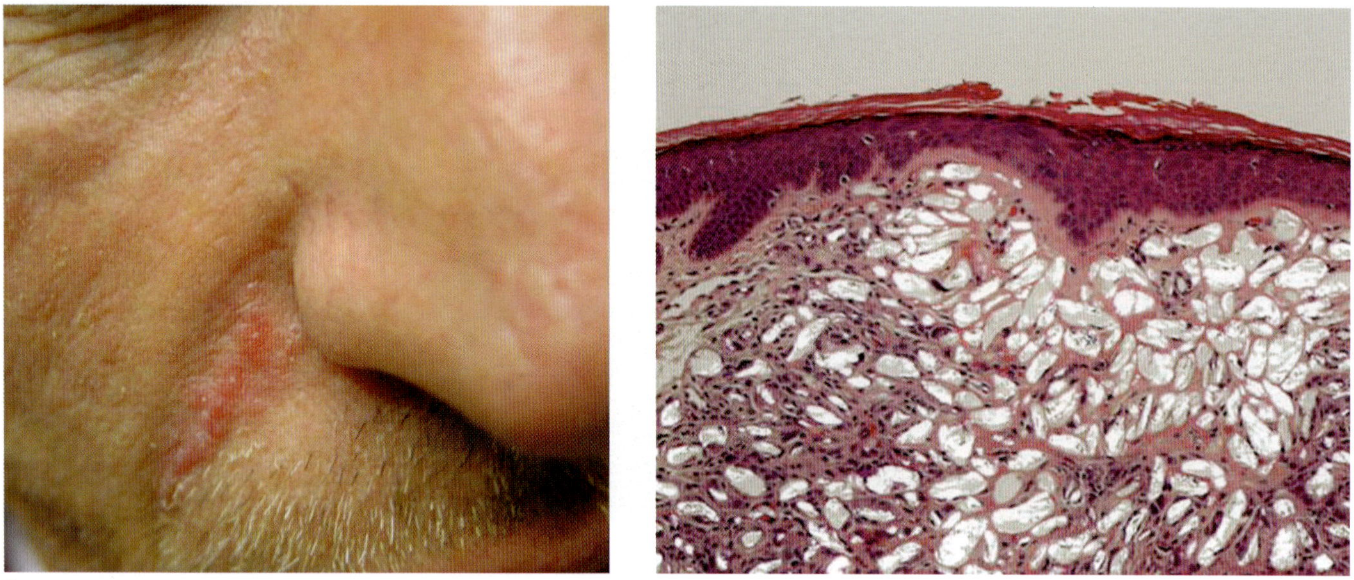

A B

FIGURE 25-11 Granulomatous papules after intradermal Sculptra injection. Clinical image (**A**) and histopathology stained for hematoxylin and eosin (H&E) (**B**).

1 atmosphere (ie, by using small syringes). Increased suction vaporizes and breaks adipocytes.[45] Gravity layers out the supernatant fat, so it can be washed of oils, blood/serum, and anesthetic fluid. Kuran et al[54] reported good success with open system purification, but this technique may increase the risk of infection. Centrifuge separation is also an option; however, resultant trauma may decrease graft survival.[55,56] Extracted adipose can be frozen at –30°C (slow freezing, slow thawing process) and stored for as long as 12 to 18 months.[57] There are also several ways to place the fat grafts. Fat is deposited with a large-bore 16- or 18-gauge needle or cannula parallel to the target rhytides. Alternative methods include pearl fat grafting or microautologous fat transplantation.[46,54]

Postinjection massage helps mold and distribute the grafts evenly. Unlike Sculptra, patients should not continue this massaging at home and should avoid dynamic facial animation, since the motion may encourage graft migration. Systemic antibiotics and aspirin/NSAID-free pain management regimens are other frequent postoperative practices. Patients should be counseled about edema that may last for weeks.

Determining the degree and longevity of graft survival has proven difficult and unpredictable.[51,52,58] Outcomes depend on technique and experience, with new methods showing up to 50% long-term success.[45] In general, repeated, small-volume injections every 3 months are better than large-volume augmentation. If the graft is too big, then passive diffusion from the recipient bed may not sufficiently maintain its metabolic demand and revascularization is insufficient. Overcorrection anticipates some graft loss but increases the rate of failure and even necrosis. Graft migration occurs with overfilling as well—moving to areas with less tension or better blood supply.

Although there have been many developments in the field of lipotransfer, questions persist. Patients should thoroughly understand the strengths and limitations, in particular the need for two procedures (harvesting and implantation) and multiple sessions, as well as likely downtime.[40,59]

Silicone

Injection of silicone (polydimethylsiloxane [PDMS]) has a storied past, and its use as a soft-tissue implant continues to be controversial. The term *silicone* refers to a family of inert, silicon-containing synthetics. Siloxanes are members of this family, composed of silicon, oxygen, and methane. For any given compound, the siloxane chain length and polymerization determine its viscosity, measured in centristokes (cs); 1 cs equals the viscosity of water and 350 cs, mineral oil. Heavy metals, oils, and other organic substances naturally contaminate silicones, so purification is compulsory. Proponents of silicone injection for augmentation believe that many of the reported adverse reactions result from impurities and that it is safe and effective in the hands of experienced providers who administer small quantities of product.

Permanent augmentation with PDMS became popular in the 1960s with the introduction of medical-grade products. Soon, untrained practitioners began injecting industrial silicones or adulterated oils instead, which caused severe complications. Medical-grade liquid injectable silicone has a viscosity of 350 cs and is purer than industrial compounds. Despite clinical trials, it was never FDA approved for use in humans. AdatoSil (5000 cs) and Silikon (1000 cs) were approved in 1994 and 1997, respectively, for ophthalmologic indications and have been injected lawfully for soft-tissue augmentation since 1997, when the FDA passed the Modernization Act allowing off-label use of medical devices. Silikon 1000 is currently the most appropriate agent available.

Technique is paramount when administering permanent fillers. The microdroplet serial puncture method allows for more precise placement: 0.005- to 0.01-mL aliquots deposited every

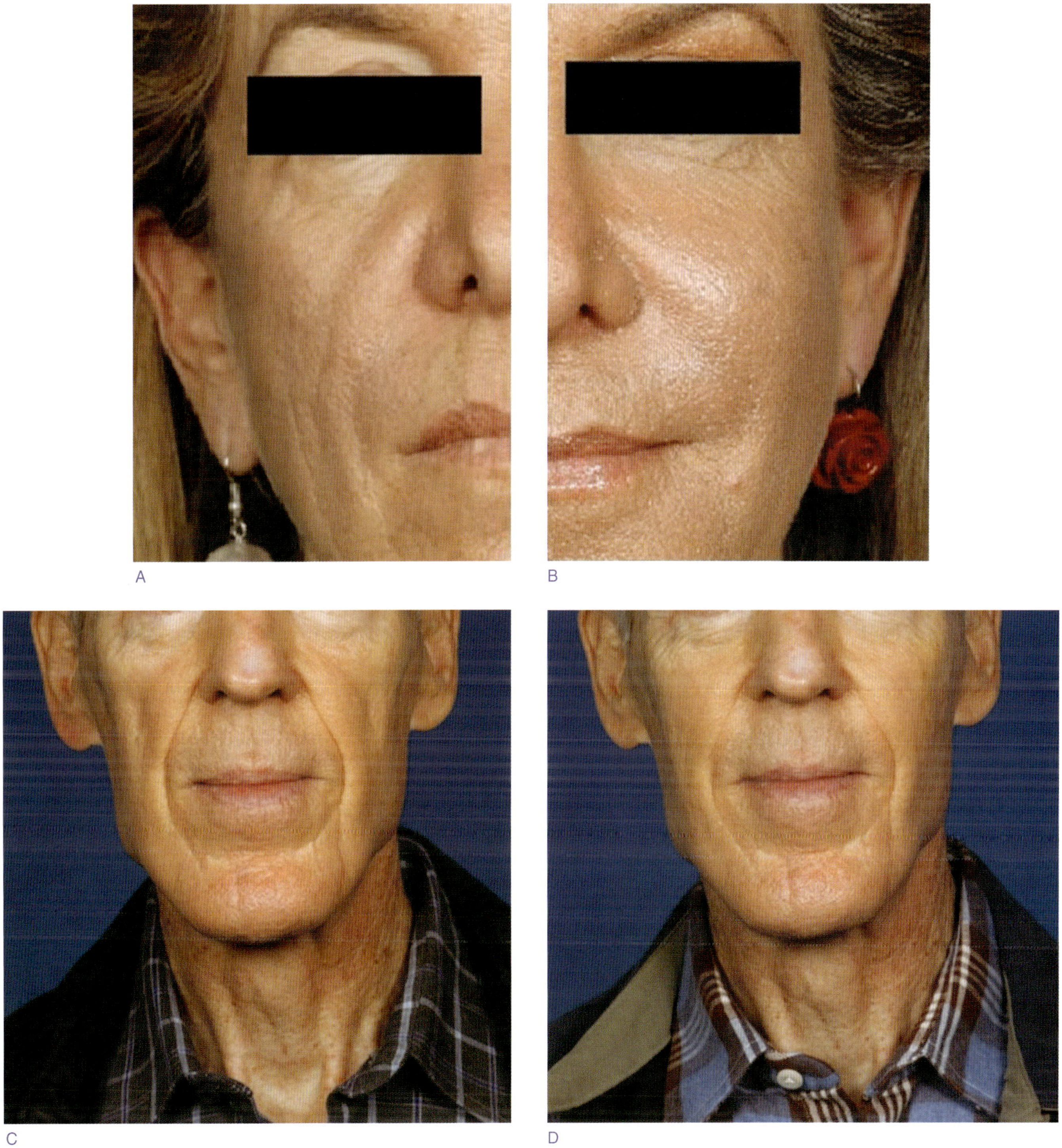

FIGURE 25-12 Treatment with Radiesse at the nasolabial folds (baseline **A**, after **B**) and midface (baseline **C**, after **D**) in immunocompetent patients.

2 to 5 mm subdermally (**Figure 25-13**). Overcorrection or multiple passes should be avoided. Relatively small volumes are recommended, and in a given treatment session, no more than 0.5 mL should be used for regions with small surface area defects (ie, the nasolabial folds), and up to 2.0 mL may be used for regions with large surface area defects (ie, facial lipoatrophy). These volumes decrease over time as the desired effect is achieved. Treatment sessions typically occur every 4 weeks initially and then can be spaced farther apart to allow sufficient time for fibroplasia to encapsulate the product.[60]

Risks related to silicone augmentation are real but often secondary to improper technique, incorrect dosage, or tainted material. Erythema, edema, and ecchymoses are common and usually resolve within days. Dermal, instead of subdermal, injection can cause rippling. Other potential complications include superficial beading from overcorrection, granuloma formation

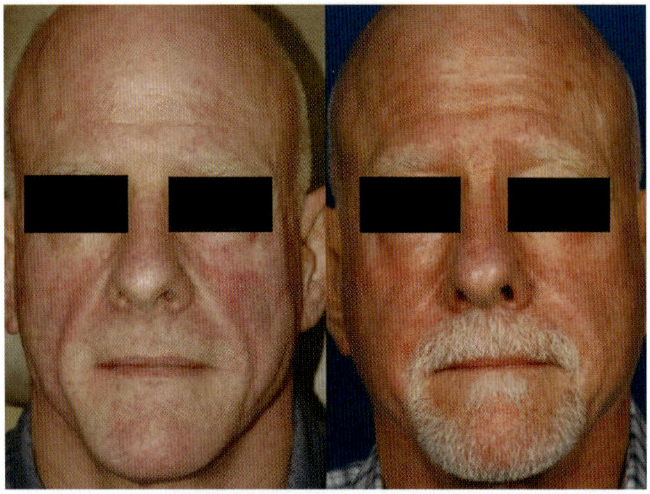

FIGURE 25-13 Silicone correction in a patient with human immunodeficiency virus (HIV).

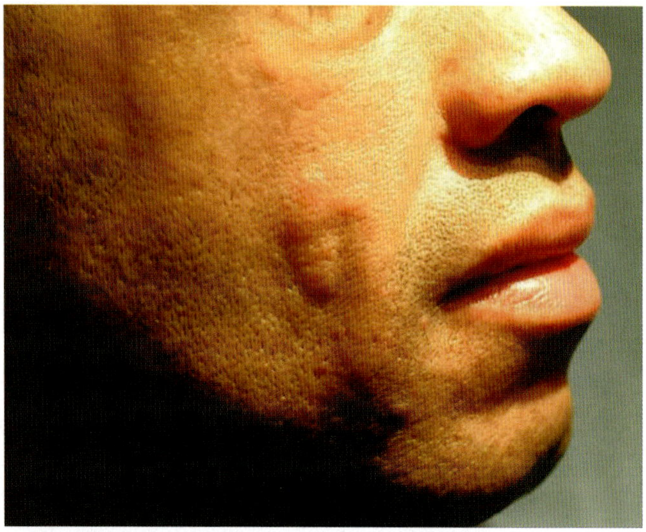

FIGURE 25-14 Nodule formation after silicone injection.

(**Figure 25-14**), and product migration, which are more likely with large amounts of less viscous oil. Meticulous treatment protocols frequently help avoid these adverse events,[61] yet delayed granulomatous reactions weeks, months, or years after treatment are possible and may require intralesional corticosteroids combined with 5-fluorouracil, and possibly systemic antibiotics

Amid decades of debate, recent studies suggest that when injected under optimal conditions, the complication rate from silicone soft tissue augmentation is less than 1%. In expert hands, highly purified injectable silicone is a reliable and reproducible option for correction of advanced HIV-associated lipoatrophy.[33,62]

COMPLICATIONS

Given that facial rejuvenation is largely an elective procedure, the safety of soft-tissue fillers is paramount. Significant adverse events are infrequent. Possible complications and methods of addressing them are listed in **Table 25-10**.

TABLE 25-10 • Complications from Soft-Tissue Fillers

Complication	Description	Prevention and Management Considerations
Injection site reactions	Generally mild and resolve in 1 week ■ Erythema ■ Edema ■ Induration ■ Pain ■ Bleeding ■ Bruising	Prevention ■ Hold anticoagulant/antiplatelet agents (eg, aspirin) if possible ■ Pretreat with local anesthetics for pain ■ Inject with small-bore needles ■ Use cannulas or fewer injection sites to limit the number of punctures and bruising ■ Avoid rigorous physical activity for 24 hours after procedure Management ■ Apply ice for edema and pain ■ Treat bruises with intense pulse light or vascular lasers
Nodules, beading, and Tyndall effect	■ Superficial injection ■ Bluish discoloration (Tyndall effect) with particulate HA derivatives	Prevention ■ Avoid superficial deposition ■ Inject smoothly and regularly without large blebs of product Management ■ Massage ■ Inject hyaluronidase if HA filler ■ Aspirate, excise
Persistent papules	■ Higher rates with specific products	■ Sculptra: increase dilution volume, dilute farther in advance of procedure, agitate solution vigorously ■ Radiesse: avoid injections around mouth due to migration from phonation ■ Bellafill/Artefill: inject smoothly ■ Silicone: use microdroplet technique

(*Continued*)

TABLE 25-10 • Complications from Soft-Tissue Fillers (Continued)

Complication	Description	Prevention and Management Considerations
Infection	▪ Acute bacterial (cellulitis, abscess)	Prevention ▪ Cleanse with antimicrobial agent (eg, alcohol, chlorhexidine) ▪ Wear clean gloves, switch after intraoral contact or injection ▪ Inject smoothly and regularly without large clumps of product Management ▪ Start antibiotics ▪ Culture and consider biopsy for histopathology ▪ Incise and drain, if indicated
Herpes simplex virus reactivation	▪ Perioral reactivation ▪ Sites of prior facial infection	Prevention ▪ Give prophylactic oral antiviral medication if history of postprocedural herpes, treating perioral region in patient with history of herpes labialis, or possibly, frequent recurrences ▪ Delay injections if evidence of active outbreak Management ▪ Start full treatment dosing of oral antiviral medication
Hypersensitivity	▪ Most common after bovine collagen fillers (up to 3%) ▪ Rare with HA fillers from contaminants, by-products of bacterial fermentation, or lower molecular weight molecules; often resolves spontaneously	Prevention ▪ Avoid injection if known sensitivity ▪ Skin testing for fillers containing bovine collagen (eg, Bellafill/Artefill) Management ▪ Consider starting tacrolimus ointment, intralesional corticosteroids ▪ Incision and drainage
Delayed nodules	▪ Inflammatory/immunologic ▪ Biofilm ▪ Infection (eg, atypical mycobacteria) ▪ Foreign body granulomas	Prevention ▪ Cleanse with antimicrobial agent (eg, alcohol, chlorhexidine) ▪ Skin testing before fillers containing bovine collagen (eg, Bellafill/Artefill) Management ▪ Incise and drain with culture and/or biopsy for histopathology ▪ Inject hyaluronidase if HA filler ▪ Start broad-spectrum antibiotics for 2-6 weeks (eg, clarithromycin, doxycycline/minocycline) ▪ Consider starting topical, oral, or intralesional corticosteroids; intralesional 5-fluorouracil; oral immunosuppressants; laser therapy ▪ Excise, if persistent
Vascular compromise	▪ Necrosis (glabella, medial cheek) ▪ Blindness, ophthalmoplegia (glabella, nasal dorsum, nasolabial folds) ▪ Extremely rarely, cerebrovascular accident	Prevention ▪ Understand thoroughly facial anatomy, especially vascular anatomy • Understand thoroughly the depth at which different fillers should be placed • Inject small aliquots, slowly, under low pressure (limits retrograde embolization) • Use cannulas or small-gauge needles in higher risk regions Management ▪ Discontinue immediately for blanching, duskiness, reticulate erythema, severe pain, vision changes ▪ Consider starting oral aspirin, prednisone, low-molecular-weight heparins, hyperbaric oxygen therapy ▪ If ulceration/necrosis, provide careful wound care ▪ In the setting of vascular compromise, apply warm compresses and nitroglycerin paste; massage; inject hyaluronidase along affected artery and its tributaries if HA filler

HA, hyaluronic acid.

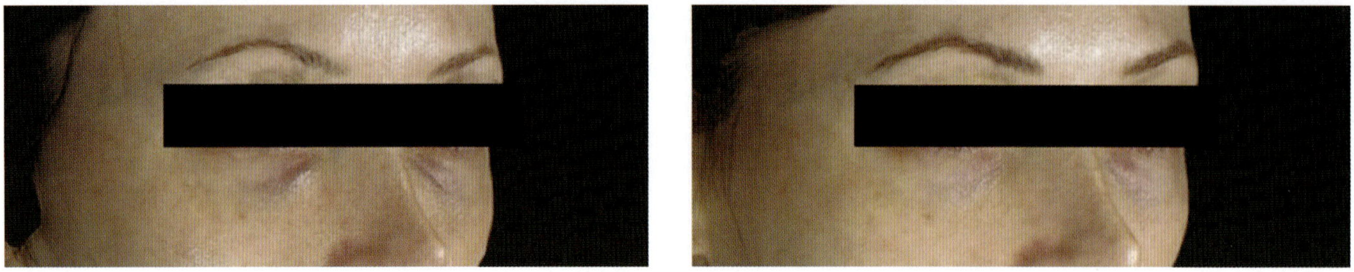

A B

FIGURE 25-15 Tyndall effect at the tear troughs from superficial deposition of hyaluronic acid filler. Baseline (**A**) and after (**B**) hyaluronidase injection.

Pain, erythema, edema, induration, bleeding, and bruising are the most common reactions. They are generally mild and resolve within 1 week. Intense physical activity that raises blood pressure may increase the incidence of ecchymoses and bleeding, so patients should abstain for 24 hours after the procedure. Limiting the number of needle sticks, using blunt-tipped cannulas or small-gauge needles, slowly injecting small volumes of product, and temporarily holding unnecessarily antiplatelet medications/supplements for the 7 to 10 days prior to treatment may help minimize these risks.[63] When bruising does develop, energy-based therapies (ie, pulsed dye or potassium titanyl phosphate lasers, intense pulsed light) may clear extravasated blood more rapidly.[64]

In addition to injection site reactions, more serious complications occur at low rates. Intradermal placement can produce ridging, beading, and palpable or visible papulonodules. Superficial HA in particular can cause a temporary bluish tint in these areas due to the Tyndall effect—differential refraction of light off particles in a colloid (**Figure 25-15**). Persistent papulonodules are more likely with Sculptra, Bellafill/Artefill, and silicone than other agents.

Infections, including cellulitis and abscesses, are another potential risk. Puncture sites can serve as portals of entry for resident skin or oral flora. Sterilizing the treatment area with isopropyl alcohol, chlorhexidine, or another appropriate antiseptic and wearing clean gloves are common practice to minimize infection rates. All suspected infections should be cultured and/or biopsied for identification and sensitivities. Patients should start broad-spectrum antibiotics with or without anaerobic coverage until the results return.[65] Incision and drainage may be needed for fluctuant lesions. Injection-related trauma can also reactivate herpes simplex virus, particularly periorally. In those with a history of frequent or postprocedural outbreak(s), prophylactic antiviral therapy may be warranted, and injection should be delayed in the case of active blistering.[64]

In the early era of soft-tissue augmentation, hypersensitivity reactions were far more frequent. Bovine collagen was the first FDA-approved soft-tissue filler in the United States, but 3% of patients developed antibodies and clinically significant allergy to the material.[66] Thus, skin testing was mandatory to decrease, albeit not fully prevent, this risk. In the United States, Bellafill/Artefill is the only currently marketed product still requiring skin testing before augmentation. Part of the appeal of HA, Sculptra, and Radiesse is their biocompatibility, a quality that eliminates the need for preprocedural allergy testing. A few cases of hypersensitivity to HA do exist and may arise from contaminants, by-products of bacterial fermentation used in production, or lower molecular weight molecules such as those in Juvederm Voluma XC.[65,67] While these reactions may subside spontaneously, topical calcineurin inhibitors, intralesional corticosteroid injections, systemic anti-inflammatory medications, incision and drainage, or hyaluronidase injection can hasten the process.[63]

Both hypersensitivity and infection with or without biofilm can contribute to the formation of delayed nodules. Foreign body reactions are another possible explanation, and distinguishing between these etiologies can be difficult. Unlike acute abscesses, biofilms lead to chronic infection. Microbial colonies adhere to the implant and secrete an extracellular polysaccharide matrix coating that is resistant to detergents, antimicrobials, and host immune responses. Clinically, nodules related to biofilms may appear inflammatory, infectious, abscess-like, or granulomatous.[65] Because conventional culturing methods frequently fail to detect the underlying bacteria, culture results may be misleading. Fluorescent in situ hybridization (FISH) detects the causative microbe in most culture-negative cases but is not routinely run.[68] Atypical mycobacteria can cause delayed infection as well, so separate histology and tissue cultures should be considered. Results from these studies should guide ongoing treatment.

Any time a foreign body is introduced into the skin, there is potential for a nonallergic granulomatous reaction, even years after treatment. The incidence after HA correction has been reported as 0.02% to 0.4%.[69,70] It is higher for non-HA materials.[69] As previously mentioned, volume injected, presence of impurities, and product type affect the rates of granuloma formation. HA and collagen typically develop cystic granulomas; silicone, paraffin, and polyacrylamide (not licensed in the United States) develop lipogranulomas; and PMMA and poly-L-lactic acid develop sclerosing granulomas.[69] Since differentiating inflammatory complications from biofilm infections is not straightforward, antibiotic treatment, such as clarithromycin or a tetracycline class medication for 2 to 6 weeks, rather than corticosteroids, should be first-line treatment, and long-term antimicrobials may be prudent in suspect infections.[71]

Fortunately, most contour irregularities, blue-gray discoloration, and acute and delayed nodules improve over time either spontaneously or with treatment. One of the appealing features of HA derivatives is the ability to reverse undesired outcomes with hyaluronidase (**Figure 25-16**). There are two

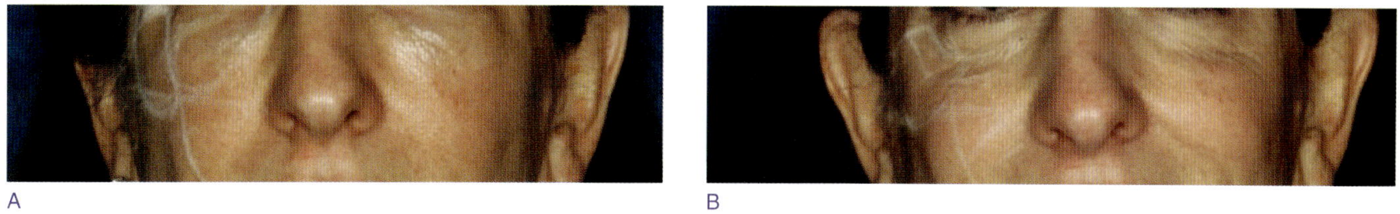

FIGURE 25-16 Correction of contour irregularities with hyaluronidase. Baseline (**A**) and after (**B**).

FDA-approved formulations, Vitrase and Hylenex, used off-label as first-line treatment to degrade injectable HA. Vitrase is a purified ovine testicular enzyme, while Hylenex is a recombinant human protein. The necessary hyaluronidase dose varies by formulation and filler. In vitro data suggest that more crosslinked HA derivatives require larger doses for optimal outcomes. It is reasonable to use 5 units of Vitrase hyaluronidase per 0.1 mL of Restylane and 10 units per 0.1 mL of Juvederm.[31] Allergic reactions to hyaluronidase are rare, estimated at 1 in 2000,[71] and the majority of these are localized. In nonemergent situations, intradermal skin testing may be considered, especially in patients with known allergies to bees, wasps, or hornets (classification order *Hymenoptera*), whose venom contains hyaluronidase. Those allergic to thimerosal are also at increased risk, since some enzyme formulations contain this preservative.[71] If intralesional hyaluronidase is ineffective or nodules occur in the setting of non-HA augmentation, other reported medical therapies include oral antibiotics (antimicrobial and anti-inflammatory effects); topical, intralesional, or systemic corticosteroids; intralesional 5-fluorouracil; oral immunosuppressants such as cyclosporine; lasers; or combination therapies.[72] Persistent or refractory nodules may require excision.

Although rare, potentially irreversible vascular complications are the most dreaded and serious adverse events following soft-tissue augmentation.[73] Vascular compromise from extravascular compression, intravascular injection, or embolism with downstream occlusion can cause tissue ischemia and necrosis. The glabella is a high-risk, watershed region due to limited collateral circulation.[74] Historically, up to 50% of patients treated with Zyplast to the glabella developed some degree of necrosis.[75] Injection at the medial cheek similarly demands care.[74] The angular artery, a terminal branch of the external carotid, runs superior to the nasolabial fold and then divides into the lateral nasal artery as well as other collateral branches that anastomose with the internal carotid system. Substantial anatomic variation in the exact course of these vessels exists. Moreover, the union of embryonic fusion planes at the alar groove prevents tissue distension, so there is little room to accommodate large quantities of filler without interrupting the vasculature.[73] Acute or excruciating pain, blanching, duskiness, and reticulate erythema (**Figure 25-17**) tracking the involved artery and its tributaries may indicate impending necrosis. Typically, these signs occur immediately but can be delayed in the case of occlusion from postprocedural edema. Once recognized, treatment should begin immediately.[63] Prompt and ongoing care decreases the risk of permanent adverse effects and disfigurement.[73] One study recently reviewed several cases of vascular compromise and outlined treatment and prevention measures.[73] Because of its ability to decrease edema and, consequently, external vessel compression, some recommend hyaluronidase injection irrespective of filler type.[76] Early reports supported infusion of up to 30 units of enzyme along the affected vasculature,[77] but now the recommendation is to exceed 100 to 200 units.[76,78,79] The more crosslinked the HA agent, the more hyaluronidase is necessary for optimal outcomes.[32] Application of warm compresses and topical nitroglycerin, as well as firm massage, are other recommended treatments. Oral aspirin, prednisone, and hyperbaric oxygen, and low-molecular-weight heparins have been employed less frequently. Meticulous wound care is important if necrosis and ulceration do develop.

Alternatively, filler implanted intravascularly can embolize retrograde into the ocular circulation, a rare cause of ophthalmoplegia or blindness.[80] Incidence of this complication was reported as 0.001% in the past, but the largest recent review of cases performed by expert physicians found a rate of 0.05%. This increased rate may be partially attributable to the introduction of newer agents designed for deeper deposition.[73] Corrections at the glabella, nasal dorsum, or nasolabial folds are highest risk,[81] since branches of the internal carotid (ie, supratrochlear and dorsal nasal arteries) either directly feed or anastomose at these anatomic locations. The internal carotid also gives rise to the ophthalmic artery and the central retinal artery; hence, injecting under high pressure can force product upstream into the ocular circulation[80]

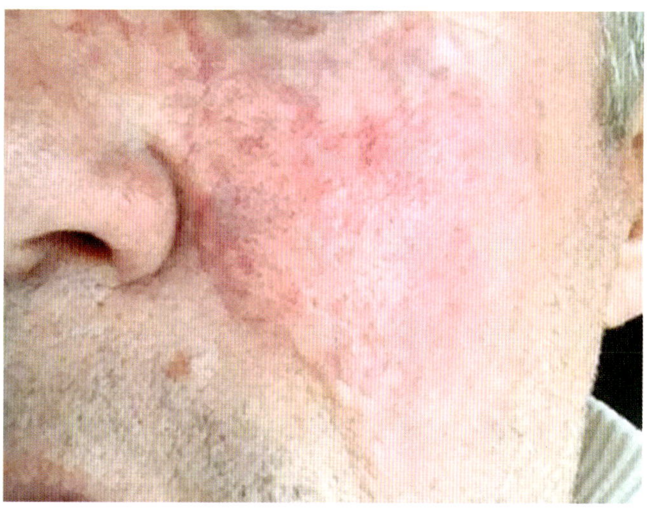

FIGURE 25-17 Evolving vascular compromise with dusky, reticulate erythema.

and produce sudden, profound pain and vision loss. More infrequently, forceful intra-arterial administration can cause cerebral artery embolism with potential infarct. Patients should undergo emergent ophthalmology and/or neurology evaluation if there is any concern for impairment; immediate retro- or peribulbar injection of at least 500 units of hyaluronidase is one technique proposed to partially reverse vision changes.[82]

Preventing vascular compromise is critical, considering that treatment of local tissue necrosis, blindness, or cerebrovascular infarct is often ineffective once it has occurred.[80] Using blunt-tipped cannulas instead of needles is one way to decrease potential risks. The cannula's flexible, dull end is less likely to pierce vessel walls and place filler intralumenally. Cannulas may be especially prudent for subdermal injection at the central cheek medial to the mid-pupillary line.

Overall, facial rejuvenation with injectable fillers and implants is a safe procedure. Understanding regional anatomy, injection techniques, and methods to prevent and manage complications ensures successful outcomes.

CONCLUSION

As the demand for minimally invasive rejuvenation procedures climbs, so does the popularity of soft-tissue fillers to correct skin folds and subcutaneous volume loss.[83] The most desirable outcomes often come from combining different agents with different properties, and a strong understanding of the relevant anatomy, available products, injection techniques, potential complications, and realistic expectations may ensure the best results for patients and clinicians alike.

REFERENCES

1. Bacigalupi R, Clark J, Lupo MP. An overview of injectable fillers with special consideration to the periorbital area. *Cosmet Dermatol.* 2012;25:421-426.
2. US Food and Drug Administration. Soft tissue fillers approved by the Center for Devices and Radiological Health. Maryland. http://www.fda.gov/MedicalDevices/ProductsandMedicalProcedures/CosmeticDevices/WrinkleFillers/ucm227749.htm. Accessed August 4, 2016.
3. Ashinoff R. Overview: soft tissue augmentation. *Clin Plast Surg.* 2000;27(4):479-487.
4. De Maio M. Ethnic and gender considerations in the use of facial injectables: male patients. *Plast Reconstr Surg.* 2015;136:40S-43S.
5. Mauricio D, Rzany B. *The Male Patient in Aesthetic Medicine.* Berlin, Germany: Springer; 2009.
6. Shaw RB Jr, Katzel EB, Koltz PF, et al. Aging of the facial skeleton: Aesthetic implications and rejuvenation strategies. *Plast Reconstr Surg.* 2011;127(1):374-383.
7. Nouveau-Richard S, Yang Z, Mac-Mary S, et al. Skin ageing: a comparison between Chinese and European populations. A pilot study. *J Dermatol Sci.* 2005;40:187-193.
8. Tsukahara K, Fujimura T, Yoshida Y, et al. Comparison of age-related changes in wrinkling and sagging of the skin in Caucasian females and in Japanese females. *J Cosmet Sci.* 2004;55:351-371.
9. Shirakabe Y, Suzuki Y, Lam SM. A new paradigm for the aging Asian face. *Aesthetic Plast Surg.* 2003;27:397-402.
10. Braun M, Braun S. Nodule formation following lip augmentation using porcine collagen-derived filler. *J Drugs Dermatol.* 2008;7(6):579-581.
11. Moers-Carpi M, Storck R, Howell DJ, Ogilvie P, Ogilvie A. Physician and patient satisfaction after use of calcium hydroxylapatite for cheek augmentation. *Dermatol Surg.* 2012;38(7 Pt 2):1217-1222.
12. Zeichner JA, Cohen JL. Use of blunt tipped cannulas for soft tissue fillers. *J Drug Dermatol.* 2012;11:70-72.
13. Sundaram H, Weinkle S, Pozner J, Dewandre L. Blunt-tipped microcannulas for the injection of soft tissue fillers: a consensus panel assessment and recommendations. *J Drug Dermatol.* 2012;11:s33-s39.
14. Tamura BM. Fascial anatomy and the applications of fillers and botulinum toxin: part 2. *Surg Cosmet Dermatol.* 2010;2(4):291-303.
15. Lohn JW, Penn JW, Norton J, Butler PE. The course and variation of the facial artery and vein: implications for facial transplantation and facial surgery. *Ann Plast Surg.* 2011;67(2):184-188.
16. Yang HM, Lee YI, Lee JG, et al. Topography of superficial arteries on the face. *Kor J Phys Anthropol.* 2013;26(4):131-140.
17. Buck DW 2nd, Alam M, Kim JY. Injectable fillers for facial rejuvenation: a review. *J Plast Reconstr Aesthet Surg.* 2009;62(1):11-18.
18. Necas JB, Brauner P, Kolar J. Hyaluronic acid (hyaluronan): a review. *Vet Med.* 2008;53(8):397-411.
19. Lin ZY, Shah V, Dhinakar A, et al. Intradermal fillers for minimally invasive treatment of facial aging. *Plast Aesthet Res.* 2016;3:72-82.
20. US Food and Drug Administration. Meeting of the General and Plastic Surgery Devices Panel FDA Advisory Committee briefing document: Juvederm Voluma XC PMA (P110033). Silver Spring, MD: FDA Maryland; 2013.
21. Bezzola AM. Esthelis acide hyaluronique de conception suisse. Premiere etude complete des caracteristiques physico-chimiques et essais cliniques. *J Med Esthet Chir Dermatol.* 2005;125:11-20.
22. Narins RS, Brandt F, Leyden J, Lorenc ZP, Rubin M, Smith S. A randomized, double-blind, multicenter comparison of the efficacy and tolerability of Restylane versus Zyplast for the correction of nasolabial folds. *Dermatol Surg.* 2003;29(6):588-595.
23. Baumann LS, Shamban AT, Lupo MP, et al. Comparison of smooth-gel hyaluronic acid dermal fillers with cross-linked bovine collagen: a multicenter, double-masked, randomized, within-subject study. *Dermatol Surg.* 2007;33(Suppl 2):S128-S135.
24. Narins RS, Coleman WP 3rd, Donofrio LM, et al. Improvement in nasolabial folds with a hyaluronic acid filler using a cohesive polydensified matrix technology: results from an 18-month open-label extension trial. *Dermatol Surg.* 2010;36(suppl 3):1800-1808.
25. Narins RS, Dayan SH, Brandt FS, Baldwin EK. Persistence and improvement of nasolabial fold correction with nonanimal-stabilized hyaluronic acid 100,000 gel particles/mL filler on two retreatment schedules: results up to 18 months on two retreatment schedules. *Dermatol Surg.* 2008;34(Suppl 1):S2-S8; discussion S9.
26. Smith SR, Jones D, Thomas JA, Murphy DK, Beddingfield FC 3rd. Duration of wrinkle correction following repeat treatment with Juvederm hyaluronic acid fillers. *Arch Dermatol Res.* 2010;302(10):757-762.

27. Micheels P, Besse S, Flynn TC, Sarazin D, Elbaz Y. Superficial dermal injection of hyaluronic acid soft tissue fillers: comparative ultrasound study. *Dermatol Surg.* 2012;38(7 Pt 2):1162-1169.

28. US Food and Drug Administration. Summary of Safety and Effectiveness Data (SSED): Restylane-L injectable Gel. Silver Spring, MD: FDA Maryland; 2012.

29. US Food and Drug Administration. Summary of Safety and Effectiveness Data (SSED): Restylane Silk Injectable GEl. Silver Spring, MD: FDA Maryland; 2014.

30. Glogau RG, Bank D, Brandt F, et al. A randomized, evaluator-blinded, controlled study of the effectiveness and safety of small gel particle hyaluronic acid for lip augmentation. *Dermatol Surg.* 2012;38(7 Pt 2):1180-1192.

31. US Food and Drug Administration. Summary of Safety and Effectiveness Data (SSED): Juvederm Voluma XC. Silver Spring, MD: FDA Maryland; 2013.

32. Jones DT, Borell M. In-vitro resistance to degradation of hyaluronic acid by ovine testicular hyaluronidase. *Dermatol Surg.* 2010;36(s1):804-809.

33. Jones D. Volumizing the face with soft tissue fillers. *Clin Plast Surg.* 2011;38(3):379-390.

34. Bauer U, Graivier MH. Optimizing injectable poly-L-lactic acid administration for soft tissue augmentation: the rationale for three treatment sessions. *Can J Plast Surg.* 2011;19(3):e22-e27.

35. US Food and Drug Administration. Summary of Safety and Effectiveness Data (SSED): Sculptra Aesthetic. Silver Spring, MD: FDA Maryland; 2009.

36. Smith S, Busso M, McClaren M, Bass LS. A randomized, bilateral, prospective comparison of calcium hydroxylapatite microspheres versus human-based collagen for the correction of nasolabial folds. *Dermatol Surg.* 2007;33(Suppl 2):S112-S121; discussion S121.

37. Carruthers A, Carruthers J. Evaluation of injectable calcium hydroxylapatite for the treatment of facial lipoatrophy associated with human immunodeficiency virus. *Dermatol Surg.* 2008;34(11):1486-1499.

38. Busso MM-C, Storck M, Ogilvie P, Ogilvie A. Multicentered, randomized trial assessing the effectiveness and safety of calcium hydroxylapatite for hand rejuvenation. *Dermatol Surg.* 2010;36:790-797.

39. Carruthers A, Liebeskind M, Carruthers J, Forster BB. Radiographic and computed tomographic studies of calcium hydroxylapatite for treatment of HIV-associated facial lipoatrophy and correction of nasolabial folds. *Dermatol Surg.* 2008;34(Suppl 1):S78-S84.

40. Tzikas TL. Autologous fat grafting for midface rejuvenation. *Facial Plast Surg Clin North Am.* 2006;14(3):229-240.

41. US Food and Drug Administration. Summary of Safety and Effectiveness Data (SSED): Artefill. Silver Spring, MD: FDA Maryland; 2003.

42. Cohen SR, Berner CF, Busso M, et al. ArteFill: a long-lasting injectable wrinkle filler material: summary of the U.S. Food and Drug Administration trials and a progress report on 4- to 5-year outcomes. *Plast Reconstr Surg.* 2006;118(3 Suppl):64S-76S.

43. Karnik J, Baumann L, Bruce S, et al. A double-blind, randomized, multicenter, controlled trial of suspended polymethylmethacrylate microspheres for the correction of atrophic facial acne scars. *J Am Acad Dermatol.* 2014;71(1):77-83.

44. Smith SR, Munavalli G, Weiss R, Maslowski JM, Hennegan KP, Novak JM. A multicenter, double-blind, placebo-controlled trial of autologous fibroblast therapy for the treatment of nasolabial fold wrinkles. *Dermatol Surg.* 2012;38(7 Pt 2):1234-1243.

45. Niechajev I, Sevcuk O. Long-term results of fat transplantation: clinical and histologic studies. *Plast Reconstr Surg.* 1994;94(3): 496-506.

46. Ellenbogen R. Free autogenous pearl fat grafts in the face: a preliminary report of a rediscovered technique. *Ann Plast Surg.* 1986;16(3):179-194.

47. Ilouz YG. L'avenir de la reutilization de la grâisee apres liposuction. *Rev Clin Esthet Lang Franc.* 1984;9:36.

48. Gamboa GM, Ross WA. Autologous fat transfer in aesthetic facial recontouring. *Ann Plast Surg.* 2013;70(5):513-516.

49. Coleman SR. Facial recontouring with lipostructure. *Clin Plast Surg.* 1997;24(2):347-367.

50. Cetinkaya A, Devoto MH. Periocular fat grafting: indications and techniques. *Curr Opin Ophthalmol.* 2013;24(5):494-499.

51. Drake LA, Dinehart SM, Farmer ER, et al. Guidelines of care for superficial mycotic infections of the skin: tinea corporis, tinea cruris, tinea faciei, tinea manuum, and tinea pedis. Guidelines/Outcomes Committee. American Academy of Dermatology. *J Am Acad Dermatol.* 1996;34(2 Pt 1):282-286.

52. Sadick NS, Hudgins LC. Fatty acid analysis of transplanted adipose tissue. *Arch Dermatol.* 2001;137(6):723-727.

53. Pinski KS, Roenigk HH Jr. Autologous fat transplantation. Long-term follow-up. *J Dermatol Surg Oncol.* 1992;18(3):179-184.

54. Kuran I, Tumerdem B. A new simple method used to prepare fat for injection. *Aesthetic Plast Surg.* 2005;29(1):18-22; discussion 23.

55. Chajchir A, Benzaquen I, Moretti E. Comparative experimental study of autologous adipose tissue processed by different techniques. *Aesthetic Plast Surg.* 1993;17(2):113-115.

56. Gerth DJ, King B, Rabach L, Glasgold RA, Glasgold MJ. Long-term volumetric retention of autologous fat grafting processed with closed-membrane filtration. *Aesthet Surg J.* 2014;34(7): 985-994.

57. Moscatello DK, Dougherty M, Narins RS, Lawrence N. Cryopreservation of human fat for soft tissue augmentation: viability requires use of cryoprotectant and controlled freezing and storage. *Dermatol Surg.* 2005;31(11 Pt 2):1506-1510.

58. Carpaneda CA, Ribeiro MT. Percentage of graft viability versus injected volume in adipose autotransplants. *Aesthetic Plast Surg.* 1994;18(1):17-19.

59. Glogau RG. Microlipoinjection. Autologous fat grafting. *Arch Dermatol.* 1988;124(9):1340-1343.

60. Narins RS, Beer K. Liquid injectable silicone: a review of its history, immunology, technical considerations, complications, and potential. *Plast Reconstr Surg.* 2006;118(3 Suppl):77S-84S.

61. Duffy DM. The silicone conundrum: a battle of anecdotes. *Dermatol Surg.* 2002;28(7):590-594.

62. Jones DH, Carruthers A, Orentreich D, et al. Highly purified 1000-cSt silicone oil for treatment of human immunodeficiency virus-associated facial lipoatrophy: an open pilot trial. *Dermatol Surg.* 2004;30(10):1279-1286.

63. Alam M, Gladstone H, Kramer EM, et al. ASDS guidelines of care: injectable fillers. *Dermatol Surg.* 2008;34(suppl 1):S115-S148.

64. Funt D, Pavicic T. Dermal fillers in aesthetics: an overview of adverse events and treatment approaches. *Clin Cosmet Investig Dermatol.* 2013;6:295-316.

65. Glashofer EC. Complications of temporary fillers. In: Carruthers JC, ed. *Soft Tissue Augmentation.* Toronto, Ontarior, Canada: Elsevier Saunders; 2013:179-187.

66. Moody BR, Sengelmann RD. Topical tacrolimus in the treatment of bovine collagen hypersensitivity. *Dermatol Surg.* 2001;27(9):789-791.

67. Jones D, Murphy DK. Volumizing hyaluronic acid filler for midface volume deficit: 2-year results from a pivotal single-blind randomized controlled study. *Dermatol Surg.* 2013;39(11):1602-1612.

68. Bjarnsholt T, Tolker-Nielsen T, Givskov M, Janssen M, Christensen LH. Detection of bacteria by fluorescence in situ hybridization in culture-negative soft tissue filler lesions. *Dermatol Surg.* 2009;35(Suppl 2):1620-1624.

69. Lee JM, Kim YJ. Foreign body granulomas after the use of dermal fillers: p9athophysiology, clinical appearance, histologic features, and treatment. *Arch Plast Surg.* 2015;42(2):232-239.

70. Lemperle G, Gauthier-Hazan N, Wolters M, Eisemann-Klein M, Zimmermann U, Duffy DM. Foreign body granulomas after all injectable dermal fillers: part 1. Possible causes. *Plast Reconstr Surg.* 2009;123(6):1842-1863.

71. Keller EC, Kaminer MS, Dover JS. Use of hyaluronidase in patients with bee allergy. *Dermatol Surg.* 2014;40(10):1145-1147.

72. Ledon JA, Savas JA, Yang S, Franca K, Camacho I, Nouri K. Inflammatory nodules following soft tissue filler use: a review of causative agents, pathology and treatment options. *Am J Clin Dermatol.* 2013;14(5):401-411.

73. Beleznay K, Humphrey S, Carruthers JD, Carruthers A. Vascular compromise from soft tissue augmentation: experience with 12 cases and recommendations for optimal outcomes. *J Clin Aesthet Dermatol.* 2014;7(9):37-43.

74. DeLorenzi C. Complications of injectable fillers, part 2: vascular complications. *Aesthet Surg J.* 2014;34(4):584-600.

75. Grunebaum LD, Bogdan Allemann I, Dayan S, Mandy S, Baumann L. The risk of alar necrosis associated with dermal filler injection. *Dermatol Surg.* 2009;35(Suppl 2):1635-1640.

76. Dayan SH, Arkins JP, Mathison CC. Management of impending necrosis associated with soft tissue filler injections. *J Drugs Dermatol.* 2011;10(9):1007-1012.

77. Hirsch RJ, Cohen JL, Carruthers JD. Successful management of an unusual presentation of impending necrosis following a hyaluronic acid injection embolus and a proposed algorithm for management with hyaluronidase. *Dermatol Surg.* 2007;33(3):357-360.

78. Landau M. Hyaluronidase caveats in treating filler complications. *Dermatol Surg.* 2015;41(Suppl 1):S347-S353.

79. DeLorenzi C. Complications of injectable fillers, part I. *Aesthet Surg J.* 2013;33(4):561-575.

80. Park SW, Woo SJ, Park KH, Huh JW, Jung C, Kwon OK. Iatrogenic retinal artery occlusion caused by cosmetic facial filler injections. *Am J Ophthalmol.* 2012;154(4):653-662.e1.

81. Ozturk CN, Li Y, Tung R, Parker L, Piliang MP, Zins JE. Complications following injection of soft-tissue fillers. *Aesthet Surg J.* 2013;33(6):862-877.

82. Carruthers J, Fagien S, Dolman P. Retro or peribulbar injection techniques to reverse visual loss after filler injections. *Dermatol Surg.* 2015;41(Suppl 1):S354-S357.

83. American Society of Plastic Surgeons. *2015 Plastic Surgery Statistics Report.* Arlington Heights, IL: American Society of Plastic Surgeons; 2015.

Chemical Peels

26

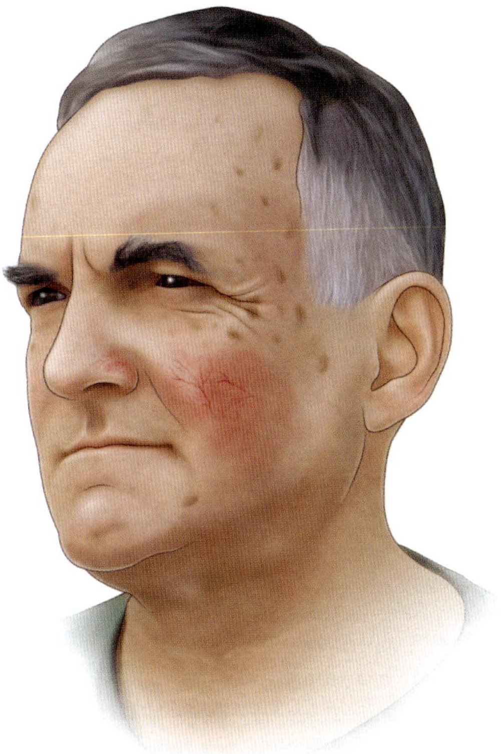

SUMMARY

- Improvement in skin quality and texture may be seen with the use of chemical peels, laser and light devices, dermabrasion, and skin needling.
- All approaches share the common mechanism of controlled wounding and stimulation of a healing response in the skin.

Beginner Tips

- Use a pre-peel regimen of either topical tretinoin or hydroquinone cream to improve efficacy and outcomes.
- Be consistent in application technique and document all the parameters of the treatment process (pre-peel regimen, degreasing regimen, and peel regimen) to achieve consistency and predictability in results.
- Feather the peels around the hairline and the chin to prevent a sharp demarcation, particularly with medium and deep peels.

Expert Tips

- Medium-depth chemical peels are an excellent modality for the treatment of diffuse actinic keratoses.
- Multiple studies have shown that a combination approach using a topical regimen with serial chemical peels can improve melasma.
- Phenol peels have also been used as an adjunct to, or a less invasive alternative to, blepharoplasty.

Don't Forget!

- When applying the peel, numerous parameters such as the pretreatment regimen, degreasing regimen, type of application, length of peel application, and end-point should all be considered and documented.
- Pretreatment with topical tretinoin daily for 2 weeks prior to the procedure results in a more rapid, uniform, and even frosting of the skin compared to no pretreatment.

Pitfalls and Cautions

- Evaluate for any areas of inflamed skin on the day of treatment. These regions will have greater uptake of the peel solution and may create a deeper than intended reaction.
- Be cautious when using newly opened chemical solution bottle for the first time. The clinician should be particularly vigilant about clinical endpoints. On rare occasions, the concentration advertised on the label may not be accurate.

Patient Education Points

- The consultation appointment is key in establishing rapport and realistic expectations, including that a series of treatments may be needed.
- Patient selection is critical given the discomfort, extensive healing process, and potential for adverse events associated with phenol peels.

26 Chemical Peels

INTRODUCTION

Chemical peels are a fast, reliable, effective, and inexpensive method of wounding the skin under controlled conditions to induce skin regeneration.[1] In trained hands, chemical peel solutions can be used to treat a diverse array of concerns including acne vulgaris, actinic keratosis, melasma, and photodamage. Scientific research on the effect of these peels is challenging given the cosmetic nature of these procedures and difficulty with obtaining biopsy samples from facial locations. The number of peels on the market also increases annually with new concentrations, formulations, and combination agents available. In addition, variations in application technique between clinicians and variations in patients' response to wounding make extrapolation of results unreliable.

Chemical peels are generally classified according to the relative depth of wounding (**Table 26-1**). Very light superficial peels penetrate only the stratum corneum, primarily acting as exfoliants, whereas superficial peels penetrate down to the basal layer of the epidermis. Medium-depth peels reach the papillary dermis, while deep peels may reach the reticular dermis. While the relative depth of penetration of each compound is generally established by its chemical properties (acidity, toxicity, and metabolic interaction with endogenous proteins), the patient's inherent skin characteristics as well as the clinician's application technique will impact penetration depth. Treatment location may also lead to variations in results. The same peel applied in the same manner may not penetrate as deeply on the forehead, where the skin is thicker and more sebaceous, compared to the preauricular cheek or the eyelid skin.

TABLE 26-1 • Chemical Peel Classification Guidelines[a]

Peel Type	Histologic Depth	Chemical Peel Solution
Very light superficial	Stratum corneum	Salicylic acid Glycolic acid 30%-50% Jessner's solution, 1-3 coats Trichloroacetic acid (TCA) 10%-20%
Superficial	Basal layer of epidermis	Glycolic acid 50%-70% Jessner's solution, 4+ coats TCA 20%-30%
Medium	Papillary dermis	TCA 35%-40% TCA 35% + Jessner's solution TCA 35% + glycolic acid 70% TCA 35% + solid CO_2
Deep	Reticular dermis	Phenol 88% Baker-Gordon phenol

[a]These are guidelines. Actual depth of penetration depends on a multitude of factors, including patient skin characteristics and application techniques

When performing chemical peels, it is best to establish a consistent technique to improve the predictability of outcomes. In general, as the ablative depth increases, so does the potential for adverse effects. When selecting a peel solution, the ablative depth of the chemical peel should correspond to the histologic depth of the targeted concern. This selection should be tailored to each patient. To minimize adverse events, appropriate screening and prepeel and postpeel regimens should also be in place.

SALICYLIC ACID SOLUTION

Salicylic acid is the most popular β-hydroxy acid used in chemical peeling. Unlike other chemical solutions, its lipophilic nature allows it to penetrate into sebaceous glands and hair follicles. It is keratolytic and comedolytic, removing intercellular lipids and desmosomes, thereby decreasing the cohesiveness between corneocytes and keratinocytes.[2] As a superficial peel, this solution is well tolerated even in patients with Fitzpatrick skin types IV to VI.[3]

There are numerous formulations for salicylic acid peels, but the most common is a 20% to 30% salicylic acid solution in an ethanol base. The skin should first be prepped with acetone to degrease the skin. The peel can then be applied in two to three coats and left on for 3 to 5 minutes starting with the forehead, then the cheeks, nose, cutaneous lip, and chin. There is no need for neutralization. The skin will develop a light frost as the ethanol evaporates and salicylic acid precipitates, signaling completion of the peel. To achieve an even peel, more solution can be applied until the faint frost is evenly distributed. The patient can then rinse and cleanse the face with a gentle and bland facial cleanser.

Patients will experience an initial mild stinging sensation, lasting around 3 minutes, which can be alleviated with a cool fan.[4] This discomfort is transient since the peel has anesthetic properties. Side effects are generally mild and transient, with the most common being dryness. Although postinflammatory hypo- and hyperpigmentation have been reported in patients, particularly in areas of inflamed skin, this is transient, even in patients with Fitzpatrick skin type IV and greater.[3] While salicylic acid is generally well tolerated, it should not be used in patients who are pregnant or breastfeeding as it is pregnancy category C. Care should also be taken to avoid using this peel with lasers or dermabrasion given the flammable ethanol base.

GLYCOLIC ACID SOLUTION

Glycolic acid is the most popular α-hydroxy acid used for chemical peels. As the α-hydroxy acid with the smallest molecular size, it is thought to have better penetration compared to other compounds. Even though it is a naturally occurring compound found in sugar cane, clinical formulations are typically synthesized. It is provided as a crystalline solid, which must first be dissolved and then applied to the skin. The formulations can vary greatly in concentration, pH, and vehicle, and the clinician should be aware of these factors as they all affect its efficacy. As the concentration of glycolic acid increases, so does penetration and tissue wounding.[5,6] The free form of glycolic acid causes greater tissue damage compared to partially neutralized or esterified formulas at the same concentration (**Table 26-2**).[5] Formulations in an aqueous solution have greater bioavailability and penetration compared to gel formulation.[7]

There are numerous formulations marketed to the consumer as part of a daily regimen, ranging in concentration from 8% to 20%.[7] In concentrations of 3% to 13% applied twice daily, glycolic acid has been shown to improve xerotic skin's texture and moisturization.[8] At these low concentrations, glycolic acid decreases corneocyte cohesiveness by reducing sulfate and phosphate groups, leading to exfoliation and a superficial peel. Stronger glycolic acid peels such as the 50% and 70% formulation are typically applied in the clinicians' office. At these higher concentrations, glycolic acid can induce subepidermal vesiculation with dermal inflammation, resulting in the induction of new dermal collagen and ground substance as the skin heals.[5,6]

No preparatory agent is used prior to applying the peeling agent. Patients will experience stinging and irritation with application of the glycolic acid peel, but tolerability can be improved with a hand-held cooling fan. The end point for this peel is a uniform level of erythema, which is typically achieved in 2 minutes, although the peel may be left in place up to a limit of 5 minutes. If regions of the skin start to blanch or frost, this may be an indication of deeper penetration and epidermolysis, and the peel should be stopped with neutralization. To neutralize the glycolic acid peel, either a bicarbonate solution or cool water can be used. If a bicarbonate solution is used, patients should be told to expect fizzing and warmth during the exothermic reaction. Glycolic acid peels can also be neutralized with water to avoid the reaction, but any remaining solution must be completely rinsed away to completely remove the acid.

Glycolic acid, like salicylic acid, is generally well tolerated and can be used in a wide range of Fitzpatrick skin types, but unlike salicylic acid, the penetration can be less predictable at higher concentrations.[9] To minimize the risk of a deeper peel than intended, patients can be asked to stop topical retinoids 3 to 7 days prior to their peel, since tretinoin can lead to a dermatitis and deeper penetration of the glycolic acid. If deeper penetration does occur, patients may experience essentially a medium-depth peel with increased erythema, edema, desquamation, and a prolonged healing time. Inflammatory conditions such as seborrheic dermatitis may cause uneven and deeper penetration, and skin affected by these conditions must be treated cautiously. Care should also be taken in how many applications and how long the solution is applied as these can both increase the wound depth. A practical approach to the treatment-naïve patient is to start with a 50% concentration with short contact time and progressively increase at subsequent treatments as tolerated. If a superficial peel is achieved, any postprocedure hyperpigmentation or hypopigmentation should be transitory. Nevertheless, patients should always be counseled on proper sun protection, as glycolic acid acts as a photosensitizer.[10] In addition to the risk for pigmentary changes, a small number of patients may experience a perioral acneiform dermatitis, in which case further peels on the chin should be avoided.[7]

TABLE 26-2 • Glycolic Acid Formulations

- Free acid
- Partially neutralized
- Buffered
- Esterified

JESSNER'S SOLUTION

Jessner's solution is composed of 14 g of salicylic acid, 14 g of resorcinol, 14 g of lactic acid, and ethanol up to total volume of 100 mL. By combining multiple peeling agents, the clinician can provide the benefits of each individual component while minimizing the risk profile from any single agent (**Figure 26-1**). As a result, Jessner's solution achieves keratolysis and exfoliation with a good safety profile. It can be used alone as a superficial peel or, more commonly, used in combination with trichloroacetic acid as a medium-depth peel. As the solution is applied, patients may experience stinging and irritation, similar to a salicylic acid peel. The clinician should look for a mild frost, likely precipitated salicylic acid, as well as mild erythema as primary end points. If applied in one to three coats, a very superficial peel is achieved. With more coats, a more pronounced frost and deeper penetration can be achieved, but the peel is generally still limited to the epidermis.[11] Overall, the peel is well tolerated, but patients may experience dryness and tightness after the peel in conjunction with the expected exfoliation. This peel is also titratable via changes to the degreasing procedure with acetone or alcohol. Variations in the intensity of the degreasing scrub or length of time allows for further customization of the peel depth.

TRICHLOROACETIC ACID SOLUTION

Trichloroacetic acid (TCA) solutions are versatile and can be used as superficial or medium-depth peels, depending on the concentration and regimen used. Solutions of TCA vary in concentration between 10% and 35%. TCA exists in a crystalline form and needs to be dissolved in water in the appropriate weight-to-volume ratio. To create a 35% solution, 35 g of crystal are dissolved in 100 mL of water. This solution is not sensitive to light and is stable at room temperature.[7] Even though higher concentrations of TCA have been used in the past to achieve deep peels comparable to Baker-Gordon phenol, modern concentrations are generally less than 40% to decrease the risk of scarring, hypopigmentation, and erythema.[12]

To achieve a superficial peel, TCA is applied as monotherapy. The skin should be degreased appropriately, followed by application of a thin layer of TCA at 10% to 30%. Like other peel

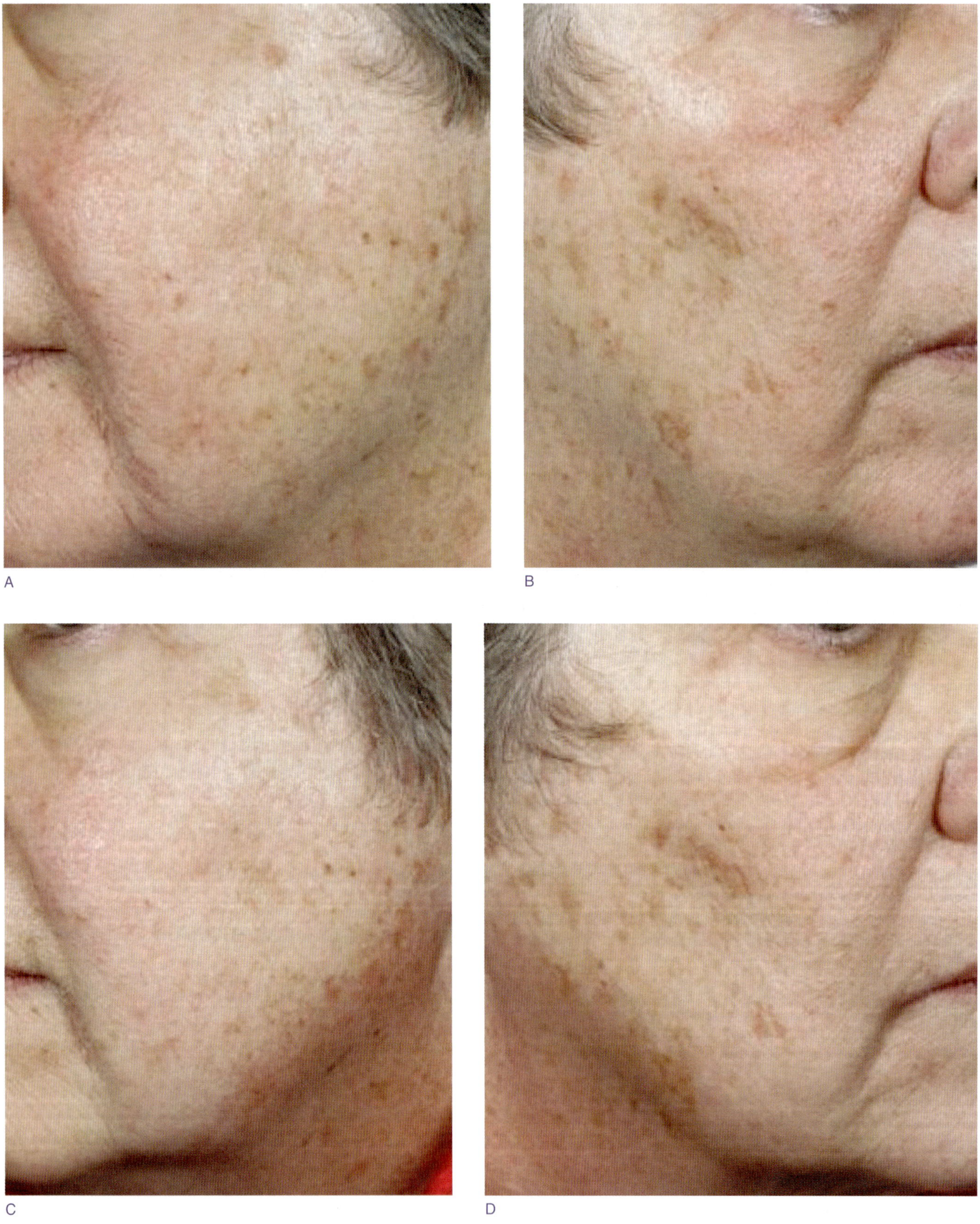

FIGURE 26-1 Jessner's peel: Before treatment (**A, B**); 1 month after treatment (**C, D**).

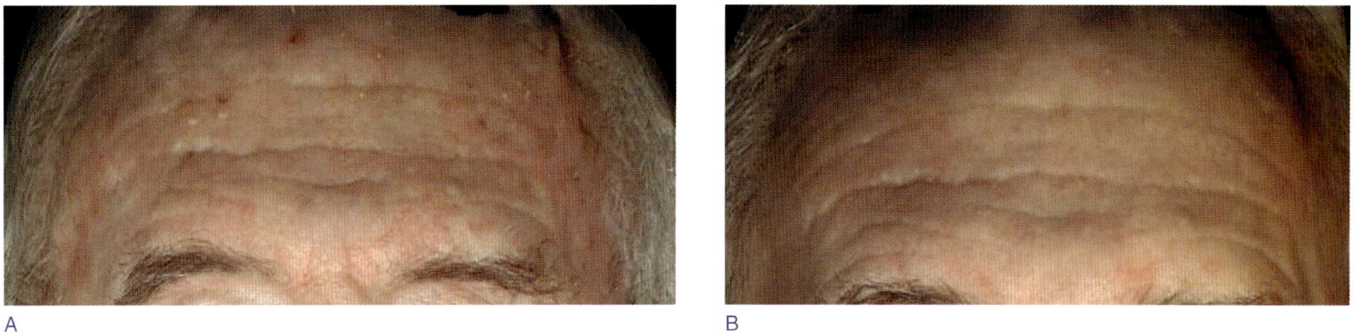

FIGURE 26-2 Jessner's + 35% TCA medium-depth peel: Treatment of actinic damage—before treatment (**A**) and after treatment (**B**).

solutions, the higher the concentration, the deeper is the penetration. The clinician should use a speckled white frost as the clinical end point for a light peel, at which point cool wet gauze is applied to neutralize the peel. Unlike salicylic acid or Jessner's peel, the frosting results from coagulation of skin proteins and can be used to gauge the patient's response to the peel.

To achieve a medium-depth peel, 35% TCA can be combined with other superficial peeling agents such as Jessner's solution, solid carbon dioxide (CO_2), or 70% glycolic acid to target more pronounced photodamage, dyschromia, lentigines, and seborrheic keratoses. The Jessner's and 35% TCA combination (Monheit combination) is popular because both peel solutions are commercially available (**Figures 26-2 and 26-3**). The skin is degreased with acetone or alcohol and then treated with Jessner's solution. Once the patient achieves a speckled frost and mild erythema with Jessner's solution, gauze soaked in cool water is applied to the skin. This initial peel removes the stratum corneum and decreases cohesiveness between keratinocytes, allowing greater penetration of the TCA solution. Since the skin has already been prepped and treated, a second degreasing step is not needed between the Jessner's and TCA steps. TCA 35% can be applied in light strokes or with more vigorous rubbing. The clinician should be aware that each successive application and deeper application pressure cause deeper penetration of the solution. The clinician should look for a moderate frosting and erythema as the primary end points, followed by cool compresses. Patients can expect postpeel erythema, edema, and peeling, with re-epithelialization within 7 to 10 days.[12]

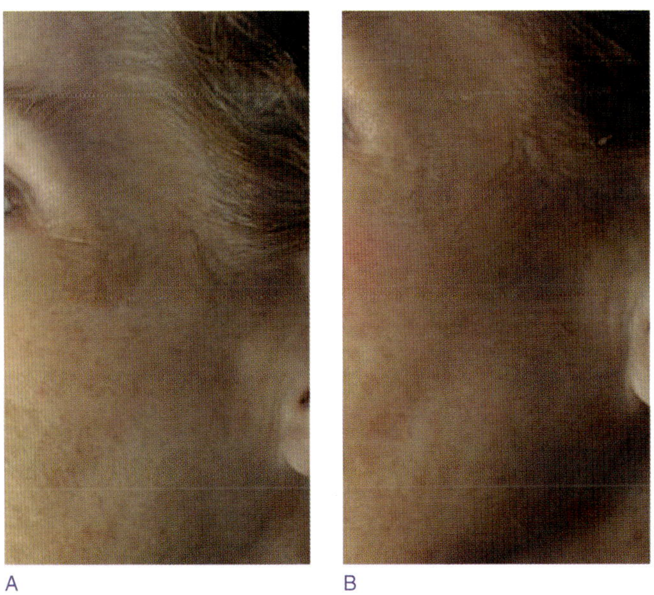

FIGURE 26-3 Jessner's + 35% TCA medium-depth peel: Treatment of a thin seborrheic keratosis—before treatment (**A**) and after treatment (**B**).

Biopsies taken from the skin after peeling with four coats of Jessner's solution showed changes limited to the epidermis without dermal changes. In contrast, when Jessner's is combined with a single coat of 35% TCA, dermal edema and an inflammatory infiltrate could be seen shortly postoperatively.[11] One month later, new collagen fibers can be seen in the upper reticular dermis. When Jessner's solution is followed by three coats of 35% TCA, the result is more prominent postoperative epidermal necrosis and edema followed by robust collagen generation as well as an increase in ground substance in the upper reticular dermis.[11]

In addition, 35% TCA can be applied following an initial treatment with solid CO_2 (Brody combination). This achieves a more robust medium-depth peel, similar to Jessner's, with three coats of 35% TCA.[11] To apply solid CO_2, a small piece is broken off to fit the clinician's hand and then dipped in a 3:1 solution of acetone and alcohol and glided over the skin. Solid CO_2 removes the stratum corneum and physically damages the epidermis, creating epidermal vesiculation. As the CO_2 is applied with increasing pressure, the epidermal damage also increases, allowing greater penetration of the TCA solution.[11] This can be helpful when customizing treatment for hyperkeratotic regions.

When solid CO_2 is followed by a single coat of 35% TCA, biopsies show more prominent epidermal necrosis, similar to that achieved by Jessner's and three coats of 35% TCA. When solid CO_2 is combined with three coats of 35% TCA, new collagen fibers can be seen in the upper reticular dermis, accompanied by an increase in ground substance extending to the reticular dermis.[11]

Similar to the concepts behind the Monheit and Brody combinations, 35% TCA can also be applied following 70% glycolic acid to achieve a deeper peel (Coleman combination). In this technique, free 70% glycolic acid can be applied directly to the skin without degreasing for 2 minutes. After 2 minutes, the skin is rinsed, followed by application of the 35% TCA solution. Biopsies taken after treatment have demonstrated a thickened papillary dermis, but less than that achieved by the Brody technique.[13] Like the Monheit combination, glycolic acid is readily available in the clinician's office. However, 70% glycolic acid is less predictable than Jessner's solution, and care must be taken to avoid inadvertently causing greater penetration in areas of inflamed skin.

Aside from full-face TCA peels, high concentrations of TCA have also been used in the treatment of depressed ice-pick acne scars using the chemical reconstruction of skin scars (CROSS) method, discussed in detail later in this chapter.

PHENOL-BASED SOLUTION

Phenol-based peels provide the deepest chemical ablations and can be used for etched-in wrinkles resistant to all other peels. The most common formulation used is the Baker-Gordon phenol solution (**Table 26-3**).[14] This formulation should be freshly prepared and frequently stirred to ensure an exact and even concentration is applied. There have been many modifications to this original formulation, including the Exoderm and Venner-Kellson solutions, which are better tolerated with an improved safety profile and less penetration.[15,16] As with the previously discussed peels, penetration is not solely determined by the formulation. Whereas increasing concentrations of phenol and croton oil lead to greater tissue damage, the application technique itself is important; more vigorous application with greater coats leads to a deeper peel and more inflammation.[17-19]

Patient selection is critical given the discomfort, extensive healing process, and potential for adverse events associated with phenol peels. Patients are commonly put under sedation for their comfort, as the process can otherwise be painful. Patients should also have cardiac monitoring and intravenous hydration throughout the procedure to minimize the risk of cardiotoxicity. The patient's face is first cleansed and degreased with acetone. This is followed by application of a thin layer of freshly mixed Baker's formula using cotton-tipped applicators, taking care to avoid excess solution. This is applied first to the forehead, then the cheeks and perioral and nasal skin. The entire procedure should be performed slowly over 60 to 90 minutes to slow the systemic absorption of phenol and decrease the risk of cardiotoxicity. The skin will immediately frost due to protein coagulation as each site is treated. To delay the absorption, the clinician should wait 15 minutes between each cosmetic unit. Each zone should be feathered out into the surrounding skin to avoid sharp demarcation between treated and untreated regions. Patients should have cardiac monitoring throughout the procedure and for 1 hour postoperatively. Once completed, the peel can either be left open or placed under occlusion with waterproof zinc oxide tape. If left open, patients should be counseled to expect erythema and edema and to apply petrolatum ointment liberally twice daily. Unoccluded phenol peels have penetration similar to medium-depth peels, so patients should expect faster healing times. For deeply etched wrinkles, patients will need a phenol peel occluded by waterproof zinc oxide tape placed in overlapping strips over the entire treated surface. This should be left on for 24 to 48 hours. At the return visit, any drainage or excess exudate can be gently removed. A second mask formed from bismuth subgallate powder can then be applied with reapplication of the powder at home as needed for the next week. By the end of the week, the skin will have re-epithelialized, and this second mask is removed with petrolatum ointment and warm compresses.[7,16]

When performing deep peels, the clinicians should be aware of potential complications. In a study of 43 consecutive patients undergoing phenol-based peels, half of the patients who had their peels completed within 30 minutes developed cardiac arrhythmias compared to none of the patients who had their peel completed over at least 60 minutes.[20] The arrhythmias included premature ventricular contraction (n = 4), bigeminy (n = 2), paroxysmal atrial tachycardia (n = 2), and ventricular tachycardia (n = 2), with no correlation with age (range: 24-73 years old). In the 10 patients who developed arrhythmias, 9 had unremarkable preoperative electrocardiograms.[20] The incidence of cardiac arrhythmias can be reduced when precautions such as intravenous hydration, proper ventilation, and prophylactic propranolol are given. In a retrospective case series of 181 patients treated with a full-face Exoderm phenol peel, which slows the absorption of phenol compared to the traditional Baker-Gordon formula, 6.6% of patients still developed an arrhythmia when the treatment was completed over 30 minutes despite concurrent treatment with

TABLE 26-3 • Phenol Peel Formulations

Baker-Gordon Solution	Exoderm Solution	Venner-Kellson Solution
3 mL of 88% phenol	1 mL 91% phenol	8 oz melted loose phenol crystals
2 mL of distilled water	1 mL phenol crystal	1 oz concentrated Lysol
8 drops of Septisol	0.5 mL distilled water	0.5 oz olive oil
3 drops of croton oil	0.5 mL mixture (alcohol, olive oil, glycerin oil, sesame oil)	1.5 oz distilled water
	2 drops croton oil	10 drops croton oil
	0.3 mL resorcinol	
	10 drops soap	
	0.2 mL citric acid	
	Buffer tris	

intravenous hydration, 1 mg of prophylactic propranolol, and an electric fan and air-conditioned room to improve ventilation.[21]

Aside from cardiac complications, phenol peels are also susceptible to hyperpigmentation, hypopigmentation, prolonged erythema, and scarring. Even though the Exoderm modified phenol peel decreases the risk of adverse events, a case series involving Asian patients still showed frequent side effects including postinflammatory hyperpigmentation (74%) and prolonged erythema of more than 3 months (11%).[22] Hypopigmentation was rare but did occur in 1 of 46 patients (2%).

Similar to TCA solutions, phenol can also be applied as monotherapy at high concentration in the treatment of depressed acne scars. Because the application area is limited, this targeted treatment method has low absorption and an improved risk profile, but patients should still be counseled on the risk of dyschromias and erythema.

PREOPERATIVE EVALUATION OF THE PATIENT

Skin Characteristics

When assessing the patient for a chemical peel, the first and foremost consideration should be the patient's skin type and characteristics. Even with the same application technique, differences between patients can significantly alter the penetration of chemical peels and affect their safety and efficacy. In selecting the appropriate peel, the clinician must first consider the patient's tendency for postinflammatory hyperpigmentation. Patients with Fitzpatrick skin type IV to VI (**Table 26-4**) have a greater risk of postinflammatory dyschromia. While superficial peels carry less risk for adverse events such as hyperpigmentation, hypopigmentation, or scarring, patients should still be given an appropriate prepeel regimen (see Prepeel Regimen section) and practice sun protection after peel.[2] Test spots in less cosmetically sensitive locations can also be performed prior to a full procedure. In addition to patients' natural tendencies toward pigmentation, inherent skin texture can also affect the efficacy of the peel (**Table 26-5**). Areas of active inflammation allow deeper penetration of chemical solutions compared to surrounding skin, leading to deeper ablation. Patients with rosacea, in particular, may experience greater inflammation and are at greater risk of prolonged erythema after the peel. Patients with thin and translucent skin will similarly experience greater ablation with greater risk for adverse events. In contrast, patients with thick sebaceous skin or those with hyperkeratotic lesions will experience less penetration and must be prepped appropriately to elicit the intended reaction. Similarly, with the same peeling regimen, areas of the face with thinner skin will experience greater penetration compared to areas of thicker skin.[5]

TABLE 26-4 • Fitzpatrick Skin Type Classification Scale

Skin Type	Characteristics
Type I	Always burns, never tans
Type II	Usually burns, tans with difficulty
Type III	Sometimes burns, gradually tans
Type IV	Rarely burns, tans with ease
Type V	Very rarely burns, tans very easily
Type VI	Never burns, tans very easily

TABLE 26-5 • Patient Evaluation

Patient Characteristics	Skin Characteristics
Patient's desired results	Tendency for postinflammatory hyperpigmentation – Fitzpatrick skin type
Tolerability for postoperative management and downtime	Areas of active inflammation – Rosacea, dermatitis, etc
Willingness for multiple treatments	Skin texture – Thin, translucent vs sebaceous or hyperkeratotic skin Glogau classification

Medical and Surgical History

When taking a medical history, the clinician should probe for any risk factors associated with poor healing and poor outcomes (**Table 26-6**). Patients with a history of hypertrophic scars or keloid formation should be limited to very light superficial peels to avoid dermal damage. Those with an active herpes simplex virus infection should wait until active sores are healed and then be treated prophylactically prior to their procedure to avoid triggering another outbreak and dissemination of the virus on resurfaced skin. If a history of HIV or nicotine use is elicited, the patient should be counseled regarding the potential for delayed wound healing. Patients with recent isotretinoin use should also be counseled regarding the

TABLE 26-6 • Factors to Elicit from Past Medical and Surgical History

Medical History	Surgical History
Keloid/hypertrophic scars	Prior radiation exposure
Recent isotretinoin use (previous 6-12 months)	Prior facial surgery
Herpes simplex virus	
HIV or other immunosuppression	
Nicotine use	
Pregnancy and breastfeeding status	
Oral contraceptive or other photosensitizers	
Staphylococcus infection	
Hypersensitivity to any peel components	

risk for delayed healing and abnormal scarring, even with superficial peels. While there have been case series questioning the need to delay peels for 6 or 12 months after completion of isotretinoin therapy, there are case reports of scarring and prolonged hyperpigmentation and erythema in patients with recent low-dose isotretinoin use, even when treated with superficial peels.[23,24] In one such case, the patient had previously tolerated 70% glycolic acid while on isotretinoin without any adverse events, suggesting that reactions may be unpredictable and idiosyncratic.[23]

When eliciting surgical history, the clinician should probe for any history of radiation or prior facelift or browlift. Radiation decreases the vasculature and density of pilosebaceous units from which the skin regenerates, thereby delaying healing. Similarly, if the patient has had prior facial surgery with extensive undermining, the superficial plexus may be disrupted in the immediate postoperative period, delaying healing. Finally, female patients of childbearing age should also be questioned about any possibility of being pregnant or if they are breastfeeding.

EVIDENCE-BASED TECHNIQUE CONSIDERATIONS

When performing chemical peels, selecting the appropriate agent is important, but this must be combined with the appropriate technique to obtain the intended effect. When applying the peel, numerous parameters such as the pretreatment regimen, degreasing regimen, type of application, length of peel application, and end point should all be considered and documented (**Table 26-7**). If the patient returns for a repeat treatment and is happy with their previous response, the clinician can then reproduce the same results. In contrast, if the patient had adverse events from previous applications, the clinician can then adjust the application technique to modulate the effects.

Prepeel Regimen

The chemical peel procedure begins even before application of the chemical solution itself. Pretreatment with topical tretinoin daily for 2 weeks prior to the procedure results in a more rapid, uniform, and even frosting of the skin compared to no pretreatment. Tretinoin helps reduce sebum and thins the stratum corneum prior to the peel, improving the efficacy of the peel without an appreciable increase in adverse events.[25] Pretreatment with topical tretinoin also speeds re-epithelialization. In a double-blind, placebo-controlled, prospective, randomized, split-face study evaluating pretreatment with tretinoin 0.1% cream versus a placebo vehicle, 75% of the hemifaces pretreated prior to a 35% TCA peel showed complete re-epithelialization at 1 week, compared to only 31% of the placebo-treated hemifaces.[25]

In patients at risk of postinflammatory hyperpigmentation, pretreatment for 2 weeks with hydroquinone decreases postprocedure hyperpigmentation compared to no pretreatment or pretreatment with 0.025% tretinoin cream.[26] In a single-blind, randomized prospective study of patients assigned to glycolic acid treatment alone (group I), glycolic acid preceded by 2 weeks of 0.025% tretinoin cream (group II), or glycolic acid preceded by 2% hydroquinone cream (group III) for the treatment of melasma, both patients' subjective response and objective observer's response indicated better outcomes in group III. Whereas 20% of patients in the glycolic acid–only group developed postinflammatory hyperpigmentation, this was decreased to 14.3% and 5.5% in the groups pretreated with tretinoin and hydroquinone, respectively.[26] These results were corroborated by another double-blind, randomized controlled trial comparing pretreatment with 2% hydroquinone versus 0.025% tretinoin for 2 weeks prior to a medium-depth TCA peel in patients with Fitzpatrick skin type III and greater.[27] Postinflammatory hyperpigmentation was limited to the group of patients pretreated with tretinoin and not seen in those pretreated with hydroquinone. Although no studies evaluated the benefit of hydroquinone pretreatment prior to deep peels, a randomized controlled trial evaluating pretreatment (10% glycolic acid twice daily, hydroquinone 4% cream nightly, and tretinoin 0.025% cream twice daily) for 2 weeks prior to ablative CO_2 resurfacing showed no benefit in decreasing posttreatment hyperpigmentation compared to the group that received no pretreatment.[28] Since ablative laser resurfacing wounds the skin to the dermis, similar to a deep chemical peel, while hydroquinone pretreatment may be effective for superficial and medium-depth peels, it will likely be ineffective in preventing postinflammatory hyperpigmentation after deep chemical peels.

For patients with Fitzpatrick skin types I and II, tretinoin 0.025% cream can be used nightly for 2 weeks prior to peel. In patients with Fitzpatrick skin type III or higher, hydroquinone 4% cream can be used twice daily for 2 weeks prior to superficial and medium-depth peels. Care must be taken, however, to evaluate for any dermatitis on the day the patients present for their peel. Since areas of inflammation allow greater and unpredictable penetration of chemical peel solutions, delay peels if the dermatitis is deemed too exuberant.

TABLE 26-7 • Surgical Techniques Affecting Peel Depth

Priming regimen
Degreasing regimen
Chemical peel scrub intensity
Number of coats applied
Length of peel application

Peel Technique

The peel application starts with degreasing the skin to remove excess sebum and to even the stratum corneum to allow equal penetration of the peel solution (**Figures 26-4 to 26-8**). Sebum is lipophilic, and lipophobic solutions will not penetrate areas with residual sebum. Patients with oily or sebaceous skin can benefit from more vigorous degreasing scrubs. Numerous degreasing agents have been used in the literature, including alcohol, Septisol, ether, and acetone. Degreasing the skin with ether results in a deeper peel compared to milder cleansers such as acetone.[14] Many clinicians prefer using acetone. Hyperkeratotic lesions prevent penetration of the peel; appropriate areas can be targeted for a more vigorous scrub to thin the stratum corneum appropriately.

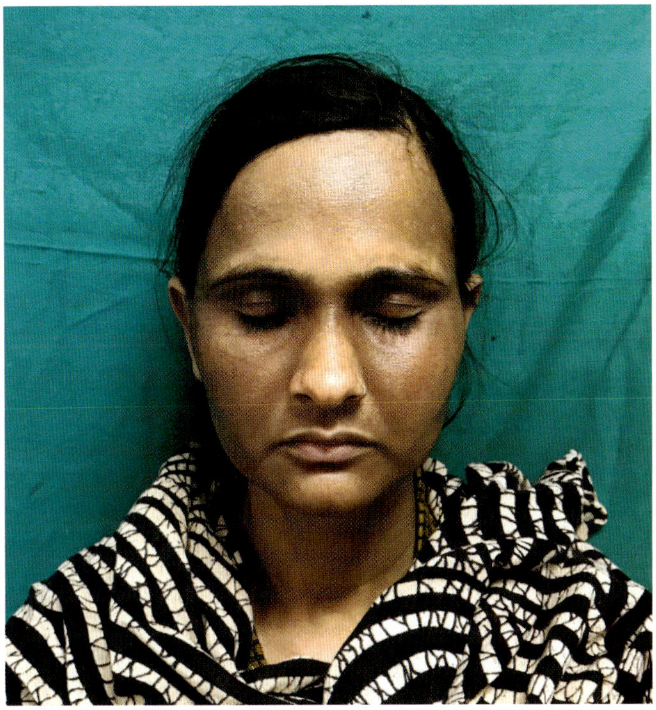

FIGURE 26-4 A 24-year-old adult female with diffuse slate-gray pigmentation over entire face (lichen planus pigmentosus) and localized brown-black–speckled pigmentation over nose (melasma).

Once the degreasing is complete, the appropriate chemical solution is chosen and applied. The method of application (brush, gauze pad, cotton tip) should be standardized and documented since different techniques deliver different quantities of these solutions, altering their effects. The number of applications

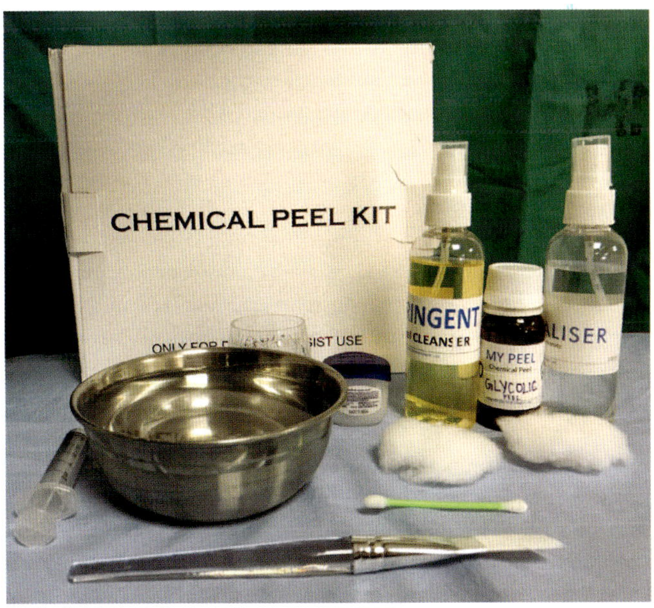

FIGURE 26-5 Equipment required for peel: The chemical peel along with prepeel cleanser, postpeel neutralizer, glass peel cup, brush applicator, petrolatum jelly, cotton bud, eye pads, and bowl of water.

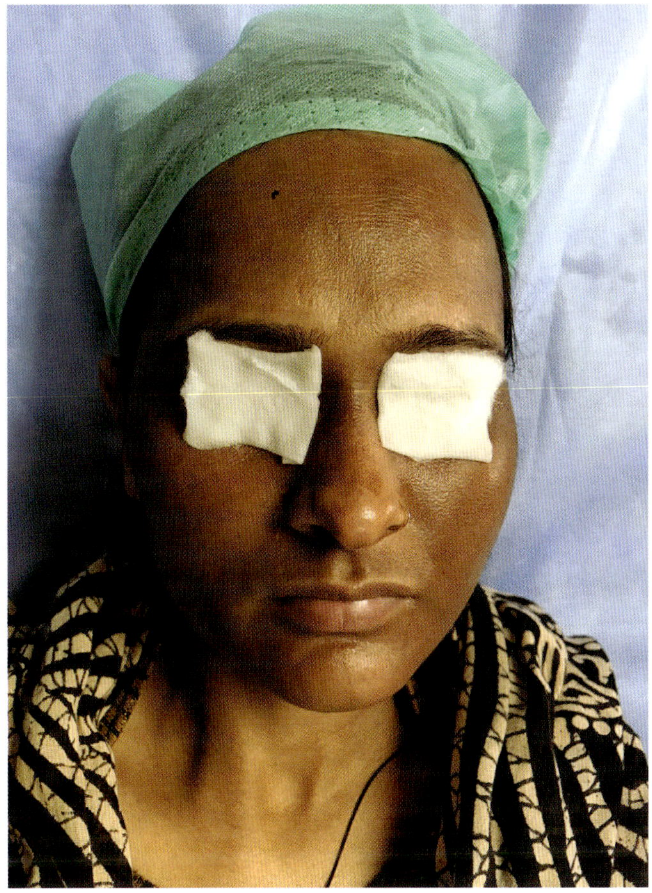

FIGURE 26-6 Patient preparation: The patient lies down with head elevated to 45 degrees, hair pulled back with a cap, and eyes closed and covered with moist eye pads; skin is cleaned and then degreased with acetone-based cleanser. Sensitive areas like the inner and outer canthus of the eyes, nasolabial folds, and angles of mouth are protected with petroleum jelly.

of the peel will also affect the peel's penetration. As the number of coats of the peel increases, so does the peeling depth, potential healing time, and risk for adverse events.[11,19] The strength with which the peel is applied can also affect penetration depth. More vigorous applications with a back-and-forth motion deposit more solution. When using solid CO_2, increasing the strength with which the CO_2 is applied also results in deeper penetration.[11]

Postpeel Regimen

Patients should be counseled to expect erythema, edema, and either exfoliation or peeling depending on the chemical depth of their treatment. To help the skin heal, patients should limit their skin care regimen to a bland facial cleanser and a bland topical emollient. Occlusion is not recommended, unless specifically intended, after phenol peels. The patient should also avoid picking at the skin or using abrasive products such as scrubs, masks, toners, tretinoin, or hydroquinone until the skin has fully re-epithelialized. Erythema is normal after a peel, but if persistent erythema is seen at more than 3 weeks, it may be a sign of contact dermatitis or an impending hypertrophic scar and should be evaluated by the clinician.[29]

STEP-BY-STEP CHEMICAL PEELING PROTOCOL

Before a Jessner's peel, every patient is started on a 2-week regimen of tretinoin 0.025% cream nightly. If there is concern for postinflammatory hyperpigmentation, 4% hydroquinone can be used instead. On the day of the chemical peel, the patient is assessed to make sure the topical prepeel regimen has not induced a severe dermatitis. Mild erythema and exfoliation are to be expected, but more severe inflammation makes the peel less predictable and would prompt a delay of treatment.

1. Lay out all the supplies needed on a Mayo tray (clean and dry 2×2 gauze, 4×4 gauze thoroughly soaked in a bucket of ice water, a stainless-steel cup, 4×4 dry gauze, Q-tip dipped in petrolatum ointment, acetone, appropriate solution bottles). Provide a hand-held fan to the patient or an assistant to blow toward the face throughout the procedure.
2. Take a 2×2 gauze with acetone and scrub the skin to degrease it. Start with the forehead and temples (one gauze pad), cheeks (one gauze pad per cheek), and chin/nose/cutaneous lips (one gauze pad). Take 2 minutes to degrease the entire face and document the vigorousness of the scrub (gentle, moderate, vigorous).
3. Take petrolatum ointment on a Q-tip and apply a small amount to the corners of the nose and lips.
4. Take one 2×2 gauze and thoroughly soak this in a stainless-steel cup containing Jessner's solution and then wring it out. Use one gauze pad to wipe the forehead and temples while covering the eyes with the nondominant hand.
5. Take a fresh 2×2 gauze that has been soaked with Jessner's solution and then wring it out and apply on one cheek.
6. Repeat step 4 on the other cheek.
7. Take another fresh 2×2 gauze soaked in Jessner's solution and then wring out and apply to the chin, cutaneous lips, and nose. By this time, mild to moderate erythema as well as scattered mild frosting on the previously treated areas should be visible.
8. Take the 4×4 gauze pads soaking in cold ice water. Gently squeeze to remove excess water and then unfold and place on the patient, starting on the forehead and then moving to the subsequent areas that have been treated. Apply more cool compresses as needed for the patient's comfort.
9. After a few minutes, the cool compresses can be removed, revealing scattered frosting and erythema.
10. The patient can wash their face with a bland facial cleanser and is instructed to continue using bland moisturizers and practice sun protection until complete resolution of the peel.

Patients may return in 1 week and 1 month to evaluate their progress and address any concerns.

EVIDENCE-BASED INDICATIONS

Acne

Medical management remains the first-line treatment for active acne, although chemical peels can be used as adjuvant therapy. Treatment of acne can be divided into therapies for active acne lesions and those for acne scars. Treatment and application regimens may differ between practitioners and are often not documented in detail in published case series, making extrapolation of results difficult. However, the superficial peeling agents (salicylic acid, Jessner's, glycolic acid, and low-concentration TCA) have all demonstrated efficacy in treating active acne lesions.

Salicylic acid peels, in particular, with their lipophilic and keratolytic properties, ease of application, and excellent safety profile, are commonly used. In a randomized single-blind prospective study comparing 30% salicylic acid peel versus Jessner's solution applied every 2 weeks for 12 weeks in patients with mild and moderate acne, salicylic acid was significantly more effective at reducing comedone count (53.4% vs 26.3%, $P = .001$).[30] For papules, the overall difference at the end of 12 weeks was not statistically significant, although the group treated with salicylic acid peels saw improvement earlier.[30] Patients from both groups experienced erythema and postinflammatory hyperpigmentation, but this was more frequent in the group treated with Jessner's solution. This study was corroborated by a separate group that found that 30% salicylic acid improved both comedonal and inflammatory acne and showed greater efficacy versus Jessner's solution for comedonal lesions.[31] In this second study, no change in inflammatory lesions was seen with Jessner's solution, but these results were only assessed after three peels, in contrast to six peels in the previous study.[31] In another prospective, double-blind, randomized split-face study comparing 30% salicylic acid versus 25% TCA in patients with Fitzpatrick skin types III to V, both treatments improved comedonal and inflammatory lesions with no statistical difference between the two group. The authors noted no complications on the hemifaces treated with salicylic acid but did note prolonged erythema (25%) and hyperpigmentation (20%) in the group treated with TCA.[32]

Glycolic acid has also been found to be efficacious in the treatment of inflammatory and noninflammatory acne lesions. In one study using 70% glycolic acid applied for 2 to 8 minutes on the skin and repeated every 10 days as needed, the authors observed improvement with all stages of acne lesions, with comedonal acne improving the fastest, followed by papulopustular acne and then nodulocystic lesions (average of 3 treatments, 6 treatments, and 8-10 treatments, respectively). While nodulocystic lesions required more treatment sessions, the authors noted an additional benefit of improvement in superficial acne scars.[33] In a separate prospective, single-blind, split-face study comparing 70% glycolic acid applied for 2 minutes versus Jessner's solution, the authors saw improvement in both arms with no clear superiority for either treatment.[34] Glycolic acid has also been compared to salicylic acid in a head-to-head prospective, randomized, double-blind, split-face study of mild to moderately severe acne. In this study, 30% glycolic acid was applied to one hemiface for 4 to 5 minutes, while 30% salicylic acid was applied for 4 to 5 minutes to the other side. Both treatments decreased the number of acne lesions without clear superiority at 1-month follow-up. At 2-month follow-up, however, the side treated with salicylic acid had

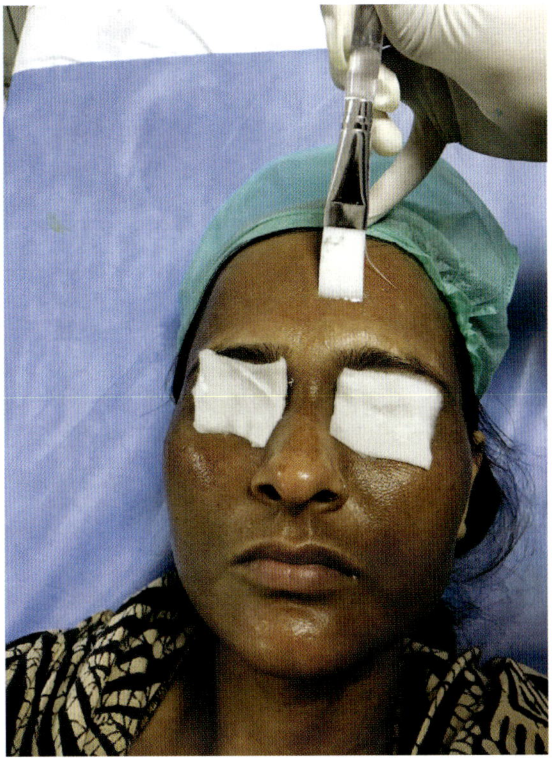

FIGURE 26-7 Peel application: The peeling agent is applied with a brush applicator on the entire face, beginning from the forehead proceeding to both cheeks, chin, nose, and malar area in that order, with care taken to maintain uniform pressure and perform feathering strokes at the edges.

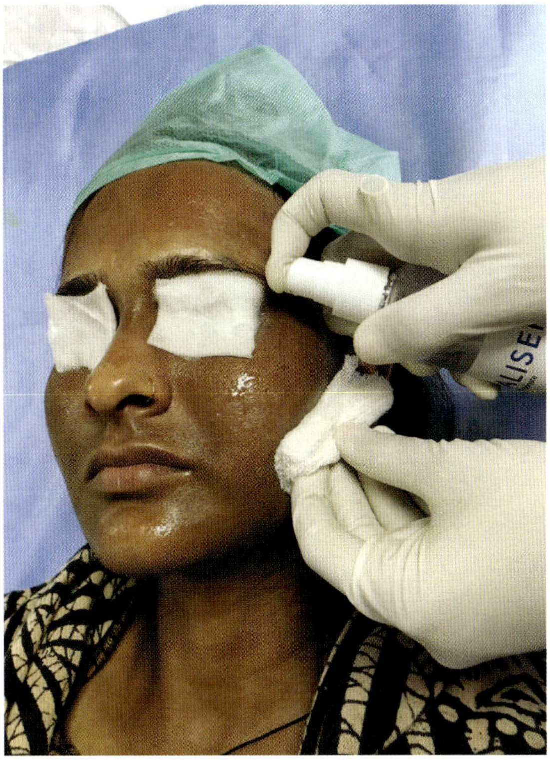

FIGURE 26-8 Neutralization: The glycolic acid peel is neutralized after the predetermined duration of time with 10% sodium bicarbonate solution and washed off with water. However, if erythema or epidermolysis occurs, the peel must be neutralized immediately, irrespective of the duration.

sustained this improvement, while the side treated with glycolic acid demonstrated a trend toward more new lesions.[35]

Acne scars are another common condition that have been studied by the chemical peel community. In 2002, the chemical reconstruction of skin scars (CROSS) technique was introduced.[36] A solution of high concentration of TCA (65% or 100%) is applied focally into the base of depressed acne scars using a sharpened wooden applicator to induce collagen regeneration (**Figures 26-9 and 26-10**). Because the solution is focally applied, local anesthesia and sedation are not needed, and healing is faster than with traditional full-face peels. In the original 2002 case series, two blinded physicians evaluated pretreatment photos against those taken 6 months after treatment, and 15 of 15 patients receiving six or more treatment courses were deemed to have a good or excellent results (>50% improvement). In the group treated with 100% TCA, all patients receiving five or six courses showed excellent results (>70% improvement).[36] In this Asian population, both groups experienced equal frequency of posttreatment erythema and transient postinflammatory hyperpigmentation. Studies involving the CROSS technique using 70% TCA, 90% TCA, and 88% phenol have all been reported and demonstrated efficacy for ice-pick scars.[37,38] In a split-face trial of 90% TCA versus 88% phenol, both sides showed significant improvement in scar grades before and after treatment, but patients rated phenol as more painful (5.3 vs 4.4) on a 10-point pain scale. Persistent erythema and hyperpigmentation were seen in both treatment sides, but hypopigmentation and widening of scars were seen only in the 90% TCA group (two patients each, 14.3%).[37] A similar case report of widening and atrophy of a scar was reported in a patient treated with an 80% TCA CROSS technique, suggesting that care must be taken in the application technique to limit the solution only to the scar depth.[39]

Actinic Keratoses

Chemical peels are an excellent modality for the treatment of diffuse actinic keratoses. In a head-to-head, nonrandomized, split-face trial, patients were treated with a single application of Jessner's/35% TCA medium-depth peel on the left side of the face and a traditional 3-week regimen of topical 5-fluorouracil on the right side of the face and then evaluated at 1, 6, and 12 months. Both sides received pretreatment with tretinoin 0.025% cream nightly for 2 weeks. Both hemifaces showed a significant reduction in the number of actinic keratoses (75%), with neither showing superiority at any follow-up end point.[40] This was confirmed histologically by biopsies taken at the 1-month follow-up, which showed significant reduction in hyperkeratosis and parakeratosis compared to pretreatment biopsies. In a questionnaire completed at the 6-month visit, all but one of the respondents reported preference for the chemical peel due to the convenience of a single treatment and the shorter healing time.[40]

In contrast to medium-depth peels, superficial peels alone are often inadequate in the treatment of actinic keratoses. In a prospective, randomized, controlled, split-face study evaluating weekly application of glycolic acid alone versus glycolic acid with 5-fluorouracil over 8 weeks, the sides treated with the combination (fluor-hydroxy pulse peel) demonstrated a 92% (range:

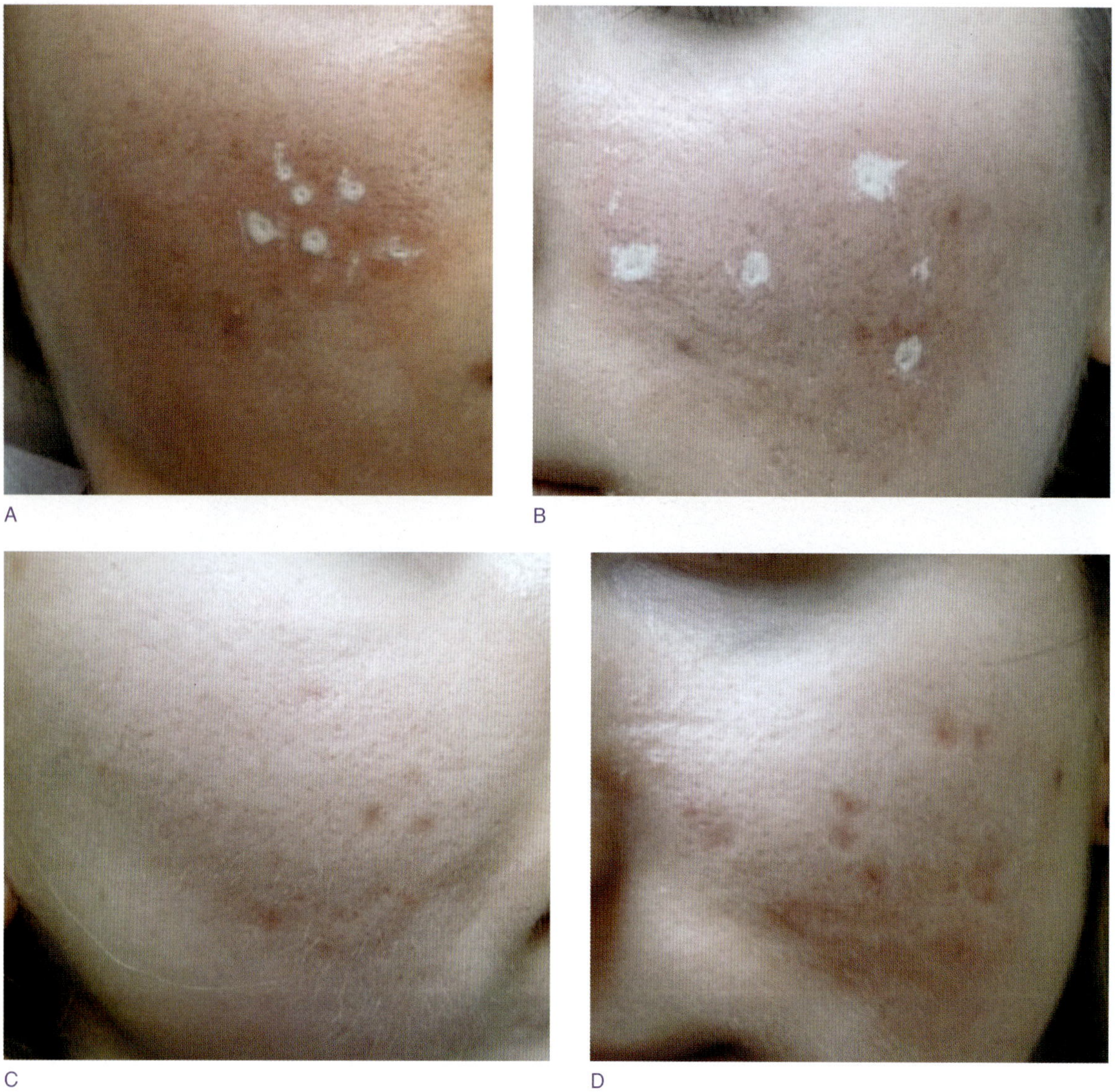

FIGURE 26-9 CROSS technique: Frosting immediately upon application (**A, B**); early postoperative erythema (**C, D**).

81%-100%) reduction in actinic keratoses compared to only 20% in the monotherapy group ($P < .05$).[41] Both investigators and patients reported preference for the side treated with the combination therapy. In addition to the reduction in actinic damage, there was also improvement in the overall cosmesis with reduction of solar lentigines, telangiectasias, and rhytides.

Melasma

Melasma is an acquired hyperpigmentation disorder that is challenging to treat. Medical therapy remains first line and consists of sun protection with some combination of hydroquinone, tretinoin, and a topical steroid, but patients often show variable results, and recurrence is high. Chemical peels can be used as an adjunct therapy, and numerous variations in treatment regimen have been reported in the literature. In general, serial treatments are needed to prevent relapse, combination treatments are better than monotherapies, and postinflammatory hyperpigmentation remains a risk factor.

Melasma is commonly divided into epidermal, dermal, and mixed types with the aid of a Wood's lamp. Most studies use superficial peeling agents to target the epidermal and dermal pigmentation and deeper peels to target mixed pigmentation. In a split-face trial comparing Jessner's solution versus 70% glycolic acid applied for 2 minutes applied 1 month apart over 3 months, both sides achieved improvement, with an average Melasma Area and Severity Index (MASI) score decrease of 8.61, with no superiority in either arm.[42] Although this decrease is on par with what has been reported with medical therapy alone, the improvement occurred over 3 months as opposed to 10 months. Interestingly, however, Wood's lamp illumination to determine the depth of pigment was not useful in predicting clinical response. Another study investigating the effect of 55% to 70% glycolic acid and 10% to 15% TCA in 100 patients showed that half of the patients required fewer than five peels, whereas half required 5 to 10 peels. While the patients treated with TCA required fewer number of peels (4.1 vs 6.1), this group also experienced higher rates of relapse and hyperpigmentation (25% vs 5.9%).[43] Of note, no discussion was made of a priming regimen.

Multiple studies have shown that a combination approach using a topical regimen with serial chemical peels can improve

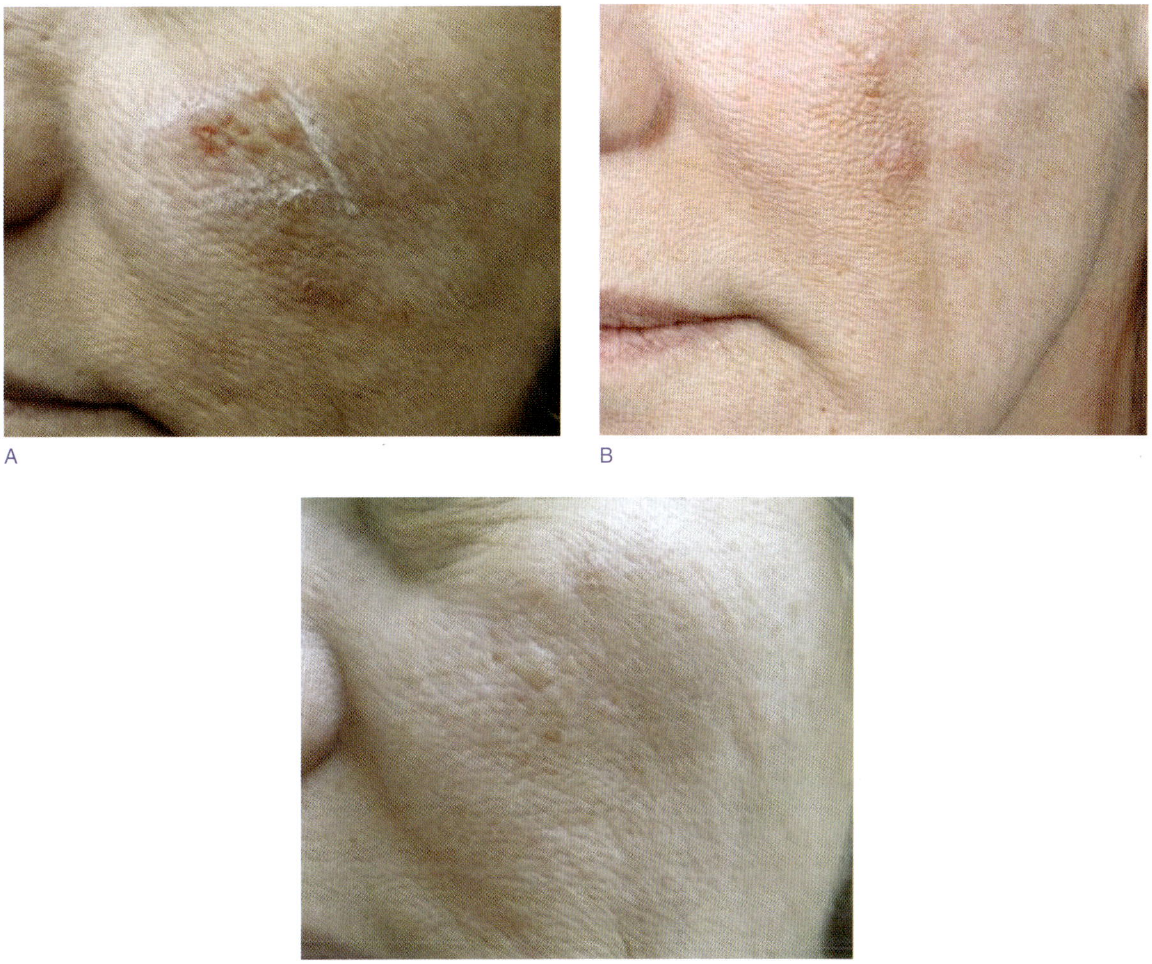

FIGURE 26-10 CROSS technique: Before treatment (**A**); 3 months after treatment (**B**); 2 years postop (**C**).

melasma. In two independent studies, when patients were primed with hydroquinone 2% or tretinoin 0.025% cream nightly for 2 weeks prior to a series of six peels (10% TCA in one study, 20%+ glycolic acid in the second), both groups showed an initial improvement that was comparable, but the group treated with hydroquinone experienced longer duration of their effect with less relapse.[26,27] In another study evaluating the additional benefit of serial glycolic acid peels, patients were randomized to either medical therapy alone (topical azelaic acid 20% cream and adapalene 0.1% gel) or medical therapy with a series of eight glycolic acid peels (35%-70%). The combination treatment group achieved an 83% decrease in mean MASI score, compared to 69% in the medical treatment group.[44]

Other peels have also been studied in the use of melasma. The data on serial salicylic acid are mixed, with one study reporting efficacy and another finding no improvement. A randomized, single-blind study divided 60 patients with epidermal melasma into two groups treated with either Jessner's solution (n = 34) or 30% salicylic acid (n = 26). Patients were primed with 0.05% tretinoin cream for 2 weeks and counseled to use SPF 60 sunscreen and then treated biweekly over 12 weeks (six treatments) with their respective chemical agents. Both groups saw statistically significant improvement, as measured by their MASI score at the end of the treatment period and at the 4- and 12-week follow-up visits.[45] No superiority in either arm was detected. A more recent prospective, randomized, controlled, split-face trial of epidermal melasma compared a series of four salicylic acid peels applied biweekly in conjunction with 4% hydroquinone cream versus hydroquinone cream monotherapy. Although both treatment regimens showed improvement by the treatment end, no superiority was seen with the addition of salicylic acid peels.[46]

Melasma is a difficult condition to treat. It is difficult to conceptualize the mechanism for superficial peels to improve dermal melasma. It may be that the majority of melasma is mixed and the improvement seen in dermal melasma is that of the epidermal component. To offer patients the best chance of success, patients should be primed and maintained on a topical regimen that includes hydroquinone with an expectation that serial peels will be needed to achieve improvement but that relapse will likely recur.

Facial Rejuvenation

Facial rejuvenation and improvement of photoaging are two of the primary applications for chemical peels. To guide clinicians in the assessment of photodamage, the Glogau classification can be used in assessing the patient (**Table 26-8**). Superficial peels can improve skin texture and mild hyperpigmentation, whereas

TABLE 26-8 • Glogau Classification for Photoaging

Group	Severity	Age Group	Wrinkles	Other Features
I	Mild	20-35	Minimal wrinkling	No keratoses No to little makeup No pigmentation changes
II	Moderate	35-50	Easy wrinkling	Early palpable actinic keratoses Few seborrheic keratoses Small amounts of makeup
III	Advanced	51-65	Wrinkles at rest	Obvious actinic keratoses Obvious seborrheic keratoses Always wears makeup
IV	Severe	66+	Deep wrinkles and wrinkles throughout	Yellow-gray skin color History of skin cancers Makeup "cakes and cracks"

Adapted with permission from Tung R, Rubin M: Procedures in Cosmetic Dermatology Series: Chemical Peels, 2nd ed. Philadelphia, PA: Elsevier/Saunders; 2011.

medium-depth peels target more extensive actinic damage and fine lines. For deeper etched-in lines, however, deep peels should be used. Glycolic acid is one of the most popular superficial peels for facial rejuvenation. Patients can be given a prepeel regimen of tretinoin and/or low concentration glycolic acid cream and then peeled with serial glycolic acid treatments with increasing concentration (50%-70%) as their skin tolerance allows. For the treatment of wrinkles and solar lentigines, 70% glycolic acid may be left on for 4 to 8 minutes.[47] The beneficial effects of glycolic acid have also been tested and confirmed in a prospective, placebo-controlled, split-patient study evaluating a 50% glycolic acid gel formulation applied for 5 minutes on the face, forearm, and hands compared to a vehicle control. After 4 consecutive weekly treatments, patients were evaluated by blinded evaluators both clinically and by biopsy. Across the three site locations, glycolic acid significantly improved rough skin texture, the number of actinic keratoses, and fine wrinkling, as compared to control ($P < .0001$ for all parameters).[48] Coarse wrinkling, however, was unaffected. Clinical improvement correlated with changes in biopsy as well, with a more compact stratum corneum and a thicker epidermis with a more prominent stratum granulosum.

Other superficial peeling agents have also been reported to be efficacious in the treatment of mild photodamage. In the original report of 30% salicylic acid peel, the authors describe their experience in a case series of 50 patients with mild to moderate photodamage. The majority of patients experienced subjective improvements in skin texture, light pigmentation, and fine lines.[49] A single application of 35% TCA peel has also been compared against a series of five peels with 30% glycolic acid in a split-face study. While the improvements at 3 months were small and not visible to naïve judges, patients subjectively reported better outcomes with the 35% TCA peel and an image analysis software detected fewer fine lines on the 35% TCA treatment side.[50] While this is not the full Jessner's/35% TCA medium-depth treatment regimen, this study does show that patients unwilling to undergo a deeper peel may need serial treatments with a superficial peeling agent to obtain a similar result.

For patients with severe photoaging with less tendency toward pigmentation, deeper phenol-based peels are preferred due to their dermal penetration. To "tighten" wrinkles, the peel needs to penetrate into the reticular dermis so that collagen regeneration can occur.[51,52] Of the various phenol-based formulations, the original Baker-Gordon solution has the greatest penetration.[15] In their 1974 publication, Baker et al[53] followed patients they had previously treated for clinicopathologic correlation. The histologic changes after treatment that they had reported earlier, including increased dermal collagen and elastic tissue, were visible in patients up to 13 years after treatment, leading the authors to conclude that the architectural and clinical changes induced by deep peels are permanent.[53] Since then, modifications in phenol peels have been used in treating photoaging. In a recent publication, a group of patients were treated with 88% phenol applied focally every 3 mm along fine wrinkles using a punctuated method similar to the CROSS technique. Since the application was limited, the authors reported no downtime and patients were not sedated. The clinical improvement in wrinkle appearance correlated with a thicker dermis, like that seen in a full-face peel, without the associated recovery time and risk profile.[54]

Phenol peels have also been used as an adjunct to, or a less invasive alternative to, blepharoplasty. In postblepharoplasty patients treated with a modified phenol formulation, a majority of patients noted improvement in wrinkling and pigmentation. While some wrinkling recurred after treatment, the authors reported an overall permanent improvement with the treatment.[55] In a separate study, phenol peels were used as a less invasive alternative to blepharoplasty, with good clinical outcomes. In a case series of eight patients with Fitzpatrick skin types I to III with mild to moderate upper eyelid ptosis, a Baker-Gordon phenol peel was applied to a focal region of excess skin on the upper eyelids followed by 88% phenol to the remaining periorbital skin. The peel was left unoccluded after treatment and healing time was approximately 6 to 8 days, similar to the periorbital areas treated with 88% phenol and 35% TCA applied elsewhere on the face. The authors reported no adverse effects and a significant increase in eyelid gap after treatment.[56]

TABLE 26-9 • Prevention and Management of Complications of Chemical Peels

Complication	Prevention	Management
Immediate		
Skin irritation, itching, or burning	Avoid high peel concentrations, excess amounts, irregular pressure	Emollients, topical steroids
Erythema, edema	Stop photosensitizers, sun exposure	Topical steroids, photoprotection, sunscreens
Eye problems	Eye protection, petroleum jelly around eyes, careful peel application	Saline irrigation of eye, ophthalmology referral
Late		
Infection (bacterial /candidal/ herpetic)	Avoid rubbing, itching, scratching Prophylactic antiviral therapy (history of herpetic infection)	Topical or oral antibiotics/antifungals Oral antiviral therapy
Reaction to chemical agent: (acneiform eruption, allergic reaction, and cardiac toxicity)	Test peel and meticulous pre-peel assessment	Topical antibiotics, steroids, intralesional corticosteroids Cardiopulmonary monitoring in case of phenol peel
Abnormal wound healing (hypertrophic scar/keloid/ delayed healing/milia)	Avoid itching or scratching Proper pre-peel assessment Early neutralization of peel if necessary	Occlusive dressing, intralesional steroids, surgical excision
Pigmentary alterations (hyperpigmentation/ hypopigmentation/demarcation lines)	Proper pre-peel assessment Priming, photoprotection Feathering during peel application	Topical depigmenting agents/lasers

CONCLUSIONS

Chemical peels are an excellent and powerful addition to the clinician's armamentarium, as they are generally safe and effective, with minimal side effects and a potentially profound effect on cosmesis. As with any procedure, significant attention should be given to minimizing and mitigating the risk of complications (**Table 26-9**). Unlike lasers and light devices, chemical peels require only a minimal investment on the part of the clinician, and therefore they represent a feasible approach for the clinician lacking a large cosmetic patient base.

REFERENCES

1. Brody HJ, Monheit GD, Resnik SS, Alt TH. A history of chemical peeling. *Dermatol Surg.* 2000;26(5):405-409.
2. Arif T. Salicylic acid as a peeling agent: a comprehensive review. *Clin Cosmet Investig Dermatol.* 2015;26(8):455-461.
3. Grimes PE. The safety and efficacy of salicylic acid chemical peels in darker racial-ethnic groups. *Dermatol Surg.* 1999;25(1):18-22.
4. Kligman D, Kligman AM. Salicylic acid peels for the treatment of photoaging. *Dermatol Surg.* 1998;24(3):325-328.
5. Becker FF, Langford FP, Rubin MG, Speelman P. A histological comparison of 50% and 70% glycolic acid peels using solutions with various pHs. *Dermatol Surg.* 1996;22(5):463-465.
6. Moy LS, Peace S, Moy RL. Comparison of the effect of various chemical peeling agents in a mini-pig model. *Dermatol Surg.* 1996;22(5):429-432.
7. Tung R, Rubin M. *Procedures in Cosmetic Dermatology Series: Chemical Peels* (2nd ed). New York, NY: Elsevier Saunders; 2011.
8. DiNardo JC, Grove GL, Moy LS. Clinical and histological effects of glycolic acid at different concentrations and pH levels. *Dermatol Surg.* 1996;22(5):421-424.
9. Sehgal VN, Luthra A, Aggarwal AK. Evaluation of graded strength glycolic acid (GA) facial peel: an Indian experience. *J Dermatol.* 2003;30(10):758-761.
10. Kaidbey K, Sutherland B, Bennet P, et al. Topical glycolic acid enhances photodamage by ultraviolet light. *Photodermatol Photoimmunol Photomed.* 2003;19(1):21-27.
11. Brody HJ. Variations and comparisons in medium-depth chemical peeling. *J Dermatol Surg Oncol.* 1989;15(9):953-963.
12. Monheit GD. The Jessner's + TCA peel: a medium-depth chemical peel. *J Dermatol Surg Oncol.* 1989;15(9):945-950.
13. Coleman WP 3rd, Futrell JM. The glycolic acid trichloroacetic acid peel. *J Dermatol Surg Oncol.* 1994;20(1):76-80.
14. Camacho FM. Medium-depth and deep chemical peels. *J Cosmet Dermatol.* 2005;4(2):117-128.
15. Stone PA. The use of modified phenol for chemical face peeling. *Clin Plast Surg.* 1998;25(1):21-44.
16. Fintsi Y. Exoderm: a novel, phenol-based peeling method resulting in improved safety. *Am J Cosm Surg.* 1997;14(1):49-54.
17. Stone PA, Lefer LG. Modified phenol chemical face peels: recognizing the role of application technique. *Clin Plast Surg.* 2001;28(1):13-36.
18. Hetter GP. An examination of the phenol-croton oil peel: part I. Dissecting the formula. *Plast Reconstr Surg.* 2000;105(1):227-239.

19. Stegman SJ. A study of dermabrasion and chemical peels in an animal model. *J Dermatol Surg Oncol.* 1980;6(6):490-497.

20. Truppman ES, Ellenby JD. Major electrocardiographic changes during chemical face peeling. *Plast Reconstr Surg.* 1979;63(1):44-48.

21. Landau M. Cardiac complications in deep chemical peels. *Dermatol Surg.* 2007;33(2):190-193.

22. Park JH, Choi YD, Kim SW, Kim YC, Park SW. Effectiveness of modified phenol peel (Exoderm) on facial wrinkles, acne scars and other skin problems of Asian patients. *J Dermatol.* 2007;34(1):17-24.

23. Gerber PA, Kukova G, Bolke E, et al. Severe hyperpigmentation and scarring following glycolic acid peel treatment in combination with low-dose isotretinoin. *Eur J Med Res.* 2014;19:60.

24. Picosse FR, Yarak S, Cabral NC, Bagatin E. Early chemabrasion for acne scars after treatment with oral isotretinoin. *Dermatol Surg.* 2012;38(9):1521-1526.

25. Hevia O, Nemeth AJ, Taylor JR. Tretinoin accelerates healing after trichloroacetic acid chemical peel. *Arch Dermatol.* 1991;127(5):678-682.

26. Garg VK, Sarkar R, Agarwal R. Comparative evaluation of beneficiary effects of priming agents (2% hydroquinone and 0.025% retinoic acid) in the treatment of melasma with glycolic acid peels. *Dermatol Surg.* 2008;34(8):1032-1039.

27. Nanda S, Grover C, Reddy BS. Efficacy of hydroquinone (2%) versus tretinoin (0.025%) as adjunct topical agents for chemical peeling in patients of melasma. *Dermatol Surg.* 2004;30(3):385-388.

28. West TB, Alster TS. Effect of pretreatment on the incidence of hyperpigmentation following cutaneous CO2 laser resurfacing. *Dermatol Surg.* 1999;25(1):15-17.

29. Maloney BP, Millman B, Monheit G, McCollough EG. The etiology of prolonged erythema after chemical peel. *Dermatol Surg.* 1998;24(3):337-341.

30. Dayal S, Amrani A, Sahu P, Jain VK. Jessner's solution vs. 30% salicylic acid peels: a comparative study of the efficacy and safety in mild-to-moderate acne vulgaris. *J Cosmet Dermatol.* 2017;16(1):43-51.

31. Bae BG, Park CO, Shin H, et al. Salicylic acid peels versus Jessner's solution for acne vulgaris: a comparative study. *Dermatol Surg.* 2013;39(2):248-253.

32. Abdel Meguid AM, Elaziz Ahmed Attallah DA, Omar H. Trichloroacetic acid versus salicylic acid in the treatment of acne vulgaris in dark-skinned patients. *Dermatol Surg.* 2015;41(12):1398-1404.

33. Atzori L, Brundu MA, Orru A, Biggio P. Glycolic acid peeling in the treatment of acne. *J Eur Acad Dermatol Venereol.* 1999;12(2):119-122.

34. Kim SW, Moon SE, Kim JA, Eun HC. Glycolic acid versus Jessner's solution: which is better for facial acne patients? A randomized prospective clinical trial of split-face model therapy. *Dermatol Surg.* 1999;25(4):270-273.

35. Kessler E, Flanagan K, Chia C, Rogers C, Glaser DA. Comparison of alpha- and beta-hydroxy acid chemical peels in the treatment of mild to moderately severe facial acne vulgaris. *Dermatol Surg.* 2008;34(1):45-50.

36. Lee JB, Chung WG, Kwahck H, Lee KH. Focal treatment of acne scars with trichloroacetic acid: chemical reconstruction of skin scars method. *Dermatol Surg.* 2002;28(11):1017-1021.

37. Dalpizzol M, Weber MB, Mattiazzi AP, Manzoni AP. Comparative study of the use of trichloroacetic acid and phenolic acid in the treatment of atrophic-type acne scars. *Dermatol Surg.* 2016;42(3):377-383.

38. Agarwal N, Gupta LK, Khare AK, Kuldeep CM, Mittal A. Therapeutic response of 70% trichloroacetic acid CROSS in atrophic acne scars. *Dermatol Surg.* 2015;41(5):597-604.

39. Weber MB, Machado RB, Hoefel IR, Manzoni AP, Da Silva Bastos Geler A. Complications of CROSS-technique on boxcar acne scars: atrophy. *Dermatol Surg.* 2011;37(1):93-95.

40. Lawrence N, Cox SE, Cockerell CJ, Freeman RG, Cruz PD Jr. A comparison of the efficacy and safety of Jessner's solution and 35% trichloroacetic acid vs 5% fluorouracil in the treatment of widespread facial actinic keratoses. *Arch Dermatol.* 1995;131(2):176-181.

41. Marrero GM, Katz BE. The new fluo-hydroxy pulse peel. A combination of 5-fluorouracil and glycolic acid. *Dermatol Surg.* 1998;24(9):973-978.

42. Lawrence N, Cox SE, Brody HJ. Treatment of melasma with Jessner's solution versus glycolic acid: a comparison of clinical efficacy and evaluation of the predictive ability of Wood's light examination. *J Am Acad Dermatol.* 1997;36(4):589-593.

43. Kalla G, Garg A, Kachhawa D. Chemical peeling: glycolic acid versus trichloroacetic acid in melasma. *Indian J Dermatol Venereol Leprol.* 2001;67(2):82-84.

44. Erbil H, Sezer E, Tastan B, Arca E, Kurumlu Z. Efficacy and safety of serial glycolic acid peels and a topical regimen in the treatment of recalcitrant melasma. *J Dermatol.* 2007;34(1):25-30.

45. Elaz A, Raza N, Iftikhar N, Muzzafar F. Comparison of 30% salicylic acid with Jessner's solution for superficial chemical peeling in epidermal melasma. *J Coll Physicians Surg Pak.* 2008;18(4):205-208.

46. Kodali S, Guevera IL, Carrigan CR, et al. A prospective, randomized, split-face, controlled trial of salicylic acid peels in the treatment of Latin American women. *J Am Acad Dermatol.* 2010;63(6):1030-1035.

47. Moy LS, Murad H, Moy RL. Glycolic acid peels for the treatment of wrinkles and photoaging. *J Dermatol Surg Oncol.* 1993;19(3):243-246.

48. Newman N, Newman A, Moy LS, Babapour R, Harris AG, Moy RL. Clinical improvement of photoaged skin with 50% glycolic acid. A double-blind vehicle-controlled study. *Dermatol Surg.* 1996;22(5):455-460.

49. Kligman D, Kligman AM. Salicylic acid peels for the treatment of photoaging. *Dermatol Surg.* 1998;24(3):325-328.

50. Kitzmiller WJ, Visscher MO, Maclennan S, et al. Comparison of a series of superficial chemical peels with a single midlevel chemical peel for the correction of facial actinic damage. *Aesthet Surg J.* 2003;23(5):339-344.

51. Brody HJ. Do chemical peels tighten the skin? *Dermatol Surg.* 2014;40(Suppl 12):S129-S133.

52. Stegman SJ. A comparative histologic study of the effects of three peeling agents and dermabrasion on normal and sun-damaged skin. *Anesthetic Plast Surg.* 1982;6(3):123-135.

53. Baker TJ, Gordon HL, Mosienko P, Seckinger DL. Long-term histological study of skin after chemical face peeling. *Plast Reconstr Surg.* 1974;53(5):522-525.

54. De Mendonca MC, Aarestrup FM, Aarestrup BJ. Clinical protocol for punctuated 88% phenol peels in the treatment of photoaging: a histopathological study of three cases. *Dermatol Surg.* 2012;38(12):2011-2015.

55. Gatti JE. Eyelid phenol peel: an important adjunct to blepharoplasty. *Ann Plast Surg.* 2008;60(1):14-18.

56. Parada MB, Yarak S, Gouvea LG, et al. "Blepharopeeling" in the upper eyelids: a nonincisional procedure in periorbital rejuvenation—a pilot study. *Dermatol Surg.* 2008;34(10):1435-1438.

Lasers for Pigmented Lesions and Tattoos

27

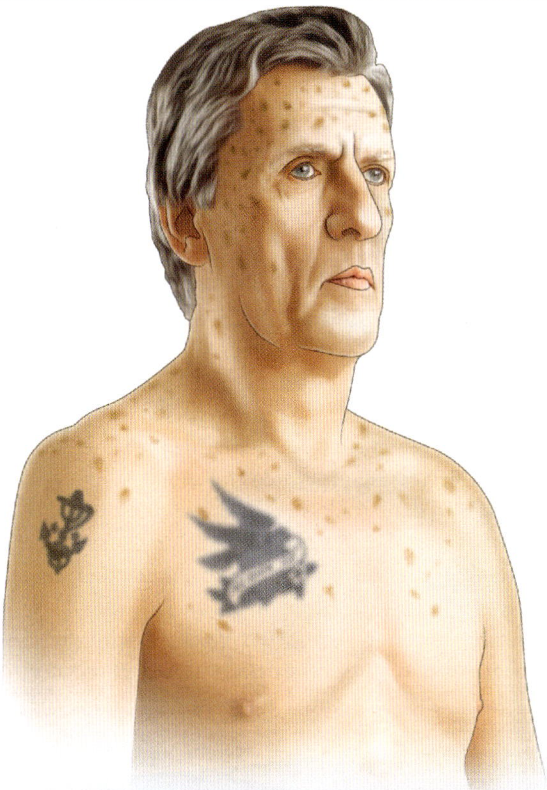

SUMMARY

- Lasers are frequently used to treat pigmented lesions and tattoos.
- Recent advances in picosecond lasers may improve both the efficacy and safety profile of these treatments.
- Depending on the depth of treatment, topical anesthesia or none at all is generally sufficient for most cases.

Beginner Tips

- Patients with a suntan or sunless tan should avoid laser treatments. The increased melanin on tanned skin acts as a competing chromophore and can increase the risk of adverse events.
- Extremely diligent sun protection is crucial after treatment of pigmented lesions such as lentigines, PIH, or melasma.
- Both UVA and UVB can trigger hyperpigmentation or hypopigmentation.

Pitfalls and Cautions

- Distinguishing a benign lentigo from lentigo maligna may be challenging. Any concerning features on examination or history should prompt a biopsy for a definitive diagnosis before laser therapy is performed.
- Allergic reactions are possible after treating tattoos, particularly red tattoos, due to breakdown and dispersal of the putative antigen.

Expert Tips

- Tattoos often require multiple lasers to treat appropriately.
- Topical steroids may be considered after treatment of melasma or PIH to help prevent an inflammatory response that may worsen the pigmentation.
- Start with a lower fluence and increase with subsequent treatments.

Patient Education Points

- Realistic expectations are critical, particularly for tattoo removal.
- Some tattoos require as many as 20 rounds of treatment, and some tattoos will never clear completely.
- Postinflammatory hyperpigmentation and melasma may worsen after laser treatment.

Don't Forget!

- Extreme caution should be used prior to treating postinflammatory hyperpigmentation or melasma with lasers, as there is a risk of exacerbating the hyperpigmentation.
- Lasers should not be used routinely to treat nevi without a preceding biopsy, and generally should not be used to treat nevi in patients with a personal or family history of dysplastic nevi.

Billing Pearls

- Almost all insurers in the United States exclude laser treatments from coverage.
- Patients may benefit from committing to a series of treatments, as this may allow significant cost savings.
- Pretreatment with occluded topical anesthesia can be started at home, and prescription plans may cover the cost of this medication.

27 Lasers for Pigmented Lesions and Tattoos

INTRODUCTION

The principle of selective photothermolysis has revolutionized laser treatment for pigmented lesions and tattoos.[1] This principle describes the mechanism by which specific wavelengths of light are preferentially absorbed by a chromophore, leading to targeted destruction. There are three main components of selective photothermolysis. The laser wavelength must be preferentially absorbed by the target chromophore; the fluence, or energy per unit area, must be sufficient to destroy the target; and the pulse duration should be equal to or less than the thermal relaxation time (TRT) of the target.

FUNDAMENTAL CONSIDERATIONS

The three main chromophores in the skin are oxyhemoglobin, melanin, and water, and each preferentially absorbs different wavelengths of light. Ideally, a laser should emit a wavelength of light that is selectively absorbed by the target chromophore and that is not absorbed by the surrounding tissue. The absorption spectrum of melanin spans from 250 to 1200 nm,[2] although the amount of absorption decreases as the wavelength increases (**Figure 27-1**). Longer wavelengths penetrate deeper into the dermis and are considered to be safer in darker skinned patients as they are associated with less epidermal damage.

The TRT is the amount of time required for the target to lose half of its heat. The TRT is related to the size of the target; overall, the smaller the chromophore, the shorter the TRT. If the pulse duration is equal to or less than the TRT of the target, the heat generated is confined to the target itself, and little energy diffuses into nearby tissue, thus minimizing unwanted destruction. The TRTs of melanosomes and tattoo particles are in the nanosecond or picosecond range.[3] Therefore, Q-switched (QS) lasers that deliver pulse durations in the nanosecond range and, more recently, picosecond lasers, which deliver pulse durations in the picosecond range, have improved both the efficacy and safety of these treatments. By delivering high energy with very short pulse durations, the pigment is broken down into particles that are phagocytized by macrophages and easily eliminated from the body. The most common QS lasers are the 694-nm QS ruby, 755-nm QS alexandrite, 1064-nm QS Nd:YAG, and 532-nm frequency-doubled QS Nd:YAG. Picosecond lasers include 532-, 755-, and 1064-nm wavelengths. The photomechanical effects dominate over the photothermal effects, shattering the target into smaller particles and decreasing unwanted diffusion.[4] With even shorter pulse durations than traditional QS lasers, picosecond lasers are able to use lower fluences for successful treatment.[5] By treating with lower fluences, the risk of epidermal injury and dyspigmentation is minimized.

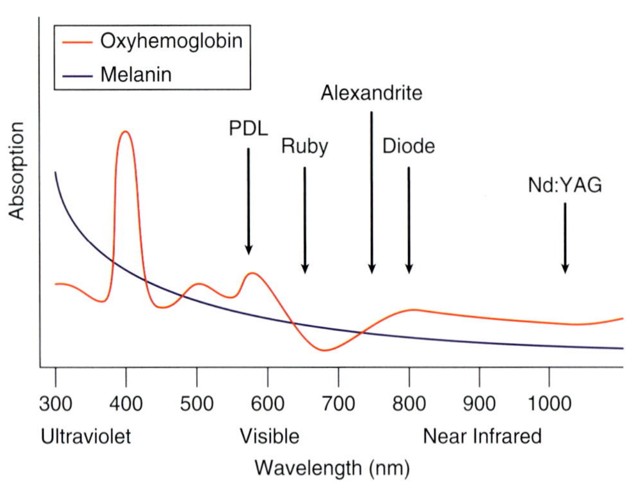

FIGURE 27-1 When choosing the appropriate laser for pigmented lesions, the different absorption spectra for hemoglobin and melanin should be considered.

Long-pulsed ruby, alexandrite, or Nd:YAG lasers with pulse durations in the millisecond range have demonstrated efficacy for the treatment of superficial pigmented lesions. By delivering the energy over a longer duration, they are thought to gently heat the tissue and decrease the rate of adverse events.[6]

Fractional lasers, both ablative and nonablative, are gaining popularity as a treatment alternative for benign pigmented lesions. The ablative fractional lasers include the 10,600-nm carbon dioxide (CO_2) and the 2940-nm erbium:yttrium aluminum garnet (Er:YAG). Nonablative fractional lasers include the 1550-nm erbium-doped laser, the 1565-nm fiber laser, and the 1927-nm thulium laser. These lasers target water as opposed to melanin. The fractional lasers create microscopic injury zones, or microthermal zones, in the epidermis and dermis. It has been suggested that the unwanted melanocytes and melanin are eliminated through these microthermal zones.[7] Since only a portion of the epidermis and dermis is affected during each treatment, multiple treatments may be needed for satisfactory results.[8]

PATIENT SELECTION

A thorough medical history must be taken before initiation of treatment. Allergies, medical history, and medications should be reviewed. A history of treatment with gold therapy is a contraindication to treatment with QS lasers, as localized chrysiasis may be induced.[9] For patients on isotretinoin, many recommend that treatment with lasers be deferred until after the medication is discontinued for 6 months, as there may be an increased risk of scar formation and delayed wound healing.[10,11] However, recent publications have failed to show an increased rate of side effects when patients are treated with lasers while on isotretinoin therapy.[12-14] The possibility of scar development should be reviewed and appropriately documented in all patients, especially those with a history of keloid or hypertrophic scar formation. Antiviral prophylaxis may be necessary when treating areas with a history of herpes simplex outbreak.

Fitzpatrick skin type (FST) must be considered in patients undergoing laser therapy. The increased melanin in higher FSTs may absorb laser energy, leading to increased thermal injury to surrounding tissue and an ensuing increased risk of dyspigmentation and scarring.

Additionally, treatment efficacy decreases in patients with higher FST, as the increased pigment content of normal background skin competitively absorbs laser energy.[15] Thus, a patient should not have a suntan or a sunless tan when receiving laser treatment. To reduce the risk of adverse events in dark-skinned patients, longer wavelengths, lower treatment fluences, and cooling devices may be used.[16]

Realistic patient expectations must be set prior to the initiation of therapy. Patients should be aware that multiple treatments will likely be necessary, and complete resolution is not always possible. Photographs should ideally be taken prior to treatment.

SAFETY AND PATIENT PREPARATION

Certain practices must be employed to ensure both the safety of the patient and the treating staff. Lasers used to treat tattoos and pigmented lesions are of the same wavelengths that can damage the retina. Therefore, all individuals in the room must wear goggles that protect against the specific wavelength being used. The patient should also be wearing protective eyewear. When treating an eyeliner tattoo or a pigmented lesion on the eyelid, a metal corneal shield must be placed under the patient's eyelid to protect the globe. Ophthalmic tetracaine is inserted onto the conjunctiva, and the concave aspect of the shield is coated with an ophthalmic lubricating ointment. While the patient is gazing up, the lower lid is retracted and the bottom aspect of the shield is inserted below the lower lid. The patient is then asked to gaze down and the top of the shield is placed below the upper eyelid. Reflective surfaces and all windows should be covered. A sign should be placed on the door to prevent accidental entry during treatment.

All makeup, creams, and topical anesthetics should be removed before treatment initiation, as they may alter the efficacy of the laser therapy. Chlorhexidine or alcohol may be used to clean the skin; if alcohol is used, it must be completely dry and residue free, as this may lead to an accidental fire. Caution should be taken that any flammable items are removed.

The need for anesthesia will vary depending on the location, size, and depth of the target. Treatment of superficial lesions with QS lasers often does not require anesthesia. For deeper lesions, sensitive areas, or fractional resurfacing lasers, topical anesthetics are generally sufficient and should be applied for approximately 30 minutes under occlusion and completely removed prior to therapy. Local infiltrative anesthesia may be used for the treatment of dermal lesions, such as nevus of Ota, or tattoos.

TATTOOS

As the percentage of the population with tattoos grows, the number of patients requesting the removal of unwanted tattoos has steadily increased.[17] Pigment-specific nanosecond QS lasers and picosecond lasers are widely accepted as the gold standard for tattoo removal, although long pulsed and ablative lasers have also been studied.

Nanosecond QS Lasers

Traditional QS lasers provide a combination of a high peak power along with a nanosecond pulse duration allowing for effective destruction of the tattoo ink particle without destruction of nearby tissue.[18] Common QS lasers used for tattoo removal include the 694-nm ruby, 755-nm alexandrite, 1064-nm Nd:YAG, frequency-doubled 532-nm Nd:YAG, and 532-nm KTP. The different wavelengths preferentially target certain colors (**Table 27-1**). If a tattoo is multicolored, several lasers with different wavelengths must be used for the best results.[19] Transient skin whitening is the desired treatment end point and represents cavitation and the formation of gas bubbles in the epidermis from heating of the target.[3] If whitening is not observed, then the fluence is likely insufficient. If excessive fluence is used, breakdown of the epidermis or significant bleeding may occur.[8] Lower fluences are recommended initially for dark, dense pigment as they have abundant target chromophore, and the fluence may be increased as the tattoo fades.[8] Typically, treatments are spaced 6 to 8 weeks apart, as more frequent treatments interfere with macrophage ink clearance and are associated with more adverse reactions.[20] Treatment risks include scarring, pigmentary alteration, and incomplete removal.

Laser selection will vary depending on the color of the tattoo ink. The QS ruby, alexandrite, and Nd:YAG lasers (**Figure 27-2**) have been shown to be effective for the treatment of dark blue and black tattoos.[19] While the QS ruby and alexandrite may

TABLE 27-1 • Laser Options for Tattoo Removal Based on Tattoo Ink Color

Color	Pigment	Laser
Yellow	Cadmium sulfide	QS 510-nm pulsed-dye, QS KTP, QS Nd:YAG (frequency doubled)
Red	Cinnabar Cadmium red	QS 510-nm pulsed-dye, QS KTP, QS Nd:YAG (frequency doubled)
Green	Chromium oxide	QS ruby, QS alexandrite, picosecond alexandrite
Blue	Cobalt blue Azure	QS ruby, QS alexandrite, QS Nd:YAG, picosecond alexandrite, picosecond Nd:YAG
Black	Carbon Iron oxide	QS ruby, QS alexandrite, QS Nd:YAG, picosecond alexandrite, picosecond Nd:YAG

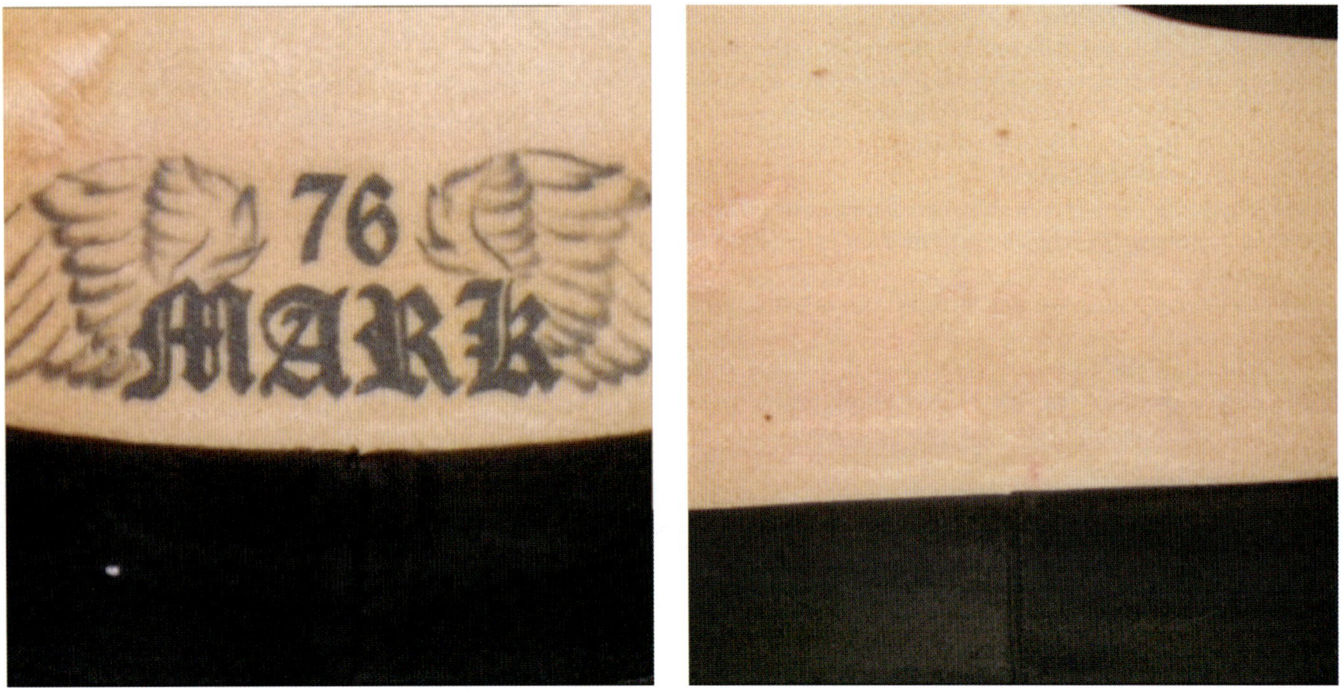

A B

FIGURE 27-2 Black tattoo (A) before and (B) after eight treatments with the QS 1,064-nm Nd:YAG laser. (Used with permission from D. Rainone, MD).

be effective in clearing dark ink, they are absorbed by melanin and are associated with unwanted pigmentary changes.[21,22] The QS Nd:YAG has less absorption by epidermal melanin and keratinocytes and is generally preferred for dark tattoos in darkly pigmented individuals.[17,23] Both the QS ruby and alexandrite have also been shown to clear green tattoos.[24,25] The frequency-doubled 532-nm Nd:YAG and the 532-nm KTP are often recommended for the treatment of yellow, orange, and red ink.[22,26] Due to the risk of pigmentary alterations, especially in higher FSTs, a test spot treatment may be advisable. The test spot should be examined approximately 1 month later for both dyspigmentation and efficacy.

Despite the significant progress with QS lasers, tattoo removal can be frustrating, time consuming, and costly. The number of required treatments varies greatly depending on the color, composition, density, depth, tattoo age, body location, and the quantity of tattoo ink present.[17] For some tattoos, as many as 20 treatments may be necessary,[27] and satisfactory clearance may never be achieved.

In an attempt to optimize outcomes and enhance clearance, one study examined the combination of fractional resurfacing immediately following treatment with the QS ruby laser.[28] In this small series of three patients, the investigators reported that both ablative and nonablative fractional resurfacing following QS laser of unwanted tattoos enhances tattoo clearance.[28] In another study, the use of daily 5% imiquimod cream as an adjunct to QS laser therapy was investigated, which demonstrated no improvement in efficacy but an increased rate of adverse events with the combination therapy.[29]

In an effort to decrease the total number of treatment sessions with QS lasers, investigators have studied the feasibility of a multipass technique. Normally, immediately after treatment, cutaneous whitening is observed. This whitening is due to the formation of gas bubbles or vacuoles in the skin, limiting the penetration of the laser into the dermis. These intradermal vacuoles resolve after 20 minutes and allow for repeat treatment. Kossida et al[30] demonstrated superior tattoo clearance with four passes with a QS alexandrite laser with 20 minutes between each pass ("R20" method) compared with a single treatment with the QS alexandrite laser. To eliminate the need to wait 20 minutes between each treatment, the "R0" method was created. By applying topical perfluorodecalin (PFD), the whitening reaction resolves almost immediately, allowing for repeat successive treatments. Reddy et al[31] recently reported the safety and efficacy of this method.

Clinical research trials are currently examining the role of acoustic wave technology in combination with traditional QS lasers. An acoustic wave device is applied to the tattoo after laser treatment to help disrupt the pigment containing macrophages and clear the intradermal vacuoles that are formed immediately after laser therapy. By rapidly dissipating the laser-induced vacuoles, multiple laser passes may be performed in a single treatment session.

Picosecond Lasers

Picosecond lasers deliver pulse durations that are approximately 100 times shorter than traditional QS lasers and are closer to the TRT of tattoo pigment. This ultra-short pulse width allows for

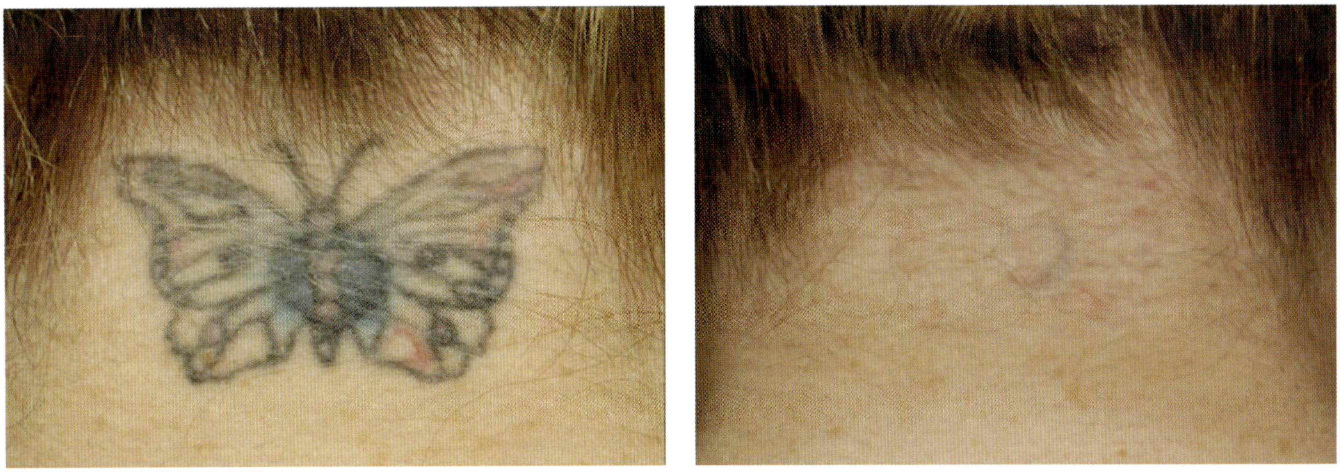

A B

FIGURE 27-3 Multicolored tattoo (**A**) before and (**B**) after six treatments with the 755-nm alexandrite picosecond laser. (Used with permission from R. Geronemus, MD).

more significant photomechanical effects and efficient breakup of the tattoo ink.[5] More effective destruction of the target means that lower fluence is required,[5] decreasing the rate of unwanted side effects. Currently, picosecond lasers are available in 532-, 755-, and 1064-nm wavelengths (**Figures 27-3 to 27-5**). Ross et al[32] compared 1064-nm picosecond and nanosecond lasers for the treatment of black tattoos. With all other parameters constant, they demonstrated greater lightening with the picosecond pulses.[32] One study by Brauer et al[33] reported at least 75% clearing of blue and/or green ink tattoos after one or two treatments with 755-nm picosecond laser. More recently, they reported clearing of yellow tattoos, which are notoriously difficult to treat, with a frequency-doubled Nd:YAG 532-nm picosecond laser (**Figure 27-6**).[34]

Clinical Considerations

For tattoo removal, several factors should be considered that will help estimate the number of treatments required. These include FST, tattoo color, location, amount of ink, layering of ink, and presence of scarring.[35] Lower FST, darker colors, and older tattoos

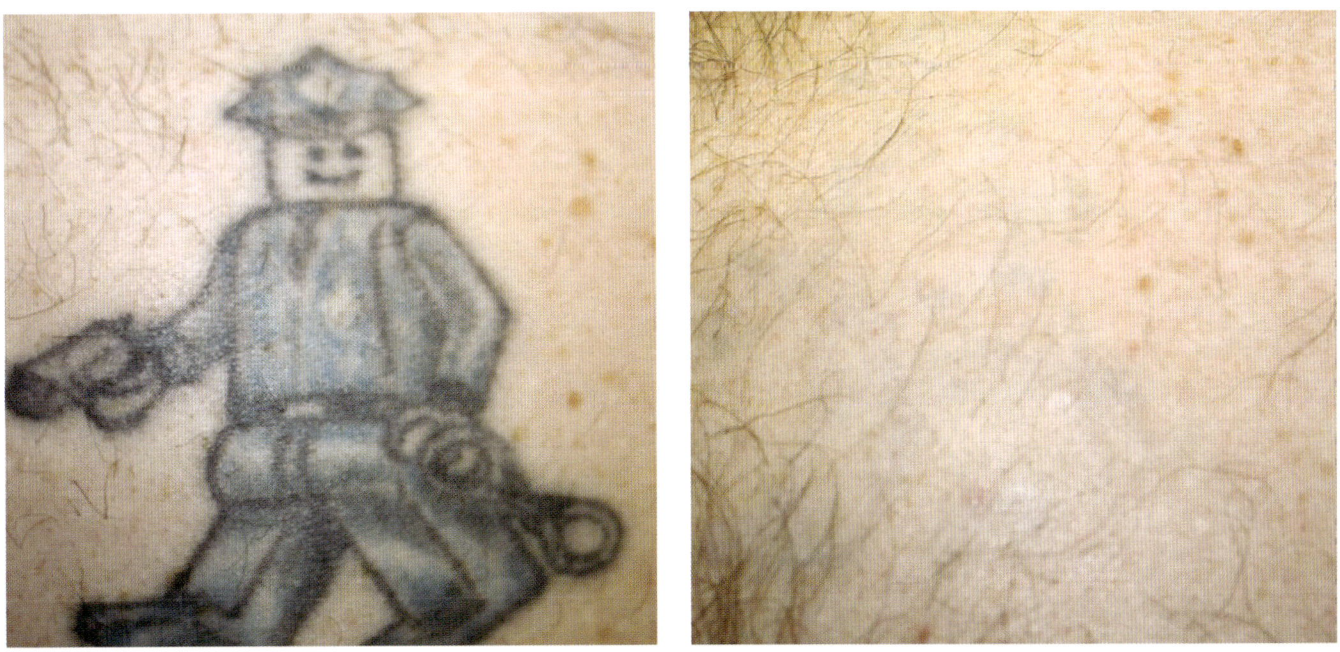

A B

FIGURE 27-4 Blue tattoo (**A**) before and (**B**) after five treatments with the 755-nm alexandrite picosecond laser. (Used with permission from Clean Slate Laser).

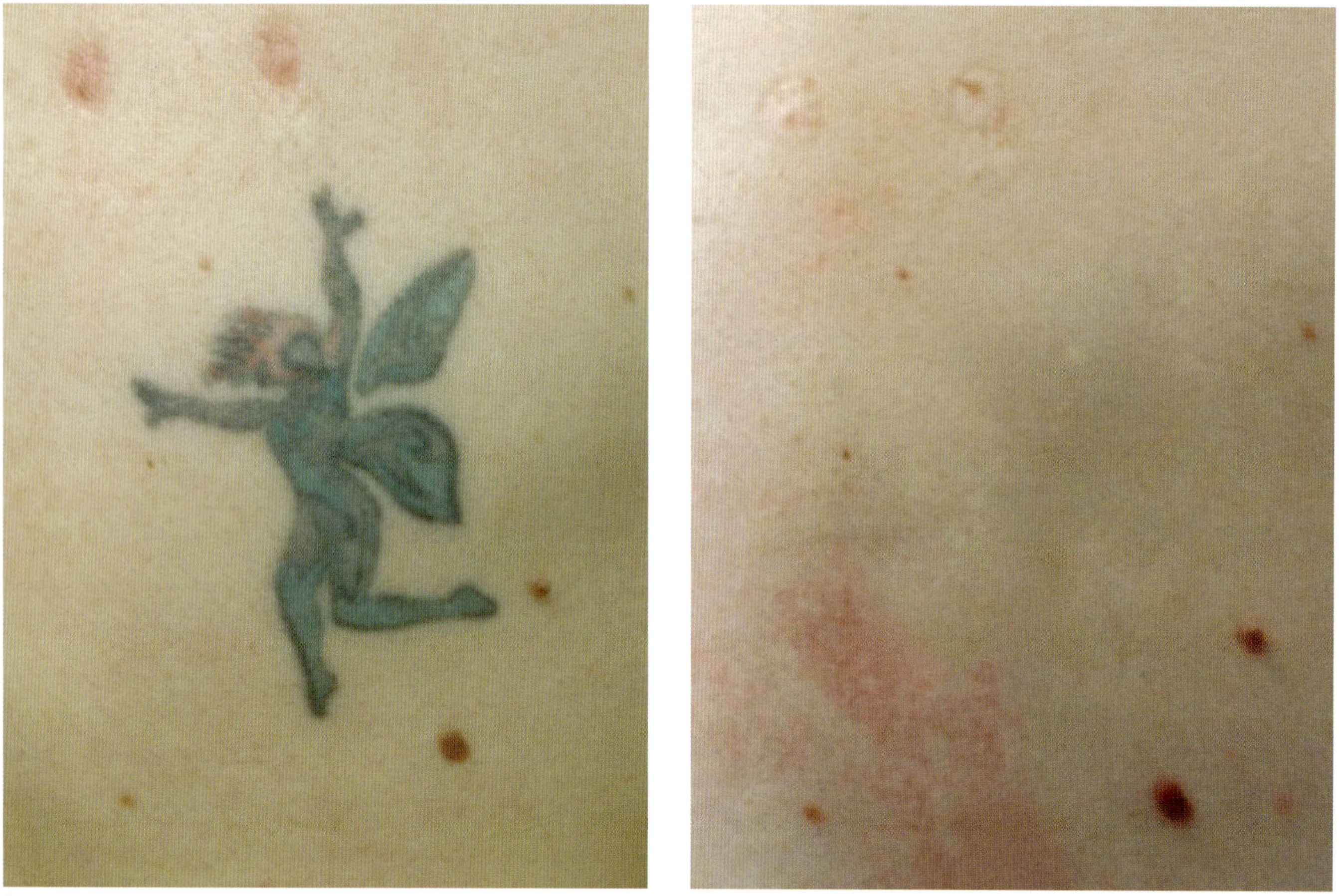

A B

FIGURE 27-5 Green tattoo (**A**) before and (**B**) after five treatments with the 755-nm alexandrite picosecond laser.

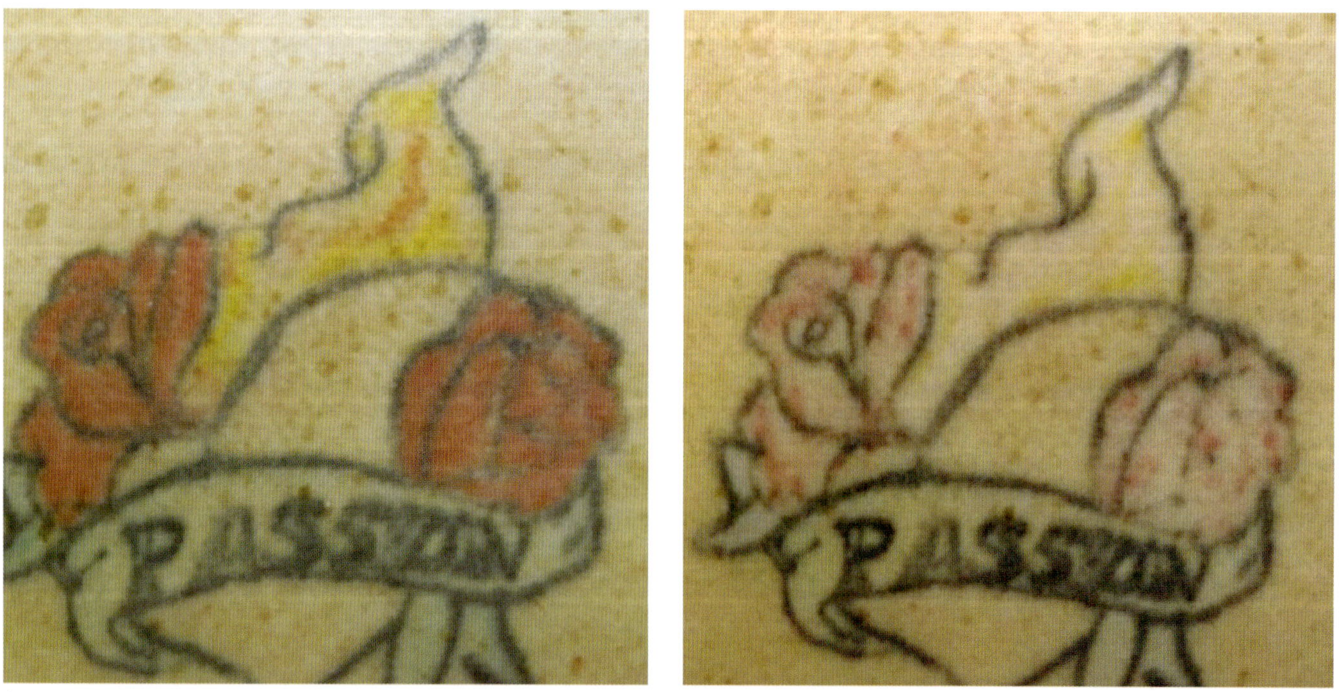

A B

FIGURE 27-6 Red, orange, and yellow pigment treated with the 532-nm picosecond laser (**A**) before and (**B**) after two treatments. (Used with permission from Cynosure, Inc.)

tend to have a better treatment response.[36] Multicolored tattoos, cover up tattoos, and sleeve tattoos may be challenging to treat, and the use of several different lasers may be needed. Amateur tattoos tend to have less ink and are located in all layers of the epidermis. In contrast, professional tattoos place high concentrations of ink at the transition from papillary to reticular dermis.[37] Therefore amateur tattoos tend to require fewer treatments.[37]

Caution must be taken when treating cosmetic tattoos with pink, tan, white, red, or brown pigment. Immediate and permanent darkening may occur after treatment with the QS lasers.[38,39] The treatment of these cosmetic tattoos may reduce white ink composed of titanium dioxide ($Ti0_2$, Ti^{4+}) to blue Ti^{2+} or rust-colored ferric oxide (Fe_2O_3) to black ferrous oxide (FeO). If paradoxical darkening does occur, subsequent treatments with a resurfacing laser[40] or additional QS laser treatments targeting the darker color may be helpful.

Tattoo pigment is a foreign substance and thus can cause an allergic or granulomatous response. The most common color to cause allergic reaction is red, as it may contain mercury-related compounds. Treatment of the ink with a laser may disperse the antigen, triggering a widespread allergic reaction.[41] While safe treatment of red tattoo reactions with the QS 532-nm Nd:YAG in combination with topical steroids has been reported,[42] many advise against the use of QS lasers in such cases and recommend treatment with the Er:YAG or CO_2 laser.[43,44]

PIGMENTED LESIONS

Prior to treating pigmented lesions, it is imperative to ensure that the lesion has no atypical features. If there is any question regarding the diagnosis or there are concern for melanocytic atypia, a biopsy must be performed prior to laser therapy. After ensuring that the lesion in question is benign, determining whether the pigment is located in the epidermis, dermal-epidermal junction, or dermis will help determine the appropriate laser wavelength. For melasma, which can have pigment in the epidermis, dermis, or both, evaluation with a Wood's lamp may be helpful in determining pigment depth. If the pigment is located in the epidermis, it will be accentuated under Wood's lamp examination, while dermal melasma will not demonstrate color accentuation. This distinction is very difficult to make in skin types V and VI.

As with tattoo removal, the desired treatment end point is transient skin whitening. For patients with FST IV to VI, it may be worthwhile to perform test spots to ensure the correct fluence is being used, as excessive fluences can lead to scarring, dyspigmentation, and burns.[8] Many clinicians will pretreat darker skin types with a bleaching agent such as hydroquinone 4% for 1 week prior to treatment and a low- to mid-potency topical steroid for 3 to 4 days after treatment.[36] The size and number of lesions must also be considered when estimating the number of treatments.

Epidermal Lesions

Commonly treated epidermal lesions include lentigines, ephelides, café-au-lait macules (CALMs), and nevus spilus. Anesthesia is usually not needed for the treatment of epidermal lesions. Any laser treatment that removes the epidermis will improve epidermal pigmented lesions. The ablative carbon dioxide and argon lasers were some of the earlier lasers used to treat epidermal pigment disorders, although because of their high rate of adverse events, they have become less popular.[45] Pigment-specific nanosecond and picosecond QS lasers are generally considered the gold standard.

Lentigines and Ephelides: Since the pigment is located superficially, lasers with a short wavelengths that have a high absorption by melanin and do not penetrate deeply are effective. Although studies for ephelides are limited, the most commonly used lasers for lentigines and ephelides are the QS frequency-doubled Nd:YAG,[46] QS ruby,[47] and QS alexandrite (**Figure** 27-7).[48,49] The long-pulse alexandrite laser has demonstrated efficacy and safety for the treatment of dark lentigines.[50] Usually, two to three treatments can completely clear lentigines, and there is a low rate of recurrence, although recurrences tend to be more common with ephelides.[49]

For widespread lesions or diffuse photodamage, fractional ablative or nonablative lasers and intense pulsed light (IPL) can be effective alternatives. Studies have reported improvement in

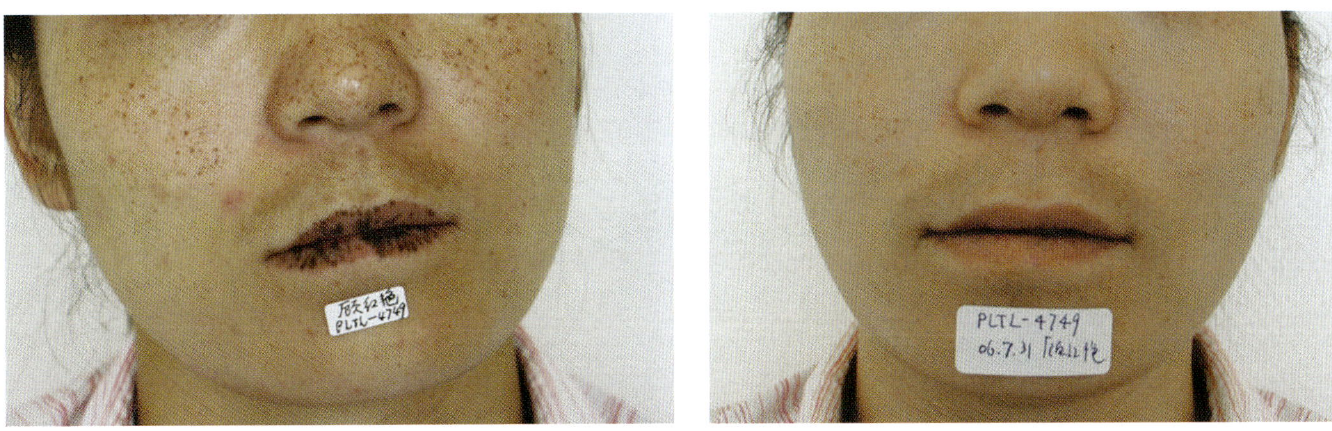

A B

FIGURE 27-7 Ephelides (**A**) before and (**B**) after five treatments with the QS 755-nm alexandrite laser. (Used with permission from L. Zhong, MD).

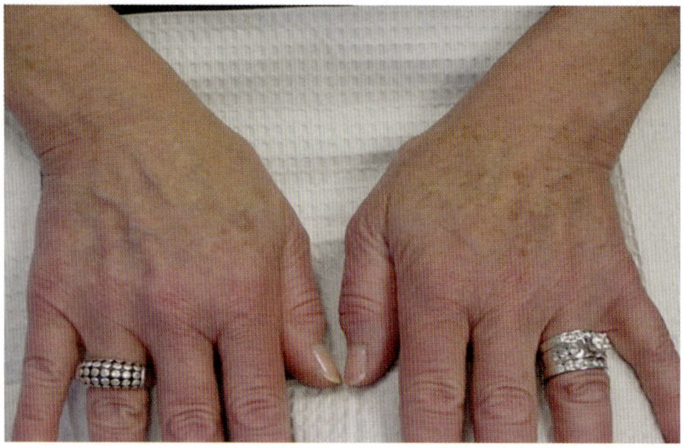

FIGURE 27-8 Treatment of lentigines with the IPL laser. (Used with permission from Robert and Margaret Weiss, MD.)

photodamage and dyspigmentation with the 1550-nm erbium-doped fractional device.[51,52] For the treatment of lentigines, a 2010 a consensus panel recommended three to five treatments at monthly intervals with fluences between 10 and 20 mJ and treatment levels from 7 to 11 for FST I to III and 4 to 7 for higher FSTs with the 1550-nm erbium-doped fractional device.[53] More recently, the 1927-nm thulium fiber fractionated laser has demonstrated efficacy for the treatment of photopigmentation and lentigines.[54,55] The 1927-nm wavelength has a higher affinity for water than the 1550-nm erbium-doped fiber laser and, therefore, more effectively targets epidermal processes.[56] IPL uses broadband visible light emitted from a noncoherent, nonlaser, filtered flashlamp, and has been shown to improve superficial pigmented lesions, with a low rate of postinflammatory hyperpigmentation (**Figure 27-8**).[57,58]

Although large-scale studies are needed, picosecond lasers may represent alternative treatment options for lentigines and pigmentary alterations from photodamage. More recently, a specialized optical hand attachment composed of approximately 120 diffractive lenses that release high levels of energy to focused areas has been developed for the 755-nm picosecond laser. Less than 10% of the skin is exposed to a high fluence while the surrounding skin is treated with lower fluence. Treatment with a 755-nm picosecond laser with the focus lens array has demonstrated efficacy for photoinduced dyspigmentation (**Figures 27-9 and 27-10**).[59]

CALMs and Nevus Spilus: Before initiating laser treatment of CALMs, if numerous lesions are present, a thorough history must be taken to rule out neurofibromatosis. Treatment of CALMs may be challenging, as multiple treatments may be required, and incomplete removal and recurrence are common. QS lasers, including the ruby, alexandrite, and Nd:YAG, have successfully treated CALMs and nevus spilus.[60-62] Although additional larger studies need to be performed, improvement of CALMs with the 755-nm picosecond laser has been demonstrated (**Figure 27-11**).[4,63]

Mixed Dermal-Epidermal Lesions

Pigment can be found in both the epidermis and the dermis in postinflammatory hyperpigmentation (PIH), melasma, Becker nevus, and melanocytic nevi.

PIH: PIH is a result of hemosiderin or melanin deposition in the skin after epidermal or dermal injury or inflammation and is more common in darker skin types. Although epidermal melanin tends to be more responsive to 532-nm than 1064-nm wavelengths, there is a higher risk of hyperpigmentation and worsening of

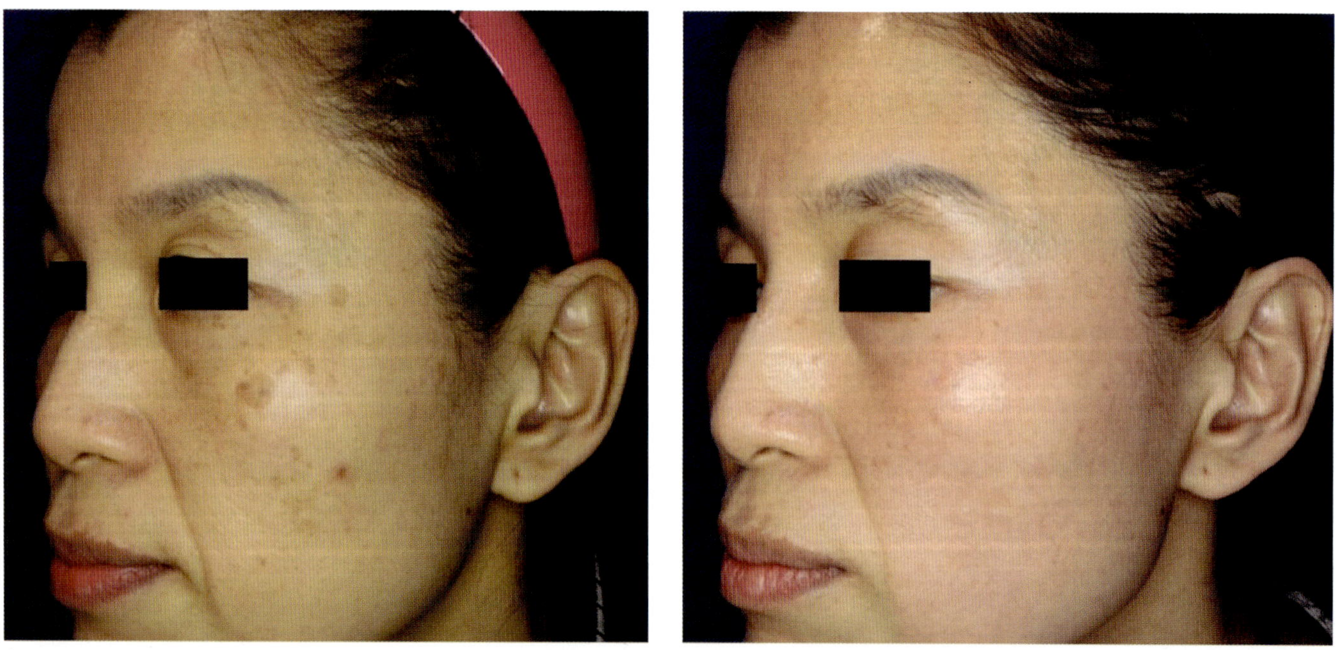

A B

FIGURE 27-9 Lentigines (**A**) before and (**B**) after five treatments with the 755-nm picosecond laser with the focus array. (Used with permission from S. Shin, MD.)

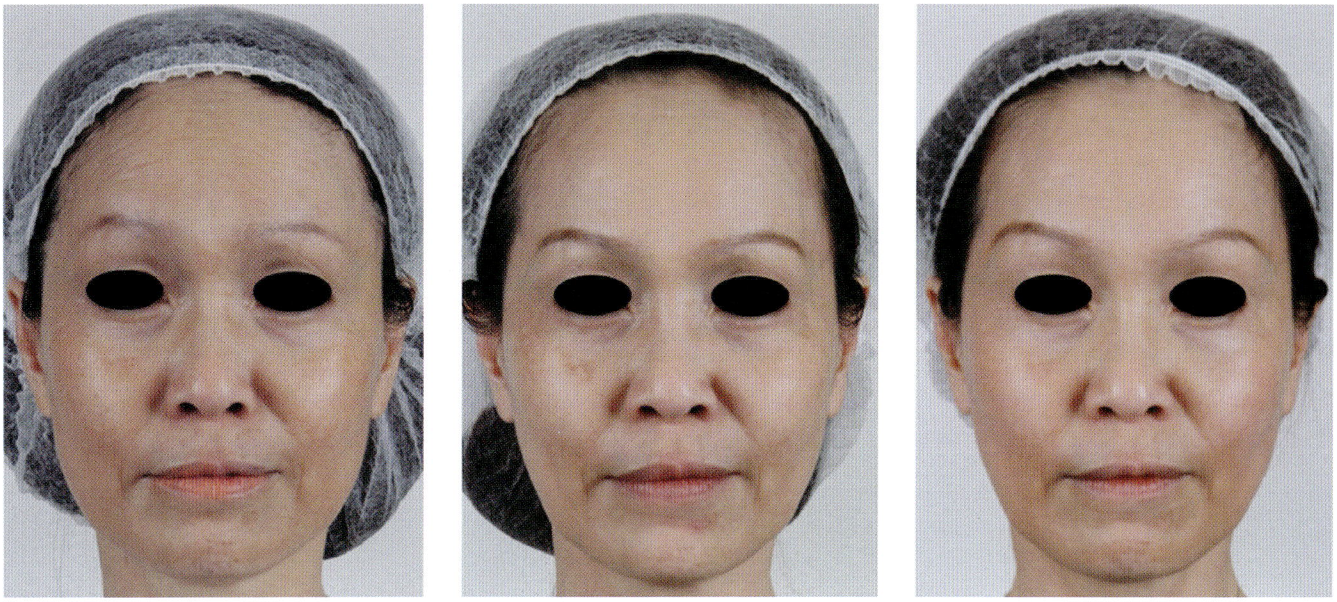

A B C

FIGURE 27-10 Photoaging (**A**) before, (**B**) after one treatment, and (**C**) 6 months after three treatments with the 755-nm picosecond laser with the focus array. (Used with permission from C. Cheng, MD.)

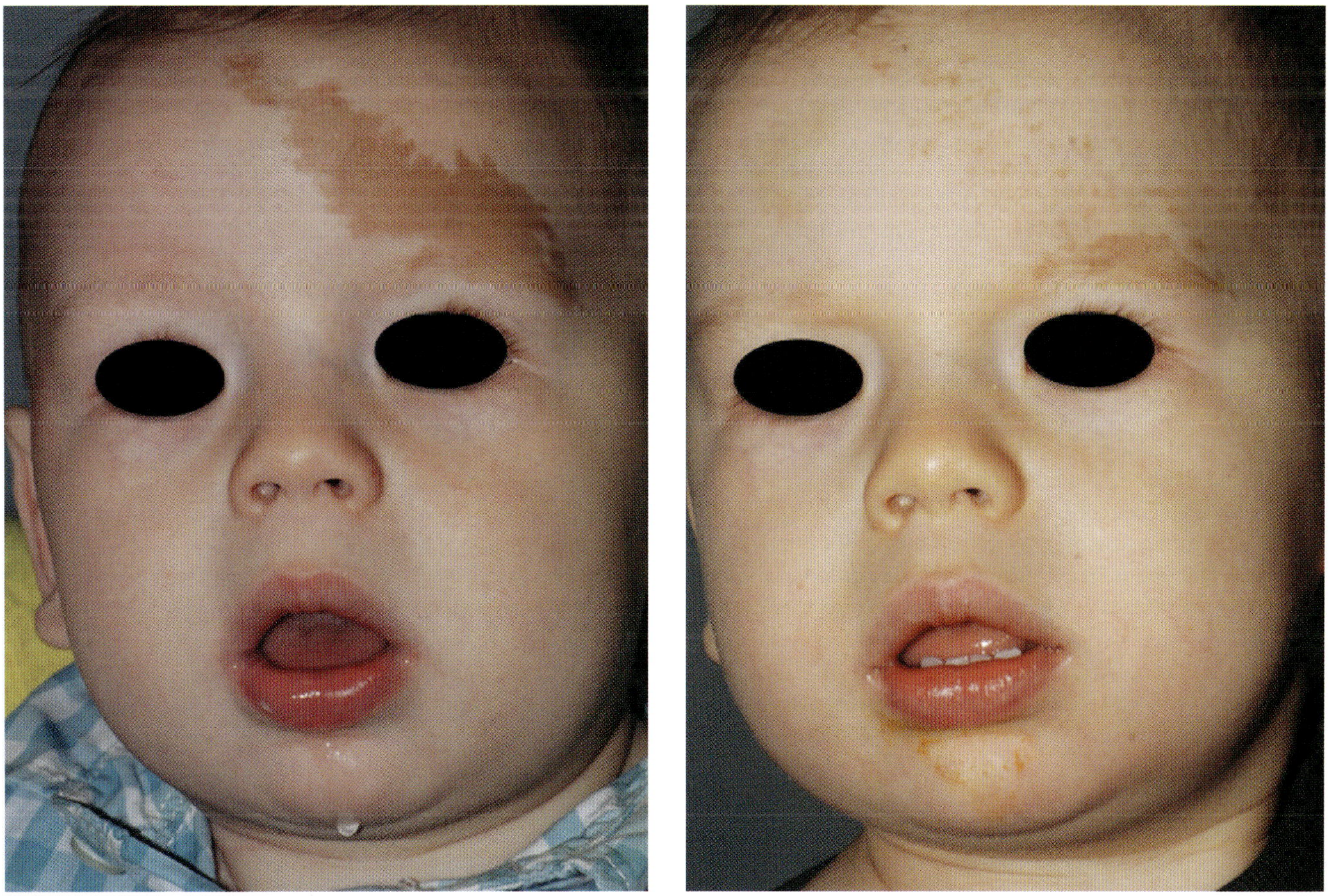

A B

FIGURE 27-11 Café-au-lait macule (**A**) before and (**B**) after two treatments with the 755-nm picosecond laser. (Used with permission from M. Taylor, MD.)

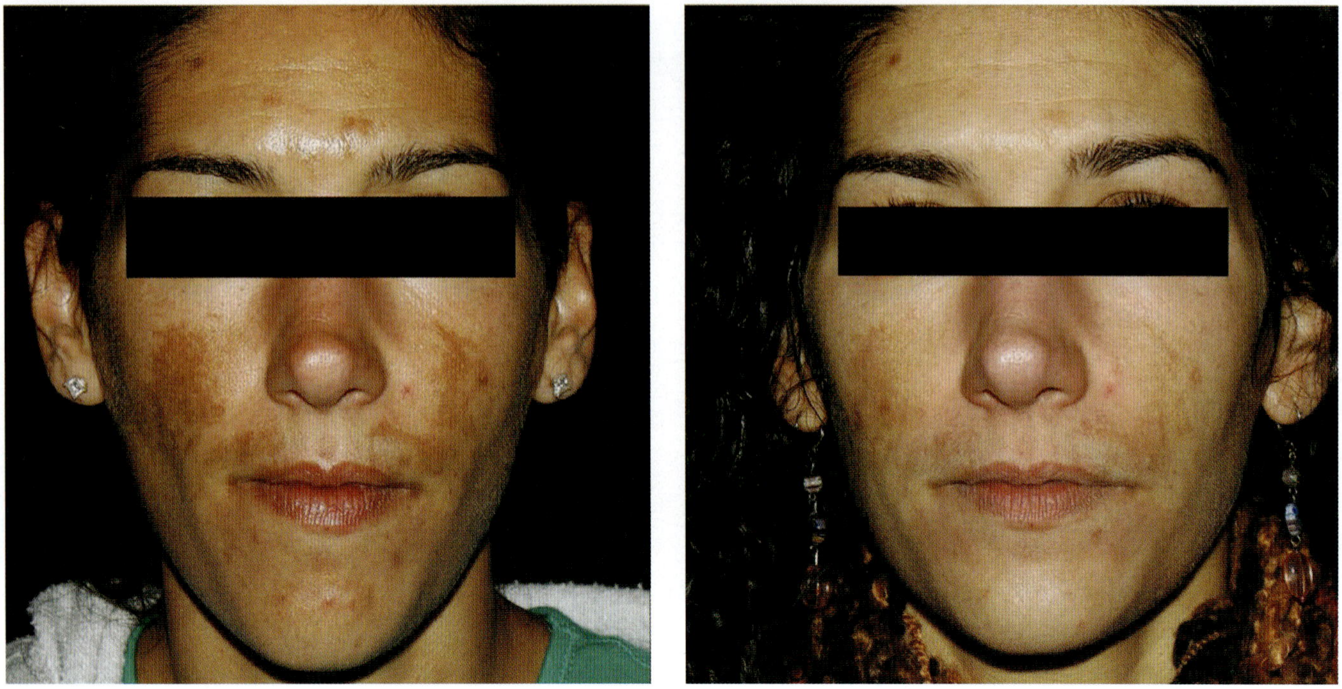

A B

FIGURE 27-12 Melasma (**A**) before and (**B**) after four treatments with the 755-nm alexandrite picosecond laser with the focus array. (Used with permission from L. Espinoza, MD.)

PIH with shorter wavelengths, particularly in darker skinned patients. Studies have reported improvement of PIH with the 1064-nm QS Nd:YAG laser with low fluence in patients with higher FSTs.[64,65] Nonablative fractional lasers have some efficacy in the treatment of PIH.[66,67] However, care must be taken, as laser treatment of PIH may exacerbate the hyperpigmentation. Many dermatologists do not recommend the use of lasers for PIH at this time. Although additional studies must be performed, picosecond technology may be employed for PIH due to its favorable side effect profile and low rates of dyspigmentation.

Melasma: Melasma, which can be epidermal, dermal, or mixed, can be extremely challenging to treat. Although controversial, factors that have been suggested to play a role in the pathogenesis of melasma include hormonal therapy, pregnancy, ultraviolet light radiation, irritating cosmetics, phototoxic medications, and genetic factors.[68] The response rate is inconsistent, and recurrence is very common. Like PIH, care must be taken, as any associated inflammation can trigger melanocytic activity and worsen the dyschromia. First-line treatments for melasma include broad-spectrum sunscreens and bleaching agents. Patients must be counseled on the use of sunscreen at all times and that even minimal sun exposure can trigger melasma. Lightening agents such as hydroquinone, topical retinoids, kojic acid, azelaic acid, and Kligman's formula (5% hydroquinone, 0.1% tretinoin, 0.1% dexamethasone) should be attempted prior to laser therapy and as maintenance. Chemical peels with glycolic acid, lactic acid, and trichloroacetic acid may be helpful, although caution must be taken to prevent inflammation and PIH especially in darker skin types. While improvement with the QS ruby, QS alexandrite, and QS Nd:YAG lasers, 1,550-nm erbium-doped fractional laser, CO_2 fractional laser, and IPL has been shown, worsening and recurrence have been a challenge.[69-74] The method of repeated treatments with the 1064-nm QS Nd:YAG laser with a low fluence has become popular to treat melasma. Kauvar[75] treated 27 patients at 4-week intervals with microdermabrasion followed by QS Nd:YAG at 1.6 to 2.0 J/cm^2 and topical hydroquinone and reported continued improvement in melasma after 1 year. Multiple treatments are often necessary, there is high rate of recurrence,[76] and guttate hypopigmentation has been reported with this technique.[77] Improvement in melasma has also been seen with the 755-nm picosecond laser with the focus lens array (**Figure 27-12**). The 1927-nm thulium fiber laser, with a high absorption coefficient for water, targets epidermal processes; it has had some efficacy with the treatment of melasma and has a low side effect profile.[54,78,79]

Becker Nevus: A Becker nevus (BN) is a benign hamartoma that presents most commonly in adolescence as a brown patch with overlying dark hair. Laser treatment of BN is variable and often disappointing.[80] Improvement in pigmentation has been reported with the QS ruby and QS Nd:YAG. A comparative study showed the QS ruby to be superior to the QS 1064-nm Nd:YAG.[60] The QS lasers do not decrease hair density, and recurrence of pigment is frequent. Ablative lasers, such as the Er:YAG and CO_2 laser,[81,82] and the nonablative 1550-nm fractional erbium-doped fiber laser have reported improvement in pigmentation but no effect on hypertrichosis.[83] Terminal hair reduction and pigment lightening have been demonstrated with long pulsed ruby and alexandrite lasers.[84,85]

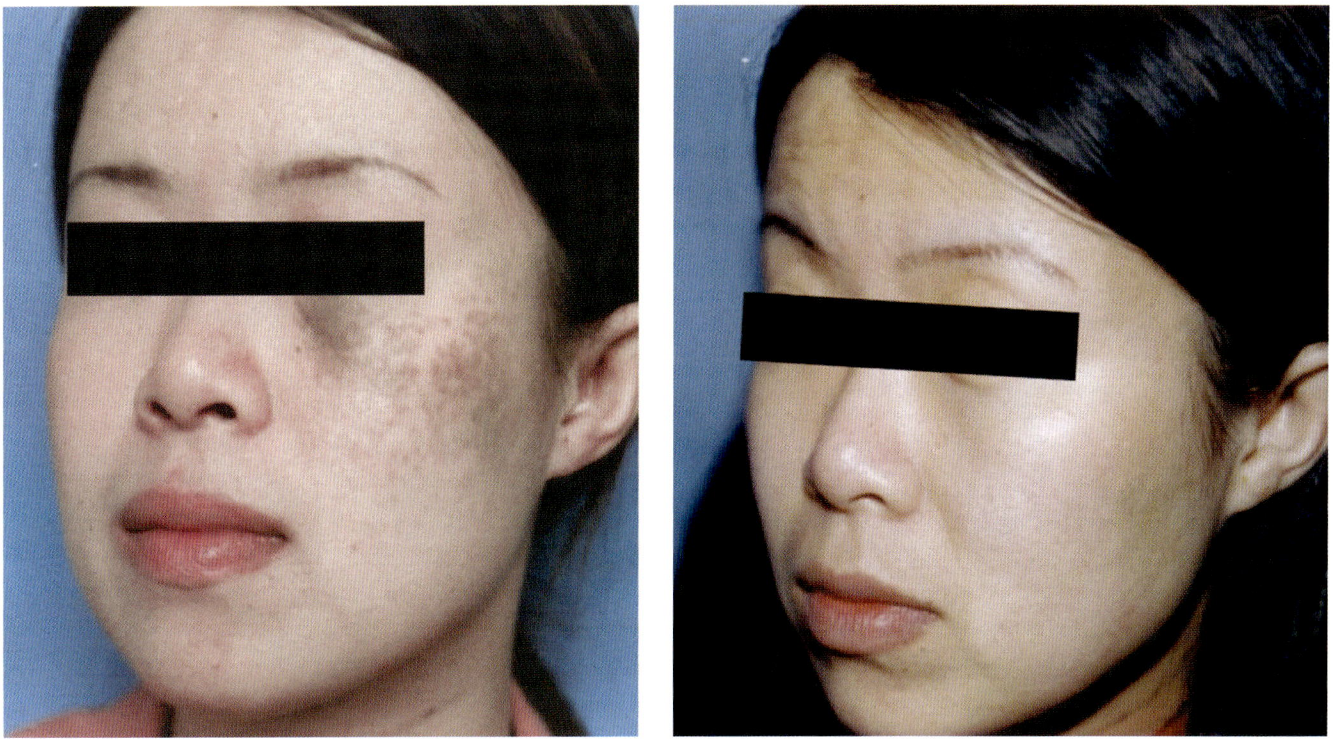

A B

FIGURE 27-13 Nevus of Ota (**A**) before and (**B**) after seven treatments with the QS 755-nm alexandrite laser. (Used with permission from H. Wang, MD.)

Melanocytic Nevi: Surgical excision is the standard of care for removal of benign melanocytic nevi. There are select cases in which a scar resulting from excision of a benign nevus may be undesirable or near a vital structure, and therefore, laser therapy may be considered. A biopsy should be considered prior to laser therapy to ensure the benign nature of a nevus, and those with a personal or family history of melanoma should not have their nevi treated with laser therapy. There is a theoretical concern that laser irradiation has the ability to promote malignant change, although this is controversial.

Junctional melanocytic nevi that are present in the epidermis and superficial dermis have been treated successfully with the QS ruby laser, QS alexandrite laser, and frequency-doubled QS Nd:YAG laser.[45] Congenital nevi often have melanocytes in the deep dermis and surrounding adnexae and do not respond consistently to QS lasers. Combining treatment with both the QS ruby laser and normal mode ruby laser has produced favorable results.[86] However, multiple treatments are often necessary, and the patient must be aware that dermal nevus cells often persist, so lifelong follow-up is necessary.[87] Ablative resurfacing lasers, such as the Er:YAG and the CO_2, may improve pigmentation,[88,89] although scarring may develop.[88]

Dermal Lesions

Dermal lesions, such as nevus of Ota, nevus of Ito, Hori nevus, and congenital dermal melanocytosis, often require treatment with lasers with longer wavelengths that have the ability to penetrate deeply into the dermis. A topical or intralesional anesthetic may be helpful. Dermal lesions may slowly improve over months as phagocytosis of the dermal pigment and gradual clearance occur.[8]

Nevus of Ota, Ito, and Hori: QS lasers, including the QS Nd:YAG, QS alexandrite, and the QS ruby, have been used to treat nevus of Ota, Ito, and Hori (**Figures 27-13 and 27-14**).[48,90-92] Although QS lasers are helpful, adverse events such as permanent hypopigmentation and textural changes can occur, and many lesions do not completely respond.[93] The picosecond alexandrite laser has recently been shown to be an effective therapy for nevus of Ota and is associated with a lower rate of PIH (**Figure 27-15**).[4,63]

POSTOPERATIVE CARE

After treatment with QS lasers, the treated site becomes darker and often develops a crust that lasts approximately 1 to 3 weeks. The areas should be cleansed gently daily with a mild soap and water, and an occlusive ointment should be applied regularly. Strict sun avoidance must be practiced. Immediate posttreatment pain is common and is often alleviated by ice packs and cold compresses. Urticaria may also be seen after treatment. Vesicles may develop after treatment of tattoos with QS lasers, although this is generally not seen after treatment of epidermal or dermal lesions.

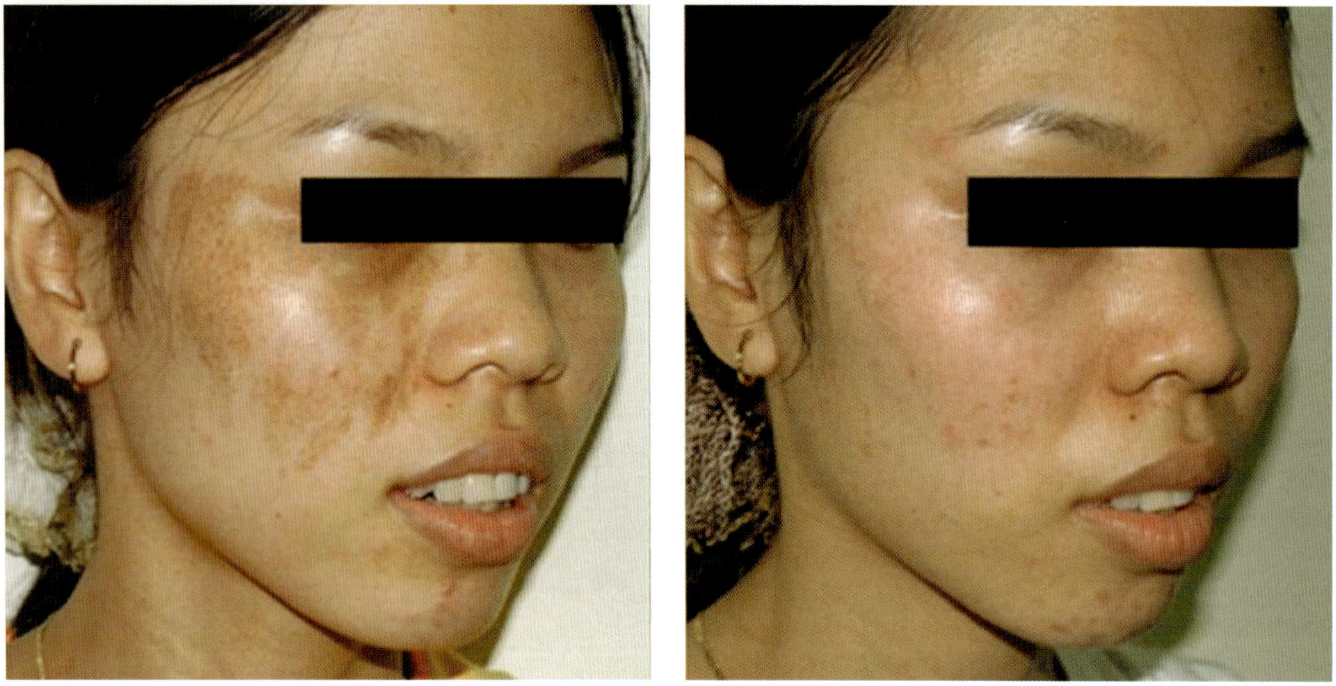

A B

FIGURE 27-14 Hori nevus (**A**) before and (**B**) after five treatments with the QS 1,064-nm Nd:YAG laser. (Used with permission from T. Tu, MD.)

Transient erythema, edema, and pain may be seen after treatment with picosecond lasers and should resolve within 1 week.

In patients treated with fractional lasers or IPL, erythema, edema, crusting, and peeling are expected. Use of sunscreens and moisturizers is usually sufficient. A sunburned sensation may develop, which can usually be controlled with cool compresses. As with QS lasers, initial darkening of pigmented lesions may occur.

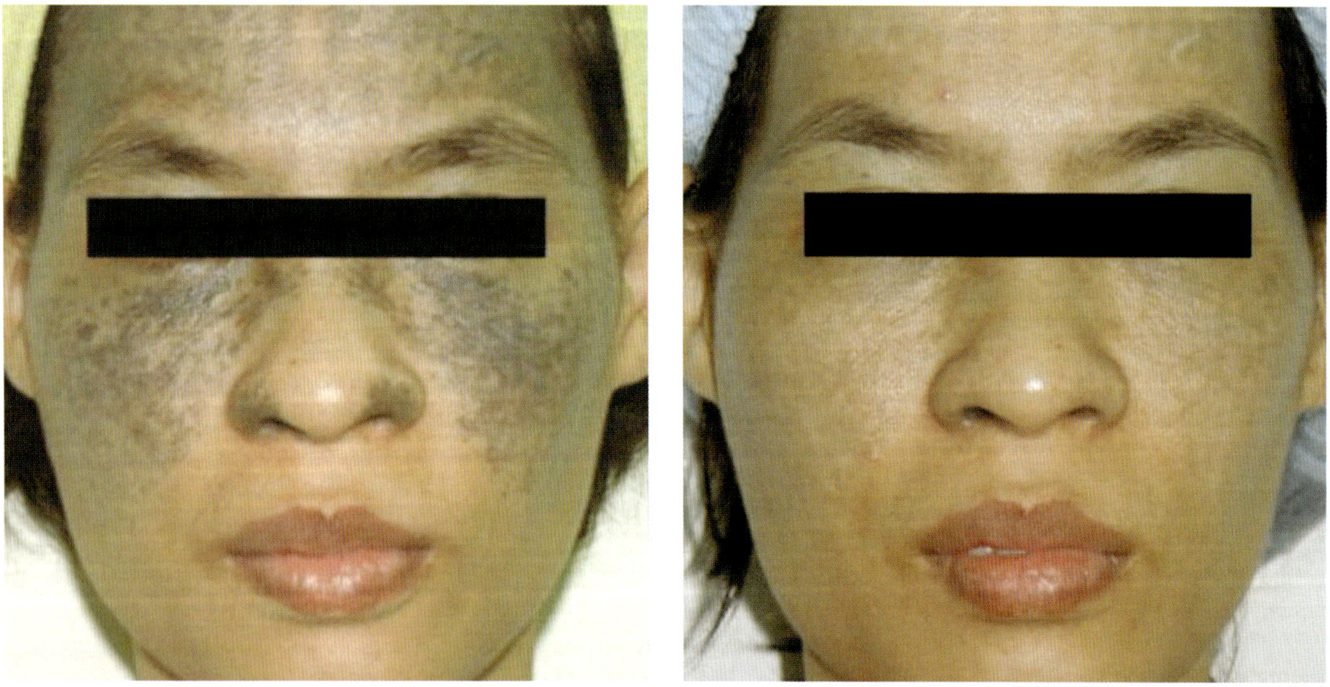

A B

FIGURE 27-15 Nevus of Ota (**A**) before and (**B**) after one treatment with the 755-nm alexandrite picosecond laser. (Used with permission from H. Chan, MD.)

CONCLUSIONS

As laser technology evolves and lasers become more selective, the removal of unwanted tattoos and pigmented lesions is becoming increasingly common. The clinician must be aware of nuances in laser therapy to ensure safe and effective treatments. Appropriate patient selection and strict adherence to protocols are crucial. Importantly, correct diagnosis of pigmented lesions is essential prior to initiation of laser therapy, as the clinician should always avoid treating a pigmented lesion with a laser when the diagnosis is not known definitively.

REFERENCES

1. Anderson RR, Parrish JA. Selective photothermolysis: precise microsurgery by selective absorption of pulsed radiation. *Science.* 1983;220:524-527.
2. Patil UA, Dhami LD. Overview of lasers. *Indian J Plast Surg.* 2008;41:S101-S113.
3. Sarnoff DS. Therapeutic update: using lasers for tattoo removal. *J Drugs Dermatol.* 2014;13:108-109.
4. Chan JC, Shek SY, Kono T, Yeung CK, Chan HH. A retrospective analysis on the management of pigmented lesions using a picosecond 755-nm alexandrite laser in Asians. *Lasers Surg Med.* 2016;48:23-29.
5. Saedi N, Metelitsa A, Petrell K, Arndt KA, Dover JS. Treatment of tattoos with a picosecond alexandrite laser: a prospective trial. *Arch Dermatol.* 2012;148:1360-1363.
6. Trafeli JP, Kwan JM, Meehan KJ, et al. Use of a long-pulse alexandrite laser in the treatment of superficial pigmented lesions. *Dermatol Surg.* 2007;33:1477-1482.
7. Hantash BM, Bedi VP, Sudireddy V, et al. Laser-induced transepidermal elimination of dermal content by fractional photothermolysis. *J Biomed Opt.* 2006;11:41115.
8. Pritzker R, Iyengar V, Rohrer T, Arndt K. Laser treatment of tattoos and pigmented lesions. In: *Surgery of the Skin.* New York, NY: Elsevier; 2015:524-535.
9. Trotter MJ, Tron VA, Hollingdale J, Rivers JK. Localized chrysiasis induced by laser therapy. *Arch Dermatol.* 1995;131:1411-1414.
10. Katz BE, Mac Farlane DF. Atypical facial scarring after isotretinoin therapy in a patient with previous dermabrasion. *J Am Acad Dermatol.* 1994;30:852-853.
11. Bernestein LJ, Geronemus RG. Keloid formation with the 585-nm pulsed dye laser during isotretinoin treatment. *Arch Dermatol.* 1997;133:111-112.
12. Kim HW, Chang SE, Kim JE, Ko JY, Ro YS. The safe delivery of fractional ablative carbon dioxide laser treatment for acne scars in Asian patients receiving oral isotretinoin. *Dermatol Surg.* 2014;40:1361-1366.
13. Yoon JH, Park EJ, Kwon IH, et al. Concomitant use of an infrared fractional laser with low-dose isotretinoin for the treatment of acne and acne scars. *J Dermatol Treat.* 2014;25:142-146.
14. Khatri KA. Diode laser hair removal in patients undergoing isotretinoin therapy. *Dermatol Surg.* 2004;30:1205-1207; discussion 1207.
15. Shah S, Alster TS. Laser treatment of dark skin: an updated review. *Am J Clin Dermatol.* 2010;11:389-397.
16. Alexis AF. Lasers and light-based therapies in ethnic skin: treatment options and recommendations for Fitzpatrick skin types V and VI. *Br J Dermatol.* 2013;169(Suppl 3):91-97.
17. Luebberding S, Alexiades-Armenakas M. New tattoo approaches in dermatology. *Dermatol Clin.* 32:2014;91-96.
18. Anderson RR, Margolis RJ, Watenabe S, Flotte T, Hruza GJ, Dover JS. Selective photothermolysis of cutaneous pigmentation by Q-switched Nd: YAG laser pulses at 1064, 532, and 355 nm. *J Invest Dermatol.* 1989;93:28-32.
19. Kent KM, Graber EM. Laser tattoo removal: a review. *Dermatol Surg.* 2012;38:1-13.
20. Kirby W, Chen CL, Desai A, Desai T. Causes and recommendations for unanticipated ink retention following tattoo removal treatment. *J Clin Aesthet Dermatol.* 2013;6:27-31.
21. Leuenberger ML, Mulas MW, Hata TR, Goldman MP, Fitzpatrick RE, Grevelink JM. Comparison of the Q-switched alexandrite, Nd:YAG, and ruby lasers in treating blue-black tattoos. *Dermatol Surg* 1999;25:10-14.
22. Kilmer SL, Anderson RR. Clinical use of the Q-switched ruby and the Q-switched Nd:YAG (1064 nm and 532 nm) lasers for treatment of tattoos. *J Dermatol Surg Oncol.* 1993;19:330-338.
23. Jones A, Roddey P, Orengo I, Rosen T. The Q-switched ND:YAG laser effectively treats tattoos in darkly pigmented skin. *Dermatol Surg.* 1993;22:999-1001.
24. Goyal S, Arndt KA, Stern RS, O'Hare D, Dover JS. Laser treatment of tattoos: a prospective, paired, comparison study of the Q-switched Nd:YAG (1064 nm), frequency-doubled Q-switched Nd:YAG (532 nm), and Q-switched ruby lasers. *J Am Acad Dermatol.* 1997;36:122-125.
25. Zelickson BD, Mehregan DA, Zarrin AA. Clinical, histologic, and ultrastructural evaluation of tattoos treated with three laser systems. *Lasers Surg Med.* 1997;15:364-372.
26. Guedes R, Leite L. Removal of orange eyebrow tattoo in a single session with the Q-switched Nd:YAG 532nm laser. *Lasers Med Sci.* 2010;25:465-466.
27. Alster TS. Q-switched alexandrite laser treatment (755 nm) of professional and amateur tattoos. *J Am Acad Dermatol.* 1995;33:69-73.
28. Weiss ET, Geronemus RG. Combining fractional resurfacing and Q-switched ruby laser for tattoo removal. *Dermatol Surg.* 2011;37:97-99.
29. Ricotti CA, Colaco SM, Shamma HN, Trevino J, Palmer G, Heaphy MR Jr. Laser-assisted tattoo removal with topical 5% imiquimod cream. *Dermatol Surg.* 2007;33:1082-1091.
30. Kossida T, Rigopoulos D, Katsambas A, Anderson RR. Optimal tattoo removal in a single laser session based on the method of repeated exposures. *J Am Acad Dermatol.* 2012;66:271-277.
31. Reddy KK, Brauer JA, Anolik R, et al. Topical perfluorodecalin resolves immediate whitening reactions and allows rapid effective multiple pass treatment of tattoos. *Lasers Surg Med.* 2013;45:76-80.
32. Ross V, Naseef G, Lin G, et al. Comparison of responses of tattoos to picosecond and nanosecond Q-switched neodymium: YAG lasers. *Arch Dermatol.* 1998;134:167-171.
33. Brauer JA, Reddy KK, Anolik R, et al. Successful and rapid treatment of blue and green tattoo pigment with a novel picosecond laser. *Arch Dermatol.* 2012;148:820-823.

34. Alabdulrazzaq H, Brauer JA, Bae YS, Geronemus RG. Clearance of yellow tattoo ink with a novel 532-nm picosecond laser. *Lasers Surg Med.* 2015;47:285-288.

35. Kirby W, Desai A, Desai T, Kartono F, Geeta P. The Kirby-Desai scale: a proposed scale to assess tattoo-removal treatments. *J Clin Aesthet Dermatol.* 2009;2:32-37.

36. Mariwalla K, Hurza G. *Lasers and Lights: Procedures in Cosmetic Dermatology.* New York, NY: Elsevier; 2013.

37. Fitzpatrick RE, Goldman MP. Tattoo removal using the alexandrite laser. *Arch Dermatol.* 1994;130:1508-1514.

38. Ross EV, Yashar S, Michaud N, et al. Tattoo darkening and nonresponse after laser treatment: a possible role for titanium dioxide. *Arch Dermatol.* 2001;137:33-37.

39. Anderson RR, Geronemus R, Kilmer SL, Farinelli W, Fitzpatrick RE. Cosmetic tattoo ink darkening. A complication of Q-switched and pulsed-laser treatment. *Arch Dermatol.* 1993;129:1010-1014.

40. Mafong EA, Kauvar AN, Geronemus RG. Surgical pearl: removal of cosmetic lip-liner tattoo with the pulsed carbon dioxide laser. *J Am Acad Dermatol.* 2003;48:271-272.

41. Ashinoff R, Levine VJ, Soter NA. Allergic reactions to tattoo pigment after laser treatment. *Dermatol Surg.* 1995;21:291-294.

42. Antony FC, Harland CC. Red ink tattoo reactions: successful treatment with the Q-switched 532 nm Nd:YAG laser. *Br J Dermatol.* 2003;149:94-98.

43. De Argila D, Chaves A, Moreno JC. Erbium:Yag laser therapy of lichenoid red tattoo reaction. *J Eur Acad Dermatol Venereol.* 2004;18:332-333.

44. Ibrahimi OA, Syed Z, Sakamoto FH, Avram MM, Anderson RR. Treatment of tattoo allergy with ablative fractional resurfacing: a novel paradigm for tattoo removal. *J Am Acad Dermatol.* 2011;64:1111-1114.

45. Polder KD, Landau JM, Vergilis-Kalner IJ, et al. Laser eradication of pigmented lesions: a review. *Dermatol Surg.* 2011;37:572-595.

46. Rashid T, Hussain I, Haider M, Haroon TS. Laser therapy of freckles and lentigines with quasi-continuous, frequency-doubled, Nd:YAG (532 nm) laser in Fitzpatrick skin type IV: a 24-month follow-up. *J Cosmet Laser Ther.* 2002;4:81-85.

47. Sadighha A, Saatee S, Muhaghegh-Zahed G. Efficacy and adverse effects of Q-switched ruby laser on solar lentigines: a prospective study of 91 patients with Fitzpatrick skin type II, III, and IV. *Dermatol Surg.* 2008;34:1465-1468.

48. Kagami S, Asahina A, Watanabe R, et al. Treatment of 153 Japanese patients with Q-switched alexandrite laser. *Lasers Med Sci.* 2007;22:159-163.

49. Jang KA, Chung EC, Choi JH, et al. Successful removal of freckles in Asian skin with a Q switched alexandrite laser. *Dermatol Surg.* 2000;26:231-234.

50. Redbord KP, Hanke CW. Case reports: clearance of lentigines in Japanese men with the long-pulsed alexandrite laser. *J Drugs Dermatol.* 2007;6:653-656.

51. Manstein D, Herron GS, Sink RK, Tanner H, Anderson RR. Fractional photothermolysis: a new concept for cutaneous remodeling using microscopic patterns of thermal injury. *Lasers Surg Med.* 2004;34:426-438.

52. Wanner M, Tanzi EL, Alster TS. Fractional photothermolysis: treatment of facial and nonfacial cutaneous photodamage with a 1,550-nm erbium-doped fiber laser. *Dermatol Surg.* 2007;33:23-28.

53. Sherling M, Friedman PM, Adrian R, et al. Consensus recommendations on the use of an erbium-doped 1,550nm fractionated laser and its applications in dermatologic laser surgery. *Dermatol Surg.* 2010;36:461-469.

54. Polder KD, Harrison A, Eubanks LE, Bruce S. 1,927 nm fractional thulium fiber laser for the treatment of nonfacial photodamage: a pilot study. *Dermatol Surg.* 2011;37:342-348.

55. Brauer JA, McDaniel DH, Bloom BS, et al. Nonablative 1927 nm fractional resurfacing for the treatment of facial photopigmentation. *J Drugs Dermatol.* 2014;13:1317-1322.

56. Polder KD, Mithani A, Harrison A, Bruce S. Treatment of macular seborrheic keratoses using a novel 1927-nm fractional thulium fiber laser. *Dermatol Surg.* 2012;38:1025-1031.

57. Wang CC, Sue YM, Yang CH, Chen CK. A comparison of Q-switched alexandrite laser and intense pulsed light for the treatment of freckles and lentigines in Asian persons: a randomized, physician-blinded, split-face comparative trial. *J Am Acad Dermatol.* 2006;54:804-810.

58. Kawada A, Shiraishi H, Asai M, et al. Clinical improvement of solar lentigines and ephelides with an intense pulsed light source. *Dermatol Surg.* 2002;28:504-508.

59. Khetarpal S, Desai S, Kruter L, et al. Picosecond laser with specialized optic for facial rejuvenation using a compressed treatment interval. *Lasers Surg Med.* 2016;48(8):723-726.

60. Tse Y, Levine VJ, McClain SA, Ashinoff R The removal of cutaneous pigmented lesions with the Q-switched ruby laser and the Q-switched neodymium: yttrium- aluminum-garnet laser. A comparative study. *J Dermatol Surg Oncol.* 1994;20:795-800.

61. Grevelink JM, González S, Bonoan R, Vibhagool C, Gonzalez E. Treatment of nevus spilus with the Q-switched ruby laser. *Dermatol Surg.* 1997;23:365-369; discussion 369-370.

62. Moreno-Arias GA, Bulla F, Vilata-Corell JJ, CampsFresneda A Treatment of widespread segmental nevus spilus by Q-switched alexandrite laser (755 nm, 100 nsec). *Dermatol Surg.* 2001;27:841-843.

63. Levin MK, Ng E, Bae YS, Brauer JA, Geronemus RG. Treatment of pigmentary disorders in patients with skin of color with a novel 755 nm picosecond, Q-switched ruby, and Q-switched Nd:YAG nanosecond lasers: a retrospective photographic review. *Lasers Surg Med.* 2016;48:181-187.

64. Kim S, Cho K. Treatment of procedure-related postinflammatory hyperpigmentation using 1064-nm Q-switched Nd:YAG laser with low fluence in Asian patients: report of five cases. *J Cosmet Dermatol.* 2010;9:302-306.

65. Kim S, Cho K. Treatment of facial postinflammatory hyperpigmentation with facial acne in Asian patients using a Q-switched neodymium-doped yttrium aluminum garnet laser. *Dermatol Surg.* 2010;36:1374-1380.

66. Katz TM, Goldberg LH, Firoz BF, Friedman PM. Fractional photothermolysis for the treatment of postinflammatory hyperpigmentation. *Dermatol Surg.* 2009;35:1844-1848.

67. Rokhsar CK, Ciocon DH. Fractional photothermolysis for the treatment of postinflammatory hyperpigmentation after carbon dioxide laser resurfacing. *Dermatol Surg.* 2009;35:535-537.

68. Grimes PE. Etiologic and therapeutic considerations. *Arch Dermatol.* 1995;131:1453-1457.

69. Yoshimura K, Sato K, Aiba-Kojima E, et al. Repeated treatment protocols for melasma and acquired dermal melanocytosis. *Dermatol Surg.* 2006;32:365-371.

70. Suh KS, Sung JY, Roh HJ, Jeon YS, Kim YC, Kim ST. Efficacy of the 1064-nm Q-switched Nd:YAG laser in melasma. *J Dermatol Treat.* 2011;22:233-238.
71. Angsuwarangsee S, Polnikorn N. Combined ultrapulse CO2 laser and Q-switched alexandrite laser compared with Q-switched alexandrite laser alone for refractory melasma: split-face design. *Dermatol Surg.* 2003;29:59-64.
72. Trelles MA, Velez M, Gold MH. The treatment of melasma with topical creams alone, CO2 fractional ablative resurfacing alone, or a combination of the two: a comparative study. *J Drugs Dermatol.* 2010;9:315-322.
73. Lee HS, Won CH, Lee DH, et al. Treatment of melasma in Asian skin using a fractional 1,550-nm laser: an open clinical study. *Dermatol Surg.* 2009;35:1499-1504.
74. Rokhsar CK, Fitzpatrick RE. The treatment of melasma with fractional photothermolysis: a pilot study. *Dermatol Surg.* 2005;31:1645-1650.
75. Kauvar AN. Successful treatment of melasma using a combination of microdermabrasion and Q-switched Nd:YAG lasers. *Lasers Surg Med.* 2012;44:117-124.
76. Gokalp H, Akkaya AD, Oram Y. Long-term results in low-fluence 1064-nm Q-Switched Nd:YAG laser for melasma: is it effective? *J Cosmet Dermatol.* 2016;15(4): 420-426.
77. Wong Y, Lee SS, Goh CL. Hypopigmentation induced by frequent low-fluence, large-spot-size QS Nd:YAG laser treatments. *Ann Dermatol.* 2015;27:751-755.
78. Massaki N, Eimpunth S, Fabi SG, et al. Treatment of melasma with the 1,927-nm fractional thulium fiber laser: a retrospective analysis of 20 cases with long-term follow-up. *Lasers Surg Med.* 2013;45:95-101.
79. Lee HM, Haw S, Kim JK, Chang SE, Lee MW. Split-face study using a 1,927-nm thulium fiber fractional laser to treat photoaging and melasma in Asian skin. *Dermatol Surg.* 2013;39:879-888.
80. Momen S, Mallipeddi R, Al-Niaimi F. The use of lasers in Becker's naevus: an evidence-based review. *J Cosmet Laser Ther.* 2016;18:188-192.
81. Trelles MA, Allones I, Moreno-Arias GA, Vélez M. Becker's naevus: a comparative study between erbium: YAG and Q-switched neodymium:YAG; clinical and histopathological findings. *Br J Dermatol.* 2005;152:308-313.
82. Meesters AA, Wind BS, Kroon MW, et al. Ablative fractional laser therapy as treatment for Becker nevus: a randomized controlled pilot study. *J Am Acad Dermatol.* 2011;65:1173-1179.
83. Glaich AS, Goldberg LH, Dai T, Kunishige JH, Friedman PM. Fractional resurfacing: a new therapeutic modality for Becker's nevus. *Arch Dermatol.* 2007;143:1488-1490.
84. Nanni CA, Alster TS. Treatment of a Becker's nevus using a 694-nm long-pulsed ruby laser. *Dermatol Surg.* 1998;24:1032-1034.
85. Choi JE, Kim JW, Seo SH, et al. Treatment of Becker's nevi with a long-pulse alexandrite laser. *Dermatol Surg.* 2009;35:1105-1108.
86. Kono T, Erçöçen AR, Chan HHL, Kikuchi Y, Nozaki M. Effectiveness of the normal-mode ruby laser and the combined (normal-mode plus q-switched) ruby laser in the treatment of congenital melanocytic nevi: a comparative study. *Ann Plast Surg.* 2002;49:476-485.
87. Bray FN, Shah V, Nouri K. Laser treatment of congenital melanocytic nevi: a review of the literature. *Lasers Med Sci.* 2016;31:197-204.
88. Horner BM, El-Muttardi NS, Mayou BJ. Treatment of congenital melanocytic naevi with CO_2 laser. *Ann Plast Surg.* 2005;55:276-280.
89. Ostertag JU, Quaedvlieg PJ, Kerckhoffs FE, et al. Congenital naevi treated with erbium:YAG laser (Derma K) resurfacing in neonates: clinical results and review of the literature. *Br J Dermatol.* 2006;154:889-895.
90. Taylor CR, Flotte TJ, Gange RW, Anderson RR. Treatment of nevus of Ota by Q-switched ruby laser. *J Am Acad Dermatol.* 1994;30:743-751.
91. Lam AY, Wong DS, Lam LK, Ho WS, Chan HH. A retrospective study on the efficacy and complications of Q-switched alexandrite laser in the treatment of acquired bilateral nevus of Ota-like macules. *Dermatol Surg.* 2001;27:937-941.
92. Polnikorn N, Tanrattanakorn S, Goldberg DJ. Treatment of Hori's nevus with the Q-switched Nd:YAG laser. *Dermatol Surg.* 2000;26:477-480.
93. Shah VV, Bray FN, Aldahan AS, Mlacker S, Nouri K. Lasers and nevus of Ota: a comprehensive review. *Lasers Med Sci.* 2016;31:179-185.

28 Lasers for Erythema and Telangiectasias

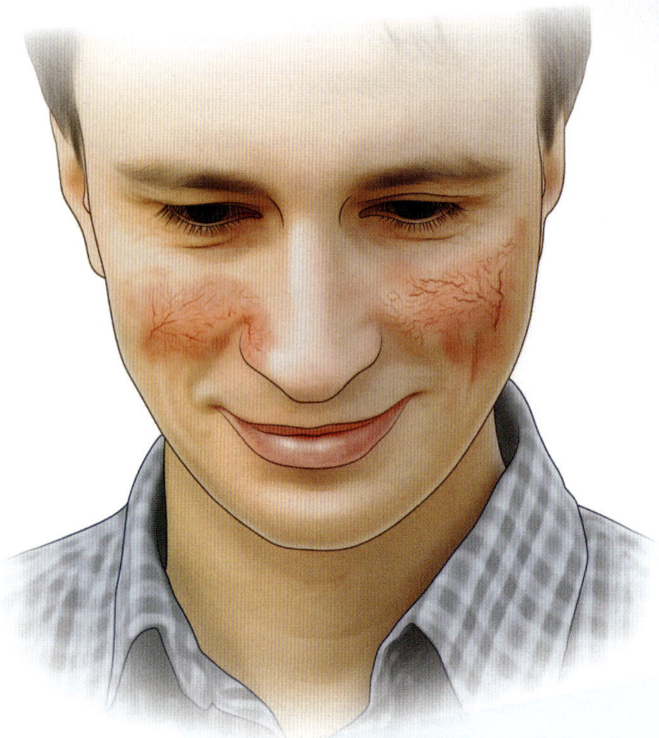

SUMMARY

- Erythema and telangiectasias are a common patient complaint.
- The mainstay of therapy is laser and IPL treatments; IPL confers the advantage of larger spot sizes, and thus more efficient treatments.
- Patients should always understand that multiple treatments will be needed, and maintenance therapy is generally required.

Beginner Tips

- Regardless of the device chosen, a slight amount of overlap of pulses is necessary to achieve uniform improvement of the treated area.
- KTP causes more swelling and bruising compared to PDL and IPL.
- PDL is safer than KTP in those with darker skin types given increased depth of penetration.
- Do not use IPL on those with tanned or sunburned skin.
- There should be approximately 10% overlap with IPL to avoid a "stamping" appearance following treatment..

Don't Forget!

- The neck has a thinner epidermis and dermis compared to the chest and back, so typically gentler settings should be used.
- It is important to become familiar with the device you choose to use. Devices of the same wavelength do not necessarily have interchangeable settings, and the time to development of erythema or purpura following a single pulse varies between devices. Also, service of the laser (such as replacement of a dye kit) may influence the performance and actual energy delivered.

Expert Tips

- Telangiectasias of the nose can be very treatment resistant; recurrence rates are quite high, necessitating maintenance treatments.
- In many patients, it can be difficult to permanently eliminate alar telangiectasias altogether; caution patients from the outset that maintenance treatments are often necessary.

Pitfalls and Cautions

- Do not pulse stack with a 1,064-nm laser, which increases the risk for scarring.
- 1,064 nm has the greatest risk for causing retinal damage because of its deep penetration, so caution should be exercised near the eye with appropriate shielding.
- Many laser experts avoid 1,064-nm laser treatments on the nasal ala due to an increased risk for depressed scarring.

Lasers for Erythema and Telangiectasias

28

INTRODUCTION

Prominent erythema and telangiectasia of the face, neck, and chest are frequent complaints and reasons for presentation to the cosmetic office. The most common etiologies of these signs are rosacea and photodamage, with less common reasons being medication use, connective tissue diseases, and genetic disorders, such as hereditary hemorrhagic telangiectasia syndrome. Sun exposure damages and weakens collagen and elastin and, with cumulative exposure, results in vascular ectasias and physical signs of erythema and telangiectasias.

Ultraviolet photodamage is believed to contribute to the development of rosacea. Rosacea symptoms typically include frequent flushing associated with facial erythema, telangiectasias, papules, and pustules. Patients with CREST (calcinosis, Raynaud phenomenon, esophageal dysmotility, sclerodactyly, and telangiectasia) often present with what are classically referred to as matlike telangiectasias. These are most prominent on the face, neck, and hands.

Connective tissue disease and other systemic illnesses may cause facial erythema and telangiectasias; patients with polycythemia vera have been referred in the past for laser treatments. Medications that can cause erythema include niacin (rather than nicotinamide), calcium channel blockers, cyclosporine, rifampin, vasodilators such as nitroglycerin, and others. It is also important to keep in mind that topical and intralesional steroids can cause telangiectasias and erythema. Intrinsic aging of the skin causes collagen breakdown and visible telangiectasias. Lastly, repeated trauma to the face will also induce localized erythema and ultimately vascular dilation. Telangiectasias frequently develop in and around surgical scars, particularly those that are under tension.

Currently the most effective treatment of erythema and telangiectasias is using lasers and intense pulsed light (IPL); however, other therapies play a role as well. Patients with erythema and telangiectasias should be instructed on a gentle skin care routine of using lukewarm water, mild cleansers, and moisturizers. Prescription topical agents for erythematotelangiectatic rosacea include metronidazole gel, lotion, and cream; azelaic acid foam and gel; and ivermectin cream. Although the former agents are more effective for papulopustular rosacea than erythema and flushing, topical agents may be included as adjunctive anti-inflammatory approaches for rosacea patients.

Brimonidine gel (Mirvaso; Galderma, Lausanne, Switzerland) is an α_2-adrenergic agonist that causes vasoconstriction and can be used for erythema of varying etiologies. When this agent was initially on the market, there was much enthusiasm for its potential efficacy, although in clinical practice, marked rebound erythema has occurred with cessation of use, even after 1 to 2 days of application; such rebound erythema may extend to areas beyond the area of direct application. Because of these side effects, the popularity of brimonidine has declined. Results of studies on topical oxymetazoline are currently under review by the US Food and Drug Administration.

Cosmeceuticals may be used to reduce erythema and telangiectasias.[1] Topical and oral nicotinamide, green tea, feverfew, and licorice root have been used to treat erythema, though there is little high-quality research in this area.

Historically, electrocautery was used to treat telangiectasias. This has fallen out of favor given the damage to the epidermis when trying to reach underlying vessels and the risk of resultant scarring. In addition, although the immediate response to cautery appears successful, recurrence is common.

BACKGROUND

Laser treatment of erythema and telangiectasias is based on the theory of selective photothermolysis: the chosen wavelength of light should correspond to the absorption peak of the target structure, and the pulse duration should be equal to or less than the thermal relaxation time of the target structure. This principle dictates that selective destruction of the target takes place with minimal damage to surrounding structures.

For erythema and telangiectasias, the target structure is usually oxyhemoglobin within the vessels, as this composes the majority of total hemoglobin. To understand the best wavelengths to treat superficial red vessels, one must know that oxyhemoglobin's primary absorption peaks are in the blue-yellow-green portion of the visible light range (418, 545, and 577 nm); the lowest wavelength peak of 418 nm is strongly absorbed by melanin, however, and therefore should not be used for vascular lasers (**Figure 28-1**). Even light with wavelengths at the peak of 542 nm will have too much absorption by melanin and therefore fail to be photoselective for hemoglobin, resulting in probable epidermal damage, unless cooling is used to protect the epidermis.

The fourth broadband hemoglobin absorption peak from 700 to 1100 nm becomes more important when targeting deeply seated vessels. In general, longer wavelengths penetrate more deeply into the skin with less scattering of photons and greater penetration to a deeper target. Not only do longer wavelengths penetrate more deeply, but they also heat the target more uniformly.

The pulse duration is determined by the thermal relaxation time; larger-diameter telangiectasias require a longer pulse duration to allow sufficient time for diffusion of heat evenly throughout the cylindrical vessel (**Table 28-1**). Shorter pulse durations may be needed for smaller vessels but can result in excessive heat and vessel rupture and thus increased risk for purpura. In general,

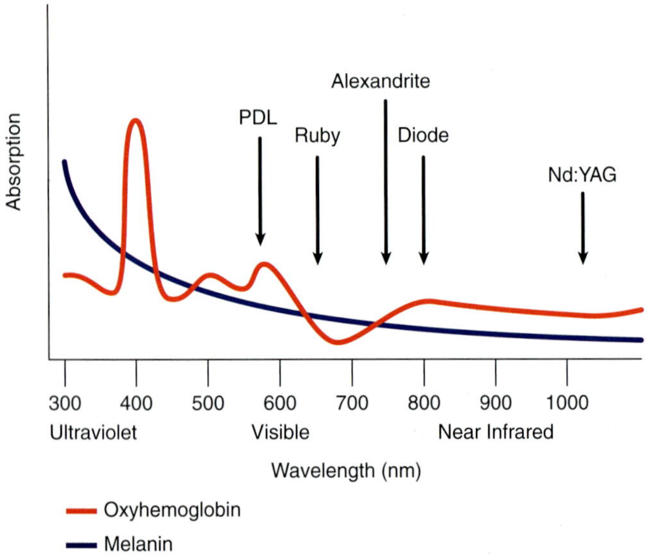

FIGURE 28-1 Absorption peaks for oxyhemoglobin and deoxyhemoglobin and relevant lasers.

longer pulse durations of at least 6 ms (and up to 40 ms) are used for telangiectasias to decrease risk for purpura. Larger spot sizes result in less scattering and deeper penetration.

While delivering a sufficient quantity of energy to thermocoagulate the target vessel, the overlying epidermis should be unharmed. This requires minimization of absorption by melanin and some mode of protective epidermal cooling. A number of different laser and IPL systems have been developed with this goal in mind. Cooling may be applied by direct contact, cold gel, cold air blowing, or spray cryogen. Cooling may also be applied before, after, or continuously during the laser pulse. In patients with higher Fitzpatrick skin types, there is a risk of depigmentation, hypopigmentation, and postinflammatory hyperpigmentation with cryogen spray if excessive. Contact cooling can be achieved via sapphire crystal, quartz, or copper. Sapphire crystal maintains cold temperatures better than the others. With contact cooling, it is important to maintain proper contact with the skin; otherwise, the risk of epidermal damage increases. Fluence needs to be adjusted on the basis of baseline vessel temperature; the colder the vessel from prechilling, the higher the fluence required.

Table 28-2 lists the most commonly used lasers to treat erythema and telangiectasias. Pulsed dye, potassium titanyl phosphate (KTP), alexandrite, neodymium:yttrium-aluminum-garnet (Nd:YAG), and infrared diode lasers, as well as IPL devices, are typically used. There are several caveats when considering a laser of choice. KTP laser is actually a laser beam generated by an Nd:YAG laser, which is then directed through a KTP crystal to produce a coherent light in the visible green portion of the spectrum. The 532-nm wavelength is one of several hemoglobin absorption peaks. Absorption of melanin is significant, and thus KTP lasers are not recommended for those with Fitzpatrick skin types greater than III or patients who are significantly tanned.

Pulsed dye laser (PDL) produces light in the yellow spectrum and has less absorption by melanin. The alexandrite laser is significantly absorbed by epidermal melanin and so is best for patients with lower Fitzpatrick skin types. Because the 1064-nm wavelength's interaction with melanin is much less than that of other laser wavelengths used for hemoglobin, its use allows treatment of skin types up to Fitzpatrick V, something not possible with other wavelengths. Because the Nd:YAG laser heats water within the epidermis and dermis, there is a higher risk of overheating the skin with possible resultant epidermal/dermal injury and eventual hypopigmentation, depigmentation, atrophy, and scarring. Therefore, the smallest spot size and lowest energy should be initiated when using this wavelength. In addition, clinical end points, such as blurring of vessels, can be less clearly visible, so there is a risk of overtreatment and thus increased risk of side effects. Lastly, diode lasers have varying wavelengths in the infrared region, which pick up the fourth peak of hemoglobin, but are infrequently used to treat vascular lesions because there is a risk of epidermal damage. Historically, they were used more often, but with the advent of lasers specific for hemoglobin, their use has declined.

An IPL device consists of a noncoherent flashlamp that delivers controlled amounts of yellow, red, and infrared wavelengths to the skin. Theoretically, a device that produces a noncoherent

TABLE 28-1 • Thermal Relaxation Times According to Vessel Diameter

Diameter (μm)	Thermal Relaxation Time (ms)
10	0.048
20	0.19
50	1.2
100	4.8
200	19.0
300	42.6

TABLE 28-2 • Commonly Used Lasers and Energy Devices for Erythema and Telangiectasias

Laser or Energy Device	Wavelength (nm)
Pulsed dye laser (PDL)	595
Potassium titanyl phosphate (KTP)	532
Intense pulsed light (IPL)	Varying and multiple
Alexandrite	755
Neodymium:yytrium-aluminum garnet (Nd:YAG)	1064
Diode	Infrared wavelengths, ie, 800, 810, 900, 940, 980

TABLE 28-3 • Principles of Laser Treatment for Telangiectasias and Erythema

Smaller, superficial, bright red vessels need shorter wavelengths of green or yellow	■ Green: 532 nm (KTP) ■ Yellow: 585-595 nm (PDL) ■ Multiple (IPL): 500-670, 870-1200 nm
Deeper blood vessels require longer wavelengths of infrared	■ Alexandrite: 755 nm ■ Diode: 800-980 nm ■ Nd:YAG: 1064 nm
Other points	■ Larger blood vessels need longer pulse durations ■ Spot size diameter should be double the size of target vessel ■ Pigmented skin will be damaged by visible light wavelengths ■ Skin types greater than type III should only be treated by infrared wavelengths

light as a continuous spectrum longer than 550 nm should have multiple advantages over a single-wavelength laser system. First, both oxygenated and deoxygenated hemoglobin should simultaneously absorb at these wavelengths. Second, larger blood vessels should be affected more than with a single wavelength. Third, thermal absorption by the exposed blood vessels should occur with less overlying epidermal absorption, as the longer wavelengths will penetrate deeper. Other advantages of this device are large spot sizes and the ability to control pulse duration and the length of the intervals between pulses, the latter of which is only possible with certain devices.

For IPL treatment of erythema and telangiectasias, shorter cutoff wavelength filters should be chosen; the value on the filter designates the shortest wavelength within it. Multiple filters may be employed to gain more selectivity, and notched filters are also now available with select systems. IPL devices satisfy the criteria for selective photothermolysis, permitting blood vessels to be selectively heated over the surrounding tissue. Pulses are typically separated to allow thermal relaxation time and cooling of the epidermis in between pulses. Modern IPL units include contact cooling and sapphire crystals to protect the skin.

The principles of laser treatment of erythema and telangiectasias are outlined in **Table 28-3**. Lasers should be analyzed in terms of the color of light they produce.

DISCUSSION

Telangiectasias

For the treatment of telangiectasias of the face, including the nose, the most commonly used lasers are PDL and KTP, as these are specific for targeting intravascular oxyhemoglobin. The pulse duration should reflect the size of the vessel; the smaller the diameter of the telangiectasia, the shorter is the pulse duration. The VBeam Perfecta (Syneron-Candela, Irvine, CA), a PDL, has a spot size of 3 × 10 mm, which is useful for treating the linear shape of telangiectasias, although a 10- or 7-mm spot size can be used as well, particularly when treating telangiectatic matting. Cooling is achieved by a patented dynamic cryogen spray cooling just before the laser pulse. The pulse durations, longer than with the original PDL, can extend from 10 to 40 ms, which allows treatment of facial vessels with less purpura. Treatment results can be enhanced by partial overlapping of pulses and pulse stacking, as appropriate.

The KTP 532-nm laser is also very effective.[2] A comparative study of 532-nm versus 595-nm laser for treatment of telangiectasias and erythema demonstrated that the KTP is slightly more effective than PDL, although it is also associated with more swelling and redness.[3] After one treatment, the KTP achieved 62% clearing versus 49% with the PDL. In the study, the settings for the PDL (Candela) were 10 mm, 7.5 J/cm^2, and 10 ms, and those for the KTP (from Laserscope, now Cutera), were 5 to 10 mm, 9 to 10 J/cm^2, and 10 to 23 ms.

With regard to energy settings, it is best to start at the lower range of recommended energy settings that are programmed into the lasers and increase as needed, because the preset parameters were established by company-sponsored clinical evaluations. The end point is constriction of the vessel or a brief purplish to grayish color of the vessel. Settings with the Excel V (Cutera) range from 5 to 7 mm, 8.6 to 9 J/cm^2, and 8 to 10 ms, with contact cooling.

The alexandrite and diode are infrequently used for treatment of telangiectasias. At 755 nm, the alexandrite laser demonstrated strong absorption by melanin, explaining its infrequent use; while it is beneficial for the treatment of larger and deeply placed telangiectasias, it can only be used in those with lower Fitzpatrick skin types. Ross et al[4] published a study using a 755-nm laser for treatment of facial telangiectasias in 19 patients with Fitzpatrick skin types I and II; a 6-mm spot size was used with a mean fluence of 88 J/cm^2 and pulse durations ranging from 20 to 80 ms. After one treatment, there was 48% clearance of vessels; of note, one patient developed a scar, demonstrating that this risk exists with these lasers. The diode laser has a similar risk for epidermal damage. Tierney et al[5] compared a 532-nm to a 940-nm diode for treatment of facial telangiectasias. They found similar efficacy in resolution of small telangiectasias, but the diode was better for larger-diameter telangiectasias.

IPL can be used for treating telangiectasias and is often the treatment of choice when larger areas need to be treated on the face, neck, or chest due to larger available spot sizes. Equivalent efficacy to the PDL has been demonstrated.[6] Purpura is uncommon, and when it does occur, it typically fades quickly. A similar end point of vessel constriction and mild to moderate erythema should be achieved; there should not be a gray "footprint" of the IPL crystal, as that indicates epidermal injury. IPL device choice is based in part on the spot size; some devices, such as the Starlux Icon Max G or Y (Cynosure, Westford, MA), have large spots sizes (4.5 × 1 cm and 1.5 × 1 cm, respectively), which work well for treating larger areas. The Lumenis M22 (Lumenis Aesthetics, Yokneam, Israel) also has both large and small spot sizes (3.5 × 1.5 cm and 1.5 × 0.8 cm) available. Smaller spot sizes are useful on the nose or forehead, where avoiding the eyebrows is needed. Both devices use a sapphire crystal cooling system.

For telangiectasias that have a diameter of 1 mm or larger, a longer wavelength, such as the 755- or 1064-nm laser, may be used; start with a lower fluence and spot size and increase as needed.[4,7] The Excel V and CoolTouch Varia (Syneron-Candela, Roseville, CA) are often used for 1064-nm treatments. With Excel V, a spot size of 5 mm, 110 J/cm^2, and 30 ms may be used; the cooling on this device is contact cooling via a sapphire crystal, and ultrasound gel may be used as well. For the CoolTouch Varia, a spot size of 3.5 mm, energies of 160 to 175 J/cm^2, and 30 ms may be used; cooling is via cryogen spray. With blue 2- to 3-mm veins, greater fluences may be necessary.

Telangiectasias of the nose can be very treatment resistant; recurrence rates are quite high, necessitating maintenance treatments. IPL has a good success rate with minimal side effects when using adequate gel and contact cooling with skin. The VBeam Perfecta with longer pulse durations and a 3 × 10 mm spot size is also very effective.[8] Although the Nd:YAG is sometimes used for nasal vessels, particularly purple telangiectasias, caution should be exercised because excessive heat buildup may occur, leaving pockmarks and linear depressions on the nasal ala. At least 2 seconds should elapse between each 1064-nm laser pulse, and skin cooling needs to be effective to reduce the risk of overheating and subsequent collagen overcontraction. Stacked pulsing should never be used. This can lead to undissipated heat from excess nonspecific heating of the water in the dermis and result in necrosis. For this reason, Nd:YAG is rarely used on the nose. In many patients, it can be difficult to permanently eliminate alar telangiectasias altogether; caution patients from the outset that maintenance treatments are often necessary.

Diffuse Erythema

For the treatment of erythema of varying etiologies on the face, neck, and chest, the PDL, KTP, and IPL are most commonly used. All have demonstrated reproducible efficacy.[9] A study comparing IPL to PDL for treatment of erythematotelangiectatic rosacea demonstrated similar efficacy after three treatments spaced 1 month apart (**Figures 28-2 and 28-3**). For the PDL, the settings were 10 mm, 7 J/cm^2, and 6 ms, and for the IPL, a 560-nm filter, a pulse train of 2.4 and 6.0 ms in duration separated by a 15-ms delay, and a starting fluence of 25 J/cm^2 were used.[10] Again, for practical purposes, the IPL is typically used for the chest and neck, although any device may be used. Longer pulse durations for the KTP and PDL may be used to avoid purpura. With the Excel V 532 nm, energies of

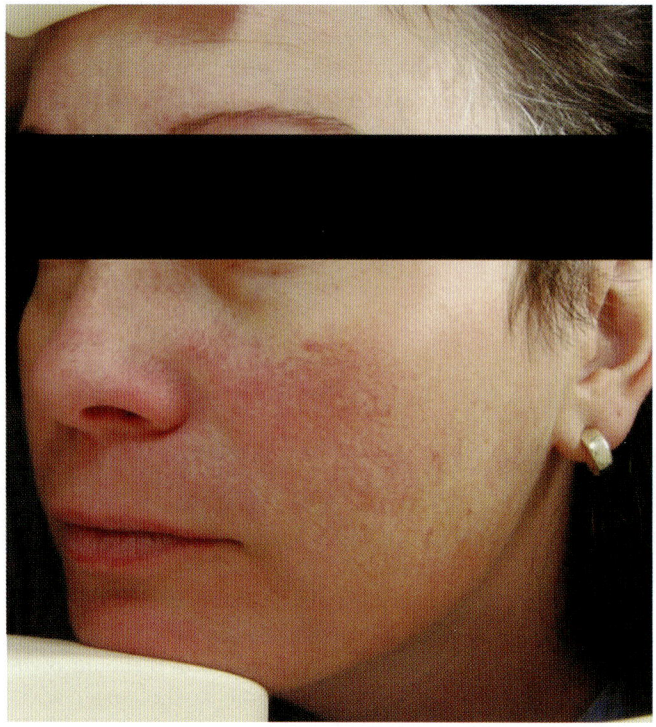

FIGURE 28-2 A 38-year-old woman with erythematotelangiectatic rosacea at baseline.

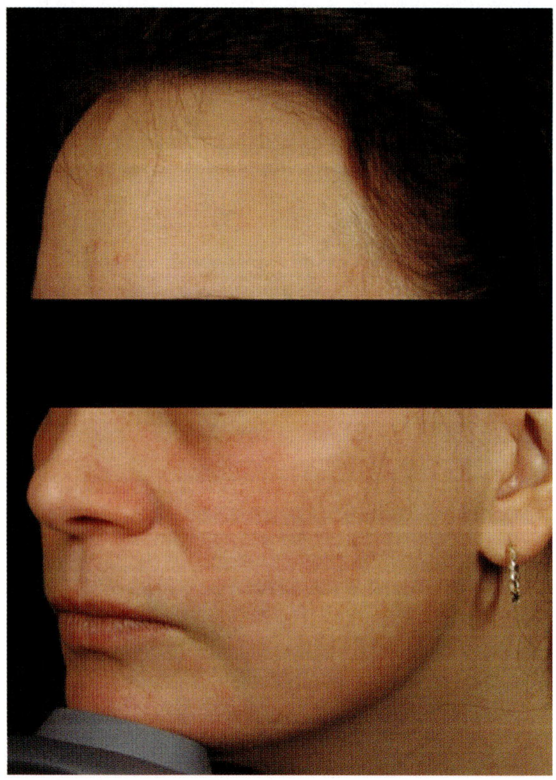

FIGURE 28-3 The same patient 2 years later after undergoing intense pulsed light (IPL) treatments every 6 to 12 months to control her signs and symptoms.

7 to 9 J/cm^2, pulse durations of 8 to 20 ms, and a 10-mm spot size may be used.

Poikiloderma of Civatte

Poikiloderma of Civatte is a combination of epidermal and dermal atrophy, increased pigmentation, and enhanced vascularity. Its occurrence is strongly associated with a history of excessive sun exposure. Patients typically present in the third to fifth decade and are usually of lower Fitzpatrick skin types. Invariably, poikiloderma of Civatte is located on the lateral and anterior neck and upper chest with sparing of sun-protected sites, such as the submentum. Because this is a combination of hyperpigmentation and increased vascularity, treatment with the noncoherent, multiple-wavelength IPL is very effective. Weiss et al[11] published data on 135 patients with poikiloderma of the neck and chest treated with IPL, with over 75% of patients achieving clearance; there were minimal side effects. These results have been reproduced in other studies.[12] In addition, both patients and treating clinicians have noted an improvement in skin texture and fine lines when using IPL. This initially was an incidental finding in early studies, but given the concomitant atrophy typically seen with poikiloderma, it is a significant additional benefit. Lastly, IPL confers the added advantage of having larger spot sizes, increasing treatment efficiency. Therefore, IPL is generally the first choice for poikiloderma treatment.

KTP and PDL can be used as well, but care must be taken to use larger spot sizes and reduced energies. PDL is best reserved for poikiloderma that is primarily composed of dilated blood vessels without hyperpigmentation. Some of the "brown" hyperpigmentation perceived with the naked eye may actually be deoxygenated hemoglobin.[13] PDL is generally more painful for patients. Another factor for the clinician to consider when treating large areas is the wear and tear to the laser itself—larger areas consume more of the dye kit and cryogen.

Regardless of the device chosen, a slight amount of overlap of pulses is necessary to achieve uniform improvement of the treated area. Skip areas can lead to visible "footprinting," which may be in the shape of the device treatment head. This can be reduced by performing more than one pass in different directions or by changing the orientation of a rectangular crystal at subsequent treatment sessions. This improves with repeated treatments, but patients should be warned ahead of time of the risk of "footprinting" or blotchy improvement. Poikiloderma requires a series of treatments, typically between three and five, and strict sun protection should be advised.

STEP-BY-STEP GUIDE

Every procedure should be preceded by patient education and informed consent. A good outcome depends on both an adequate medical response to therapy and a satisfied patient. Patient satisfaction depends not only on the technical success of the procedure, but also, and sometimes more so, on their expectations. The expectations of the patient and the doctor should be the same before beginning any treatment.

Patients should be educated that there are risks associated with every procedure and that no procedure guarantees an excellent outcome every time. The patient must understand that medicine is not an exact science and that there is no guarantee he or she will be satisfied with the end results. Patients should be given time to ask questions and to receive complete answers. One should not proceed with treatment until one feels comfortable with the patient's understanding and expectations. It is difficult to establish the appropriate clinician–patient relationship with patients who are unreasonable, overly demanding, or unable to comprehend the basics of treatment planning and outcomes. These types of patients are also the most likely to complain about any aspect of their treatment.

For the treatment of erythema and telangiectasias, standardized photos with proper and consistent lighting should be taken. Patient consents should be signed and dated prior to procedures. Potential risks include, but are not limited to, purpura, edema, blistering, pigmentary changes, and scarring. Clarification of patient expectations and review of the likely need for multiple treatments and possible maintenance treatments are necessary and ultimately enhance the patient experience. In addition, patients should be instructed on proper sun-protective measures, particularly for erythema caused by rosacea and actinic damage.

On the face, neck, or chest, patients may or may not receive topical anesthesia. In general, vascular lasers and IPL are well tolerated, so topical anesthesia is not necessarily indicated. Some patients find treatment of large areas of the face sufficiently painful with PDL that they request topical anesthetic. If topical anesthesia is to be used, it is important that it not contain phenylephrine, as this will cause vasoconstriction of the target vessels. If necessary, using a device that blow cold air or applying chilled rollers (Cynosure, Westford, MA) allows comfortable treatment without topical anesthetic. As with any procedure, the skin should be clear of makeup, lotions, creams, or other topical products prior to commencing laser treatment. Patients may clean with soap and water followed by wiping the skin with alcohol pads.

Proper eye protection for patients, assisting staff, and the treating provider is critical. Laser goggles should have an optical density (OD) of at least 4. When treating on the face, it is best for patients to use metal goggles or disposable laser or IPL-rated eye adhesive pads. Treatment within the orbital rim requires the use of intraocular eye shields. Do not use the deeply penetrating Nd:YAG wavelength within the orbital rim.

A laser warning sign should be visible on the outside of the door. Prior to commencing the laser treatment, ensure that the proper foot pedal is in place and recheck the laser settings and cooling. For lasers that have more than one wavelength, recheck the selected wavelength and that glasses are appropriate. Patients should be instructed to call if they have unexpected swelling or bruising. If patients experience significant swelling following treatment, there are a number of adjunctive agents that may be used, including topical steroids, antihistamines, oral prednisone, and diuretics.

TABLE 28-4 • Treatment Parameters for Facial, Chest, and Neck Telangiectasias Using PDL and KTP

	Pulse Duration (ms)	Energy (J/cm²)	Spot size (mm)	Cooling
Excel V	Facial: 8-10 Neck/chest: 10-15	Facial: 8.6-9 Neck/chest: 6-8	Facial: 5 Neck/chest: 12	5°C and ultrasound gel
Excel V: skin type III	8-12	7-10	5-7	5°C and ultrasound gel
VBeam Perfecta	6-10	11-14	3 × 10	Cryogen
VBeam Perfecta	6-10	5.5-8	10	Cryogen
VBeam Perfecta	6-10	7-12	7	Cryogen
VBeam Perfecta	6-10	7.5-12.5	5	Cryogen

Telangiectasias

For a patient presenting with nasal or facial telangiectasias, the long-pulsed PDL, VBeam Perfecta, KTP/Nd:YAG, or IPL may be used. For telangiectasias of the neck or chest, the larger spot–sized IPL devices allow more efficient treatment, with appropriate judicious adjustment of fluence.

1. Most laser devices for treatment of vascular lesions are based on a fiber delivery system with a contact or dynamic cooling device. For contact cooling devices, a water-based gel is placed directly on the skin, and the crystal or spacing device is held directly against the skin. In contrast, for dynamic cooling, no gel should be used because the cryogen cools the skin. Gel is not necessary with PDL and may introduce water that diminishes the fluence before reaching the target vessels. Minimal pressure is placed against the skin, as the target may be compressed with excessive hand pressure. Treatment parameters are outlined in **Tables 28-4 and 28-5**.

2. If using an IPL device, use the filter with cutoffs at 560 to 590 nm. Rarely, the 515-nm cutoff filter can be used in patients with type I or II skin. For devices that have fixed filters, use an IPL head that produces green or yellow wavelengths. If a contact cooling device is used, a small layer of water-based or coupling gel is placed on the skin. With minimal pressure, the cooling device with crystal is placed directly onto the skin overlying the targeted area. No pressure is applied, as the target vessels collapse with compression, leaving very little target. **Figure 28-4** shows placement of the IPL crystal with gel on the skin. An immediate gray tone to the skin in the shape of the crystal is not desirable; pronounced erythema and urtication in the shape of the crystal should be avoided as well. The Cynosure ICON MaxG for the face and MaxY for the neck and chest may be used at 10 to 20 ms and 25 to 42 J/cm² and the Lumenis One at 3 ms, double pulse, with 10 to 20 ms off time between pulses at total fluence of 14 to 20 J/cm². The ICON has the added advantage of the SkinTel, which determines the patient's melanin index and suggests a range of safe treatment parameters based upon that index. Extended pulse durations may be used for larger-nasal telangiectasias

TABLE 28-5 • Treatment Parameters for Nasal Telangiectasias Using PDL and KTP

	Pulse Duration (ms)	Energy (J/cm²)	Spot Size (mm)	Cooling
Excel V	8-10	8.6-9	5	5°C and ultrasound gel
Excel V: Skin type III	8-12	7-10	5-7	5°C and ultrasound gel
VBeam Perfecta	10-40	10-13.5	3 × 10	Cryogen
VBeam Perfecta	10-40	6.5-8.5	10	Cryogen
VBeam Perfecta	10-40	8-12	7	Cryogen
VBeam Perfecta	10-40	8-12	5	Cryogen

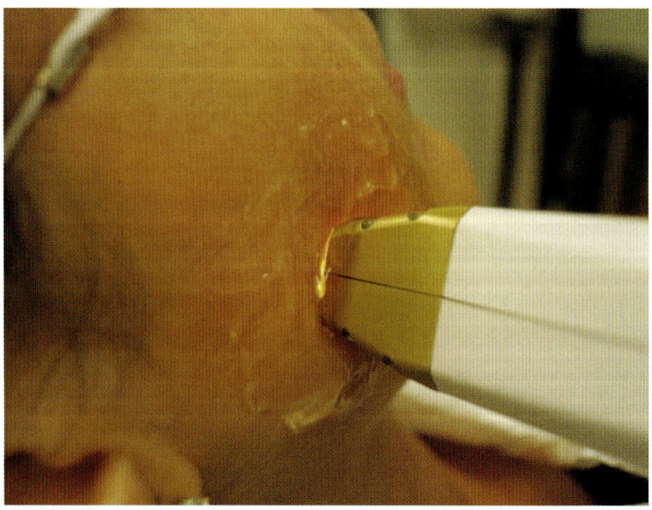

FIGURE 28-4 Intense pulsed light (IPL) device with cooling gel on the skin.

TABLE 28-6 • Treatment Parameters for Facial, Nose, Neck, and Chest Telangiectasias Using IPL

For vessels <0.2 mm in diameter	■ Lumenis One: 3.0 ms, 560-nm filter, 14-20 J/cm^2 ■ Starlux Max G: 5-10 ms, 20-36 J/cm^2
For vessels 0.2-0.4 mm in diameter	■ Lumenis One: 2.5/2.5 ms (10-ms delay), 560-nm filter, 14-22 J/cm^2 ■ Starlux Max G: 10 ms, 30-40 J/cm^2
For vessels 0.4-0.8 mm in diameter	■ Lumenis One: 2.4/7.0 ms (10- to 15-ms delay), 590-nm filter, 15-24 J/cm^2 ■ Starlux Max G: 10-20 ms, 30-46 J/cm^2

with pulse durations of 40 to 50 ms. Pulse stacking can be done on the face, nose, neck, and chest and enhances efficacy. During a lengthy treatment, some device crystals may start to warm up; one must be alert for this. Treatment parameters are outlined in **Table 28-6**.

3. Regardless of the light source or laser used, there are some features and pitfalls common to all devices. Typical end points include immediate vessel contraction; visible intravascular photodarkening, which represents intravascular coagulation; and rupture of the vessel causing immediate purpura. In general, purpura may be avoided without compromise of efficacy, and purpura causes significant patient downtime. The pulse duration should be extended when purpura is encountered. If vessel constriction is not noted, either the energy needs to be increased or the pulse duration may need to be increased, as the entire vessel may not be heating. The risk of hyper- or hypopigmentation from overcooling the skin with cryogen also exists. Blanching is to be avoided with all devices. For the PDL and KTP lasers and IPL, up to three passes may be performed over the treated area.
4. With the 1064-nm lasers, the Cutera ExcelV or CoolTouch Varia are commonly used; there are multiple lasers available with similar wavelengths. For telangiectasias of the nose (not ala), face, neck, or chest, a pulse duration of 30 ms, fluences of 110 to 120 J/cm^2, spot size of 5 mm, and cooling at 5°C may be used. Lateral spread of thermal effects within the vessel beyond the point of treatment is frequently noted so that overlap is not necessary; pulses should be spaced out by at least 1 mm. Stacked pulsing, which can be performed with PDL and KTP, should never be used for infrared lasers, particularly 1064-nm lasers. The 1064-nm laser is especially effective at treating blue 1- to 3-mm telangiectasias of the forehead.

Poikiloderma of Civatte

For the treatment of poikiloderma of Civatte, IPL is used most frequently, although PDL or KTP may be used as well, particularly if there are clearly visible telangiectasias. If the latter situation is present, two to three passes may be performed with an IPL followed by treatment of the larger vessels using PDL, KTP, or Nd:YAG. The large telangiectasias may also be treated first, followed by the IPL.

TABLE 28-7 • Treatment Parameters for Facial, Nose, Neck, and Chest Poikiloderma of Civatte and Erythema Using IPL

Poikiloderma and erythema	■ Lumenis One: 2.5-3.0 ms, 10- to 15-ms delay, 560- or 590-nm filter, 14-22 J/cm^2 ■ Starlux Max G: 10-20 ms, 22-46 J/cm^2

1. When using the IPL for treatment of poikiloderma, similar settings are used as to when treating telangiectasias (**Table 28-6**). At least two passes may be performed at each visit. One pass can be done at 20 ms to target larger vessels, and the second at 10 ms to target dyspigmentation. If the vessels are particularly large, the pulse duration can be increased to 50 to 60 ms and the energy increased to around 50 J/cm^2 or even higher, depending on the patient's skin type and response. Devices such as the Lumenis One and newer IPL sources typically have preset or recommended settings for clinical findings such as poikiloderma of Civatte.
2. If using the VBeam Perfecta, a spot size of 10 or 12 mm, pulse durations of 6 to 10 ms, and energies of 5 to 7 J/cm^2 can be used. Although quicker pulse durations may decrease the number of total treatments, the resulting purpura on the neck and chest is usually not well liked by patients. Purpura is frequent with the 2-ms pulse duration.
3. For KTP, a spot size of 10 or 12 mm, energies of approximately 7 to 9 J/cm^2, and pulse duration of 8 to 10 ms should be used.

For patients presenting with facial, neck, or chest erythema, PDL, KTP, or IPL devices may be used on the face, with IPL alone used on the neck and chest. See **Tables 28-7 and 28-8** for treatment parameters.

TABLE 28-8 • Treatment Parameters for Erythema of Face, Nose, Neck, and Chest Using KTP or PDL

	Pulse Duration (ms)	Energy (J/cm^2)	Spot size (mm)	Cooling
Excel V	8-20, typically start with 10	7-9, typically start at 7.4	10	5°C and ultrasound gel
Excel V: skin type III	8-20, typically start at 12	7-9, typically start at 7	10	5°C and ultrasound gel
VBeam Perfecta	6-10	5-8	10	Cryogen
VBeam Perfecta	6-10	8-11	7	Cryogen

CONCLUSIONS

Erythema and telangiectasias are a common problem, and patients frequently present to the clinician eager to address these concerns. Most telangiectasias can be managed using laser and light devices without causing significant purpura, although immediate post-procedure edema, as well as other local reactions, may be seen. An array of devices may be used, although IPL is the mainstay of therapy for telangiectasias and is an efficient and cost-effective approach to telangiectasia management.

REFERENCES

1. Fowler JF Jr, Woolery-Lloyd H, Waldorf H, Saini R. Innovations in natural ingredients and their use in skin care. *J Drugs Dermatol.* 2010;9(6 Suppl):S72-S81; quiz s82-s83.
2. Clark C, Cameron H, Moseley H, Ferguson J, Ibbotson SH. Treatment of superficial cutaneous vascular lesions: experience with the KTP 532 nm laser. *Lasers Med Sci.* 2004;19(1):1-5.
3. Uebelhoer NS, Bogle MA, Stewart B, Arndt KA, Dover JS. A split-face comparison study of pulsed 532-nm KTP laser and 595-nm pulsed dye laser in the treatment of facial telangiectasias and diffuse telangiectatic facial erythema. *Dermatol Surg.* 2007;33(4):441-448.
4. Ross EV, Meehan KJ, Domankevitz Y, Trafeli JP, Annandono J, Jacoby M. Use of a variable long-pulse alexandrite laser in the treatment of facial telangiectasia. *Dermatol Surg.* 2010;36(4):470-474.
5. Tierney E, Hanke CW. Randomized controlled trial: comparative efficacy for the treatment of facial telangiectasias with 532 nm versus 940 nm diode laser. *Lasers Surg Med.* 2009;41(8):555-562.
6. Tanghetti EA. Split-face randomized treatment of facial telangiectasia comparing pulsed dye laser and an intense pulsed light handpiece. *Lasers Surg Med.* 2012;44(2):97-102.
7. Ozyurt K, Colgecen E, Baykan H, Ozturk P, Ozkose M. Treatment of superficial cutaneous vascular lesions: experience with the long-pulsed 1064 nm Nd:YAG laser. *Sci World J.* 2012;2012:197139.
8. Madan V, Ferguson J. Using the ultra-long pulse width pulsed dye laser and elliptical spot to treat resistant nasal telangiectasia. *Lasers Med Sci.* 2010;25(1):151-154.
9. Jasim ZF, Woo WK, Handley JM. Long-pulsed (6-ms) pulsed dye laser treatment of rosacea-associated telangiectasia using subpurpuric clinical threshold. *Dermatol Surg.* 2004;30(1):37-40.
10. Neuhaus IM, Zane LT, Tope WD. Comparative efficacy of nonpurpuragenic pulsed dye laser and intense pulsed light for erythematotelangiectatic rosacea. *Dermatol Surg.* 2009;35(6):920-928.
11. Weiss RA, Goldman MP, Weiss MA. Treatment of poikiloderma of Civatte with an intense pulsed light source. *Dermatol Surg.* 2000;26(9):823-827; discussion 828.
12. Rusciani A, Motta A, Fino P, Menichini G. Treatment of poikiloderma of Civatte using intense pulsed light source: 7 years of experience. *Dermatol Surg.* 2008;34(3):314-319; discussion 319.
13. Stamatas GN, Kollias N. Blood stasis contributions to the perception of skin pigmentation. *J Biomed Opt.* 2004;9(2):315-322.

29 Laser Resurfacing

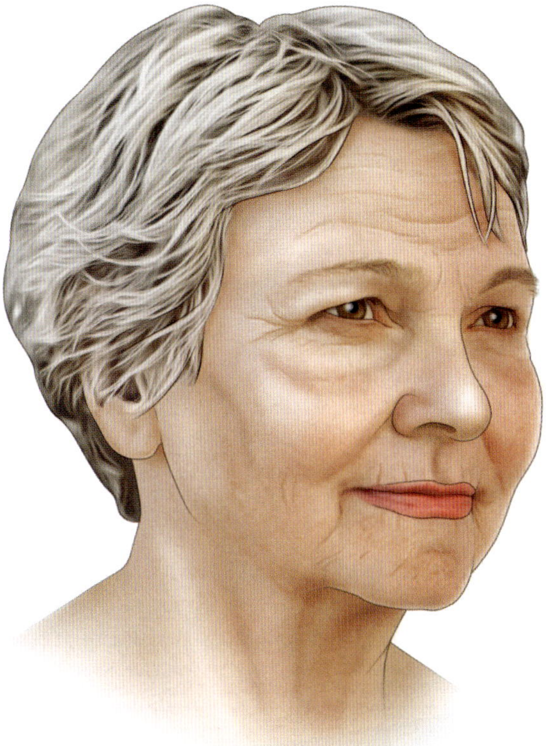

SUMMARY

- Skin resurfacing is a common aesthetic procedure, and can result in improvement in rhytides, skin texture, dyspigmentation, and skin tightening.
- Several laser and energy devices are available, and they can broadly be divided into ablative nonfractional lasers, nonablative nonfractional lasers, ablative fractional lasers, and nonablative fractional lasers.

Beginner Tips

- There is generally a tradeoff between efficacy, or number of required treatments, and the amount of downtime that a patient can expect.
- Ablative nonfractional lasers have the most dramatic effect for resurfacing, but also the greatest downtime. At the other end of the spectrum are nonablative fractional lasers, which require the most treatments but have the least downtime.

Pitfalls and Cautions

- Ablative nonfractional lasers should generally not be used in skin types V to VI, given the risk of dyspigmentation and scarring.
- The rate of acneiform eruptions and milia formation for laser resurfacing remains fairly high, and this should be discussed with patients preprocedure.

Expert Tips

- Closely overlapping fractional laser pulses can lead to the MTZs blending together, resulting in a nonfractional result.
- Needed treatment energy and density is not uniform across the face; select areas may require increased fluence or an increased density.

Patient Education Points

- For all treatments other than ablative nonfractional lasers, patients should be told to expect several treatment sessions before seeing meaningful results.
- Patients should have realistic expectations regarding the healing process, and should be warned that they will be out of commission for up to 2 weeks with ablative nonfractional lasers.

Don't Forget!

- Ablative nonfractional lasers may lead to dramatic improvement after a single treatment, but other approaches generally require a series of multiple treatments.
- When combining PDL or IPL and resurfacing lasers, be sure to treat for erythema before resurfacing so that the immediate postprocedure erythema is not the target of the PDL or IPL.

Billing Pearls

- Almost all insurers in the United States exclude laser treatments from coverage.
- Patients may benefit from committing to a series of treatments, as this may allow significant cost savings.
- Pretreatment with occluded topical anesthesia can be started at home, and prescription plans may cover the cost of this medication.

29 Laser Resurfacing

INTRODUCTION

Skin resurfacing with energy-based devices decreases dyspigmentation, reduces rhytids, and improves texture. Tighter skin is made possible through thermal damage to dermal collagen bundles and stimulation of dermal fibroblasts. To produce dermal collagen damage, energy is transmitted through the epidermis and into the dermis at a minimum temperature of 65°C, the temperature required to damage collagen.

Originally, energy devices required destruction of the epidermis along with the dermis. These ablative lasers are effective at collagen destruction but also cause full epidermal destruction, requiring a significant recuperation period. Lasers that do not destroy the epidermis, but produce heat in the dermis, are referred to as nonablative lasers. They do not require the same duration of recovery but necessitate a greater number of treatments to achieve appreciable results. The abbreviated recovery time following fractionated laser resurfacing reflects the creation of microscopic treatment zones (MTZs) that allow faster epidermal healing while thermally heating dermal collagen. Radiofrequency devices are not lasers but use the same premise as resurfacing laser devices. Using radiofrequency, the dermis is heated to a temperature that damages collagen and stimulates fibroblasts, while avoiding epidermal destruction. Each energy-based device has benefits and drawbacks. One device may produce faster results but require extensive downtime, while another may have an increased risk of hypopigmentation when used to treat a patient with a darker skin type.

ABLATIVE NONFRACTIONATED LASERS

Since their 1964 invention at Bell Laboratories until the 1990s, the only dermatologic energy-based device for the treatment of scars, rhytids, dyspigmentation, and surface texture was an ablative nonfractionated carbon dioxide (CO_2) laser.[1] Ablative lasers are excellent at resurfacing, as they instantly heat epidermal cells to greater than 100°C, leading to vaporization of the surface cells, and produce coagulation necrosis of the residual cellular layer. In the dermis, the energy emitted from the laser creates nonfatal damage to dermal fibroblasts, stimulating collagen production and resulting in decreased rhytids, resolution of dyspigmentation, and smoother skin. Currently available laser platforms for ablative lasers are CO_2, which emits energy at 10,600 nm, and erbium:yttrium-aluminum-garnet (Er:YAG), which emits at 2940 nm.

In their nonfractionated form, ablative lasers vaporize the entire field of skin on which they are projected. As with other skin rejuvenation lasers, the thermal damage produced denatures the existing dermal collagen and stimulates production of new collagen. New collagen synthesis may continue 4 to 6 months after treatment.[1] As collagen is generated, the wound heals with subsequent tightening of the dermis and epidermis, resulting in improved skin texture.[2]

Nonfractionated ablative CO_2 lasers produce excellent improvement in skin texture, dyspigmentation, and rhytids,[3] but require a 2-week recovery period from edema, burning, and crusting, and result in an average of 4 months of treatment site erythema.[1,4] There is also a risk of permanent hypopigmentation, herpes simplex virus (HSV) outbreak, scarring, milia formation, and acne flare.[5,6] Ablative nonfractionated Er:YAG lasers, which were developed after ablative nonfractionated CO_2 lasers, when used with longer pulse duration, produce results equal to their CO_2 counterparts but with less unintentional tissue destruction, shortening the patient's recovery period.

CO_2 and Er:YAG nonfractionated ablative lasers are used only for patients with light skin types. Dyspigmentation risk and scarring among Fitzpatrick skin types V and VI are considered too great to consider this group for nonfractionated ablative resurfacing treatment[7] (**Figures 29-1 and 29-2**).

NONABLATIVE NONFRACTIONATED LASERS

The development of nonablative nonfractionated lasers near the end of the 20th century provided an alternative to ablative laser devices. Devices include the 1450-nm diode (Candela Smoothbeam), 1320-nm Nd:YAG (CoolTouch CT3Plus and Alma Harmony XL), and 1319-nm pulsed energy (Sciton Thermascan). Nonablative lasers use milder heat that will not vaporize tissue but will denature target proteins, such as dermal collagen. In contrast to their ablative brethren, nonablative nonfractionated lasers produce less radical cosmetic results per treatment but have drastically reduced healing times, which may limit erythema to a single post\treatment afternoon.[8,9] As with ablative nonfractionated lasers, 80% of patients treated with nonablative nonfractional lasers will develop a transient acneiform eruption, and 14% develop transient milia.[10] An additional benefit of nonablative lasers is a decreased risk of hypopigmentation in darker skin types (Fitzpatrick skin types V and VI), as compared to ablative lasers.[11]

NONABLATIVE FRACTIONAL LASER

In 2005, nonablative fractional laser resurfacing (NAFR) entered the market.[12] Unlike nonfractionated lasers, fractionated lasers produce MTZs one-tenth of the diameter of a hair follicle scattered throughout the treatment field. The MTZ depth may be set between 0 and 550 µm with diameter ranging from 50 to 150 µm. As a nonablative laser, the heat targets the dermis and does not vaporize the stratum corneum, leaving a natural bandage covering the coagulated tissue of the damaged epidermis and dermis. The creation of MTZ leaves surrounding keratinocytes uninjured and promotes faster healing than full-field ablative lasers, while still stimulating dermal fibroblasts and collagen formation.

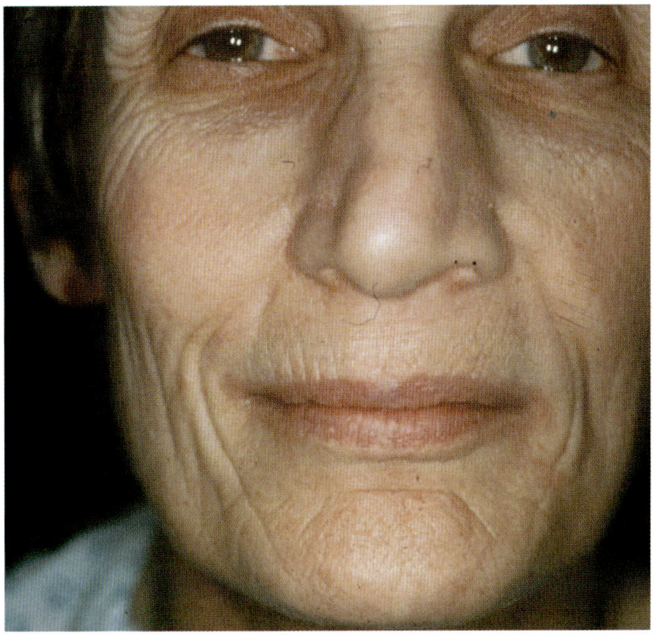

FIGURE 29-1 Before ablative carbon dioxide laser resurfacing.

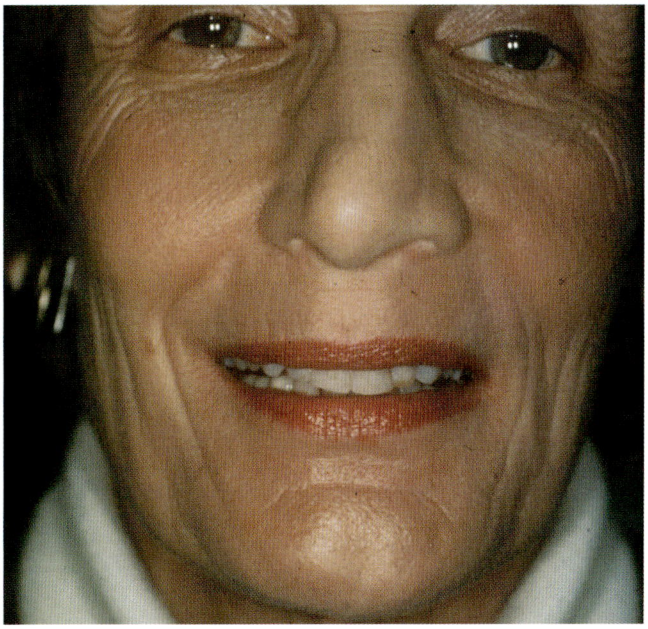

FIGURE 29-2 Six months after laser resurfacing.

There is an increased desire for resurfacing technologies for patients of skin types V and VI.[7] Those with darker skin types have increased epidermal melanin, larger melanosomes that are widely distributed within epidermal keratinocytes, and more reactive fibroblasts and melanocytic responses. These features increase the tendency to develop dyspigmentation after exposure to laser light.[7] As with the nonablative nonfractionated devices, nonablative fractionated lasers are safer in Fitzpatrick skin types up to VI than ablative lasers and allow patients a more rapid posttreatment recovery.[6] Current devices on the market include 1440-nm Nd:YAG (Cynosure Affirm, Palomar StarLux), 1550-nm erbium glass (Solta Fraxel re:store), 1565-nm fiber (Lumenis ResurFx), and 1927-nm thulium fiber (Solta Fraxel re:store Dual). Erbium-doped 1550-nm nonablative lasers (Fraxel re:store Dual 1550-nm) have been successful in resurfacing acne scars in Fitzpatrick skin types IV to VI,[13] but with a significant incidence of self-limited postinflammatory hyperpigmentation among patients with these skin types. Preoperative treatment with hydroquinone does not diminish this risk.[13] Unlike nonfractionated lasers, only 10% of patients treated with NAFR will develop an acneiform eruption, and 19% will develop milia.[10] In addition to rhytids, NAFR has been successfully used in treatment of hypertrophic scars, including those resulting from surgical procedures such as Mohs surgery.[14] When treating scars with an erythematous component, it is recommended to initially treat with a vascular laser, such as a pulsed dye laser (PDL), and then NAFR, to ensure that the PDL is treating the vascular component of the scar, not the erythema from the NAFR.[15] For erythematous surgical scars, a protocol of PDL treatments every 4 weeks followed by NAFR has been suggested. Eilers et al[15] recommend settings of 30 to 50 mJ and 20% to 39% density for NAFR resurfacing of hypertrophic surgical scars (**Figures 29-3 to 29-6**).

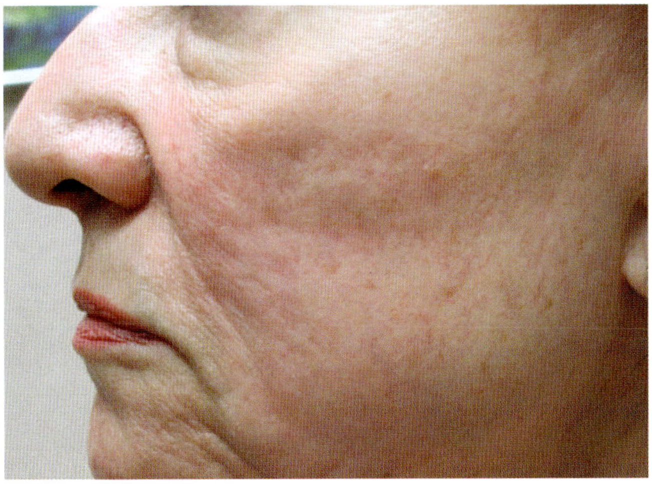

FIGURE 29-3 Before nonablative fractional resurfacing.

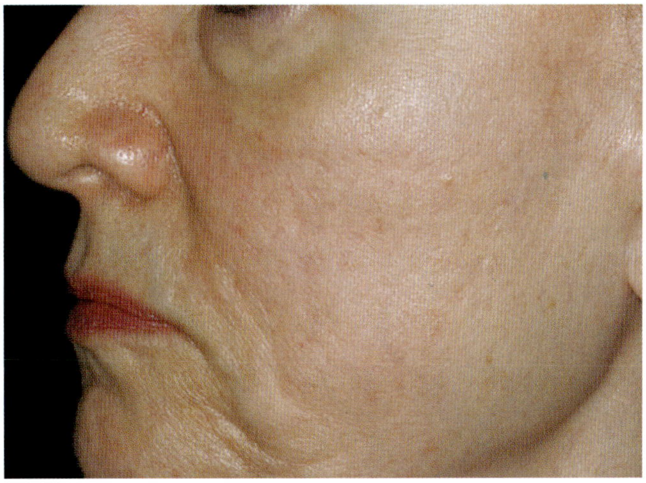

FIGURE 29-4 Six months after four sessions of nonablative fractional resurfacing.

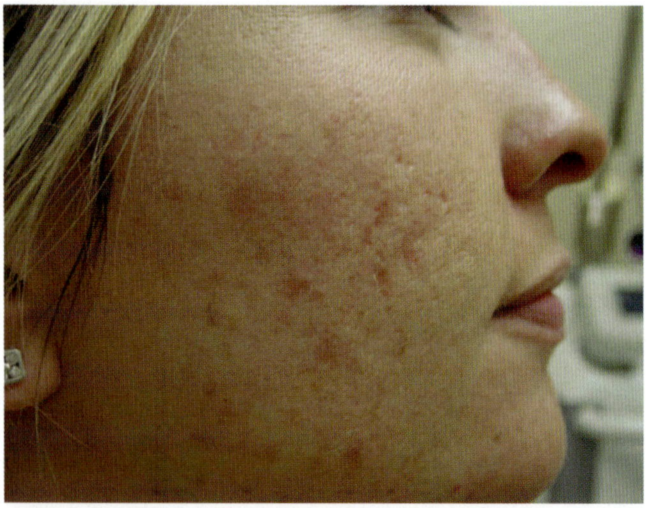

FIGURE 29-5 Before nonablative fractional resurfacing.

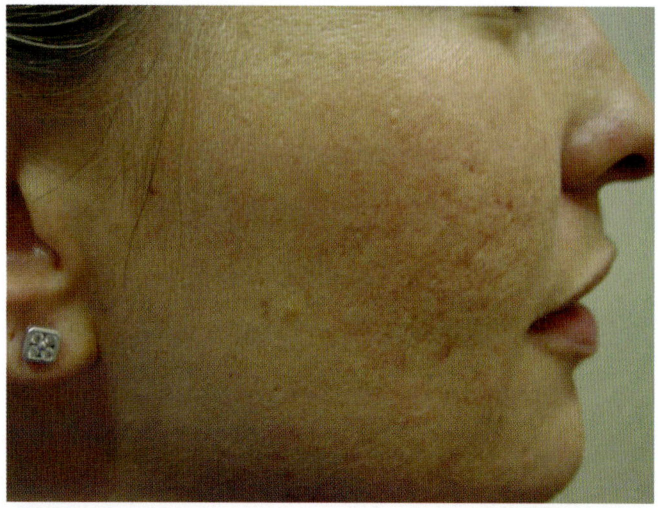

FIGURE 29-6 Six months after four sessions of nonablative fractional resurfacing.

ABLATIVE FRACTIONATED LASERS

Use of ablative fractionated lasers (AFLs) began in 2007. These lasers create MTZs while sparing surrounding tissue, allowing for rapid healing and little downtime. Both nonablative fractionated lasers and AFLs are able to penetrate to the same depth, dependent on settings, with the ablative form vaporizing tissue. Most patients develop postprocedural edema and erythema, lasting up to 3 days.[1] Studies have demonstrated significant improvement of acne scars from both CO_2 and Er:YAG AFL devices[16] (**Figures 29-7 to 29-14**).

Ablative fractional CO_2 has successfully been used in the treatment of smooth elevated surgical scars in patients with skin types I to IV.[16,17] Ciocon et al[18] performed a split-face trial comparing efficacy, efficiency, and tolerability between a device with a stamping handpiece (UltraPulse Encore Deep FX, Lumenis) and a device with a rolling handpiece (Fraxel Repair, Solta Medical). Results demonstrated equal efficacy, but the rolling handpiece was reported to produce less pain and be more efficient for the operator.[18]

In another study, Korean patients with skin types III and IV were treated with either a 2940-nm Er:YAG (Matrixell, Medro), with 10 to 20 passes per lesion at 2.5 to 3.0 J at 3- to 4-week intervals for a total of two to seven treatments, or a 10,600-nm CO_2 (eCO_2, Lutronic), at 40 to 60 mJ with 150 spots/cm^2 and three to five passes in static mode for a total of one to nine treatments every 4 to 8 weeks.[19] Among the AFL lasers tested, Er:YAG improved the scars an average of 28.2%, and the CO_2 improved scars by an average of 49.8%.[19] Adjuvant therapies such as the addition of autologous platelet-rich plasma have been studied but have not been shown to improve resurfacing when used in conjunction with CO_2 AFL.[20]

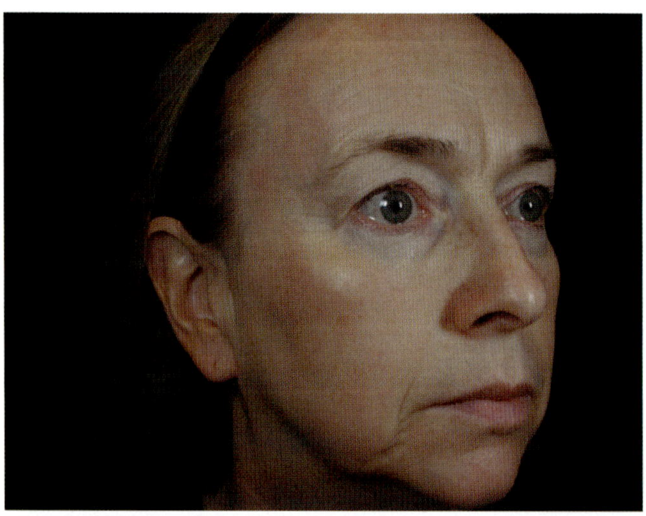

FIGURE 29-7 Before ablative fractional carbon dioxide laser resurfacing.

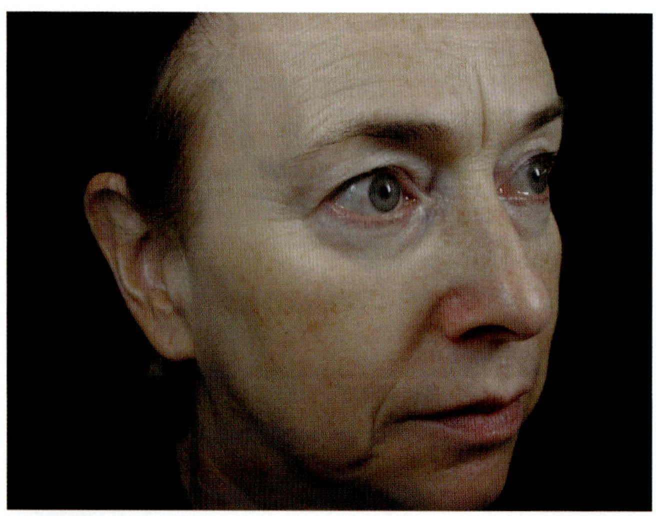

FIGURE 29-8 Six months after ablative fractional carbon dioxide laser resurfacing.

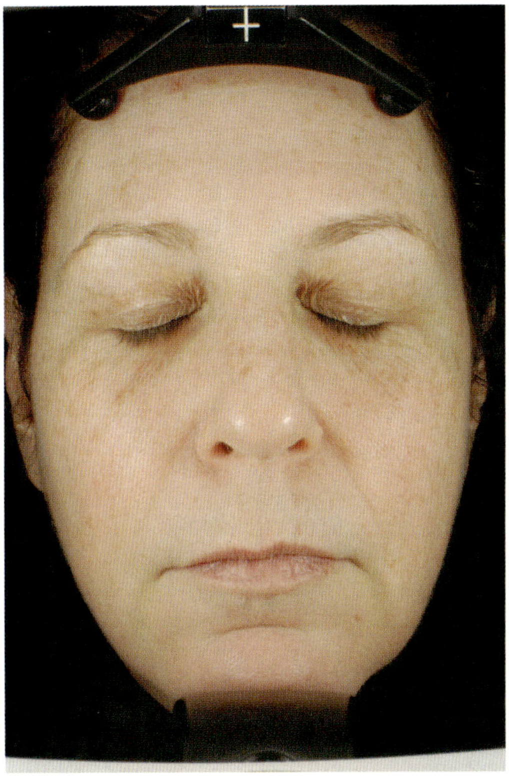

FIGURE 29-9 Before ablative fractional carbon dioxide laser resurfacing.

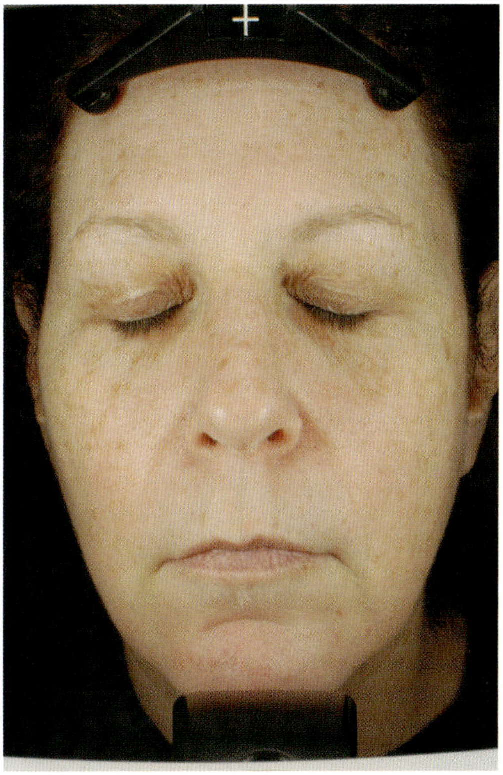

FIGURE 29-10 Six months after ablative fractional carbon dioxide laser resurfacing.

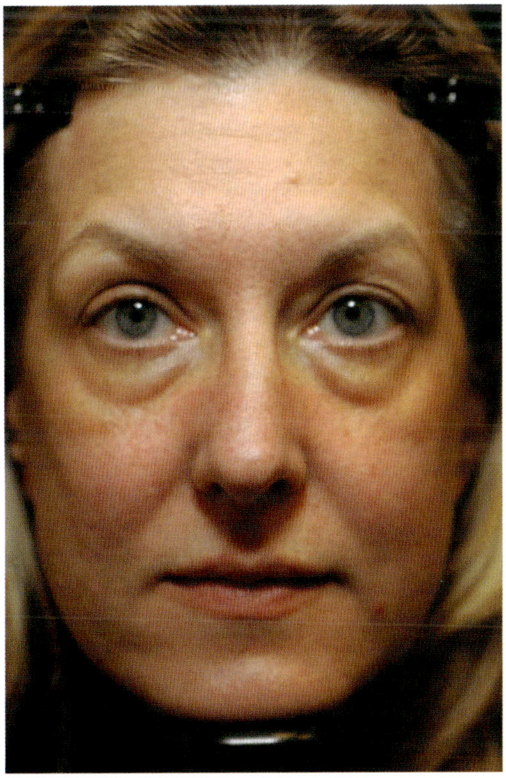

FIGURE 29-11 Before ablative fractional carbon dioxide laser resurfacing.

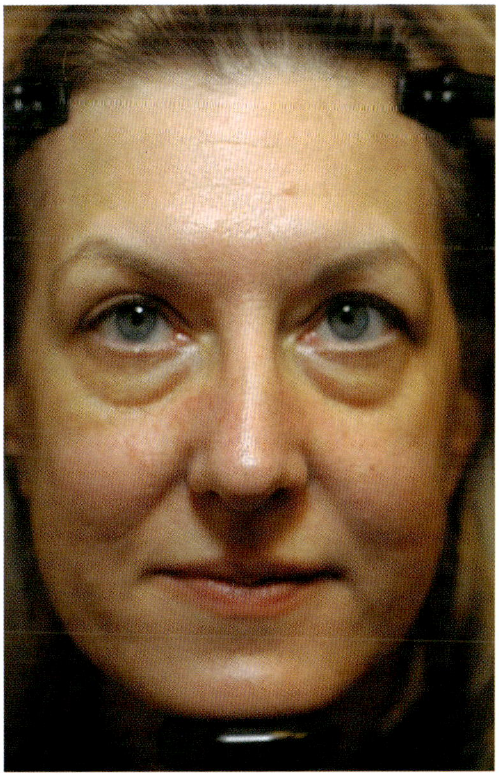

FIGURE 29-12 Six months after ablative fractional carbon dioxide laser resurfacing.

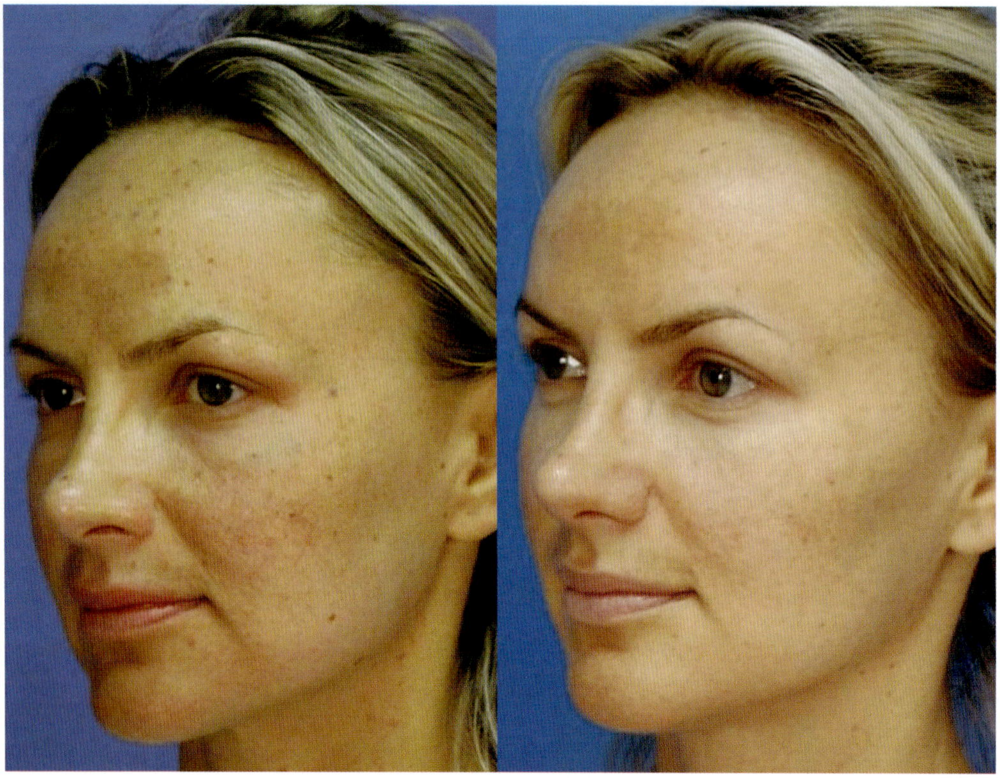

FIGURE 29-13 Before and 6 months after ablative fractional Er:YAG laser resurfacing.

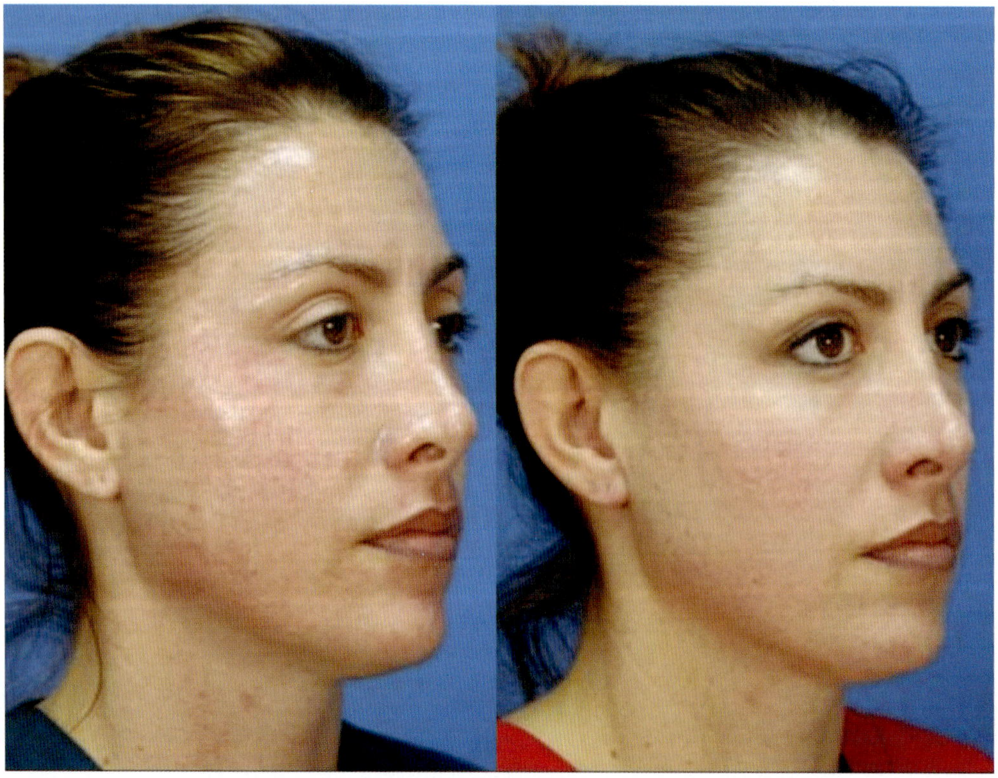

FIGURE 29-14 Before and 6 months after ablative fractional Er:YAG resurfacing.

ER:YSGG

Both CO_2 and Er:YAG lasers are effective at ablative tissue resurfacing and require a similar re-epithelialization time of 8 to 14 days.[21,22] In addition to downtime from re-epithelialization, there may be associated psychological distress resulting from treatment area erythema. Er:YAG lasers produce energy at a wavelength of 2940 nm, with 10 times more water absorption than CO_2 lasers. This allows a reduction in thermal damage, correlating to a reduction in scarring, while maintaining high superficial tissue ablation. In contrast, the efficacy of the CO_2 laser in the treatment of deep rhytids, resulting from its production of deeper coagulation with fewer passes, is superior to the Er:YAG.[22]

The erbium-yttrium-scandium-gallium-garnet (Er:YSGG), a 2790-nm mid-infrared laser, originally tested in the 1990s,[23] is between the CO_2 and Er:YAG.[24] The Er:YSGG laser destroys the epidermis 10 to 30 µm in depth and coagulates the epidermis with heat. The Er:YSGG has a tissue absorption coefficient five times greater than CO_2 but one-third that of Er:YAG, thus producing greater thermal damage and neocollagenesis and elastinogenesis in the proliferative stage of wound healing than an Er:YAG laser, but its limited depth of thermal injury produces less postoperative pain compared to a 10,600-nm CO_2 laser.[24,25] The remodeling phase that follows the proliferative stage results in a tighter dermis and removal of epidermal wrinkles.[26] The Er:YSGG laser has successfully been tested for scar treatment, pore treatment, wrinkle reduction, and skin tone improvement.[26] In a single-blinded trial of 10 subjects with skin type II or III, a two-pass facial treatment, first at 226 J/cm^2 and then at 283 J/cm^2, at a total density of 16% to 24% demonstrated moderate or greater improvement among 60% of subjects' perioral wrinkles and 50% of subjects' full-face wrinkles and fine lines.[27] There was persistent erythema in 20% of patients at the 6-month mark but no serious adverse events.[27] In a split-face trial of 920 µb/cm^2 fractional ablative Er:YSGG and Er:YAG, Er:YAG demonstrated greater periorbital wrinkle reduction with fewer required passes.[28] With regard to perioral wrinkle reduction, the Er:YSGG demonstrated no improvement after a single pass that was greater than a 2 on a 0 to 9 scale, whereas the Er:YAG, using a one to two stacked pass technique, demonstrated a 57% improvement greater than 2 on a 0 to 9 wrinkle scale.[28]

The benefit of the fractional ablative treatment is rapid healing after treatments, but it is important to minimize the number of passes because if the MTZs merge or overlap, then the procedure is similar to an ablative resurfacing. In a blinded study by Munavalli et al,[25] subjects were treated with an Er:YSGG laser with combined ablative and fractional ablative capabilities for study of treatment of superficial and deep skin changes from photoaging. Among 10 enlisted subjects, limited to skin types I to III, 80% of patients were rated as having a moderate to very significant improvement of their wrinkles and overall photoaging at 6 months after the procedure.[25] An 11-patient 6-week follow-up study of the Er:YSGG laser found that 56% of patients had an improvement of between 26% and 75% in dyschromia and 18% had improvement in that range of wrinkles.[29] No patient had greater than 51% improvement in their overall appearance 6 weeks after Er:YSGG laser.[29] The Er:YSGG results in minimal downtime, 5 days of erythema at treatment sites, and a 50% to 89% reduction in acne scars in 70% of Fitzpatrick skin type IV or V patients.[30]

RADIOFREQUENCY

Radiofrequency (RF) devices are an important tool in photofacial resurfacing. Their energy penetrates into the reticular dermis, but unlike lasers, avoids heating the skin surface. Similar to lasers, the energy transferred to the dermis stimulates denaturation of existing collagen and promotes generation of new, shorter collagen bundles.[31] Collagen, which denatures after 10 minutes at 65°C, shrinks by 10%, resulting in tightening of the skin. This is independent of chromophore interaction and does not interfere with melanin in the epidermis.[32] Approved by the US Food and Drug Administration in 2008 for atrophic acne scars, RF has shown acne scar improvement in split-face studies.[33] A study among 30 Thai subjects with skin types III to V demonstrated significant acne scar reduction with either 60 or 100 mJ/pin. Subjects were not provided anesthetic and noted increased procedural pain with the higher energy setting. Neither group developed postinflammatory hyperpigmentation lasting longer than 4 weeks.[33] Similar findings have been demonstrated in skin types I to III.[34] Another study of skin types III and IV found that 80% of subjects demonstrated a 50% or greater improvement of acne scars when treated every 4 weeks for 12 weeks with combined microneedling and fractional RF.[35]

Bipolar RF devices deliver energy to the skin in fractionated thermal zones with a pyramid-shaped output, thereby minimizing heat within the epidermis.[6,36] Among those treated with bipolar RF devices, 61%, 35%, 78%, 87%, and 83% of all treated patients have reported a 50% improvement or greater of their fine lines, pores, tightness, brightness, and overall appearance, respectively, 6 weeks after treatment.[37] Some RF devices, called fractional RF systems, create microablative resurfacing of the epidermis and enhance collagen and elastin production in the dermis.[30,39] As with other RF devices, there is stimulation of collagen production with minimal downtime.[6] Adverse events are typically limited to posttreatment erythema and crusting.[40] Microneedling has become increasingly used for treatment in facial resurfacing. Microneedles placed into dermal collagen induce collagen production and the addition of fractional ablative needle RF.[41,42] A study from Egypt among patients with Fitzpatrick skin types III to IV used a monopolar RF device with cryogen unit or cooling (Biorad, Shenzhen GSD Tech Co.) with two passes of 150 J to the face (except for 200 J applied to the periorbital, nasolabial, and forehead areas). After 3 months, there was 70% to 75% improvement in skin tightening and 90% to 95% improvement in facial rhytides.[42] The researchers observed new collagen synthesis on histologic analysis in those treated. Repeated studies have demonstrated that multiple passes are more beneficial than a single pass at denaturation of collagen. The most common side effect was erythema lasting less than 24 hours and mild edema, which may last up to 1 week.[43] RF allows for treatment of patients with any skin type. In one study, 15 subjects with skin types V or VI were treated with 30 to 50 mJ from a fractionated bipolar RF device (e-Matrix, Syneron Medical Inc).[32] After three monthly treatments, greater than 85% of subjects had improved tone and texture and a decrease in fine lines and wrinkles[32] (**Figures 29-15 to 29-18**).

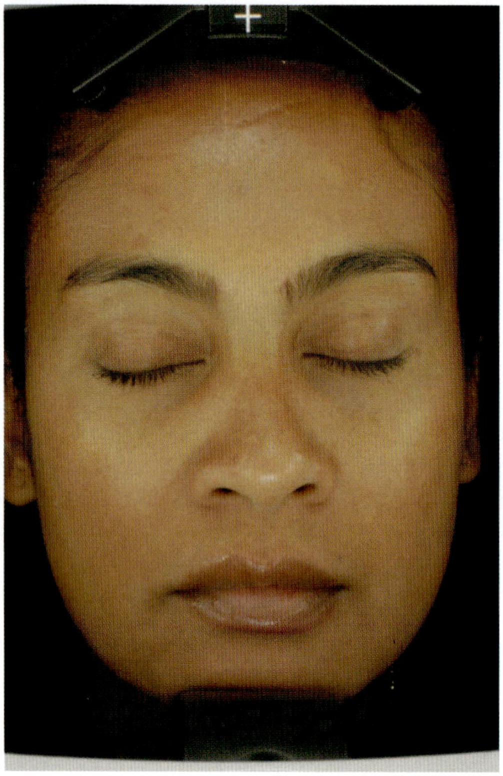

FIGURE 29-15 Before fractional radiofrequency resurfacing.

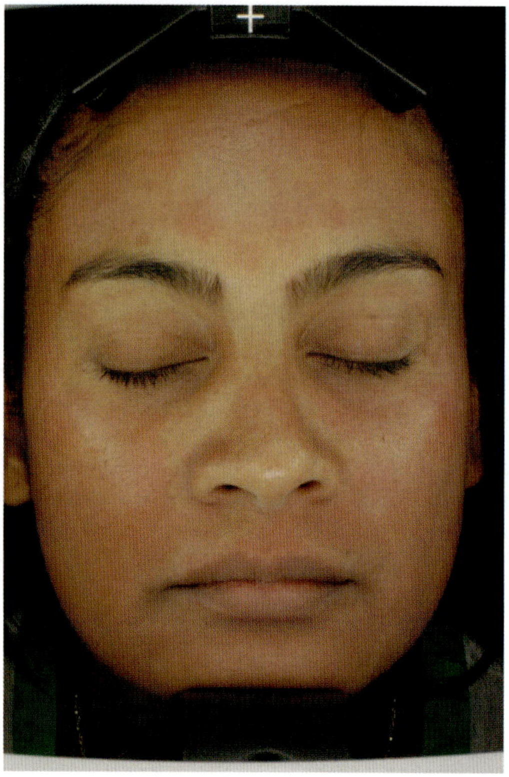

FIGURE 29-16 Immediately after fractional radiofrequency resurfacing. Note minimal erythema in darker-skinned patient.

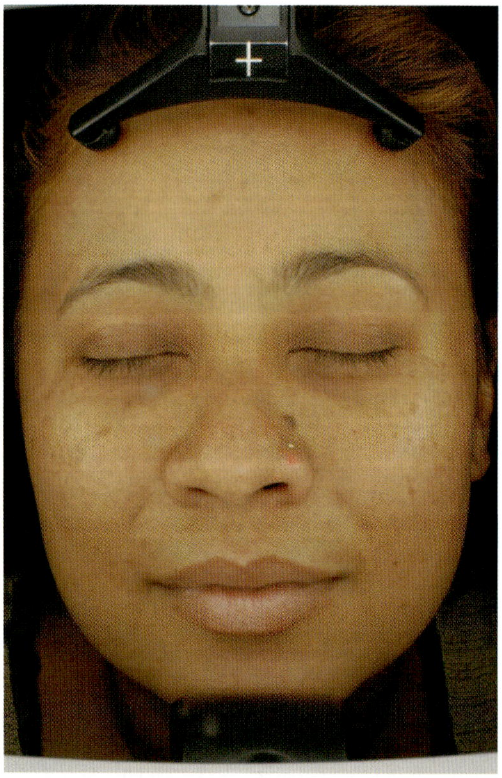

FIGURE 29-17 Before fractional radiofrequency resurfacing.

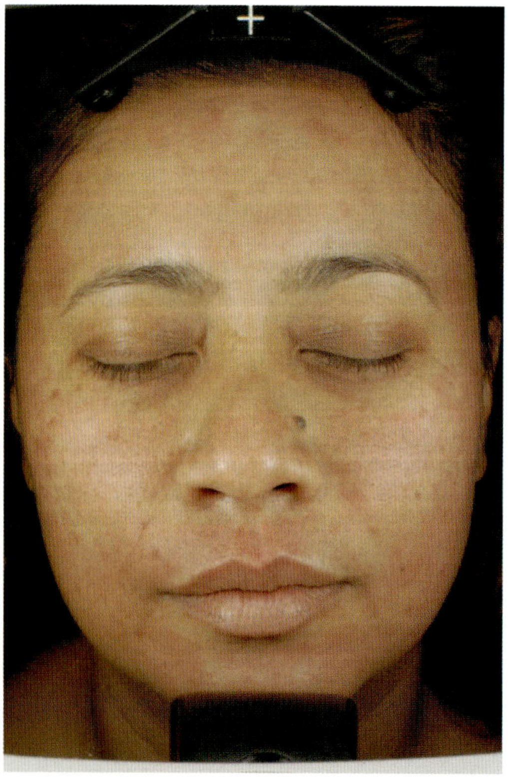

FIGURE 29-18 Six months after fractional radiofrequency resurfacing. Note tightened skin and improved nasolabial folds in darker-skinned patient.

POSTPROCEDURE CARE

After laser treatment, patients should apply noncomedogenic moisturizers to mitigate the risk of acneiform eruptions and milia. In patients with anticipated severe acne flares, oral tetracycline may be provided.[44] If the patient was treated with a nonablative fractionated laser, erythema should be expected for up to 4 days.[45] If the laser was ablative, erythema may last 4 weeks. Postinflammatory hyperpigmentation is most commonly observed in those with Fitzpatrick skin types III to VI.[44,46] The risks of treating a patient with a skin type of III to VI with a nonfractional ablative laser typically outweigh the benefits.[10,46,47] Additional recommendations are to minimize sun exposure 2 weeks before and after treatment and be religious with sunscreen use. Development of HSV reactivation occurs in up to 2% of those treated with nonablative fractionated lasers.[48] Among those treated with nonfractionated ablative lasers, the incidence may be as high as 7%.[49] To reduce the risk of an HSV eruption, oral antivirals may be given for 5 to 7 days, beginning the day of, or the day prior to, the procedure.

Patients treated with fractional lasers may rarely experience delayed purpura 3 days after treatment. For this reason, anticoagulants such as aspirin and other nonsteroidal anti-inflammatory agents are not recommended.[50] Rarely reported recall phenomena have been described with patients treated with fractional lasers. A transient, benign, erythematous patch may appear after a hot shower or sunlight exposure in the previously treated areas.[51] In those treated with RF devices, erythema and scabs may develop, in addition to pain that is experienced by up to 88% of patients.[37] A reported side effect of monopolar RF treatment is loss of adipose tissue due to heating, which may lead to contour irregularities.[52,53]

CONCLUSIONS

There have been significant advances in energy-based resurfacing devices over the past three decades. Five major classes of resurfacing devices are available, including ablative fractionated, ablative nonfractionated, nonablative fractionated, nonablative nonfractionated and radiofrequency devices. Combination devices have been studied and have demonstrated efficacy in facial skin resurfacing.[54] Choice of device depends on a patient's skin type, acceptance of postoperative downtime, and desired outcome. Technologic advancements continue to be made in energy-based resurfacing with a focus on maximizing cosmetic efficacy while minimizing subsequent postoperative pain, dyspigmentation, desquamation, and erythema.

REFERENCES

1. van Aardt R. Lasers and pulsed-light devices. In: *Pfenninger and Fowler's Procedures for Primary Care.* Vol 1. 3rd ed. Philadelphia, PA: Saunders; 2010:313-320.
2. Ross EV, McKinlay JR, Anderson RR. Why does carbon dioxide resurfacing work? A review. *Arch Dermatol.* 1999;135(4):444-454.
3. Manuskiatti W, Fitzpatrick RE, Goldman MP. Long-term effectiveness and side effects of carbon dioxide laser resurfacing for photoaged facial skin. *J Am Acad Dermatol.* 1999;40(3):401-411.
4. Ratner D, Tse Y, Marchell N, Goldman MP, Fitzpatrick RE, Fader DJ. Cutaneous laser resurfacing. *J Am Acad Dermatol.* 1999;41(3 Pt 1):365-389; quiz 390-362.
5. Ward PD, Baker SR. Long-term results of carbon dioxide laser resurfacing of the face. *Arch Facial Plast Surg.* 2008;10(4):238-243; discussion 244-245.
6. Preissig J, Hamilton K, Markus R. Current laser resurfacing technologies: a review that delves beneath the surface. *Semin Plast Surg.* 2012;26(3):109-116.
7. Alexis AF. Lasers and light-based therapies in ethnic skin: treatment options and recommendations for Fitzpatrick skin types V and VI. *Br J Dermatol.* 2013;169(Suppl 3):91-97.
8. Ciocon DH, Doshi D, Goldberg DJ. Non-ablative lasers. *Curr Probl Dermatol.* 2011;42:48-55.
9. Kirkland EB, Gladstone HB, Hantash BM. What's new in skin resurfacing and rejuvenation? *G Ital Dermatol Venereol.* 2010;145(5):583-596.
10. Metelitsa AI, Alster TS. Fractionated laser skin resurfacing treatment complications: a review. *Dermatol Surg.* 2010;36(3):299-306.
11. DeHoratius DM, Dover JS. Nonablative tissue remodeling and photorejuvenation. *Clin Dermatol.* 2007;25(5):474-479.
12. Khan MH, Sink RK, Manstein D, Eimerl D, Anderson RR. Intradermally focused infrared laser pulses: thermal effects at defined tissue depths. *Lasers Surg Med.* 2005;36(4):270-280.
13. Alexis AF, Coley MK, Nijhawan RI, et al. Nonablative fractional laser resurfacing for acne scarring in patients with Fitzpatrick skin phototypes IV-VI. *Dermatol Surg.* 2016;42(3):392-402.
14. Pham AM, Greene RM, Woolery-Lloyd H, Kaufman J, Grunebaum LD. 1550-nm nonablative laser resurfacing for facial surgical scars. *Arch Facial Plast Surg.* 2011;13(3):203-210.
15. Eilers RE Jr, Ross EV, Cohen JL, Ortiz AE. A combination approach to surgical scars. *Dermatol Surg.* 2016;42(Suppl 2):S150-S156.
16. Baca ME, Neaman KC, Rapp DA, Burton ME, Mann RJ, Renucci JD. Reduction of post-surgical scarring with the use of ablative fractional CO lasers: a pilot study using a porcine model. *Lasers Surg Med.* 2017;49(1):122-128.
17. Jared Christophel J, Elm C, Endrizzi BT, Hilger PA, Zelickson B. A randomized controlled trial of fractional laser therapy and dermabrasion for scar resurfacing. *Dermatol Surg.* 2012;38(4):595-602.
18. Ciocon DH, Engelman DE, Hussain M, Goldberg DJ. A split-face comparison of two ablative fractional carbon dioxide lasers for the treatment of photodamaged facial skin. *Dermatol Surg.* 2011;37(6):784-790.
19. Choi JE, Oh GN, Kim JY, Seo SH, Ahn HH, Kye YC. Ablative fractional laser treatment for hypertrophic scars: comparison between Er:YAG and CO2 fractional lasers. *J Dermatolog Treat.* 2014;25(4):299-303.
20. Faghihi G, Keyvan S, Asilian A, Nouraei S, Behfar S, Nilforoushzadeh MA. Efficacy of autologous platelet-rich plasma combined with fractional ablative carbon dioxide resurfacing laser in treatment of facial atrophic acne scars: a split-face randomized clinical trial. *Indian J Dermatol Venereol Leprol.* 2016;82(2):162-168.

21. Adrian RM. Pulsed carbon dioxide and long pulse 10-ms erbium-YAG laser resurfacing: a comparative clinical and histologic study. *J Cutan Laser Ther.* 1999;1(4):197-202.

22. Adrian RM. Pulsed carbon dioxide and erbium-YAG laser resurfacing: a comparative clinical and histologic study. *J Cutan Laser Ther.* 1999;1(1):29-35.

23. Kaufmann R, Hartmann A, Hibst R. Cutting and skin-ablative properties of pulsed mid-infrared laser surgery. *J Dermatol Surg Oncol.* 1994;20(2):112-118.

24. Ross EV, Swann M, Soon S, Izadpanah A, Barnette D, Davenport S. Full-face treatments with the 2790-nm erbium:YSGG laser system. *J Drugs Dermatol.* 2009;8(3):248-252.

25. Munavalli GS, Turley A, Silapunt S, Biesman B. Combining confluent and fractionally ablative modalities of a novel 2790nm YSGG laser for facial resurfacing. *Lasers Surg Med.* 2011;43(4): 273-282.

26. Rhie JW, Shim JS, Choi WS. A pilot study of skin resurfacing using the 2,790-nm erbium:YSGG laser system. *Arch Plast Surg.* 2015;42(1):52-58.

27. Ciocon DH, Hussain M, Goldberg DJ. High-fluence and high-density treatment of perioral rhytides using a new, fractionated 2,790-nm ablative erbium-doped yttrium scandium gallium garnet laser. *Dermatol Surg.* 2011;37(6):776-781.

28. Dierickx CC, Khatri KA, Tannous ZS, et al. Micro-fractional ablative skin resurfacing with two novel erbium laser systems. *Lasers Surg Med.* 2008;40(2):113-123.

29. Walgrave SE, Kist DA, Noyaner-Turley A, Zelickson BD. Minimally ablative resurfacing with the confluent 2,790 nm erbium:YSGG laser: a pilot study on safety and efficacy. *Lasers Surg Med.* 2012;44(2):103-111.

30. Kim S. Treatment of acne scars in Asian patients using a 2,790-nm fractional yttrium scandium gallium garnet laser. *Dermatol Surg.* 2011;37(10):1464-1469.

31. Kaplan H, Gat A. Clinical and histopathological results following TriPollar radiofrequency skin treatments. *J Cosmet Laser Ther.* 2009;11(2):78-84.

32. Man J, Goldberg DJ. Safety and efficacy of fractional bipolar radiofrequency treatment in Fitzpatrick skin types V-VI. *J Cosmet Laser Ther.* 2012;14(4):179-183.

33. Phothong W, Wanitphakdeedecha R, Sathaworawong A, Manuskiatti W. High versus moderate energy use of bipolar fractional radiofrequency in the treatment of acne scars: a split-face double-blinded randomized control trial pilot study. *Lasers Med Sci.* 2016;31(2):229-234.

34. Verner I. Clinical evaluation of the efficacy and safety of fractional bipolar radiofrequency for the treatment of moderate to severe acne scars. *Dermatol Ther.* 2016;29(1):24-27.

35. Park JY, Lee EG, Yoon MS, Lee HJ. The efficacy and safety of combined microneedle fractional radiofrequency and sublative fractional radiofrequency for acne scars in Asian skin. *J Cosmet Dermatol.* 2016;15(2):102-107.

36. Brightman L, Goldman MP, Taub AF. Sublative rejuvenation: experience with a new fractional radiofrequency system for skin rejuvenation and repair. *J Drugs Dermatol.* 2009;8(11 Suppl):s9-s13.

37. Lee HS, Lee DH, Won CH, et al. Fractional rejuvenation using a novel bipolar radiofrequency system in Asian skin. *Dermatol Surg.* 2011;37(11):1611-1619.

38. Gold MH, Adelglass J. Evaluation of safety and efficacy of the Tri-Fractional RF technology for treatment of facial wrinkles. *J Cosmet Laser Ther.* 2014;16(1):2-7.

39. Hantash BM, Ubeid AA, Chang H, Kafi R, Renton B. Bipolar fractional radiofrequency treatment induces neoelastogenesis and neocollagenesis. *Lasers Surg Med.* 2009;41(1):1-9.

40. Lanoue J, Goldenberg G. Acne scarring: a review of cosmetic therapies. *Cutis.* 2015;95(5):276-281.

41. El-Domyati M, Barakat M, Awad S, Medhat W, El-Fakahany H, Farag H. Microneedling therapy for atrophic acne scars: an objective evaluation. *J Clin Aesthet Dermatol.* 2015;8(7):36-42.

42. el-Domyati M, el-Ammawi TS, Medhat W, et al. Radiofrequency facial rejuvenation: evidence-based effect. *J Am Acad Dermatol.* 2011;64(3):524-535.

43. Polder KD, Bruce S. Radiofrequency: thermage. *Facial Plast Surg Clin North Am.* 2011;19(2):347-359.

44. Alster TS, Tanzi EL, Lazarus M. The use of fractional laser photothermolysis for the treatment of atrophic scars. *Dermatol Surg.* 2007;33(3):295-299.

45. Fisher GH, Geronemus RG. Short-term side effects of fractional photothermolysis. *Dermatol Surg.* 2005;31(9 Pt 2):1245-1249; discussion 1249.

46. Chan HH, Manstein D, Yu CS, Shek S, Kono T, Wei WI. The prevalence and risk factors of post-inflammatory hyperpigmentation after fractional resurfacing in Asians. *Lasers Surg Med.* 2007;39(5):381-385.

47. Kono T, Chan HH, Groff WF, et al. Prospective direct comparison study of fractional resurfacing using different fluences and densities for skin rejuvenation in Asians. *Lasers Surg Med.* 2007;39(4):311-314.

48. Setyadi HG, Jacobs AA, Markus RF. Infectious complications after nonablative fractional resurfacing treatment. *Dermatol Surg.* 2008;34(11):1595-1598.

49. Alster TS, Nanni CA. Famciclovir prophylaxis of herpes simplex virus reactivation after laser skin resurfacing. *Dermatol Surg.* 1999;25(3):242-246.

50. Fife DJ, Zachary CB. Delayed pinpoint purpura after fractionated carbon dioxide treatment in a patient taking ibuprofen in the post-operative period. *Dermatol Surg.* 2009;35(3):553.

51. Foster KW, Fincher EF, Moy RL. Heat-induced "recall" of treatment zone erythema following fractional resurfacing with a combination laser (1320 nm/1440 nm). *Arch Dermatol.* 2008;144(10):1398-1399.

52. Dawson E, Willey A, Lee K. Adverse events associated with nonablative cutaneous laser, radiofrequency, and light-based devices. *Semin Cutan Med Surg.* 2007;26(1):15-21.

53. Narins RS, Tope WD, Pope K, Ross EV. Overtreatment effects associated with a radiofrequency tissue-tightening device: rare, preventable, and correctable with subcision and autologous fat transfer. *Dermatol Surg.* 2006;32(1):115-124.

54. Gotkin RH, Sarnoff DS. A preliminary study on the safety and efficacy of a novel fractional CO(2) laser with synchronous radiofrequency delivery. *J Drugs Dermatol.* 2014;13(3):299-304.

Laser- and Light-Based Approaches to Hair Removal

30

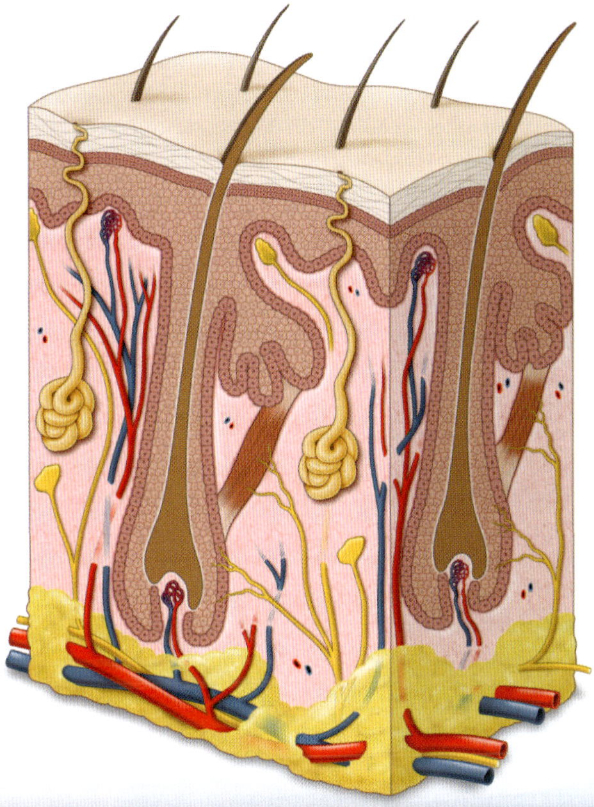

SUMMARY

- Hair removal is one of the most common aesthetic procedures performed in the United States, and the number of procedures performed each year continues to increase.
- A full treatment course for hair reduction typically consists of six to eight treatment sessions, commonly spaced 3 to 6 weeks apart.

Beginner Tips

- Light-based therapies shown to be effective for LHR include ruby lasers, alexandrite lasers, diode lasers, Nd:YAG lasers, and intense pulsed light (IPL).
- The long-pulsed Nd:YAG is the most appropriate laser in darker-skinned patients because the longer wavelength and greater depth of penetration reduces the risk of epidermal injury when combined with appropriate epidermal cooling measures. IPL can also be used for hair removal in lighter-skinned patients (skin types I–III) depending on the filter used.
- The desired clinical endpoint for LHR is perifollicular erythema and edema.

Pitfalls and Cautions

- Signs of tissue necrosis include immediate or delayed blistering, and/or graying or blackening of the skin. If tissue necrosis occurs, adjustment of the treatment parameters to increase the pulse duration and decrease the fluence should be strongly considered.
- Additional warning endpoints include a positive Nikolsky sign indicating epidermal necrosis; second- or third-degree "stamping burns," indicating inadequate cooling, possibly from skin or charred hair residue on the skin contact window; crescent-shaped burns suggesting misalignment of the laser or cryogen cooling spray; or charring caused by tissue carbonization and burning.

Expert Tips

- The hair should be freshly shaved, so that it is <1 mm in length, and so that exposed hair shafts do not lead to inadvertent epidermal burns.
- A dark-colored pen has an absorption spectrum similar to melanin, and can cause inadvertent burns and scarring, so white pencil is best used if marking the treatment site.

Patient Education Points

- Multiple treatments will be needed to attain significant clinical improvement. It is important to review this with patients prior to initiating therapy so that they understand that a single treatment will likely yield only minimal improvement.
- While some patients (and laser systems) do not regularly need topical local anesthesia prior to treatment, this is variable, and many patients may benefit from anesthetics, particularly in sensitive locations.

Don't Forget!

- Physicians treating a patient with a history of recurrent herpes simplex virus (HSV) infections in the area of treatment should consider providing a course of anti- HSV medication such as valacyclovir.
- With IPL, posttreatment effects (perifollicular erythema) are not always apparent.

Billing Pearls

- Almost all insurers in the United States exclude laser treatments from coverage.
- Patients may benefit from committing to a series of treatments, as this may allow significant cost savings.
- Pretreatment with occluded topical anesthesia can be started at home, and prescription plans may cover the cost of this medication.

30 Laser- and Light-Based Approaches to Hair Removal

INTRODUCTION

Hair removal is one of the most common aesthetic procedures performed in the United States, and the number of procedures performed each year continues to increase. Hair removal is most commonly performed to reduce cosmetically unwanted hair, although it is occasionally performed for medical purposes to treat hirsutism.

Laser, light, and energy-based devices may all be used to remove hair. Laser hair reduction (LHR) was introduced in 1996.[1] The US Food and Drug Administration (FDA) terms this removal of hair as *hair reduction* to help guide patient expectations and to accurately portray outcomes because the decrease in hair may not be permanent and all of the hairs in a treated area may not be fully removed even after several treatments. A full treatment course for hair reduction typically consists of six to eight treatment sessions, commonly spaced 3 to 6 weeks apart. The term laser hair *reduction* is also used because hair may spontaneously regrow (often several years after completion of treatment with satisfactory hair reduction), and women who become pregnant and patients on hormonal therapy may experience a regrowth of previously successfully removed hair.

Background

LHR functions based on the theory of selective photothermolysis. Drs. R.R. Anderson and J. Parrish pioneered the concept of the theory of selective photothermolysis in 1983,[2] which specified that specific wavelengths of light and pulse durations can be selectively used to target different chromophores, which are color-based or water-based structures in the skin. Effective LHR treatments use permutations of the following key parameters: (1) wavelengths that selectively target the hair follicle as a chromophore, (2) enough fluence (energy) to lead to destruction; and (3) a pulse duration short enough to confine energy to the hair follicle to selectively destroy the hair follicle without damaging the surrounding tissue (based on the thermal relaxation time). A key consideration when performing hair reduction is sparing damage to the surrounding tissue. Selective treatment of the hair follicle and sparing of injury to the surrounding skin are achieved based on the *thermal relaxation time* of the hair follicle, which is based on the diameter of the hair follicle. To account for the width of the hair follicle and to safely confine the treatment laser energy within the hair follicle, the duration of each laser pulse is spread over milliseconds (ms). The typical pulse duration range is from 30 to 50 ms.

History and Evolution of Technology

LHR was introduced in 1996. Over the years, LHR technology has expanded to include lasers that were pioneered to be safely used in skin of color with the advent of the neodymium-doped yttrium-aluminum-garnet (Nd:YAG) 1064-nm long-pulsed laser. Diode lasers allow for the largest treatment spot sizes on the commercial market, enabling the fastest treatment of large surface areas. In recent years, other nonlaser energy-based devices have been found to reduce hair, such as radiofrequency and microwave technology.

Mechanism of Action

The mechanism of action associated with LHR is based on the theory of selective photothermolysis, wherein the laser wavelength used for treatment can selectively target a chromophore in the skin—in this case, melanin in the hair follicle—to heat the hair follicle and cause selective destruction of the follicle. Clinically, hair reduction works best with dark hair (black) on a background of fair skin. White hair is a challenge to remove, as the hairs and hair follicle lack sufficient melanin for the laser to selectively target the hair follicle for destruction. Radiofrequency and microwave technology work to remove hair follicles by bulk heating the dermis to a temperature that is hot enough to induce hair follicle death and ultimate reduction in hair.

LASER HAIR REDUCTION METHODS

Lasers used for LHR use wavelengths of 600 to 1200 nm in the red and near-infrared portion of the electromagnetic spectrum to target melanin as their primary chromophore. Light-based therapies shown to be effective for LHR include ruby lasers, alexandrite lasers, diode lasers, Nd:YAG lasers, and intense pulsed light (IPL).[3] The pulse durations used depend on the thermal relaxation time of a hair follicle and typically range from 30 to 50 ms. In certain circumstances, a wider range of pulse durations is used, which range from 10 to 100 ms, and pulse durations of up to 1000 ms have been used, although they are uncommon in routine clinical practice.[4] There are myriad potential indications for LHR, including aesthetic reasons, hirsutism, inflammatory conditions (pilonidal sinus disease, hidradenitis suppurativa, pseudofolliculitis barbae), congenital conditions, aberrant hair growth from surgical intervention, reduction of hair in those undergoing hormonal therapy, and treatment of scrotal skin prior to gender reassignment vaginoplasty.[5,6]

The choice of laser for hair removal depends mainly on skin type. The long-pulsed Nd:YAG is the most appropriate laser in darker skinned patients because the longer wavelength and greater depth of penetration reduce the risk of epidermal injury when combined with appropriate epidermal cooling measures. IPL can also be used for hair removal in lighter skinned patients (skin types I to III) depending on the filter used.[3]

PATIENT SELECTION AND SAFETY

Clinicians should employ safety precautions when using lasers and light-based devices. Laser treatment rooms should have opaque windows and warning signs to indicate when the laser is in use. The patient and all personnel involved in the procedure should wear wavelength-specific eye protection. Laser hair removal within the orbital rim should be avoided due to risk of pinhole vision defects.[7,8] A plume evacuator may be used, as the plume may contain infectious viral particles and contains carcinogenic matter.[9,10]

Because the target chromophore of LHR is melanin, the ideal patient for the LHR procedure is someone with light skin and thick, dark hair. Patients with darker skin tend to have a decreased contrast between the color of the hair and the skin, leading to a higher risk of inadvertent energy absorption in the surrounding skin. For this reason, a laser test spot in an inconspicuous area may be employed. It is also helpful to perform a laser test spot in the area being treated, as the skin response to laser therapy may vary and differ in different anatomic sites.

Initial evaluation of a patient should including a detailed medical history, including screening for endocrinologic and menstrual irregularities that may signal a treatable medical cause of hirsutism.[1] Clinicians should evaluate patients with sudden-onset lanugo-type hypertrichosis for a paraneoplastic syndrome or eating disorders.[11-13] They should also screen for potential contraindications or relative contraindications of treatment, including photosensitivity, photosensitizing medications, daily use or recent use (within 1 week before or after) of facial cleansing brushes, koebnerizing conditions such as psoriasis and vitiligo,[14] recently tanned skin, history of poor wound healing or increased risk of skin infections, and a history of keloidal scars.

Clinicians treating a patient with a history of recurrent herpes simplex virus (HSV) infections in the area of treatment should consider providing a course of anti-HSV medication such as valacyclovir or acyclovir. There is evidence for the safety of LHR during isotretinoin therapy,[15-18] suggesting that the prior recommendation against LHR for 6 to 12 months after isotretinoin treatment should be reconsidered.

PREPARATION

Prior to initiation of the LHR procedure, the clinician should discuss the risks, benefits, alternatives, potential side effects, and expected results of the procedure. A discussion of expected results should include mention that hair reduction may not be permanent; the potential for poorer response in thinner or lighter colored hairs; potential for no response for red, gray, or white hairs; and the need for multiple treatments, often in a range of six to eight treatments. Alternatives to LHR should be reviewed, including trimming, shaving, bleaching, waxing, tweezing, threading, use of chemical depilatory agents, electrolysis, and thermolysis.[19]

Clinicians should familiarize themselves with the appearance of both therapeutic and warning end points to appropriately tailor the laser settings to achieve clinical efficacy while minimizing adverse effects.[20,21] These visual signs are evidence of early tissue reactions that are either desirable, such as perifollicular erythema and edema, or undesirable, such as epidermal necrosis. The desired clinical end point for LHR is perifollicular erythema and edema.[21] Signs of tissue necrosis include immediate or delayed blistering and/or graying or blackening of the skin. If tissue necrosis occurs, adjustment of the treatment parameters to increase the pulse duration and decrease the fluence should be strongly considered. Additionally, reassessment of the treatment device is recommended to ensure compatibility with the patient's skin type. It is also important to exercise medical caution in treating patients with recently tanned skin. Additional warning end points for LHR include a positive Nikolsky sign indicating epidermal necrosis; second- or third-degree "stamping burns," indicating inadequate cooling, possibly from skin or charred hair residue on the skin contact window; crescent-shaped burns suggesting misalignment of the laser or cryogen cooling spray; or charring caused by tissue carbonization and burning.[20]

The patient's skin should be prepared by cleaning with soap and water and degreasing the relevant areas with alcohol wipes or a similar compound. The skin should be free of personal care products such as deodorant, makeup, lotions, or self-tanner. The hair should be freshly shaved, so that it is less than 1 mm in length and so that exposed hair shafts do not lead to inadvertent epidermal burns. Since much of the targeted melanin is in the hair shaft, patients should also avoid procedures that remove the hair shaft such as waxing, plucking, or electrolysis for at least 6 weeks. Depending on the type of laser used, a layer of either refrigerated or room-temperature transparent, water-based gel may be applied to act as a heat sink for epidermal protection.[22]

The use of topical anesthesia is not universally required for laser hair removal but may be indicated depending on patient tolerance of discomfort and the anatomic site.[23] Sensitive regions of the body such as the upper lip or groin area may benefit from a 30-minute to 1-hour incubation of a topical anesthetic such as lidocaine, prilocaine, Betacaine, or tetracaine.[1,24] Forced cooled air can be soothing to the patient during and after the procedure.

The laser and cooling device should be tested to make sure the system is working appropriately. The clinician should choose appropriate settings based on the patient's prior treatments and skin type. Some clinicians recommend marking the site, but it is important to remember that a dark colored pen has an absorption spectrum similar to melanin and can cause inadvertent burns and scarring, so white pencil is best used if marking the treatment site.[25] Many others have not found a need to mark the treatment site.

TYPES OF TREATMENTS

Alexandrite Laser

Introduction: Finkel et al[22] first used the long-pulsed alexandrite laser for laser hair removal in 1997. This laser has a wavelength of 755 nm, which allows for deep penetration into the dermis, with a relatively low affinity for hemoglobin.[22] This laser has several convenient features that explain why it is one of the most widely used lasers for LHR. It has a flexible optical fiber arm that allows maneuverability across different body sites. These lasers are generally compact machines that can fit into smaller rooms as long as there is adequate ventilation, and the large spot sizes (up to 18 mm) also make it easier to treat large surface areas.[26] The cooling systems for these lasers vary depending on the model and include cold air cooling, contact cooling, and dynamic cooling.[7] Long-term efficacy for LHR varies based on number of treatments and ranges from 4% hair reduction at 6 months after one treatment[27] to 40% to 74% hair reduction at 6 months after three treatments[28,29] to 78% to 85% hair reduction at 1 year after four to five treatments.[30,31]

Several studies comparing the alexandrite laser to other lasers and light devices have found alexandrite to be noninferior to diode,[29,30,32,33] IPL,[34-36] and Nd:YAG lasers.[32] Another study comparing the efficacy of alexandrite versus a combination of alexandrite and Nd:YAG found no additional benefit to Nd:YAG over alexandrite alone.[32] A study of 18 patients found no significant difference in efficacy or side effects between long-pulse and short-pulse alexandrite laser, although the short-pulse alexandrite procedure was about five times faster than the long-pulse procedure.[37] In a study of 389 patients comparing long-pulse alexandrite, short-pulse alexandrite, and IPL, Marayiannis et al[36] found that the efficacy of the different lasers was the same, although the long-pulse alexandrite had a higher risk of transient erythema, edema, crusting, dyspigmentation, and hair induction.

Procedure: Using the flexible handpiece, an appropriate spot size, fluence, and pulse duration are selected. It is recommended that an inconspicuous test spot be performed before treating the full area to check the settings and ensure an appropriate therapeutic end point of skin erythema without erosion, char, or sloughing. One study of 36 patients showed equivalent 6-month efficacy for pulse durations of 5, 10, and 20 ms using a 10-mm spot size and fluences ranging from 15 to 20 J/cm². Hyperpigmentation occurred in all treatment groups but was less severe and more transient in the 20-ms pulse duration group.[27]

Special Considerations: An alexandrite laser is a good choice for LHR in type I to III skin (although it can be used up to skin type IV) and is generally fairly effective and well tolerated. Caution should be exercised in using alexandrite lasers in darker skinned patients due to the increased risk of adverse events.

Diode

Introduction: Diode lasers are based on the use of semiconductors such as gallium arsenide and aluminum gallium arsenide and have wavelengths of 755,[38] 800 to 810, 940, and 980 nm.[7,39] Laser hair removal is usually performed with 800- to 810-nm diode lasers, although a newer 755-nm diode laser has been developed and was shown to have efficacy in a single-patient study comparable to a 755-nm alexandrite laser.[38] The advantages of diode lasers are that they are relatively small and compact and generally lower cost.[39] The longer wavelength allows deeper penetration into the skin, which allows improved treatment of the hair follicle while limiting damage to the epidermal melanin.[40] This laser type can be used to treat patients with Fitzpatrick skin types I to IV or V.[7] The hair count reduction of the long pulse diode laser ranges from 22% to 74%, depending on the study and number of treatments administered.[4,29,41-45] Grunewald et al[46] saw hair reduction rates of 74% that persisted after 18 months using a fluence of 24 to 30 J/cm², a pulse duration of 12 ms, and a spot size of 50 mm × 12 mm for a total of six treatments.

Like the other hair removal modalities, repeat treatments are important for success. One study found that after two treatments, the mean hair reduction was 28%, which increased to 78% after three treatments.[47] Studies on the appropriate interval between treatments are lacking, but one study found that shorter treatment intervals led to more hair reduction, with 45-day intervals performing better than 60-day and 90-day intervals.[47]

Procedure: The clinician should choose appropriate settings based on the patient's skin type, prior experience, and settings available on the particular machine. Spot size may affect efficacy in addition to speed of treatment. One study that kept fluence, pulse duration, and epidermal cooling constant between groups found that a larger spot size of 10 × 30 mm had a 50% mean hair clearance compared to 39% for a spot size of 10 × 10 mm.[48]

If there is a cooling tip, the handpiece should be placed firmly and directly on the area to be treated for about 0.5 seconds to allow the epidermis to cool, and the laser pulse should then be delivered. Firm pressure also compresses the skin, effectively decreasing the depth of follicular structures and concomitantly blanching the underlying vasculature, which helps minimize laser energy absorption of the competing chromophore oxyhemoglobin.[42]

Although the diode is not the laser of choice for patients with types V or VI skin, for patients with medium skin tones, the clinician should start with lower fluences and wider pulse widths for patients with darker colored skin. The use of a diode laser with darker skin types is associated with a higher risk of blistering and either temporary or permanent dyspigmentation than in lighter skinned patients.[49] If blistering occurs, standard skin wound care measures are recommended.

Special Considerations: Classic diode lasers are appropriate for treatment of types I to IV skin. With some newer contact cooling technologies, diode lasers may be safe for treatment of type V skin, although a test spot should always be performed. Ensuring complete skin contact is important when using contact-based cooling. It is important to note that patients may sometimes inadvertently move and create distance between the cooled tip and the skin and increase the risk of blister formation.

Nd:YAG

Introduction: The Nd:YAG laser emits 1064-nm light in the infrared spectrum. Of all the laser systems used for hair removal, the 1064-nm Nd:YAG is considered the safest laser for hair removal in darker skin types[50] and can be used in all skin types.[51-53] The Nd:YAG has the deepest depth of penetration and a wavelength that is at the tail end of the melanin absorption curve, so it better bypasses epidermal melanin. However, it is also one of the least effective of the hair removal light-based therapies.[32,52] In one study comparing alexandrite, diode, and

Nd:YAG, the percentage of hair reduction was 70.3%, 59.7%, ad 47.4% respectively.[32] One study specifically looking at the use of IPL versus Nd:YAG in patients with type IV to VI skin found better efficacy and patient satisfaction with the Nd:YAG laser.[54]

Overall, the Nd:YAG laser has been found to have hair reduction rates ranging from 27% to 79%,[32,54,55] with more treatments (five to six) associated with more hair reduction.[56] One study also found that treatment for laser hair removal also incidentally led to a decrease in sweating in the axillae.[57]

Procedure: After ensuring that all the equipment is functioning appropriately, cleaning the skin, and making sure the hair is shaved to less than 1 mm, the clinician should next conduct a test spot. A test spot is particularly important in patients with darker skin who are undergoing laser hair removal to avoid using settings that will lead to adverse effects. The test spot should show appropriate perifollicular erythema and edema without signs of overtreatment (eg, immediate graying, blistering, vesiculation, or induced epidermal sloughing). When the appropriate settings are chosen, proceed with covering the area with slightly overlapping pulses to achieve uniform treatment.

Special Considerations: The Nd:YAG laser is appropriate for hair removal in all skin types, although care should be taken to reduce the fluence and perform a test spot prior to treating the whole area. Repeat treatments are typically necessary, with the amount of hair removal proportional to the number of treatments administered. While this laser is the best choice for hair removal in patients with darker colored skin, treatment of fine hairs in these patients is still difficult because the fluences required for hair reduction may be associated with increased risk of adverse effects in this population.[58]

Intense Pulsed Light

Introduction: In contrast to the traditional lasers discussed so far, IPL is a xenon polychromatic broadband flashlamp that emits wavelengths from 500 to 1200 nm. With IPL, energy stored in a computer-controlled capacitor bank is released and passed through xenon gas, leading to conversion of electrical energy into optical energy and the emission of a bright light.[59] Optical filters are used to further restrict noncoherent light beams to a therapeutic range. Both lasers and IPL operate based on the concept of photothermolysis, although IPL emits a spectrum of light rather than a single wavelength. IPL therefore allows the treatment of several different chromophores at one time. For instance, melanin has an absorption spectrum from 250 to 1200 nm. Oxyhemoglobin has absorption peaks at 418, 542, and 577 nm, and collagen fibers absorb light in the 400- to 600-nm range.[60] Because of the competing chromophores, filters for light below 620 nm are often used with IPL for hair removal to more selectively target melanin. The broad range of wavelengths emitted allows versatility in treatments and the ability to target multiple different problems at once. However, this feature also requires well-trained clinicians to avoid inadvertently causing nonspecific thermal damage.[1] In most IPL systems, the pulse duration ranges from 0.2 to 100 ms, and it should generally be set to be less than the thermal relaxation time of the intended target.[60]

IPL has several advantages and disadvantages compared to lasers. IPL is relatively lower cost and has a large handpiece that can be used to quickly treat large surface areas. However, that large handpiece can also be heavy and cumbersome, and the need for direct skin contact makes it more difficult to see the site and immediate effects of the area that is being treated. IPL also does not typically yield the same immediate local visible skin changes as lasers, so it is more difficult to delineate treated from untreated areas, leading to potential treatment gaps or pulse stacking. Lastly, depending on the unit used, the emitted spectrum and fluence can vary from pulse to pulse, particularly if the capacitor bank is small. This variation can potentially lead to inconsistent or less predictable results.[59]

Efficacy of IPL ranges from 34% to 85% hair reduction at 6- to 12-month follow-up.[61-67] In comparisons with diode,[61-64,68] alexandrite, and Nd:YAG, IPL was found to lead to the same or inferior results. Of the studies comparing diode and IPL, two studies found that patients had more pain with diode treatment,[61,64] and the other showed greater pain with IPL treatment.[63]

The use of filters for IPL depend on the treatment indication, and in laser hair removal, wavelengths below 620 nm are typically filtered out. Because of the broad spectrum of light applied with IPL, it is most appropriate for patients with skin types I to III, although it can be used with caution in patients with skin type IV. Higher skin types require longer wavelengths, longer pulse durations, and effective epidermal cooling to help prevent adverse effects.

Procedure: After appropriate equipment checks, skin preparation, and safety checks, the procedure may be started. Both the clinician and patient should wear broad-spectrum eye protection appropriate for IPL. An optical coupling gel should be placed on the surface of the skin. A test spot in an inconspicuous location may be performed in order to evaluate for potential adverse effects as well as therapeutic efficacy of the chosen settings. When treating an area, there should be less than 10% overlap between spots, and melanocytic lesions or tattoos that are incidentally in the treatment area should be avoided or covered with nonabsorbent white paper.[59]

Special Considerations: With IPLs that use dichroic filters to filter out unwanted wavelengths of light, 10% to 15% of the filtered wavelengths can still pass through and have the potential to cause epidermal damage. Therefore, methods of protecting the epidermis, such as cooling, are very important regardless of the filter used.[69]

Postprocedure Considerations

The clinician should look for immediate perifollicular edema and erythema as a therapeutic end point (**Figure 30-1**), except for the IPL, where posttreatment effects are not always apparent. The area can be cooled for comfort with wet gauze, cool compresses, ice packs, cold gel packs, or forced cool air. The use of a lower to medium-potency topical corticosteroids is dependent on the clinician's preference and treatment site, but should be more strongly considered in case of burns, blistering, erosions, or more inflammatory reactions in darker skinned patients. The patient

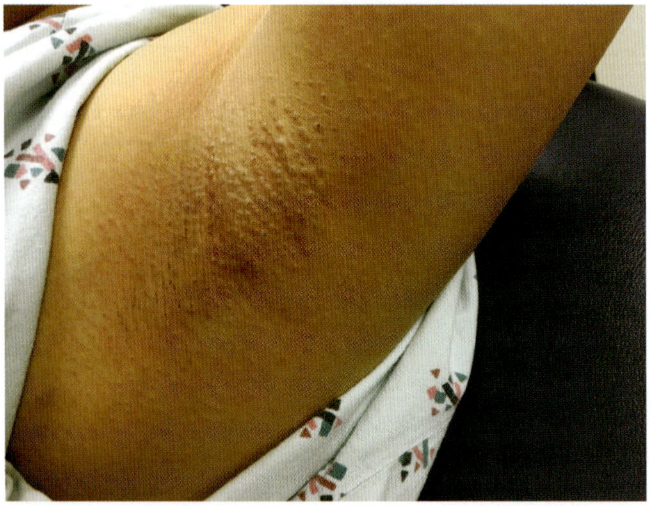

FIGURE 30-1 The clinician should look for immediate perifollicular edema and erythema as a therapeutic end point.

should be informed that it may take several weeks for the hair to shed and to take care with sun avoidance to decrease the risk of postinflammatory hyperpigmentation. Repeat treatments should be performed in 4 to 6 weeks.

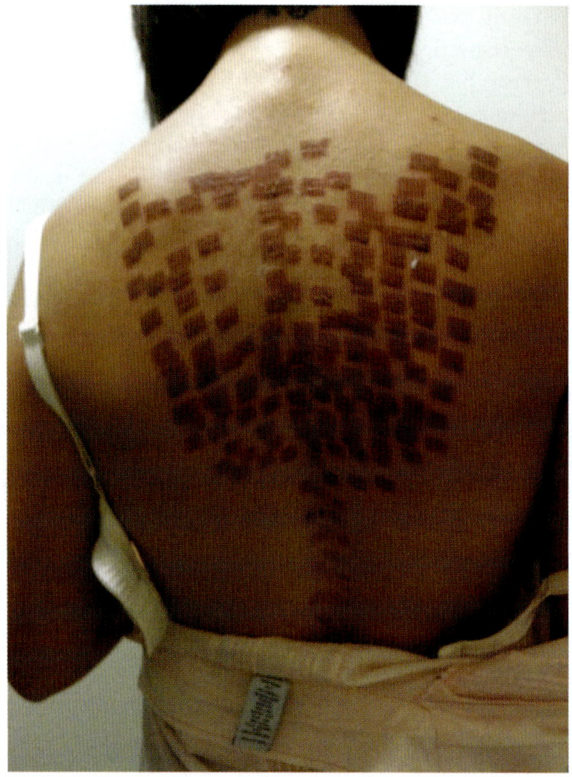

FIGURE 30-2 Intense pulsed light (IPL) treatment for hair reduction in skin of color may result in burns that present as linear erythema and subsequent postinflammatory dyspigmentation and/or scarring.

Complications

Despite the frequency of laser hair removal, significant or severe side effects are still rare. Many of the complications that can be seen with laser therapy are common to different types of lasers and light-based therapies. Patients can experience pain, blistering, erosions, hyperpigmentation, hypopigmentation, folliculitis, crusting, and very rarely permanent scarring.[70-72] Epidermal damage can occur with inadequate or dysfunctional cooling. This complication can also occur if hair is not adequately shaved. The charred hair can accumulate on the cooling tip during treatment without being recognized, interfering with the functionality of the cooling tip. Unwanted side effects may arise from choosing a laser or light device with inadequate cooling or light wavelengths that compete for melanin in darkly pigmented patients. For example, IPL treatment for hair reduction in skin of color may result in burns that present as linear erythema and subsequent postinflammatory dyspigmentation and/or scarring (**Figure 30-2**).[73]

Although rare, there have been reports of patients experiencing paradoxical hypertrichosis within or near treatment sites, also termed terminalization, induction, and terminal hair growth.[74-80] All lasers are thought to have the potential to induce terminalization of hairs, with an estimated incidence ranging from 0.6% to 10% (although the 10% estimate was found in a nonrepresentative patient population).[75] In situations where there is increased hair growth at adjacent, untreated sites, the causal relationship between laser treatment and terminal hair growth is undetermined, since it seems unlikely that the optical energy is directly responsible for changes in the dermal papillae that ultimately determine hair type.[76] Risk factors for paradoxical hypertrichosis include obesity, polycystic ovarian syndrome, androgen hormonal irregularities, darker skin phenotype, and middle age.[76] The mechanism of this phenomenon is unknown. Increasing fluences and changing laser wavelengths can sometimes successfully reverse paradoxical hypertrichosis, but some cases do not respond and only continue to worsen.

The development of Fox-Fordyce disease (FFD) or apocrine miliaria is a newly described complication of LHR therapy.[81-85] Patients typically present with monomorphic skin-colored to yellowish, pruritic, follicular or perifollicular papules that are classically limited to apocrine areas. The pathogenesis of FFD is unknown, but it is thought that keratinocyte dysfunction leads to follicular plugging with subsequent dilation and extravasation of sweat into the surrounding tissues, leading to a chronic inflammatory response.[81]

While performing laser hair removal, the clinician should try to avoid the treatment of melanocytic nevi in the field. The long-term sequelae and effects of laser therapy on melanocytic nevi are unknown, and there have been reports of changing nevi following diode laser treatment for hair removal.[86] The treatment of melanocytic nevi is controversial, and there have been several cases reported of melanoma either arising or discovered after laser therapy, arguing that laser clinicians should be cautious in their use of lasers on pigmented lesions.[87-90] In addition, treatment over a tattoo can lead to burns because of pigment absorption of laser energy.[91]

OTHER TECHNOLOGIES: RADIOFREQUENCY AND MICROWAVES

There have been other technologies based on electromagnetic energy that have been used for laser hair removal, such as radiofrequency and microwaves.

Radiofrequency Hair Reduction

In one study, researchers used a combination of IPL and radiofrequency in patients with white or light-colored hairs. The concept behind the combination of energy sources was the ability to apply a level of optical energy that is safe for all skin types while compensating for the reduced laser intensities with the additional radiofrequency energy. They used fluences of 24 to 30 J/cm^2 and radiofrequency energy of 20 J/cm^3. They found an average of 52% clearance with blonde hair, a 44% clearance of white hair, and overall an 80% to 85% clearance in darker haired patients after four treatments. However, the study lacked a control or other comparison group.[92,93]

Microwave Hair Reduction

A new device using microwaves (MiraSmooth) was recently cleared by the FDA for hair reduction. It uses microwaves to heat the area of treated skin, which leads to destruction of sweat glands and hair follicles and concurrent decrease in sweating, as well as hair reduction. Although long-term and larger studies are lacking so far, one small study of seven people found an average hair reduction of 43%.[94]

CONCLUSIONS

Hair reduction is the most common laser and energy-based device treatment performed in the United States. There are a variety of laser and energy-based device methods to reduce hair, and technical innovations in hair reduction continue to occur. These methods are generally safe for patients and yield excellent outcomes, and an appreciation of the range of devices and their appropriate application to the desired patient population are of significant value to the clinician.

REFERENCES

1. Gan SD, Graber EM. Laser hair removal: a review. *Dermatol Surg.* 2013;39(6):823-838.
2. Anderson RR, Parrish JA. Selective photothermolysis: precise microsurgery by selective absorption of pulsed radiation. *Science.* 1983;220(4596):524-527.
3. Husain Z, Alster TS. The role of lasers and intense pulsed light technology in dermatology. *Clin Cosmet Investig Dermatol.* 2016;9:29-40.
4. Rogachefsky AS, Silapunt S, Goldberg DJ. Evaluation of a new super-long-pulsed 810 nm diode laser for the removal of unwanted hair: the concept of thermal damage time. *Dermatol Surg.* 2002;28(5):410-414.
5. Zhang WR, Garrett GL, Arron ST, Garcia MM. Laser hair removal for genital gender affirming surgery. *Transl Androl Urol.* 2016;5(3):381-387.
6. Koch D, Pratsou P, Szczecinska W, Lanigan S, Abdullah A. The diverse application of laser hair removal therapy: a tertiary laser unit's experience with less common indications and a literature overview. *Lasers Med Sci.* 2015;30(1):453-467.
7. Ibrahimi OA, Avram MM, Hanke CW, Kilmer SL, Anderson RR. Laser hair removal. *Dermatol Ther.* 2011;24(1):94-107.
8. Robinson JK. *Surgery of the Skin: Procedural Dermatology.* Philadelphia, PA: Elsevier Mosby; 2014.
9. Garden JM, O'Banion MK, Bakus AD, Olson C. Viral disease transmitted by laser-generated plume (aerosol). *Arch Dermatol.* 2002;138(10):1303-1307.
10. Capizzi PJ, Clay RP, Battey MJ. Microbiologic activity in laser resurfacing plume and debris. *Lasers Surg Med.* 1998;23(3):172-174.
11. Slee PH, van der Waal RI, Schagen van Leeuwen JH, et al. Paraneoplastic hypertrichosis lanuginosa acquisita: uncommon or overlooked? *Br J Dermatol.* 2007;157(6):1087-1092.
12. Vulink AJ, ten Bokkel Huinink D. Acquired hypertrichosis lanuginosa: a rare cutaneous paraneoplastic syndrome. *J Clin Oncol.* 2007;25(12):1625-1626.
13. Schulze UM, Pettke-Rank CV, Kreienkamp M, et al. Dermatologic findings in anorexia and bulimia nervosa of childhood and adolescence. *Pediatr Dermatol.* 1999;16(2):90-94.
14. Mavilia L, Mercuri SR. Koebner's phenomenon induced vitiligo following Nd:YAG laser epilation treatment in a woman with a past history of a Sutton nevus. *Dermatol Ther.* 2014;27(6):355-356.
15. Khatri KA. Diode laser hair removal in patients undergoing isotretinoin therapy. *Dermatol Surg.* 2004;30(9):1205-1207; discussion 1207.
16. Khatri KA. The safety of long-pulsed Nd:YAG laser hair removal in skin types III-V patients during concomitant isotretinoin therapy. *J Cosmet Laser Ther.* 2009;11(1):56-60.
17. Khatri KA, Garcia V. Light-assisted hair removal in patients undergoing isotretinoin therapy. *Dermatol Surg.* 2006;32(6):875-877.
18. Chandrashekar BS, Varsha DV, Vasanth V, Jagadish P, Madura C, Rajashekar ML. Safety of performing invasive acne scar treatment and laser hair removal in patients on oral isotretinoin: a retrospective study of 110 patients. *Int J Dermatol.* 2014;53(10):1281-1285.
19. Wanitphakdeedecha R, Alster TS. Physical means of treating unwanted hair. *Dermatol Ther.* 2008;21(5):392-401.
20. Wanner M, Sakamoto FH, Avram MM, Anderson RR. Immediate skin responses to laser and light treatments: warning endpoints: how to avoid side effects. *J Am Acad Dermatol.* 2016;74(5):807-819.
21. Wanner M, Sakamoto FH, Avram MM, et al. Immediate skin responses to laser and light treatments: therapeutic endpoints: how to obtain efficacy. *J Am Acad Dermatol.* 2016;74(5):821-833.
22. Finkel B, Eliezri YD, Waldman A, Slatkine M. Pulsed alexandrite laser technology for noninvasive hair removal. *J Clin Laser Med Surg.* 1997;15(5):225-229.
23. Aimonetti JM, Ribot-Ciscar E. Pain management in photoepilation. *J Cosmet Dermatol.* 2016;15(2):194-199.
24. Ballin AC, França K, Nouri K. Anesthesia for lasers. In: Nouri K, ed. *Handbook of Lasers in Dermatology.* New York, NY: Springer; 2014:37-54.

25. Lee SJ, Yeo IK, Park KY, Seo SJ. Second-degree burns on skin marked for photoepilation: the need for white pencil use in cutaneous marking. *J Am Acad Dermatol.* 2014;71(1):e13.
26. Al-Dhalimi MA, Kadhum MJ. A split-face comparison of facial hair removal with the long-pulsed alexandrite laser and intense pulsed light system. *J Cosmet Laser Ther.* 2015;17(5):267-272.
27. Nanni CA, Alster TS. Long-pulsed alexandrite laser-assisted hair removal at 5, 10, and 20 millisecond pulse durations. *Lasers Surg Med.* 1999;24(5):332-337.
28. Gorgu M, Aslan G, Akoz T, Erdogan B. Comparison of alexandrite laser and electrolysis for hair removal. *Dermatol Surg.* 2000;26(1):37-41.
29. Handrick C, Alster TS. Comparison of long-pulsed diode and long-pulsed alexandrite lasers for hair removal: a long-term clinical and histologic study. *Dermatol Surg.* 2001;27(7):622-626.
30. Eremia S, Li C, Newman N. Laser hair removal with alexandrite versus diode laser using four treatment sessions: 1-year results. *Dermatol Surg.* 2001;27(11):925-929; discussion 929-930.
31. Lloyd JR, Mirkov M. Long-term evaluation of the long-pulsed alexandrite laser for the removal of bikini hair at shortened treatment intervals. *Dermatol Surg.* 2000;26(7):633-637.
32. Khoury JG, Saluja R, Goldman MP. Comparative evaluation of long-pulse alexandrite and long-pulse Nd:YAG laser systems used individually and in combination for axillary hair removal. *Dermatol Surg.* 2008;34(5):665-670; discussion 670-661.
33. Bouzari N, Tabatabai H, Abbasi Z, Firooz A, Dowlati Y. Laser hair removal: comparison of long-pulsed Nd:YAG, long-pulsed alexandrite, and long-pulsed diode lasers. *Dermatol Surg.* 2004;30(4 Pt 1): 498-502.
34. McGill DJ, Hutchison C, McKenzie E, McSherry E, Mackay IR. A randomised, split-face comparison of facial hair removal with the alexandrite laser and intense pulsed light system. *Lasers Surg Med.* 2007;39(10):767-772.
35. Amin SP, Goldberg DJ. Clinical comparison of four hair removal lasers and light sources. *J Cosmet Laser Ther.* 2006;8(2):65-68.
36. Marayiannis KB, Vlachos SP, Savva MP, Kontoes PP. Efficacy of long- and short-pulse alexandrite lasers compared with an intense pulsed light source for epilation: a study on 532 sites in 389 patients. *J Cosmet Laser Ther.* 2003;5(3-4):140-145.
37. Boss WK Jr, Usal H, Thompson RC, Fiorillo MA. A comparison of the long-pulse and short-pulse alexandrite laser hair removal systems. *Ann Plast Surg.* 1999;42(4):381-384.
38. Paasch U, Wagner JA, Paasch HW. Novel 755-nm diode laser vs. conventional 755-nm scanned alexandrite laser: side-by-side comparison pilot study for thorax and axillary hair removal. *J Cosmet Laser Ther.* 2015;17(4):189-193.
39. Jelínková H. *Lasers for Medical Applications: Diagnostics, Therapy, and Surgery.* New York, NY: Elsevier; 2016.
40. Mustafa FH, Jaafar MS, Ismail AH, Mutter KN. Comparison of alexandrite and diode lasers for hair removal in dark and medium skin: which is better? *J Lasers Med Sci.* 2014;5(4):188-193.
41. Baugh WP, Trafeli JP, Barnette DJ, Jr., Ross EV. Hair reduction using a scanning 800 nm diode laser. *Dermatol Surg.* 2001;27(4): 358-364.
42. Campos VB, Dierickx CC, Farinelli WA, Lin TY, Manuskiatti W, Anderson RR. Hair removal with an 800-nm pulsed diode laser. *J Am Acad Dermatol.* 2000;43(3):442-447.
43. Fiskerstrand EJ, Svaasand LO, Nelson JS. Hair removal with long pulsed diode lasers: a comparison between two systems with different pulse structures. *Lasers Surg Med.* 2003;32(5):399-404.
44. Lou WW, Quintana AT, Geronemus RG, Grossman MC. Prospective study of hair reduction by diode laser (800 nm) with long-term follow-up. *Dermatol Surg.* 2000;26(5):428-432.
45. Williams RM, Gladstone HB, Moy RL. Hair removal using an 810 nm gallium aluminum arsenide semiconductor diode laser: a preliminary study. *Dermatologic Surgery.* 1999;25(12):935-937.
46. Grunewald S, Bodendorf MO, Zygouris A, Simon JC, Paasch U. Long-term efficacy of linear-scanning 808 nm diode laser for hair removal compared to a scanned alexandrite laser. *Lasers Surg Med.* 2014;46(1):13-19.
47. Bouzari N, Tabatabai H, Abbasi Z, Firooz A, Dowlati Y. Hair removal using an 800-nm diode laser: comparison at different treatment intervals of 45, 60, and 90 days. *Int J Dermatol.* 2005;44(1):50-53.
48. Jo SJ, Kim JY, Ban J, Lee Y, Kwon O, Koh W. Efficacy and safety of hair removal with a long-pulsed diode laser depending on the spot size: a randomized, evaluators-blinded, left-right study. *Ann Dermatol.* 2015;27(5):517-522.
49. Richter AL, Barrera J, Markus RF, Brissett A. Laser skin treatment in non-Caucasian patients. *Facial Plast Surg Clin North Am.* 2014;22(3):439-446.
50. Breadon JY, Barnes CA. Comparison of adverse events of laser and light-assisted hair removal systems in skin types IV-VI. *J Drugs Dermatol.* 2007;6(1):40-46.
51. Chan CS, Dover JS. Nd:YAG laser hair removal in Fitzpatrick skin types IV to VI. *J Drugs Dermatol.* 2013;12(3):366-367.
52. Tanzi EL, Alster TS. Long-pulsed 1064-nm Nd:YAG laser-assisted hair removal in all skin types. *Dermatol Surg.* 2004;30(1):13-17.
53. Nanda S, Bansal S. Long pulsed Nd:YAG laser with inbuilt cool sapphire tip for long term hair reduction on type IV and V skin: a prospective analysis of 200 patients. *Indian J Dermatol Venereol Leprol.* 2010;76(6):677-681.
54. Ismail SA. Long-pulsed Nd:YAG laser vs. intense pulsed light for hair removal in dark skin: a randomized controlled trial. *Br J Dermatol.* 2012;166(2):317-321.
55. Goldberg DJ, Silapunt S. Hair removal using a long-pulsed Nd:YAG laser: comparison at fluences of 50, 80, and 100 J/cm. *Dermatol Surg.* 2001;27(5):434-436.
56. Lorenz S, Brunnberg S, Landthaler M, Hohenleutner U. Hair removal with the long pulsed Nd:YAG laser: a prospective study with one year follow-up. *Lasers Surg Med.* 2002;30(2):127-134.
57. Letada PR, Landers JT, Uebelhoer NS, Shumaker PR. Treatment of focal axillary hyperhidrosis using a long-pulsed Nd:YAG 1064 nm laser at hair reduction settings. *J Drugs Dermatol.* 2012;11(1): 59-63.
58. Woolery-Lloyd H, Viera MH, Valins W. Laser therapy in black skin. *Facial Plast Surg Clin North Am.* 2011;19(2):405-416.
59. Babilas P, Schreml S, Szeimies RM, Landthaler M. Intense pulsed light (IPL): a review. *Lasers Surg Med.* 2010;42(2):93-104.
60. Ciocon DH, Boker A, Goldberg DJ. Intense pulsed light: what works, what's new, what's next. *Facial Plast Surg.* 2009;25(5):290-300.
61. Ormiga P, Ishida CE, Boechat A, Ramos ESM. Comparison of the effect of diode laser versus intense pulsed light in axillary hair removal. *Dermatol Surg.* 2014;40(10):1061-1069.

62. Chen J, Liu XJ, Huo MH. Split-leg comparison of low fluence diode laser and high fluence intense pulsed light in permanent hair reduction in skin types III to IV. *Australas J Dermatol.* 2012;53(3):186-189.

63. Haak CS, Nymann P, Pedersen AT, et al. Hair removal in hirsute women with normal testosterone levels: a randomized controlled trial of long-pulsed diode laser vs. intense pulsed light. *Br J Dermatol.* 2010;163(5):1007-1013.

64. Klein A, Steinert S, Baeumler W, Landthaler M, Babilas P. Photoepilation with a diode laser vs. intense pulsed light: a randomized, intrapatient left-to-right trial. *Br J Dermatol.* 2013;168(6):1287-1293.

65. El Bedewi AF. Hair removal with intense pulsed light. *Lasers Med Sci.* 2004;19(1):48-51.

66. Sadick NS, Weiss RA, Shea CR, Nagel H, Nicholson J, Prieto VG. Long-term photoepilation using a broad-spectrum intense pulsed light source. *Arch Dermatol.* 2000;136(11):1336-1340.

67. Troilius A, Troilius C. Hair removal with a second generation broad spectrum intense pulsed light source: a long-term follow-up. *J Cutan Laser Ther.* 1999;1(3):173-178.

68. Cameron H, Ibbotson SH, Dawe RS, Ferguson J, Moseley H. Within-patient right-left blinded comparison of diode (810 nm) laser therapy and intense pulsed light therapy for hair removal. *Lasers Med Sci.* 2008;23(4):393-397.

69. Ross EV. Laser versus intense pulsed light: Competing technologies in dermatology. *Lasers Surg Med.* 2006;38(4):261-272.

70. Aldraibi MS, Touma DJ, Khachemoune A. Hair removal with the 3-msec alexandrite laser in patients with skin types IV-VI: efficacy, safety, and the role of topical corticosteroids in preventing side effects. *J Drugs Dermatol.* 2007;6(1):60-66.

71. Goldberg DJ. Laser- and light-based hair removal: an update. *Expert Rev Med Devices.* 2007;4(2):253-260.

72. Toosi P, Sadighha A, Sharifian A, Razavi GM. A comparison study of the efficacy and side effects of different light sources in hair removal. *Lasers Med Sci.* 2006;21(1):1-4.

73. Kacar SD, Ozuguz P, Demir M, Karaca S. An uncommon cause of laser burns: the problem may be the use of gel. *J Cosmet Laser Ther.* 2014;16(2):104-105.

74. Bernstein EF. Hair growth induced by diode laser treatment. *Dermatol Surg.* 2005;31(5):584-586.

75. Desai S, Mahmoud BH, Bhatia AC, Hamzavi IH. Paradoxical hypertrichosis after laser therapy: a review. *Dermatol Surg.* 2010;36(3):291-298.

76. Town G, Bjerring P. Is paradoxical hair growth caused by low-level radiant exposure by home-use laser and intense pulsed light devices? *J Cosmet Laser Ther.* 2016;9:1-8.

77. Bukhari IA. Pili bigemini and terminal hair growth induced by low-fluence alexandrite laser hair removal. *J Cutan Med Surg.* 2006;10(2):96-98.

78. Moreno-Arias G, Castelo-Branco C, Ferrando J. Paradoxical effect after IPL photoepilation. *Dermatol Surg.* 2002;28(11):1013-1016; discussion 1016.

79. Moreno-Arias GA, Castelo-Branco C, Ferrando J. Side-effects after IPL photodepilation. *Dermatol Surg.* 2002;28(12):1131-1134.

80. Vlachos SP, Kontoes PP. Development of terminal hair following skin lesion treatments with an intense pulsed light source. *Aesthetic Plast Surg.* 2002;26(4):303-307.

81. Sammour R, Nasser S, Debahy N, El Habr C. Fox-Fordyce disease: an under-diagnosed adverse event of laser hair removal? *J Eur Acad Dermatol Venereol.* 2016;30(9):1578-1582.

82. Tetzlaff MT, Evans K, DeHoratius DM, Weiss R, Cotsarelis G, Elenitsas R. Fox-Fordyce disease following axillary laser hair removal. *Arch Dermatol.* 2011;147(5):573-576.

83. Yazganoglu KD, Yazici S, Buyukbabani N, Ozkaya E. Axillary Fox-Fordyce-like disease induced by laser hair removal therapy. *J Am Acad Dermatol.* 2012;67(4):e139-e140.

84. Helou J, Maatouk I, Moutran R, Obeid G. Fox-Fordyce-like disease following laser hair removal appearing on all treated areas. *Lasers Med Sci.* 2013;28(4):1205-1207.

85. Bernad I, Gil P, Lera JM, Gimenez de Azcarate A, Irarrazaval I, Idoate MA. Fox Fordyce disease as a secondary effect of laser hair removal. *J Cosmet Laser Ther.* 2014;16(3):141-143.

86. Soden CE, Smith K, Skelton H. Histologic features seen in changing nevi after therapy with an 810 nm pulsed diode laser for hair removal in patients with dysplastic nevi. *Int J Dermatol.* 2001;40(8):500-504.

87. Dvorackova J, Sterba J, Ceganova L, et al. [Problems of suitability laser's excision of pigmented dermal lesions: case report of minimal deviation melanoma]. *Cesk Patol.* 2007;43(2):64-67.

88. Boer A, Wolter M, Kaufmann R. [Pseudomelanoma following laser treatment or laser-treated melanoma?]. *J Dtsch Dermatol Ges.* 2003;1(1):47-50.

89. Dummer R, Kempf W, Burg G. Pseudo-melanoma after laser therapy. *Dermatology.* 1998;197(1):71-73.

90. Zipser MC, Mangana J, Oberholzer PA, French LE, Dummer R. Melanoma after laser therapy of pigmented lesions–circumstances and outcome. *Eur J Dermatol.* 2010;20(3):334-338.

91. Riml S, Larcher L, Grohmann M, Kompatscher P. Second-degree burn within a tattoo after intense-pulsed-light epilation. *Photodermatol Photo.* 2013;29(4):218-220.

92. Sadick NS, Laughlin SA. Effective epilation of white and blond hair using combined radiofrequency and optical energy. *J Cosmet Laser Ther.* 2004;6(1):27-31.

93. Sadick NS, Shaoul J. Hair removal using a combination of conducted radiofrequency and optical energies–an 18-month follow-up. *J Cosmet Laser Ther.* 2004;6(1):21-26.

94. Brauer JA, Brightman LA, Hale EK, et al. Reduction of axillary hair of all colors after single treatment with microwave technology. https://miramarlabs.com/wp-content/uploads/ASLMS-2013-Axillary-Hair-Reduction-eposter-3.19.13.pdf. Accessed March 6, 2020.

31 Body Contouring Devices and Noninvasive Fat Removal

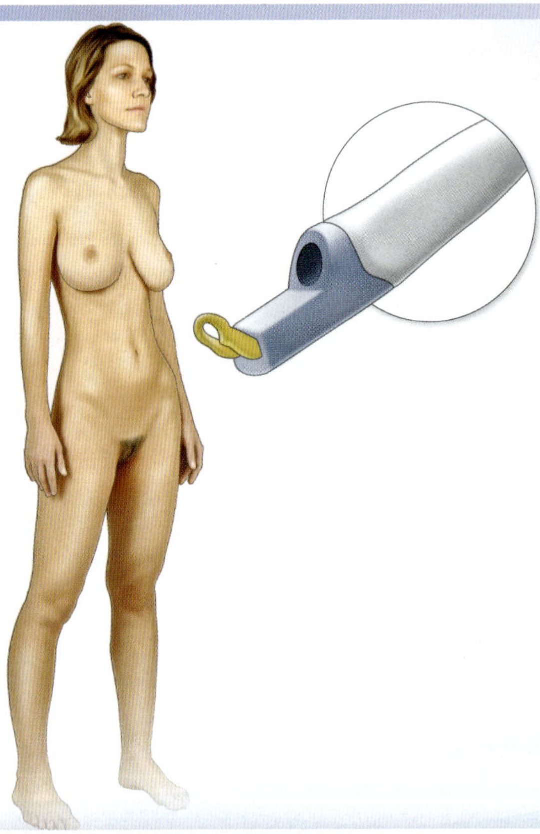

SUMMARY

- Liposuction is now the second most frequently performed cosmetic procedure in the United States.
- Approaches to noninvasive body contouring include cryolipolysis, high-intensity focused ultrasound (HIFU), low-level laser therapy (LLLT), hyperthermic lasers, radiofrequency, and infrared lasers.
- These approaches to noninvasive fat removal all selectively target components of adipose tissue.
- All minimally invasive body-contouring technologies fall far short of liposuction in terms of clinical efficacy and rapidity of response.

Beginner Tips

- No head-to-head studies have been performed comparing various technologies for body contouring.
- Be sure to closely investigate the various options before purchasing a device, as some systems require a significant ongoing expenditure on consumables, while others do not.

Expert Tips

- Patient selection is critical, as the degree of response seen with body contouring may be relatively modest.
- Most body-contouring approaches should only be used for patients with a BMI in the normal range.
- Combination therapies are a reasonable option for many patients..

Don't Forget!

- Some treatments, such as cryolipolysis, take several months to demonstrate complete benefit. Therefore, appropriate planning is important for patients aiming to improve their body profile before a major event.
- While all treatments are minimally invasive, some lead to more significant postoperative edema and ecchymosis.

Pitfalls and Cautions

- Paradoxical adipose hyperplasia may be rarely seen after cryolipolysis.
- If it occurs, spontaneous resolution is not expected; therefore patients should always be warned of this rare possibility.
- While there is a theoretical risk of LFT and lipid changes during the fat resorption phase, this has not been reported clinically.

Patient Education Points

- Multiple treatments may be required.
- No minimally invasive treatment can match liposuction in terms of efficacy, flexibility, and rapidity of response.
- Realistic expectations are critical, and patients who expect a dramatic response should probably be warned against this approach.

Body Contouring Devices and Noninvasive Fat Removal

31

INTRODUCTION

The number of cosmetic procedures has soared over the past decades, with liposuction the second most popular cosmetic surgical procedure performed in the United States.[1] Despite its popularity and overall safety, liposuction is an invasive surgical procedure with risks including infection and complications from anesthesia. Therefore, there is demand for noninvasive approaches that may lead to the ideal physique with less risk and downtime. Multiple body-contouring devices have been created over recent years to meet these demands such as cryolipolysis, low-level laser therapy, high-intensity focused ultrasound, radiofrequency, and infrared lasers.[2,3] These new approaches to noninvasive fat removal all selectively target components of adipose tissue that differentiate it from the overlying epidermis and dermis.[4]

CRYOLIPOLYSIS

Cryolipolysis dates back to the 1970s, when Epstein and Oren[5] observed a red indurated nodule followed by transient fat necrosis on the cheek of an infant who had been sucking on a popsicle. They termed this phenomenon *popsicle panniculitis*, which led to the discovery that adipose tissue is more susceptible to cold injury than surrounding tissue, a concept now referred to as *cold-induced panniculitis*.[5] This idea was first exploited by Manstein et al[6] in 2007, when they performed the initial studies exploring the selective destruction of fat. Using black Yucatan pigs, copper plates were applied at various temperatures (–8, –7, –5, –3, –1, and 20°C) to a test site for 10 minutes. These areas were studied grossly and histologically at different time points, with the longest one being 3.5 months. They found that cooling induced a lobular panniculitis, and the amount of fat damage increased up to a month after exposure. This study was followed up by Zelickson et al[7] in 2009 using three pigs that underwent a single cryolipolysis treatment. They assessed the results histologically and by ultrasound and found a 50% and 33% reduction, respectively, in the thickness of the superficial fat.

The mechanism of action for cryolipolysis and how it produces selective apoptosis in adipocytes remains unclear. One possible mechanism is that adipocyte death is caused by reperfusion injury, which triggers free radicals, oxidative stress, and ensuing cell death. Under histologic analysis, there are no notable changes immediately after treatment. However by day 3, an inflammatory process occurs and adipocytes become encircled by histiocytes, neutrophils, and lymphocytes. By 7 days, a lobular panniculitis is noticed. This process peaks at day 14, and between days 14 and 30, macrophages engulf the adipocytes and the inflammation decreases slowly over a 90-day period. Histologically, interlobular septae are thickened, and the fat volume is decreased by 2 to 3 months after treatment. In addition, the epidermis, dermis, nerves, blood vessels, and muscles remain unharmed.[2,4,8]

In 2010, the first cryolipolysis device (CoolSculpting, Zeltiq Aesthetics) was approved by the US Food and Drug Administration (FDA) for the reduction of abdominal and flank fat. Since then, its clinical indications have expanded to include fat reduction of the abdomen, flanks, upper arm, brassiere rolls, lumbar rolls, banana roll, thigh, and submental area in individuals with a body mass index (BMI) of 30 kg/m^2 or less.[9] During a typical 60-minute session, the area of fat is vacuum suctioned into a cup-shaped applicator, which is attached to a central console via an umbilical cable. The console maintains a preset temperature, below 0°C, using sensors implanted in cooling plates on the sides of the applicator. The suction allows for maximum contact with the cooling plates and causes some vasoconstriction, allowing more rapid cooling of the skin.[2,3,10,11]

There have been numerous human clinical trials performed demonstrating the efficacy of cryolipolysis for selective fat reduction. In 2009, Dover et al[12] performed a trial using cryolipolysis on the flanks of 32 subjects. They assessed improvement using photography, physician assessment, and subject satisfaction. Ten subjects were further assessed by ultrasound of the treatment area. They found that all subjects had a reduction in the fat layer, with an average reduction of 22.4% seen by ultrasound. Another study by Kaminer et al[13] in 2009 treated 50 subjects, with each serving as their own control. Each patient underwent cryolipolysis treatment of one flank, and photography and three blinded physicians were used to assess the subjects. The physicians could differentiate with an 82% accuracy rate between the treated and untreated side. The evidence from these two studies led to FDA approval for treatment of the flanks by cryolipolysis. Further studies include those by Sasaki et al,[3] who in 2014 treated six patients in a pilot study and then went on to treat 112 patients in the clinical treatment group. This study demonstrated similar findings to previous studies, with an average fat reduction at 6 months of 21.5% by caliper measurements and 19.6% by ultrasound measurements (**Figure 31-1**). They also found that massage in one patient after treatment led to more rapidly increased temperatures. In 2015, Ingargiola et al[4] published a review article evaluating 19 cryolipolysis clinical trials in humans. They found that average fat reduction ranged from 14.67% to 28.5%, as measured by caliper and 10.3% to 25.5% as measured by ultrasound.

Adverse events from cryolipolysis are generally mild and include erythema, ecchymosis, swelling, sensitivity, and pain. Erythema is most common, occurs immediately, and can last for several hours after treatment (**Figure 31-2**).[11] Ecchymosis can be observed for days after treatment due to the vacuum suction used during the procedure and is worse in patients taking anticoagulants.[2,4] Transient numbness is another finding that was studied by Coleman et al[14] in 2009. They reported that six of nine subjects experienced decreased sensation assessed by neurologic evaluation; however, this completely resolved after a mean

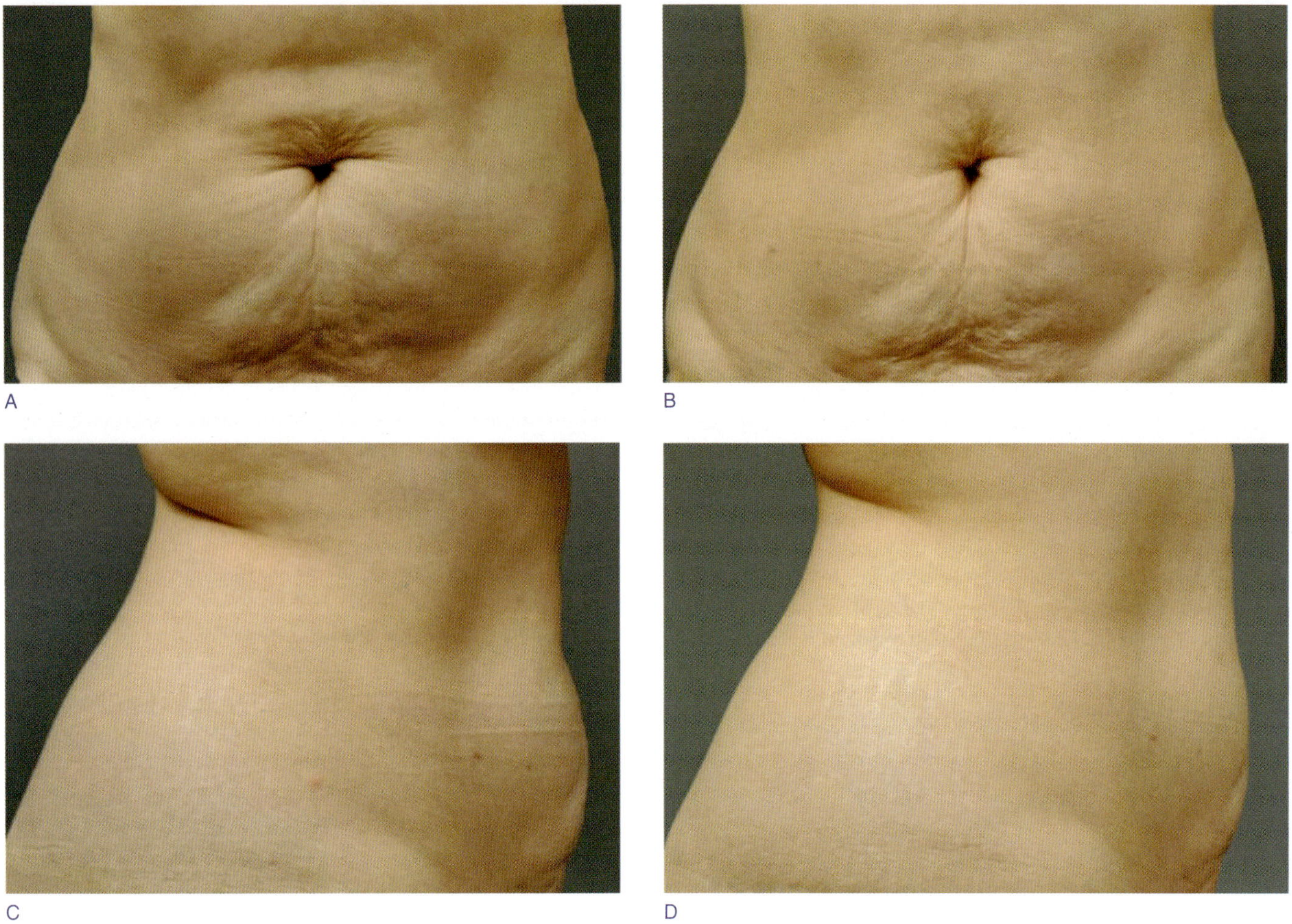

FIGURE 31-1 A 51-year-old woman from the pilot study. (**A, C**) Subject's pretreatment photographs. (**B, D**) Subject's photographs 6 months after cryolipolysis treatment of her entire lower abdomen with a large applicator in a single session.

of 3.6 weeks posttreatment. On biopsy, there were no long-term changes observed in the nerve structure. Another very common complaint is pain. Most subjects experience a "shooting" or "cramping" pain within 1 week after treatment. This is most likely due to the cold-induced panniculitis, and studies have found a correlation between increased pain and larger surface area treated. Most subjects reported that the pain was tolerable, could be controlled with oral analgesics, and resolved spontaneously over 1 to 4 weeks.[2,8]

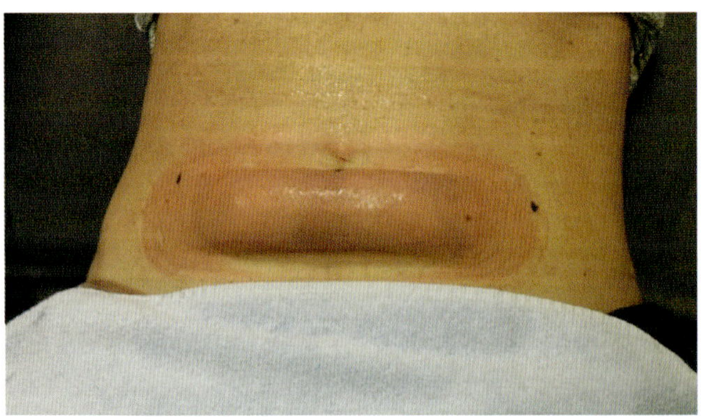

FIGURE 31-2 "The butter stick" erythema and swelling of the abdomen immediately after treatment.

In addition, there is a theoretical risk that lipid levels and liver function tests could possibly be increased due to the absorption of adipocytes by macrophages. However, multiple studies evaluating lipid levels and liver function tests (including aspartate aminotransferase, alanine aminotransferase, alkaline phosphatase, total bilirubin, and albumin) after treatment found no evidence of a significant increase in levels.[15-18] One very rare side effects that has been observed is paradoxical adipocyte hyperplasia. This has been reported in 33 cases, and the exact mechanism of action is unknown. No spontaneous resolution has been reported, and the only treatment is liposuction or abdominoplasty.[19] Contraindications to cryolipolysis include cold-induced conditions such as cold urticaria, cryoglobulinemia, and paroxysmal cold hemoglobinuria. It also should not be performed in areas with edema, dermatitis, varicose veins, or other cutaneous conditions.[4] As far as patient satisfaction, Dierickx et al[20] performed a study in 2013 that reported 73% of 518 subjects were satisfied with their treatment and 82% would recommend the procedure to a friend. In that study, only 6 of 528 subjects were dissatisfied and 4 of the 6 were satisfied after a second treatment was performed.

Overall, cryolipolysis has proved to be an effective means of selective noninvasive fat reduction, with the best results seen in individuals close to their ideal body weight. Most people can expect to see an estimated 25% reduction in the fat layer with final results seen 3 months after treatment. Sometimes, a second treatment can be beneficial for targeting thicker areas, such as the abdomen.[2]

HIGH-INTENSITY FOCUSED ULTRASOUND

High-intensity focused ultrasound (HIFU) is another method used for noninvasive fat reduction. Although the device for body contouring was approved in 2011 (LipoSonix by Medicis), HIFU has been used for decades to noninvasively treat kidney stones, for epicardial tissue ablation for arrhythmias, to destroy uterine fibroids, and to destroy tumors of various organs. This device was first used in the cosmetic field as an adjunct to liposuction; however, when highly focused, it can be used effectively as a stand-alone procedure.[2,21] HIFU works by a thermomechanical process in which the acoustic waves are precisely focused on the subcutaneous fat layer, bypassing the overlying epidermis and dermis. This quickly heats the area to a temperature above 56°C to cause a coagulative necrosis of the adipocytes in 1 to 2 seconds. The mechanical action is achieved through microscopic shear forces that generate additional frictional heating. Histologic examination after treatment identifies adipocyte necrosis immediately after treatment. After 2 weeks, a localized inflammatory response with mostly lipid-laden macrophages can be seen within the treatment area, which completely dissipates by 14 weeks after treatment when maximum clinical effects can be observed.[2,22,23]

Jewell et al[22] performed some of the first clinical trials in 2011 targeting abdominal fat in 26 Yorkshire pigs. They found that, during treatment, the targeted subcutaneous fat layer approached 70°C with no damage seen histologically to the surrounding tissues, vasculature, or nerve fibers. Microscopic examination showed the accumulation of macrophages at the damaged tissue with no evidence of fat emboli or fat accumulation. No significant changes were seen either in serum lipid levels or liver function tests. Initial clinical studies involving humans were performed by Fatemi et al.[24,25] In 2009, they published a retrospective case series involving 282 subjects who underwent a single HIFU treatment of their abdomen and flanks. The treatment took approximately 1 to 1.5 hours to perform and resulted in an average waist circumference decrease of 4 to 5 cm.[24] Then, in 2010, they reported on an additional 85 subjects who underwent a single session of HIFU to the same treatment areas. They found an average waist circumference decrease of 4.6 cm 3 months after treatment.[25] Subject satisfaction was found to be greater than 70% 3 months after treatment in both series. Jewell et al[26] published another clinical trial in 2011 in which 180 adults (aged 18-65 years) with subcutaneous abdominal fat greater than or equal to 2.5 cm thick were selected to be in one of three groups in a 1:1:1 randomized fashion. There were two treatment groups that differed in energy levels (47 J/cm and 59 J/cm) and one sham treatment control group that had an energy level of 0 J/cm. After 12 weeks, statistically significantly decreased waist circumference was achieved for both treatment groups compared to the control group, with greater efficacy noticed in the 59 J/cm group (–2.52 cm vs –2.10 cm in the 47 J/cm group). However, a 1.2-cm decrease was also seen in the sham-treated group at 12 weeks.

Common adverse events are reported in roughly 12% of subjects who have received HIFU and include prolonged tenderness, edema, ecchymosis, and hard lumps. These have been found to spontaneously resolve within 1 to 3 months after treatment. Some patients also report excessive pain during the process, but this resolves after the procedure is completed.[2,27] A study by Lee et al[27] published in 2016 used a contact cooling system during the HIFU procedure, which appeared to provide a less painful experience without loss of efficacy. Further trials exploring adjunctive cooling methods may make the HIFU procedure a more comfortable experience in the future.

LOW-LEVEL LASER THERAPY

Low-level laser therapy (LLLT), or cold laser therapy, was first reported by Endre Mester in 1968 when he noticed hair regrowth in mice after exposure to a ruby laser for stimulation of wound healing.[28] Since then, LLLT has been used for multiple purposes including pain relief, decreasing inflammation and edema, and regenerating tissue growth.[29] In 2002, Neira et al[30] introduced the concept of using LLLT for fat removal as an adjunct to liposuction. Using a 635-nm, 10-mW diode laser, tissue from 12 subjects after liposuction was collected and irradiated for 0, 2, 4, and 6 minutes. The type of laser chosen was based on previous evidence that wavelengths between 630 and 640 nm were optimal for biomodulation. Their results showed that, at 4 minutes, 80% of the fat was released from adipose cells and, at 6 minutes, 99% of the fat had been released. The mechanism of action remains somewhat controversial. In the report by Neira et al,[30] the tissue was examined under an electron microscope, and transitory pores were discovered in the cell membrane, presumably caused by the laser. This allowed the lipid content to leave the cell into the interstitial space, resulting in adipocyte deflation. Therefore, unlike other methods of noninvasive fat removal, the adipocyte is not destroyed using LLLT, but decreased in size. The pore is hypothesized to be induced by the photoexcitation of cytochrome C oxidase, a terminal enzyme within the mitochondria.[29,30] Other hypothesized mechanisms include the formation of increased reactive oxygen species (ROS), initiating a process known as lipid peroxidation, where ROS causes pores due to reactions with lipids found in the cell membrane. Some report that they do not see microscopic pores and believe that that LLLT causes activation of the complement cascade, resulting in adipocyte apoptosis followed by release of lipids. These theories are the subject of active investigation.[29]

An LLLT device (Zerona by Erchonia) was first approved in 2010 by the FDA for noninvasive selective fat reduction of the waist, hips, and thighs, and in 2012, it gained approval for fat reduction of the arms. It was the first noninvasive aesthetic device approved by the FDA for circumferential reduction of the waist, hips, and thighs in the United States. The device consists of five low-power laser diode modules (one central unit and four suspended by adjustable arms) that each emit 17 mW of 635-nm laser light. Generally, treatment of an area requires six to eight sessions lasting around 30 minutes each.[2,29,31]

Multiple studies have been performed assessing LLLT for noninvasive fat reduction. The first study conducted, which helped to gain approval by the FDA for Zerona, was performed by Jackson et al.[32] and published in 2009. This double-blind, randomized, placebo-controlled trial evaluated 67 adults assigned to receive either LLLT or matching sham treatments three times a week for 2 weeks. Subjects in the treatment arm demonstrated an average reduction of 0.98 inches at the waist, 1.05 inches at the hip, and 0.85 and 0.65 inches across the right and left thighs, respectively. In 2011, Caruso-Davis et al[33] used a similar but different device, the LAPEX 2000 LipoLaser System by Meridian, with wavelengths between 635 and 680 nm, to evaluate its effectiveness for body contouring. With 40 subjects randomized 1:1 into the treatment arm or the control group, treatment occurred for 30 minutes twice a week for 4 weeks. Cumulative circumference loss at the end of 4 weeks was –2.15 cm, showing significant improvement compared to the control group. However, this system has not been approved by the FDA for body contouring and is currently only indicated for pain associated with carpal tunnel syndrome. In 2012, Nestor et al[34] published a clinical trial in which 40 subjects were randomized 1:1 to a treatment group (Zerona) or a sham treatment group. They received treatment sessions three times per week for 2 weeks to the upper arm area. After six treatments, the treatment group showed a combined arm circumference reduction of 3.7 cm versus 0.2 cm in the control group (**Figure 31-3**). In 2016, Thornfeldt et al[35] tested a different treatment protocol using the Zerona device. A total of 54 subjects were treated once weekly with LLLT to the waist, hips, thighs, and abdomen for 6 weeks. Findings showed an average decrease in combined body circumference of 5.4 inches. They compared their data to previous studies using the 2-week protocol consisting of three treatments per week and found that the 6-week method may be more effective. However, there was no control group in this study, and the mean BMI of subjects in the 2-week versus the 6-week protocol differed.

Researchers are investigating other frequencies of LLLT, such as green laser light, for body contouring. Although green laser light has previously been used for tattoo removal, low-level green laser is now being studied for its role in noninvasive fat removal. In 2013, Jackson et al[36] performed one of the first trials using a green laser called Verjú by Erchonia.[37] This system was approved by the FDA in 2013 and was the first green laser to use six 532-nm green diodes instead of five 635-nm red diodes typical of other LLLT models. In this double-blind clinical trial, 68 subjects were randomized into either a treatment or sham treatment group to primarily evaluate the reduction in the appearance of cellulite, but also to evaluate the combined reduction of thigh circumference. Subjects received six treatments (15 minutes to the anterior abdomen and 15 minutes to the lower back area) over a 2-week period. After 6 weeks, 19 subjects in the treatment group saw reduction in the appearance of cellulite compared to three subjects in the sham-treated group. In addition, a significant decrease was found in the mean combined thigh circumference at 6 weeks (44.77 inches) compared to baseline measurements (47.13 inches). Since then, two other studies have been performed testing the efficacy of the Verjú laser for fat reduction. In 2014, Suarez et al[38] conducted a similar study using 67 subjects randomized to receive six treatments or sham treatments over a 2-week period. After 2 weeks, the total mean combined circumference measurements decreased by 3.9 inches over the waist, hips, and upper abdomen in the treatment group versus 1.1 inches for the sham-treated group. Likewise in 2016, Roche et al[39] randomized 53 obese subjects (BMI between 30 and 40 kg/m^2) into either a treatment or sham treatment group to receive three weekly treatments over a 4-week period. After 4 weeks, 71.43% of subjects in the LLLT group achieved a 7.2-cm or greater decrease in combined measurements over the hip, waist, and upper abdomen compared to three subjects in the sham-treated group. In addition, the mean decrease in combined

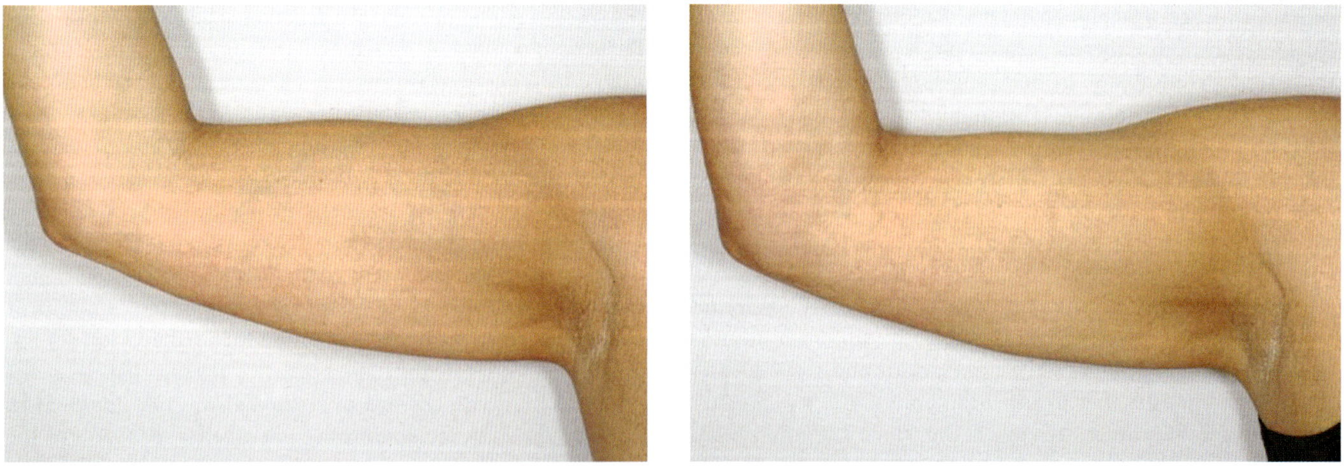

A B

FIGURE 31-3 (**A**) Before treatment of the arm. (**B**) Two weeks after six treatments of low-level laser therapy over a 2-week period.

measurements for the LLLT group was 10.52 cm, compared with 1.80 cm in the sham-treated group.

LLLT appears to be not only an effective means for fat reduction, but also a very safe alternative. There have been no adverse events reported to date, and results can be seen sooner—within 2 weeks—compared to other methods of noninvasive body contouring.[31,34,35,36,38,39]

HYPERTHERMIC LASERS, RADIOFREQUENCY, AND INFRARED LASERS

Other modalities to achieve noninvasive body contouring are continuing to be explored. In 2015, a hyperthermic laser (SculpSure by CynoSure) was approved by the FDA for noninvasive fat removal. It is a 1060-nm diode laser that heats the subcutaneous adipose tissue to a temperature between 42°C and 47°C. This causes destruction of adipocytes, which are later reabsorbed by the lymphatic system. The epidermis and dermis are spared due to a contact cooling system, which is used during the typical 25-minute procedure. In 2017, Decorato et al[40] published a study using the SculpSure device. They enrolled 17 subjects and performed a single session on either their abdomen or flank. The only side effects observed were mild pain, stinging, and numbness, which all resolved by 2 weeks. After 12 weeks, with the aid of photographs, ultrasound, and magnetic resonance imaging, they found overall fat reduction similar to results using cryolipolysis (24%).

Radiofrequency (RF) waves provide another approach to noninvasive fat reduction. When RF waves irradiate tissue, they generate an oscillating electrical field, which generates an electrical current. This current causes collisions between charged molecules and ions, generating molecular friction, which is then transformed into heat. When targeted at adipose tissue, RF destroys fat by causing apoptosis within the cells. Skin and muscle have different conductivity and relative permittivity than fat, which allows for fat to be selectively targeted without destroying the overlying epidermis, dermis, and surrounding tissues. RF has been FDA approved for reduction in the appearance of cellulite, skin tightening, and circumference reduction when paired with infrared light and suctioning.[31,41]

Infrared lasers, using infrared vibrational absorption bands, also work by heating adipose tissue. Selective photothermolysis is the mechanism of choosing a specific wavelength of light and pulse duration to target a tissue without impairing the surrounding structures.[2] In 2006, Anderson et al[42] found that the absorption peaks of lipids were at 1210 and 1720 nm. This is where the absorption of lipids is greater than that of water, allowing targeting of the fat layer without damage to the overlying skin. In 2009, a human pilot study was conducted by Wanner et al[43] exploring the effectiveness of a 1210-nm laser using a 10-mm spot size with a 3-second exposure time on the abdomen of 24 adults. After the treatment, punch biopsies were taken at 1 to 3 days or 4 to 6 weeks later. Results showed dose-dependent damage to the subcutaneous fat and dermis. Subjects also reported that the treatment was painful, although it was well tolerated in most subjects. Although significant results were observed, there has not been evidence to support treating larger surface areas. The ability to target the reticular dermis may provide a future role for the treatment of cellulite by infrared lasers.

These two modalities have been combined to provide more effective results. In 2014, Addato et al[44] published a study looking at the effectiveness of a device (Velashape, Syneron Medical Ltd.) that incorporates four treatment modalities including bipolar RF, infrared light, pulsed vacuum, and mechanical massage. This device is indicated to not only reduce fat, but also to cause skin tightening. Throughout the study, 35 subjects received once-weekly treatment to their abdomen, flank, buttock, or thigh area for 6 weeks and were followed for up to 3 months after treatment. At 3 months, subjects showed an average reduction of 1.4, 0.5, and 1.2 cm to their abdomen/flank, buttocks, and thighs, respectively, compared to baseline. Combining modalities like these in future studies may provide enhanced efficacy of current treatments.

CONCLUSION

Noninvasive fat removal has come a long way in the past decades and has expanded the cosmetic field of body contouring. That said, large-scale head-to-head studies have not been conducted to directly compare the effectiveness of different modalities. Further studies are needed to better delineate the ideal treatment approach, although to date all minimally invasive body contouring technologies fall far short of liposuction in terms of clinical efficacy and rapidity of response.

REFERENCES

1. The American Society of Plastic Surgeons. 2015 Plastic surgery statistics. 2015 https://www.plasticsurgery.org/news/plastic-surgery-statistics. Accessed January 20, 2017.
2. Jalian HR, Avram MM. Body contouring: the skinny on noninvasive fat removal. *Semin Cutan Med Surg.* 2012;31(2):121-125.
3. Sasaki GH, Abelev N, Tevez-Ortiz A. Noninvasive selective cryolipolysis and reperfusion recovery for localized natural fat reduction and contouring. *Aesthet Surg J.* 2014;34(3):420-431.
4. Ingargiola MJ, Motakef S, Chung MT, Vasconez HC, Sasaki GH. Cryolipolysis for fat reduction and body contouring. *Plast Reconstr Surg.* 2015;135(6):1581-1590.
5. Epstein EH, Oren ME. Popsicle panniculitis. *N Engl J Med.* 1970;282(17):966-967.
6. Manstein D, Laubach H, Watanabe K, Farinelli W, Zurakowski D, Anderson RR. Selective cryolysis: a novel method of non-invasive fat removal. *Lasers Surg Med.* 2008;40(9):595-604.
7. Zelickson B, Egbert BM, Preciado J, et al. Cryolipolysis for noninvasive fat cell destruction: initial results from a pig model. *Dermatol Surg.* 2009;35(10):1462-1470.
8. Krueger N, Mai SV, Luebberding S, Sadick NS. Cryolipolysis for noninvasive body contouring: clinical efficacy and patient satisfaction. *Clin Cosmet Invest Dermatol.* 2014;7:201-205.
9. US Food and Drug Administration. Premarket notification 510(k). http://www.accessdata.fda.gov/scripts/cdrh/cfdocs/cfpmn/pmn.cfm?ID = K162050. Accessed January 20, 2017.
10. Landman B. CoolSculpting your way to a better beach body. 2014. https://hamptons-magazine.com/coolsculpting-your-way-to-a-better-beach-body. Published June 4, 2014.

11. Dumitru A. Zwivel's complete guide to Coolsculpting. 2017. https://www.zwivel.com/blog/the-complete-guideto-coolsculpting. Accessed February 1, 2017.

12. Dover J, Burns J, Coleman S, et al. A prospective clinical study of noninvasive cryolipolysis for subcutaneous fat layer reduction: interim report of available subject data. *Lasers Surg Med.* 2009;41(21):43.

13. Kaminer M, Weiss R, Newman J, Allison J. Visible cosmetic improvement with cryolipolysis: photographic evidence. Presented at the Annual Meeting of the American Society for Dermatologic Surgery, 2009, Phoenix, AZ.

14. Coleman SR, Sachdeva K, Egbert BM, Preciado J, Allison J. Clinical efficacy of noninvasive cryolipolysis and its effects on peripheral nerves. *Aesthetic Plast Surg.* 2009;33(4):482-488.

15. Ferraro GA, De Francesco F, Cataldo C, Rossano F, Nicoletti G, D'Andrea F. Synergistic effects of cryolipolysis and shock waves for noninvasive body contouring. *Aesthetic Plast Surg.* 2012;36:666-679.

16. Lee KR. Clinical efficacy of fat reduction on the thigh of Korean women through cryolipolysis. *J Obes Weight Loss Ther.* 2013;3(6):1-5.

17. Riopelle JT, Kovach B. Lipid and liver function effects of the cryolipolysis procedure in a study of male love handle reduction. *Lasers Surg Med.* 2009;41:82.

18. Klein KB, Zelickson B, Riopelle JG, et al. Noninvasive cryolipolysis for subcutaneous fat reduction does not affect serum lipid levels or liver function tests. *Lasers Surg Med.* 2009;41:785-790.

19. Jalian HR, Avram MM, Garibyan L, Mihm MC, Anderson RR. Paradoxical adipose hyperplasia after cryolipolysis. *JAMA Dermatol.* 2014;150(3):317-319.

20. Dierickx CC, Mazer J, Sand M, Koenig S, Arigon V. Safety, tolerance, and patient satisfaction with noninvasive cryolipolysis. *Dermatol Surg.* 2013;39(8):1209-1216.

21. Kes Laser. New liposonix operation system ultrasonic HIFU machine for cellulite reduction. 2017. http://www.best-laser.com/sale-7686328-new-liposonix-operation-system-ultrasonic-hifu-machine-for-cellulitereduction.html. Accessed January 24, 2017.

22. Jewell ML, Desilets C, Smoller BR. Evaluation of a novel high-intensity focused ultrasound device: preclinical studies in a porcine model. *Aesthet Surg J.* 2011;31(4):429-434.

23. Leslie TA, Kennedy JE. High-intensity focused ultrasound principles, current uses, and potential for the future. *Ultrasound Q.* 2006;22(4):263-272.

24. Fatemi A. High-intensity focused ultrasound effectively reduces adipose tissue. *Semin Cutan Med Surg.* 2009;28(4):257-262.

25. Fatemi A, Kane MA. High-intensity focused ultrasound effectively reduces waist circumference by ablating adipose tissue from the abdomen and flanks: a retrospective case series. *Aesthetic Plast Surg.* 2010;34(5):577-582.

26. Jewell ML, Baxter RA, Cox SE, et al. Randomized sham-controlled trial to evaluate the safety and effectiveness of a high-intensity focused ultrasound device for noninvasive body sculpting. *Plast Reconstr Surg.* 2011;128(1):253–262.

27. Lee HJ, Lee M, Lee SG, Yeo U, Chang SE. Evaluation of a novel device, high-intensity focused ultrasound with a contact cooling for subcutaneous fat reduction. *Lasers Surg Med.* 2016;48(9): 878-886.

28. Mester E, Szende B, Gartner P. The effect of laser beams on the growth of hair in mice. *Radiobiol Radiother (Berl).* 1968;9(5):621-626.

29. Avci P, Nyame TT, Gupta GK, Sadasivam M, Hamblin MR. Low-level laser therapy for fat layer reduction: a comprehensive review. *Lasers Surg Med.* 2013;45(6):349-357.

30. Neira R, Arroyave J, Ramirez H, et al. Fat liquefaction: effect of low-level laser energy on adipose tissue. *Plast Reconstr Surg.* 2002;110(3):912-922.

31. Nestor MS, Newburger J, Zarraga MB. Body contouring using 635-nm low level laser therapy. *Semin Cutan Med Surg.* 2013;32(1):35-40.

32. Jackson RF, Dedo DD, Roche GC, Turok DI, Maloney RJ. Low-level laser therapy as a non-invasive approach for body contouring: a randomized, controlled study. *Lasers Surg Med.* 2009;41(10):799-809.

33. Caruso-Davis MK, Guillot TS, Podichetty VK, et al. Efficacy of low-level laser therapy for body contouring and spot fat reduction. *Obes Surg.* 2010;21(6):722-729.

34. Nestor MS, Zarraga MB, Park H. Effect of 635 nm low-level laser therapy on upper arm circumference reduction: a double-blind, randomized, sham-controlled trial. *J Clin Aesthet Dermatol.* 2012;5(2):42-48.

35. Thornfeldt CR, Thaxton PM, Hornfeldt CS. A six-week low-level laser therapy protocol is effective for reducing waist, hip, thigh, and upper abdomen circumference. *J Clin Aesthet Dermatol.* 2016;9(6):31-35.

36. Jackson RF, Roche GC, Shanks SC. A double-blind, placebo-controlled randomized trial evaluating the ability of low-level laser therapy to improve the appearance of cellulite. *Lasers Surg Med.* 2013;45:141-147.

37. Erchonia Corporation. Verjú laser system. 2017. http://www.erchonia.com/verju-laser-system. Accessed February 2, 2017.

38. Suarez DP, Roche GC, Jackson RF. A double-blind, sham-controlled study demonstrating the effectiveness of low-level laser therapy using a 532-nm green diode for contouring the waist, hips, and thighs. *Am J Cosmet Surg.* 2014;31(1):34-41.

39. Roche GC, Shanks S, Jackson RF, Holsey LJ. Low-level laser therapy for reducing the hip, waist, and upper abdomen circumference of individuals with obesity. *Photomed Laser Surg.* 2016;35(3):142-149.

40. Decorato JW, Chen B, Sierra R. Subcutaneous adipose tissue response to a non-invasive hyperthermic treatment using a 1,060 nm laser. *Lasers Surg Med.* 2017;49(5):480-489.

41. Hayre N, Palm M, Jenkin P. A clinical evaluation of a next generation, non-invasive, selective radiofrequency, hands-free, body-shaping device. *J Drugs Dermatol.* 2016;15(12):1557-1561.

42. Anderson RR, Farinelli W, Laubach H, et al. Selective photothermolysis of lipid-rich tissues: a free electron laser study. *Lasers Surg Med.* 2006;38(10):913-919.

43. Wanner M, Avram M, Gagnon D, Mihm MC, Zurakowski D, Watanabe K. Effects of non-invasive, 1,210 nm laser exposure on adipose tissue: results of a human pilot study. *Lasers Surg Med.* 2009;41(6):401-407.

44. Adatto MA, Adatto-Neilson RM, Morren G. Reduction in adipose tissue volume using a new high-power radiofrequency technology combined with infrared light and mechanical manipulation for body contouring. *Lasers Med Sci.* 2014;29(5):1627-1631.

Photodynamic Therapy for Acne, Actinic Keratoses, and Nonmelanoma Skin Cancer

32

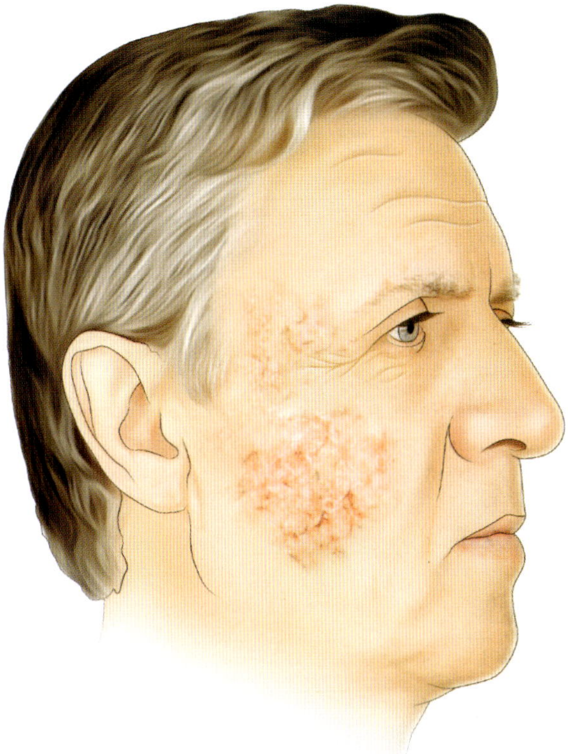

SUMMARY

- PDT combines the use of a photosensitizer, a light source within the absorption spectrum of the photosensitizer, and molecular oxygen which, when stimulated, destroys a specific target tissue.
- PDT is a common procedure, and is used for the treatment of actinic keratoses, superficial nonmelanoma skin cancers, acne, and photodamage, among other indications.

Beginner Tips

- While both ALA and MAL are effective photosensitizers for PDT, currently only ALA is available in the United States.
- The ideal time from ALA application to activation ranges broadly, and while the FDA-approved indication calls for ALA application the day before activation, in practice many clinicians wait only 1 hour prior to light activation.

Pitfalls and Cautions

- Stripping may occur due to uneven light or photosensitizer application, and can be treated by retreating the entire area.
- In the United States, PDT is generally not used for the treatment of skin cancers as monotherapy.

Expert Tips

- Daylight PDT is becoming increasingly popular due to both convenience and comfort, though further studies are needed to better quantify the amount of exposure needed for different geographic locations and different times of the year.
- Both blue LED and IPL have been used with significant success for activation.

Patient Education Points

- Patients should be warned that they will need to not only practice religious sun protection, but that they will also have significant erythema for at least several days after the procedure. Work and social schedules should be planned accordingly.

Don't Forget!

- Sun protection, including indirect sun protection, is absolutely critical to avoid overactivating the photosensitizer.
- Consider HSV prophylaxis in all patients with a history of HSV in the treated area.

Billing Pearls

- Insurance coverage for PDT is variable, and generally the only indication for coverage in the United States is nonhypertrophic actinic keratoses on the face and scalp.
- ALA is currently only available from a single manufacturer in the United States and in single-use stick form.
- Since physicians bill directly for the photosensitizing drug, extreme caution is warranted in assuring the amount of coverage available for a given insurance company, as the physician risks spending more on purchasing the medication than they will be reimbursed.

32 Photodynamic Therapy for Acne, Actinic Keratoses, and Nonmelanoma Skin Cancer

INTRODUCTION

Photodynamic therapy (PDT) involves a chemical reaction, where a photosensitive chemical (photosensitizer) is activated by a light source in target tissue. The chemical reaction produces singlet oxygen and other cytotoxic free radicals. PDT thus combines the use of a photosensitizer, a light source within the absorption spectrum of the photosensitizer, and molecular oxygen, which, when stimulated, will destroy a specific target tissue.

HISTORY

Modern PDT was initially described by Raab[1] in the early 1900s, who highlighted the phototoxic effects of natural dyes. Later, Jesionek and Tappeiner[2] used eosin dye to successfully treat skin cancer. In the early 1960s, Lipson and Schwartz injected hematoporphyrins into neoplastic tissue and demonstrated fluorescence in tumors.[3,4]

PDT has been used in the field of oncology, where porfimer sodium injected as an intravenous (IV) infusion has been used for esophageal and non–small-cell lung cancer,[5,6] and was the first photosensitizer for PDT to gain approval for human use. Its photosensitizing properties allowed tumors to be illuminated in the gastrointestinal, genitourinary, and pulmonary tracts, as well as skin, to help surgeons better localize neoplasms,[7-9] although it was also noted to lead to severe cutaneous photosensitivity for weeks after treatment. An IV infusion PDT procedure using the photosensitizer verteporfin has also been used in ophthalmology to treat the wet form of macular degeneration, which causes central serous retinopathy.[10]

One of the noted side effects of the early photosensitizers was that actinic keratoses (AKs) were activated by porfimer sodium. Later, a topically applied PDT procedure was developed with the photosensitizer 5-aminolevulinic acid.[11] PDT was approved in the United States in the late 1990s for nonhyperkeratotic AKs of the face and scalp.[12] PDT has subsequently been used to treat a wide variety of cutaneous conditions, from acne to hidradenitis to cosmetic conditions.

SCIENCE OF PDT

Cutaneous Photosensitizers

US Food and Drug Administration (FDA)–approved photosensitizers include 5-aminolevulinic acid (ALA) and methyl aminolevulinate (MAL), used to treat AKs. MAL is not currently on the market in the United States, whereas ALA is absorbed preferentially by actinically damaged skin, skin cancers, and pilosebaceous glands. ALA acts as a prodrug and penetrates the stratum corneum and becomes localized in target tissue.[13]

Mechanism of Action

ALA itself is not photosensitive, but after penetrating into the underlying tissue it is converted to protoporphyrin IX (PpIX), a photosensitive compound.[14] A source that emits light at wavelengths within the PpIX absorption spectrum (spectrum peaks: 409, 509, 544, 584, 634, 636, and 708 nm) is then exposed to the treated skin. Since all absorption spectrum peaks are greater than 400 nm (ie, no longer in the ultraviolet [UV] spectrum), light exposure itself is not carcinogenic (**Figure 32-1**).

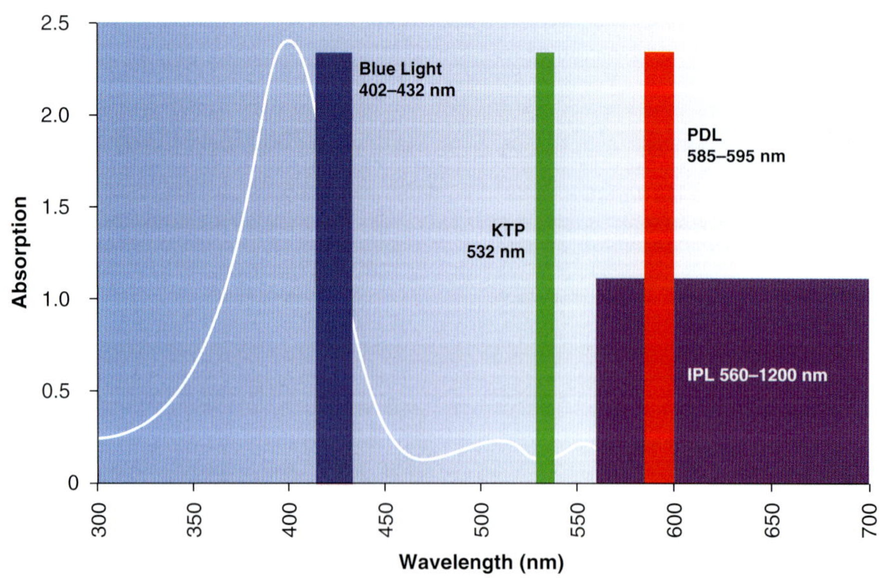

FIGURE 32-1 Protoporphyrin IX absorption spectrum in vivo for photodynamic therapy. IPL, intense pulsed light; KTP, potassium titanyl phosphate; PDL, pulsed-dye laser.

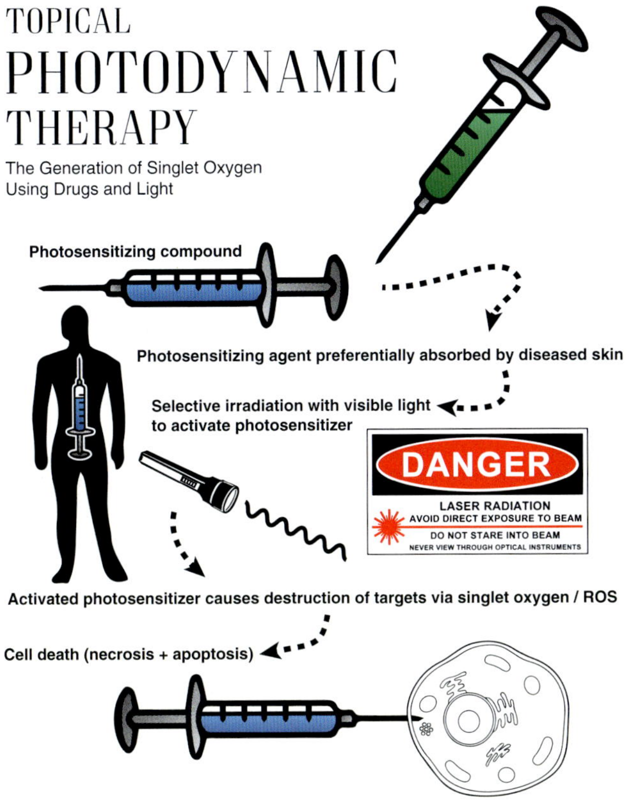

FIGURE 32-2 Photodynamic therapy leads to apoptosis.

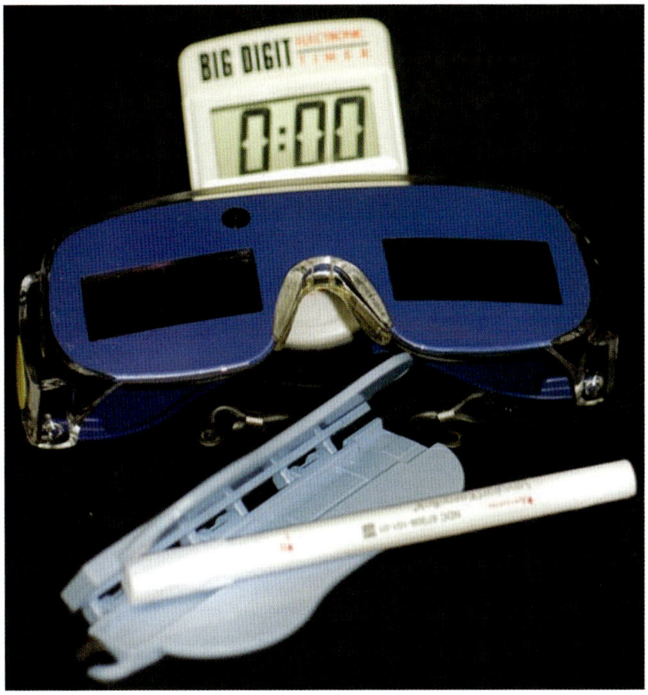

FIGURE 32-3 Necessary equipment, including safety eye protection, a timer, and ALA.

The ideal time between ALA administration and light activation has been studied, with suggested ranges between 30 minutes and 24 hours. Penetration is proportional to wavelength of light used for activation, so the longer the wavelength of light source used, the deeper it penetrates into tissue. Light around 630 nm penetrates to a depth of 5 mm, whereas longer wavelengths of 700 to 800 nm may penetrate as deep as 2 cm. However, with increasing depth, there is decreased energy transmitted, and so longer wavelengths lead to a lesser activation of PpIX into toxic metabolites (**Figure 32-2**).

PDT PROCEDURE

Pretreatment Considerations

Preprocedure consultation is critical, including a detailed history regarding underlying conditions that may be exacerbated by light, photosensitizing medications, history of herpes simplex virus or methicillin-resistant *Staphylococcus aureus*, and whether the patient is able to modify his or her lifestyle to accommodate the amount of downtime needed after the procedure (**Figure 32-3**).

Before the procedure, the area is cleansed well with an acetone scrub. In the United States, ALA is sold as a stick applicator for single use. The applicator tip is affixed to plastic tubing, which contains one vial of ALA in powder form and one vial of ethanol solvent. When ready to use, the glass vials are broken with light pressure, and the contents are mixed by rotating the stick back and forth for a recommended 3 minutes. The ALA solution must be used immediately following preparation to avoid instability of the activated product. The dry applicator tip should be dabbed on a gauze pad until uniformly wet with solution. Apply the solution directly to the target area by dabbing gently with the wet applicator tip. Two passes are recommended to ensure even ALA application to treatment areas. After application is complete, the area may be covered with plastic wrap to prevent ALA evaporation. Occlusive plastic wrap is very helpful during the incubation time period for optimal efficacy.

ALA is incubated on the treatment area for a predetermined time, and the patient is reminded to avoid sun exposure during incubation. This includes indirect sun exposure, so the patient should stay away from windows and remain indoors to prevent premature activation. The conversion of ALA into PpIX is heat dependent, and thus optimal room temperature during incubation of ALA is 80°F to 83°F. This may not always be feasible, although electric space heaters may be used and can be monitored via a digital thermometer.

Light and Laser Selection

The effective light dose depends on the quantity of delivered light and the extent that it includes wavelengths that are absorbed by PpIX. Significant PpIX absorption bands are around 410, 505, 540, 580, and 635 nm. The Soret band absorption at 410 nm is up to 15- to 30-fold greater than the longer wavelengths. Both laser and nonlaser light sources have been used with success in PDT.[15] The light sources that have been studied include incoherent light sources such as halogen/tungsten, xenon, and LED light sources, as well as lasers such as argon dye (630 nm), excimer (630 nm), pulsed-dye laser (PDL, 595 nm), and intense pulsed light (IPL) devices.

Blue light, with a spectral output at 417 nm, has 40 times greater potency than red light in activating ALA, although its depth of penetration is more modest. Augmenting penetration with other lasers before treatment may result in greater efficacy and downtime.

The FDA-approved protocol uses 20% ALA solution without occlusion to nonhypertrophic AKs on the face and scalp with a 14- to 18-hour delay between application of ALA and blue light exposure. Pain from ALA-PDT is proportional to the PDT dose rate and may be mediated by direct injury to cutaneous nerves. To mitigate this pain, incubation times as low as 1 hour have been suggested and have demonstrated acceptable efficacy.[16,17]

Other frequently used approaches include IPL, which has been used for AK and photoaging with a clearance rate of 50% to 90%. In addition, PDL is also very effective at PDT activation, using a 100-mm spot size, fluence of 7.5 J/cm^2, pulse duration of 10 to 20 ms, and double pulsed. Finally, 635-nm LED light sources may be used with an exposure time of 10 minutes.

Laser-Assisted Drug Delivery

The effectiveness of ALA is contingent on how deeply and selectively it penetrates the skin. ALA penetration is influenced by baseline skin thickness and lesion type (deeper penetration with AKs, sun damage, abrasions, and inflammation). Thicker lesions are more resistant to PDT due to the limited depth of penetration of topical photosensitizers. A study by Sandberg et al[18] revealed that both ALA and MAL often fail to permeate to tissue depths greater than 1 mm, in part due to the polar and hydrophilic nature of these compounds.

Curettage and laser-assisted drug delivery have been explored to improve ALA penetration. Laser pretreatment of the skin has been shown to increase the penetration of these photosensitizers. In an ex vivo porcine skin model, both continuous and fractional ablative Er:YAG lasers increased the penetration of topically applied ALA[19] using a fluence of 4 J/cm^2 corresponding to a pore depth of approximately 12.5 μm localized to the stratum corneum.

Another in vitro study showed that skin pretreatment using the fractional ablative Er:YAG laser increased the flux of ALA 27- to 124-fold in nude mouse skin and 3- to 260-fold in porcine skin, independent of the number of passes.[20] The skin received one to six passes (169 pores per pass) at a fluence of 2 or 3 J/cm^2, which corresponded to penetration depths of 8 and 12 μm, respectively. These investigators suggested that laser pretreatment of the skin could potentially reduce the required dose of topically applied ALA by 20%.

The fractional carbon dioxide (CO_2) laser has also been shown to enhance the delivery of photosensitizing agents used in PDT. Fractional CO_2 laser pretreatment of in vivo porcine skin significantly enhanced the penetration of topically applied MAL, along with the subsequent PDT response throughout the superficial and deep layers of the skin at fluences of 37 and 200 J/cm^2.[21,22]

Haak et al[23] investigated the importance of depth of ablation and incubation time for fractional CO_2 laser-assisted delivery of MAL in porcine skin and demonstrated that pretreatment with the laser significantly reduced incubation times required for a given accumulation of MAL from the skin surface to the deep dermis, compared to skin that was not treated with the laser.

Depth of ablation did not affect drug delivery, as the drug dispersed equally within the dermis for both shallow and deep MTZs, suggesting that once the epidermis is breached, MAL and other drugs may disperse readily within the dermis.

Daylight PDT

Daylight PDT is emerging as an effective treatment for AK, particularly for patients who require treatment of large areas of chronic actinic damage that can be exposed easily to daylight sun. Conventional PDT for AKs is associated with inconveniently lengthy clinic visits and discomfort during therapy. Three randomized controlled studies have shown that daylight-mediated PDT is an effective treatment of thin AKs. Benefits over traditional PDT include an almost pain-free experience, improved convenience, and the ability to easily treat large areas. Further investigation is needed to determine at which time of the year and in which weather conditions daylight-mediated PDT will be possible in different geographical locations,[24] although in Australia this has already become an effective and popular treatment option given the abundance of adequate daylight.[25]

Postoperative Considerations

After treatment, ice packs may be applied to the treated areas, although ice should not be placed in direct contact with the skin. Patients should avoid all sunlight exposure for at least 48 hours. Over-the-counter analgesics such as acetaminophen or ibuprofen may be used as needed (**Figure 32-4**).

MEDICAL INDICATIONS FOR PDT

Actinic Keratoses and Nonmelanoma Skin Cancers

PDT is an attractive therapy for AKs because it allows treatment of large areas, has a high response rate, and results in excellent cosmesis. Because of the risk of transformation of AK to invasive squamous cell carcinoma (SCC), consensus guidelines recommend that AKs be treated to prevent progression to invasive disease. High-risk patients include those with a significant history of sun exposure, who reside in sunny climates, or who have extensive outdoor work or recreational exposure. In addition, solid organ transplant recipients and others with chronic immunosuppression are also at greater risk for developing AKs and for progression to SCC; 97% of SCCs are associated with a nearby AK.[26] One randomized controlled trial of PDT for nonhyperkeratotic AKs on the face and scalp using a 14- to 18-hour incubation period demonstrated an AK clearance rate of 72% to 85%.[27] In Europe, ALA and MAL research has focused on treating superficial cutaneous malignancies including SCC in situ and basal cell carcinoma. PDT has also been studied as a primary preventive technique for skin cancer (**Figures 32-5 and 32-6**).

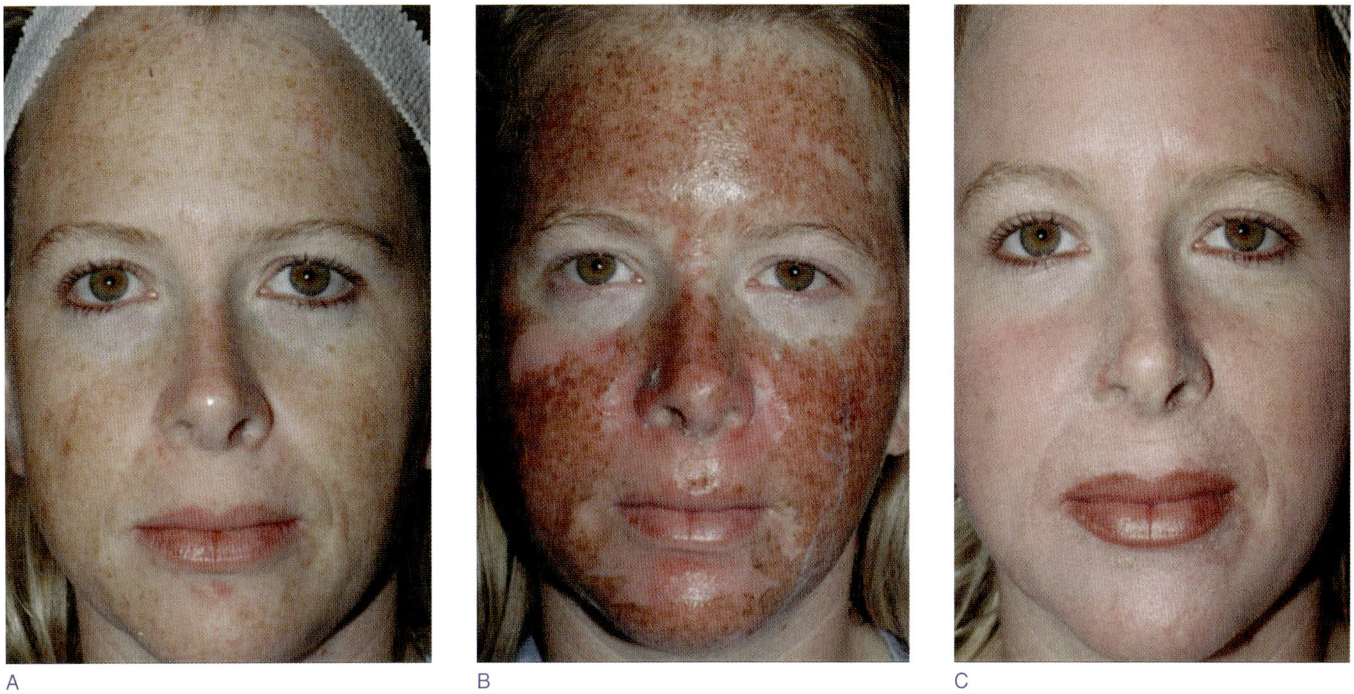

FIGURE 32-4 (**A**) A 38-year-old Caucasian woman with Fitzpatrick skin type II with photodamage on her face prior to photodynamic therapy. (**B**) Patient 2 days after photodynamic therapy in the office. (**C**) Patient approximately 1 month after photodynamic therapy completed.

Acne Vulgaris

Acne vulgaris is estimated to affect 70% to 96% of all individuals in their lifetime. Acne is primarily a disease of the pilosebaceous gland and is sometimes hormonally mediated and associated with *Propionibacterium acnes*. Challenges associated with medical treatment options are that conventional topical and systemic agents are associated with adverse effects, partial response, contraindications, and recurrence.

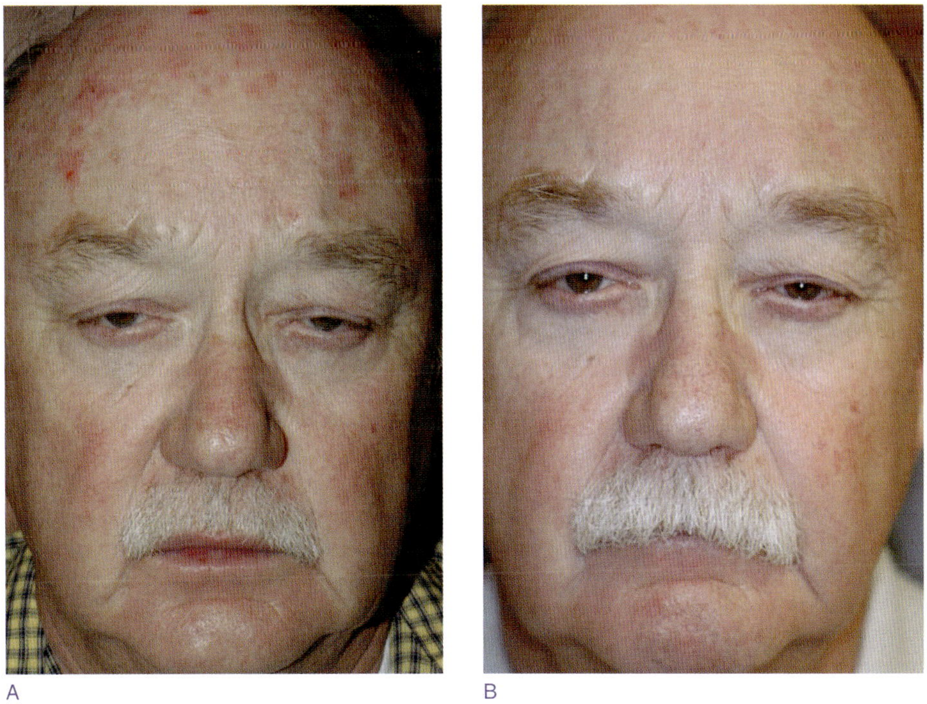

FIGURE 32-5 (**A**) A 69-year-old Caucasian man with Fitzpatrick skin type II with several actinic keratoses on the forehead prior to receiving photodynamic therapy. (**B**) Same patient approximately 1 month after receiving photodynamic therapy for actinic keratoses.

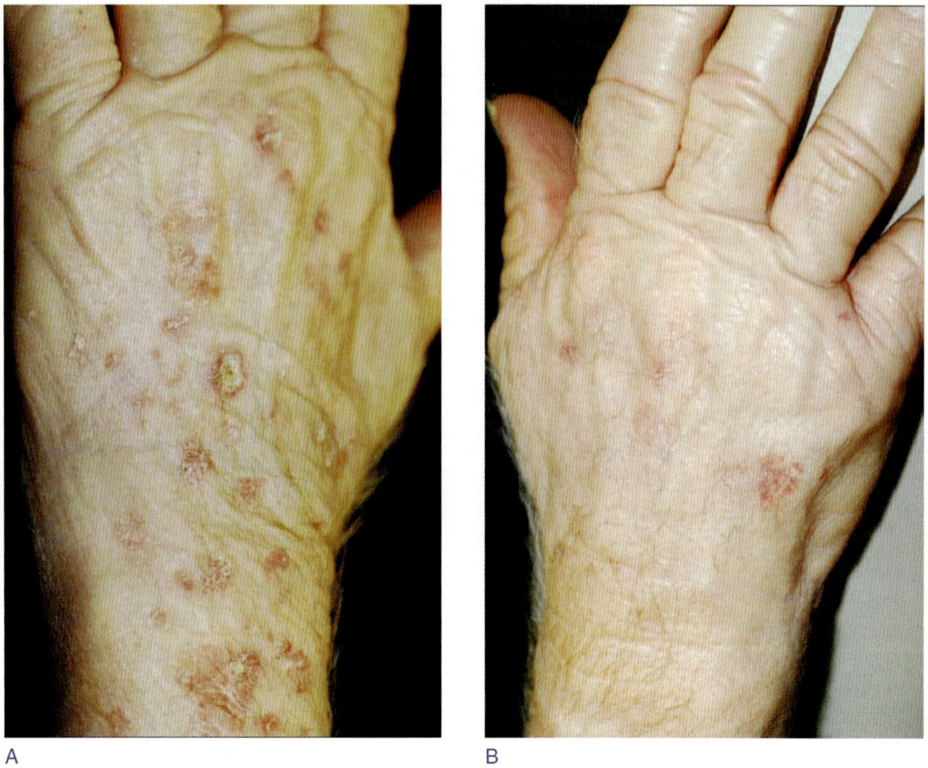

FIGURE 32-6 (**A**) A 72-year-old Caucasian woman with Fitzpatrick skin type II with several actinic keratoses prior to curettage and photodynamic therapy. (**B**) Same patient approximately 1 month after a single treatment of photodynamic therapy.

P acnes produces endogenous protoporphyrins, including PpIX and coproporphyrin III, both of which have an absorption spectrum in the near ultraviolet range of light, with peak absorption seen at 415 nm. Thus, exposure to blue light alone may be effective for acne, as photoactivation ultimately destroys *P acnes*. Indeed, 63% of acne lesions responded to blue light alone, and 45% of comedonal acne also demonstrated a response. A variety of vascular lasers and IPL devices are also being used to treat acne vulgaris.[28]

A recent review included 36 studies on the use of PDT.[29] These studies largely supported the role for PDT in acne management, although further research is needed to better define an ideal treatment protocol (**Figure 32-7**).

Hidradenitis Suppurativa

Hidradenitis suppurativa (HS) is a challenging disease, and there are reports of successful use of ALA-PDT using a blue light source. One study evaluated patients with recalcitrant HS who were treated with short-contact ALA for three to four sessions with a blue light source over 1- to 2-week intervals. Seventy-five percent of the HS lesions responded and remained clear during a 3-month follow-up.

AESTHETIC INDICATIONS FOR PDT

The aesthetic effects of PDT for photoaged skin are well documented, and improvement of lentigines, skin roughness, sallow complexion, and fine wrinkles has been demonstrated. A reduction in the histologic signs of photoaging, manifested as a decrease in solar elastosis and expression of p53, together with induction of neocollagenesis, has been shown as well.[30] One study evaluated IPL/PDT versus IPL alone for photoaging, and better results were achieved for the global score, fine lines, and coarse wrinkles on the IPL/PDT-treated side than on the IPL-only side at the final visit.[31] In another split-face trial of IPL/PDT versus IPL alone, similar efficacy of PDT treatment for the clinical signs of photoaging was seen.[32] In another randomized trial, patients received three PDT treatments at 3-week intervals applied to half of the face 30 to 60 minutes prior to IPL treatment. The IPL/PDT group showed better results for global score for photoaging, improvement of fine lines, and pigmentation. The final cosmetic evaluation by the investigator and subject satisfaction scores were both significantly superior on the IPL/PDT sides. However, there was also a higher incidence of side effects, including more intense erythema, scaling and dryness, edema, crusting, and vesiculation on the IPL/PDT side.

The molecular effects of ALA-PDT using a PDL for photoaged forearm skin have also been evaluated.[33]PDL/PDT was shown to induce collagen production, as there were elevated levels of procollagen I and III mRNA and procollagen I protein in the dermis. Other findings included an upregulated marker of keratinocyte proliferation (Ki67) and increased epidermal thickness. However, immunostaining for p53 did not show a decrease following PDL/PDT. Moreover, in comparison with PDL treatment alone, dermal remodeling was more pronounced with PDL/PDT (**Figure 32-8**).

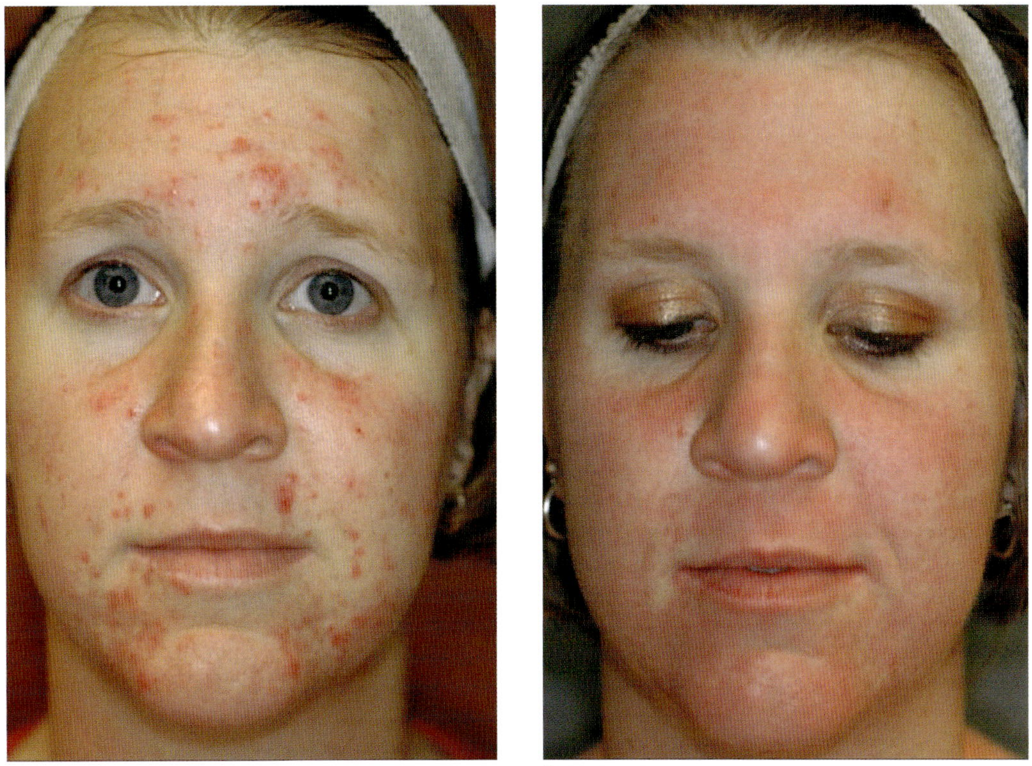

A B

FIGURE 32-7 (**A**) A 34-year-old Caucasian woman with Fitzpatrick skin type II before receiving blue light treatment for facial acne. (**B**) Same patient after several treatments of blue light for acne vulgaris on face.

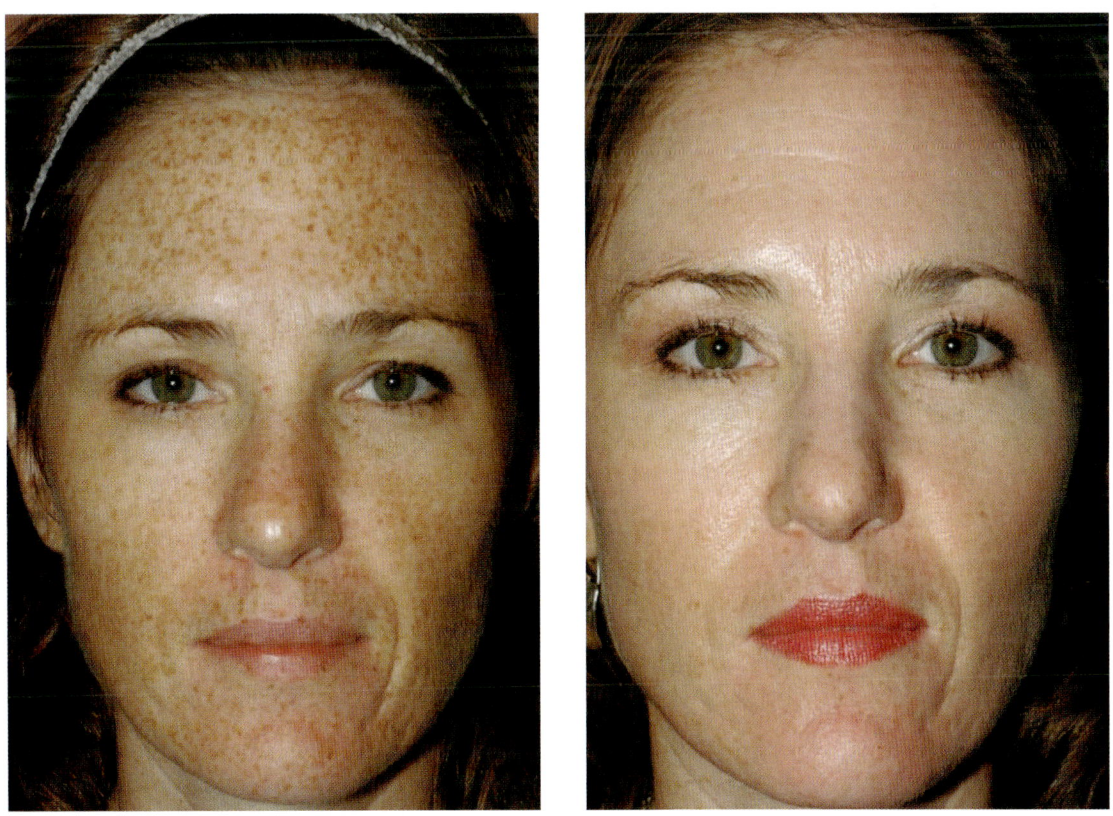

A B

FIGURE 32-8 (**A**) A 36-year-old Caucasian woman with Fitzpatrick skin type II before receiving photodynamic therapy (PDT) and intense pulsed light (IPL) on face for photodamage. (**B**) Same patient 1 month after receiving one treatment of PDT and IPL on face for photodamage.

COMPLICATIONS

Treated areas may become edematous and erythematous, and tissue response is directly correlated with the amount of photodamage. In some patients, a histamine reaction may occur with significant surrounding erythema. Patients may also develop superficial erosions accompanied by weeping and crusting. Infection during the postoperative period should be managed aggressively to mitigate the risk of scarring. In the event of moderate to severe pain or pruritus, patients should be seen and cultures may be performed. Prophylactic treatment may be initiated to prevent bacterial, viral, and yeast infections. Patients should always be instructed to avoid sun exposure for 48 hours after ALA application due to cutaneous phototoxicity associated with increased sun exposure after treatment.

The most common complication of PDT is phototoxicity, presenting clinically as an exaggerated sunburn. Phototoxicity is most likely due to inadvertent outdoor exposure after PDT and typically occurs within hours of excess photoactivation manifested as intense erythema, edema, and burning. Treatment includes rest, application of ice, and elevation (sleep on two pillows). Topical corticosteroid ointments, oral corticosteroids, and occlusive moisturizers may also offer some relief.

Another frequently seen complication is "stripping" caused by nonuniform ALA application or uneven laser activation. If stripping occurs, it can be easily corrected by a second treatment to clear the entire area. This should be distinguished from scarring caused by overly aggressive laser parameters or infection (**Figure 32-9**).

Cutaneous viral and bacterial infections after PDT are uncommon but may occur due to the impaired skin barrier after the procedure. Prophylactic antiviral agents are recommended in patients with a history of recurrent herpes simplex virus infection within the treatment area. These medications are generally started 1 day prior to PDT treatment and continued for 7 days. Patients with active herpetic lesions should not be treated due to the risk of diffuse spread and subsequent risk of scarring.

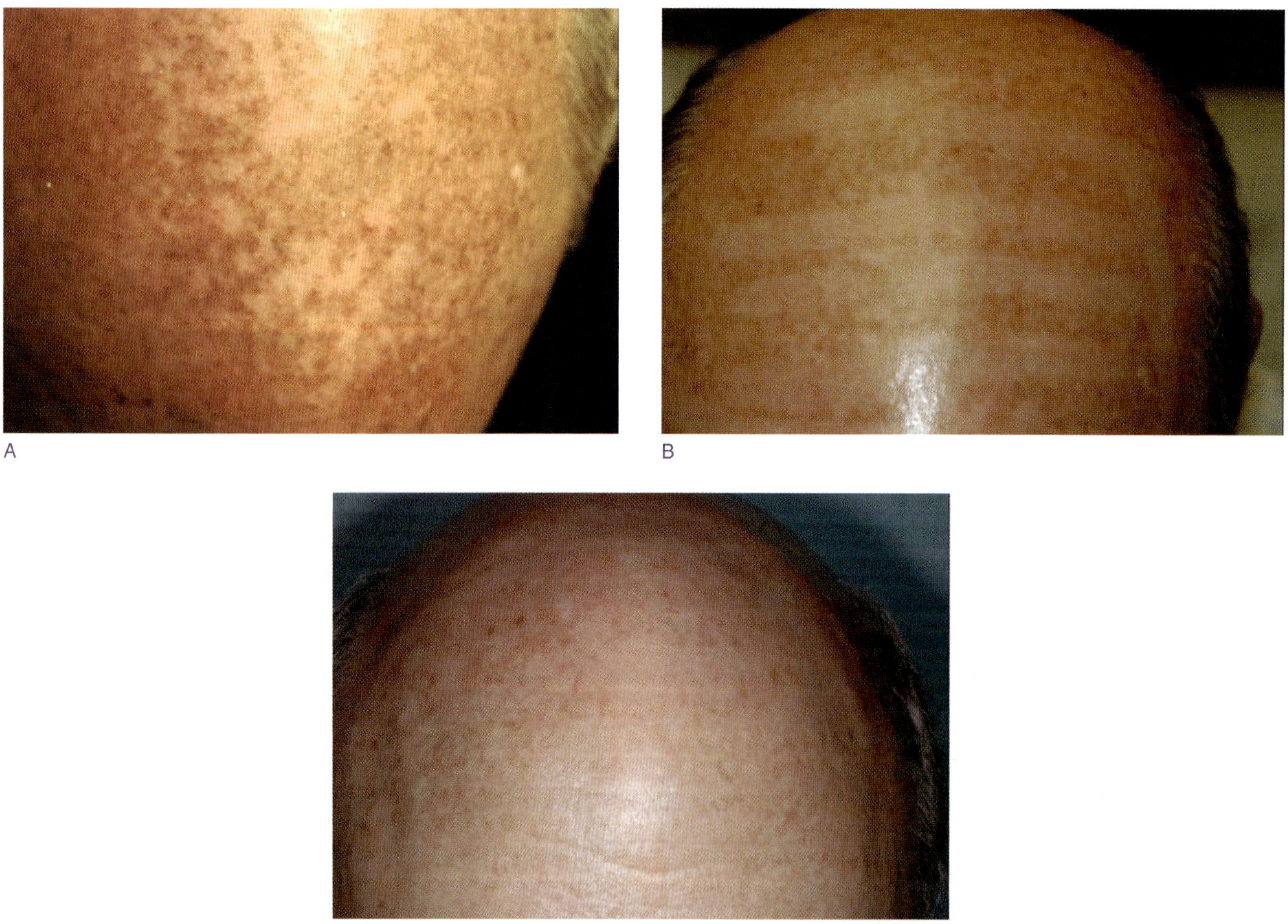

A B C

FIGURE 32-9 (**A**) A 75-year-old Caucasian man with Fitzpatrick skin type II with moderate to severe photodamage on the scalp prior to receiving photodynamic therapy (PDT) and intense pulsed light (IPL) laser. (**B**) Same patient approximately 1 month after PDT and IPL on scalp for photodamage; note the clinical appearance of stripping. (**C**) Same patient approximately 1 month after a second treatment of PDT and IPL on the scalp. Note the complete resolution of the stripping appearance.

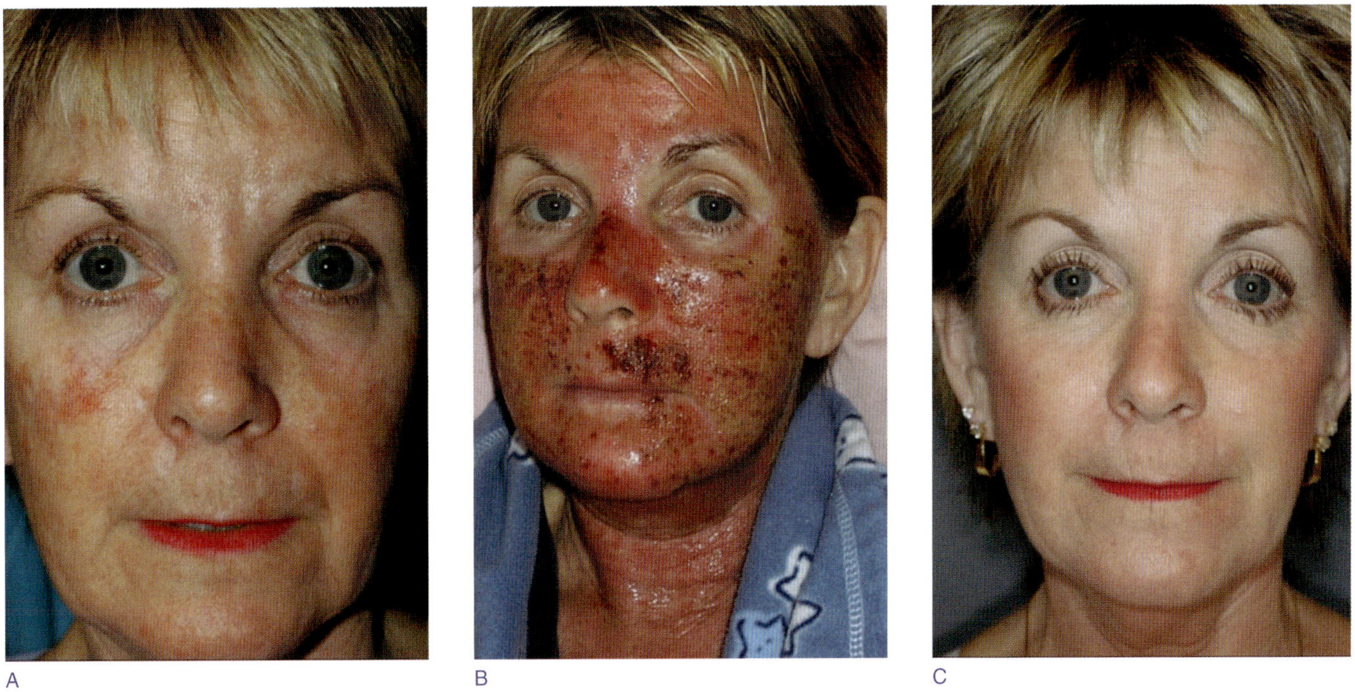

FIGURE 32-10 (**A**) A 59-year-old Caucasian woman with Fitzpatrick skin type II before receiving photodynamic therapy (PDT) and intense pulsed light (IPL) treatment on the face for photodamage and actinic keratoses. (**B**) Same patient 1 week after PDT and IPL with erythema and edema caused by candidiasis. (**C**) Same patient after applying topical nystatin ointment on the affected area twice a day for 10 days, along with taking oral antibiotics for 10 days.

Patients are told to gently wash the face twice daily with a mild soap during the healing period. In addition, washing and an acetone scrub prior to PDT may decrease periprocedural infections. However, superficial bacterial infections such as impetigo or cellulitis may still be seen due to impaired skin barrier function and may cause significant pain or pruritus. Patients should return for culture and appropriate topical and/or systemic antibiotic coverage if pain and itching increase, especially after day 2. Topical and oral antibiotics should be used until symptoms resolve. Rarely, patients may develop candidiasis associated with intense erythema and edema, which should be treated appropriately (**Figure 32-10**).

Acute postoperative hypertension has also been reported after PDT for nonmelanoma skin cancer.[34] In this study, blood pressure was taken twice at 2-minute intervals before and after MAL-PDT. Prevalence of post–MAL-PDT acute postoperative hypertension was 22%, and 11% of patients developed hypertensive crisis. Therefore, blood pressure may be monitored in high-risk patients receiving MAL-PDT.

FUTURE DIRECTIONS

Future PDT light sources include LED[35] portable light sources, handheld devices, and an increased reliance on daylight PDT.

Third-generation photosensitizers (not yet approved) include lutetium texaphyrin and antibody-conjugated photosensitizers. These drugs have absorptions of 700 to 800 nm, allowing deeper penetration into tissues, and therefore, they can be delivered selectively to the tumor tissue.[36,37]

Other directions include combination of PDT with other therapies and improved drug delivery technology. New studies with combination therapy using antiangiogenic agents (eg, VEGF or COX2 inhibitors) with PDT resulted in a significant reduction of PDT-induced expression of prostaglandin E2 and VEGF, as well as a marked improvement in tumoricidal response.[38,39]

CONCLUSIONS

PDT is a noninvasive method of treating AKs, nonmelanoma skin cancers, acne, and cosmetic conditions. A variety of light sources may be used for activation, and daylight PDT is a promising area. PDT targets specific skin cells while leaving surrounding tissue unharmed. This treatment may be used in patients with nonmelanoma skin cancer, although additional studies are needed and it lacks margin control. Pretreating the tumor to make it more susceptible to PDT may be another promising direction, although further research is needed.

REFERENCES

1. Raab O. On the effect of fluorescent substances on infusoria (in German). *Z Biol.* 1900;39:524.
2. Jesionek A, Von Tappeiner H. On the treatment of skin cancers with fluorescent substances. *Arch Klin Med.* 1905;82:223-227.
3. Lipson RL, Baldes EJ, Olsen AM. The use of a derivative of hematoporphyrin in tumor detection. *J Natl Cancer Inst.* 1961;26:1-11.

4. Zelickson B. *Photodynamic Therapy: Mechanism of Action of Topical Aminolevulinic Acid.* Philadelphia, PA: Elsevier Saunders; 2005.
5. Hunter J. QLT PhotoTherapeutics. Maclean's. 1999. https://www.thecanadianencyclopedia.ca/en/article/qlt-phototherapeutics. Accessed March 8, 2020.
6. Drabkin DL. Selected landmarks in the history of porphyrins and their biologically functional derivatives. In: Dolphin D, ed. *The Porphyrins.* Cambridge, MA: Academic Press; 1978:31-84.
7. Wagnieres GA, Star WM, Wilson BC. In vivo fluorescence spectroscopy and imaging for oncological applications. *Photochem Photobiol.* 1998;68(5):6030-6032.
8. Pass HI. Photodynamic therapy in oncology: mechanisms and clinical use. *J Natl Cancer Inst.* 1993;85:443-456.
9. Overholt B, Lightdale C, Wang K, et al. International multicenter, partially-blinded, randomized study of the efficiency of photodynamic therapy using porfimer sodium for the ablation of high grade dysplasia in Barrett's esophagus: results of 24-month follow up. *Gastroenterology.* 2003;124(abstr):A20.
10. Verteporfin in Photodynamic Therapy Study Group. Verteporfin therapy of subfoveal choroidal neovascularization in age-related macular degeneration: two-year results of a randomized clinical trial including lesions with occult with no classic choroidal neovascularization—Verteporfin in Photodynamic Therapy Report 2. *Am J Ophthalmol.* 2001;131(5):541-560.
11. McLoone N, Donnelly RF, Walsh M, et al. Aminolevulinic acid diffusion characteristics in "in vitro" normal human skin and actinic keratosis: implications for topical photodynamic therapy. *Photodermatol Photoimmunol Photomed.* 2008;24(4):183-190.
12. Tschen EH, Wong DS, Pariser DM, et al. Photodynamic therapy using aminolevulinic acid for patients with nonhyperkeratotic actinic keratoses of the face and scalp: phase IV multicentre clinical trial with 12-month follow up. *Br J Dermatol.* 2006;155:1262-1269.
13. Wachowska M, Muchowicz A, Firczuk M, et al. Aminolevulinic acid (ALA) as a prodrug in photodynamic therapy of cancer. *Molecules.* 2011;16:1440-4164.
14. Rollankanti K, Kanick S, Davis S, Pogue B, Maytin E. Techniques for fluorescence detection of protoporphyrin IX in skin cancers associated with photodynamic therapy. *Photonics Lasers Med.* 2013;2(4):287-303.
15. Mallidi S, Anbil A, Bulin A, Obaid G, Ichikawa M, Hasan T. Beyond the barriers of light penetration: strategies, perspectives and possibilities for photodynamic therapy. *Theranostics.* 2016;6(13):2458-2487.
16. Smith S, Piacquadio D, Morhenn V, et al. Short incubation PDT versus 5-FU in treating actinic keratoses. *J Drugs Dermatol.* 2003;2(6):629-635.
17. Touma D, Yaar M, Whitehead S. A trial of short incubation, broad-area photodynamic therapy for facial actinic keratoses and diffuse photodamage. *Arch Dermatol.* 2004;140(1):33-40.
18. Sandberg C, Halldin CB, Ericson MB, Larko O, Krogstad AL, Wennberg AM. Bioavailability of aminolevulinic acid and methylaminolaevulinate in basal cell carcinomas: a perfusion study using microdialysis in vivo. *Br J Dermatol.* 2008;159:1170-1176.
19. Forster B, Klein A, Szeimies RM, Maisch T. Penetration enhancement of two topical 5-aminolaevulinic acid formulations for photodynamic therapy by erbium:YAG laser ablation of the stratum corneum: continuous versus fractional ablation. *Exp Dermatol.* 2010;19:806-812
20. Lee WR, Shen SC, Pai MH, Yang HH, Yuan CY, Fang JY. Fractional laser as a tool to enhance the skin permeation of 5-aminolevulinic acid with minimal skin disruption: a comparison with conventional erbium:YAG laser. *J Control Release.* 2010;145:124-133.
21. Haedersdal M, Katsnelson J, Sakamoto FH, et al. Enhanced uptake and photoactivation of topical methyl aminolevulinate after fractional CO2 laser pretreatment. *Lasers Surg Med.* 2011;43:804-813.
22. Haedersdal M, Sakamoto FH, Farinelli WA, Doukas AG, Tam J, Anderson RR. Fractional CO_2 laser-assisted drug delivery. *Lasers Surg Med.* 2010;42:113-122.
23. Haak CS, Farinelli WA, Tam J, Doukas AG, Anderson RR, Haedersdal M. Fractional laser-assisted delivery of methyl aminolevulinate: impact of laser channel depth and incubation time. *Lasers Surg Med.* 2012;44:787-795.
24. Wiegell SR, Wulf HC, Szeimies RM, et al. Daylight photodynamic therapy for actinic keratosis: an international consensus: International Society for Photodynamic Therapy in Dermatology. *J Eur Acad Dermatol Venereol.* 2012;26(6):673-679.
25. See JA, Shumack S, Murrell DF, et al. Consensus recommendations on the use of daylight photodynamic therapy with methyl aminolevulinate cream for actinic keratoses in Australia. *Australas J Dermatol.* 2016;57(3):167-174.
26. Hurwitz RM, Monger LE. Solar keratosis: an evolving squamous cell carcinoma. Benign or malignant? *Dematol Surg.* 1995;21(2):184.
27. Jeffes EW, McCullough JL, Weinstein GD, et al. Photodynamic therapy of actinic keratosis with topical aminolevulinic acid hydrochloride and fluorescent blue light. *J Am Acad Dermatol.* 2001;45(1):96-104.
28. Papageorgiou P, Katsambas A, Chu A. Phototherapy with blue (415 nm) and red (660 nm) light in the treatment of acne vulgaris. *Br J Dermatol.* 2000;142:973-978.
29. Keyal U, Bhatta AK, Wang XL. Photodynamic therapy for the treatment of different severity of acne: a systematic review. *Photodiagnosis Photodyn Ther.* 2016;14:191-199.
30. Kohl E, Karrer S. Photodynamic therapy for photorejuvenation and non-oncologic indications: overview and update. *G Ital Dermatol Venereol.* 2011;146(6):473-485.
31. Xi Z, Shuxian Y, Zhong L, et al. Topical 5-aminolevulinic acid with intense pulsed light versus intense pulsed light for photodamage in Chinese patients. *Dermatol Surg.* 2011;37(1):31-40.
32. Dover JS, Bhatia AC, Stewart B, Arndt KA. Topical 5-aminolevulinic acid combined with intense pulsed light in the treatment of photoaging. *Arch Dermatol.* 2005;141(10):1247-1252.
33. Orringer JS, Hammerberg C, Hamilton T, et al. Molecular effects of photodynamic therapy for photoaging. *Arch Dermatol.* 2008;144(10):1296-1302.
34. Borroni RG, Carugno A, Rivetti N, Arbustini E, Brazzelli V. Risk of acute postoperative hypertension after topical photodynamic therapy for non-melanoma skin cancer. *Photodermatol Photoimmunol Photomed.* 2013;29(2):73-77.
35. Sadick NS. A study to determine the efficacy of a novel handheld light-emitting diode device in the treatment of photoaged skin. *J Cosmet Dermatol.* 2008;263-267.
36. Young SW, Woodburn KW, Wright M, et al. Lutetium texaphyrin (PCI-0123): a near-infrared, water-soluble photosensitizer. *Photochem Photobiol.* 1996;63(6):892-897.

37. Woodburn KW, Fan Q, Kessel D, Luo Y, Young SW. Photodynamic therapy of B16F10 murine melanoma with lutetium texaphyrin. *J Invest Dermatol.* 1998;110(5):746-751.

38. Zhou Q, Olivo M, Lye KY, Moore S, Sharma A, Chowbay B. Enhancing the therapeutic responsiveness of photodynamic therapy with the antiangiogenic agents SU5416 and SU6668 in murine nasopharyngeal carcinoma models. *Cancer Chemother Pharmacol.* 2005;56(6):569-577.

39. Ferrario A, Von Tiehl K, Wong S, Luna M, Gomer CJ. Cyclooxygenase-2 inhibitor treatment enhances photodynamic therapy-mediated tumor response. *Cancer Res.* 2002;62(14):3956-3961.

33 Sclerotherapy and Management of Varicose Veins

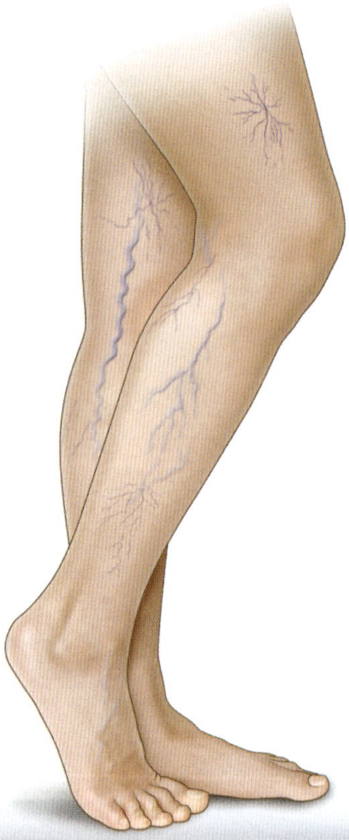

SUMMARY

- Sclerotherapy is a highly effective technique for the treatment of varicose veins.
- Sclerosants may be divided based on whether they exert osmotic or detergent effects on the vessels.
- Both liquid and foam sclerotherapy may be used, depending on vessel caliber.

Beginner Tips

- Common sclerosants include sodium tetradecyl sulfate (STS), polidocanol, and hypertonic saline.
- Larger caliber vessels may benefit from foam sclerotherapy, which can be prepared immediately prior to use.

Pitfalls and Cautions

- Microemboli are frequently seen after foam sclerotherapy, and vision changes, while rare, are possible.
- DVT is a significant risk post treatment, and patients should be warned of this risk.

Expert Tips

- Vessels should be treated from deep to superficial.
- Treating with Nd:YAG laser after sclerotherapy may be helpful and lead to markedly increased levels of response.

Patient Education Points

- The risk of DVT and vision changes, while unusual, should be discussed at length with all patients.
- Compression stockings are very helpful in the postoperative period, and ace wraps should be avoided.

Don't Forget!

- Maintaining or increasing activity in the postprocedure period is of vital importance.
- Superficial thrombophlebitis is common after surgery, and localized urticarial reactions may be seen as well.

Billing Pearls

- In the United States, insurance generally does not cover sclerotherapy, even when performed for symptomatic patients. Motivated patients with symptomatic disease may wish to contact their insurer to assess coverage.

Sclerotherapy and Management of Varicose Veins

33

INTRODUCTION

Primary care clinicians are presented with varicose veins on a daily basis. They represent a symptom of chronic venous disease that encompasses a wide spectrum of morphologic (venous dilation) and functional (venous reflux) abnormalities.[1-3] Vein-related problems may be symptomatic and range from minimal superficial venous dilation to chronic skin changes with ulceration.

Depending on associated signs and symptoms, chronic venous disease manifestations have been stratified in classes from C0 to C6 based on the Clinical-Etiology-Anatomy-Pathophysiology (CEAP) classification (**Table 33-1**). Using this classification, chronic venous insufficiency is generally restricted to disease of greater severity (ie, classes C4 to C6).[4] Thus, varicose veins (CEAP category 2) in the absence of skin changes are not indicative of true chronic venous insufficiency. They are dilated, elongated, tortuous, subcutaneous veins 3 mm or greater in diameter that may involve the saphenous veins (great or small), saphenous tributaries, or nonsaphenous superficial leg veins (**Figure 33-1**). Varicose veins are present in 10% to 30% of the general population, with increasing rates in older individuals.[5,6] Although they are generally thought to be more common in women than men, depending on the population evaluated, men may have a higher rate of disease.[5-7]

Treatment of varicose veins depends on symptoms, extent of lower extremity disease, patient expectations, and likelihood of providing a durable benefit with respect to either appearance or improvement in symptoms. Typical strategies include excision, laser therapy, sclerotherapy, or combination approaches.

Sclerotherapy is a minimally invasive procedure wherein veins are injected with a sclerosing agent that causes endothelial damage by either detergent or osmotic action. After treatment, the target vein shrinks, and over a period of weeks, the treated vein is gradually resorbed. The procedure itself usually lasts no more than 10 minutes, and compared to true surgical vein removal, the downtime is minimal. Currently, sclerotherapy is considered the gold standard and preferred strategy to treat small varicose leg veins.[8] Sclerotherapy is also superior to laser ablation in its ability to close feeder veins or complex venous networks, thus reducing the rate of potential recurrence.

Two main types of sclerotherapy exist, liquid and foam, and both have been successfully used to treat varicose veins.[9-11] Liquid sclerosant preparations are typically used to treat small varicose veins. Foam preparations are available to increase the surface area of the sclerosant and decrease the volume of sclerosant needed when applied to the treatment of larger varicosities, incompetent saphenous veins, and perforators. Multiple injections of dilute sclerosant are injected into the abnormal surface veins of the involved leg. Ultrasound-guided sclerotherapy, with the injection of the sclerosant at the level of refluxing perforator veins, has also been used to treat the associated clusters of varicose veins with good long-term results and without significant complications, but requires an experienced practitioner.

TABLE 33-1 • CEAP Classification

Clinical classification	
C0	No visible or palpable signs of venous disease
C1	Telangiectasias, reticular veins, malleolar flares
C2	Varicose veins
C3	Edema without skin changes
C4	Skin changes ascribed to venous disease (eg, pigmentation, venous eczema, lipodermatosclerosis)
C4a	Pigmentation or eczema
C4b	Lipodermatosclerosis or atrophie blanche
C5	Skin changes as defined above with healed ulceration
C6	Skin changes as defined above with active ulceration
S	Symptomatic, including ache, pain, tightness, skin irritation, heaviness, and muscle cramps, and other complaints attributable to venous dysfunction
A	Asymptomatic
Etiologic classification	
Ec	Congenital
Ep	Primary
Es	Secondary (postthrombotic)
En	No venous cause identified
Anatomic classification	
As	Superficial veins
Ap	Perforator veins
Ad	Deep veins
An	No venous location identified
Pathophysiologic classification	
Pr	Reflux
Po	Obstruction
Pr,o	Reflux and obstruction
Pn	No venous pathophysiology identifiable

Data from Eklöf B, Rutherford RB, Bergan JJ, et al: Revision of the CEAP classification for chronic venous disorders: consensus statement. J Vasc Surg. *2004 Dec;40(6):1248-1252.*

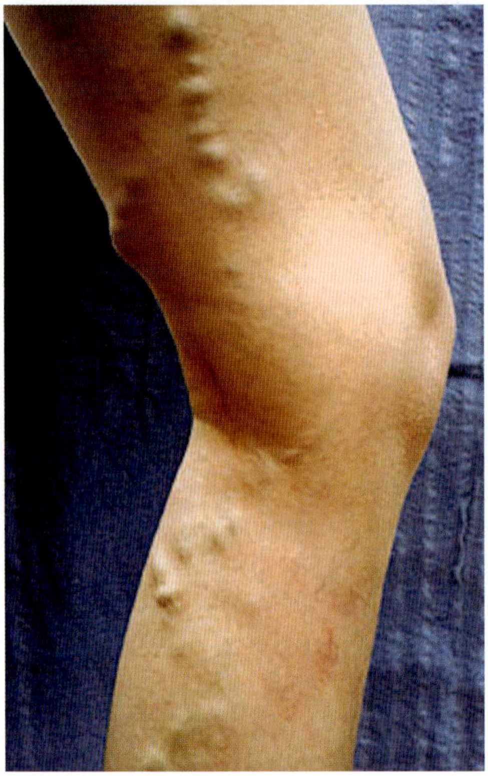

FIGURE 33-1 Varicose vein (CEAP: C2).

ETIOLOGY

Veins are responsible for ensuring blood return to the heart, and a series of valves close between heartbeats to prevent retrograde flow. A varicose vein occurs when a valve weakens, putting more pressure on other valves and causing blood to stagnate. The vein then becomes distended and endothelial walls stretch, allowing the vein to swell locally into a miniature balloon near the surface of the skin. There are several risk factors for varicose vein formation, including advancing age, family history of venous disease, ligamentous laxity such as hernia, platypodia, prolonged standing, increased body mass index, smoking, sedentary lifestyle, lower extremity trauma, prior venous thrombosis (superficial or deep), the presence of an arteriovenous shunt, some hereditary conditions, high-estrogen states, and pregnancy.[5,12-17]

Many studies have suggested a strong familial component to the development of varicose veins.[18] In a case-control study of 67 patients and their parents, the risk for varicose veins was 90% when both parents were affected, 25% for men and 62% for women when one parent was affected, and 20% if neither parent had varicose veins.[19] A recent genetic study demonstrated that polymorphisms of matrix metalloproteinase 9 (MMP9) and specific tissue inhibitors of MMP (TIMP2) genes were associated with susceptibility to varicose vein formation, and individuals with specific genotypes may have a lower risk for varicose vein formation.[20]

Because prevalence rates appear to be lower in non-Western populations, it has been widely thought that factors related to Western lifestyle, such as prolonged standing and sitting, increase the likelihood of the development of varicose veins.[21] A longitudinal study from 1999 to 2004 in 38,036 patients found that risk of surgery for varicose veins was associated with prolonged standing/walking and heavy lifting, with more than 60% of cases seen in those with high-risk occupations.[22] Several other studies in individuals with occupations that require prolonged standing, such as midwives and hairdressers, have confirmed these results.[23-25] Increased body mass appears to be a significant aggravating factor.[26]

Pregnancy is also presumed to be a major contributory factor in the increased incidence of varicose veins in women, affecting about 40% of pregnant women. Moreover, multiparous women have a higher incidence of varicose veins compared with nulliparous women.[27,28] Both the increased blood volume, which increases venous pressure, and hormones such as progesterone, which relax the muscular walls of blood vessels, aggravate the venous ability to ensure blood flow back to the heart. Moreover, the increasing weight of the growing uterus puts pressure on the pelvic veins and on the inferior vena cava, increasing blood pressure in the leg veins and thus influencing the development of varicose veins. Estrogen and progesterone receptors have been found in saphenous veins, and although their function is not yet known, it has been hypothesized that they may provoke venous dilation and valvular failure in pregnancy.[29]

INDICATIONS

Varicose veins may occur in the presence or absence of either symptoms or an underlying functional venous disorder, such as reflux.[30] Candidates for sclerotherapy manifest persistent symptoms (eg, pain, aching, and swelling) and signs (eg, telangiectasias, reticular veins, varicose veins, pigmentary changes, and ulceration) of venous disease after 6 months of medical therapy.

Sclerotherapy techniques to achieve perforator and saphenous closure are available for patients with documented reflux (ie, retrograde flow >0.5 seconds in duration) as a source of their symptoms. For patients with ulceration refractory to medical management or those who manifest recurrent ulceration, ultrasound-guided sclerotherapy of perforators can lead to significant reduction of symptoms and signs. For small varicosities that are mostly a cosmetic concern, sclerotherapy can be performed following physical examination without additional diagnostic studies, as these patients are not as likely as symptomatic patients to have underlying venous reflux.[30,31] Patients with complaints of recurrent bleeding and stigmata of recent venous hemorrhage may benefit from sclerotherapy of that vein site.[32,33] Sclerotherapy is often successful even in the presence of venous insufficiency.[32]

ANATOMIC CONSIDERATIONS

Intimate knowledge of the venous system and interconnections between the veins is a prerequisite prior to performing sclerotherapy. The axial veins of the venous system of the lower extremity

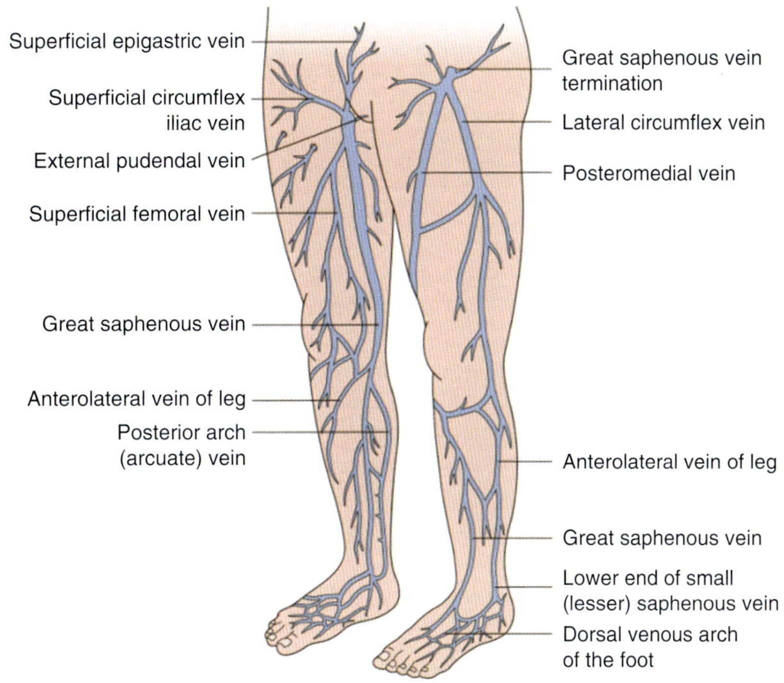

FIGURE 33-2 Superficial veins of the lower extremity. (Reproduced with permission from Bolognia JL, Jorizzo JL, Rapini RP: *Dermatology*, 2nd ed. Philadelphia, PA: Elsevier; 2008.)

are divided into the superficial and deep systems. Veins that traverse the same system are termed communicating veins, whereas veins that connect the superficial to the deep system are called perforating veins. The superficial veins are contained in the subcutaneous tissue of the lower extremity within a superficial space that is bounded deeply by the muscular fascia and superficially by the dermis. The major axial superficial veins of the lower extremity include the great and small saphenous veins. Other lower extremity superficial veins with more variant anatomy include the anterior, posterior, and superficial accessories of the great saphenous vein; the superficial accessory of the small saphenous vein; intersaphenous veins; and the lateral venous system (**Figures 33-2 and 33-3**).

The deep veins of the lower extremity are contained within the deep muscle compartments bounded by the muscle fascia (**Figure 33-3**). The deep veins of the lower extremity are classified as intramuscular (within a single muscle) or intermuscular (between muscle groups). The intermuscular veins are more important in the development of chronic venous disease. Sclerotherapy is effective in destroying a segment or length of vein that is usually axially oriented, although it cannot safely and predictably eradicate a circumferential finite point of reflux, such as a junction at which two veins converge, without the potential risk of concomitantly obliterating some length of vein distal and proximal to this point of reflux. As an example, injection of a sclerosant at the point of an incompetent saphenofemoral junction could produce destruction of the adjacent segments of the femoral vein and the greater saphenous vein. Injection of a sclerosant seldom obliterates incompetent perforating veins, but merely the varicosity of the superficial venous system into which these perforating veins empty. It is

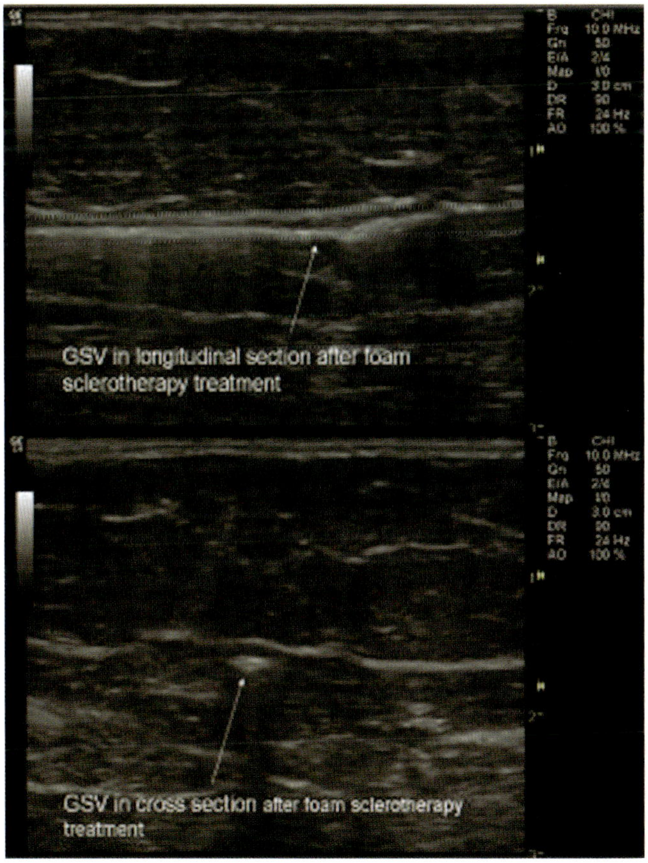

FIGURE 33-3 Cross and longitudinal sections from ultrasound-guided foam sclerotherapy (UGFS) after treatment of great saphenous vein.

advised that all sites of reflux from the deep venous system into the superficial varicosities should be surgically treated before sclerotherapy, as this would diminish the development of new varicosities by preventing retrograde flow, as well as associated elevated venous pressure, into adjacent competent veins. It also aids in minimizing retrograde flow into existing varicosities that are the targets of treatment.[34]

CONTRAINDICATIONS

Sclerotherapy should not be performed in patients who have signs of acute thrombosis or phlebitis due to the increased risk of deep venous thrombosis. Pregnant patients should defer treatment until after delivery. Diabetes and peripheral arterial occlusive disease (ankle-brachial index <0.9) are relative contraindications, as they pose a risk for wound healing complications, but this depends on the nature and extent of sclerotherapy being considered. A history of migraine headache and patent foramen ovale are also relative contraindications to sclerotherapy due to the risk for microembolism.[35-39] Those with a history of hypersensitivity and allergic reactions to any of the sclerosants should be pretested to mitigate the risk of anaphylaxis. Sclerotherapy should not be performed in individuals with active infections due to the risk of bacterial spread. Immunocompromised patients and cancer patients receiving chemotherapy should not be treated due to an increased risk of thromboembolic events. Women treated with tamoxifen are at a higher risk for thromboembolic complications during the first 2 years after exposure.[40]

WORKUP

Inspection and palpation are important elements necessary to identify venous disease. Photography can be critical because patients undergoing treatment for varicose veins often forget the original appearance of their legs and frequently report that preexisting lesions were caused by treatment. Inspection is performed in an organized manner, usually progressing from proximal to distal and from anterior to posterior. The perineum, groin, and abdominal wall must also be inspected. Normal veins typically are visibly distended at the foot and ankle and occasionally in the popliteal fossa, but dilated veins above the ankle usually are evidence of venous pathology. Inspection may reveal findings such as stasis dermatitis, lipodermatosclerosis, ulceration, atrophie blanche, interdigital mycosis, acrocyanosis, eczematous lesions, flat angiomata, clusters of telangiectatic veins, corona phlebectatica, hemosiderin deposition, prominent varicose veins, scars from a prior surgical operation, or evidence of previous sclerotherapy. Skin discoloration or ulceration along the medial aspect of the lower leg often is a sign of chronic venous stasis. Skin changes or ulcerations that are localized only to the lateral aspect of the ankle are more likely to be related to prior trauma or to arterial insufficiency, although small saphenous venous insufficiency may present in this manner as well. Palpation should begin along the anteromedial surface of the lower limb proceeding to the lateral and then finally to the posterior surface of both lower limbs. The location and course of all varicosities should be carefully noted. The great saphenous vein may be palpated in thin patients without varicose veins, but it is particularly well appreciated in patients with truncal reflux at the saphenofemoral junction. If reflux is present, a forced cough or Valsalva maneuver may produce expansion at this level. The small saphenous vein may be palpable below the gastrocnemius muscle in some slender or muscular patients. Other superficial veins above the feet are usually not palpable even after prolonged standing.

Currently used technologies such as duplex imaging have revealed that the great saphenous vein is often not the refluxing vessel causing varicosities. Accessory veins, circumflex veins, or even small groin veins, such as the superficial epigastric vein, may be the source. It should be emphasized that ultrasound technicians are often unfamiliar with superficial venous anatomy and its many variations. The treating clinician must therefore be self-sufficient with regard to handling an ultrasound probe and recognizing the nuances of venous anatomy. The diagnosis of varicose veins is confirmed by the presence of venous reflux, which is diagnosed by duplex ultrasound as retrograde or reversed flow of greater than 0.5 second in duration.[41,42]

SCLEROSANTS AND SCLEROTHERAPY

The most common agents used in the treatment of varicose veins are sodium tetradecyl sulfate (STS), polidocanol, glycerin, and hypertonic saline. These substances cause endothelial damage by their actions as either osmotic or detergent agents. Osmotic agents achieve their effect by dehydrating endothelial cells through osmosis. Detergents are surface-active agents that damage the endothelium by interfering with cell membrane lipids.[43] In vitro, detergent agents also exhibit procoagulant activity at lower concentrations and anticoagulant activity in higher concentrations.[44] When comparing the two agents in terms of short-term success of sclerotherapy for varicosities, several systematic reviews have failed to support the use of one sclerosant over another (**Table 33-2**).[45-47]

STS is the most commonly studied sclerosant.[45] The maximum recommended dosage is 10 mL of a 3% solution in the United States and Canada, but the volume used varies worldwide depending on formulation. Dilutions between 0.1% and 3.0% are used depending on the size of the vein treated; narrower diameter veins are treated with lower concentrations. A systematic review comparing various sclerotherapy agents for the treatment of small varicosities found that STS was more likely to cause adverse reactions at a concentration of 1% compared with polidocanol at 0.5%.[47,48]

Polidocanol, also known as aethoxysklerol, is another detergent sclerosant available for commercial use in the United States, where it is marketed as Asclera. The maximum dosage is dependent on the weight of the patient. Dilutions between 0.25% and 5% are used depending on the size of the vein. In a systematic review comparing various sclerotherapy agents for the treatment of small varicosities, polidocanol was no more painful than placebo.[47]

TABLE 33-2 • Concentrations of Sclerosants According to Vessel Diameter

Type of Varicose Veins	Polidocanol Liquid	Sotradecol Liquid	Polidocanol Foam	Sotradecol Foam
Small varices up to 4 mm in diameter, visual or duplex-guided injections (subdermal veins)	0.5%-1% Up to 1 mL per injection point	0.25%-0.5% Up to 1 mL per injection point	0.5% Up to 1 mL per injection point. In case of inefficacy of liquid	0.25% Up to 1 mL per injection point In case of inefficacy of liquid
4-6 mm in diameter extrafascial varices, under duplex guidance	1%-2% Up to 1 mL per injection point	1%-2% Up to 1 mL per injection point	1%-2% Up to 2 mL per injection point, compress and massage to fill desired network, and trigger spasm	0.5%-1.5% Up to 2 mL per injection point, compress and massage to fill desired network, and trigger spasm

Hypertonic saline is the most commonly used osmotic agent for lower extremity sclerotherapy. The dilution used to treat lower extremity vessels ranges from 11.7% to 23.4%. Hypertonic saline (20%) mixed with heparin 100 units/mL constitutes Heparsal. Hypertonic saline is frequently mixed with local anesthetic to reduce the pain associated with injection (eg, 20% saline plus 2% lidocaine).

Chromated glycerin (eg, Chromex, Skermo) is a potent osmotic agent with dilutions that range from 25% to 72%. The maximum recommended amount per session is 10 mL.[49] While very popular worldwide, it is not commercially available in the United States.

Liquid sclerotherapy can be used to treat telangiectasias, reticular veins, small nonsaphenous varicose veins (<5 mm), residual or recurrent varicosities following endovenous ablation or surgery, and perforator veins.[45,50] Liquid injection sclerotherapy is the gold standard for the treatment of the majority of lower extremity varicosities as the results are usually superior to those of cutaneous laser/light therapy.

When vessels are treated sequentially from deep to superficial and from larger to smaller veins, over 90% of vessels can be successfully treated. Due to the risk of longstanding hypopigmentation from laser and light treatments, liquid sclerotherapy is a more appropriate choice for patients with Fitzpatrick skin types IV, V, and VI. Laser/light treatments are recommended for patients who have failed sclerotherapy or experienced a poor outcome, patients with postsclerotherapy matting, needle-phobic patients, and patients allergic to sclerosant agents. Laser/light treatment is also preferred for vessels located at or below the ankle regions, which are more prone to ulceration with sclerotherapy.

Sclerosant foams were developed from liquid detergent sclerosant agents to increase the surface area of exposure and are more commonly used for the treatment of larger varicosities.[51] The foam can be produced manually just prior to injection using the Tessari method (**Figure 33-4**).[19] Foam prepared according to the Tessari technique has a half-life of approximately 90 seconds. Thus, the procedure should be completed within 1 minute, before the foam separates. An alternative consists of a product that dispenses a low-nitrogen gas and sclerosant liquid under pressure to produces polidocanol foam with appreciably smaller and consistently sized bubbles compared with a foam/air mixture made by hand.[52] Sclerosant foam is echogenic due to the tiny air bubbles in the foam, which are easily seen with duplex ultrasound. The expanded volume of the foam compared with liquid agents provides more surface contact and a more uniform vessel closure and permits the use of smaller volumes of sclerosant. In principle, all calibers of veins are suitable for foam sclerotherapy; however, foams are not generally used for the treatment of telangiectasias or reticular veins because there is no significant advantage over liquid sclerotherapy in small vessels and, therefore, ultrasound-guided foam sclerotherapy is predominantly used for the treatment of saphenous incompetence (great or small) and incompetent perforating veins (**Figure 33-3**).[51]

PREOPERATIVE EVALUATION

Prior to the procedure, a careful review of the patient's medical file, including personal and family medical history, current medical treatments, previous phlebo-surgical and sclerosing treatments and outcomes, allergies, and contraindications, should be performed. Review of complete and recent duplex ultrasound scanning of both limbs, including superficial, deep, and perforating veins, and the patient's signed informed consent forms should also be done.

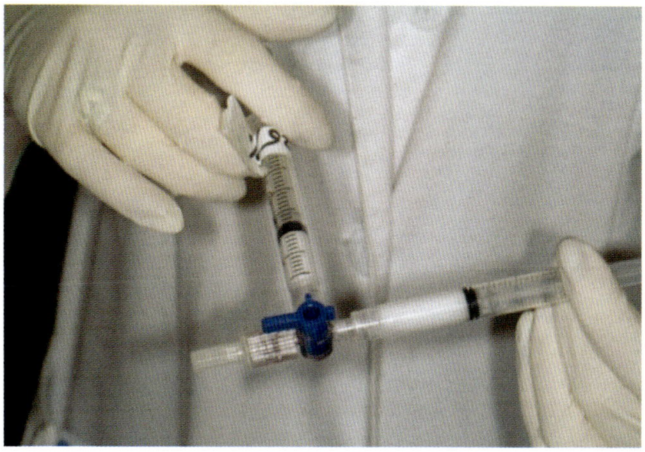

FIGURE 33-4 Tessari method.

TECHNIQUE: LIQUID SCLEROTHERAPY SESSION

- Position the patient on the table:
    - Half sitting for treatment on the anterior aspect of limb
    - Prone for treatment of the posterior leg
    - On the side for lateral and medially located lesions
- Prepare the skin with alcohol or chlorhexidine.
- Don new gloves.
- Prepare syringes and needles for the tray:
    - For subcutaneous varicose veins up to 4 mm: 2.5-mL syringe, 25- to 28-gauge needle, liquid polidocanol 0.5% to 2%, or STS 0.5% to 1%. If necessary: foamed polidocanol 0.5% to 1% or STS 0.25% to 0.5%.
    - Larger varicose veins injected without duplex guidance: liquid polidocanol 1% to 3% or STS 1% to 3%. Preferably foam if no contraindication.
- Localize, puncture, and inject larger varices first, then reticular varices, and finally telangiectasias. Check appropriate needle tip placement by usual means (reflux of blood in the needle when aspirating, absence of visible or palpable bump or swelling at the injection site, blanching of catheterized veins). Use magnifying goggles, transillumination (**Figures 33-5 and 33-6**), or other visualization devices when needed. Favor multiple injections of low volumes. In telangiectasias, avoid blanching areas bigger than 2.5 cm × 2.5 cm from a single injection point.
- Report injection sites, volume used, concentrations, immediate outcomes, and side effects in patient's chart.
- Microthrombectomy of previously treated varicose veins may be necessary during the session (**Figures 33-7, 33-8, and 33-9**).

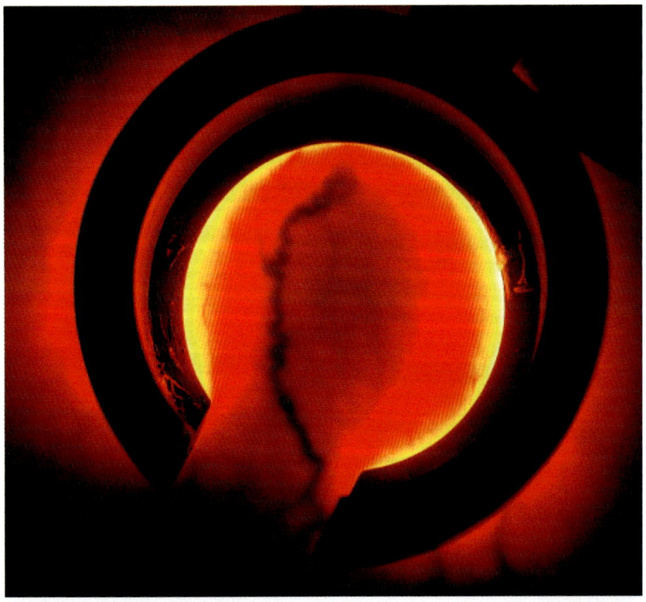

FIGURE 33-5 Handheld transilluminator to facilitate vein access and treatment.

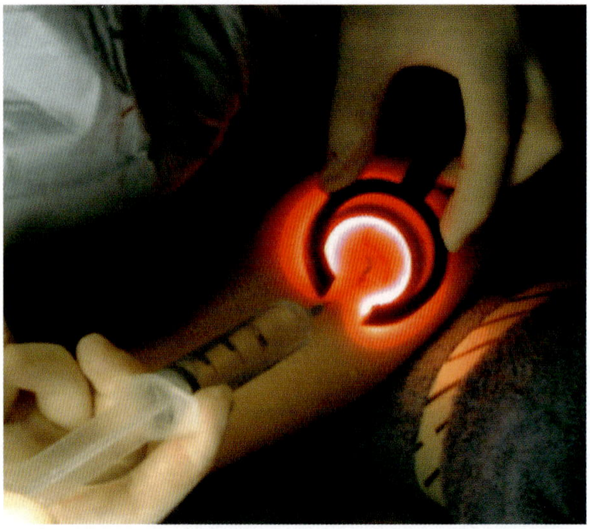

FIGURE 33-6 Handheld transilluminator used during sclerotherapy.

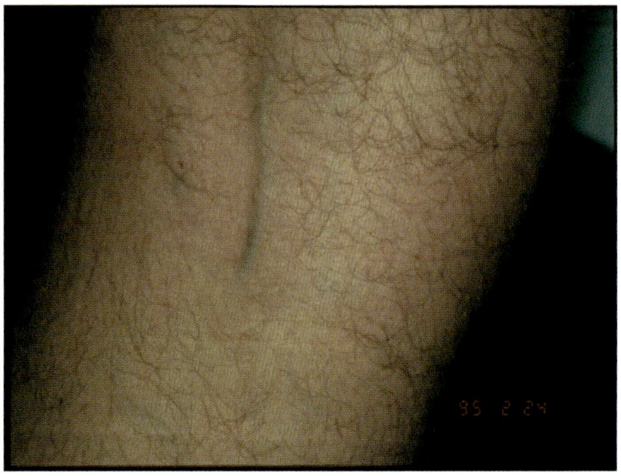

FIGURE 33-7 A 40-year-old male in good physical condition and an occupation that involved prolonged standing presented with a varicose vein on his right leg. Symptoms included pain and "heaviness" that intensified at night and during warm weather.

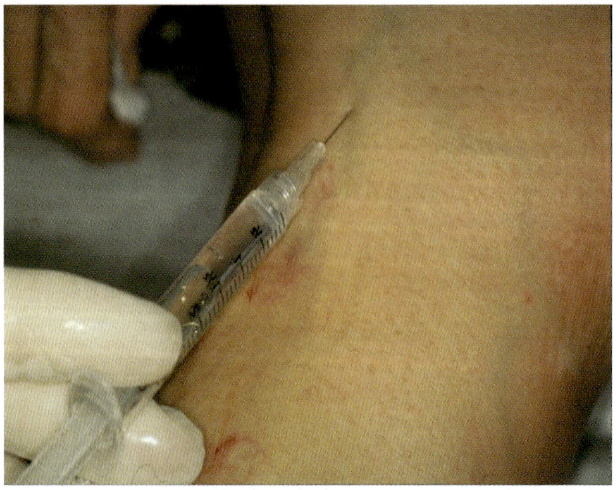

FIGURE 33-8 Duplex ultrasound did not reveal reflux, thus liquid sclerotherapy with polidocanol was prescribed.

TECHNIQUE: FOAM SCLEROTHERAPY SESSION

- Locate target vein in longitudinal or transverse view according to local conditions and preferred technique. Measure depth to compute needle length, and measure diameter to estimate volumes to inject.
- Prepare foam with two syringes and a female-female connector (Tessari method):
  - In one 2.5-mL syringe, aspirate 2 mL of gas: room air, sterile air, other gas mix (if using 5-mL syringes, aspirate 4 mL of gas).
  - In the other syringe, aspirate 0.5 mL of sclerosing agent (polidocanol or STS) at the desired concentration (0.5%-3%).
  - Unite syringes with connector.
  - Pass contents back and forth from one syringe to the other 20 times. Foam is now ready and must be used in less than 2 minutes (**Figures 33-10 and 33-11**).
- If open vein access is ready, connect foam syringe to access, aspirate to check blood reflux, inject a few bubbles, check their presence in vein lumen on duplex screen, and proceed to injection of desired amount of foam according to planned protocol (predetermined volume or sufficient volume to induce venous spasm).
- If no open vein access has been inserted previously, attach a needle to the foam syringe (no smaller than 25 gauge, sufficient length is two to three times the depth of the vein). Puncture the vein and check presence of tip in the middle of the vein lumen. Aspirate to verify blood reflux in syringe, inject a few bubbles to verify their presence on duplex screen, and proceed to inject the desired volume.
- Check progression of sclerosing foam in target varices. If necessary, massage foam into remote veins, observe venous spasm, and observe progression of scattered bubbles into perforating and deep system if any.
- Report injection sites, volumes, concentrations, diffusion, immediate outcomes, side effects, and all relevant information in patient's chart (**Figures 33-12** and **33-13**).

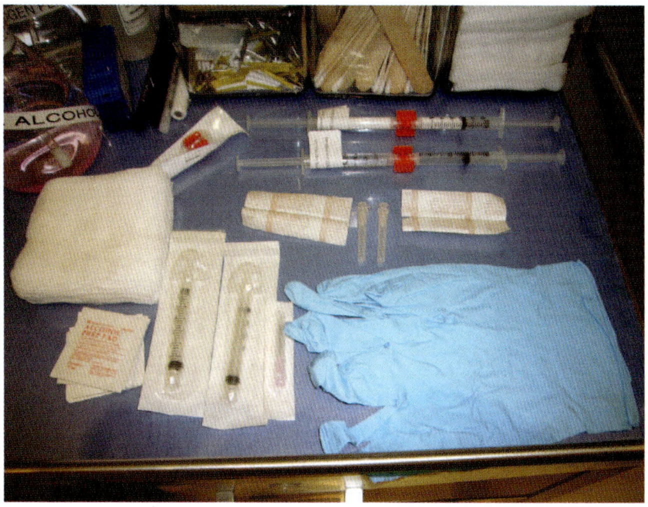

FIGURE 33-10 Preparation of tray for foam sclerotherapy.

POSTOPERATIVE CARE

After treatment of large varicose veins by any method, a 30- to 40-mm Hg gradient compression stocking is applied, and patients are instructed to maintain or increase their normal activity levels (**Figure 33-14**). Many clinicians also recommend the use of gradient compression stockings even after treatment of smaller varicose veins. In a randomized trial of patients undergoing foam sclerotherapy for primary uncomplicated varicose veins, no significant difference was noted in vein occlusion, phlebitis, skin discoloration, or pain at 2 and 6 weeks with the two techniques.[53] Ace wraps and other long-stretch bandages should not be used. These elastic bandages fail to maintain adequate compression for more than a few hours. They often slip or are misapplied by patients, with a resulting tourniquet effect that causes distal swelling and increases the risk of deep vein thrombosis (DVT). Activity is particularly important after treatment

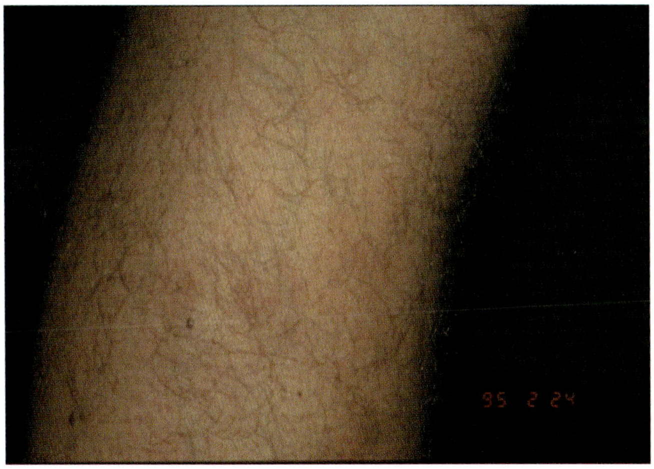

FIGURE 33-9 A 2-year follow-up showed complete clearance.

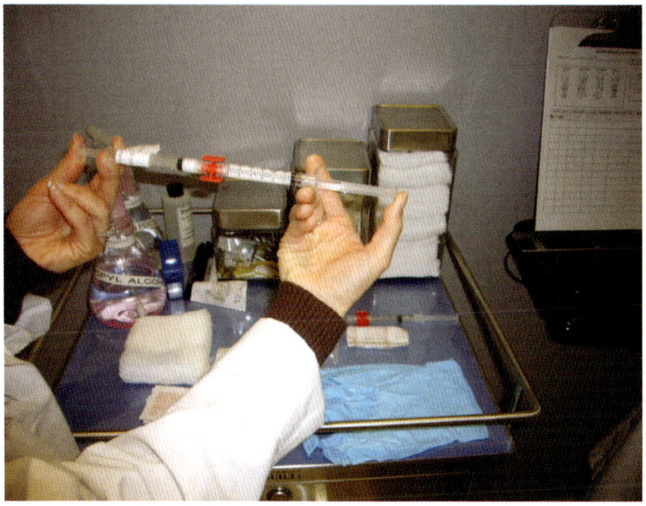

FIGURE 33-11 Preparation of foam sclerosant.

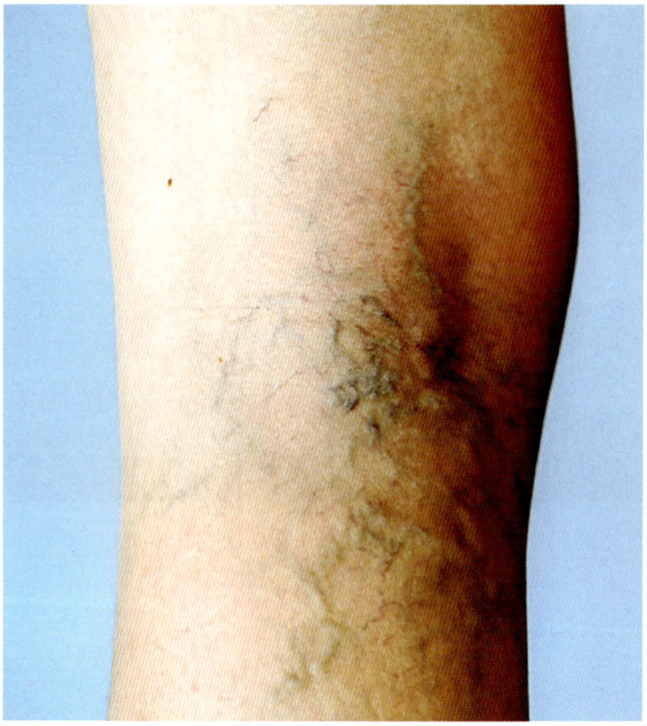

FIGURE 33-12 A 42-year-old woman presented with networked varicose veins in her left leg after her third pregnancy. She had an unremarkable medical history and took no medications. Her main concern was the aesthetic appearance. As part of the routine investigation protocol, a thorough lower limb duplex venous mapping scan was performed that revealed no great or small saphenous vein incompetence. The patient was treated conservatively with ultrasound-guided foam sclerotherapy (UGFS) with sodium tetradecyl sulfate (STS) solution foamed with air (three parts air and one part 1.5% STS). Six milliliters foam utilizing six separated injections of 1-mL foam were injected in the leg vein. Class 2 compression stockings were applied, and the patient was asked to wear a firm pair of cotton underwear and walk for half an hour immediately after completion of the treatment. She returned 1 week post treatment for a left lower limb follow-up duplex scan, which demonstrated that all the treated veins were well sclerosed and the deep veins were patent with normal flows. The patient did not report any adverse symptoms.

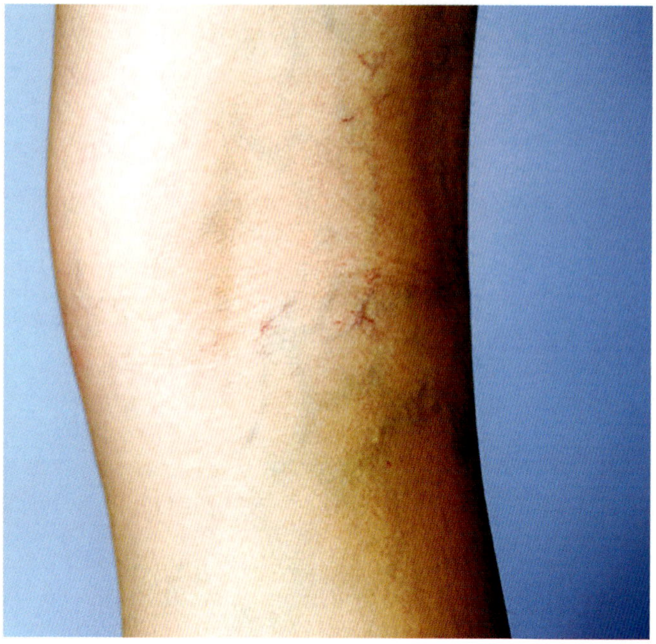

FIGURE 33-13 Subject post sclerotherapy session.

DVT

A systematic review of foam sclerotherapy reported DVT in 0.02% to 5.7% of patients.[54] Although DVT can occur after sclerotherapy of telangiectasias, it is more likely to occur after sclerotherapy of the saphenous veins.[55] Popliteal vein thrombosis by any technique, as all treatments for varicose disease have the potential to increase the risk of DVT. Activity is a strong protective factor against venous stasis. Indeed, many venous specialists will not treat a patient who is unable to remain active following treatment.

COMPLICATIONS

Superficial Thrombophlebitis

A mild inflammatory response is expected after sclerotherapy, and some patients may have urticaria at the site of injection. A more intense superficial thrombophlebitis with erythema, warmth, and pain can extend to veins neighboring the injection site.

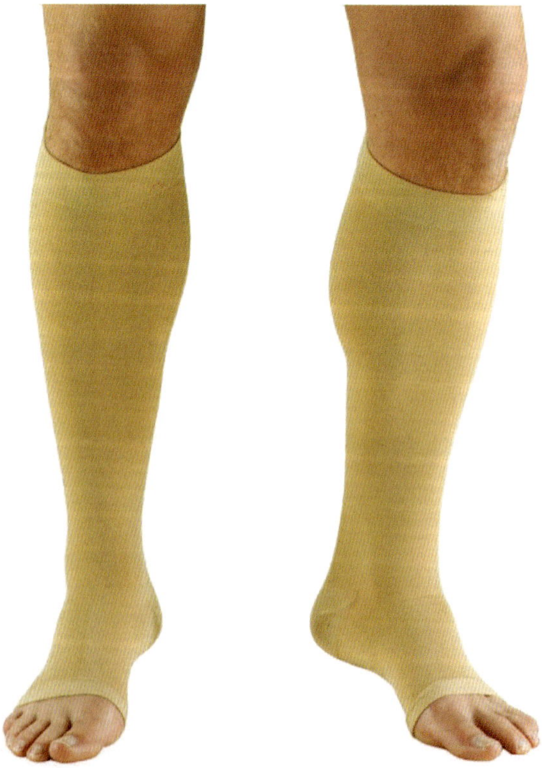

FIGURE 33-14 Compression stockings for sclerotherapy.

has been reported with foam sclerotherapy of the small saphenous vein.[56,57] Patients are diagnosed and treated for DVT following standard protocols.

Visual and Other Neurologic Disturbances

Visual or neurologic disturbance is uncommon during or following sclerotherapy. In a systematic review, the incidence of visual disturbance following sclerotherapy ranged from 0.09% to 2%.[58] These disturbances are usually transient; permanent deficits are rare.[54] Symptoms include visual disturbance (scotoma), migraine-like headache, and neurologic deficits. These appear to be more common with foam compared with liquid sclerotherapy.[59] Visual disturbances reported following sclerotherapy of telangiectasias and reticular veins are strongly associated with the use of air-block and foam techniques, suggesting that the etiology is air microembolization. Most visual disturbances occur during or immediately after the procedure when the patient ambulates, possibly due to rising microbubbles in the bloodstream. In one study, 20 (0.16%) of 12,173 patients treated with sclerotherapy experienced visual disturbances, 70% of which were following sclerotherapy of small varicosities.[55] Visual disturbances were associated with nausea, headache, or vasovagal episodes; all cases regressed spontaneously.

During foam sclerotherapy of the great saphenous vein, microbubbles can be detected in the right heart and pulmonary circulation and, in patients with a patent foramen ovale, in the left heart as well.[38] Coughing following foam sclerotherapy has been attributed to air microembolization into the pulmonary circulation. In a prospective study of 33 patients, cardiac echocardiography was performed during foam sclerotherapy and cardiac microemboli were detected in every patient studied. Microemboli were also seen in the left ventricle of five patients, and each was subsequently found to have a patent foramen ovale; however, none of these patients experienced neurologic symptoms.[38] Given the significant prevalence (25%-30%) of patent foramen ovale in the general population, it is apparent that the incidence of significant neurologic sequelae following foam sclerotherapy is low.

COMBINATION WITH LASERS

Several studies have demonstrated the clinical superiority and patient preference of sclerotherapy compared with laser therapy for the treatment of varicosities.[60] However, given the need for repeat sclerotherapy sessions in order to achieve complete clearance of varicose veins, combination therapy with lasers has been evaluated to improve clinical results while minimizing patient discomfort and time investment. In an early study, combination treatment with pulsed-dye laser (585 nm) followed by sclerotherapy with polidocanol (0.1-0.25 mL per injection site) in 30 female patients with varicosities showed that the treatments were efficacious for the larger varicose veins rather than for smaller vessels.[61] In a later study of 14 patients with leg varicosities that were treated with long-pulsed Nd:YAG alone, sclerotherapy alone, laser then sclerotherapy, or sclerotherapy then laser, results demonstrated that combination approaches may increase response to treatment.[62] The best sequence appeared to be sclerotherapy followed by laser, as this demonstrated a higher clearance compared to laser then sclerotherapy. A recent randomized, polidocanol-controlled clinical trial compared the results between 79 legs treated with polidocanol and 517 treated with polidocanol together with long-pulsed Nd:YAG laser and showed that the combination treatment was much more effective than polidocanol microfoam alone in clearing varicosities with a diameter under 4 mm. The 3-year follow-up showed clearing percentages of 89% (class I veins), 94% (class II veins), and 95% (class III veins) in the combination treatment cohort in comparison to 15%, 18%, and 17% when only polidocanol was applied.[63]

CONCLUSIONS

In-office sclerotherapy is a highly effective technique for varicose vein management and can lead to marked cosmetic and quality-of-life improvement. Attention to detail in the preoperative, intraoperative, and postoperative periods may improve outcomes. Smaller vessels may be treated with liquid sclerosants, whereas foam approaches are helpful for the treatment of larger vessels. Considering combination approaches with both laser and sclerotherapy may represent a promising approach as well. Ultimately, the goal is to balance the risks of the procedure with the desired outcome by the patient.

REFERENCES

1. Gloviczki P, Comerota AJ, Dalsing MC, et al. The care of patients with varicose veins and associated chronic venous diseases: clinical practice guidelines of the Society for Vascular Surgery and the American Venous Forum. *J Vasc Surg*. 2011;53(5 Suppl):2S-48S.
2. Wittens C, Davies AH, Baekgaard N, et al. Editor's choice: management of chronic venous disease: clinical practice guidelines of the European Society for Vascular Surgery (ESVS). *Eur J Vasc Endovasc Surg*. 2015;49(6):678-737.
3. O'Donnell TF Jr, Passman MA. Clinical practice guidelines of the Society for Vascular Surgery (SVS) and the American Venous Forum (AVF): management of venous leg ulcers. Introduction. *J Vasc Surg*. 2014;60(2 Suppl):1S-2S.
4. Bergan JJ, Schmid-Schonbein GW, Smith PD, Nicolaides AN, Boisseau MR, Eklof B. Chronic venous disease. *N Engl J Med*. 2006;355(5):488-498.
5. Callam MJ. Epidemiology of varicose veins. *Br J Surg*. 1994;81(2):167-173.
6. Evans CJ, Fowkes FG, Ruckley CV, Lee AJ. Prevalence of varicose veins and chronic venous insufficiency in men and women in the general population: Edinburgh Vein Study. *J Epidemiol Community Health*. 1999;53(3):149-153.
7. Carpentier PH, Maricq HR, Biro C, Poncot-Makinen CO, Franco A. Prevalence, risk factors, and clinical patterns of chronic venous disorders of lower limbs: a population-based study in France. *J Vasc Surg*. 2004;40(4):650-659.
8. Sadick N, Sorhaindo L. Chapter 16: Laser treatment of telangiectasias and reticular veins. In: Bergan JJ, ed. *The Vein Book*. San Diego, CA: Elsevier; 2007:157-166.

9. Fegan WG. Continuous compression technique of injecting varicose veins. *Lancet.* 1963;2(7299):109-112.
10. Meissner MH. What is effective care for varicose veins? *Phlebology.* 2016;31(1 Suppl):80-87.
11. Marsden G, Perry M, Bradbury A, et al. A cost-effectiveness analysis of surgery, endothermal ablation, ultrasound-guided foam sclerotherapy and compression stockings for symptomatic varicose veins. *Eur J Vasc Endovasc Surg.* 2015;50(6):794-801.
12. Brand FN, Dannenberg AL, Abbott RD, Kannel WB. The epidemiology of varicose veins: the Framingham study. *Am J Prev Med.* 1988;4(2):96-101.
13. Chiesa R, Marone EM, Limoni C, Volonte M, Petrini O. Chronic venous disorders: correlation between visible signs, symptoms, and presence of functional disease. *J Vasc Surg.* 2007;46(2):322-330.
14. Scott TE, LaMorte WW, Gorin DR, Menzoian JO. Risk factors for chronic venous insufficiency: a dual case-control study. *J Vasc Surg.* 1995;22(5):622-628.
15. Fowkes FG, Lee AJ, Evans CJ, Allan PL, Bradbury AW, Ruckley CV. Lifestyle risk factors for lower limb venous reflux in the general population: Edinburgh vein study. *Int J Epidemiol.* 2001;30(4):846-852.
16. Sadick NS. Predisposing factors of varicose and telangiectatic leg veins. *J Dermatol Surg Oncol.* 1992;18(10):883-886.
17. Iannuzzi A, Panico S, Ciardullo AV, et al. Varicose veins of the lower limbs and venous capacitance in postmenopausal women: relationship with obesity. *J Vasc Surg.* 2002;36(5):965-968.
18. Criqui MH, Denenberg JO, Bergan J, Langer RD, Fronek A. Risk factors for chronic venous disease: the San Diego population study. *J Vasc Surg.* 2007;46(2):331-337.
19. Cornu-Thenard A, Boivin P, Baud JM, De Vincenzi I, Carpentier PH. Importance of the familial factor in varicose disease. Clinical study of 134 families. *J Dermatol Surg Oncol.* 1994;20(5):318-326.
20. Kunt AT, Isbir S, Gormus U, et al. Polymorphisms of MMP9 and TIMP2 in patients with varicose veins. *In Vivo.* 2015;29(4):461-465.
21. Stanhope JM. Varicose veins in a population of lowland New Guinea. *Int J Epidemiol.* 1975;4(3):221-225.
22. Tabatabaeifar S, Frost P, Andersen JH, Jensen LD, Thomsen JF, Svendsen SW. Varicose veins in the lower extremities in relation to occupational mechanical exposures: a longitudinal study. *Occup Environ Med.* 2015;72(5):330-337.
23. Azma K, Mottaghi P, Hosseini A, Salek S, Bina R. Venous insufficiency after prolonged standing: is joint hypermobility an important risk factor? *Adv Biomed Res.* 2015;4:98.
24. Joseph N, B A, Faizan Thouseef M, Devi MU, Abna A, Juneja I. A multicenter review of epidemiology and management of varicose veins for national guidance. *Ann Med Surg (Lond).* 2016;8:21-27.
25. Randall S. Looking after your health. 3. Avoiding varicose veins. *Pract Midwife.* 2015;18(2):32-34.
26. Kohno K, Niihara H, Hamano T, et al. Standing posture at work and overweight exacerbate varicose veins: Shimane CoHRE study. *J Dermatol.* 2014;41(11):964-968.
27. Rabhi Y, Charras-Arthapignet C, Gris JC, et al. Lower limb vein enlargement and spontaneous blood flow echogenicity are normal sonographic findings during pregnancy. *J Clin Ultrasound.* 2000;28(8):407-413.
28. Beebe-Dimmer JL, Pfeifer JR, Engle JS, Schottenfeld D. The epidemiology of chronic venous insufficiency and varicose veins. *Ann Epidemiol.* 2005;15(3):175-184.
29. Mashiah A, Berman V, Thole HH, et al. Estrogen and progesterone receptors in normal and varicose saphenous veins. *Cardiovasc Surg.* 1999;7(3):327-331.
30. Langer RD, Ho E, Denenberg JO, Fronek A, Allison M, Criqui MH. Relationships between symptoms and venous disease: the San Diego population study. *Arch Intern Med.* 2005;165(12):1420-1424.
31. Criqui MH, Jamosmos M, Fronek A, et al. Chronic venous disease in an ethnically diverse population: the San Diego population study. *Am J Epidemiol.* 2003;158(5):448-456.
32. Labas P, Cambal M. Profuse bleeding in patients with chronic venous insufficiency. *Int Angiol.* 2007;26(1):64-66.
33. Hamahata A, Yamaki T, Osada A, Fujisawa D, Sakurai H. Foam sclerotherapy for spouting haemorrhage in patients with varicose veins. *Eur J Vasc Endovasc Surg.* 2011;41(6):856-858.
34. Green D. Sclerotherapy for the permanent eradication of varicose veins: theoretical and practical considerations. *J Am Acad Dermatol.* 1998;38(3):461-475.
35. Forlee MV, Grouden M, Moore DJ, Shanik G. Stroke after varicose vein foam injection sclerotherapy. *J Vasc Surg.* 2006;43(1):162-164.
36. Gillet JL, Guedes JM, Guex JJ, et al. Side-effects and complications of foam sclerotherapy of the great and small saphenous veins: a controlled multicenter prospective study including 1,025 patients. *Phlebology.* 2009;24(3):131-138.
37. Raymond-Martimbeau P. Transient adverse events positively associated with patent foramen ovale after ultrasound-guided foam sclerotherapy. *Phlebology.* 2009;24(3):114-119.
38. Ceulen RP, Sommer A, Vernooy K. Microembolism during foam sclerotherapy of varicose veins. *N Engl J Med.* 2008;358(14):1525-1526.
39. Hanisch F, Muller T, Krivokuca M, Winterholler M. Stroke following variceal sclerotherapy. *Eur J Med Res.* 2004;9(5):282-284.
40. Hernandez RK, Sorensen HT, Pedersen L, Jacobsen J, Lash TL. Tamoxifen treatment and risk of deep venous thrombosis and pulmonary embolism: a Danish population-based cohort study. *Cancer.* 2009;115(19):4442-4449.
41. Coleridge-Smith P, Labropoulos N, Partsch H, Myers K, Nicolaides A, Cavezzi A. Duplex ultrasound investigation of the veins in chronic venous disease of the lower limbs-UIP consensus document. Part I. Basic principles. *Eur J Vasc Endovasc Surg.* 2006;31(1):83-92.
42. Labropoulos N, Tiongson J, Pryor L, et al. Definition of venous reflux in lower-extremity veins. *J Vasc Surg.* 2003;38(4):793-798.
43. Goldman MP. Treatment of varicose and telangiectatic leg veins: double-blind prospective comparative trial between aethoxyskerol and sotradecol. *Dermatol Surg.* 2002;28(1):52-55.
44. Parsi K, Exner T, Connor DE, Ma DD, Joseph JE. In vitro effects of detergent sclerosants on coagulation, platelets and microparticles. *Eur J Vasc Endovasc Surg.* 2007;34(6):731-740.
45. Tisi PV, Beverley C, Rees A. Injection sclerotherapy for varicose veins. *Cochrane Database Syst Rev.* 2006;4:CD001732.
46. Tisi PV, Beverley CA. Injection sclerotherapy for varicose veins. *Cochrane Database Syst Rev.* 2002;1:CD001732.
47. Schwartz L, Maxwell H. Sclerotherapy for lower limb telangiectasias. *Cochrane Database Syst Rev.* 2011;12:CD008826.
48. Sadick NS. Choosing the appropriate sclerosing concentration for vessel diameter. *Dermatol Surg.* 2010;36(Suppl 2):976-981.
49. Leach BC, Goldman MP. Comparative trial between sodium tetradecyl sulfate and glycerin in the treatment of telangiectatic leg veins. *Dermatol Surg.* 2003;29(6):612-614; discussion 615.

50. Galland RB, Magee TR, Lewis MH. A survey of current attitudes of British and Irish vascular surgeons to venous sclerotherapy. *Eur J Vasc Endovasc Surg*. 1998;16(1):43-46.

51. Breu FX, Guggenbichler S. European consensus meeting on foam sclerotherapy, April, 4-6, 2003, Tegernsee, Germany. *Dermatol Surg*. 2004;30(5):709-717; discussion 717.

52. Eckmann DM. Polidocanol for endovenous microfoam sclerosant therapy. *Expert Opin Investig Drugs*. 2009;18(12):1919-1927.

53. O'Hare JL, Stephens J, Parkin D, Earnshaw JJ. Randomized clinical trial of different bandage regimens after foam sclerotherapy for varicose veins. *Br J Surg*. 2010;97(5):650-656.

54. Jia X, Mowatt G, Burr JM, Cassar K, Cook J, Fraser C. Systematic review of foam sclerotherapy for varicose veins. *Br J Surg*. 2007;94(8):925-936.

55. Guex JJ, Allaert FA, Gillet JL, Chleir F. Immediate and midterm complications of sclerotherapy: report of a prospective multicenter registry of 12,173 sclerotherapy sessions. *Dermatol Surg*. 2005;31(2):123-128; discussion 128.

56. Darvall KA, Bate GR, Silverman SH, Adam DJ, Bradbury AW. Medium-term results of ultrasound-guided foam sclerotherapy for small saphenous varicose veins. *Br J Surg*. 2009;96(11):1268-1273.

57. Gillet JL, Lausecker M, Sica M, Guedes JM, Allaert FA. Is the treatment of the small saphenous veins with foam sclerotherapy at risk of deep vein thrombosis? *Phlebology*. 2014;29(9):600-607.

58. Willenberg T, Smith PC, Shepherd A, Davies AH. Visual disturbance following sclerotherapy for varicose veins, reticular veins and telangiectasias: a systematic literature review. *Phlebology*. 2013;28(3): 123-131.

59. Hill DA. Neurological and chest symptoms following sclerotherapy: a single centre experience. *Phlebology*. 2014;29(9):619-627.

60. Lupton JR, Alster TS, Romero P. Clinical comparison of sclerotherapy versus long-pulsed Nd:YAG laser treatment for lower extremity telangiectasias. *Dermatol Surg*. 2002;28(8):694-697.

61. Goldman MP, Fitzpatrick RE. Pulsed-dye laser treatment of leg telangiectasia: with and without simultaneous sclerotherapy. *J Dermatol Surg Oncol*. 1990;16(4):338-344.

62. Levy JL, Elbahr C, Jouve E, Mordon S. Comparison and sequential study of long pulsed Nd:YAG 1,064 nm laser and sclerotherapy in leg telangiectasias treatment. *Lasers Surg Med*. 2004;34(3):273-276.

63. Moreno-Moraga J, Smarandache A, Pascu ML, Royo J, Trelles MA. 1064 nm Nd:YAG long pulse laser after polidocanol microfoam injection dramatically improves the result of leg vein treatment: a randomized controlled trial on 517 legs with a three-year follow-up. *Phlebology*. 2014;29(10):658-666.

34 Approaches to Neck Rejuvenation

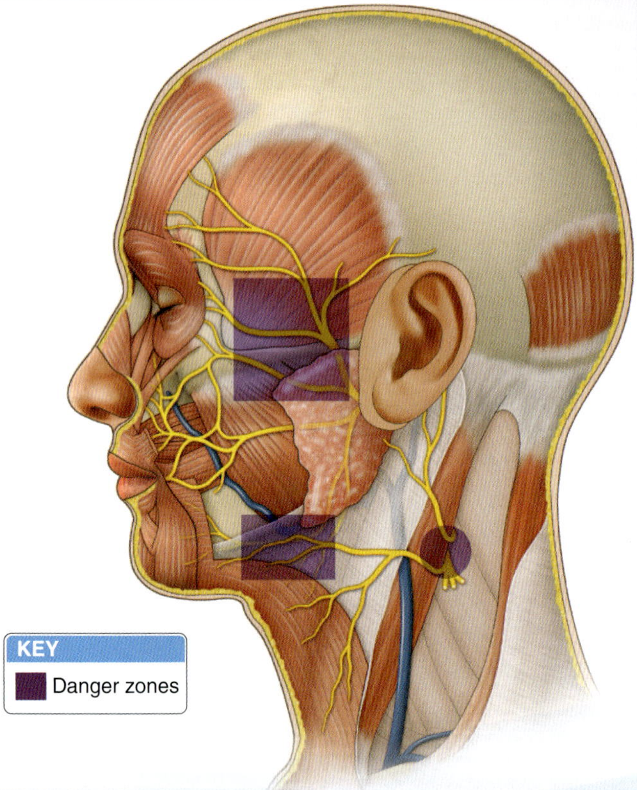

SUMMARY

- Restoration of a youthful neckline is arguably one of the most critical aspects of achieving overall aesthetic balance.
- Multiple intrinsic and extrinsic factors including genetics, photodamage, and gravity contribute to aging in the neck.
- Combination treatments may ultimately yield better outcomes for many patients.

Beginner Tips

- Loss of definition along the jaw—an invariable effect of changing anatomy over time—may be improved via the Nefertiti Lift.
- Microbotox is another useful technique for improving the overall appearance of the neck.

Pitfalls and Cautions

- Laser resurfacing on the neck should be performed with caution due to the lack of pilosebaceous units and the attendant increased risk of scarring.
- There have been reports of scarring even with a fractional CO_2 laser.

Expert Tips

- For optimal restoration and multilevel cosmetic revitalization, dilute fillers are frequently combined with light- or energy-based modalities that stimulate tissue contraction and subsequent tightening.

Patient Education Points

- There is typically a tradeoff between the amount of downtime associated with a procedure and its efficacy.
- Patients should understand that many treatments used for neck rejuvenation will need to be repeated on a regular basis.
- Patients should ideally see neck rejuvenation as one component of a global approach to facial rejuvenation.

Don't Forget!

- Combination treatments may offer the best solution for neck rejuvenation.
- Plication sutures may be very useful to maximize and maintain lift.

Approaches to Neck Rejuvenation

34

INTRODUCTION

Treatment of the aging neck presents a special challenge for the cosmetic clinician. Thin, fragile skin; the small number of cutaneous adnexal and pilosebaceous units; variable accumulation of submental fat; and hypertrophied and separated platysmal bands require careful planning and a comprehensive approach.[1] Restoration of the youthful neckline is arguably one of the most critical aspects of achieving overall aesthetic balance, particularly as the increasing popularity of procedures in facial aesthetics gives rise to greater disparity between the smooth contours of the treated face and a neck that appears skeletonized and distinctly aged.

NECK ANATOMY

While the overall anatomy of the neck is complex, the superficial anatomy most commonly addressed by cosmetic procedures includes the skin, subcutaneous fat, superficial cervical fascial system, and the platysma. Neck skin is very thin, only slightly thicker than upper eyelid skin. Subcutaneous fat distribution is variable, although it is thinly layered over the platysmal muscle but tends to accumulate in the submentum. There is a deeper submental fat pad.

The platysma is a thin shield-like muscle. It originates on pectoralis fascia. Its anterior border is the risorius muscle at the oral commissure. Posteriorly, it inserts into the superficial muscular aponeurotic system (SMAS). The platysma is innervated by the cervical branch of the facial nerve. Its vascular supply stems from branches of the facial artery. The function of the platysma is not clear. In animals such as horses, contraction of the platysma helps to ward off insects. In humans, it depresses the corners of the mouth and acts as a stabilizing force.

The sternocleidomastoid (SCM) is a major muscle of the neck, but generally, it is not manipulated cosmetically. However, the greater auricular nerve (C2, C3) travels superficial to the SCM and is very superficial as it terminates inferior to the auricle around the lobule. It is susceptible to injury during a surgical neck lift. The spinal accessory nerve (cranial nerve XI) lies in the posterior triangle, and although less likely to be compromised in many superficial neck rejuvenation procedures, it is also susceptible to injury during a neck lift. Anteriorly, the marginal mandibular branch of the facial nerve courses inferior to the angle of the mandible and then runs in the superficial layer of the deep cervical fascia just superficial to the submandibular gland and the anterior facial vein. It continues its course over the mandible where the nerve is very superficial and terminates lateral to the anterior commissure. In a small percentage of individuals, its thin rami anastomose with those of the buccal branch of the facial nerve. Extreme care must be taken in these areas.

THE YOUTHFUL NECK

The youthful neck is characterized by a uniform skin tone, a smooth texture and contour, tautness of the skin, and defined fullness that is in harmony with the face. The neck is bounded by a sharp jawline superiorly and, inferiorly, by a smooth transition at the sternal notch. Structurally, the youthful neck including the submentum is distinguished by a cervicomental angle of between 105 and 120 degrees and a submental SCM angle of 90 degrees. Male necks typically are more muscular with a greater circumference with a more defined and larger submentum than the female. The female neck generally has smoother skin. Michelangelo's *David* epitomizes the youthful neck.

THE AGED NECK

Multiple intrinsic and extrinsic factors, including genetics, photodamage, and gravity, contribute to aging in the neck. A decrease in collagen and elasticity throughout the face and neck leads to loss of subcutaneous support and results in sagging and ptotic submandibular glands. Skin becomes lax, and fat accumulates in the submental region, softening the mandibular contour and creating jowls.[2] Regular twisting and swivelling motions and contraction of the platysma muscle result in prominent banding and horizontal rhytides, whereas chronic exposure to ultraviolet (UV) radiation wreaks havoc on skin texture and pigmentation and accelerates the course of natural aging.[3] Platysmal bands—longitudinal cords in the neck midline—appear. There is mostly likely a dual etiology for this phenomenon—genetics and anterior platysmal hypertrophy. It is estimated that 39% of the population has undecussated (separated) midline platysmal muscle fibers. These are hidden in youth, but as fat diminishes with age, they become more apparent. Relaxation of surrounding tissue also contributes to this separation. Decades of vigorous muscle contraction result in hypertrophy in some individuals. Clinically, this contributes to the "turkey gobbler" neck.

TREATMENT PHILOSOPHY

When evaluating the neck, it is paramount to evaluate all layers including skin, fat, and muscle, and to accurately diagnose the pathophysiology, which will lead to the appropriate treatments. It is uncommon that neck rejuvenation can be maximized with one type of treatment. During the consultation, it is important to examine the patient from all angles. When examining the neck, it is important to have the patient bite down and smile since this will help identify platysma banding. It is helpful to take photos and then show the patient. Often, a patient will not realize the extent of their aged neck since they look at their neck from the frontal view. When developing a plan, it is important to remember that if liposuction is an appropriate treatment for submental fat, then it may unmask platysmal bands, which will also need to be treated. It is also important to determine if the patient has a prominent hyoid bone, which can create the effect of a less acute cervicomental angle, and standard aesthetic procedures will not be appropriate. It is also important to understand that surgical neck procedures will not improve jowling—unlike a full facelift. Aesthetic restoration of the neck aims to improve laxity, skin quality, and texture; reduce wrinkling and the appearance of prominent bands; and define the cervicomental angle formed by the horizontal plane of the submental region and the vertical plane of the neck. Although surgery remains the gold standard and often provides the best outcomes, nonsurgical options are in high demand. Because they target individual aspects of aging, noninvasive or minimally invasive alternatives are frequently used in combination to achieve optimal results.

COSMECEUTICALS

Topical formulations are crucial components of an ongoing, preventative, or restorative skin care regimen, although care must be taken: the thin, crepey skin of the neck is delicate and prone to irritation or injury that can be slow to heal. There are a staggering number of day and night formulations on the market that contain additives designed to improve skin texture and appearance: moisturizing agents to smooth and hydrate, antioxidants (eg, vitamins C and E) to reduce oxidative stress and free radical damage, and topical growth factors and peptides to boost collagen and elastin production for improvements in laxity and fine rhytides.[4,5] Retinoid acid—the active form of vitamin A and considered the gold standard treatment for photodamage—induces neocollagenesis for marked improvements in elasticity, fine lines, and hyperpigmentation but is more likely to cause significant irritation in the neck and should be used cautiously and at low strength. Nonprescription retinol—the weaker version—may produce similar efficacy with better tolerability.[6]

NEUROTOXINS

Botulinum toxin (BoNT) is the most widely used treatment for platysmal bands and dynamic rhytides.[7-9] Deep intradermal injections using small doses placed equidistantly across multiple sites along the length of each vertical band produce a gentle anterior neck lift and consistently soften the prominence of the cords on animation. Injecting the bands may also diminish horizontal "necklace" lines in some patients, but this is inconsistent. Guidelines recommend a total dose of 30 to 60 units of onabotulinumtoxinA divided among all injection points, as determined by patient assessment and clinical experience.[10]

Loss of definition along the jaw—an invariable effect of changing anatomy over time—may be improved via the so-called Nefertiti lift, in which small doses of BoNT (15 units of onabotulinumtoxinA per side) are injected in multiple sites under the mandible and intradermally into the upper half of the actively contracting posterior platysmal band to sharpen the contours of the jaw and raise the corners of the mouth.[10,11]

Not everyone is a good candidate for neurotoxin injections in the neck; some precautions are advised. BoNT works best on younger patients with good skin elasticity or postoperatively for residual bands.[12] In individuals with extensive cutaneous laxity, poor cervical skin elasticity, and flaccid platysmal cords, injections can worsen the appearance of the neck. Large doses—in excess of 50 units onabotulinumtoxinA in one session—can produce weakness in the neck flexors and dysphagia and should be avoided.[9,11]

Alternatively, microbotox—the injection of multiple microdroplets of diluted onabotulinumtoxinA into the dermis or the interface between the dermis and superficial layer of facial muscles—is a simple alternative for patients with early signs of aging in the neck.[13] Microinjections target the superficial fibers under the surface of the skin, decreasing sweat and sebaceous gland activity for an intradermal effect. In the neck, tiny blebs injected as superficially as possible across the entire sweep of the platysma muscle improve skin texture, color, and smoothness; reduce the appearance of horizontal necklace lines and vertical banding; and create a lifting effect of the jowls and jawline for better cervicomental contouring.[13]

FILLERS

Residual wrinkling and skin laxity in the neck can be improved with soft-tissue fillers, such as hyaluronic acid, calcium hydroxylapatite, or poly-L-lactic acid, especially when used in combination with other aesthetic procedures. Fillers can be used in neck rejuvenation to soften necklace lines and redefine the jawline, which can improve the submental contour, and as intradermal injections for improvement of skin quality. Although the neck was once considered unsuitable for particulate fillers due to the scarcity of subcutaneous tissue and consequent risk of complications,[14,15] increasing the dilution ratios raises the safety profile and provides visible improvement in texture, skin thickness, and wrinkles.[1,16] For optimal restoration and multilevel cosmetic revitalization, fillers are frequently combined with light- or energy-based modalities that stimulate tissue contraction and subsequent tightening.[3,17,18]

CRYOLIPOLYSIS

Submental fat accumulation contributes to an obtuse cervicomental angle and can age a patient or make the patient appear overweight. Widely used in all areas of the body, cryolipolysis selectively reduces fat cells with controlled, localized cooling and is a promising procedure for nonsurgical fat reduction, and it may also be a viable alternative to liposuction.[19,20] Although there are limited data for use of cryolipolysis in the neck, a pivotal study of 60 patients demonstrated visible improvements in the neck contour and high patient satisfaction, with a mean fat layer reduction of 2 mm.[21] Cryolipolysis of submental fat may require multiple sessions to achieve the desired effect.[3]

SODIUM DEOXYCHOLATE

Recently approved by the US Food and Drug Administration, deoxycholic acid injection (ATX-101) is the first minimally invasive, nonsurgical treatment for the reduction of submental fullness. Subcutaneous injection of deoxycholic acid into submental fat results in adipocyte lysis, leading to significant localized fat reduction.[22-24] Four phase III trials have demonstrated significant clinical efficacy[25-28] with only minimal side effects, such as pain, swelling, bruising, and erythema. Although increased skin laxity is normally a concern after removal of targeted subcutaneous fat, secondary or adjunctive procedures for skin tightening have not been routinely required after injection, suggesting that deoxycholic acid may induce concomitant skin retraction (**Figure 34-1**).[29]

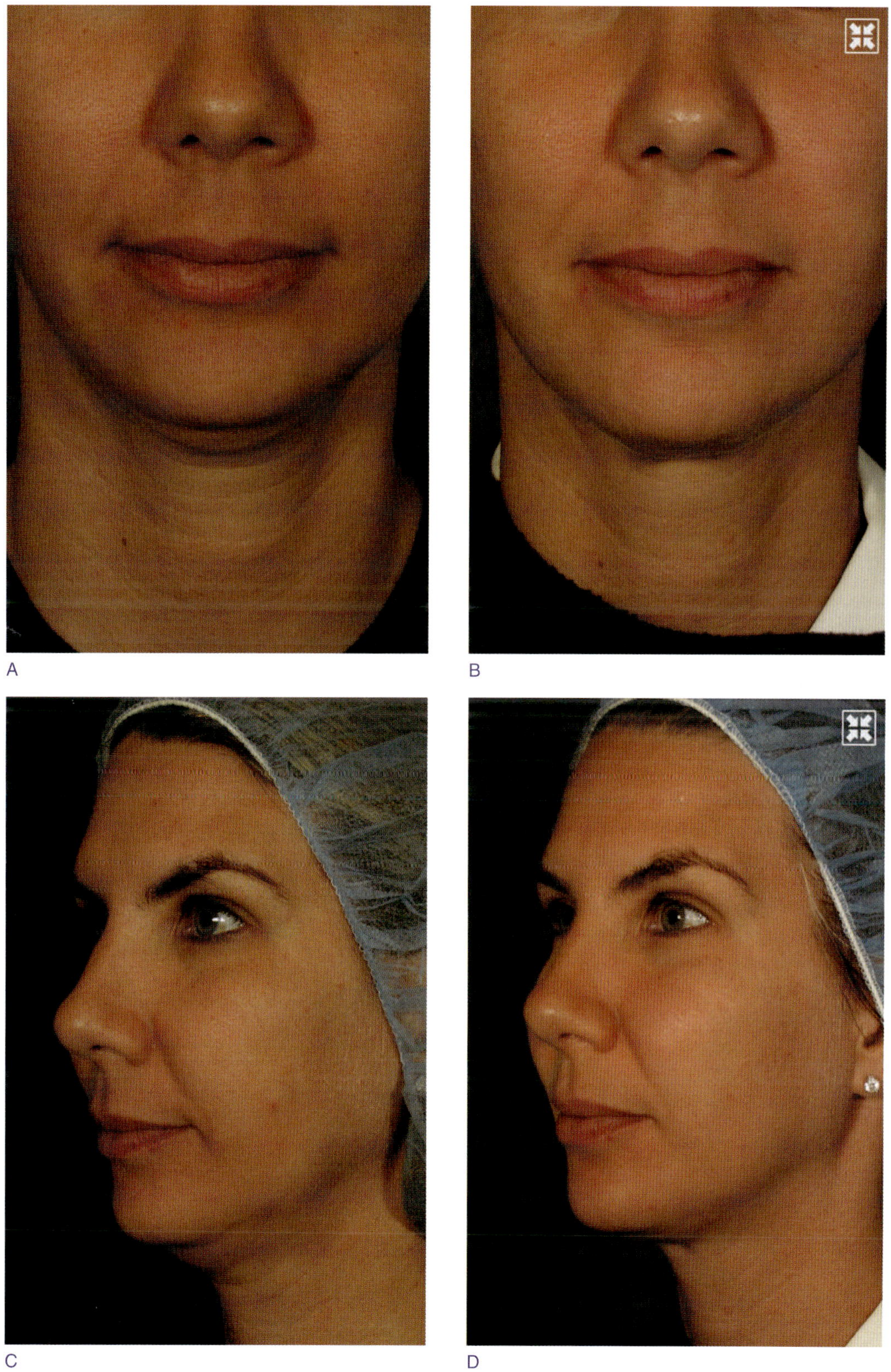

FIGURE 34-1 Sodium deoxycholate for submental contouring. (**A/C**) A 41-year-old woman before treatment. (**B/D**) Six months after two treatments with sodium deoxycholate for submental fullness (total dose 6 mL).

NEEDLING

Percutaneous collagen induction (PCI) therapy, or collagen induction therapy, is a minimally invasive procedure involving the physical trauma of needle penetration to promote regeneration.[30] Microneedling devices equipped with fine needles applied to the skin create controlled-depth skin injury and are believed to induce the tissue-repair cascade of inflammation, proliferation, and remodeling for continued improvements in overall skin quality, thickness, and superficial wrinkling over a period of several months.[31] Histologic examination of skin treated over multiple sessions has shown significant increases in collagen deposition and epidermal thickness at 6 months.[32-34] A variety of devices and systems are on the market, with needles ranging in length from 0.5 to 3 mm; increasing needle depth demonstrates improved results but is associated with longer downtime and greater swelling, bruising, and bleeding.[33] Because treatment does not ablate the epidermis or create open wounds, PCI therapy is slowly gaining ground as treatment for photoaged skin, particularly in areas considered unsuitable for resurfacing with lasers or chemical peels.[32,35] The procedure is well tolerated, with minimal downtime, although multiple sessions are required to produce a visible response. The evidence to guide best practices in the use of microneedling for neck rejuvenation is scant.

ENERGY DEVICES

Although one must proceed carefully with laser resurfacing due to the lack of pilosebaceous units and the increased risk of scarring, it was first demonstrated that short-pulsed carbon dioxide laser was safe and effective for the skin of the neck. It can be used to improve mottled pigmentation, texture, mild rhytides, and the necklace line. One retrospective study demonstrated a 39% reduction in rhytides in 308 subjects without any pigmentation or scarring.[36] The erbium laser on lower depth settings was also found to be safe and effective for the neck. The advent of nonablative and ablative fractional laser resurfacing has also created more options for neck skin rejuvenation. Nonablative fractional laser has minimal downtime but requires multiple treatments to be effective. Fractional carbon dioxide can be used but with low-energy settings and one pass. There have been reports of scarring with the fractional carbon dioxide laser[19] and an increased risk of hypopigmentation. Recently, hybrid lasers, where the clinician can use mostly the nonablative component and then add an ablative component for rhytides, have shown great promise.

For moderate lifting and tightening with minimal downtime, high-intensity focused ultrasound can be moderately effective for the appropriate patient. This technology penetrates deeper into the skin and remodels collagen and possibly the SMAS. It improves jowls and will improve the cervicomental angle. Although it is tempting to treat the neck only, there will be better results if the lower face is also treated since this will provide additional lift, tightening, and harmony. High-intensity ultrasound can be painful. Some clinicians will perform micro field blocks with 1% lidocaine and 1/100,00 epinephrine and then wait for 15 to 20 minutes so there is no swelling and the liquid has been absorbed, so it does not modify the effectiveness of the treatment. Patients are uniformly comfortable with this technique. Generally, there is no downtime with this procedure, and results may require 6 to 12 months. Using multiple treatments, this modality can also be used to reduce neck circumference.[37]

Fractional radiofrequency (RF) needling is another novel energy device that can improve neck contour. The RF generates heat transmitted fractionally by small needles into the dermis. In studies, these devices have been shown to lift, tighten, smooth, and volumize. In one study, fractional RF was determined to have the equivalent effectiveness of one-third of rhytidectomy.[38] For the neck, some of these RF microneedling devices have modified the angle and depth of their needles for deeper penetration. This resulted in fat reduction and improved cervicomental angle in one unpublished study. This modality will result in downtime. There can be extensive swelling of the neck that may last 1 week. Similar to ultrasound, optimal results may require 6 to 12 months. Another RF-based technology—thermistor-regulated—has been shown to significantly increase neck tightening with minimal recovery time (**Figure 34-2**).

COMBINATION PROCEDURES

Although surgically based procedures are effective, results can be maximized by combining these approaches with the energy-based devices. Following liposuction, high-intensity ultrasound, RF needling or thermistor-regulated RF technology can be performed on the neck to aid in further contraction of the skin.

Recently, the synergistic effect of combination BoNT injections (using both a microbotox approach and a Nefertiti lift) and sodium deoxycholate injections has been described.[39-43] The Bellatox technique led to significant aesthetic improvement after a single treatment, although further studies are needed. Ultimately, complete rejuvenation of the neck is rewarding and requires many different devices and techniques in the clinician's armamentarium (**Figures 34-3 and 34-4**).

CONCLUSIONS

The neck is a critical cosmetic area that has historically been overlooked by aesthetic clinicians. As patients increasingly expect rejuvenation of not just the face, but also the neck, hands, and other areas as well, neck rejuvenation is increasingly becoming a focus of patient concern. Indeed, perhaps related in part to the new availability of minimally invasive approaches to neck rejuvenation, a significant proportion of patients are now interested in such procedures.

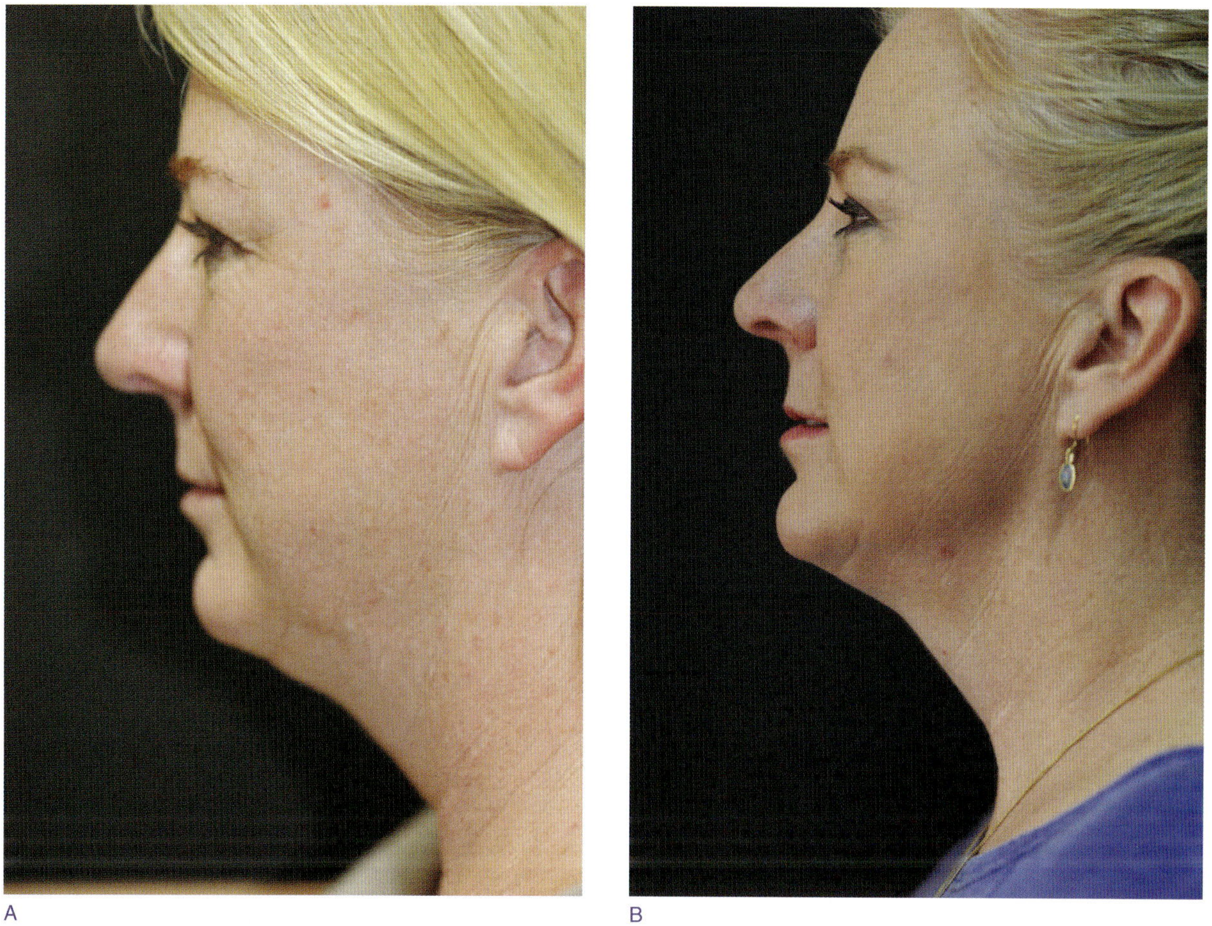

FIGURE 34-2 Profound RF. (**A**) Before. (**B**) Three months post submental Profound using the SubQ handpiece.

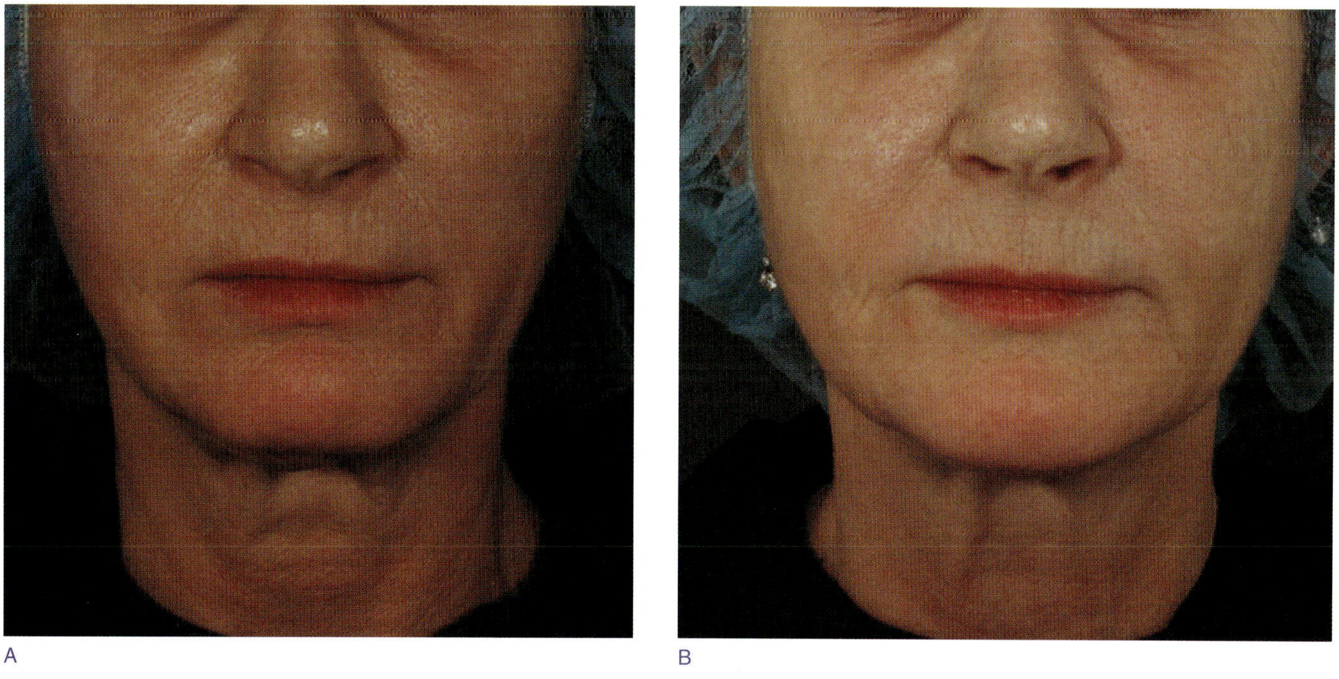

FIGURE 34-3 Combination treatment with high intensity–focused ultrasound, onabotulinum toxin A, and sodium deoxycholate. (**A**) A 58-year-old woman before treatment. (**B**) Three months after treatment with high intensity–focused ultrasound to the lower face and neck and 60 units of onabotulinum toxin A to the platysma.

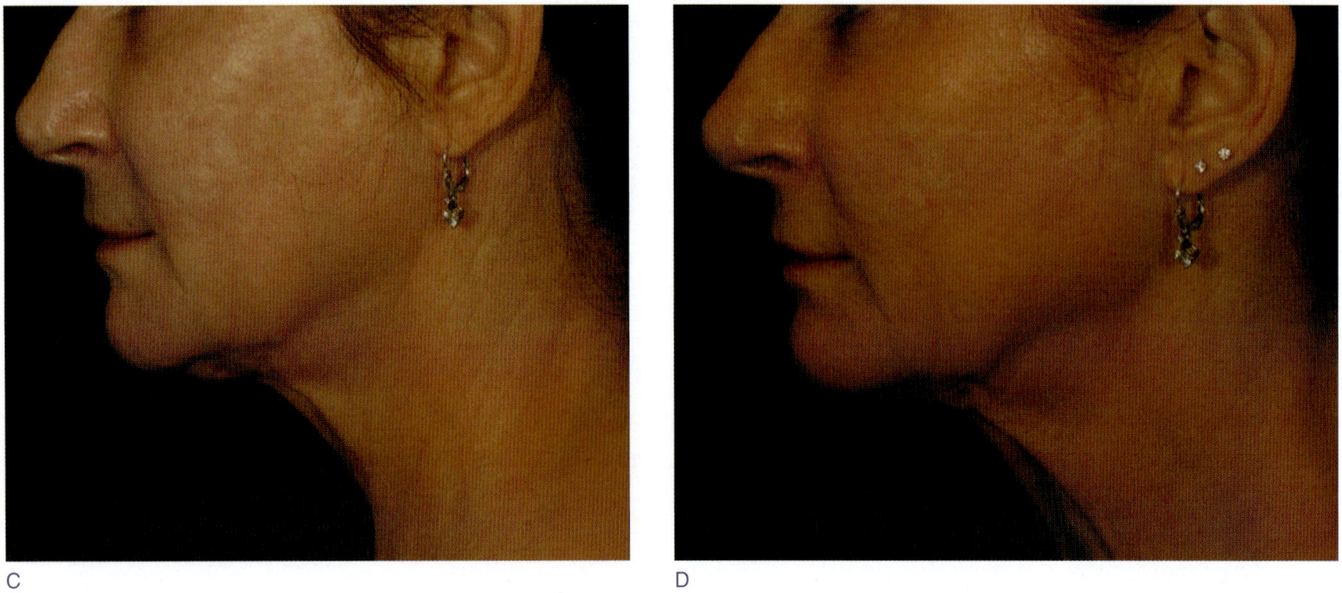

FIGURE 34-3 (*Continued*) (**C**) Four months after previous treatment, no additional intervention. (**D**) Three months after a single treatment with sodium deoxycholate for submental contouring (4 mL); note improvement in submental region and worsening of platysmal bands as onabotulinum toxin is no longer active.

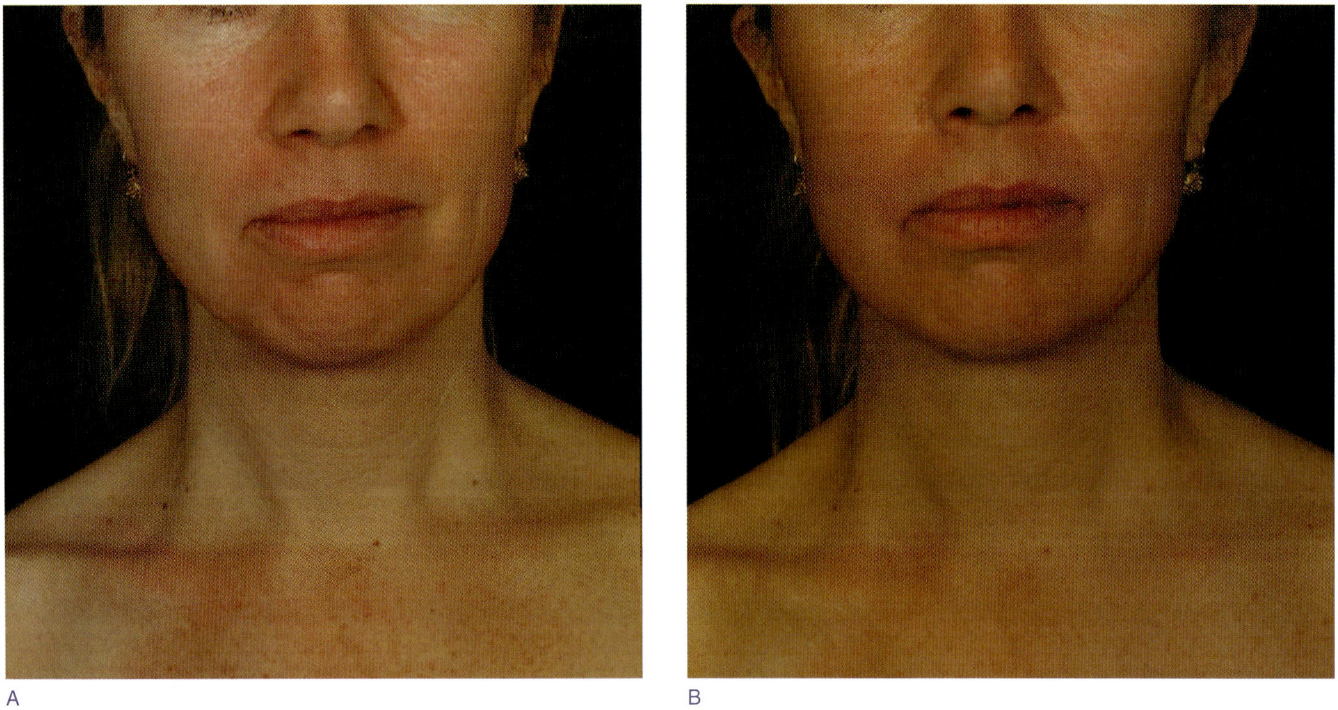

FIGURE 34-4 Combination treatment with intense pulsed light and nonablative fractional laser. (**A**) A 49-year-old woman before treatment. (**B**) After a single treatment of intense pulsed light and 1,927 nm fractional laser.

REFERENCES

1. Mazzuco R, Hexsel D. Poly-L-lactic acid for neck and chest rejuvenation. *Dermatol Surg.* 2009;35:1228-1237.
2. Dayan SH, Arkins JP, Chaudhry R. Minimally invasive neck lifts: have they replaced neck lift surgery? *Facial Plast Surg Clin North Am.* 2013;21:265-270.
3. Vanaman M, Fabi SG, Cox SE. Neck rejuvenation using a combination approach: our experience and a review of the literature. *Dermatol Surg.* 2016;42(Suppl 2):S94-S100.
4. Visscher MO, Pan BS, Kitzmiller WJ. Photodamage: treatments and topicals for facial skin. *Facial Plast Surg Clin North Am.* 2013;21:61-75.
5. Sherber NS. Topicals in skin rejuvenation: prescription topicals. *Facial Plast Surg.* 2014;30:12-15.
6. Babcock M, Mehta RC, Makino ET. A randomized, double-blind, split-face study comparing the efficacy and tolerability of three retinol-based products vs. three tretinoin-based products in subjects with moderate to severe facial photodamage. *J Drugs Dermatol.* 2015;14:24-30.
7. Brandt FS, Bellman B. Cosmetic use of botulinum A exotoxin for the aging neck. *Dermatol Surg.* 1998;24:1232-1234.
8. Matarasso A, Matarasso SL, Brandt FS, Bellman B. Botulinum A exotoxin for the management of platysma bands. *Plast Reconstr Surg.* 1999;103:645-652.
9. Carruthers J, Carruthers A. Aesthetic botulinum A toxin in the mid and lower face and neck. *Dermatol Surg.* 2003;29:468-476.
10. Carruthers J, Fournier N, Kerscher M, et al. The convergence of medicine and neurotoxins: a focus on botulinum toxin type A and its application in aesthetic medicine—a global, evidence-based botulinum toxin consensus education initiative. Part II: Incorporating botulinum toxin into aesthetic clinical practice. *Dermatol Surg.* 2013;39:510-525.
11. Levy PM. The "Nefertiti lift": a new technique for specific recontouring of the jawline. *J Cosmet Laser Ther.* 2007;9:249-252.
12. Carruthers J, Fagien S, Matarasso SL. Consensus recommendations on the use of botulinum toxin type A in facial aesthetics. *Plast Reconstr Surg.* 2004;114(Suppl):1S-22S.
13. Wu WT. Microbotox of the lower face and neck: evolution of a personal technique and its clinical effects. *Plast Reconstr Surg.* 2015;136(5 suppl):92S-100S.
14. Lowe NJ. Dispelling the myth: appropriate use of poly-L-lactic acid and clinical considerations. *J Eur Acad Dermatol Venereol.* 2006;20(Suppl 1):2-6.
15. Vleggaar D. Soft-tissue augmentation and the role of poly-L-lactic acid. *Plast Reconstr Surg.* 2006;118(3 Suppl):46S-54S.
16. Raedaelli A, Forte R. Cosmetic use of polylactic acid: report of 568 patients. *J Cosmet Dermatol.* 2009;8:239-248.
17. Casabona G, Michalany N. Microfocused ultrasound with visualization and fillers for increased neocollagenesis: clinical and histological evaluation. *Dermatol Surg.* 2014;40(Suppl 12):S194-S198.
18. Hart DR, Fabi SG, White WM, Fitzgerald R, Goldman MP. Current concepts in the use of PLLA: clinical synergy noted with combined use of microfocused ultrasound and poly-L-lactic acid on the face, neck, and décolletage. *Plast Reconstr Surg.* 2015;136(5 Suppl):180S-187S.
19. Avram MM, Harry RS. Cryolipolysis for subcutaneous fat layer reduction. *Lasers Surg Med.* 2009;41:703-708.
20. Ingargiola MJ, Motakef S, Chung MT, Vasconez HC, Sasaki GH. Cryolipolysis for fat reduction and body contouring: safety and efficacy of current treatment paradigms. *Plast Reconstr Surg.* 2015;135:1581-1590.
21. Kilmer SL, Burns AJ, Zelickson BD. Safety and efficacy of cryolipolysis for non-invasive reduction of submental fat. *Lasers Surg Med.* 2016;48:3-13.
22. Rotunda AM, Suzuki H, Moy RL, Kolodney MS. Detergent effects of sodium deoxycholate are a major feature of an injectable phosphatidylcholine formulation used for localized fat dissolution. *Dermatol Surg.* 2004;30:1001-1008.
23. Rotunda AM, Ablon G, Kolodney MS. Lipomas treated with subcutaneous deoxycholate injections. *J Am Acad Dermatol.* 2005;53:973-978.
24. Thuangtong R, Bentow JJ, Knopp K, et al. Tissue-selective effects of injected deoxycholate. *Dermatol Surg.* 2010;36:899-908.
25. Ascher B, Hoffmann K, Walker P, et al. Efficacy, patient-reported outcomes and safety profile of ATX-101 (deoxycholic acid), an injectable drug for the reduction of unwanted submental fat: results from a phase III, randomized, placebo-controlled study. *J Eur Acad Dermatol Venereol.* 2014;28:1707-1715.
26. Humphrey S, Brandt F, Walker P, et al. REFINE-2: a multicenter, double-blind, randomized, placebo-controlled pivotal phase 3 study with ATX-101, an injectable drug for submental contouring. *J Am Acad Dermatol.* 2014;70:AB20.
27. Rzany B, Griffiths T, Walker P, et al. Reduction of unwanted submental fat with ATX-101 (deoxycholic acid), an adipocytolytic injectable treatment: results from a phase III, randomized, placebo-controlled study. *Br J Dermatol.* 2014;170:445-453.
28. Jones DH, Carruthers J, Joseph JH, et al. REFINE-1, a multicenter, randomized, double-blind, placebo-controlled, phase 3 trial with ATX-101, an injectable drug for submental fat reduction. *Dermatol Surg.* 2016;42:38-49.
29. Dayan SH, Humphrey S, Jones DH, Lizzul PF, Gross TM, Beddingfield FC. Overview of ATX-101 (deoxycholic acid injection): a nonsurgical approach for reduction of submental fat. *Dermatol Surg.* 2016;42(Suppl 1):S263-S270.
30. Lee JC, Daniels MA, Roth MZ. Mesotherapy, microneedling, and chemical peels. *Clin Plast Surg.* 2016;43:583-595.
31. El-Domyati M, Medhat W. Minimally invasive facial rejuvenation: current concepts and future expectations. *Expert Rev Dermatol.* 2013;8:565-580.
32. Aust MC, Fernandes D, Kolokythas P, Kaplan HM, Vogt PM. Percutaneous collagen induction therapy: an alternative treatment for scars, wrinkles, and skin laxity. *Plast Reconstr Surg.* 2008;121:1421-1429.
33. Fernandes D, Signorini M. Combating photoaging with percutaneous collagen induction. *Clin Dermatol.* 2008;26:192-199.
34. Zeitter S, Sikora Z, Jahn S, et al. Microneedling: matching the results of medical needling and repetitive treatments to maximize potential for skin regeneration. *Burns.* 2014;40:966-973.
35. Aust MC, Reimers K, Gohritz A, et al. Percutaneous collagen induction: scarless skin rejuvenation: fact or fiction? *Clin Exp Derm.* 2010;35:437-439.
36. Behroozan DS, Christian MM, Moy RL. Short-pulse carbon dioxide laser resurfacing of the neck. *J Am Acad Dermatol.* 2000;43(1 Pt 1):72-76.

37. Robinson DM, Kaminer MS, Baumann L, et al. High-intensity focused ultrasound for the reduction of subcutaneous adipose tissue using multiple treatment techniques. *Dermatol Surg.* 2014;40: 641-651.

38. Alexiades-Armenakas M, Rosenberg D, Renton B, Dover J, Arndt K. Blinded, randomized, quantitative grading comparison of minimally invasive, fractional radiofrequency and surgical face-lift to treat skin laxity. *Arch Dermatol.* 2010;146:396-405.

39. Kantor J. Synergistic effect of combination deoxycholic acid and botulinum toxin (the Bellatox technique) for the treatment of submental fullness. *J Am Acad Dermatol.* 2017;76(6):e209-e211.

40. Wu WT. Microbotox of the lower face and neck: evolution of a personal technique and its clinical effects. *Plast Reconstr Surg.* 2015;136(5 Suppl):92S-100S.

41. Levy PM. Neurotoxins: current concepts in cosmetic use on the face and neck: jawline contouring/platysma bands/necklace lines. *Plast Reconstr Surg.* 2015;136(5 Suppl):80S-83S.

42. Liew S. Discussion: microbotox of the lower face and neck: evolution of a personal technique and its clinical effects. *Plast Reconstr Surg.* 2015;136(5 Suppl):101S-103S.

43. Carruthers J, Carruthers A. Aesthetic botulinum A toxin in the mid and lower face and neck. *Dermatol Surg.* 2003;29(5):468-476.

Approaches to Hand Rejuvenation

35

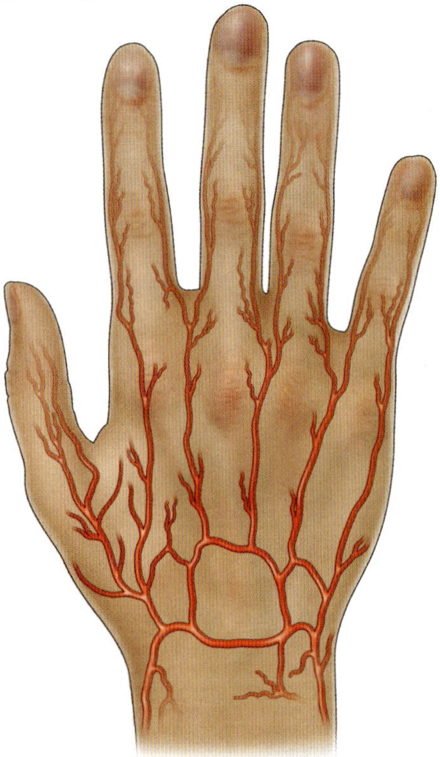

SUMMARY

- As many patients seek facial cosmetic procedures, a discrepancy forms between the rejuvenated look of their face and the aged appearance of their hands.
- Hand rejuvenation addresses both surface changes and volume loss, and combination multimodality approaches may be best.

Beginner Tips

- A thorough understanding of hand anatomy is a prerequisite for procedural intervention.
- IPL and lasers are highly effective at improving surface changes on the hands.
- When using CaHA fillers, the scrape skin threading technique may help to avoid overly deep product placement.

Pitfalls and Cautions

- When performing chemical peels on the hand, it is important to remember that treatments should be limited to superficial and medium depth peels because of the risk of impaired wound healing.
- Since the dorsal hand skin is thinner, has decreased vascularity, and fewer pilosebaceous units than the face, the fluence, density, and number of passes should generally be reduced to minimize recovery time.

Expert Tips

- If nodule formation occurs after filler injections: antibiotics -> hyaluronidase/ILK -> excision.
- Overcorrect when performing autologous fat transfer.
- Consider sclerotherapy if volumization does not solve vein prominence.

Patient Education Points

- Patients should understand that they will likely require multiple treatments.
- Remember the 5–5–5 rule after filler injection: massage for 5 minutes at a time, 5 times per day, for a total of 5 days.
- As always, appropriate patient selection and assuring adequate motivation are of vital importance.

Don't Forget!

- Sclerotherapy and autologous fat transfer should be performed separately.
- Vein treatments should be performed at least 1 month prior to other procedures.

35 Approaches to Hand Rejuvenation

INTRODUCTION

The face, neck, and hands are not only the most visible parts of the human body, but they are also the areas most susceptible to environmental factors that accelerate the aging process. As many patients seek facial cosmetic procedures, a discrepancy forms between the rejuvenated look of their face and the aged appearance of their hands. Therefore, both clinicians and patients have become more aware of the need to treat the hands (**Figures 35-1 to** 35-3).

APPROACH TO HAND REJUVENATION

When examining the hand, it is important to consider the different layers that contribute to the aged appearance of the skin (**Table 35-1 and Figure** 35-4). First, looking at the epidermis and dermis, one should note the presence of superficial rhytids, solar lentigines, telangiectasias, and keratoses. Light-based devices or chemical peels that target the epidermis and dermis will most effectively treat these changes.

Next, the clinician should note the amount of volume loss contributing to skin laxity and the visibility of veins and tendons in the dorsal hand. Adding volume to the dorsal hand, via filler or fat grafting, will best mask the prominence of these changes. Alternatively, the veins themselves can be selectively targeted through sclerotherapy, endovenous laser ablation, or phlebectomy.

Many patients benefit from a multimodality approach. Some clinicians perform epidermal and dermal treatments prior to filling of the subcutaneous tissue, theorizing that energy from light-based treatments may lead to degradation of the filler.[1] This theory has never been supported, and a study by Goldman et al[2] failed to show any difference in wrinkle severity or global improvement scores in 36 patients treated with hyaluronic acid filler alone or filler followed by nonablative laser, intense pulsed light (IPL), or radiofrequency (RF). The only procedures that should always be performed separately are vein treatments such as sclerotherapy and endovenous laser ablation, because of their more complicated postoperative management regimens. Vein treatments should be performed at least 1 month prior to other procedures.

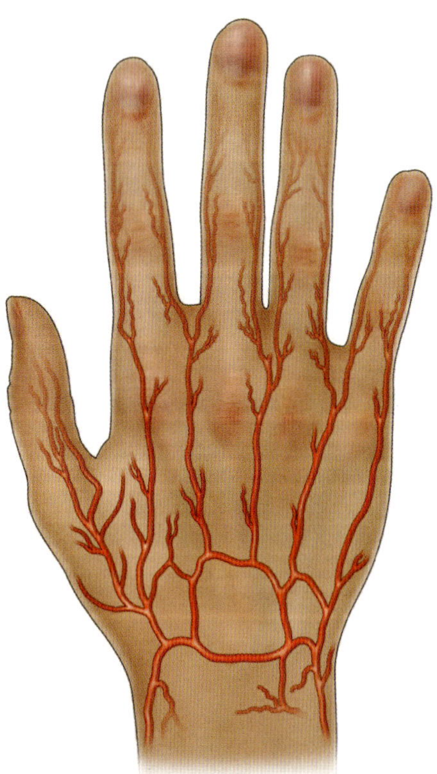

FIGURE 35-1 Dorsal hand arterial supply.

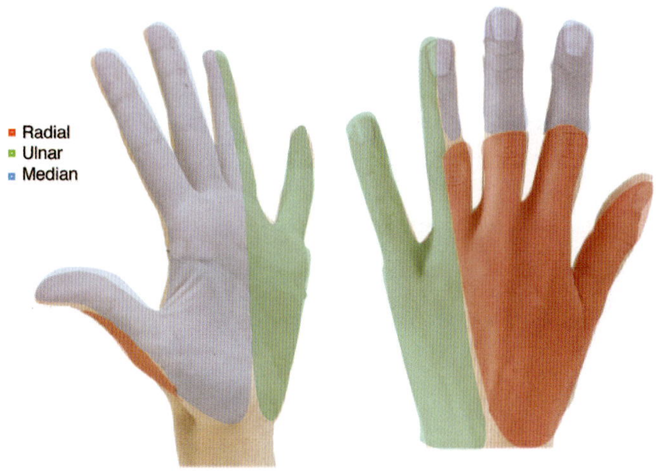

FIGURE 35-2 Sensory innervation of the hand.

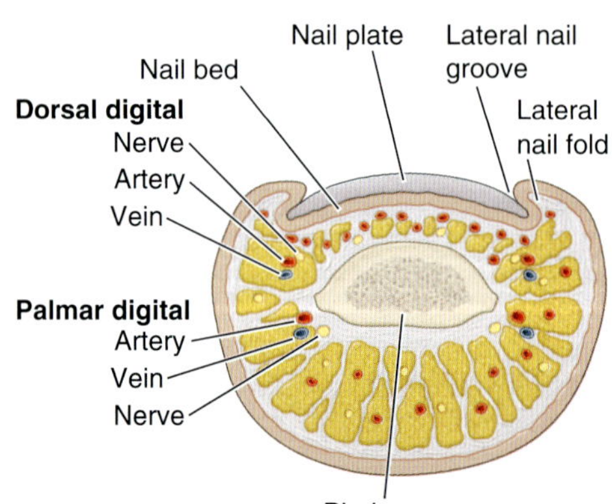

FIGURE 35-3 Cross-sectional anatomy of the digit.

TABLE 35-1 • Signs of Aging

Extrinsic Aging	Intrinsic Aging
Solar lentigines	Rhytids
Telangiectasias	Dermal atrophy
Solar purpura	Fat atrophy
Guttate hypomelanosis	Visibility of tendon color
Actinic keratoses	Prominent and tortuous veins
Seborrheic keratoses	Visible bony contour

During the pretreatment consultation, the aesthetic goals, expectations, downtime, and possible adverse events of each procedure need to be discussed. The clinician should inquire about the patient's usual scope of hand activity, as temporary swelling and dressings may interfere with function. Baseline photographs should be taken with the patient's hands relaxed on a flat surface to capture the appearance of prominent hand veins at rest that commonly disappear when the hand is positioned upright. Additionally, the patient should be educated about the regular use of sun protection and possibly topical retinoids and other cosmeceuticals to potentially better maintain their results.

FILLER INJECTIONS

During the patient evaluation, the clinician should obtain a thorough medical, drug, and allergy history. Each dorsal hand must be examined for areas of volume loss and tendon and vein visibility, and the clinician should formulate a plan as to which specific filler will be used and the volume necessary. Specific techniques vary depending on the filler used and clinician preference (**Table 35-2**).

Topical anesthetics applied for 30 to 45 minutes may help reduce pain, although this is typically unnecessary. The patient is then asked to wash their hands with soap and water, and chlorhexidine is used as a sterile prep for the entire hand, from wrist to fingertips. It is helpful to identify and mark entry points for the injections. The treatment area should be bounded by the hand-wrist crease, metacarpophalangeal (MCP) joints, and the first and fifth metacarpals.[3] The hand can be placed horizontally on a stand, or the injector may choose to hold the hand in order to have greater control. Some clinicians place the patient in Trendelenburg position or elevate the hands above the level of the heart in order to reduce venous return, which can potentially minimize edema and ecchymosis.[4]

Once the treatment is complete, ice can be applied to the hands for at least 10 minutes. Some clinicians advise patients to sit on their hands immediately following the procedure in order to decrease edema.[5] The hands are often wrapped with a compressive dressing, and the patient is instructed to keep the hands elevated as often as possible. Exercise and other physical activities are generally avoided until the edema has decreased. Many fillers have been used for hand rejuvenation. Because of the paucity of data supporting the use of polymethyl methacrylate (PMMA) and bovine collagen for hand rejuvenation, they are not frequently used for this purpose.

Calcium Hydroxyapatite

Calcium hydroxyapatite (CaHA), or Radiesse (Merz Aesthetics, Franksville, WI), is the only dermal filler approved by the US Food and Drug Administration (FDA) for hand rejuvenation. CaHA microspheres, which are made of substances identical to human bone, are suspended in a polysaccharide carrier made of glycerin and sodium carboxymethylcellulose. This filler is biodegradable (broken down into calcium and phosphate over time) and biostimulatory (stimulates collagen deposition by fibroblasts) (**Figure 35-5**).

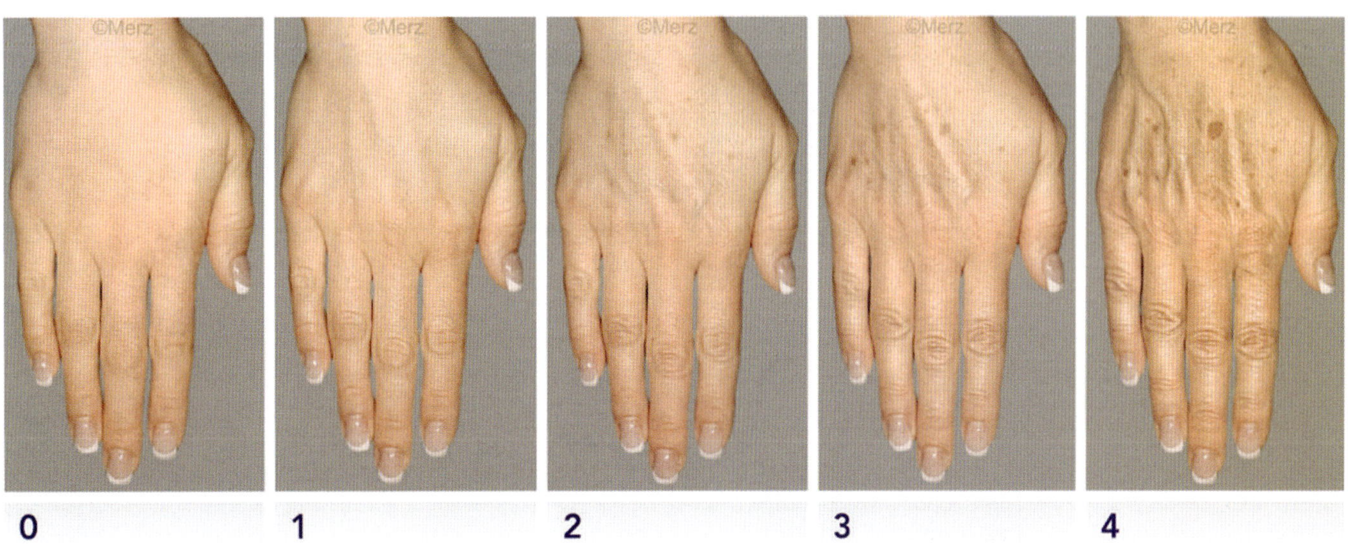

FIGURE 35-4 Merz Hand Grading Scale. 0 = No loss of fatty tissue; 1 = mild loss of fatty tissue, slight visibility of veins; 2 = moderate loss of fatty tissue, mild visibility of veins; 3 = severe loss of fatty tissue, moderate visibility of veins; and 4 = very severe loss of fatty tissue, marked visibility of veins bands.

TABLE 35-2 • Most Commonly Used Fillers for Hand Rejuvenation

Filler	Advantages	Disadvantages
Calcium hydroxyapatite	■ Only FDA-approved filler ■ Biostimulatory and biodegradable ■ Lasts 12-24 months	■ Not reversible ■ Requires dilution
Hyaluronic acid	■ Reversible with hyaluronidase ■ Does not require dilution	■ Tyndall effect if placed too superficially ■ Lasts <12 months
Poly-L-lactic acid	■ Biostimulatory ■ Lasts 18-24 months	■ Dilution is recommended ■ Higher risk of nodule formation ■ Multiple treatments are needed
Autologous fat	■ No risk of foreign body reaction	■ Requires a donor site ■ Causes more significant edema ■ Final results more unpredictable

FDA, US Food and Drug Administration.

When used on the dorsal hand, CaHA has been shown to last 12 to 24 months.[6-9] Previously published literature has reported the use of different dilutions, filler volume, and injection techniques. Overall, dilution of CaHA with lidocaine or saline reduces the viscosity and facilitates an even distribution of the filler.[9] Additionally, lidocaine makes the procedure more comfortable for the patient. The various options for injection include the bolus method, linear retrograde, fanning, serial puncture, microdroplets, and cannula.

In a pivotal US trial, no more than two syringes of product were used per hand (1 syringe = 1.5 mL of CaHA mixed with 0.26 mL of 2% lidocaine).[10] Using a 27-guage needle, boluses of up to 0.5 mL were introduced via a skin tenting technique in the area bounded by the first and fifth metacarpals, dorsal wrist crease, and MCP joints.[4] The needle is inserted parallel to the bone, and a bolus is placed within the center of the tented skin.[4] The bolus is thoroughly massaged into the areas of volume loss until an even surface is achieved. Massage is most easily performed with the hand in a flexed position. Topicals such as emollients, hand soap, chlorhexidine, ultrasound gel, and vitamin K cream may aid in the massage.[5]

In the scrape skin threading technique (SSTT), a soft tip, blunt, 21- or 23-guage cannula is used. First, a needle slightly larger than the cannula creates an entry point in the webspace between the MCPs. Next, the cannula is inserted through the entry point with the bevel facing up toward the dermis. The cannula is gently guided toward the wrist; the injector should feel the cannula scraping the underside of the dermis. Then, filler can be slowly and evenly injected as the cannula is withdrawn. The cannula can then be repositioned through the entry point and a

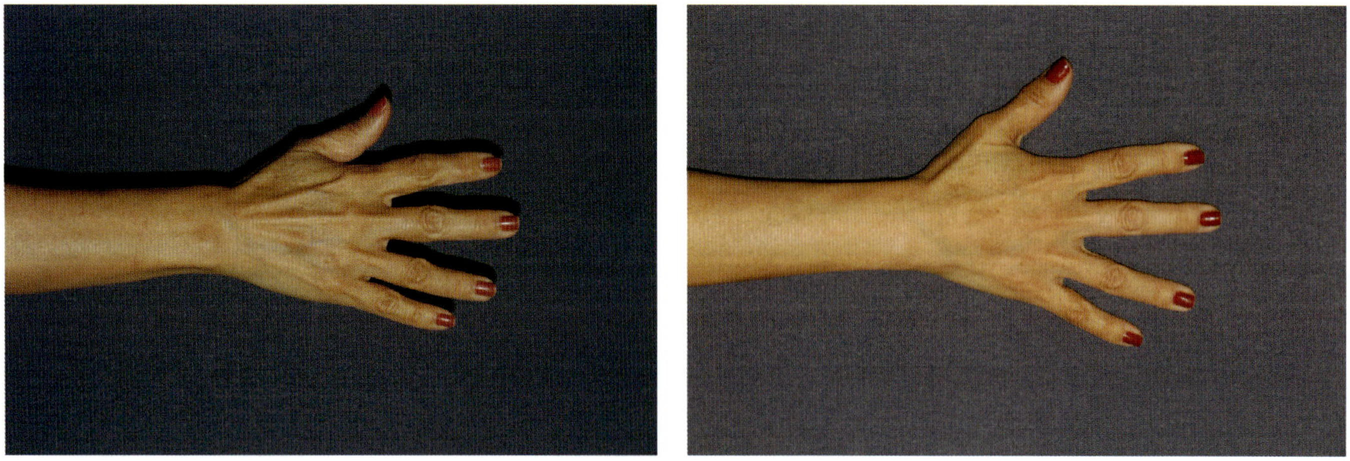

FIGURE 35-5 A 58-year-old woman presented to clinic worried about the aged appearance of the hands, specifically her prominent veins, and wanted sclerotherapy of her hands. Upon inspection, it was noted the patient had prominent dorsal hand tendons in addition to veins. Patients are always encouraged to restore dorsal hand volume prior to treating veins alone. Adding volume to the dorsal hands typically minimizes the appearance of the prominent veins while also addressing tendons and improving the quality of skin. Using 1.5 mL of CaHA diluted with 0.5 mL of lidocaine, 1.0 mL of product was injected into each hand. When injecting, it is important to remember that the safest plane of filler injection is the potential space between the dermis and superficial fascia. This plane can be accessed via the scrape skin threading technique. Before (left) and 14 weeks after (right) 1.5 mL of CaHA mixed with 0.5 mL of lidocaine, 1.0 mL to each hand.

fan-shaped configuration used to fill the triangular area of volume loss corresponding to the interosseous spaces. If necessary, additional entry points can be made and the same technique can be used to fill more proximal areas of volume loss. Gentle massage is used to correct unevenness. This approach may also be used with entry points on the proximal hand near the hand-wrist crease, pointing the cannula toward the MCPs (**Figure 35-6**).

On occasion, a patient may also desire volume correction of the space between the MCPs and proximal interphalangeal (PIP) joints. Lefebvre-Vilardabo et al[4] recommend injecting only dorsally between the MCP and PIP and avoiding injecting over the joint or laterally as the arteries and veins run on both sides of the digit. After injection, the filler can be blended with the hand in palmar flexion.

The expected adverse events of CaHA injection include transient edema, erythema, pain, and ecchymosis lasting up to 2 weeks. In the pivotal trials, pain and edema were the most common adverse events, with 89% of symptoms developing within 14 days.[3] Seven (6.2%) of the patients developed palpable nodules, all of which resolved without intervention by day 268. In certain cases, the onset of swelling can be delayed by 30 days. Busso et al[10] note that CaHA mixed with lidocaine can produce more prominent edema than using undiluted CaHA. Ice, hand elevation, gentle compression, and light massage can help reduce the edema. Another study evaluated the use of triamcinolone to minimize adverse events associated with CaHA injections.[11] Twenty subjects were injected with one syringe of CaHA diluted with 0.3 mL of 1% lidocaine and 1.2 mL of bacteriostatic normal saline. Following treatment, each hand was randomized to receive injections of either 5 mL of 2 mg/mL triamcinolone acetate or 5 mL of bacteriostatic normal saline. A blinded investigator noted a decrease in edema at days 7 and 14 after injection in the triamcinolone treated hands ($P < .10$). This was corroborated by a statistically significant increase in swelling from days 6 to 19 in the placebo hand, documented in the subjects' daily diary. No statistically significant difference in treatment efficacy was noted between those treated with triamcinolone or placebo.

Hyaluronic Acid

Hyaluronic acid (HA), a naturally occurring glycosaminoglycan, can also be used for hand rejuvenation. Man et al[12] and Brandt et al[13] demonstrated the efficacy of Restylane (Medicis Aesthetics Inc., Scottsdale, AZ), a small gel-particle (SGP) non–animal-derived stabilized HA (NASHA) made of 20 mg of

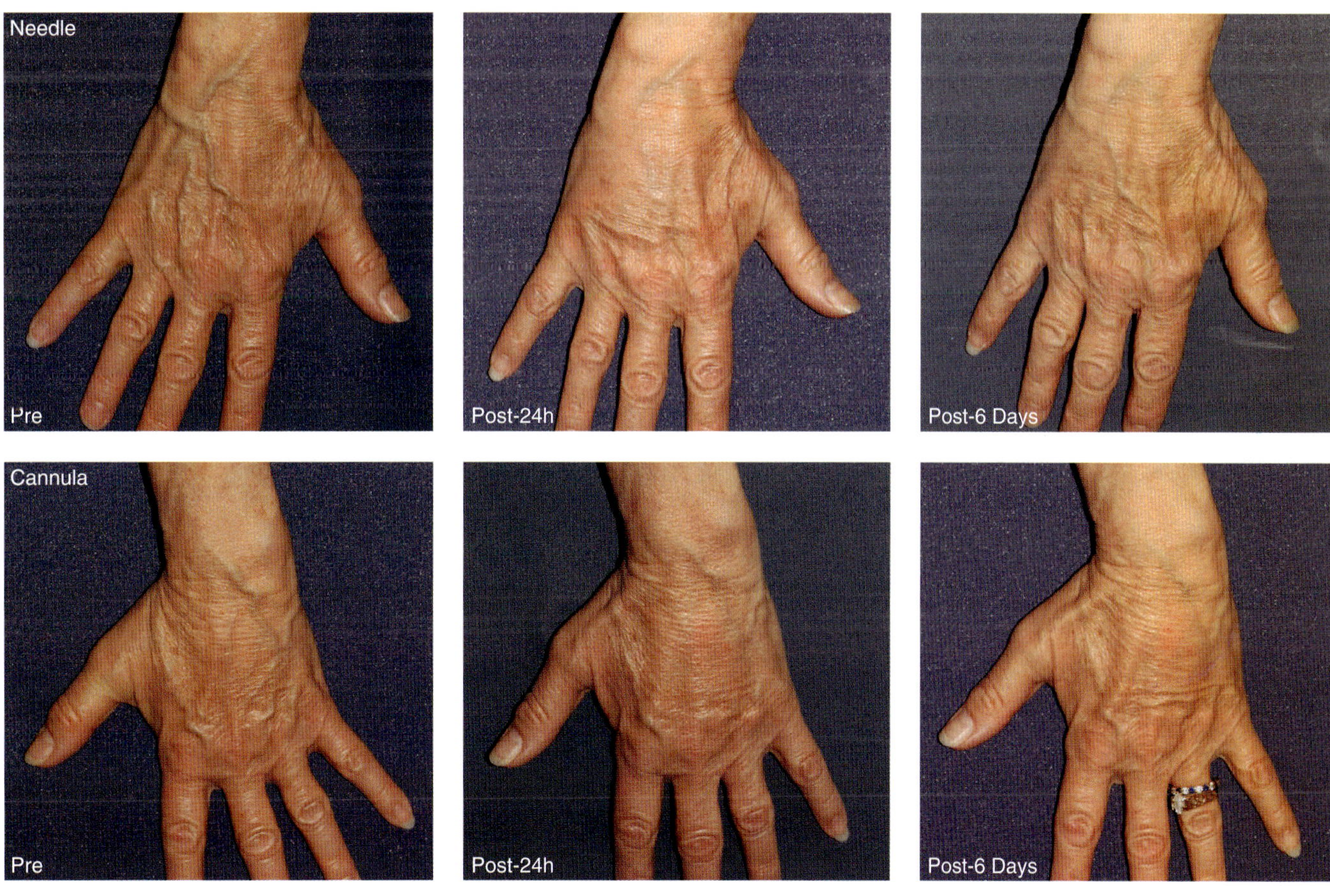

FIGURE 35-6 A 66-year-old woman had CaHA injections using two techniques. One hand was injected with 1.5 mL of CaHA diluted with 0.5 mL of 1% lidocaine, using a 1.5-inch 25-guage blunt-tipped cannula and a linear threading technique. The other hand was injected with 1.5 mL of CaHA diluted with 1.5 mL of bacteriostatic normal saline, using a 1.0-inch 27-gauge cannula and a multiple bolus technique.

HA per milliliter, for volume augmentation in a total of 48 patients (10 and 38, respectively). In their study, Man et al[12] compared two vials of SGP-NASHA to two vials of human collagen. With the patient in Trendelenburg position, filler was injected subcutaneously, inserting the needle at an oblique angle adjacent to the dorsal hand veins. Gentle massage was then performed with the hand in a flexed position. HA was found to be more painful (likely due to the presence of lidocaine in human collagen) but produced greater patient satisfaction; it was also more efficacious at improving the clinician-assessed visibility of dorsal hand veins. In order to decrease pain during massage, NASHA can be premixed with lidocaine.[9]

SGP-NASHA (20 mg/mL) was used on 16 patients by Brandt et al.[13] This study found substantial improvement in the prominence of vessels, tendons, and bones; in skin turgor; and in patient and investigator global aesthetic improvement and satisfaction scales. Using a single entry point, the material was threaded along the dorsum of the hand. The authors did not indicate whether a needle or cannula was used. The mean volume used for both hands was 7.38 mL, with a maximum of 4 mL per hand. Five patients underwent a touch-up treatment at 2 weeks, using a mean volume of 1.96 mL for both hands.

A European study treated 99 patients with Juvéderm (Allergan, Inc., Irvine, CA).[14] Juvéderm Ultra 3, with a volume of 0.8 to 1.6 mL, was injected into the mid to deep dermis at the first visit. Injections were performed via cannula in 54.3% of patients, and the rest through needle. Juvéderm Hydrate, with a volume of 0.5 to 1.0 mL, was injected into the superficial dermis at day 15. Injections were performed via needle in 79.3% of patients, and the rest through cannula. The study demonstrated a significant improvement in patient and investigator assessments. Interestingly, the proportion of injections rated as "very easy" was significantly higher with needle for Juvéderm Ultra 3 than with cannula for Juvéderm Hydrate. Edema, hematoma, redness, and pain were experienced by 13.2% of patients. Of these 32 adverse events, 26 were reported with cannula and 6 with needle. Additionally, subject discomfort was found to be significantly greater with cannula injections (**Figure 35-7**).

Another study compared 27-guage hypodermic needles to blunt-tip microcannulas (using either a 25-guage 50-mm flexible microcannula or 18-guage 70-mm semi-rigid microcannula) on the dorsal hands.[15] A total of 95 patients were injected with 20 to 28 mg/mL of HA. In both methods, the filler was placed in a linear retrograde fanning technique. The authors found that although there was no difference in the Global Aesthetic Improvement Scale (GAIS) score between the two techniques, pain and bruising were greater with the use of a hypodermic needle.

In a placebo-controlled study, Gubanova et al[16] used a multipuncture, microinjection technique to assess NASHA versus saline in 30 patients. A 30-guage needle was introduced 3 to 4 mm into the dermal layer, delivering 0.02 mL of product. Approximately 50 injections were placed at even intervals along the dorsal hand until the desired outcome was achieved. Patients received 1.0 mL of HA or 1.0 mL of saline monthly, for a total of three treatments. HA resulted in a significant improvement in patient and investigator questionnaires and measurements of skin hydration and elasticity.

Restylane Vital or Vital Light (Q-Med, Uppsala, Sweden) has been used for hand rejuvenation in parts of Europe and Asia. Unlike other Restylane products, Restylane Vital contains 12 mg/mL of HA. Streker et al[17] used the Restylane Injector (Q-Med) to deliver a controlled volume of 10 µL per injection into the mid dermis, using a 30-guage needle. Injections were spaced 0.5 to 1.0 cm apart. A mean of 2.8 mL of NASHA was injected per hand. All patients demonstrated aesthetic improvement and increased satisfaction through the 36-week follow-up. Lacarrubba et al[18] also applied an autoinjector to dispense aliquots of approximately 17 µL of either 16 or 20 mg/mL HA salts (Viscoderm; Bigpharma, Seixal, Portugal) per injection. Each hand received 30 microdroplets at a maximum volume of 1.0 mL. Patients received treatment every week for 4 weeks. Ultrasound was performed prior to each treatment and 1 week following the fourth

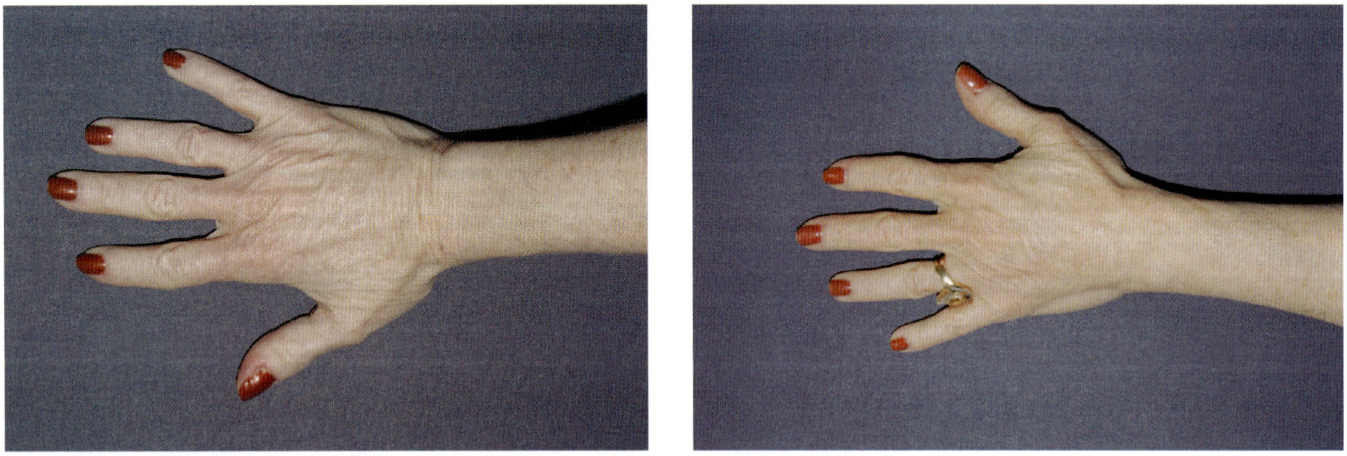

FIGURE 35-7 Patient was going to undergo liposculpture of her flanks. She was also bothered by the volume loss in her hands. Fat transfer to the hands was elected to restore volume to the patient's hands as she was already planning to undergo liposculpture. Otherwise, CaHA would have been the filler of choice to avoid undergoing a costly harvesting procedure that adds a different set of side effects from simply using a synthetic filler. Before (left) and 30 days after (right) 8 mL of autologous fat to the dorsal hand.

injection. Fifteen of 19 subjects demonstrated a statistically significant increase in subepidermal low-echogenic band echogenicity, which the authors believed to represent an increased density of collagen fibers produced by activated fibroblasts.

Side effects of HA injection in these studies included pain, edema, and ecchymosis. The results produced by HA are expected to last 6 to 12 months.[9] HA has the advantage of being reversible with hyaluronidase. However, it has a shorter duration, requires more syringes per hand to achieve a significant improvement, and has the potential for causing the Tyndall effect if placed too superficially; no studies have reported the Tyndall effect with the use of HA on the hands.

Poly-L-Lactic Acid

Another well-studied product is poly-L-lactic acid (PLLA), or Sculptra Aesthetic (Galderma Laboratories, Fort Worth, TX), which is a biodegradable and biostimulatory filler. The first use of PLLA for hand rejuvenation was described in 27 patients by Redaelli[19] in 2006. A 150-mg vial of PLLA was diluted with 0.5 mL of 3% mepivacaine and sterile water to achieve a volume of 5 to 8 mL, typically using higher concentrations in the first session. The dilution is made 12 hours before injection and stored at room temperature. With each treatment, a maximum of 2 mL of the 5- to 8-mL solution was used per hand. Injections were made with a 2.5-mL syringe and 25- to 27-gauge needle, entering the skin parallel to the metacarpal bones, although at times in various directions. With each injection, volumes of 0.05 to 0.1 mL of product were placed into the deep subcutaneous tissue. During the procedure, patients were kept in a Trendelenburg position in order to decrease venous pressure. Immediately following treatment, each hand was massaged for 15 minutes, and the patient was encouraged to continue massage at home at least twice a day for 3 days. Patients receiving PLLA had a measurable decrease in the visibility of veins and tendons, in addition to an improvement in patient and investigator satisfaction scores. In the study, patients required between three and six sessions about 1 month apart. One patient developed a nontender, nonvisible palpable deep nodule noticed at the last follow-up visit. PLLA with dilutions of 5, 6, and 7 mL were used at the first, second, and last session, respectively. Redaelli[19] believed the nodule was likely due to errors in injection and massage done during the first two sessions.

In a 2008 study, Sadick et al[20] treated 26 patients with PLLA. A 367.5-mg vial was reconstituted with an 8- to 10-mL mixture of sterile water and 1% lidocaine. Using a 1- or 3-mL syringe attached to a 25-gauge 1.5-inch needle, the product was introduced into the deep subcutaneous space using a tenting maneuver. One-half vial, or 5 mL, was used per hand. Apart from massage done immediately after injection, patients were asked to massage for 5 minutes at a time, five times per day, for a total of 5 days ("5-5-5" rule). Patients received an average of 2.38 treatments 1 to 2 months apart. No papules or nodules were reported.

Eight patients had their hands treated with PLLA by Palm et al.[21] A 367.5-mg vial of PLLA was reconstituted with 1 mL of 1% lidocaine (with or without epinephrine) and 5 mL of bacteriostatic water the day before treatment. The day of treatment, a Vortex Genie (Scientific Industries, Inc., Bohemia, NY) was used to agitate the product. Then, 1.5 mL of agitated product and 1.5 mL of bacteriostatic water were drawn into a 3-mL syringe. The final reconstituted product should equal 12 mL, with 6 mL used per hand. Using a 25-gauge, 1.5-inch syringe, the product was injected into the subcutaneous tissue plane in a retrograde fanning technique. Subjects were instructed to perform vigorous massage and keep to the 5-5-5 rule. Patients received an average of 2.5 treatments. One (12.5%) of the eight patients who received PLLA to the hands developed a nodule; this patient had been treated once with a 9-mL dilution.

When treating off the face with this product, one approach is to reconstitute one vial of PLLA overnight with 1 mL of 1% lidocaine and 7 mL of bacteriostatic water. Although the manufacturer recommends sterile water for reconstitution, the vast majority of clinicians use preserved (bacteriostatic) water, as the preservative decreases patient discomfort during cosmetic injections.[22] The reconstituted product is agitated with the Vortex Genie mixing device immediately prior to injection, and then 1.5 mL is withdrawn into a 3-mL syringe. Next, another 1.5 mL of bacteriostatic water is drawn into the syringe, resulting in a combined total volume of 3 mL. This step is repeated until a final total of 16 mL is mixed and drawn into the syringes. A 16-mL dilution cannot be done at the outset, as the vial can only hold up to 10 mL of diluent. Half of the PLLA vial (or 8 mL) is used per hand. The length of correction with PLLA has been reported to last 18 to 24 months, but requires multiple treatments spaced 4 to 6 weeks apart.[22]

Besides developing edema, ecchymoses, and hematomas, PLLA can lead to the formation of nodules.[23] Because of this and the availability of other filler agents, PLLA should be used with caution for hand augmentation. A 10-year retrospective review by Park et al[24] published in 2012 identified 15 patients who developed foreign body granulomas. Four patients had been treated with PMMA, three with CaHA, three with HA, two with PLLA, and three with "other" material. Subjects had been symptomatic from 1 month to 9 years, with 12 of the 15 having symptoms for more than 1 year. Four patients (two with PMMA and two with other fillers) had sensory dysfunction, and four (two with other fillers, one with PMMA, and one with CaHA) developed hand stiffness.

In their article, Park et al[24] recommended an algorithm for dealing with nodule formation. First, the authors started an antibiotic trial consisting of a second-generation cephalosporin combined with a third-generation macrolide. If the nodule persisted despite antibiotics, hyaluronidase was used for HA fillers, excision for CaHA, and intralesional triamcinolone for other types of filler. Excision was reserved as an intervention of last resort.

For those who use PLLA, there are techniques that can decrease nodule formation: using dilutions greater than 5 mL (16 mL is advised), using smaller volumes, not overcorrecting, spacing treatments at least 4 weeks apart, reconstituting the product the night prior, and performing massage after treatment.[9] Although the Sculptra product insert recommends reconstitution with 5 mL of sterile water at least 2 hours before treatment, dilutions less than 5 mL are associated with an increased risk of nodule formation.[20]

TREATMENT OF VISIBLE VEINS

Dorsal hand veins become more visible in the aging hand. Their visibility can often be minimized with revolumization of the dorsal hand. For patients who decline dermal fillers or for those who still have prominent veins despite revolumization, treatment of dorsal hand veins alone may be an option. Although sclerotherapy, endovenous vein ablation, and phlebectomy are not well studied, sclerotherapy is the most commonly used technique on the dorsal hands.

Sclerotherapy

In sclerotherapy, a liquid or foam is injected into a vein in order to produce endothelial cell damage and resultant vessel sclerosis. Various agents can be used to perform sclerotherapy. On the hand, the detergents sodium tetradecyl sulfate (STS) (Sotradecol Elkins-Sin, Inc., Cherry Hill, NJ) and polidocanol (POL) (Asclera; Kreussler, Chemische-Fabrik, Wiesbaden, Germany) are most commonly used. Both are FDA approved for small varicosities of the lower extremity. Thus, their use on dorsal hand veins is off-label.

Good candidates for sclerotherapy are patients with bulging dorsal hand veins who do not have known contraindications to sclerotherapy. For the hands specifically, sclerotherapy should be avoided in patients with a history of hand surgery, need for frequent intravenous access, hand arthritis, chronic edema or pain of the hands, functional abnormalities of the hands, carpal tunnel syndrome, or dialysis shunts.[25]

Prior to starting the treatment session, the patient is seated with the arms positioned perpendicular to the upper body. The entire hand and wrist are prepped with chlorhexidine. A tourniquet or pressure from an assistant's hand is applied to the mid-forearm in order to increase the prominence of the veins, making them easier to inject.

Concentrations of 0.5% to 3% liquid STS or 1.5% to 3% liquid POL are most commonly used. In general, lower concentrations should be used for smaller veins, and higher concentrations for larger veins. Duffy et al[26] treated 100 patients with dorsal hand veins ranging from 1 to 6 mm in diameter (mean, 3 mm) with liquid 0.5% STS, 1.5% POL, or 3% POL. They observed higher success rates in patients treated with 3% POL (95% vs 20% success rate). The authors concluded that 3% POL is more effective in vessels larger than 3 mm or vessels of any diameter in younger patients. It is important to note that 14.5% of the patients treated with 3% POL developed telangiectatic matting in the treatment area, a side effect that was not observed with 0.5% STS or 1.5% POL. Bowes et al[27] reported complete resolution of 3- to 6-mm dorsal hand veins in 11 (79%) of 14 hands treated with 1 to 4 mL of liquid 1.5% to 3% STS.

With foam sclerotherapy, the sclerosing solution is mixed with either room air or carbon dioxide gas. Foaming allows for longer contact between the sclerosant and the endothelium, increasing the efficacy of the procedure and allowing the clinician to use lower concentrations and smaller volumes of sclerosant.[28] Rao and Goldman[28] attach a 3-mL syringe filled with 1 mL of the sclerosant to a 5-mL syringe containing 4 mL of room air. A female-to-female connector is used to attach the two syringes. The liquid and room air are mixed together approximately 10 times until a homogenous consistency is achieved. Either 0.5% STS or 1% POL, with a total of 3 to 5 mL of foamed sclerosant per hand, is frequently used.[28] In a retrospective review of 38 hands, Tremaine et al[25] used 2.5 to 10 mL of foamed 0.25% to 1% STS per hand, with 0.5% and 0.25% predominating.

For practical purposes, a single hand is treated per day, generally using a 30-gauge, 0.5-inch needle connected to a 3-mL syringe of sclerosant. The vein should be entered at its most distal aspect and canalized in a proximal direction. With the bevel of the needle facing up, the vein is directly punctured, entering at an angle of 30 to 45 degrees to the skin. The sclerosant is injected slowly. Once all the desired vessels are treated, the tourniquet is released, the hand is elevated, and gentle massage is performed to the treated area from a distal to proximal direction. Cotton swabs are then applied to each treatment site, and the hand and distal forearm are wrapped in an elastic bandage. The patient is asked to keep the bandage on for 24 hours and can return for treatment of the second hand the following day so that the other hand is free to assist with daily function. Signs of excessive compression from the bandage include paresthesias, decreased motion, or changes in temperature or color of the fingers. Some authors recommend keeping continued compression for 2 weeks.[29]

Common side effects due to sclerotherapy include pain during the injection, ecchymosis, edema, and soreness. Tremaine et al[25] noted pain lasted an average of 7.4 days, edema and erythema 3 to 4 days, and ecchymosis 3.7 days. Less frequently, patients may develop hyperpigmentation, neovascularization, localized hypertrichosis (never reported in the hands), urticaria, and allergic reactions. In their study, Tremaine et al[25] reported that 61.9% of 38 treated hands developed posttreatment coagulum. A 22-gauge needle can be used to pierce the center of the coagulum, and its contents can be gently expressed; all coagula in the study resolved within 2 months. Patients should be seen for follow-up at 2 weeks to assess for this complication. Neovascularization, or telangiectatic matting, more often occurs in patients with high levels of estrogen, as seen during pregnancy and the use of oral contraceptives or estrogen supplementation.[30,31] High volume of sclerosant, high injection pressure, large treatment areas, extensive blanching upon injection, and lack of posttreatment compression are also associated with the development of neovascularization.[32]

Rare adverse events include local skin necrosis, arterial injection resulting in distal skin necrosis, thrombophlebitis, deep vein thrombosis, wheezing in asthmatics, and angina in cardiac patients.[33] Duffy et al[26] reported one patient who, after treatment of vessels located on the thenar web, developed blanching of the thumb, index, and middle fingers for 10 minutes. The patient then experienced 2 weeks of numbness and paresthesia. These symptoms were thought to be secondary to neuropraxia caused by extravasation of the sclerosing agent. Although never reported in treatment of the dorsal hand, the microbubbles introduced into the circulation by foam sclerotherapy can cause visual changes, headache, chest tightness, coughing, migraine with or without aura, and transient ischemic attacks (**Figure 35-8**).

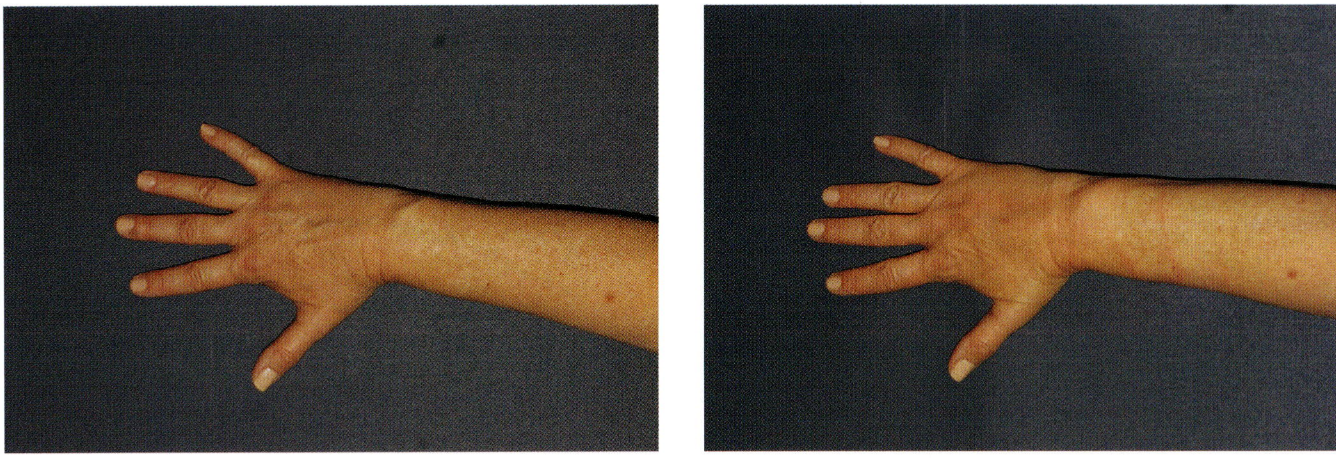

FIGURE 35-8 A patient was extremely bothered by her prominent hand veins. She had no history of diabetes or kidney disease and denied need for frequent intravenous access. The patient did not want to have any fillers injected and was not bothered by prominent tendons or the quality of skin. She subsequently underwent sclerotherapy. For dorsal hand veins 3 mm in diameter or greater, use 3% liquid POL, 1% foamed POL, 1.5% to 3% liquid STS, or 0.5% foam STS. Before (left) and 24 hours after (right) foam sclerotherapy to the dorsal hand.

Endovenous Laser Ablation and Phlebectomy

Endovenous laser ablation and phlebectomy are other methods of treating prominent dorsal hand veins. While widely used for leg veins, these procedures have not been well studied in the dorsal hand.

In endovenous laser ablation, a laser fiber is introduced percutaneously into a vein through a catheter and guidewire. The energy emitted by the laser causes damage to the vessel wall, causing obliteration of the treatment area. In a 2007 article, Shamma and Guy[34] detailed their methods for endovenous laser ablation in 54 hands. While wavelengths of 810 to 1320 nm have been used in the legs, Shamma and Guy[34] used a Dornier MedTech 940-nm diode laser (Medilas Compact; Dornier MedRech Laser GmbH, Germering, Germany). After tumescent anesthesia, a 600-micron laser fiber was introduced through a 4-F laser sheath, tracked over a 0.018-inch guidewire. An average of four veins were treated per hand, and a compressive dressing was applied postoperatively. All patients were satisfied with their treatment. Hand swelling was a common side effect that lasted up to 2 weeks. One patient developed a 3-mm burn at a laser exit site.

Phlebectomy involves the removal of a desired length of the vein through 2- to 3-mm incisions in the skin. Only one case report has been published on this procedure for dorsal hand veins in the literature.[35] Because endovenous laser ablation and phlebectomy require specialized instrument, materials, and staff in order to be performed safely and effectively, sclerotherapy remains a first-line option for the treatment of dorsal hand veins.

LIGHT-BASED THERAPIES

Various light, laser, and energy devices have been used for hand rejuvenation. These include IPL, photodynamic therapy (PDT), Q-switched (QS) lasers, 1320-nm neodymium-doped yttrium-aluminum-garnet (Nd:YAG) laser, fractionated 1550-nm erbium-doped laser, fractionated 1927-nm thulium laser, 2940-nm erbium-doped YAG (Er:YAG) laser, and fractionated 10,600-nm carbon dioxide (CO_2) laser (**Table 35-3**). Since the dorsal hand skin is thinner, has a decreased vascularity, and has fewer pilosebaceous units than the face, the fluence, density, and number of passes should generally be reduced to minimize recovery time.[9]

TABLE 35-3 • Summary of Light-Based Therapy Indications and Disadvantages

Treatment	Indications	Disadvantages
Q-switched laser	Pigmented lesions	Dyschromia, erythema, scarring, textural change, bleeding, bullae formation
Intense pulsed light	Pigmented and vascular lesions can be treated simultaneously	Requires multiple treatment sessions
Photo-dynamic therapy	Actinic keratoses	Pruritus, erosions, erythema, edema, and pain
Nonablative laser resurfacing	Neocollagenesis	Subtle and mild improvement, cost, requires multiple treatments
Nonablative fractionated laser	Photoaging and neocollagenesis	Erythema, edema, and pruritus, less noticeable improvement than fractionated laser
Ablative resurfacing	Photoaging and neocollagenesis	Infection, dyschromia, scarring

TABLE 35-4 • Q-Switched (QS) Lasers Used to Treat Epidermal Pigmented Lesions (in order of decreasing effectiveness)

- QS ruby
- Frequency doubled 532-nm Nd:YAG
- QS alexandrite
- 1064-nm QS Nd:YAG

A frequent patient complaint about their hands is the development of solar lentigines and macular seborrheic keratoses. These rarely resolve permanently with topical superficial peeling agents. Selective photothermolysis of the pigment within melanosomes, such as that employed by QS lasers, is highly effective.[36] Melanin has a broad spectrum of wavelength absorption across the optical spectrum. Preferred lasers have wavelengths from approximately 500 to 755 nm. Since the thermal relaxation time of melanosomes is only 0.25 μs, short pulse durations are optimal.[36] For this reason, the QS ruby laser (694 nm), QS or picosecond alexandrite laser (755 nm), and the frequency-doubled QS or picosecond Nd:YAG laser (532 nm) are most often employed (**Table 35-4**).[37,38] These devices deliver pulse durations in the nanosecond and picosecond range. Usually a one-time treatment is required, and the fluence should result in epidermal whitening without vesiculation or pinpoint bleeding. A single pass is typically performed, but pulses may be stacked over macular seborrheic keratoses (**Figure 35-9**).

In a study comparing three lasers and liquid nitrogen (Medlite II frequency-doubled QS Nd:YAG laser, Continuum Biomedical, Livermore, CA; HGM K1 krypton laser, HGM Medical Laser Systems Inc., Salt Lake City UT; DioLite 532-nm diode-pumped vanadare laser, Iridex Corp, Mountain View, CA), a single treatment with the frequency-doubled QS Nd:YAG laser was the most effective technique at destroying melanin and preserving the surrounding tissue.[39]

For QS and picosecond lasers, patients should be counseled that they may see urticarial-like papules for 24 hours followed by 7 to 10 days of purpura or coffee-ground–appearing macules, followed by temporary hypopigmented macules, which can be seen after the lesion sloughs superficially (**Table 35-5**). Purpura is more frequently encountered with the QS Nd:YAG (532 nm) or pulsed-dye lasers because the competing chromophore, deoxyhemoglobin, causes immediate rupture of small vessels. The use of the QS ruby laser is not recommended in darker skin types. These can be more safely treated with the 1064-nm QS or picosecond Nd:YAG laser.[40]

TABLE 35-5 • Frequent Adverse Events of Laser Therapy

- Erythema
- Hypopigmentation and hyperpigmentation
- Scarring
- Textural change
- Crusting
- Bleeding
- Bullae formation

IPL therapy has been used as a nonablative photorejuvenating device for the hand. IPL systems are high-intensity pulsed sources emitting light between 515 and 1200 nm. This broad spectrum facilitates the selective targets of vessels with hemoglobin (580 nm) or deoxyhemoglobin and melanin (400-755 nm). Its largest advantage is that it allows simultaneous correction of vascular and pigmented lesions with little to no downtime.[41] Additionally, dermal heating from IPL therapy, which spares the epidermis, has been shown histologically to induce collagen production in the papillary and reticular dermis.[42] Filters can be added to select for wavelengths only above a certain range. Fitzpatrick skin types IV to VI require cutoff filters at higher wavelengths, triple pulsing, and longer pulse delays between pulses in order to prevent damage or epidermal compromise (**Table 35-6**). Optimal correction of erythema and vascular lesions, where oxygenated hemoglobin predominates, can be achieved using 515- to 590-nm cutoff filters (based on patient skin type and extent of erythema). Purpuric

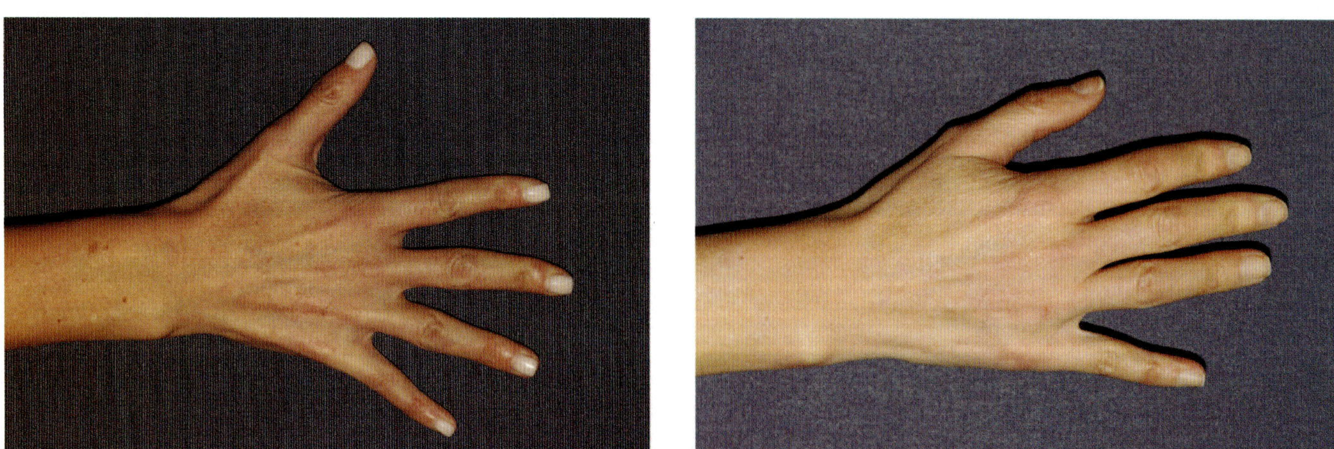

FIGURE 35-9 A 42-year-old woman demonstrated scattered and few solar lentigines and macular seborrheic keratosis on the dorsal hand. One treatment of Q-switched alexandrite to the lesions resulted in complete clearance of the lesions. Before (left) and 7 weeks after (right) one treatment of Q-switched alexandrite.

TABLE 35-6 • Fitzpatrick Skin Type and Intense Pulsed Light Filter

- I to III: 560 nm
- IV: 590 nm
- V: 695 nm
- VI: 755 nm

patches (rich in deoxygenated hemoglobin) are better targeted with filters of 590 nm or higher.

Settings using the Lumenis 1 or the Lumenis M22 IPL (Lumenis Ltd., Yokneam, Israel) are optimized with a 560-nm cutoff filter for skin types I to III and a 590-nm filter for skin type IV. Patients with predominantly mottled hyperpigmentation and solar lentigines benefit from a double-pulse technique with a 3-ms pulse duration. If there is a combination of pigment and vascular structures, a 3.5-ms pulse duration for both pulses is used, and a 4-ms pulse duration is used if only fine telangiectasias and erythema predominate. A 10- to 30-ms delay is set between pulses in skin types I to III and a 30- to 40-ms delay in skin type IV. The fluence is set between 15 and 18 J/cm^2. Treatments are performed monthly for two or three sessions.

In a study by Goldman et al,[43] 23 patients with dermatoheliosis and solar lentigines on the dorsal hands were treated with four IPL sessions at 3- to 4-week intervals. In 100% of cases, investigators noted good to excellent results in the improvement of lentigines and skin quality. Subjective patient self-assessments showed similar results. Twenty (87%) of 23 subjects noted good to excellent improvement. No significant side effects were observed (**Figure 35-10**).

PDT is an effective photoaging treatment, especially in the presence of precancerous conditions. PDT uses a photosensitizer, such as 20% aminolevulinic acid solution (ALA) or 16% methyl aminolevulinate cream (MAL), which is converted in vivo into protoporphyrin IX. PDT is indicated for the treatment of nonhyperkeratotic actinic keratoses, with the advantageous side effect of improving the appearance of fine lines and rhytids, mottled hyperpigmentation, and texture.[34] To increase efficacy from a single PDT treatment, patients may apply other topicals (imiquimod or 5-fluorouracil) for 7 to 10 days prior to PDT treatment to the area to be treated. ALA or MAL may be applied after the dorsal hand skin has been exfoliated with a vibrating microdermabrasion system (if available) and degreased with an acetone wash. On the hands, photosensitizer may be left in place for 3 hours occluded and ideally under a warming blanket or in a warm dimly lit room. After the photosensitizer has been washed off with soap and water and a baby wipe has been used to remove any additional residue, any light source within the visible light spectrum can be used to activate the photosensitizer. Friedman et al[44] found a sequential combination of laser and light sources to be superior to using a single light source.

The sequence is as follows: initial activation with a PDL (Cynergy, Cynosure, Westford, MA) 595 nm with a 7-mm spot size, 40-ms pulse width, and 10 to 12 J/cm^2 targeting individual actinic keratoses so that the end point is subpurpuric. This is followed by the IPL using the treatment parameters outlined earlier. Lastly, the treatment area is concomitantly illuminated with a blue light source (Blu-U, DUSA Pharmaceuticals, Inc., Wilmington, MA) positioned 25 to 50 mm from the skin for an illumination period of 16 minutes and 40 seconds at a light dose of 10 J/cm^2 and a red light source (Aktilite CL 128, PhotoCure ASA, Oslo, Norway) positioned 50 to 80 mm from the skin for a total of 8 minutes and 49 seconds at a standardized fluence of 37 J/cm^2. Prior to discharge home, a mineral-based sunscreen is applied and the patient is told to stay indoors with strict sunlight avoidance for the remainder of the treatment day and the following day. Using this combination, generally one PDT treatment is sufficient. Orringer et al[45] examined the histologic effects of PDT on the hand and found an increase in expression of procollagen

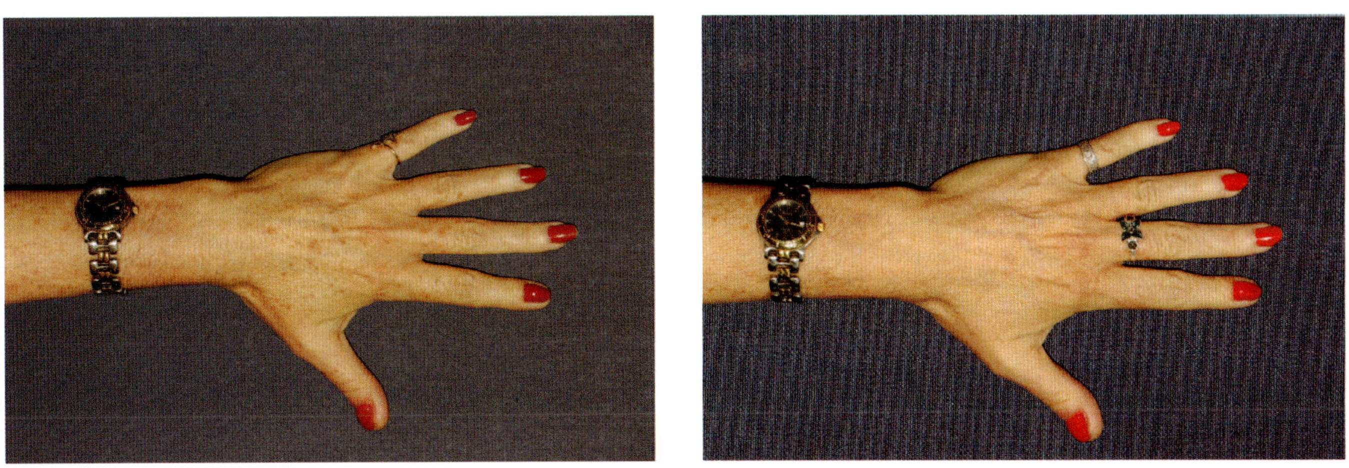

FIGURE 35-10 A 57-year-old patient presented with fine wrinkling, solar lentigines, and macular seborrheic keratoses of the dorsal hands and digits. She underwent one session of intense pulsed light and Q-switched alexandrite to the hands, with improvement in texture and pigmentation. Because the dorsal hand skin is thinner, has a decreased vascularity, and has fewer pilosebaceous units than the face, the fluence, density, and number of passes used for all light-based therapies should be reduced. Before (left) and 4 weeks after (right) one session of intense pulsed light and Q-switched alexandrite to the hands

types I and III, epidermal thickening, and Ki-67, a keratinocyte differentiation marker, after PDT using a 595-nm PDL for activation of the photosensitizer.

Nonablative laser resurfacing also improves the appearance of photodamaged skin of the hand. These lasers emit longer wavelengths, in the mid-infrared range, that penetrate into the deep dermis, stimulating fibroblasts while avoiding injury to the epidermis.

The 1320-nm Nd:YAG laser been employed as a treatment modality in hand rejuvenation. Sadick and Schecter[46] performed a study involving seven patients using the 1320-nm Nd:YAG laser (CoolToughII, New Star Lasers, Roseville, CA). These patients received six treatments separated by 4 weeks and were followed for 3 months after the last treatment. Patient assessment scores were higher than objective measures, with six of seven patients reporting a mean improvement score of 2 (range, 1-6), corresponding to 1% to 19% improvement from baseline. Results are mild to moderate at best, and patients should be warned of the slow progress and subtle improvement that can be expected.

Nonablative fractional lasers treat a fraction of the skin as compared with traditional nonablative lasers, leaving up to a maximum of 95% of the skin uninvolved. Microthermal treatment zones (MTZs) are delivered to the dermis, causing coagulation necrosis followed by collagen remodeling. The selected wavelength should correspond to the cosmetic target; the 1550-nm wavelength is best for stimulating collagen production and improving skin texture, whereas the 1927-nm wavelength and 1927-nm thulium lasers are best for pigmentation (**Table 35-7**).[47] Jih et al[48] employed fractional resurfacing technology for hand rejuvenation using the 1550-nm diode-pumped erbium fiber laser (Fraxel SR, Reliant Technologies) on a series of 10 patients. Patients received a total of five treatments 2 to 3 weeks apart using a setting of 8 to 9 mJ/MTZ with 10 passes at 250 MTZ/cm^2 to achieve a final treatment density of 2500 MTZ/cm^2. The study reported a subjective patient improvement of 51% to 75% in skin pigmentation and 25% to 50% improvement in skin roughness and wrinkling. Biopsies of the skin showed an increase in density of dermal collagen. It may be best to use one wavelength per session to allow a more focused treatment and include a greater number of passes.

Ablative laser skin resurfacing using the CO_2 or Er:YAG laser is the standard for facial rejuvenation. When employing this modality for hand rejuvenation, great caution should be taken because of the reduced number of pilosebaceous structures and vasculature. This leads to a lengthier recovery period, a higher risk of infection, and a greater risk for scarring and dyschromia. Optimal treatment parameters using the Er:YAG laser that have been reported in the literature include the use of two passes at 15 J/cm^2 and 30% intensity, followed by cleaning and a third pass at the same settings.[34] A single-pass resurfacing technique has also been described using decreased fluence (150-200 mJ/pulse) with a computer-generated pattern of 6, leaving the epidermal debris in place to serve as a biologic dressing.[45]

Fractional thermolysis can also be employed using ablative fractional lasers. This creates columns of vaporized tissue and coagulation necrosis. Because only a small portion of the skin is affected, neighboring untreated tissue aids in the healing process, promoting a favorable side effect profile and minimal posttreatment recovery. Stebbins et al[49] treated the hand with a single pass of the Dermal Optical Thermolysis ablative fractional CO_2 laser (DEKA, Calenzano, Italy) and noted transient erythema and edema, with no long-term scarring or pigmentary alterations. After three treatments at 4- to 6- week intervals, investigators rated a mean improvement of 26% to 50% for wrinkles, 51% to 75% for pigment, and 26% to 50% for texture, with subjects reporting similar results.

Before treatment, a topical anesthetic such as bupivacaine/lidocaine/tetracaine anesthetic cream is applied for 30 minutes preoperatively.[34] After the removal of the cream, the area is treated with a nonsequential fractional CO_2 laser using 75 mJ, 100 Hz, and a 0.3-second repeat delay (Active FX, Lumenis Ltd., Yokneam, Israel). A computer pattern generator with settings of 3 pattern, 5 size, and 1 density (corresponding to <10% overlap) is used. After the procedure, cool sterile saline compresses and ointment are applied. In skin types III or greater, a class VI topical corticosteroid ointment is started daily for 5 days on postoperative day 2 to minimize the occurrence of postinflammatory pigmentary alteration. The use of fractionated ablative laser is generally not recommended in patients of skin types V and VI unless performed by a highly experienced laser surgeon.

TABLE 35-7 • Common Settings for Nonablative Fractional Laser

Laser Wavelength	Number of Passes	Fluence	Coverage/ Fitzpatrick Skin Type
1550-nm	8	20-35 mJ	14%-28% (I-III), 14%-20% (IV-VI)
1927-nm	8	10-20 mJ	40%-50% (I-IV)

Data from Fraxel Re:Store Dual system, Solta Medical, Inc. https://www.fraxel.com/hcp#home.

RADIOFREQUENCY

RF uses an alternating electrical current to deliver energy to the skin. The purpose of RF devices used for minimally invasive cosmetic treatments of the face and body is to produce selective dermal injury, leading to a responsive wound repair while keeping the overlying epidermis intact.[50,51] The electrical current heats the deep dermis, fat, fibrous septae, and (with internally applied monopolar RF devices) fascia. RF energy is not reflected or absorbed by epidermal melanin or vasculature as it passes through the skin, making it safer to use in all skin types. This volumetric heating of the dermis and subcutaneous fibrous septae is associated with collagen denaturation and subsequent thickening and shortening of the collagen fibers leading to increased fibroblast activity and new collagen formation and resulting in skin tightening over 4 to 6 months. An advantage this technique employs over fractional lasers is a low risk of postinflammatory hyperpigmentation.[52]

In a prospective multicenter study using a monopolar RF device for moderate to severe hand wrinkles, 31 patients receiving three RF treatments at 2-week intervals showed a 50% improvement from baseline with no adverse effects reported.[53] For the treatment, the RF device (Pelleve S5 Wrinkle Treatment Generator; Ellman International Inc., Oceanside, NY; 4.0 MHz, 120 W) with a 20-mm handpiece (GlideSafe; Ellman International Inc.) was set at a level of energy based on verbal feedback about tip warmth from the patient. The handpiece was moved in continuous overlapping corkscrew patterns to completely cover each of the three gel-coated treatment zones. When the skin surface temperature of the treated areas reached 40°C to 42°C, the treatment was continued for an additional 3 minutes. This sequence was then repeated for a total of two passes in each zone.

Microneedle fractional RF systems generate precise ovoid areas of coagulation in the dermis and subcutaneous tissue, bypassing the epidermis. The location of the thermal injury depends on needle depth and conduction times. The technology has been studied on the face and neck for skin rejuvenation and treatment of acne scars. While no studies have yet to evaluate its use on the dorsal hands, keeping the intensity low and the depth of needle penetration shallow is advisable.

CHEMICAL PEELS

The aged appearance of the hand can be improved with chemical peeling, although there are few reports in the literature. Much like the concerns noted for laser therapy, the reduced number of pilosebaceous units and decreased vasculature can often lead to impaired wound healing. Chemical peels are classified as superficial, medium, or deep based on their depth of penetration into the epidermis and dermis. In general, a light or medium-depth peel should be employed to minimize the risk of postprocedure complications. Swinehart[54] employed a 50% salicylic acid paste for photoaging on the forearms and hands in a cohort of 11 patients. Maceration and desquamation followed, and recovery took up to 4 weeks. While rare, salicylism is a potential side effect when treating large areas. The process should be employed conservatively, and patients should be warned that numerous treatment sessions may be required before the gradual and mild improvement in skin texture is noticeable.

Superficial chemical peels penetrate to the level of the epidermis and include 70% glycolic acid, salicylic acid, 50% resorcinol, Jessner's solution, solid CO_2 slush, and 10% to 25% trichloroacetic acid (TCA) peel. Medium-depth peels penetrate through the papillary dermis and include TCA peels at concentrations greater than 30%. The results of the chemical peels vary greatly and are dependent on the concentration, contact time, and the manner in which the skin is prepared. Although more likely with deeper peels, all chemical peels confer a risk of dyschromia, prolonged erythema, a discrete line at the treatment border of the arm and hand, and scarring. Cox[55] reported the development of multiple keratoacanthomas following a 70% glycolic acid gel and 40% TCA chemical peel to the forearms.

COMBINATION TREATMENTS FOR HAND REJUVENATION

Patients who exhibit more than one sign of aging often require several therapeutic modalities, some of which can be completed on the same day. Sclerotherapy and autologous fat transfer should be performed separately. When combining treatments on the same day, start with modalities that target the epidermis and dermis, followed by those that remedy volume loss.

For patients with extrinsic sings of aging (pigmentation, vascular lesions, actinic keratosis), various energy devices can be used. For those with mild pigmentation and photoaging, the entire dorsal hand can be treated with IPL followed by a QS or picosecond 755- or 1064-nm laser to individual solar lentigines or seborrheic keratoses. For skin types IV to VI, IPL can be substituted by the 1927-nm diode laser (Clear + Brilliant Perméa). If the degree of photodamage is more severe, one can perform a fractionated 1550-nm or fractionated CO_2 laser treatment after the use of a QS or picosecond pigment laser for individual lentigines and keratoses.

PDT can be used in patients with photodamage and actinic keratoses. Subsequent to epidermal and dermal procedures, the filler of choice can be injected to address skin laxity, volume loss, and the visibility of tendons, bones, and veins. Some clinicians may use RF instead of fillers for patients with skin laxity and volume loss.

CONCLUSIONS

Hand rejuvenation is becoming increasingly popular as both patients and clinicians appreciate its aesthetic impact. Most procedures require minimal downtime and produce excellent aesthetic results. Dermal fillers minimize the prominence of tendons, bones, and veins, while improving the appearance of skin laxity. Sclerotherapy and endovenous laser ablation can minimize the appearance of dorsal hand veins. Chemical peels, IPL, QS and picosecond lasers, and both nonablative, and ablative lasers can improve dyschromia and skin texture. A multimodality approach to treat the multiple causes of visible hand aging is often necessary, and most procedures may be performed sequentially on the same day or spaced over multiple treatment visits.[56]

REFERENCES

1. Beer KR. Combined treatment for skin rejuvenation and soft-tissue augmentation of the aging face. *J Drugs Dermatol.* 2011;10:125-132.
2. Goldman MP, Alster TS, Weiss R. A randomized trial to determine the influence of laser therapy, monopolar radiofrequency treatment, and intense pulsed light therapy administered immediately after hyaluronic acid gel implantation. *Dermatol Surg.* 2007;33:535-542.
3. RADIESSE injectable implant instruction for use. http://www.radiesse.com/wp-content/uploads/RADIESSE_Wrinkle_Filler_Instructions_for_Use.pdf. Accessed December 18, 2017.
4. Lefebvre-Vilardabo M, Trevidic P, Moradi A, Busso M, Sutton AB, Bucay VW. Hand: clinical anatomy and regional approaches with injectable fillers. *Plast Reconstr Surg.* 2015;136(5s):258-275.

5. Fathi R, Cohen JL. Challenges, considerations, and strategies in hand rejuvenation. *J Drugs Dermatol.* 2016;15(7):809-815.
6. Edelson KL. Hand recontouring with calcium hydroxylapatite (Radiesse®). *J Cosmet Dermatol.* 2009;8:44-51.
7. Sadick NS. A 52-week study of safety and efficacy of calcium hydroxylapatite for rejuvenation of the aging hand. *J Drugs Dermatol.* 2011;10:47-51.
8. Gargasz SS, Carbone MC. Hand rejuvenation using Radiesse. *Plast Reconstr Surg.* 2010;125:259-260.
9. Fabi SG, Goldman MP. Hand rejuvenation: a review and our experience. *Dermatol Surg.* 2012;38:1112-1127.
10. Busso M, Moers-Carpi M, Storck R, Ogilvie P, Ogilve A. Multicenter, randomized trial assessing the effectiveness and safety of calcium hydroxylapatite for hand rejuvenation. *Dermatol Surg.* 2010;36:790-797.
11. Wu DC, Goldma MP. A prospective double-blinded randomized bilateral comparison study of injectable calcium hydroxylapatite with and without triamcinolone acetate for the treatment of volume loss to the dorsum areas of the hands. Accepted abstract at American Surgical Dermatologic Society Annual Meeting, November 2016, New Orleans, LA.
12. Man J, Rao J, Goldman M. A double-blind, comparative study of nonanimal-stabilized hyaluronic acid versus human collagen for tissue augmentation of the dorsal hands. Dermatol Surg. 2008;34:1026-1031.
13. Brandt FS, Cazzaniga A, Strangman N, Coleman J, Axford-Gatley R. Long-term effectiveness and safety of small gel particle hyaluronic acid for hand rejuvenation. *Dermatol Surg.* 2012;38:1128-1135.
14. Dallara JM. A prospective, noninterventional study of the treatment of the aging hand with Juvederm Ultra 3 and Juvederm Hydrate. *Aesthet Plast Surg.* 2012;36:949-954.
15. Fulton J, Caperton C, Weinkle S, Dewandre L. Filler injections with the blunt-tip microcannula. *J Drugs Dermatol.* 2012;11(9):1098-1103.
16. Gubanova EI, Starovatova PA, Rodina MY. 12-month effects of stabilized hyaluronic acid gel compared with saline for rejuvenation of aging hands. *Drugs Dermatol.* 2015;14(3):288-298.
17. Streker M, Reuther T, Krueger N, Kerscher M. Stabilized hyaluronic acid-based gel of non-animal origin for skin rejuvenation: face, hand, and décolletage. *J Drugs Dermatol.* 2013;12(9):990-994.
18. Lacarrubba F, Tedeschi A, Nardone B, Micali G. Mesotherapy for skin rejuvenation: assessment of the subepidermal low-echogenic band by ultrasound evaluation with cross-sectional B-mode scanning. *Dermatol Ther.* 2008;21(Suppl 3):S1-S5.
19. Redaelli A. Cosmetic use of polylactic acid for hand rejuvenation: report on 27 patients. *J Cosmet Dermatol.* 2006;5:233-238.
20. Sadick NS, Anderson D, Werschler WP. Addressing volume loss in hand rejuvenation: a report of clinical experience. *J Cosmet Laser Ther.* 2008;10:237-241.
21. Palm MD, Woodhall KE, Butterwick KJ, Goldman MP. Cosmetic use of poly-l-lactic acid: a retrospective study of 130 patients. *Dermatol Surg.* 2010;36:161-170.
22. Bolton J, Fabi SG, Peterson J, Goldman M. Poly-L-lactic acid for chest rejuvenation: a retrospective study of 28 cases using a 5-point chest wrinkle scale. *Cos Dermatol.* 2011;24:278-284.
23. Vleggaar D. Soft-tissue augmentation and the role of poly-L-lactic acid. *Plast Reconstr Surg.* 2006;118:46S-54S.
24. Park TH, Yeo KK, Seo SW, et al. Clinical experience with complications of hand rejuvenation. *Plast Reconstr Aesthet Surg.* 2012;65(12):1627-1631.
25. Tremaine AM, Friedmann DP, Goldman MP. Foam sclerotherapy for reticular veins of the dorsal hands: a retrospective review. *Dermatol Surg.* 2014;40(8):892-898.
26. Duffy DM, Garcia C, Clark RE. The role of sclerotherapy in abnormal varicose hand veins. *Plast Reconstr Surg.* 1999;104:1474-1479.
27. Bowes LE, Goldman MP. Sclerotherapy of reticular and telangiectatic veins of the face, hands, and chest. *Dermatol Surg.* 2002;28:46-51.
28. Rao J, Goldman MP. Stability of foam in sclerotherapy: differences between sodium tetradecyl sulfate and polidocanol and the type of connector used in the double-syringe system technique. *Dermatol Surg.* 2005;31:19-22.
29. Butterwick K, Sadick N. Hand rejuvenation using a combination approach. *Dermatol Surg.* 2016;42(Suppl 2):S108-S118.
30. Goldman MP, Sadick NS, Weiss RA. Cutaneous necrosis, telangiectatic matting, and hyperpigmentation following sclerotherapy. *Dermatol Surg.* 1995;21:19-29.
31. Sadick NS, Urmacher C. Estrogen and progesterone receptors. Their role in postsclerotherapy angiogenesis telangiectatic matting (TM). *Dermatol Surg.* 1999;25:339-343.
32. Weiss RA, Sadick NS, Goldman MP, Weiss MA. Post-sclerotherapy compression: controlled comparative study of duration of compression and its effects on clinical outcome. *Dermatol Surg.* 1999;25:105-108.
33. Goldman MP, Bergan JJ, Geux JJ, Weiss RA. *Sclerotherapy: Treatment of Varicose and Telangiectatic Leg Veins.* 5th ed. Philadelphia, PA: Elsevier; 2011.
34. Shamma AR, Guy RJ. Laser ablation of unwanted hand veins. *Plast Reconstr Surg.* 2007;120:2017-2024.
35. Lee BJ. The role of sclerotherapy in abnormal varicose hand veins. *Plast Reconstr Surg.* 2000;106:227-229.
36. Taylor CR, Anderson RR. Treatment of benign pigmented epidermal lesions by Q-switched ruby laser. *Int J Dermatol.* 1993;32:908.
37. Lee M. Combination 532-nm and 1064-nm laser for noninvasive skin rejuvenation and toning. *Arch Dermatol.* 2003;139:1265-1276.
38. Jang KA, Chung EC, Choi JH, et al. Successful removal of freckles in Asian skin with a Q-switched alexandrite laser. *Dermatol Surg.* 2000;26:231-234.
39. Todd MM, Rallis TM, Gerwels JW, Hata TR. A comparison of 3 lasers and liquid nitrogen in the treatment of solar lentigines: a randomized, controlled, comparative trial. *Arch Dermatol.* 2000;136:841-846.
40. Butterwick, KJ. Rejuvenation of the aging hand. *Dermatol Clin.* 2005;23:515-527.
41. Raulin C, Greve B, Grema H. IPL technology: a review. *Lasers Surg Med.* 2003;32:78-87.
42. Prieto VG, Sadick NS, Lloreta J, et al. Effects of intense pulsed light on sun-damaged human skin, round and ultrastructural analysis. *Lasers Surg Med.* 2002;30:82-85.
43. Goldman A, Prati C, Rossato F. Hand rejuvenation using intense pulsed light. *J Cutan Med Surg.* 2008;12:107-113.
44. Friedmann D, Goldman MP, Fabi SG, Guiha I. The effect of multiple sequential light sources to activate aminolevulanic acid in the treatment of actinic keratoses. *J Clin Aesthet Dermatol.* 2014;7(9):20-25.

45. Orringer JS, Hammerberg C, Hamilton T, et al. Molecular effects of photodynamic therapy for photoaging. *Arch Dermatol.* 2008;144:1296-1302.

46. Sadick N, Schecter AK. Utilization of the 1320-nm Nd:Yag laser for the reduction of photoaging of the hands. *Dermatology.* 2004;30:1140-1144.

47. Allemann I, Kaufman J. Fractional photothermolysis: an update. *Lasers Med Sci.* 2010;25:137-144.

48. Jih MH, Goldberg LH, Kimyai-Asadi A. Fractional photothermolysis for photoaging of hands. *Dermatol Surg.* 2008;34(1):73-78.

49. Stebbins WG, Hanke CW. Ablative fractional CO2 resurfacing for photoaging of the hands: pilot study of 10 patients. *Dermatol Ther.* 2011;24:62-70.

50. Sadick N, Rothaus KO. Minimally invasive radiofrequency devices. *Clin Plast Surg.* 2016;43(3):567-576.

51. Carruthers J, Fabi SG, Weiss R. Monopolar radiofrequency for skin tightening. *Derm Surg.* 2014;40(Suppl 12):S168-S173.

52. Fritz K, Salavastru C. Ways of noninvasive facial skin tightening and fat reduction. *Facial Plast Surg.* 2016;32(03):276-282.

53. Vega JM, Bucay VW, Mayoral FA. Prospective, multicenter study to determine the safety and efficacy of a unique radiofrequency device for moderate to severe hand wrinkles. *J Drugs Dermatol.* 2013;12:24-26.

54. Swinehart JM. Salicylic acid ointment peeling of the hands and forearms. Effective nonsurgical removal of pigmented lesions and actinic damage. *J Dermatol Surg Oncol.* 1992;18:495-498.

55. Cox SE. Rapid development of keratoacanthomas after a body peel. *Dermatol Surg.* 2003;29:201-203.

56. Fabi SG, Carruthers J. A single modality approach to rejuvenate the aging face and body: a thing of the past? *Derm Surg.* 2016;42(Suppl 2): S73-S76.

Index

Page references for figures are indicated by *f*, for tables by *t*, and for boxes by *b*.

J

K

L

T